THE LOWER EXTREMITY & SPINE
IN SPORTS MEDICINE

THE LOWER EXTREMITY & SPINE
IN SPORTS MEDICINE

Edited by

JAMES A. NICHOLAS, M.D.

Founder and Director
Nicholas Institute of Sports Medicine and Athletic Trauma
Director Emeritus, Department of Orthopaedic Surgery, Lenox Hill Hospital
Consultant in Orthopaedic Surgery, Hospital for Special Surgery
Chairman, Medical Staff, New York Jets Football Club
New York, New York

ELLIOTT B. HERSHMAN, M.D.

Assistant Director, Department of Orthopaedic Surgery
Consultant, Nicholas Institute of Sports Medicine and Athletic Trauma
Lenox Hill Hospital
Team Orthopaedist, New York Jets Football Club
Team Physician, Hunter College Athletic Program
New York, New York

SECOND EDITION

with 2633 illustrations and 15 color plates

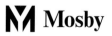 Mosby

St. Louis Baltimore Berlin Boston Carlsbad Chicago London Madrid
Naples New York Philadelphia Sydney Tokyo Toronto

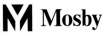

Mosby

Dedicated to Publishing Excellence

Publisher: Alison Miller
Acquisition Editor: Robert Hurley
Developmental Editor: Kathryn H. Falk
Project Manager: Patricia Tannian
Production Editor: Suzanne C. Fannin
Manufacturing Supervisor: Betty Richmond
Book and Cover Designer: Gail Morey Hudson

SECOND EDITION

Printed in the United States of America
Composition by Clarinda Company
Printing/binding by Maple-Vail Book Mfg. Group

Mosby–Year Book, Inc.
11830 Westline Industrial Drive
St. Louis, Missouri 63146

Library of Congress Cataloging in Publication Data
The Lower extremity and spine in sports medicine / edited by James A.
    Nicholas, Elliott B. Hershman. – – 2nd ed.
        p.   cm.
    Includes bibliographical references and index.
    ISBN 0-8151-6391-6
    1. Leg– –Wounds and injuries.   2. Spine– –Wounds and injuries.
3. Sports injuries.   I. Nicholas, James A., 1921-
II. Hershman, Elliott B.
    [DNLM: 1. Leg Injuries. 2. Spinal Injuries. 3. Athletic
Injuries.   WE 850 L917 1995]
RD560.L69   1995
617.5′8044--dc20
DNLM/DLC
for Library of Congress

94 95 96 97 98 / 9 8 7 6 5 4 3 2 1

Contributors

WAYNE H. AKESON, MD

Professor and Chairman
Department of Orthopaedics
University of California, San Diego
San Diego, California

STEVEN ALBERT, MD

Assistant Clinical Professor of Radiology
Cornell University Medical Center-New York Hospital
New York, New York

D. AMIEL, PhD

Professor
Department of Orthopaedics
University of California, San Diego
La Jolla, California

ELIZABETH A. ARENDT, MD

Orthopaedic Consultant and Head Medical Director
for Men's and Women's Varsity Athletics
Director of Sports Medicine Institute
Assistant Professor
Department of Orthopaedic Surgery
University of Minnesota
Minneapolis, Minnesota

STEVEN PAUL ARNOCZKY, DVM, Dipl ACVS

Wade O. Brinker Endowed Professor of Surgery
Director
Laboratory for Comparative Orthopaedic Research
College of Veterinary Medicine
Professor of Surgery
College of Human Medicine
Michigan State University
East Lansing, Michigan

EVAN J. BACHNER, MD

Orthopaedic Surgeon
West Valley Orthopaedics and Sports Medicine
West Hill, California
Former Fellow in Sports Medicine and Arthroscopy
Southern California Orthopedic Institute
Van Nuys, California

GORDON R. BELL, MD

Director, Spine Fellowship Program
Surgical Consultant to Spine Center
Department of Orthopaedic Surgery
Cleveland Clinic Foundation
Consultant
Cleveland Browns and Cleveland Cavaliers
Cleveland, Ohio

JACK R. BENEDICK, MS

Director of Disabled Skiing
United States Ski Team
Park City, Utah

KEVIN P. BLACK, MD

Associate Professor and Associate Chairman
Department of Orthopaedics
Milton S. Hershey Medical Center
Pennsylvania State University College of Medicine
Team Physician
Hershey Bears Professional Hockey Club
Hershey, Pennsylvania

ARTHUR L. BOLAND, Jr, MD

Assistant Clinical Professor of Orthopaedic Surgery
Harvard Medical School-Massachusetts General Hospital
Consultant
New England Patriots Professional Football Team
Boston Bruins Professional Hockey Team
Boston, Massachusetts

MARK K. BOWEN, MD

Assistant Professor of Orthopaedic Surgery
Department of Orthopaedic Surgery
Northwestern University Medical School
Team Physician
Chicago Bears Football Team
Orthopaedic Consultant
Chicago Cubs Baseball Team
Chicago, Illinois

CLIVE E. BREWSTER, MS, PT

Director
Department of Physical Therapy
Kerlan-Jobe Orthopaedic Clinic
Inglewood, California

DAVID M. BRODY, MD

Senior Orthopaedic Attending
Department of Orthopaedic Surgery
Norwalk Hospital
Norwalk, Connecticut

ROBERT D. BRONSTEIN, MD

Assistant Professor, Section of Athletic Medicine
Department of Orthopaedics
University of Rochester School of Medicine
Team Physician
Rochester Americans Hockey Team (AHL)
Rochester Redwings Baseball Team (AAA)
University of Rochester
St. John Fisher College
Rochester, New York

T. PEPPER BURRUSS, ATC, RPT, EMT

Head Athletic Trainer
Green Bay Packers Football Team
Green Bay, Wisconsin

FRANK P. CAMMISA, Jr, MD

Assistant Professor of Surgery
Cornell University Medical College
Assistant Attending Surgeon
The Hospital for Special Surgery
New York, New York

JEROME V. CIULLO, MD

Assistant Clinical Professor, Department of Orthopaedic
Surgery
Director of Sports Medicine
Wayne State University
Detroit, Michigan
Michigan State University
East Lansing, Michigan

DENIS R. CLOHISY, MD

Assistant Professor
Department of Orthopaedic Surgery
University of Minnesota Hospital and Clinic
Minneapolis, Minnesota

MARK D. CONNELL, MD

Post-Doctoral Associate
Department of Orthopaedics and Rehabilitation
Yale University School of Medicine
New Haven, Connecticut

KENNETH E. DeHAVEN, MD

Professor and Associate Chairman
Department of Orthopaedics
Director, Athletic Medicine
University of Rochester School of Medicine
Team Physician
Rochester Americans Hockey Team (AHL)
Rochester Redwings Baseball Team (AAA)
University of Rochester
St. John Fisher College
Rochester, New York

MICHAEL F. DILLINGHAM, MD

Sports, Orthopedic, and Rehabilitation Medicine
Associates
Clinical Professor
Stanford University Medical School
Team Orthopaedic Surgeon
San Francisco 49ers
Team Physician
Stanford University
Stanford, California
Team Physician
Santa Clara University
Santa Clara, California

VINCENT DISTEFANO, MD

Chairman
Department of Orthopaedic Surgery
The Graduate Hospital
Clinical Associate Professor of Orthopaedic Surgery
Hospital of the University of Pennsylvania
Orthopaedic Consultant
Philadelphia Eagles
Philadelphia, Pennsylvania

DAVID DREZ, Jr, MD

Director
Louisiana State University Knee and Sports Medicine
Fellowship
New Orleans, Louisiana
Team Physician
Department of Knee, Shoulder, and Sports Medicine
Center
McNeese State University
Lake Charles, Louisiana, Calcasieu (Parish)

JOSEPH F. FETTO, MD

Associate Clinical Professor
Department of Orthopaedics
New York University Medical Center
Medical Director, Sports Medicine
Consultant to United States Judo Team
New York University Intercollegiate Athletics
New York University
New York, New York

HENRY FEUER, MD

Indianapolis Neurosurgical Group
Clinical Associate Professor of Neurosurgery
Indiana University Medical Center
Neurosurgical Consultant
Indianapolis Colts, Indiana Hoosiers,
and Purdue Boilermakers
Indianapolis, Indiana

DANIEL N. FISH, MD

Former Clinical Fellow in Orthopaedic Surgery and Sports
Medicine
Massachusetts General Hospital
Boston, Massachusetts
Private Practice
Danburg, Connecticut

DEAN FOCHIOS

Former Fellow
Nicholas Institute of Sports Medicine and Athletic Trauma
Lenox Hill Hospital
New York, New York
Attending Staff
Maimonides Hospital
Brooklyn, New York

JAMES M. FOX, MD

Attending Surgeon
Southern California Orthopaedic Institute
Van Nuys, California

VICTOR H. FRANKEL, MD, PhD

Chairman, Department of Orthopaedic Surgery
Hospital for Joint Diseases
Orthopaedic Institute
Professor of Orthopaedic Surgery
New York University School of Medicine
Lecturer, Mount Sinai School of Medicine
New York, New York

MARC J. FRIEDMAN, MD

Clinical Instructor
Division of Orthopedics
University of California, Los Angeles School of Medicine
Los Angeles, California
Attending Surgeon
Southern California Orthopaedic Institute
Van Nuys, California

FREDDIE H. FU, MD

Professor of Orthopaedic Surgery
Vice Chairman, Clinical Services
Department of Orthopaedic Surgery
Chief, Division of Sports Medicine
University of Pittsburgh Medical Center
Team Physician
University of Pittsburgh
Pittsburgh, Pennsylvania

GREGORY G. GALLANT, MD

Department of Orthopaedic Surgery
University of Connecticut Medical School
Farmington, Connecticut

WILLIAM E. GARRETT, Jr, MD, PhD

Associate Professor of Orthopaedic Surgery and Cell
Biology
Department of Orthopaedic Surgery and Anatomy
Duke University Medical Center
Team Physician, Duke Athletics, Duke University
Medical Director, United States Soccer Federation
Durham, North Carolina

BENJAMIN GELFAND, BS, PT

Supervisor, Physical Therapy
Nicholas Institute of Sports Medicine and Athletic Trauma
Lenox Hill Hospital
Adjunct Faculty
School of Education, Health, Nursing, and Art Professions
New York University
New York, New York

BERNARD GHELMAN, MD

Attending Radiologist
The Hospital for Special Surgery
Associate Professor
Department of Radiology
New York Hospital-Cornell University Medical Center
New York, New York

GILBERT W. GLEIM, PhD

Director of Research
Nicholas Institute of Sports Medicine and Athletic Trauma
Lenox Hill Hospital
Adjunct Associate Professor
New York University
New York, New York

JAMES M. GLICK, MD

Associate Clinical Professor
Department of Orthopaedic Surgery
University of California, San Francisco
Team Physician
San Francisco State University
Chief, Department of Orthopaedic Surgery
Mount Zion Medical Center of the University of
California, San Francisco
San Francisco, California

DOUGLAS L. GOLLEHON

Corporate Associate
Cary Orthopaedic and Sports Medicine Specialist
Team Physician
Raleigh Flyers Soccer Team
Attending Physician
Western Wake Medical Center
Raleigh, North Carolina

ALISON B. HAIMES, MD

Assistant Clinical Professor of Radiology
Cornell University Medical Center-New York Hospital
Memorial-Sloan Kettering Cancer Center
New York, New York

CHARLES E. HENNING, MD†

Mid-America Center for Sports Medicine
Associate Professor
Kansas University Medical School
Department of Orthopaedics
Wichita, Kansas

JACK H. HENRY, MD

Columbia Presbyterian Medical Center
New York Orthopaedic Hospital Associates, PC
New York, New York
Former Team Physician
San Antonio Spurs
San Antonio, Texas

STANLEY A. HERRING, MD

Puget Sound Sports and Spine Physicians
Clinical Associate Professor
Department of Rehabilitation Medicine
Clinical Associate Professor
Department of Orthopaedics
University of Washington
Consultant
Seattle Seahawks
Seattle, Washington

ELLIOTT B. HERSHMAN, MD

Assistant Director
Department of Orthopaedic Surgery
Consultant, Nicholas Institute of Sports Medicine and
Athletic Trauma
Lenox Hill Hospital
Team Orthopaedist
New York Jets Football Club
Team Physician
Hunter College Athletic Program
New York, New York

JAMES C. HOLMES, MD

Orthopaedic Surgeon
Western Orthopaedics
Team Orthopaedist
United States Cycling Team
Denver, Colorado

MICHAEL J. HULSTYN, MD

Assistant Professor of Orthopaedic Surgery
Brown University School of Medicine
Rhode Island Hospital
Team Physician
Providence Bruins Professional Hockey Team
Brown University Bears
Providence, Rhode Island
Bryant Bulldogs
Bryant College
Smithfield, Rhode Island

LETHA Y. HUNTER-GRIFFIN, MD, PhD

Staff Physician, Peachtree Orthopaedic Clinic
Team Physician
Georgia State University
Atlanta Georgia
Agnes Scott College
Decatur, Georgia

DOUGLAS W. JACKSON, MD

Medical Director, Southern California Center for Sports
Medicine
Medical Director, Orthopaedic Research Institute
Long Beach, California

JONATHAN S. JAIVIN, MD

Attending Surgeon
Southern California Orthopaedic Institute
Van Nuys, California
Team Physician
St. Genevieve High School
Panorama City, California

PETER JOKL, MD

Professor
Department of Orthopaedics and Rehabilitation
Chief, Section of Sports Medicine
Yale University School of Medicine
New Haven, Connecticut

DONALD C. JONES, MD

Orthopaedic Consultant
Athletic Department
University of Oregon
Orthopaedic and Fracture Clinic
Eugene, Oregon

LAWRENCE I. KARLIN, MD

Chief, Pediatric Orthopaedics
New England Medical Center
Boston, Massachusetts

RICHARD KATZ, MD

Assistant Clinical Professor of Radiology
Cornell University Medical Center-New York Hospital
New York, New York

---

†Deceased.

MARK T. KIRCHER, MD

Former Fellow
Nicholas Institute of Sports Medicine and Athletic Trauma
Lenox Hill Hospital
New York, New York
North Country Sports Medicine
Queensbury, New York

AMY L. KRUMHOLZ, PT, BA, BS

Senior Physical Therapist
Nicholas Institute of Sports Medicine and Athletic Trauma
Lenox Hill Hospital
New York, New York

JOE LEE, MD, BE, ME

Department of Orthopaedics and Rehabilitation
University of California, San Diego
La Jolla, California

MATTHEW P. LOREI, MD

Chief Resident
Department of Orthopaedic Surgery
Lenox Hill Hospital
New York, New York

WYLIE D. LOWERY, Jr, MD

Assistant Professor
Department of Orthopaedic Surgery
George Washington University
Washington, DC
Family Orthopaedics and Sports Medicine of Northern
Virginia
Woodbridge, Virginia

MARY A. LYNCH, MD

Director
The Center for Sports Medicine
Associate Director
St. Joseph Medical Center
Sports Medicine Department
Wichita, Kansas

ANTHONY V. MADDALO, MD

Orthopaedic Consultant
New York Rangers Hockey Team
Hudson Valley Bone and Joint Surgeons
North Tarrytown, New York

S. PETER MAGNUSSON, PT

Project Coordinator
Team Danmark Test Center
Copenhagen, Denmark

ROGER A. MANN, MD

Director, Foot Fellowship Program
Private Practice
Oakland, California
Associate Clinical Professor of Orthopaedic Surgery
University of California
San Francisco, California

MALACHY McHUGH, MA

Fitness Specialist
Nicholas Institute of Sports Medicine and Athletic Trauma
Lenox Hill Hospital
Adjunct Clinical Assistant Professor
Department of Physical Therapy
School of Education
New York University
New York, New York

DUANE G. MESSNER, MD

Associate Clinical Professor
Orthopaedics
University of Colorado School of Medicine
Head Team Physician
United States Disabled Ski Team
Denver, Colorado

LYLE J. MICHELI, MD

Director, Division of Sports Medicine
The Children's Hospital
Associate Clinical Professor of Orthopaedic Surgery
Harvard Medical School
Attending Physician
Boston Ballet
Boston, Massachusetts

DAVID L. MILBAUER, MD

Medical Director
Regency MRI, PC
New York, New York

THEODORE T. MILLER, MD

Assistant Professor
Department of Radiology
Division of Musculoskeletal Radiology
Columbia Presbyterian Medical Center
New York, New York

MATTHEW C. MORRISSEY, MA, PT

Clinical Assistant Professor
Physical Therapy Program
Department of Physical Therapy
Boston University
Boston, Massachusetts

MICHAEL NEUWIRTH, MD

Chief Spine Services
Hospital for Joint Diseases
New York, New York

KENNETH E. NEWHOUSE, MD

Idaho Orthopaedics and Sports Clinic
Team Physician
Idaho State University
Pocatello, Idaho

JAMES A. NICHOLAS, MD

Founder and Director
Nicholas Institute of Sports Medicine and Athletic Trauma
Director Emeritus, Department of Orthopaedic Surgery
Lenox Hill Hospital
Consultant in Orthopaedic Surgery
Hospital for Special Surgery
Chairman, Medical Staff
New York Jets Football Club
New York, New York

STEPHEN J. NICHOLAS, MD

Associate Director
Nicholas Institute of Sports Medicine and Athletic Trauma
Department of Orthopaedic Surgery
Lenox Hill Hospital
Associate Team Physician
New York Jets Football Club
New York, New York

BARTON NISONSON, MD

Section Chief, Division of Arthroscopy
Department of Orthopaedic Surgery
Lenox Hill Hospital
Associate Clinical Professor
Orthopaedic Surgery
Mount Sinai Medical Center
Team Physician and Orthopaedic Surgeon
New York Rangers
New York, New York

GORDON W. NUBER, MD

Associate Professor of Orthopaedic Surgery
Vice Chairman, Department of Orthopaedic Surgery
Director of Orthopaedic Surgery Residency Program
Northwestern University Medical School
Team Physician
Chicago Bears Football Team
Orthopaedic Consultant
Chicago Cubs Baseball Team
Chicago, Illinois

PATRICIA A. O'CONNOR, PT

Senior Physical Therapist
Nicholas Institute of Sports Medicine and Athletic Trauma
Lenox Hill Hospital
New York, New York

PATRICK F. O'LEARY, MD

Clinical Associate Professor of Surgery
Cornell University Medical College
Director, Spine Service
The Hospital for Special Surgery
Chief, Spine Service
Lenox Hill Hospital
New York, New York

MICHAEL J. PAGNANI, MD

Attending Orthopaedic Surgeon
The Lipscomb Clinic
Clinical Assistant Professor
Department of Orthopaedics and Rehabilitation
Vanderbilt University School of Medicine
Associate Team Physician
Tennessee State University
Orthopaedic Consultant
Nashville Sounds Baseball
Nashville, Tennessee

JIM PAPPAS

Fellow in Sports Medicine
Department of Orthopaedics and Rehabilitation
Vanderbilt University Medical Center
Nashville, Tennessee

SHASHIKANT A. PATEL, MD, FRCS, FRCR

Attending Radiologist
Department of Radiology
St. James Hospital
Newark, New Jersey

JOSEPH PATTEN, ATC

Assistant Athletic Trainer
New York Jets Football Club
Hempstead, New York

LONNIE E. PAULOS, MD

Medical Director
Orthopaedic Biomechanics Institute
The Orthopaedic Specialty Hospital
Salt Lake City, Utah

MARK I. PITMAN, MD

Director
Department of Sports Medicine
Hospital for Joint Diseases
Team Physician
Long Island University College of the City of New York
Consultant
Public School Athletic League of New York City
New York, New York

HOLLIS G. POTTER, MD

Assistant Attending Radiologist
The Hospital for Special Surgery
Assistant Professor
Department of Radiology
New York Hospital-Cornell University Medical Center
New York, New York

ANDREW L. PRUITT, EDD, ATC

Director, Sports Medicine
United States Cycling Team
Director, Western Orthopaedic Sports Medicine and
Rehabilitation
Denver, Colorado

WILLIAM G. RAASCH, MD

Assistant Professor of Orthopaedic Surgery
Director, Sports Medicine
Medical College of Wisconsin
Head Team Physician
Milwaukee Mustangs Arena Football Team
Company Physician
Milwaukee Ballet
Milwaukee, Wisconsin

LOUIS H. RAPPOPORT, MD

Orthopaedic Multispeciality Medical Group of San Diego
San Diego, California

ROBERT C. REESE, Jr, ATC

Head Athletic Trainer
New York Jets Football Club
Hempstead, New York

STUART REMER, MD

Spine Surgeon
St. Barnabas Hospital and The Center for Orthopaedic
Surgery and Sports Medicine
Bronx, New York

MICHAEL G. ROCK, MD

Consultant and Professor
Department of Orthopaedic Surgery
Mayo Clinic, Mayo Foundation
Rochester, Minnesota

JEFFREY A. SAAL, MD, FACP

Sports, Orthopedic, and Rehabilitation Medicine
Associates
Clinical Associate Professor
Stanford University Medical School
Team Physician
Stanford University
Stanford, California
Team Physician
Santa Clara University
Santa Clara, California

G. JAMES SAMMARCO, MD, FACS

Volunteer Professor
Department of Orthopaedics
University of Cincinnati
Director
Foot and Ankle Fellowship
The Center for Orthopaedic Care, Inc.
Cincinnati, Ohio

THOMAS G. SAMPSON, MD

Associate Clinical Professor
Department of Orthopaedic Surgery
University of California, San Francisco
Department of Orthopaedic Surgery
Mount Zion Medical Center of the University of
California, San Francisco
Team Physician
San Francisco State University
San Francisco, California

FRANK SANTOPIETRO, DPM

Affiliate in Orthopaedic Surgery (Podiatry)
Children's Hospital
Boston, Massachusetts
Podiatry Consultant to New England Patriots Football
Team
Foxborough, Massachusetts

MICHAEL F. SCHAFER, MD

Ryerson Professor and Chairman
Department of Orthopaedic Surgery
Northwestern University Medical School
Orthopaedic Consultant
Chicago Cubs Baseball Team
Team Physician
Chicago Bears Football Team
Chicago, Illinois

STEPHEN C. SCHARF, MD

Chief, Division of Nuclear Medicine
Lenox Hill Hospital
New York, New York

ROBERT SCHEINBERG, MD

Clinical Assistant Professor
Department of Orthopaedic Surgery
University of Texas Southwestern Medical Center
Dallas, Texas
Orthopaedic Associates
Steadman Hawkins Clinics
Team Physician
United States Ski Team Physician
Vail, Colorado

DANIEL W. SCHMOLL, MD

Trinity Lutheran Family Practice
Kansas City, Missouri

MORTON SCHNEIDER, MD

Consultant in Radiology
Lenox Hill Hospital
New York, New York

STEVEN G. SCOTT, DO

Consultant
Department of Physical Medicine and Rehabilitation
James A. Haley Veterans Hospital
University of Southern Florida
Department of Internal Medicine
Tampa, Florida

JUDY L. SETO, MA, PT

Coordinator of Physical Therapy Research
Department of Physical Therapy
Kerlan-Jobe Orthopaedic Clinic
Inglewood, California

CLARENCE L. SHIELDS, Jr, MD

Associate
Kerlan-Jobe Orthopaedic Clinic
Inglewood, California
Associate Clinical Professor
Department of Orthopaedics
University of Southern California School of Medicine
Orthopaedic Consultant, Los Angeles Rams
Los Angeles, California

FRANKLIN H. SIM, MD

Orthopaedic Surgeon
Department of Orthopaedics
Mayo Clinic
Rochester, Minnesota

KENNETH M. SINGER, MD

Clinical Assistant Professor of Surgery
Division of Orthopaedics and Rehabilitation
Oregon Health Sciences University
Portland, Oregon
Associate Team Physician
University of Oregon
Private Practice
Orthopaedic Fracture Clinic
Eugene, Oregon

ANGELA D. SMITH, MD

Assistant Professor
Department of Orthopaedic Surgery
Case Western Reserve University
Chair, Sports Medicine
United States Figure Skating Association
Cleveland, Ohio

ROGER SOHN, MD

Medical Staff
Century City Hospital
Cedars Sinai Medical Center
Los Angeles, California

KURT SPINDLER, MD

Team Physician and Assistant Professor
Department of Orthopaedics and Rehabilitation
Vanderbilt University Medical Center
Nashville, Tennessee

J. RICHARD STEADMAN, MD

Clinical Professor
University of Texas Southwestern Medical School
Dallas, Texas
Chairman, Medical Group United States Ski Team
Orthopaedic Surgeon
Steadman Hawkins Clinic
Vail, Colorado

DAVID A. STONE, MD

Assistant Professor of Orthopaedics
Division of Sports Medicine
Department of Orthopaedic Surgery
University of Pittsburgh Medical Center
Assistant Team Physician
University of Pittsburgh
Team Physician
Point Park College
Pittsburgh, Pennsylvania

ALAN M. STRIZAK, MD

Clinical Assistant Professor of Pediatrics
University of California at Los Angeles School of Medicine
Los Angeles, California
Clinical Assistant Professor
Department of Orthopaedic Surgery
University of California, Irvine School of Medicine
Irvine, California

MARIO R. TAILLON, MD, FRCS(C)

Calgary, Alberta, Canada

MALCOLM D. THOMAS, MB, BS, FRACS

Consultant Orthopaedic Surgeon
Department of Orthopaedics
Latnobe Valley Hospital
Traralgon, Victoria, Australia

PETER A. TORZILLI, PhD

Associate Professor of Applied Biomechanics
Cornell University Medical College
Senior Scientist and Director
Laboratory for Soft Tissue Research
New York, New York

VINCENT J. TURCO, MD

Director, Orthopaedic Resident Training
Department of Orthopaedic Surgery
St. Francis Hospital and Medical Center
Team Physician Emeritus
Hartford Whalers Hockey Team (NHL)
Hartford, Connecticut
Professor of Orthopaedic Surgery
University of Connecticut Medical School
Farmington, Connecticut

DANIEL M. VELTRI, MD, MAJOR USAF MC

Chief of Orthopaedic Services
Luke Air Force Base
Litchfield Park, Arizona

THOMAS W. VORDERER, DPM

Affiliate in Orthopaedic Surgery (Podiatry)
Division of Sports Medicine
The Children's Hospital
Boston, Massachusetts

JOHN F. WALLER, MD

Associate Attending Physician
Orthopaedic Department
Mount Sinai Hospital
Orthopaedic Department
Mount Sinai School of Medicine
New York, New York

RUSSEL F. WARREN, MD

Surgeon-in-Chief
The Hospital for Special Surgery
Professor of Orthopaedic Surgery
Cornell University Medical College
Team Physician
New York Giants
New York, New York

STUART M. WEINSTEIN, MD

Puget Sound Sports and Spine Physicians
Clinical Assistant Professor
Department of Rehabilitation Medicine
University of Washington
Seattle, Washington

NINA J. WHALEN, RN, ANP

Research Coordinator
Western Orthopaedics
Western Orthopaedic Sports Medicine
Denver, Colorado

THOMAS L. WICKIEWICZ, MD

Associate Attending Orthopaedic Surgeon
Chief, Sports Medicine and Shoulder Service
The Hospital for Special Surgery
Associate Professor of Orthopaedic Surgery
Cornell University Medical College
New York, New York

SAVIO L-Y WOO, PhD

Ferguson Professor of Orthopaedics and Vice Chairman
for Research
Department of Orthopaedic Surgery
Professor of Mechanical Engineering
Department of Orthopaedic Surgery
University of Pittsburgh
Pittsburgh, Pennsylvania

JOHN L. XETHALIS, MD

Adjunct, Department of Orthopaedic Surgery
Lenox Hill Hospital
Team Physician
New York Cosmos Soccer Club
New York, New York

JOHN G. YOST Jr, MD

Associate Clinical Professor of Orthopaedic Surgery
Truman Medical Center
University of Missouri
Kansas City, Missouri
Team Physician
Baker University
Baldwin City, Kansas
Orthopaedic Consultant
Northwest Missouri State University
Maryville, Missouri

PAUL M. ZABETAKIS, MD

Research Physician
Nicholas Institute of Sports Medicine and Athletic Trauma
Associate Chief, Nephrology
Department of Medicine
Lenox Hill Hospital
Clinical Associate Professor of Medicine
Department of Medicine
New York University School of Medicine
New York, New York

BERTRAM ZARINS, MD

Assistant Clinical Professor of Orthopaedic Surgery
Harvard Medical School
Chief, Sports Medicine Unit
Massachusetts General Hospital
Team Physician
Boston Bruins and New England Patriots
Boston, Massachusetts

To
Kiki
my lifelong love, who has made our days together wonderful
James A. Nicholas

To
Todd and Daniel
the shining light of every day
Elliott B. Hershman

Foreword

Just as the field of sports medicine has become popular over the past 20 years, so have textbooks relating to sports injuries. Beginning with Dr. O'Donoghue's textbook on *Treatment of Injuries to Athletes*, texts are now increasingly available. However, in this second edition of *The Lower Extremity and Spine in Sports Medicine,* Dr. Nicholas and Dr. Hershman have undertaken and fulfilled the task of providing us with a comprehensive, well-illustrated, and well-referenced text.

Well-known and respected authors from across the United States have written 66 chapters that present information ranging from basic science considerations and individual regional topics to sports-specific injuries. Each chapter, preceded by an outline, thoroughly discusses its topic with comprehensive references before the author's preferred methods are discussed. The majority of the chapters from the first edition have been completely rewritten, providing us with an up-do-date text. Twenty entirely new chapters have been added, extending the comprehensive coverage of sports medicine.

Coordinating a textbook of this magnitude is not an easy task, especially with as many topics and authors as Dr. Nicholas and Dr. Hershman have selected. I am sure that the individual authors were happy to contribute, as I am, because of our admiration for Dr. Nicholas and his unquestionable status as one of the fathers of sports medicine in this country. Dr. Hershman has worked extensively with Dr. Nicholas, and the contributors have come to respect Dr. Hershman for his dedication to the field of sports medicine and are pleased to have this opportunity to present their perspective.

Lenox Hill Hospital is a well-known center for excellence in treating all phases of athletic injuries, and the editors have lived up to their reputation by publishing a "must have" book for all sports medicine physicians, fellowships, and sports medicine libraries.

K. Donald Shelbourne, M.D.

Preface
to the second edition

The popularity of sports reflects society's abiding interest in them, both as entertainment and leisure time activities. The pursuit of sports is integrated into daily life to such a degree that sports medicine has become an important ingredient in successful and safe athletic participation.

The technology explosion is progressing so rapidly that constant updates are needed in the diagnostic, surgical, clinical, and rehabilitative aspects of sports medicine. Advances in these areas over the past few years, coupled with technologic breakthroughs in imaging, have yielded earlier and more accurate diagnoses. Surgical techniques improve as many procedures give way to arthroscopic or minimally invasive protocols. Nonoperative care and rehabilitation benefit from well-controlled research, with improved and accelerated rehabilitation techniques forming part of the routine care of athletes. Clinical and basic science research enables athletes to safely and successfully extend their careers. New procedures and techniques should be viewed with healthy skepticism until meaningful data to support them are available; therefore sports medicine practitioners should continue to base their treatment on generally accepted principles. This text makes available to the sports medicine clinician the most current information extant in the field. We have added extensive material on the latest techniques in im-aging, surgical procedures, nonoperative treatment, and rehabilitation.

The health care reform debate seeks to emphasize the role of primary care professionals as the initial contact to the injured athlete. As health care changes, up-to-date reference texts are vital to the ability of providers to care for athletes. Costs may be controlled by accurate diagnosis and early treatment. We have attempted to make our text a resource to meet the needs of the primary care provider and the specialist in sports medicine. The prevention of athletic trauma, given its high cost, cannot be stressed enough; we have included new information in this area as well.

We continue to emphasize the linkage relationship of movement. Integration of the entire musculoskeletal system into prevention and treatment is an integral part of sports medicine. The entire text is written with these concepts in mind.

We hope the reader finds these books a useful reference for the prevention, diagnosis, and treatment of injuries in athletes. If safe participation, speedy and successful recovery from injury, and enhanced quality of life from sports are achieved, we have met our goal—for our athletes.

James A. Nicholas
Elliott B. Hershman

Preface
to the first edition

Within the last two decades, sports medicine has emerged to become a rapidly expanding, multilayered discipline. The increased participation in athletics by millions of individuals, coupled with demand for knowledge about prevention, care, and treatment of athletic injuries, led to the development of the Institute of Sports Medicine and Athletic Trauma (ISMAT),* a special section of the Department of Orthopaedic Surgery at Lenox Hill Hospital in New York City. Indeed, ISMAT was the first hospital-based sports medicine institute of its type in the country. The Institute is currently a national center devoted to research, education, and clinical service, supported in part by an endowment fund.

The exponential growth and explosion of interest has contributed to the development of the sports medicine physician. Although a number of medical specialities are involved in the care of the athlete, the orthopaedic surgeon is at the core of sports medicine because of the fundamental importance of the musculoskeletal system in athletic endeavors. The role of the sports medicine physician is clear: to provide scientifically based intervention to all athletes, male or female, young or old, novice or professional, that will enable individuals to participate to their fullest potential so as to enjoy recreation and enhance physical fitness and ability. This should include disabled persons who wish to indulge in recreational activities.

We feel that the musculoskeletal system is of primary importance in the acquisition of fitness by an individual. It provides part of the fuel system as well as the motors, levers, and joints that move the body through space. For this reason, injuries to this finely coordinated and conditioned system demand a special emphasis, with rehabilitation being an integral part of treatment. The economy of motion and efficiency in overcoming inertia decide, to a large extent, the impact of sports on the ability of the individual to train and enjoy sports without danger.

The human musculoskeletal system is highly integrated, and its malfunctioning parts are inextricably related to the whole spectrum which comprises the integrated human system. The brain can be likened to a giant emotional computer, the heart to a pump, the kidneys to a waste system, and the musculoskeletal system to a leverage system, which overcomes inertia when we move about. Sports medicine must therefore emphasize how injury and pathology affect the body, encompassing areas such as anatomy, biochemistry, biomechanics, histopathology, pharmacology, and physiology.

With this in mind, this text has been written to emphasize the complex interrelationship between various parts of the musculoskeletal system, as well as the physiologic and psychologic implications of musculoskeletal injury. Every substantial injury to the body leaves a residual effect. Subsequently, the ability to meet maximal demands of sport at a later date, perhaps even years later, may be compromised. Musculoskeletal derangement, pathology, or physiologic malfunction can occur far from the site of the initial injury. Tunnel vision of a malfunctioning part must not occur. To exclude the implications of such a pathologic condition on the rest of the body may lead to further defects in the musculoskeletal system. Interrelationships between body segments and systems are emphasized by the concepts inherent in the linkage system. Throughout the text, the reader should relate each joint and its injury in relation to the linkage system. Assessment and treatment of the entire proximal and distal links of the spine and lower extremity then must always be kept in mind in treating athletic injuries.

We have attempted to relate clinical situations to some basic scientific knowledge. Hence significant sections of the text have been devoted to the basic sciences. Coupling basic science with clinical experience yields basic patterns of intervention firmly grounded on scientific inquiry, an approach now possible in sports medicine as a result of the excellent research being done in the basic sciences.

The text has been written by a talented cadre of health care professionals who are heavily involved or interested in the care of athletes. Our aim is to have them describe their opinions as to the mechanisms of injuries in the lower extremity and in the spine, their recognition, treatment, and rehabilitation, and how they may be prevented. Because of this comprehensive approach, we have limited the text to the lower extremity and entire spine to allow complete discussion of the areas covered. We have also included a number of chapters on some sports-specific injuries, which will enable the reader to consider injuries directly in light of the demands of specific sports. Moreover, the skeletally immature athlete is considered in a separate section of the text, because treatment of these individuals is significantly different from their adult counterparts. Because of the rapidly changing nature of the way upper extremity work is be-

*Now referred to as Nicholas Institute of Sports Medicine and Athletic Trauma (NISMAT).

ing done, such as diagnostic and surgical arthroscopy of the shoulder, elbow, and hand, the use of scanning techniques, and the early, less-defined studies of upper body training on the entire linkage system, we thought it wise to defer the upper extremity volume until more clinical material becomes readily available.

We think that the young field of sports medicine will continue to advance with the assistance of computerized study into the linkage phenomena. In particular, it is important that we recognize and understand the relationship of motions used in various sports and how these motions are directly related to the causes of injury, and the subsequent effects of recurring injury on the body. We do not believe in any "average individual," and we are confident that future research will substantiate this premise. With time, the concept of profiling—the interrelationship between physical and psychologic attributes of athletes and the demands of sport—will be better understood by those professionals responsible for the pre-

vention, diagnosis, and treatment of injuries. Exercise programs will then be specifically adapted to each athlete's profile, pathology, and performance demands.

Although this text has been written primarily for practicing orthopaedic surgeons, orthopaedic residents, and sports medicine specialists, it is also intended for allied health professionals, including the athletic trainer, health and physical educator, exercise physiologist, physical therapist, and others who are part of the sports medicine team. Understanding the mechanisms of injuries in sports, the diagnosis, treatment, and rehabilitation of injuries, and the subsequent course of an individual following an injury is an immense task, but a great challenge. This book will hopefully integrate the multidisciplinary concepts of sports medicine and provide the reader with an understanding of the importance of the musculoskeletal system and the concept of linkage.

James A. Nicholas
Elliott B. Hershman

Acknowledgments

Our deep appreciation and gratitude:

To our contributing authors, who continue to write up-to-date, authoritative, and well-researched chapters. We cannot thank them enough for their efforts in completing this project.

To Suzanne VanderSanden whose unsurpassed organizational and leadership skills enabled clinical schedules and responsibilities to mesh with didactic, research, and writing commitments. Her daily administrative efforts keep the office afloat.

To Trish Naso and Pat Kennemur, who ably and diligently handled our correspondence and communication.

To Jeannette Gudino, Peggy Pappas, Shirley Bekas, Pat Taleb, Sylvia Melendez, and Mary DiRado for their energetic and gracious assistance throughout the publication process.

To George Tanis and Sophie Bedmarz of the Lenox Hill Hospital Department of Medical Photography for their outstanding work in the production of many of the fine photographs used throughout the text.

To our editors at Mosby–Year Book, Bob Hurley, Kathy Falk, Ellen Baker-Geisel, and Suzanne Fannin. They continued to guide and work untiringly on this text. Their patience and understanding are invaluable.

Contents

CHAPTER 45

Thigh Injuries

Jonathan S. Jaivin
James M. Fox

Thigh injuries are a relatively uncommon sports injury. However, the prompt recognition and treatment of these injuries are critical to prevent prolonged disability. Recent advances in the treatment of these injuries has deepened our awareness and understanding of this clinical problem. Despite the comparatively simple anatomic configuration of the thigh, this region is a finely tuned muscular mechanism with both anterior and posterior muscles crossing two joints. Consequently, contracture of the thigh musculature can result in decreased flexion or extension of the knee or flexion or extension contractures at the hip. Thigh injuries can result in local problems and dysfunction, both proximally and distally. The pelvis and lower back may be affected in a similar fashion. Therefore a systematic and thorough approach to thigh injuries is necessary to identify, treat, and rehabilitate this region. The purpose of this chapter is to discuss some of the more common thigh injuries and their recommended treatments. This chapter is divided into sections on anatomy, physical examination, descriptions of common injuries and suggested treatment programs, and rehabilitative techniques.

ANATOMY

Compartments

The human thigh can be divided into a posterior, or flexor, compartment and an anterior, or extensor, compartment that are divided by a lateral intermuscular septum. There is no medial intermuscular septum. The inner aspect of the thigh contains the adductor muscles. The flexor and adductor compartments fuse at the adductor magnus. The thigh muscles overlie the largest and longest bone in the body, the femur. Because of the extensive soft-tissue envelope that surrounds the femur, the femur is only palpable under the subcutaneous tissue at its most distal and proximal aspects.

Cutaneous Sensory Innervation

The inner aspect of the thigh includes the L1, L2, L3, and L4 dermatomes progressing from the proximal to the distal level. Sensation on the lateral aspect of the thigh is provided by the L5 dermatome. The central portion of the posterior thigh is supplied by the S1 and S2 dermatomes (Fig. 45-1). The posterior thigh is innervated by the **posterior femoral cutaneous nerve.** Laterally, sensation to the thigh is via the **lateral femoral cutaneous** nerve. The posterior femoral cutaneous nerve runs vertically down the thigh just beneath the tensor fasciae latae and ends halfway down the calf. The anterior aspect of the thigh is supplied by three major cutaneous nerves: the **medial femoral cutaneous** nerve,

---

Cutaneous nerves of the thigh

- Posterior femoral cutaneous nerve
- Medial femoral cutaneous nerve
- Intermediate femoral cutaneous nerve
- Lateral femoral cutaneous nerve

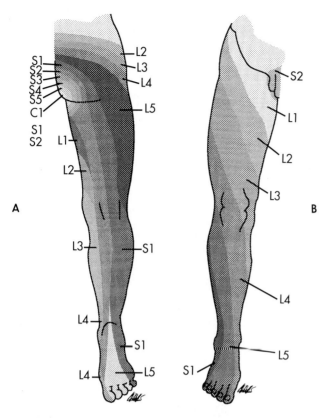

FIG. 45-1. Dermatomes of the thigh. **A,** Posterior view. **B,** Anterior view.

the **intermediate femoral cutaneous** nerve, and the **lateral femoral cutaneous nerve.** The lateral femoral cutaneous nerve is incorporated within the substances of the inguinal ligament near the anterior superior iliac crest and continues distally and laterally (Fig. 45-2).

Fascia and Subcutaneous Tissue

Subcutaneous fat in the well-trained athlete may be minimal. Beneath the subcutaneous fat layer is the **fascia lata,** a fascial envelope that surrounds the entire thigh musculature. The fascia lata originates at the level of the pelvis and attaches distally to the patella, the distal margins of the tibial condyles, and the head of the fibula. It becomes thicker and less expansive distally, and its fibers run in a longitudinal fashion from proximal to distal.

Posterior Structures

The hamstring muscles form the bulk of the posterior thigh and include the **biceps femoris,** the **semitendinosus,** and the **semimembranosus** (Fig. 45-3). These muscles originate from the ischial tuberosity. The biceps femoris has two distinct muscle bellies. The long head of the biceps femoris arises from the ischial tuberosity and the sacrotuberal ligament. It inserts into the head of the fibula and the lateral condyle of the proximal tibia. The short head of the biceps femoris arises from the lateral linea aspera and the lateral intermuscular septum. It inserts into the lateral condyle of the proximal tibia. The semitendinosus arises from the ischial tuberosity

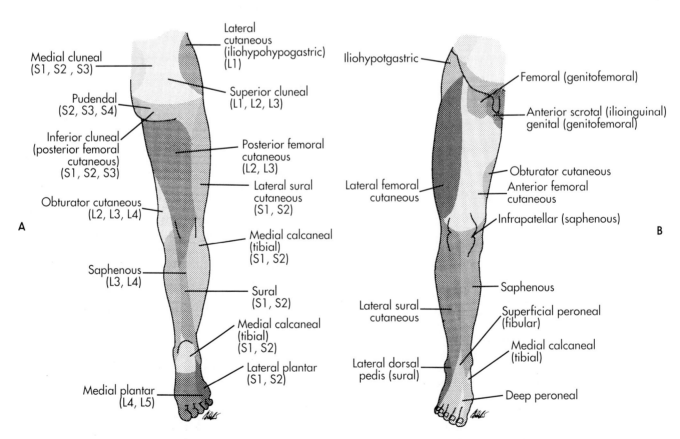

FIG. 45-2. Cutaneous nerves of the thigh. **A,** Posterior view. **B,** Anterior view.

and inserts into the medial portion of the proximal tibia. The semimembranosus arises from the ischial tuberosity and inserts into the posteromedial aspect of the proximal tibial condyle. This insertion is diffuse in nature and includes ramifications into the posterior aspect of the knee joint and the capsular area. All of these muscles are innervated by the tibial portion of the sciatic nerve. The ischial fibers of the adductor magnus muscle may also be included as part of the hamstring.

In the proximal one third of the thigh the sciatic nerve lies on the adductor magnus, approximately 1 cm from the lateral margin of the semimembranosus tendon deep

to the proximal portions of the biceps femoris and semitendinosus muscles. The cordlike tendon of the semitendinosus muscle overlies the muscular portion of the semimembranosus tendon. The muscle belly of the semimembranosus is transformed at the level of the medial femoral condyle into a strong tendon that inserts onto the posterior aspect of the medial tibia.

The **semitendinosus** muscle is a bulky structure located proximally in the thigh. It decreases in size as it courses distally and lies as a thin, flat tendinous structure overlying the flat tendon of the semimembranosus muscle. The name *semitendinosus* is well suited to this

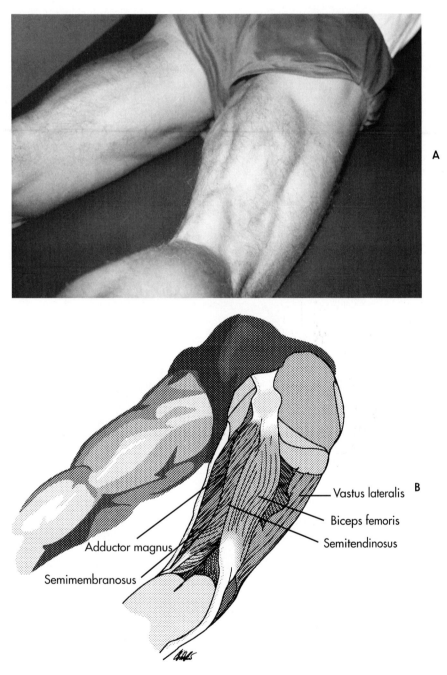

FIG. 45-3. A, Photograph of posterior anatomy of thigh. **B,** Drawing of posterior anatomy of thigh.

structure because the muscle is rapidly replaced by its long tendinous portion. The tendon passes posterior to the medial femoral condyle and continues anteriorly to insert on the medial portion of the proximal tibia as part of the pes anserinus.

The **biceps femoris** is composed of two heads. The short head originates from the linea aspera and the femur. Its muscle fibers fuse with the long head of the biceps femoris into a single tendon. This conjoined tendon inserts into the head of the fibula and the lateral condyle of the tibia.

Functional Anatomy

Actions of the hamstring muscles are reciprocal, causing flexion of the knee joint distally and extension of the hip joint proximally. With the knee held in the extended position by the action of the quadriceps muscles anteriorly, the hamstring muscles extend the hip. This complex two-joint role for the hamstrings makes them susceptible to injury. Of note, the only one-joint muscle in this group is the short head of the biceps femoris. The hamstring muscles also contribute to rotatory motion of the tibia by virtue of their insertions on the medial and lateral portions of the proximal tibia. The biceps femoris muscle externally rotates the lower leg because of its lateral insertion. Internal rotation is provided by the semitendinosus muscle by virtue of its medial insertion.

Reciprocal actions of the hamstrings

- Hip *extension*
- Knee *flexion*

These muscles receive their blood supply from the perforating branches of the profunda femoris artery.

Lateral Structures

On the lateral aspect of the thigh is the strong thickening of the tensor fasciae latae known as the **iliotibial tract** (Fig. 45-4). The iliotibial tract, or band, is composed of the distal fascial continuation of the tensor fasciae latae muscle and the distal expansion of the fascia overlying the gluteus maximus. The tract passes down the posterolateral aspect of the thigh and has attachments to the lateral intermuscular septum and to the vastus lateralis anteriorly. This tract has a major stabilizing influence on the knee with actions of both flexion and extension, depending on the angle of flexion of the knee joint.

Medial Structures

The adductor component of the thigh is contiguous with the flexor compartment. However, the adductors

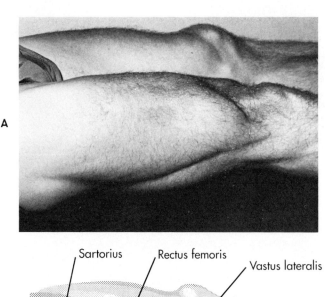

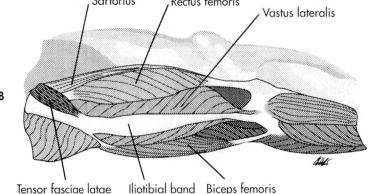

FIG. 45-4. A, Photograph of lateral anatomy of thigh. **B,** Drawing of lateral anatomy of thigh.

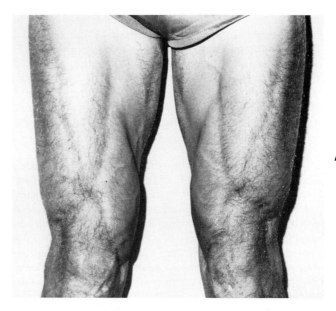

A

are separated from the quadriceps by the medial intermuscular septum. The muscles of this medial compartment consist of the gracilis muscle and the three adductors: longus, brevis, and magnus. The **gracilis** arises as a flat sheet from the edge of the pubis and extends distally to blend into the pes anserinus tendon. The **adductor longus** arises from the pubic crest and inserts by a flat aponeurotic tendon into the lower two thirds of the linea aspera. The **adductor brevis** originates from the inferior aspect of the pubis, widens, and inserts into the upper part of the linea aspera. The **adductor magnus** arises on the inferior portion of the pubis and inserts into the adductor tubercle of the distal femur. The gracilis is the most superficial of these muscles, overlying the anteriorly located adductor longus and posterior adductor magnus. The adductor brevis lies between the longus and magnus proximally.

All of these muscles are innervated by the obturator nerve. They are also supplied by the profunda femoris artery. This artery enters the adductor compartment from the lateral side of the femoral artery to pass behind the upper border of the adductor longus.

Anterior Structures

The femoral artery and vein emerge from the femoral sheath and course downward to lie deep to the sartorius muscle. The major branch of the femoral artery within the thigh is the profunda femoris. The superficial femoral artery continues distally, becoming the popliteal artery at the hiatus of the adductor magnus. Coursing with the artery and vein is the saphenous nerve, which exits at the level of the pes anserinus tendon group.

The anterior thigh musculature, bounded laterally by the lateral intermuscular septum and medially by the adductor muscles and the vascular bundle, consists of the quadriceps muscle and the sartorius muscle. The quadriceps muscle is the largest muscle in the body and has four components, as signified by its name (Fig. 45-5).

The **rectus femoris** muscle arises from the ilium by two heads: the reflected head arising immediately above the acetabulum and the straight, or direct, head arising from the upper half of the anterior inferior iliac spine. Immediately above the patella it flattens to form the anterior aspect of the quadriceps tendon. Its posterior surface has a thick, glistening aponeurosis that glides on the anterior surface of the underlying vastus intermedius.

The **vastus lateralis** muscle has an extensive origin from the upper half of the intertrochanteric line, the lateral aspect of the linea aspera, and the upper two thirds of the femoral shaft. The portion of the origin on the in-

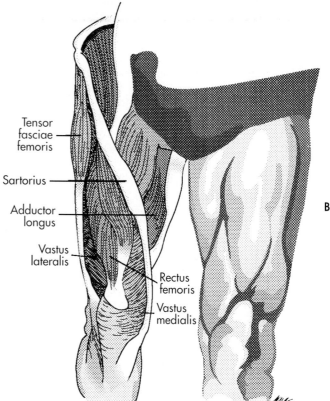

Tensor
fasciae
femoris

Sartorius

Adductor
longus

Vastus
lateralis

Rectus
femoris

Vastus
medialis

B

FIG. 45-5. A, Photograph of anterior anatomy of thigh. **B,** Drawing of anterior anatomy of thigh.

ferior and lateral margin of the greater trochanter is known as the **vastus ridge.** The vastus lateralis also inserts into the quadriceps tendon.

The **vastus intermedius** muscle, the deepest of the quadriceps muscle, takes it origin from the anterior portion of the distal two thirds of the femur. It lies deep to the rectus femoris and between the vastus medialis and vastus lateralis. Distally the tendinous expansion of the vastus intermedius forms the deep layer of the trilaminar quadriceps tendon.

The **vastus medialis** muscle arises from the medial aspect of the linea aspera and from the tendon of the adductor magnus. It slopes distally and lies on the vastus intermedius, finally inserting in a horizontal fashion directly into the medial border of the patella. The vastus medialis muscle generally consists of two parts: the vastus medialis longus and the vastus medialis obliquus. These portions of the vastus medialis muscle are identified by the direction of the muscle fibers. The vastus medialis longus fibers run parallel to the long axis of the entire quadriceps group. The vastus medialis obliquus fibers, however, are angled 30 to 45 degrees from the long axis of the quadriceps muscle. The insertion of vastus medialis obliquus is also located more distally on the patella than that of the vastus medialis longus.

An additional small muscle in the thigh is the **articularis genus** muscle, which arises beneath the vastus intermedius muscle and inserts into the upper aspect of the suprapatellar bursa. It functions to retract the suprapatellar synovium with knee extension.

All five muscles, the rectus femoris, vastus lateralis, vastus intermedius, vastus medialis, and articularis genus, are supplied by the femoral nerve.

Functional Anatomy

The main action of the quadriceps muscle is knee extension. Patellofemoral motion is guided by the complex insertion of the quadriceps muscle on the patella. The rectus femoris is the sole two-joint muscle in the quadriceps group, taking origin from the pelvis. As such, it also functions as a hip flexor. This two-joint function makes it particularly vulnerable to injury from abnormal stretch occurring with maximal knee flexion and hip extension.

Summary

A basic understanding of the gross anatomic relationships is critical to the physical examination of the thigh. In some individuals, such as the world-class miler, the muscle groups can be seen to stand out as distinct entities. In the unconditioned athlete, they may not be as dramatically defined.

PHYSICAL EXAMINATION
Observation

The patient must be examined with the area in question appropriately exposed. Simply rolling up the pant leg is not sufficient; the clothing must be removed to expose both legs for adequate inspection and palpation of the thigh. Physical examination of the thigh commences

with observation. The patient is inspected in the standing position. The patient should be viewed from the anterior, posterior, and lateral aspects (Fig. 45-6, A-C). This allows the examiner to appreciate the alignment of the extremity with the foot flat on the ground. Particular attention needs to be directed to internal and external rotation of the extremities and to visible deformities. Areas of ecchymosis and swelling are observed by simply comparing one leg with the other. Muscle bulk and symmetry are also noted. The knees should be fully extended. Flexion at the knee may be a clue to a hamstring problem. Additionally, the patient is asked to squat or kneel on the ground and place the buttocks on the heels. This facilitates observation of the anterior and medial muscle masses (Fig. 45-6, D).

Supine Examination

The patient is placed on the examining table in the supine position and inspected again for areas of deformity. Palpation is then done in an organized manner, beginning first on the anterior thigh at the pubic symphysis. Here the adductor musculature is palpated, and the presence of a spasm, soft-tissue enlargement, and asymmetric contour are noted. In a similar fashion the proximal origin of the quadriceps muscles is palpated. Continuing distally down the muscles, areas of enlargement, tenderness, or defects can be felt with careful palpation. The patient then contracts the quadriceps, and any change in the presence or size of defects is noted (Fig. 45-7, A).

Next, the ranges of motion of the hip and knee joints are evaluated. Subtle contractures of the anterior hip and thigh musculature can usually be demonstrated by the Thomas test (Fig. 45-7, B). Both hips are flexed maximally to eliminate lumbar lordosis. The patient holds one hip in the flexed position. The opposite hip is then carefully extended. Lack of complete extension is consistent with a hip flexion contracture. The angle formed by the horizontal and the incompletely extended hip is the degree of contracture.

Hamstring tightness or contracture is evaluated by lifting the legs off the examining table by the heels. In this position the hips should allow flexion to at least 60 degrees without involuntary knee flexion. Flexion of the knee that occurs at less than 60 degrees of hip flexion is consistent with tight hamstring musculature (Fig. 45-7, C).

Another test for quantifying hamstring contracture is **measuring the popliteal angle.** To test the right side, the right hip is flexed to 90 degrees from the table and a

---

Measuring the popliteal angle

- The examiner places a hand on the iliac spine to stabilize the pelvis.
- The hip of leg being tested is flexed to 90 degrees, keeping the knee flexed.
- The knee is extended from a fully flexed position to a position where the pelvis is felt to move.
- The angle of knee flexion is measured (full knee extension is 0 degrees).

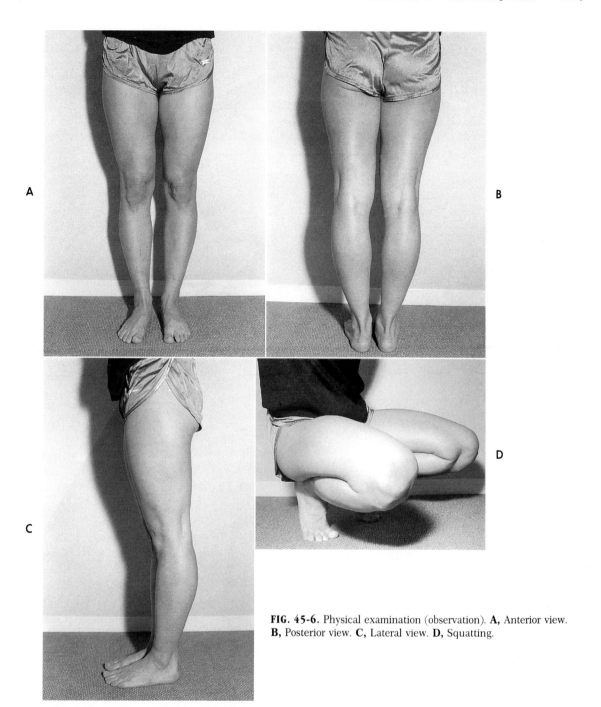

FIG. 45-6. Physical examination (observation). **A,** Anterior view. **B,** Posterior view. **C,** Lateral view. **D,** Squatting.

hand is placed on the iliac spine. The right knee is slowly extended until the pelvis moves. The amount of knee flexion at the popliteal angle is measured. By convention, if the leg is able to be extended fully, the popliteal angle measurement is 0 degrees (Fig. 45-7, *D*).

Prone Examination

The patient is placed in the prone position, and beginning proximally at the gluteal fold the examiner slowly palpates the entire proximal thigh musculature, progressing distally. Both the medial and lateral hamstring areas are carefully palpated. At times, to further delineate the anatomy, the patient is asked to flex the knee.

This brings the hamstring muscles into tension. The examiner applies resistance to maintain the muscle contraction. Defects within the muscles are often more apparent when the patient is contracting the muscles. Palpation extends into the popliteal fossa with digital confirmation of the integrity of the medial and lateral hamstring folds (Fig. 45-8, *A*).

Next the range of motion is evaluated and compared with the opposite extremity. Each leg is maximally flexed. Limitation of flexion secondary to contracture of the anterior thigh musculature **(Ely's test)** may be demonstrated as either limitation of knee flexion or compensatory hip flexion (Fig. 45-8, *B*).

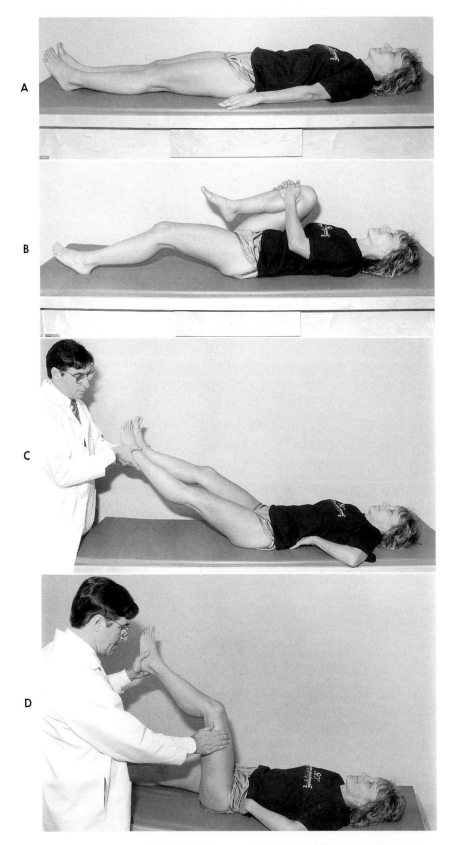

FIG. 45-7. Physical examination (supine). **A,** Maximal quadriceps contracture (normal). **B,** Positive Thomas test: left hip flexion contracture. **C,** Right hamstring contracture. **D,** Forty-five–degree popliteal angle.

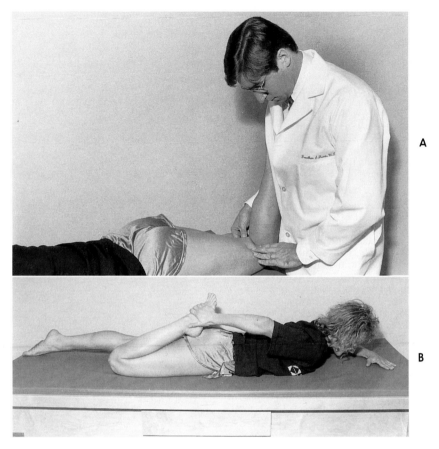

FIG. 45-8. A, Examination of hamstrings in prone position. Patient flexes gently against resistance to facilitate palpation of muscles and the hamstring folds. **B,** Flexion in prone position (Ely's test).

"Decubitus" Position

With the affected side up, flexion and extension of the hip and of the knee joint are evaluated by feeling over the greater trochanteric area for palpable snapping of the tensor fasciae latae over the underlying structure. Palpation is continued distally for any localized swelling or defects. In this position, Ober's test can be performed to evaluate for contracture of the iliotibial tract (see Fig. 41-18).

Radiographic and Additional Studies

After completion of the physical examination, additional standard diagnostic tests, including routine radiographs in the anterior and posterior planes from the hip to the knee, are obtained. Bony structure, cortical thickening, periosteal reaction, and soft-tissue calcifications are evaluated. The probability of finding an abnormality on these routine films initially is extremely low, but they serve as the baseline for subsequent studies. Follow-up radiographs may become necessary to delineate the progressive metaplastic calcification that frequently occurs within soft-tissue hematomas. If radiographs are not performed, confusion can later arise regarding the chronology of calcification.

Other studies that may provide additional information

include sedimentation rate, alkaline phosphatase, calcium and phosphorus levels, and coagulation studies. Computed tomography (CT) can be used to differentiate myositis ossificans from other lesions by demonstrating the mature bone of the outer shell of the lesion (zoning effect).

Technetium bone scan can be used to evaluate bone turnover rate for early diagnosis of stress-reactive changes and activity within myositis ossificans. Myositis ossificans may also be detected with ultrasound before the appearance of radiographic changes. Generally, ossification becomes apparent after only 2 to 5 weeks.

INJURIES
Fractures
Major Fractures

Fractures of the femoral shaft are infrequent athletic injuries, except in high-velocity or vehicular sports. However, they do occasionally occur. The principles of management of a fractured femur are beyond the scope of this chapter. It is important to recognize that high-performance athletes cannot tolerate a significant leg length or rotational discrepancy. Therefore restoring and maintaining length, rotation, and angulation are ex-

Radiographic examination of the femur

By David L. Milbauer and Shashikant Patel

Stress fractures

The femur has been recognized as a potential site of stress fracture.[4,8,11] Specifically, the femoral neck has been recognized as particularly vulnerable to this type of injury.[1,5,7,13] As in cases of stress fractures involving the lower leg and foot, initial plain radiographs are typically normal. We emphasize the importance of using radionuclide bone scanning when femoral stress fractures are clinically suspected, particularly when early diagnosis may be critical in patient management (Fig. 1).

Myositis ossificans

Myositis ossificans is characterized by localized heterotopic bone formation in soft tissues that have undergone direct trauma. Norman and Dorfman[10] have shown that the radiographic changes parallel a definable histopathologic evolution. A soft-tissue mass may be detected shortly following injury, and faint calcifications become evident in the third to fourth week. Juxtacortical lesions may be associated with a localized periosteal reaction as well. At 6 to 8 weeks a sharply circumscribed cortical periphery forms around the central lacy pattern of new bone (Fig. 2, *A*).[3] A radiolucent cleft separates the juxtacortical lesions from the adjacent bone, a finding that may require special tangential views or computed tomography for demonstration. The ossified lesions may develop cysts that may enlarge and result in an eggshell cyst.[10] Maturity is reached in 5 to 6 months (Fig. 3), and the ossified mass may regress in size, usually disappearing completely within a year, but a residual exostosis with an attachment to bone may remain.[3] Radionuclide bone imaging demonstrates an uptake of the bone tracer in the affected soft tissues (Fig. 2, *B*).

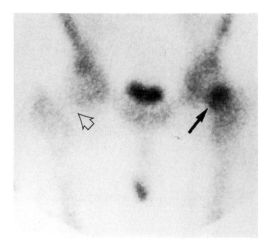

FIG. 1. Radionuclide bone scan demonstrates increased uptake in region of left femoral neck *(closed arrow)*, compared with normal appearance on right *(open arrow)*. Initial radiographs were interpreted as normal.

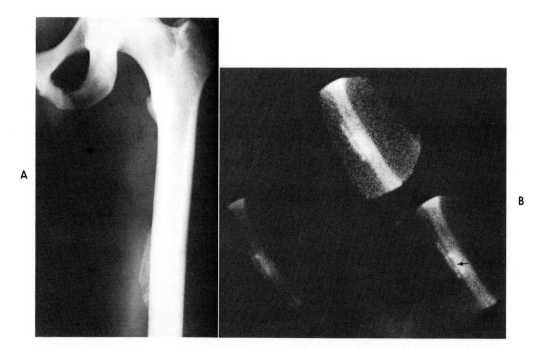

FIG. 2. A, Juxtacortical myositis ossificans. Sharply circumscribed cortical periphery with a fine, lacy central pattern. **B,** Radionuclide bone scan demonstrates increased juxtacortical soft-tissue uptake separated from femur by a thin cleft *(arrow)*.

Radiographic examination of the femur—cont'd

The pattern of calcifications may be used as a distinguishing feature from other such entities, including dermatomyositis, cartilaginous tumors, and periosteal sarcoma. Computed tomography has been advocated as a useful imaging modality in the early stages of myositis ossificans.[9] The pattern of subtle circumferential ossification in the early stages of myositis ossificans can be diagnostic. This ossification may not be visible on plain films, and even if visualized, its circumferential nature can be difficult to ascertain.

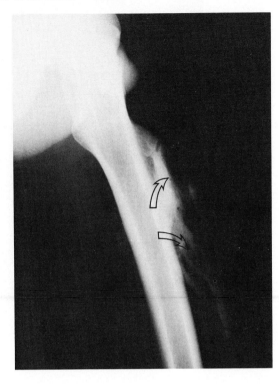

FIG. 3. Mature myositis ossificans. Note cyst development *(arrows)*.

tremely important. Angular and rotational deformities place high stress on the distal and proximal joints and are not well tolerated in repetitive competition (Fig. 45-9). For athletes, stable internal fixation permits early motion at the hip and knee. Joint contracture can be avoided, and relatively quick return to competitive activity can be accomplished.

Stress Fractures

Stress fractures of the femoral shaft are infrequent and predominantly occur either proximal or distal to the femoral shaft in areas such as the femoral neck (see Chapter 46) or condyle. Stress fractures have been encountered within the distal femoral shaft, and these fractures occur typically in serious recreational athletes who are undergoing lengthy training periods, such as training for a marathon. Typically, patients have low-grade aching in the distal thigh. There is generally no physical deformity and no evidence of intraarticular knee derangement. If the diagnosis is not suspected and patients continue to train, the pain can become present during daily ambulatory activity. Often the initial diagnosis may be iliotibial band tendinitis or quadriceps strain, and, as expected, treatment with antiinflammatory medications and rehabilitation exercises is unsuccessful. Standard radiographs may be totally within normal limits. The diagnosis of femoral stress fracture can be loosely dependent on the

radioisotope bone scan. Treatment should be cessation of athletic activity, which generally leads to healing of the stress fracture. After the fracture has healed the athlete can return to training (Figs. 45-10 and 45-11).

Another location for stress fractures of the femoral shaft is in the subtrochanteric region (Fig. 45-11). Athletes who are subsequently found to have subtrochanteric stress fractures often complain of thigh pain and invariably are initially treated for presumed muscle injury. Scintigraphy performed for further evaluation after lack of improvement in symptoms with conventional treatment demonstrates the fracture (Fig. 45-11). Treatment consists of cessation of activity until the fracture heals. Generally, healing occurs in 4 to 8 weeks. Displacement is uncommon, although it can occur. A short period of protected weight bearing is appropriate if athletes have difficulty bearing full weight. A rehabilitation program is required before allowing the athlete to return to sports. Also, the athlete should review training programs, equipment, and training conditions before being allowed to resume full athletic participation.

Soft-Tissue Injuries
Hamstring Strain

Mechanism of injury. Injuries to the soft tissues are the most common injuries in the thigh. Primarily, these occur in the posterior compartment and are strains of the

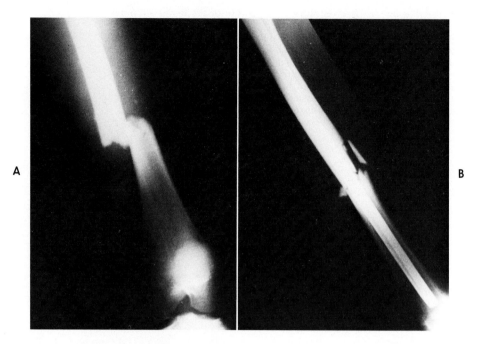

FIG. 45-9. A, Fracture of femur. **B,** Internal fixation of fracture of femur.

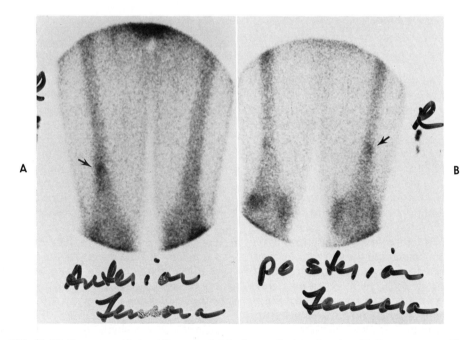

FIG. 45-10. Bone scan of stress fracture of right femur. **A,** Anterior view. **B,** Posterior view. This patient was a 45-year-old male dentist who had been running for a 7-year period, averaging 6 miles per day. Over the previous 6 months, he had been training for the Boston Marathon, increasing his mileage over the previous 6 weeks to 12 miles per day. He had a history of 3 weeks of pain of insidious onset, which originally began at approximately 6 miles into his run. The patient had tried anti-inflammatory medication and reduction of his mileage, but was experiencing pain on ambulation.

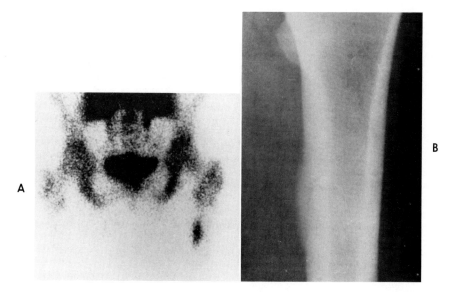

FIG. 45-11. Subtrochanteric stress fracture in a young female hurdler and high jumper. **A,** Bone scan, and **B,** radiograph taken 1 month after onset of symptoms. (From Butler JE, Brown SL, Mc-Connell BG: *Am J Sports Med* 10:228, 1982.)

hamstring muscles at the musculotendinous junctions. The hamstrings primarily are knee flexors and hip extensors. During sports, these muscles serve as antagonists to the anterior thigh musculature. In running activities, they provide decelerating forces to knee extension and hip flexion. Sudden, forced change in the musculotendinous length may result in strain or rupture at the junction. In particular, during active sprinting with forcible flexion of the hip and extension of the knee in forward striding the hamstring is placed under maximal stretch (Fig. 45-12). The sudden violent contraction with its tearing effect is well known to many athletes. During running, the hamstring muscles contract not only in extension of the hip joint, but also in flexion of the knee. During quadriceps contraction, extending the knee joint, the hamstrings continue to contract in antagonistic fashion to decelerate the extension of the knee. This injury occurs not only in the highly trained muscular individual, but also seems to have a higher frequency in the older age group. This older population generally has attrition of the musculotendinous junction and increasing muscle "tightness," which occur with the aging process.

The ultrastructural configuration of the tendinous portion of the muscle-tendon unit is a collagen fiber network

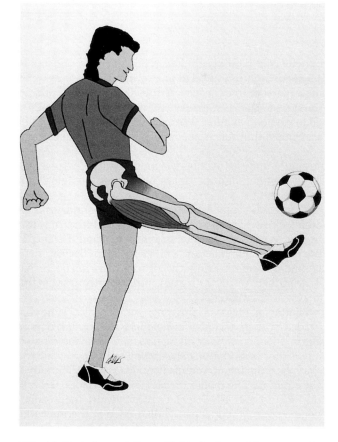

FIG. 45-12. Active sprinting with hip flexion and knee extension places hamstring at risk for strain.

Factors related to hamstring strain

- Inadequate hamstring flexibility
- Hamstring strength imbalance between legs
- Quadriceps/hamstring ratio imbalance
- External mechanical factors causing inappropriate knee extension and hip flexion (e.g., collision)
- Previous injury
- Muscle weakness
- Electrolyte depletion

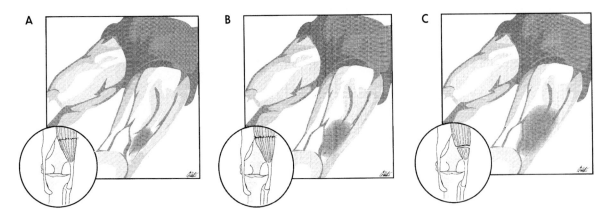

FIG. 45-13. Drawing of hamstring tears. **A,** First-degree tear. **B,** Second-degree tear. **C,** Third-degree tear.

TABLE 45-1 Hamstring strain

Degree of Injury	Pain	Spasm	Loss of Extension (Degrees)	Defect	Swelling
First	Mild	+	<20	0	+
Second	Moderate	+ +	20-45	0	+ +
Third	Severe	+ + +	>45	+*	+ + +

*Present before hematoma forms.

interspersed with elastin and reticulin fibers. All this is suspended within a gelatinous ground substance. The muscular portion consists of myofibrils encased within sarcoplasm and connective tissue. These myofilaments glide past one another. With aging, there is a buildup of scarring within this tissue and loss of its normal compliance. Scar tissue does not have the normal tensile strength, and this is in association with the normal collagen degeneration that takes place with the aging process.

The incidence of hamstring strains also increases in athletes who have not had adequate opportunity to warm up. In "cold," or unstretched, muscles, lengthening of the musclotendinous unit with its resultant development of fluid movement within the structure has not occurred. Tearing can result with pain, inhibition of movement, spasm, and swelling.

Clinical findings. Hamstring strains are generally graded by their severity (Table 45-1). With a first-degree strain, there is minimal disruption, and the symptomatology is at a level that is exacerbated only by movements that place the involved muscle under stretch. The site of the strain may be tender to palpation, but minimal swelling occurs and no defect is palpable. In the second-degree strain, there is partial disruption at the musculotendinous junction. Ecchymosis develops from bleeding, leading to increased muscle spasm and causing the patient to hold the extremity with the knee in flexion and

the hip in extension. This position alleviates the stresses on the strained area. In a third-degree strain, there is marked pain, disability, splinting of the extremity, gross ecchymosis and, if examined early, a palpable defect. This finding may be obscured by hematoma formation if the patient is examined a significant time after the injury (Fig. 45-13).

Treatment. Treatment is dictated by the degree of symptoms (Fig. 45-14). Application of ice for brief periods produces anesthesia of the area and relaxation of the muscle. Ice application for approximately 10 minutes is suggested, and reapplication is done hourly, depending on the symptoms. Compressive wraps should not be so tight as to produce peripheral edema. The wrappings should be reapplied at hourly intervals to prevent the formation of peripheral edema and to promote comfort. Splinting of the extremity with an external support such as crutches is also dependent on the degree of symptoms. When the athlete is reclining, an appropriately sized pillow should be placed under the thigh to flex the knee and shorten the musculotendinous structure. Compression in the popliteal fossa can easily be avoided with soft pillow elevation.

Rehabilitation is instituted as pain, swelling, and disability diminish. Slow and steady stretching techniques are promoted. Rapid stretching maneuvers of a ballistic nature must be avoided. Sudden stretches cause reflex contraction of the involved muscle and can lead to further tearing with continuation of symptoms. Modalities such as ice massage appear to be beneficial for the anesthetic qualities during the initial stages. However, deep massage is not recommended because it may stimulate muscle contraction and disrupt the organizing hematoma. Moist applications and deep heat, such as ultrasound at low intensities, promote relaxation of the muscular structures. The difficulty in treatment is caused by the often slow healing response of the musculotendinous unit, and a prolonged recovery often occurs. Attempts to shorten this healing time by the athlete and physician must be controlled. The first goal is the elimination of pain to allow initiation of a rehabilitation program. Once

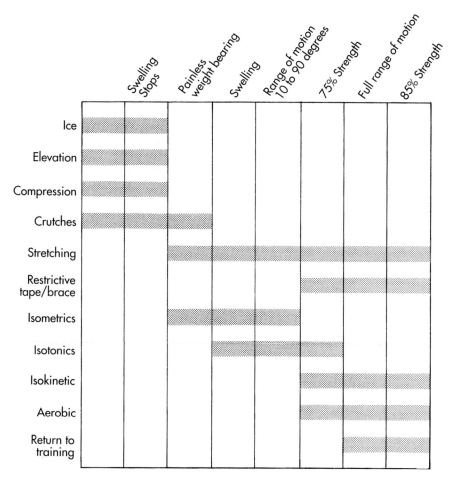

FIG. 45-14. Phases of hamstring strain rehabilitation.

the acute symptoms have stabilized the musculotendinous unit needs to be slowly stretched to reestablish its full length (Fig. 45-15). If this is not obtained before the resumption of activities, recurrent strain will occur. This is a result of healing of the musculotendinous unit in a shortened position. Extension of the knee beyond the shortened muscle length causes recurrent strain. After complete reestablishment of length has occurred, efforts at redevelopment of muscular power with a progressive resistance program, both isometrically and isokinetically, need to be performed. If adequate power and endurance of the hamstring muscles are not reestablished, the antagonist muscle group, the quadriceps, overpowers the hamstring, and reinjury can occur. After the second phase of rehabilitation (development of power and endurance) is complete, then the return to function and the performance of athletic endeavor, that is, rapid maneuvering, is brought along slowly, once again to "reeducate" the damaged structure. "Striding," a technique for progressive functional exercises to facilitate return to sports, is described in Chapter 15. Attention must be directed not only to third-degree strains, but also to first- and second-degree strains because they can have a similar prolonged recovery if adequate attention is not paid to re-

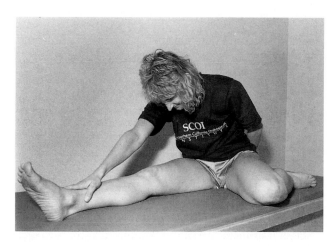

FIG. 45-15. Proper technique of stretching following hamstring strain.

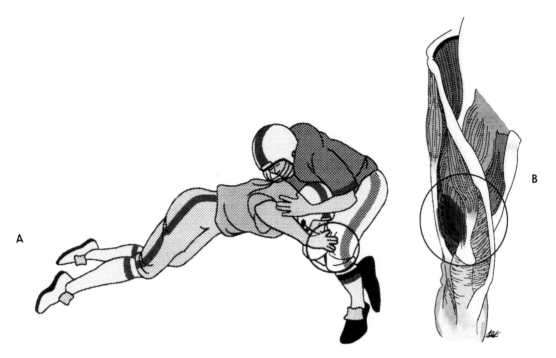

FIG. 45-16. A, Mechanism of injury in football. **B,** Region of injury.

establishment of length, flexibility, power, and endurance.

Prevention of reinjury. At the time of return to sports, the injured hamstring can be somewhat protected by an appropriate knee brace or taping. Specifically, hypertension must be prevented. Therefore a brace with an extension stop or a taping to limit extension can be useful. Hamstring stretching and a complete muscle strengthening program should be continued after the athlete returns to sports. Stretching is always performed before and after athletic participation. If during the course of participation a long period of inactivity and "cooling" occurs, stretching should be done before resuming activity. For example, athletes may lose flexibility while in the locker room between periods or while standing on the sidelines. When the time is sufficiently long, the athlete *must* stretch before "going back in the game."

Criteria for return to sports following hamstring sprain

- Equal (preferably increased) flexibility
- Hamstring strength parity
- Appropriate hamstring/quadriceps isokinetic ratio
- Equal isokinetic power and endurance
- No pain or tenderness
- Hip adductor and abductor strength parity

Quadriceps Contusion

Clinical findings. Anterior thigh musculature is at high risk in all athletic activities in which blunt trauma can occur. Most of these injuries are of minimal significance and are treated by the athlete as a bruise. But with a severe blunt force, significant hemorrhage may develop within the quadriceps muscle (Fig. 45-16). With significant bleeding into the tight fascial compartment, distension occurs, and this results in pain, spasm, and inhibition of movement. Because of anatomic exposure, most injuries occur anteriorly and anterolaterally. With injury, bleeding within this closed space causes spasm of the quadriceps muscle, and the athlete holds the extremity in extension. Ecchymosis usually becomes evident within 24 hours. The barometers of injury are pain, progressive thigh swelling, and range of motion. With moderate and severe bruises, particularly those in the distal one third of the thigh, an effusion may develop in the ipsilateral knee. It is important to document the knee laxity at the time of the initial evaluation because occasionally a knee injury can occur in conjunction with a thigh bruise. For example, a lateral blow to the distal thigh can cause a medial collateral ligament and a quadriceps contusion. Often, however, no knee injury has occurred, and the effusion is a result of the quadriceps injury. These sympathetic knee effusions resolve spontaneously as the contusion heals and the knee range of motion is restored.

Treatment. A 1991 West Point study provides a sound rationale for treatment of quadriceps contusions.[12] Contusions are first classified based on knee range of motion at 12 to 24 hours after the injury or at initial presentation (Table 45-2). A mild injury is defined as active knee motion greater than 90 degrees. Moderate contusions have 45 to 90 degrees of active knee motion, and severe contusions have less than 45 degrees of active knee motion. The treatment program differed from that of Jackson and Feagin's program[6] in that the leg is rested in flexion (vs. extension), and early flexion (vs. exten-

Treatment of quadriceps contusion

Phase I

Purpose:	Limit hemorrhage:
Treatment:	Rest
	Bear weight as tolerated
	Use crutches if limp is present
	Ice or cold whirlpool
	Compression wrap
	Elevate leg
	Lock brace at position of maximum flexion as tolerated by patient

Advance to next phase when:
- Comfortable
- Pain free at rest
- Thigh girth is stabilized

Phase II

Purpose:	Restoration of pain-free motion
Treatment:	Ice, ice massage, or cool whirlpool
	Isometric quadriceps exercises
	Supine and prone active knee flexion
	Well-leg gravity-assisted motion
	Stationary bicycle on low tension
	Discard crutches if flexion >90 degrees is present, no limp, good quadriceps control, pain-free, weight-bearing gait
	Discard compression wrap when the thigh girth is equivalent to the normal thigh
	Option: use continuous passive motion, advancing flexion range as tolerated

Advance to next phase when:
- Greater than 120 degrees of pain-free active knee motion is established
- Thigh girth is equivalent to the normal thigh

Phase III

Purpose:	Functional rehabilitation strength, flexibility, and endurance
Treatment:	Isotonic and isokinetic pain-free strengthening
	Stretch the hip flexors, iliotibial band, quadriceps, hamstrings, adductors, and calf to pain-free tolerance
	Use stationary bicycle, Stair Master, Kinetron, and Nordic Trak, when available

Advance to next phase when:
- Full active range of motion
- Full squat
- Pain-free for all activities

Phase IV

Purpose:	Safe return to sport
Treatment:	Maintain strength, flexibility, and endurance
	Wear thigh girdle with thick pad for 3 to 6 months for sports participation

Modified from Ryan JB et al: *Am J Sports Med* 19(3):299, 1991.

TABLE 45-2 Quadriceps contusion*

Degree of Injury	Pain	Swelling	Flexion (Degrees)	Average Recovery Time (Days)
First	Mild	+	>90	13
Second	Moderate	++	45-90	19
Third	Severe	+++	<45	21

From Ryan JB et al: *Am J Sports Med* 19(3):299, 1991.
*See also Jackson DW, Feagin JA: *J Bone Joint Surg* 55A:95, 1973.

sion) exercises are emphasized. The results were significantly better with respect to both disability time and development of myositis ossificans.

Treatment consists of three phases and begins with rest, ice, compression, and elevation (RICE). The goal is to limit hemorrhage, and crutches are used if a limp is present. Immobilization of the limb can begin as early as possible following the injury with the knee flexed to the patient's tolerance. A brace that can be locked at any desired point in the range of motion can be used to maintain the knee in the flexed position. This phase of treatment usually lasts 24 hours or less in mild contusions and 48 hours in moderate or severe contusions. Phase II begins when the thigh circumference has stabilized and

the patient is pain-free at rest. Ice application or immersion in a cool whirlpool is used with isometric exercises, active flexion exercises, and gravity-assisted range of motion exercises to restore pain-free motion. Crutches are discarded when the range of motion is greater than 90 degrees and there is no gait abnormality. Compression dressing is removed when the thigh circumference is equal to the normal contralateral extremity. The continuous passive motion machine was proposed as an adjunct to treatment. Given the cost, this is generally not practical. Phase III begins with greater than 120 degrees of active pain-free motion. The goal of the third phase is functional rehabilitation with emphasis on strength and endurance. Following treatment of a quadriceps contusion, a thigh girdle with a thick pad is worn for 3 to 6 months for all contact sports.

Myositis ossificans developed in 9% of the patients and was associated with five risk factors. Knee motion less than 120 degrees, football injuries, previous quadriceps injury, delayed treatment, and ipsilateral knee effusion all were associated with a higher rate of myositis ossificans. Aspiration of injectable or oral medications, femoral nerve blocks, and radiation therapy appear to decrease the incidence of myositis ossificans but are generally not used and are not recommended.

Complications. Rarely a hematoma causes **vascular or neurologic compression;** therefore appropriate moni-

---

Factors associated with development of myositis ossificans following quadriceps contusion

- Motion <120 degrees
- Football injuries
- Previous quadriceps injury
- Delayed treatment
- Ipsilateral knee effusion

Criteria for return to sports following a quadriceps contusion

- Normal quadriceps flexibility
- Quadriceps strength parity between legs
- Normal quadriceps/hamstring isokinetic ratio
- Fabrication and fitting of protective padding
- Normal hip abductor, adductor, and flexor strength and flexibility

---

toring is always indicated. If there is an abnormal amount of bleeding, clotting deficiencies, although rare, need to be considered. Routine coagulation studies help screen for this problem. Massive and increasing thigh swelling are the signs of vascular injury. Arteriography is mandatory to evaluate the vascular system in this setting. Percutaneous embolization or surgical exploration may be necessary.

Myositis Ossificans

Recurrent injuries or massive contusions can cause the formation of heterotopic bone. When this occurs, **myositis ossificans** may cause continued sensitivity in that area. A mass may be palpable, and inhibition of quadriceps mobility with continued loss of function may result. Initial radiographs of a contusion with follow-up comparison studies show the development of this heterotopic bone (Fig. 45-17). A CT scan demonstrates mature bone at the periphery of the lesion. If radiographs were not obtained initially, confusion may arise. Radiographs taken long after the initial injury may show an ossified mass that can be confused with juxtacortical osteogenic sarcoma (Fig. 45-17, *B*). At this late date the athlete may not recollect a specific event, increasing the concern of the radiologist and treating physician.

Periosteal osteogenic sarcoma can be differentiated from myositis ossificans by virtue of its predilection for patients older than 30 years. Also, pain is of a more constant nature in patients with osteogenic sarcoma as opposed to those with myositis ossificans, whose pain is related to activity. Alkaline phosphatase levels are elevated with the sarcoma; however, histologic examination may be required for differentiation. Juxtacortical osteogenic sarcoma demonstrates abnormal cells on the periphery of the mass. In myositis ossificans the abnormal cells are seen within the depth of the lesion, and the mature, well-developed cells are found at the periphery of the lesion. Careful attention to the histologic findings prevents an unnecessary amputation or other treatment modalities.

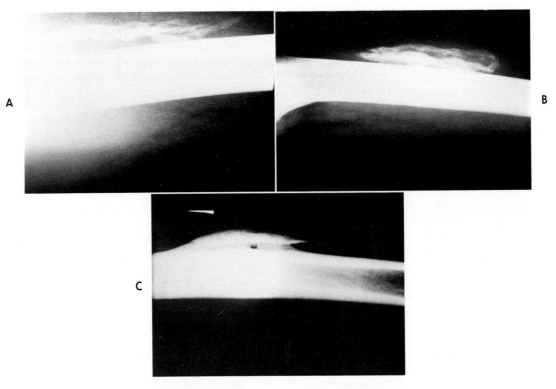

FIG. 45-17. A, Myositis ossificans. **B,** Progressive development. **C,** Remodeling.

Experience has shown that surgery on myositis ossificans needs to be delayed until the ossifying mass has reached maturity. Surgery performed early in the maturation process may stimulate an even more voluminous reaction. The natural history of myositis ossificans depends largely on its location. If the myositis ossificans is within a large muscle mass, it progressively becomes resorbed and shrinks. When based at a more proximal or distal site that has limited muscle mass, resorption becomes less likely. In this case the ossified mass may cause continued sensitivity and restriction of motion. Surgery should be delayed for at least 6 to 12 months, regardless of the location of the mass, to allow for maturation and resultant disability to become manifest (Fig. 45-17, C).

Compartment Syndrome

An uncommon but potentially devastating sequela of a quadriceps contusion is a thigh compartment syndrome. An acute compartment syndrome of the thigh is generally associated with a femur fracture but may also result from application of antishock trousers or compression after narcotic overdose. Muscle overuse and contusion are the most common injuries in athletes who develop an acute thigh compartment syndrome. If compartment syndrome of the thigh is suspected following a sports injury, compartment pressure measurements of all compartments (anterior, medial, and posterior) should be taken, and all compartments involved should have prompt decompressive fasciotomies. The threshold pressures for decompression of the thigh are variable among authors and range from 30 to 80 mm Hg. A common recommendation is to proceed with fasciotomy when clinically indicated if pressures are noted in the 50- to 60-mm Hg range with a normal diastolic blood pressure present. In general, wounds are left open for later closure. As in other parts of the body, the degree of the initial pain and increased pain with passive stretching of the involved muscles are more reliable indicators of compartment syndrome than neurologic deficits or pulselessness. Following early identification and successful decompression with delayed wound closure, athletes can expect to return to full activities following appropriate rehabilitation.

Quadriceps Strain

Mechanisms of injury. Strain of the quadriceps may occur from tensile overload. The rectus femoris and sartorius muscles are most commonly affected, although any component of the quadriceps may be involved. Susceptibility of the rectus femoris muscle is created by its role as a two-joint muscle. Forceful contraction of the quadriceps muscle with the knee flexed and hip extended is a common mechanism of injury. This may occur, for example, when kicking a ball and meeting sudden, unexpected resistance. Such a mechanism can occur in soccer, rugby, or football. Injury can also take place during sudden acceleration. Abrupt change in speed with the hip extended and the knee flexed can lead to a muscle contraction. Strain of the rectus then occurs (Fig. 45-18).

Clinical findings. Pain occurs immediately after injury in the anterior portion of the thigh. Often the athlete has a sense that "something has torn." If the athlete is evaluated immediately after the injury, a defect may be palpable in the rectus. Gentle knee flexion makes the defect more apparent. Later, swelling occurs, and a palpable hematoma obscures the defect. Limitation of active knee flexion is present as a result of pain and spasm. Inability to contract the remaining quadriceps muscle occurs. With healing and return to function, a permanent defect may be visible in the rectus (Fig. 45-19). This defect does not usually lead to restricted function.

Treatment. In the acute stage, treatment is identical to that for hamstring strain. Ice, compression, and elevation are used. In severe strains, crutches and immobilization with the knee extended are beneficial. When pain and swelling are reduced, the athlete begins with gentle stretching exercises for the quadriceps. This is combined with transcutaneous electric nerve stimulation (TENS) and ultrasound to allow effective stretching. Following stretching, ice application is beneficial. When quadriceps contraction is possible, isometric quadriceps exercising is begun. Straight leg raising, which puts added tension

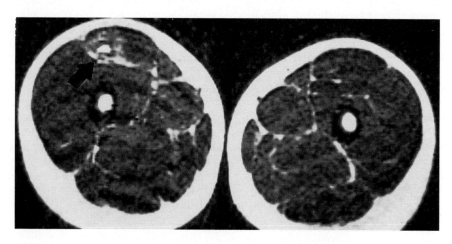

FIG. 45-18. Magnetic resonance image of quadriceps muscle strain involving one third of the muscle substance in a high school field goal kicker.

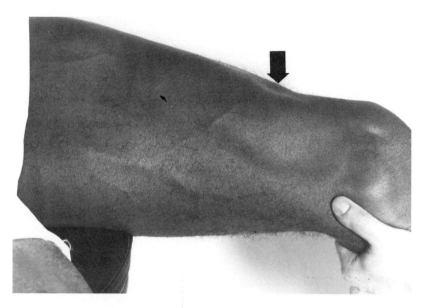

FIG. 45-19. Defect present in rectus femoris 2 years after rectus strain in collegiate football player. No functional problem accompanies defect.

on the rectus femoris, is avoided. As muscle control returns and symptoms resolve, knee flexion and extension exercises are begun, using a low-resistance isokinetic apparatus. When a full range of motion has been achieved, functional rehabilitation followed by return to sports can proceed.

Vascular Problems
Adductor Canal Syndrome

Exercise-induced vascular claudication is unusual in young athletes. A rare cause of arterial occlusion has been reported in the adductor canal. An abnormal musculoskeletal band arising from the adductor magnus and lying adjacent and superior to the adductor tendon may lead to compression of the femoral artery at the adductor hiatus. The band may extend from the adductor magnus to the vastus medialis above and across the outlet of Hunter's canal.

Symptoms in this syndrome are identical to other vascular occlusion problems. **Exercise-induced claudication** is present. On examination the pulses distal to the occlusion are diminished or absent. The workup in these patients consists of noninvasive vascular testing, such as Doppler studies and arteriography. If the arteriogram shows occlusion at the adductor hiatus, surgical intervention is indicated.

Surgery should consist of elimination of the abnormal extrinsic tissue, resection of the artery at the site of compression, and autogenous saphenous vein graft. At the site of compression the artery may be abnormal and show marked internal and medial hyperplasia, focal calcification, and chronic inflammation. Postoperatively the individual can return to sports in a graded fashion, approximately 6 to 8 weeks following surgery.*

---

*Editors' note: Invariably, in the few cases in our experience, the entire leg must be rehabilitated for strength, power, endurance, and flexibility. This may take 4 to 6 months in sports requiring both speed and endurance.

REHABILITATION

At times the physician, trainer, and, more importantly, the patient confuse the definition of rehabilitation with that of training or conditioning. It needs to be understood that rehabilitation is an effort of modalities to diminish pain, allow for healing of the damaged tissue, reestablish the musculotendinous length, and redevelop basic strength. The specificities of muscle training and conditioning cannot occur until preceding rehabilitation has been completed. The common denominator of all these injuries, whether muscle tear or contusion, is small-vessel injury with bleeding and disruption of tissue. With the hemorrhage there is pressure necrosis of the tissue beyond that of the localized area of disruption. These tissues heal with fibrosis and subsequent remodeling. However, regardless of the extent of the injury, there is residual scarring of the underlying tissue, depending on the severity of the injury. This residual scar does not have the normal elasticity that unaffected body tissues have. Therefore it is more prone to recurrent injury, and ultimate rehabilitation training needs to be reached to protect against chronic sequelae.

Injuries to the thigh have one particular dimension that must be recognized in rehabilitation efforts. This factor changes rehabilitation from certain standard techniques of reintroducing power, endurance, form, and function. This dimension is the reestablishment of the appropriate length of the muscle. With injury to the thigh, whether it be to the anterior or posterior aspect, contraction of the protagonist and relaxation of the antagonist muscle groups lead to shortening at the injured musculotendinous junction. Length must be reestablished before concentrated efforts are aimed at strength development. Mentioned earlier in this chapter are ways of determining the degree of contracture. For the quadriceps, this is best seen by evaluation of the muscle length with the patient in the prone position with the hip in extension and the knee in progressive flexion. Com-

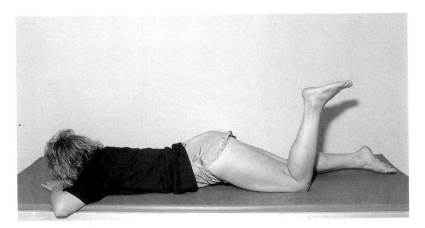

FIG. 45-20. Quadriceps contracture demonstrated by loss of hip extension occurring with flexion of knee.

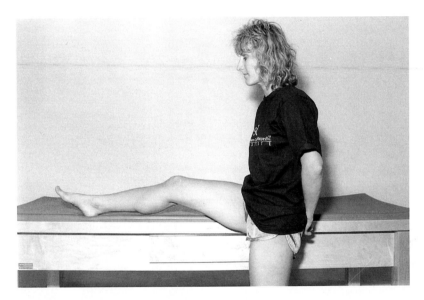

FIG. 45-21. Hamstring contracture demonstrated by limited knee extension.

parison to the opposite side is essential (Fig. 45-20). The hamstring musculature is evaluated with the involved side hip in flexion, knee in extension, and opposite side hip in extension (Fig. 45-21). This allows for relative comparison of actual length. If contracture of a particular muscle group is noted, in particular the hamstrings or the quadriceps, the first rehabilitation goal is progressive stretching. This stretching needs to be done in a slow but definitive manner, as opposed to ballistic, or "bouncing," maneuvers. Stretching must be done slowly and deliberately over repetitive, regular intervals of time. This is followed by a relaxation phase, and then stretching is repeated. If appropriate musculotendinous length is not reestablished, the individual is prone to recurrent tears and trauma. Simply confining rehabilitation to reestablishment of strength would further compromise the length characteristics of these units. Stretching also slowly realigns those cross-linkages that occurred with the injury secondary to hemorrhage, edema, and fibrosis along the muscular plane (Figs. 45-15 to 45-22).

After adequate length has been reestablished, efforts should be aimed at strengthening. Suggested first is an isometric program, which includes the athlete tightening the musculature of the extremity against resistance without arc of movement being provided. This is classically done against a fixed resistance, either the therapist's hand or a fixed-resistance block. No movement of the involved joints is allowed, and therefore the muscular contraction is confined to a basically fixed length. After the patient has demonstrated comfort within these contraction aspects, a short arc isotonic program against resistance is instituted within a comfortable arc of movement (Fig. 45-23). The guideline for this aspect was originally described by DeLorme[2] as 10 arcs of movement loaded at the maximum weight that the athlete can lift 10 times before the specific muscle group being worked fatigues. Advocated initially were three sets of 10 repetitions, the first set using one half of the maximum weight, the second set using three fourths, and the third set using the maximum weight. Rest is provided between each

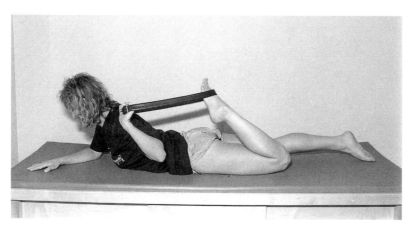

FIG. 45-22. Quadriceps (assisted) stretching.

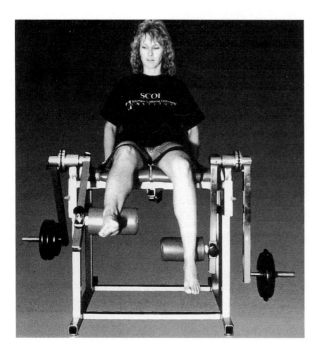

FIG. 45-23. Exercise with leg table.

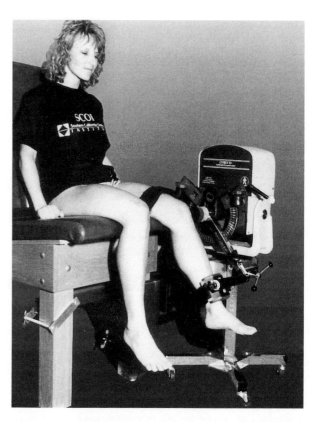

FIG. 45-24. Exercise with isokinetic motion.

set of exercises. The athlete performs a similar exercise program on the uninvolved extremity to use as a guide and also for its cross-over reflex benefits. When this set of exercises is tolerated without fatigue, feelings of weakness, or pain, the patient is advanced in appropriate increments. When the patient has obtained approximately 75% of the strength of the opposite extremity, an isokinetic exercise program may be begun.

The advantages of an isokinetic program are that the muscle groups are exercised at maximal tension over the full arc of movement. This seems to duplicate the strength required in normal training programs or competitive athletics. The main disadvantage is that the equipment may be quite expensive. Examples available at the present time include Cybex or Orthotron equipment. In isokinetic contraction, maximal tension is present within the muscle at a constant speed over the arc of movement. An additional benefit is the development of muscle endurance, which is an improvement over the initial isometric and isotonic programs (Fig. 45-24).

Modalities are available that facilitate relaxation of muscles. These include application of heat, both superficial and deep. Superficial heat is applied by metholated balms and via direct infrared heat. Available deep heat sources include ultrasound. Superficial application of cold for a brief period is also useful in obtaining muscle

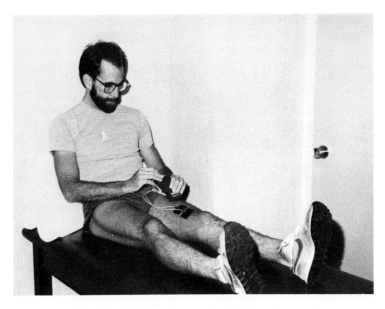

FIG. 45-25. Electric stimulation.

relaxation. Ice massage performed for approximately 5 to 10 minutes affords certain anesthetic qualities and seems to improve the athlete's ability to perform stretching maneuvers. Whether this effect is from a superficial anesthetic property or from deep biochemical and vascular interactions remains to be determined.

Use of running treadmills with variation of incline, stationary stair-climbing devices, or stationary bicycles with variable resistance help to improve muscle endurance. These modalities bring cardiopulmonary systems into play as well. These provide an overall stress to the human anatomy.* At times the patient is unaware of the benefits of cardiopulmonary exercise. It can be explained that cardiopulmonary exercise improves the general body conditioning and oxygen transport system, which enables the muscles to withstand fatigue and shortens recovery time. It can be further emphasized to the patient that with thigh injuries there is damage to the muscle tissue itself with scarring and diminution of localized blood flow. This type of general conditioning further helps to improve oxygenation of the muscle system.

Galvanic stimulation of muscle contraction appears to be of benefit during the acute rehabilitation process. Use of electric stimulation seems to allow patients to locate their muscle groups and to stimulate specific contractions. Electric impulses are also produced by muscle contraction, and sensor devices over the particular muscle group can allow for biofeedback so that the athletes can recognize their capabilities to contract muscles to various degrees (Fig. 45-25). These devices seem to be of benefit initially, but the complete rehabilitation process cannot be obtained via machine. It can only be ultimately achieved by total involvement of the patients and their commitment to their own rehabilitation.

The last factor to acknowledge is that of "warming

down" (or "cooling down"). Following any vigorous exercise, whether in the rehabilitation phase or in training, the body builds up by-products from the muscular performance. The particular product that can be modified is lactic acid. For recovery to be rapidly resolved after exercise, 3 to 5 minutes of stretching and light exercise should be performed, for example, 3 to 4 minutes on a stationary bicycle with minimal resistance or a walk-jog program. Associated stretching, once again, helps the stimulated muscle group to reestablish preexercise length. With a maximal, stressful, sustained exercise program, there is involvement with lactic acid not only in the aerobic exercise level, but also in the aerobic glycolysis level. The muscle glycogen can be resynthesized in approximately 1 to 2 hours following moderate exercise, but complete replacement usually takes between 6 and 24 hours. Therefore it is suggested that when the athlete reaches the intense exercise level, the exercise program be performed on alternate days to allow for rebuilding of maximally stressed tissue.

Education of the athlete in these principles is critical. The athlete must appreciate the importance of maintaining the stretching program, not only during the acute rehabilitation phase, but also into the future. "Warming down" must be emphasized in all sporting activities to recreate maximal muscle length and maintain the smooth gliding ability of these muscle units. Warm-up stretching exercises are performed not only before participation, but also after and even during participation if periods of inactivity occur. This is especially important during sports in which there are prolonged periods of inactivity, such as baseball and football. The situation is further compromised by climatic conditions, such as cold, damp weather, excessive heat, and dehydration. With cold and inactivity, the muscles go into a contraction phase and shorten; when called on to exceed their newly achieved length, they are at risk of injury. Dehydration affects the fluid balance, not only within the vas-

---

*Editors' note: "Linkage" to the heart is never absent in exercise. Musculoskeletal and cardiovascular deconditioning are intimately related.

cular system, but also in the interstitial tissues. Therefore adequate hydration and maintenance of mobility are essential.

Of late, there has been interest in specific muscle fiber types. Basically two separate types of skeletal muscle units are noted: the fast-twitch, which have an abundant capillary supply (often called the "red" fibers), and the slow-twitch, which have a diminished vascular supply (known as the "white" fibers). The fast-twitch fibers contract rapidly and generate maximal tension in a brief time in comparison to the slow-twitch fibers. However, the slow-twitch fibers have greater aerobic capacity. Fast-twitch fibers have been identified as taking part in short-burst activities, such as sprinting, and slow-twitch as acting in long-distance events. It is believed that each individual has a predetermined distribution of these fibers and that the activity performed recruits the appropriate motor units. Specific training does not appear to alter the ratio of fast-twitch to slow-twitch units but seems to improve the abilities of these units. The predominance of a high percentage of slow-twitch fibers in world-class distance runners is probably more related to a performance selection than the result of training. Specificity of training in the design of programs for athletes has been found to require a specific design. It is essential that athletes be specifically trained for the type of performance they are going to want. Strengthening the specific muscle groups involved in that activity, attempting to use the same patterns of movement, appears to be the most effective. Athletes may be unable to vary the ratio of slow- to fast-twitch fibers, but they may be able to improve the performance of those specific fibers and their recruitment.*

SUMMARY

Injury to the structures of the thigh does not have the dramatic qualities of other leg injuries, such as those to the knee joint, which carry resultant instability or a high risk of long-term degenerative change. However, all serious athletes have experienced the disability of a pulled muscle or a contusion with its effect on performance level during their careers.

Historically, little attention has been given to these strains and contusions. Their devastating properties have not yet been widely recognized. The attitude that such an injury should be handled by "running it off" does not adequately support efforts at rehabilitation from a psychologic viewpoint. Participants are limited in their ability to return to participation and are faced with the criticism of "poor effort." Appropriate emphasis on rehabilitation, stretching, reestablishment of muscle lengths, and redevelopment of power and endurance not only allows a higher level of participation at the time of return to sports, but also diminishes the probability of recurrent injury.

The anatomy and physical diagnosis of the thigh do not lend themselves to the dramatic qualities that are described so frequently in the literature in reference to in-

juries of the knee and ankle joints. Also, surgical intervention is rarely necessary; therefore actual inspection of the anatomic interrelationships does not occur. The same principles and relationships of superficial and deep anatomy and their physical diagnosis and total rehabilitation not only should be underscored, but also should be of paramount importance to all those involved in the care of athletes.

REFERENCES
1. Butler JE, Brown SL, McConnell BG: Subtrochanteric stress fractures in runners, *Am J Sports Med* 10:228, 1982.
2. De Lorme TL: Progressive resistance exercises. In American Academy of Orthopaedic Surgeons *Instructional course lectures,* vol 7, Ann Arbor, Mich, 1950, JW Edwards.
3. Edeiken J: *Roentgen diagnosis of diseases of bone,* ed 3, Baltimore, 1981, Williams & Wilkins.
4. Greaney RB et al: Distribution and natural history of stress fractures in US Marine recruits, *Radiology* 146:346, 1983.
5. Hajek MR, Noble HB: Stress fractures of the femoral neck in joggers, *Am J Sports Med* 10:112, 1982.
6. Jackson DW, Feagin JA: Quadriceps contusion in young athletes: relation of severity of injury to treatment and prognosis, *J Bone Joint Surg* 55A:95, 1973.
7. Lombardo SJ, Bensen DW: Stress fractures of the femur in runners, *Am J Sports Med* 10:219, 1982.
8. Meurman KOA, Elfving S: Stress fractures in soldiers: a multifocal bone disorder, *Radiology* 134:483, 1980.
9. Moss AA, Gamsu G, Gannant HK: *Computed tomography of the body,* Philadelphia, 1983, WB Saunders.
10. Norman A, Dorfman HD: Juxtacortical circumscribed myositis ossificans: evolution and radiographic features, *Radiology* 96:301, 1970.
11. Orava S, Puranen J, Ali-Ketola L: Stress fracutres caused by physical exercise, *Acta Orthop Scand* 49:19, 1978.
12. Ryan JB et al: Quadriceps contusions, *Am J Sports Med* 19(3):299, 1991.
13. Skinner HB, Cook SD: Fatigue failure stress of the femoral neck, *Am J Sports Med* 10:245, 1982.

ADDITIONAL READINGS
Anatomy
Grant JCB: *Grant's atlas of anatomy,* Baltimore, 1983, Williams & Wilkins.
Gray H: *Anatomy of the human body,* Philadelphia, 1959, Lea & Febiger.
Last RJ: *Anatomy regional and applied,* Edinburgh, 1972, Churchill Livingstone.
Verta MJ, Vitello J, Fuller J: Adductor canal compression syndrome, *Arch Surg* 119:345, 1984.
Displaced fractures
Luchini MA, Sarokhan AJ, Micheli LJ: Acute displaced femoral-shaft fractures in long-distance runners, *J Bone Joint Surg* 65A:689, 1983.
Mira AJ, Carlisle KM, Greer RB: A critical analysis of quadriceps function after femoral shaft fracture in adults, *J Bone Joint Surg* 62A:61, 1980.
Stress fractures
Blatz DJ: Bilateral femoral and tibial shaft stress fractures in a runner, *Am J Sports Med* 9:322, 1981.
Butler JE, Brown SL, McConnell BG: Subtrochanteric stress fractures in runners, *Am J Sports Med* 10:228, 1982.
Hershman EB, Lombardo J, Bergfeld JA: Femoral stress fractures in athletes, *Clin Sports Med* 9(1):111, 1990.
Hershman EB, Mailly T: Stress fractures, *Clin Sports Med* 9(1):183, 1990.
Johnson, AW, Weiss CB Jr, Wheeler DL: Stress fractures of the femoral shaft in athletes—more common than expected: a new clinical test, *Am J Sports Med* 22(2):248, 1994.
Leinberry CF et al: A displaced subtrochanteric stress in a young amenorrheic athlete, *Am J Sports Med* 20(4):485, 1992.

---

*See Chapter 3 for a more detailed discussion of muscle fiber types.

Lombardo SJ, Benson DW: Stress fractures of the femur in runners, *Am J Sports Med* 10:219, 1982.

McBryde AM Jr: Stress fractures in athletes, *Am J Sports Med* 3:212, 1975.

Provost RA, Morris JM: Fatigue fracture of the femoral shaft, *J Bone Joint Surg* 51A:487, 1969.

Rosen PR, Lyle JM, Treves S: Early scintigraphic diagnosis of bone stress and fractures in athletic adolescents, *Pediatrics* 70:11, 1982.

Hamstring and quadriceps strains

Burkett LN: Investigation into hamstring strains: the case of the hybrid muscle, *Am J Sports Med* 3:228, 1975.

Ciullo JV, Zarins B: Biomechanics of the musculotendinous unit: relation to athletic performance and injury, *Clin Sports Med* 2:71, 1983.

Jönhagen S, Németh G, Eriksson E: Hamstring injuries in sprinters: the role of concentric and eccentric hamstring muscle strength and flexibility, *Am J Sports Med* 22(2):262, 1994.

Rask MR, Lattig GH: Traumatic fibrosis of the rectus femoris muscle, *JAMA* 221:268, 1972.

Speer KP, Lohnes J, Garrett WE: Radiographic imaging of muscle strain injury, *Am J Sports Med* 21(1):89, 1993.

Taylor DC et al: Experimental muscle strain injury: early functional and structural deficits and the increased risk for reinjury, *Am J Sports Med* 21(2):190, 1993.

Zarins B, Ciullo JV: Acute muscle and tendon injuries in athletes, *Clin Sports Med* 2:167, 1983.

Muscle-fiber types

Gollnick PD, Matoba H: The muscle fiber composition of skeletal muscle as a predictor of athletic success: an overview, *Am J Sports Med* 12:212, 1972.

Smith MJ: Muscle-fiber types: their relationship to athletic training and rehabilitation, *Orthop Clin North Am* 14:403, 1983.

Thorstensson A: Muscle strength, fibre types, and enzyme activities in man, *Acta Physiol Scand Suppl* 443:1, 1976.

Thorstensson A et al: Muscle strength and fiber composition in athletes and sedentary men, *Med Sci Sports Exerc* 9:26, 1977.

Quadriceps hematoma

Garland DE: A clinical perspective on common forms of heterotopic ossification, *Clin Orthop* 263:13, 1991.

Ivey JM: Myositis ossifans of the thigh following manipulation of the knee, *Clin Orthop* 198:102, 1985.

Kalenak A et al: Treating thigh contusion with ice, *Phys Sportsmed* 3:65, 1975.

Kirkpatrick JS, Koman LA, Rovere GD: The role of ultrasound in the early diagnosis of myositis ossificans, *Am J Sports Med* 15:179, 1987.

Lipscomb AB, Thomas ED, Johnston RK: Treatment of myositis ossificans traumatica in athletes, *Am J Sports Med* 4:111, 1976.

Rothwell AG: Quadriceps hematoma: a perspective clinical study, *Clin Orthop* 171:97, 1982.

Zeanah WR, Hudson TM: Myositis ossificans: radiologic evaluation of two cases with diagnostic computed tomograms, *Clin Orthop* 168:187, 1982.

Rehabilitation

Goldberg AL et al: Mechanism of work-induced hypertrophy of skeletal muscle, *Med Sci Sports Exerc* 7:185, 1975.

Gould N et al: Transcutaneous muscle stimulation as a method to retard disuse atrophy, *Clin Orthop* 164:215, 1982.

Kulund DN, Tottossy M: Warm-up, strength, and power, *Orthop Clin North Am* 14:427, 1983.

McMaster WC: A literary review on ice therapy in injuries, *Am J Sports Med* 5:124, 1977.

Wiktorsson-Moller M et al: Effects of warming up, massage, and stretching on range of motion and muscle strength in the lower extremity, *Am J Sports Med* 11:249, 1983.

Strength

Costain R, Williams AK: Isokinetic quadriceps and hamstring torque levels of adolescent, female soccer players, *J Orthop Sports Phys Ther* 5:196, 1984.

DeLorme TL: Progressive resistance exercises. In *American Academy of Orthopaedic Surgeons instructional course lectures*, vol 7, Ann Arbor, Mich, 1950, JW Edwards.

DeLorme TL: Recent developments in progressive resistance exercises. In *American Academy of Orthopaedic Surgeons instructional course lectures*, vol 10, Ann Arbor, Mich, 1953, JW Edwards.

Knapik JJ, Ramos MU: Isokinetic and isometric torque relationships in the human body, *Arch Phys Med Rehabil* 61:64, 1980.

Stafford MJ, Grana WA: Hamstring/quadriceps ratios in college football players: a high velocity evaluation, *Am J Sports Med* 12:209, 1984.

Wyatt MP, Edward AM: Comparison of quadriceps and hamstring torque values during isokinetic exercise, *J Orthop Sports Phys Ther* 3:48, 1981.

Compartment syndrome

An HS et al: Acute compartment syndrome of the thigh, *J Orthop Trauma* 1:180, 1989.

Blasier RB, Pape JM: Simulation of compartment syndrome by rupture of the deep femoral artery from blunt trauma, *Clin Orthop* 266:214, 1991.

Clancey GJ: Acute posterior compartment syndrome in the thigh: a case report, *J Bone Joint Surg* 67A:1278, 1985.

Klasson SC, VanderSchilden JL: Acute anterior thigh compartment syndrome complicating quadriceps hematoma, *Orthop Rev* 19:421, 1990.

Rooseri D: Quadriceps contusion with compartment syndrome, *J Bone Joint Surg* 62A:286, 1980.

Rooseri D: Quadriceps contusion with compartment syndrome: evacuation of hematoma in two cases, *Acta Orthop Scand* 58:170, 1987.

Schwartz JT Jr et al: Acute compartment syndrome of the thigh: a spectrum of injury, *J Bone Joint Surg* 71A:392, 1989.

Vegas SF et al: Acute compartment syndrome in the thigh, *Clin Orthop* 234:232, 1988.

Winternitz WA, Methany JA, Wear LC: Acute compartment syndrome of the thigh in sports-related injuries not associated with femoral fractures, *Am J Sports Med* 20:476, 1992.

Vascular injury

Thompford NR, Curtiss PH, Marable SA: Injuries of the iliac and femoral arteries associated with blunt skeletal trauma, *J Trauma* 9:126, 1989.

CHAPTER 46

Pelvis and Hip Injuries in Athletes: Anatomy and Function

Franklin H. Sim
Michael G. Rock
Steven G. Scott

Regardless of the sports activity, normal function of the pelvis and hip is a prerequisite for normal athletic performance. Normal kinematics of the hip and pelvis are important in athletic endeavors, whether they involve the use of the upper extremity in throwing and racquet sports or the lower extremity in sports primarily involving kicking, skating, or jumping.[*]

The types of athletic injuries differ among children, adolescents, and adults. The young child sustains few serious injuries in sports, despite his or her musculoskeletal immaturity, whereas the adolescent is the most vulnerable to athletic injuries. The adolescent has a skeletal maturity that seems to be inadequate for the physical demands of sports. The middle-aged or senior athlete sustains a different type of sports-related injury to the pelvis and hip. Levinthal[56] indicated that the increased vulnerability of the older athlete is secondary to the cumulative effects of previous injuries, the diminished elasticity of tissue, and the diminished ability of tissues to restore themselves to normal after injury.

Because most recreational sports require certain patterns of activity that result in special risk to various parts of the body, the prevention and treatment of these injuries are facilitated by a careful analysis of the environment of the particular sport. Although most sports injuries involve many factors and multiple stresses, injuries generally involve two types of stresses. One is from persistent, repetitive, controlled stress resulting in microtrauma or overuse syndromes. This type is more typical of noncontact and endurance sports (i.e., stress fractures of the pelvis or hip in joggers). The second type is caused by excessive uncontrolled force overload, which results from blunt trauma or overstretching of the structures beyond the normal range. This mechanism of injury to the structures of the hip and pelvis is more frequent and results from contact forces in collision sports. Disability from injuries to the pelvis and hip varies among sports. For instance, a minor injury such as a muscle pull in the pelvis or hip may represent a major disability for the ballet dancer from the strenuous demands of this activity.

ANATOMIC CONSIDERATIONS

Diagnosis and treatment of traumatic and nontraumatic conditions of the pelvis and hip in athletes require

---

[*]Editors' note: The pelvis is a key link in the chain of load transmission from the foot to the spine and vice versa—in all three planes of motion.

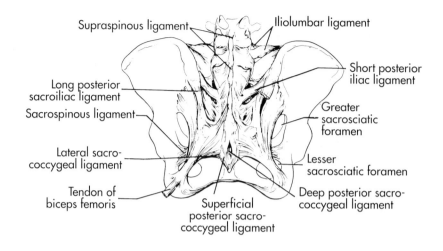

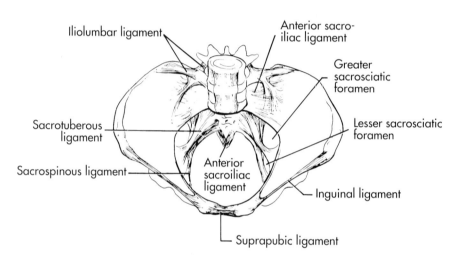

FIG. 46-1. Posterior and superior views of pelvis showing bony structures and ligamentous attachments. (From Berquist TH, Coventry MM: The pelvis and hips. In Berquist TH [ed]: *Orthopedic radiology: imaging of orthopedic trauma and surgery*, Philadelphia, 1986, WB Saunders.)

a thorough knowledge of the complex anatomy and function of these structures.

Function

The pelvis is a unique mechanism designed to support the downward and forward thrust transmitted to it by the weight of the trunk. The spine, which attaches to the pelvis through the sacrum, is anchored in all four directions by a combination of ligaments and muscles that contribute to the transfer of weight. In the erect walking position, body weight is transferred alternately to each hip joint. The weight-bearing forces are transmitted from the proximal femur to the acetabulum, hence through the ilium along the arcuate lines superior to the sciatic notch to the sacroiliac joints, then into the spinal column through the sacrum (Fig. 46-1). This region is called the **femoral sacral arch** and is augmented anteriorly by the subsidiary tie arch of the pelvis.[48] In sitting, the weight-bearing forces are transmitted through the **ischial sacral arch** with the forces transmitted from the ischial tuberosities through the ilium into the sacroiliac joint.

This region is also joined anteriorly by the subsidiary tie arch of the anterior portion of the pelvis.

In addition to its primary function as a weight bearer between the trunk and the lower extremity, the pelvis protects the lower abdominal and pelvic viscera.

Bony and Ligamentous Structures

The pelvis is formed by the two paired innominate bones, which articulate firmly with the sacrum and the pubic symphysis (Fig. 46-2). Each coxal bone consists of three separate bones—the ilium, ischium, and pubis—that meet to form the acetabulum. Within the acetabulum the junction between these components in the growing person is occupied by the triradiate cartilage, which disappears as fusion occurs at about the sixteenth year. The ilium forms the superior element of the coxal bone. On its inner surface the wing of the ilium forms the iliac fossa and posteriorly forms the articular surface for its articulation with the sacrum. The arcuate line runs downward from the anterior end of this articulation to the iliopubic eminence, which marks the junction of the

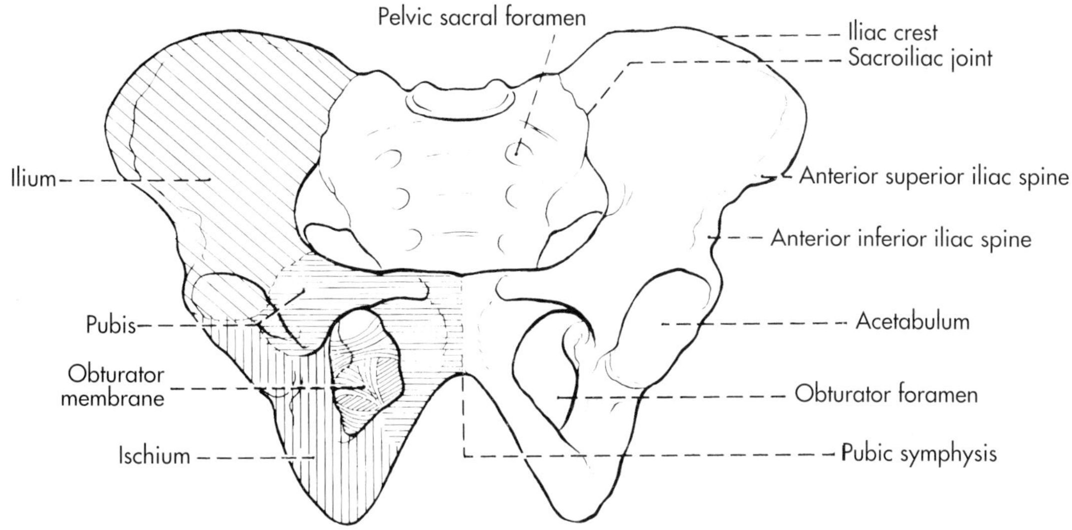

Pelvic sacral foramen

Iliac crest

Sacroiliac joint

Ilium

Anterior superior iliac spine

Anterior inferior iliac spine

Pubis

Acetabulum

Obturator
membrane

Obturator foramen

Ischium

Pubic symphysis

FIG. 46-2. Two coxal (innominate) bones articulating with sacrum. (From Hollinshead WH: *Functional anatomy of the limbs and back: a text for students of physical therapy and others interested in the locomotor apparatus*, Philadelphia, 1951, WB Saunders.)

ilium and pubis. Of the inferior elements of the coxal bone, the ischium is the more posterior; it forms the posterior half of the lower two thirds of the acetabulum. The ramus of the ischium extends forward at the lower border of the obturator foramen to join the pubis. The posterior edge of the ischium forms the ischial spine at the lower border of the greater sciatic notch. The lesser sciatic notch lies between the spine and the tuberosity that projects posterolaterally.

The pubis forms the anterior portion of the lower coxal bone. The superior ramus forms approximately the anterior half of the lower two thirds of the acetabulum. The inferior ramus of the pubis curves posteriorly and downward to the ischial ramus, completing the obturator foramen. The articular surfaces of the bodies of the two pubic bones articulate by a fibrocartilaginous disk. This interpubic fibrocartilaginous disk is reinforced by a superior ligament and inferiorly by the arch of the pubic ligament. In addition, the anterior interpubic ligament is an important structure for maintaining the integrity of the tie mechanism across the symphysis. Posteriorly the two coxal bones are firmly attached to the sacrum through the sacroiliac articulations (Fig. 46-1). This articulation consists of a small synovial joint cavity, which

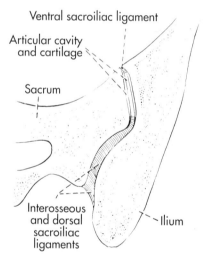

Ventral sacroiliac ligament

Articular cavity
and cartilage

Sacrum

Interosseous
and dorsal
sacroiliac
ligaments

Ilium

FIG. 46-3. Horizontal section through sacroiliac joint. (From Hollinshead WH: *Anatomy for surgeons: the back and limbs*, vol 3, ed 3, Philadelphia, 1982, Harper & Row.)

is reinforced by strong ligaments. Anteriorly the ventral sacroiliac ligament is relatively thin. However, the dorsal sacroiliac ligament is strong and blends with the extremely strong interosseous sacroiliac ligament to resist the weight of the body on the sacrum. Joint movement is also minimized by the wavy anatomic configuration of this joint (Fig. 46-3). In addition, the sacroiliac joint is strongly reinforced by the accessory ligaments (Fig. 46-1). These include the sacrotuberous ligament, which stretches from the sacrum and coccyx to the ischial tuberosity, and the sacrospinous ligament, which extends from the sacrum and coccyx to the ischial spine. The iliolumbar ligament stretches from the transverse process

---

**Ligamentous reinforcement of the
sacroiliac joint**

- Anterior
  Ventral sacroiliac ligament—thin
- Posterior
  Dorsal sacroiliac ligament—strong
  Interosseous sacroiliac ligament—strong
- Accessory
  Sacrotuberous
  Sacrospinous

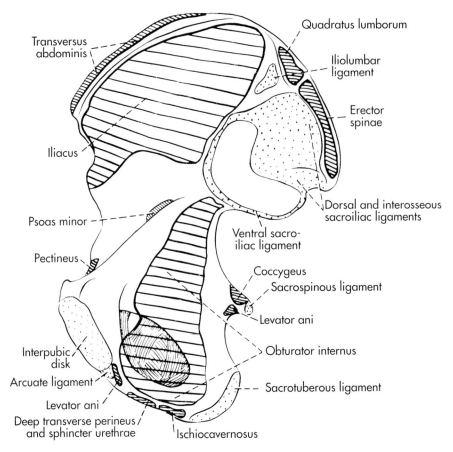

FIG. 46-4. Muscle origins and insertions on medial surface of innominate bone. (From Hollinshead WH: *Anatomy for surgeons: the back and limbs*, vol 3, ed 3, Philadelphia, 1982. Harper & Row.)

of the fifth lumbar vertebra to blend with the anterior sacroiliac ligament.

The sacroiliac joint is exceedingly strong and allows little motion. Sashin[84] described a slight upward and downward gliding with a slight anteroposterior movement, allowing for a limited amount of rotation estimated to average 4 degrees. The numerous muscular and ligamentous attachments on the pelvis are shown in Figs. 46-4 and 46-5. The relationship of these muscles to the hip joint is shown in Fig. 46-6.

Hip Joint

The hip joint is a ball-and-socket joint composed of the head of the femur and the acetabulum (Fig. 46-7). The acetabulum, which projects downward laterally and slightly forward, is deepened by the fibrocartilaginous acetabular labrum attached to its edge. Inferiorly the acetabular notch is bridged by the labrum as the transverse ligament of the acetabulum. This acetabular rim helps hold the head tightly within the acetabulum. The flattened ligamentum teres passes from the upper part of the head to the acetabular fossa. The neck of the femur projects anteriorly and is referred to as the angle of inclination. This angle has been shown to have a mean of 120.8 degrees.[48] The angle of torsion, or declination, indicates the angle of anterior projection, which is the angle made by the long axis of the femur and a line drawn through the centers of the two femoral condyles. This angle has been measured by Pick, Stack, and Anson[76] as having an average of 14 degrees in the adult.

The trabeculae are oriented along the lines of stress. The thickest trabeculae extend from the calcar inferiorly to the weight-bearing dome of the femoral head superiorly and transmit compressive forces.[99] A smaller trabecular pattern extends from the foveal region across the head and along the superior portion of the femoral neck to the trochanter. These trabeculae transmit tensile loads.

The forces acting across the articular surface of the hip joint have received increased attention in recent years because of their importance in the design of prostheses. The forces transmitted at the hip joint under conditions of dynamic equilibrium were measured by Rydell.[83] He showed that maximum force on the joints occurred at early and late periods of the stance phase of the walking cycle, reaching more than three times body weight (Table 46-1). This force increased to more than 4.3 times body weight during easy running. Morrison[69] estimated the total force acting across the hip joint and showed that this force is increased with activities such as ascending and descending a ramp.

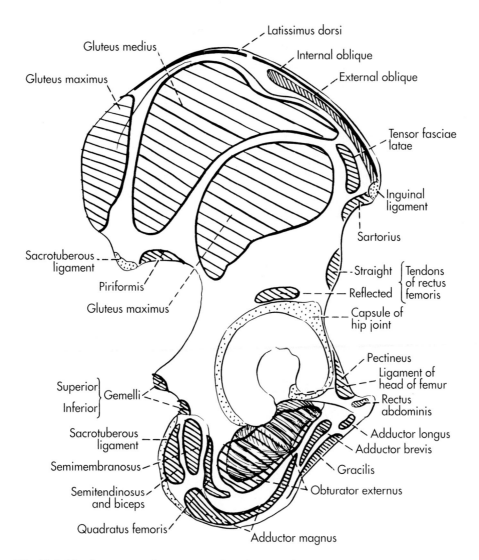

FIG. 46-5. Muscle origins and insertions in lateral aspect of innominate bone. (From Hollinshead WH: *Anatomy for surgeons: the back and limbs*, vol 3, ed 3, Philadelphia, 1982, Harper & Row.)

TABLE 46-1 Forces across the hip joint

Activity	Force
Walking (early and late stance phase)	3 times body weight
Running	4.3 times body weight

The stability and the bony anatomic configuration of the hip joint are dependent primarily on the ligaments of the joint rather than the associated muscles (Figs. 46-8 and 46-9). The articular capsule of the hip joint is strong and is reinforced by three ligamentous thickenings that extend in a spiral course from the acetabulum to the femur. The **iliofemoral ligament** is a strong ligament that covers most of the front of the joint extending from the anterior inferior iliac spine, spiraling medially in two separate bands to the intertrochanteric line. This has the configuration of an inverted **Y** and has been

referred to as the Y-shaped ligament of Bigelow. This ligament strongly resists hyperextension, and because weight-bearing stress tends to extend the hip, the ligament has the function of maintaining erect posture without constant muscle action. The **pubofemoral ligament** arises from the body of the pubis and superior ramus and extends across the anteroinferior aspect of the joint to blend with the lower portion of the iliofemoral ligament and inferior portion of the femoral neck. The fibers of this ligament help prevent excess abduction, as well as resist extension. A weak triangular area between those two anterior ligaments may allow a communication between the hip joint and the bursa that underlies the iliopsoas tendon. The third restraining ligament of the hip capsule, the **ischiofemoral ligament,** is the thinnest of the three. This ligament extends from the ischial rim of the acetabulum across the lower posterior aspect of the joint transversely toward the neck of the femur. The ligament is tightened in extension and helps in-

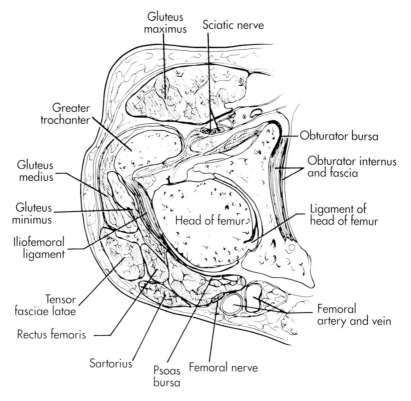

FIG. 46-6. Cross section through hip joint showing relationship of surrounding muscles. (From Berquist TH, Coventry MM: The pelvis and hips. In Berquist TH [ed]: *Orthopedic radiology: imaging of orthopedic trauma and surgery*, Philadelphia, 1986, WB Saunders.)

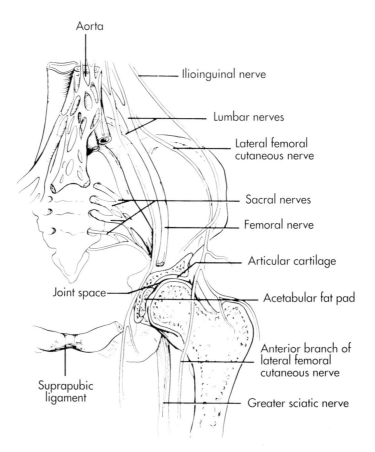

FIG. 46-7. Pelvis and hip showing relationship of lumbosacral plexus. (From Berquist TH, Coventry MM: The pelvis and hips. In Berquist TH [ed]: *Orthopedic radiology: imaging of orthopedic trauma and surgery*, Philadelphia, 1986, WB Saunders.)

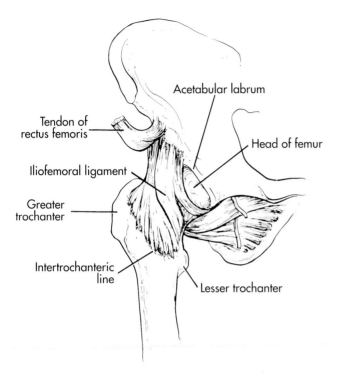

FIG. 46-8. Anterior view of hip joint showing hip capsule and ligaments. (From Berquist TH, Coventry MM: The pelvis and hips. In Berquist TH [ed]: *Orthopedic radiology: imaging of orthopedic trauma and surgery*, Philadelphia, 1986, WB Saunders.)

crease stability in the extended position. Moreover, all three stabilizing ligaments are tightened in internal rotation, limiting this motion, but they are lax in external rotation.

Nerve and Blood Supply

Innervation of the hip joint is variable, with branches arising from a number of different nerves. Gardner[32] found branches from the femoral nerve and its upper muscular branches, as well as a contribution from the obturator nerve, the nerve of the quadratus femoris, and the superior gluteal nerve.

The blood supply of the proximal femur has been studied in detail by a number of investigators because of its importance in fractures of the femoral neck and dislocations of the hip. The blood supply to the femoral head and neck is primarily derived by retinacular vessels arising from the medial and lateral femoral circumflex arteries (Fig. 46-10). Trueta and Harrison[96] indicated that the main blood supply to the femoral head is through the posterosuperior group (lateral epiphyseal vessels), which enters close to the articular surface, closely following the line of the old epiphyseal plate. The contribution of the obturator artery to the blood supply of the upper end of the femur is through its acetabular branch, supplying the acetabular fossa and ligamentum teres, through which distribution to the head is limited. Branches from the superior gluteal artery extend to the region about the greater trochanter, and a branch from the first perforating artery off the profundus supplies the posterior surfaces of the trochanters.

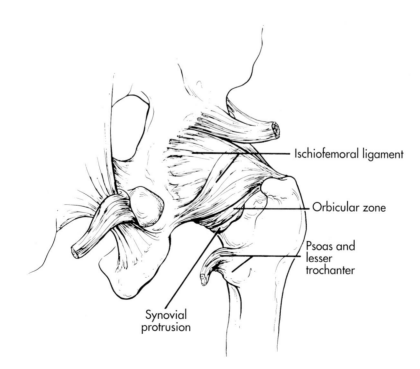

FIG. 46-9. Posterior view of hip joint showing hip capsule and ligaments. (From Berquist TH, Coventry MM: The pelvis and hips. In Berquist TH [ed]: *Orthopedic radiology: imaging of orthopedic trauma and surgery*, Philadelphia, 1986, WB Saunders.)

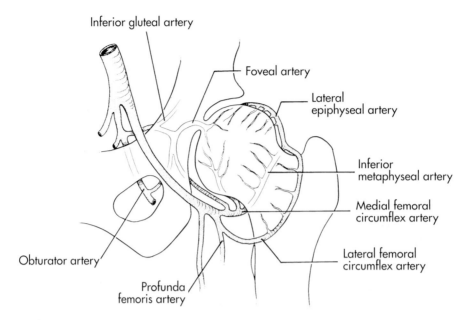

Inferior gluteal artery

Foveal artery

Lateral
epiphyseal artery

Inferior
metaphyseal artery

Medial femoral
circumflex artery

Lateral femoral
circumflex artery

Obturator artery

Profunda
femoris artery

FIG. 46-10. Blood supply to hip joints. (From Berquist TH, Coventry MM: The pelvis and hips. In Berquist TH [ed]: *Orthopedic radiology: imaging of orthopedic trauma and surgery*, Philadelphia, 1986, WB Saunders.)

Musculature of the Pelvis and Hip

The muscles of the pelvis and hip may produce different effects as the relative position of the trunk and lower extremities is altered. Analysis of these muscle actions depends on knowledge of the origins, insertions, and line of pull of the various fibers.

The pelvis acts practically as a fixed unit with coordinated motion that occurs between the lumbar spine and the hip joint as a result of muscle coordination. The muscles of the trunk and abdominal wall, which attach to the upper border of the pelvis, may act by moving the vertebral column as the pelvis is fixed, or conversely, if the thorax is fixed, the pelvis moves toward the thorax.

The spine-pelvis-hip linkage

- Fixed pelvis → Spine moves
- Fixed spine → Pelvis moves

When the pelvis is fixed, flexion of the vertebral column is achieved by the rectus abdominus muscle, which is assisted by the internal oblique and external oblique muscles acting bilaterally. Lateral flexion of the vertebral column is achieved by the lateral fibers of the external oblique and the ipsilateral internal oblique muscle. Rotation is achieved by the external oblique and contralateral internal oblique muscles.

The three motions of the pelvis that occur at the hip are anteroposterior pelvic tilting, lateral pelvic tilting, and pelvic rotation. Anteroposterior pelvic tilting is controlled by the coordinated actions of the muscles associated with both the hip and trunk regions. Anterior pelvic tilting of the pelvis occurs in the sagittal plane around a coronal axis. In anterior tilting of the pelvis, hip flexors work with the trunk extensors as a force couple to produce anterior tilting. This tilting usually occurs with contraction of the iliopsoas and the other hip flexor muscles to pull the pelvis anteriorly and inferiorly. At the same time the extensor muscles of the lumbar spine are pulling the pelvis superiorly. This combination causes the symphysis pubis to move inferiorly and results in an increase in the lordotic curve of the lumbar spine. Posterior pelvic tilting is accomplished by decreasing the lumbar lordotic curve of the spine and bringing the posterior aspect of the pelvis closer to the posterior surface of the femur, resulting in hip extension. In posterior tilting the hip extensor muscles are working with the trunk flexors (rectus and oblique muscles) to produce the posterior tilting. The rectus abdominis and the external oblique muscles bring the symphysis pubis anteriorly, whereas the gluteus maximus and hamstring muscles pull inferiorly on the posterior pelvis.

Lateral pelvic tilting occurs in the frontal plane around the anteroposterior axis (Table 46-2). The hip joint acts as the axis of rotation, and the pelvis tilts superiorly or inferiorly around this axis. Lateral tilting is accomplished by the lateral flexion and rotation of the vertebral spine and results in either adduction or abduction of the hip. The lateral pelvic tilt is controlled by eccentric or isometric contractions of the contralateral hip abductors. Pelvic rotation is the forward and backward rotation that occurs in the transverse plane around the vertical axis of the hip joint. Forward rotation of the pelvis occurs in the transverse plane around a vertical axis.

It is important, particularly for athletes, to determine

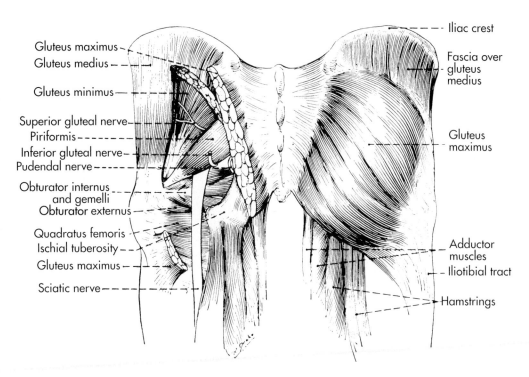

FIG. 46-11. Musculature of the buttocks. (From Hollinshead WH: *Functional anatomy of the limbs and back: a text for students of physical therapy and others interested in the locomotor apparatus,* Philadelphia, 1951, WB Saunders.)

TABLE 46-2 Pelvic motion

Motion	Muscles	Action
Anteroposterior pelvic tilt		
Anterior tilt	Hip flexors	Pull pelvis anteriorly and inferiorly
Posterior tilt	Lumbar spine extensors	Pull posterior pelvis superiorly
	Hip extensors	Pull posterior pelvis inferiorly
	Trunk flexors	Pull symphysis pubis anteriorly
Lateral pelvic tilt	Hip abductors	Coupled pelvic motion by contralateral eccentric and concentric contractions

the deficit resulting from weakness of these various muscle groups. This was well outlined by Kendall, Kendall, and Wadsworth.[52] For instance, weakness of the rectus abdominis causes an anterior pelvic tilt and secondarily an increased lumbar curvature. Moreover, when an athlete is performing double straight leg raises with abdominal muscles that are not strong enough to maintain the pelvis in a position of posterior tilt and the low back flat on the table, the abdominal muscles elongate and are subject to strain as the legs are raised.

There are many muscles that act at the hip joint (Fig. 46-6). The chief **extensors** of the hip are the gluteus maximus and the ischial portion of the adductor magnus (Fig. 46-11). The gluteus maximus, which extends over a broad origin on the sacrotuberous ligament and the posterior ilium inserting into the femur, tensor fasciae latae, and iliotibial tract, is an especially strong extensor. Because the weight of the body maintains the hip joint in extension, the gluteus maximus is of most important in walking up a grade, climbing stairs, and jumping and running activities.

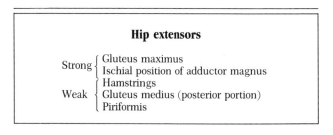

The hamstrings themselves weakly contribute to extension. They are active in the forward bending of the hips and act as postural muscles in resisting this maneuver. The posterior portion of the gluteus medius and the piriformis may also aid in extension.

The **flexors** of the thigh are shown in Fig. 46-12. Most

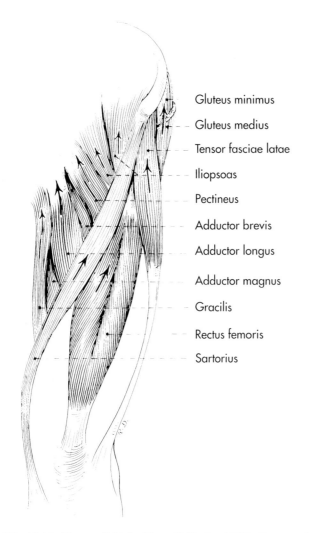

Gluteus minimus

Gluteus medius

Tensor fasciae latae

Iliopsoas

Pectineus

Adductor brevis

Adductor longus

Adductor magnus

Gracilis

Rectus femoris

Sartorius

FIG. 46-12. Flexors of thigh. (From Hollinshead WH: *Functional anatomy of the limbs and back: a text for students of physical therapy and others interested in the locomotor apparatus*, Philadelphia, 1951, WB Saunders.)

of the muscles attached to the front of the pelvis can help in flexion. The rectus femoris is a flexor primarily after flexion has been initiated by other muscles. The pectineus and tensor fasciae latae muscles assist in hip flexion. The chief flexor of the hip joint is the iliopsoas, which arises from the ventral surface of the transverse processes and sides of the lumbar vertebrae and joins the iliac portion, which arises primarily from the iliac fossa and inserts at and immediately below the lesser trochanter. Weakness results in disability in activities involving hip flexion, such as running uphill and jumping. Con-

---

Hip flexors

Strong { Iliopsoas / Rectus femoris

Weak { Adductors / Tensor fasciae latae

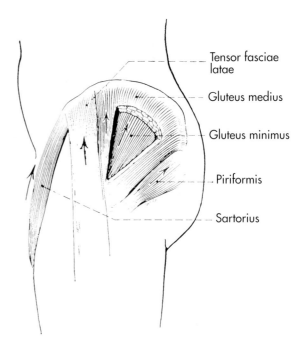

Tensor fasciae latae

Gluteus medius

Gluteus minimus

Piriformis

Sartorius

FIG. 46-13. Abductors of thigh. (From Hollinshead WH: *Functional anatomy of the limbs and back: a text for students of physical therapy and others interested in the locomotor apparatus*, Philadelphia, 1951, WB Saunders.)

tracture results in a hip flexion deformity with increased lumbar lordosis. When the patient is lying on a table, inability to bring the thigh down to touch the table while the back is held flat indicates shortness of the hip flexor muscles. However, if the knee extends as the thigh is brought down to the table, this confirms shortness of the rectus femoris.

The **abductors** of the thigh are shown in Fig. 46-13. While the tensor fasciae latae arising on the anterior part of the external portion of the iliac crest and inserting into the iliotibial tract may assist in abduction, it functions more as a flexor and medial rotator of the hip in addition to its function in knee extension. In testing of the tensor fasciae latae, with the athlete lying on his or her side, the thigh of the extended leg is able to drop in adduction below the level of the table top. With tightness of this muscle the leg fails to drop when the pelvis is fixed.

The two major abductors of the thigh are the gluteus medius and the gluteus minimus (Fig. 46-13). The former arises from the external surface of the ilium between the anterior and the posterior gluteal line and covers the gluteus minimus as it inserts on the lateral surface of the greater trochanter of the femur. The gluteus medius is the primary lateral stabilizer of the hip for

---

Hip abductors

Strong { Gluteus medius / Gluteus minimus

Weak   Tensor fasciae latae

standing. Mild weakness of the gluteus medius may be the result of a strain from postural or occupational causes, or there may be residual weakness after a prior athletic injury. Once established, the weakness further contributes to the faulty mechanics of the hip and pelvis. With the pronounced weakness the abductors are unable to keep the pelvis horizontal when weight is put on one leg, resulting in a gluteus medius limp. Slight weakness results in adduction of the hip in relationship to the pelvis with an ipsilateral high pelvis and a lumbar curvature toward the opposite side. Contracture of this muscle results in abduction deformity.

The **adductors** of the thigh, which can be divided into an anterior and a posterior group, are shown in Fig. 46-14. The anterior muscles include the pectineus, the adductors, and the gracilis. In the posterior group, the gluteus maximus, quadratus femoris, and obturator externus, as well as the hamstrings, assist in adduction.

Hip adductors

Anterior
- Pectineus
- Adductor magnus, longus, brevis
- Gracilis

Posterior
- Gluteus maximus
- Quadratus femoris
- Obturator externus
- Hamstrings

The chief **external rotators** are posteriorly located. These include the short rotators in the buttocks: the piriformis, obturator internus, and gemelli; the obturator externus; and the quadratus femoris. The gluteus maximus is the most important external rotator. Moreover, the iliopsoas has been shown electromyographically to be active in external rotation.[46]

Hip external rotators

- Piriformis
- Obturator internus
- Superior and inferior gemelli
- Obturator externus
- Quadratus femoris
- Gluteus maximus
- Iliopsoas

The tensor fasciae latae, the anterior portion of the gluteus medius, and the gluteus minimus are the most important **internal rotators** of the hip.

Hip internal rotators

- Tensor fasciae latae
- Gluteus medius (anterior portion)
- Gluteus minimus

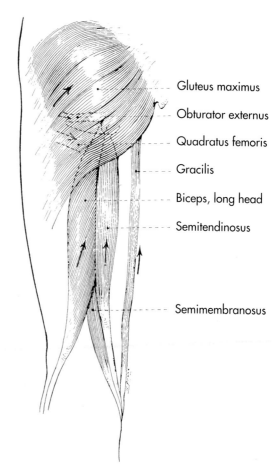

Gluteus maximus

Obturator externus

Quadratus femoris

Gracilis

Biceps, long head

Semitendinosus

Semimembranosus

FIG. 46-14. Posteriorly placed adductors of thigh. (From Hollinshead WH: *Functional anatomy of the limbs and back: a text for students of physical therapy and others interested in the locomotor apparatus,* Philadelphia, 1951, WB Saunders.)

CONDITIONS OF THE PELVIS AND HIP

Pelvic, hip, and referred thigh pain are common sources of concern in the athlete. The differential diagnosis can be complex. Pain and disability in the pelvis and hip may have many causes; these may be of local or regional musculoskeletal origin or may be referred from an extrapelvic location. Despite these difficulties the physician's responsibility is to establish a specific diagnosis.

Nontraumatic Causes

Nontraumatic causes should be considered even when the onset of pain seems to be related to a specific injury. For instance, tumor, infection, inflammatory conditions, and other causes may be responsible. The injury serves to draw attention to the underlying pathologic condition known as "traumatic predeterminism." Because pain can be referred to the pelvis and hip region from visceral conditions or from pathologic changes in the lumbar spinal column, such as spondylolisthesis, a thorough evaluation is necessary.

A number of inflammatory conditions must be considered in the evaluation of the athlete with pain of the but-

---

Nontraumatic causes of hip and pelvis pain

- Inflammatory conditions
  Ankylosing spondylitis
  Reiter's syndrome
  Rheumatoid spondylitis
- Infectious conditions
  Osteomyelitis
  Septic joint
- Tumors
  Osteoid osteoma
  Metastatic disease
  Others
- Referred pain
  Pathologic conditions of lumbar spine (e.g., spondylolisthesis)
- Metabolic bone disease with decreased bone mass

---

tocks, hip, and thigh.[47] Usually there is no problem when the patient with advanced rheumatoid spondylitis presents with obliteration of the sacroiliac joint. However, the physician must have a high index of suspicion if ankylosing spondylitis is to be diagnosed at its earliest manifestation. The presence of this condition should be considered in any young athlete who has pain in the low back, buttocks, and thigh associated with protracted stiffness. These young patients relate the onset of the pain to a traumatic incident. However, when questioned they recall prior stiffness and pain. While stiffness and muscle spasm of low back, pelvis, and hip occur frequently in traumatic disorders, protracted morning stiffness that is alleviated during the day, only to return in the evening or during the night, is characteristic of ankylosing spondylitis. The diagnosis, however, is ultimately based on the demonstration of pathognomonic radiographic findings. Usually, a careful radiographic evaluation of the sacroiliac joints reveals changes concomitant with the onset of the symptoms. However, if the initial radiographs show no abnormality, radiography should be repeated after 6 months and almost certainly shows changes if ankylosing spondylitis is present. Reiter's syndrome[47] similarly occurs in an age group of athletically active persons and can cause the erosive changes of unilateral sacroiliitis. The physician must have a high index of suspicion when these symptoms occur in a young athlete, and a complete rheumatologic evaluation should be performed.

Moreover, infectious disease must always be considered in the differential diagnosis of pelvic and hip pain. The early signs of infection in the sacroiliac joint may be obscure. Hedström and Lidgren[46] reported on acute hematogenous osteomyelitis involving the sacroiliac joint in athletes. These were active ballplayers who had small abrasions of the knee and elbows with an associated bacteremia. Septic arthritis or osteomyelitis of the sacroiliac joint is a distinctly unusual phenomenon often associated with other underlying pathologic conditions such as immunologic incompetence (human immunodeficiency virus), sexually transmitted diseases (gonorrhea), intra-

venous drug abuse, and iatrogenic introduction through therapeutic injections or operative procedures.

The broad range of benign and malignant tumors must also be considered in the differential diagnosis. Osteoid osteoma, Ewing's sarcoma, and lymphoma frequently occur in the pelvis and hip in young athletes, resulting in an obscure pain syndrome.[20] Bone scintigraphy, computed tomography (CT), and magnetic resonance imaging (MRI) are needed to assist in determining the diagnosis. Moreover, the senior athlete is in the age group in which metastatic tumors commonly occur in the pelvis and hip, and metastasis must be considered in the differential diagnosis of pain in the pelvis, hip, and leg. With such a broad range of conditions to consider, a stepwise and thorough approach to the evaluation is needed.*

The physical examination coupled with thorough history taking usually results in an accurate diagnosis. When indicated, abdominal, vaginal, and rectal examinations are useful. These may be supplemented by additional laboratory data, such as levels of serum calcium and alkaline phosphatase, blood count, sedimentation rate, and urinalysis. Specific radiographs may need to be correlated with special studies such as tomography, arthrography, and bone scan.

Traumatic Causes

Pelvis and hip injuries in the athlete may cause considerable disability. The most frequent of these, the sprain and soft-tissue contusion, are often difficult to differentiate from conditions that are potentially more disabling.

Contusions

In contact sports, a direct blow to the soft tissues from a collision injury may result in a contusion of the pelvis and hip region.[71] Such an injury causes bleeding into the deep tissue. In basketball, a violent fall to the floor may result in bleeding in the deep muscles of the buttocks. The mechanism is similar to that seen in the football player who lands forcibly on the buttocks or iliac crest when tackled or in a hockey player who is checked forcibly into the boards or onto the ice surface. These muscular contusions involving the buttocks and hip may be disabling to the athlete. In addition, the sacrum and sacroiliac joints are largely subcutaneous, and a direct blow to this region may result in a painful contusion.

Significant contusion can occur over the trochanter because of its superficial location and may result in trochanter bursitis with persistent pain and tenderness. Moreover, a blow to the ischial tuberosity in a fall may result in a painful contusion with severe pain and localized tenderness in this area. The localized pain increases on straight leg raising and on active resisted contraction

---

*Editors' note: This point cannot be overemphasized. Tumors must always be kept in mind during evaluation of athletes. A series of 30 athletes found to have tumors as the source of pain was presented by Lewis and Reilly of Lenox Hill Hospital (American Association of Orthopaedic Surgeons meeting, Las Vegas, 1985). In these patients the pathologic condition was silent until athletic activity, and the loading it involves produced pain and disability, which led to the diagnosis.

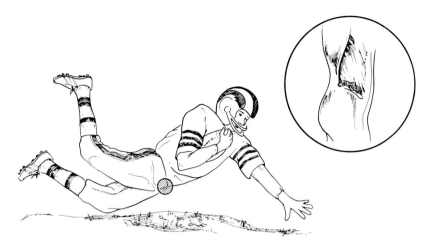

FIG. 46-15. Mechanism of hip pointer: player falls to turf, suffering a contusion to iliac crest and its muscle attachments.

of the hamstrings. This trauma may result in secondary ischial bursitis with persistent pain. The ascending ramus of the ischium or descending ramus of the pubis may be contused by a direct blow, such as a fall across a bar or a blow from the saddle while horseback riding. Contusion to the deeper structures of the perineum from falling on a hard object may result in a painful hematoma. It is important to exclude more serious injuries to the perineal structures, including labial or vaginal tears in females and urethral or prostatic injuries in males. The most disabling contusion in the pelvis is the **hip pointer**[55,71] in which a hematoma forms at the point of contact along the iliac crest (Fig. 46-15). A contusion in this area should be differentiated from a tear of the muscle aponeurosis or an avulsion of the apophysis of the iliac crest. Generally, such differentiation is not difficult because in a contusion, functional movement of the muscles attached to the crest does not increase the pain significantly.

Clinically the athlete with a hip pointer has difficulty in walking normally and in standing upright because of pain and muscle spasm; local tenderness, swelling, and ecchymosis are evident. At times, slow bleeding into the surrounding tissue occurs overnight after the initial injury, and the athlete experiences more symptoms. These include the distinct possibility of partial or complete femoral nerve palsy as a result of an expanding hematoma within the iliacus muscle called the **iliacus hematoma syndrome.** In general, this condition is rare in patients who have normal hemostasis, but it does occur and has been reported.[36] The femoral nerve dysfunction is generally noted a day or two after the original injury, implying the gradual increase in the hematoma and causation and not a traction injury on the nerve itself. This lesion is best identified by a CT scan and mandates early surgical evacuation to ensure complete recovery of nerve function. In most other cases of contusions or hematoma in the area of the iliac crest, heat, massage, and vigor-

ous physical therapy should be delayed because of the possibility of increasing the bleeding. Treatment the day after the injury should be aimed at controlling the bleeding by the use of ice, compression, and rest. Attempts to aspirate the initial hematoma of a deep muscle contusion are ineffective because the blood supply is usually spread throughout the muscle and the hematoma is not well localized. However, occasionally in a hip pointer there may be a fluctuant mass that can be aspirated. Once a muscle contusion has occurred, the use of the muscle must be restricted until function has returned to normal. Rehabilitation is aimed at strengthening the muscle and regaining adjacent joint motion. A subcutaneous hematoma along the iliac crest may remain tender and requires protective padding on return to sports activity.*

Prevention of disabling contusions to the pelvis is most important. In football and hockey, hip pads protect the iliac crest, greater trochanters, and coccyx. These pads should be kept from sliding down below the iliac crest during play, or they will predispose the athlete to further injury.

Myositis Ossificans

Myositis ossificans is the second most frequent problem in the thigh and is also seen in the musculature about the hip after a contusion.[1,47] Early radiographs show a soft-tissue mass, but within 7 to 10 days, calcific flocculations may appear and progress to heterotopic bone between the second and third week after injury. As the acute symptoms subside, a painless mass may remain, and adjacent hip motion may be lost as a result of restricted muscle function. Occasionally the mass may simulate a soft-tissue sarcoma, but differentiation is usually not difficult. Within 2 weeks the typical punctate calcification can be seen in the lesion, but even before this

---

*The technique of hard shell protective pad fabrication is described on pp. 303-306.

the peripheral capsule of the process can be seen to be composed of a thin layer of bone differentiating this process from a soft-tissue sarcoma on CT scans and MR images. Generally, surgical removal of the heterotopic bone is not indicated. If removal becomes necessary because of persistent loss of function with a contracture of the involved musculature, it must be delayed for 12 to 18 months, until the lesion is mature. Attempts to correlate maturity with bone scan activities or alkaline phosphatase levels have failed in the past, and it is now generally perceived that the myositis matures at 12 to 18 months, which can be further suggested by the typical mature appearance of the bone with contoured surfaces commensurate with the surrounding muscle activity and the mature trabecular pattern of the bone within the lesion. Treatment of myositis ossificans includes a high index of suspicion for injuries that ultimately progress to heterotopic bone deposition. These include proximal hamstring strains and direct quadriceps contusions. Acutely, these should be treated with protection from further injury, rest, ice application, compressive dressings, and graduated active exercises to regain contiguous joint function and motion rapidly. Patients with extensive injury, particularly to the quadriceps mechanism, may need to be admitted to the hospital to rule out the possibility of a compartment syndrome. The athlete should be allowed to return to competitive activities only after full strength, motion, and coordination have returned in an effort to minimize further intercurrent injuries. Additional injuries are simply additive to the original insult, resulting in prolonged muscle spasm, disuse atrophy, and marked decreased range of motion in the contiguous joint that may become intractable to therapeutic endeavors. When returning to competitive sports, particularly where contact is anticipated, the athlete must wear protective padding in the area of the previous contusion to minimize further insults.

Compartment Syndrome

Compartment syndrome of the gluteal musculature has been reported[75] following severe blunt trauma to the gluteal musculature. The classic features of compartment syndrome, severe pain and pain with passive muscle stretch, are present. Elevated compartment pressure measurements are found. Treatment is emergency surgical compartment fasciotomy. Potential complications of this problem include sciatic nerve injury and necrosis of the involved muscle.

Bursitis

Bursitis about the hip and pelvis is considered an affliction that can affect anyone, but it can be particularly disabling in an athlete.[71] Most commonly, bursitis involves the trochanteric bursa, ischial bursa, or iliopectineal bursa. In **trochanteric bursitis,** tenderness is localized over the greater trochanter, and pain is elicited with external rotation and adduction of the leg. Excessive stress in the various muscle attachments to the greater trochanter can initiate inflammation of the bursa; for instance, inflammation of the bursa is common in the female runner because of the broad configuration of her

---

Factors contributing to trochanteric bursitis

- Excessive stress in greater trochanteric muscle attachments (e.g., females with broad pelvis)
- Leg length discrepancy
- Weakness or contracture of gluteus medius or tensor fasciae femoris (positive Ober test)
- Running on banked surfaces
- Abnormal running mechanics

---

pelvis. A concentration of stress in this area may occur in runners with a leg length discrepancy, resulting in abnormal pelvic tilt. Also, a previous injury with residual weakness or a contracture of the gluteus medius may cause increased stress. The terrain may also be a factor[55] because running on banked surfaces focuses stress that may result in trochanteric bursitis. Abnormal running mechanics may be an additional factor; for instance, bursitis is more common in runners whose feet cross over the midline, increasing the adduction angle, and painful bursitis can develop from friction between the trochanter and the overlying iliotibial band.

Clinically, motion of the tensor fasciae femoris across the bursa in movement of the hip may accentuate discomfort. In addition to tenderness, crepitation, and warmth in athletes with a snapping hip in which the tensor fasciae latae slide over the trochanter, an audible and palpable snap is evident. This condition is more common in the female with a wide pelvis, prominent trochanters, and associated ligamentous laxity. Occasionally, surgical division of a portion of the iliotibial band may be necessary to correct this chronic irritation.

Ischial bursitis may result from a direct blow to the ischial bursa in a fall; however, there is often a history of prolonged sitting, especially with the legs crossed or on a hard surface. This condition is sometimes referred to as "benchwarmer's bursitis." Examination reveals tenderness over the ischial bursa.

The patient with **iliopectineal bursitis** is initially seen with acute disabling pain in the anterior aspect of the hip associated with an antalgic gait. Deep tenderness is elicited. The person assumes a position of flexion and external rotation of the hip, and stressing the iliopsoas muscle accentuates the discomfort. The differential diagnosis includes primary degenerative arthritis of the contiguous hip, labral tear of the hip, femoral direct hernia, or femoral neuritis or neuropathy, particularly if the bursa is sufficiently large enough to compromise the function of the nerve (Fig. 46-16). There may be a communication of the iliopectineal bursa and hip joint. This sometimes can be visualized or imaged with an arthrogram being performed into the hip joint with extravasation of the dye into the bursa anterior to the hip joint and underneath the iliopsoas tendon. On examination, some of these patients manifest a mass in the groin that can often be misinterpreted as a primary bone or soft-tissue malignancy.[7] Further imaging reveals the true nature of the process (Fig. 46-16). Some of these lesions reach large proportions. If the patient is embarrassed by these

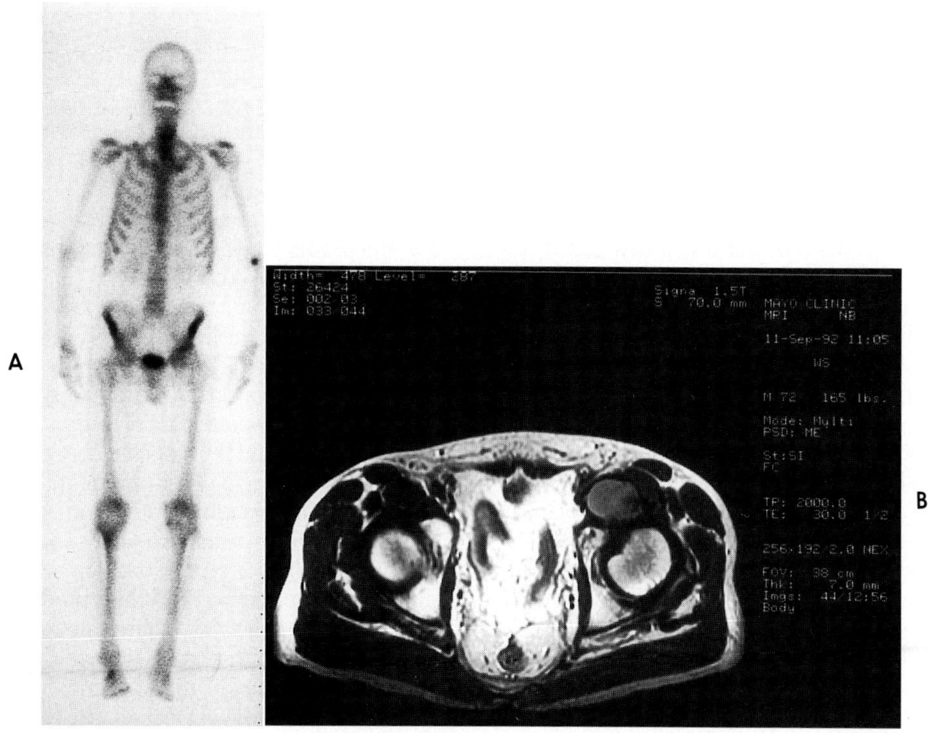

FIG. 46-16. A 55-year-old long-distance runner appears in our clinic with problems referrable to left upper thigh groin region. He noticed weakness, particularly during running up hills and even climbing stairs. Examination revealed 2½-cm discrepancy in quadriceps musculature with decreased strength in quadriceps muscles amounting to 3+ out of 5 and decreased ankle jerk. **A,** Bone scintigraphy reveals increased uptake just superior to pubic ramus and anterior column of hip joint. **B,** Magnetic resonance image reveals what appears to be a cystic process lying between iliopsoas muscle and tendon and underlying hip joint.

lesions, decompressive surgery is recommended. Chronic pain in the thigh and anterior aspect of the hip and localized tenderness and swelling may also be associated with a ganglion cyst of the hip.

Snapping Hip

Athletes can develop painful snapping in the region of the hip. External iliotibial band snapping occurs at the greater trochanter, and internal iliopsoas snapping occurs across the iliopectineal eminence.

Iliotibial band snapping. Iliotibial band snapping can occur as the hip goes from flexion to extension and as the iliotibial band crosses over the greater trochanter going from anterior to posterior. At times this snapping may be asymptomatic. If no symptoms such as pain are present, the snapping can be left alone. Trochanteric bursitis can develop in association with the snapping. Treatment should include rest, iliotibial band stretching, antiinflammatory medication, and therapeutic modalities such as ultrasound or heat. Often a series of steroid injections into the bursa may be required. If treatment is successful, the snapping may diminish and the discomfort should be relieved. At times the snapping can be recalcitrant to conservative measures, and both the snapping and bursitis can be painful and disabling. In these situations, surgery can be performed to eliminate the snapping iliotibial band. Techniques described include excision of an elliptic piece of iliotibial band centered over the trochanter,[108] Z-plasty of the iliotibial band,[12] and fixation of the iliotibial band to the trochanter.[13] Surgery can be effective for these refractory cases, allowing athletes to return to sports without snapping or pain.

Snapping of the iliopsoas muscle. Iliopsoas snapping presents as a deep anterior snapping in the groin. Often the movement that produces the snapping is extension of the hip from a flexed, adducted, and externally rotated position. Jacobson and Allen[49] studied in anatomic specimens the movement of the iliopsoas tendon and described the snapping of the iliopsoas tendon over the anterior femoral head and capsule as the tendon moves from lateral to medial with hip extension. They theorized that the bursa between the tendon and the hip capsule gets inflamed with the snapping tendon. This can be confirmed by iliopsoas bursography under fluoroscopic control.[43] A small amount of contrast injected into the bursa demonstrates the presence of the snapping in the region of the pelvic brim. Bursography is indicated only in cases that do not respond to conservative measures. By far, most cases of iliopsoas snapping respond to a program of modified activity, hip flexor stretching, and antiinflammatory medication. Surgery for this condition consists of lengthening of the iliopsoas tendon. Although the procedure may be successful, complications of the procedure include sensory loss along the anterolateral thigh and subjective hip flexor weakness.[49]

Muscle Strains

The most frequent injuries of the hip and pelvis in athletes are muscle and tendon strains. The pelvis is a site of many muscle insertions (Figs. 46-4 and 46-5). The iliac wing is the site of attachment of the abdominal muscles above and the gluteal muscles below. The ischium is the site of attachment of the hamstrings, and the pubis and anterior pelvis are the sites of insertion of the adductor muscles and accessory hip flexors. Although a strain may occur anywhere throughout the length of the muscle, in adults the injury is most common at the muscle-tendon junction. In adolescent athletes, avulsion injuries of the tendon-cartilaginous insertions are more common.[72] The muscle strains vary in degree, depending on the extent of tearing of the muscle-tendon fibers.

The aponeurosis of the **external oblique muscles** may be torn completely from the iliac crest. These strains are often caused by forceful contraction of the abdominal muscles while the trunk is being forced to the contralateral side. When initially seen, the patient has severe pain, difficulty in straightening the torso, and associated localized tenderness. The patient has pain when flexing to the opposite side, indicating damage to the muscle attachment. Moreover, aggravation of the pain by active abduction or extension of the thigh when the patient is lying on his or her side indicates damage to the gluteal insertions and the tensor fasciae femoris as well as to the lateral abdominal muscles. Most of these injuries respond to supportive treatment and restriction of activities until symptoms subside. Abdominal binders or adhesive taping is often helpful. Occasionally, surgical repair to restore anatomic continuity of the tissues has been done. When activity is resumed, protective padding over the iliac crest is required.

Strain of the **adductor** origin on the pelvis (groin strain) is a common problem in the athlete (Fig. 46-17). This muscle group is the major site of muscle strain in professional athletes, and such strain is generally seen in the older age groups.

In a study of groin strain injuries in hockey players, Merrifield and Cowan[66] indicated that a disparity in muscle strength between both hip joint adductor muscle groups is a contributing factor in these injuries. They indicated that strengthening and stretching exercises of the adductor muscle of the thigh to eliminate the power imbalance between the two groups help prevent groin strain injury in hockey players. These injuries are most common in ice hockey players because of the dynamic requirements of the skating motion. The player adducts the thigh forcibly in push-off to initiate the gliding stroke.

Groin strain injuries are also common in football and rugby. Forcible external rotation of the abducted leg, such as occurs when a football player slips on a muddy field, may result in a disabling groin strain. Forceful abduction of the thighs, as in a straddling injury, may strain the adductor muscle attachments to the ischial pubic rami (rider's strain).

Sports in which adductor strains commonly occur

- Hockey
- Football
- Rugby
- Horseback riding
- Swimming (breast stroke)
- Cricket
- Bowling

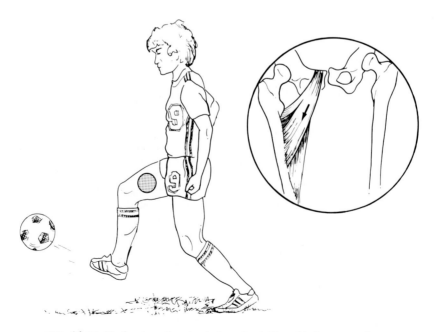

FIG. 46-17. Mechanism of groin strain and osteitis pubis in soccer player.

A breast stroker in swimming, a cricket player,[97] or a bowler who slips while delivering the ball can commonly strain the adductors. Localized tenderness is evident along the subcutaneous edge of the ramus. Pain is elicited on passive abduction of the thigh and in forced active adduction. Occasionally, complete avulsion of an adductor muscle (usually the longus) occurs. In this injury, the physician can palpate a defect and the avulsed muscle mass, and surgical repair is recommended.

The duration of treatment depends mainly on the symptoms. Initial treatment involves the use of ice, rest, protection, and antiinflammatory agents. The athlete's hip can be strapped in a spica wrap with the thigh flexed and slightly externally rotated. The athlete should avoid climbing stairs, jumping, and running. Often severe groin injuries require use of crutches or a cane to minimize pain.

After the acute period, treatment can be changed from cold to heat modalities such as ultrasound or short-wave diathermy. With the patient lying on his or her side, gentle, pain-free, active range of motion is usually started early to maintain a normal range of motion. Active resistance exercises against gravity should not begin for approximately 3 to 6 weeks after the initial injury because they may aggravate the pain. Strengthening the adductors is started first, using the hands for isometric squeezes or for squeezing a medicine ball. Also, flexion muscles of the hip can be strengthened using Therabands. A good home program of strengthening and stretching of the hip adductors should be taught to the athlete to prevent recurrence.

Conservative treatment yields satisfactory results in almost all cases. A small percentage of patients may have recurrent strains and chronic tendinitis of the adductors at their origin on the pelvis. Martens, Hansen, Mulier[62] have described a surgical technique to release the adductor from the bone in these cases. This procedure is appropriate if all conservative measures have failed for a prolonged time.

Hamstring strains are a frequent cause of disability in the athlete. The injury may occur anywhere along the muscle but is more common at the junction of the proximal muscle tendon. The mechanism involves forced flexion of the hip with the knee extended. A classic example is the hurdler who crosses the hurdle with the hip flexed maximally and the knee extended (Fig. 46-18). With a sudden overstrain in running, excessive force may be applied to the origin of the hamstring in the forward recovery phase when the hip is flexed and the knee is extended just before the heel strikes. In addition, sudden forceful straight leg raising exerts the same stress on the hamstring attachment. Hamstring strains are associated with poor flexibility, inadequate warm-up, exercise fatigue, poor coordination, and imbalance between hamstring and quadriceps strength. The athlete with a hamstring pull experiences localized tenderness and pressure over the ischial tuberosity and accentuation of the pain with straight leg raising. Active resisted extension of the hip also accentuates the pain (see Chapter 45).

Factors associated with hamstring strains

- Poor flexibility
- Inadequate warm-up
- Exercise fatigue
- Poor coordination
- Muscle imbalance

Strain of the muscle-tendon units that are **anterior** to the hip is not uncommon (Figs. 46-17 and 46-18); strain occurs primarily in kicking sports because of flexion overload against the fixed limb. Because of the proximity of these muscle attachments (Fig. 46-19), the site of injury may be difficult to localize accurately. However, determining the location of the tenderness and stressing the involved muscle-tendon unit helps distinguish the strain on the various muscle attachments, such as the rectus femoris, sartorius, and tensor fasciae latae muscles.

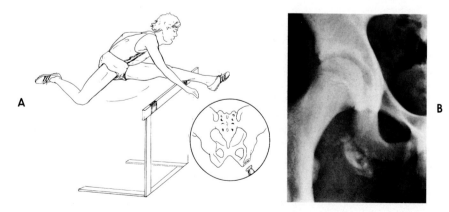

FIG. 46-18. A, Mechanism of hamstring pull or avulsion of ischial apophysis in hurdler. Athlete crosses hurdle with hip flexed and knee extended with maximum stress on hamstrings. **B,** Anteroposterior view of pelvis showing large, bony overgrowth and pseudotumor from previous avulsion of ischial apophysis.

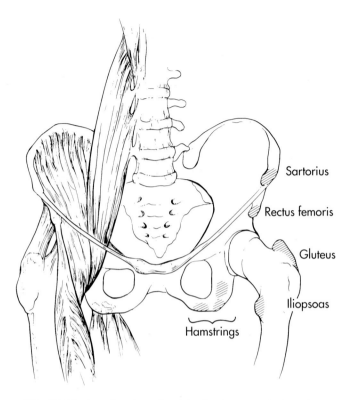

FIG. 46-19. Anterior view of pelvis showing muscle insertions. (From Berquist TH, Coventry MM: The pelvis and hips. In Berquist TH [ed]: *Orthopaedic radiology: imaging of orthopedic trauma and surgery,* Philadelphia, 1986, WB Saunders.)

Strain of the **iliopsoas tendon** is caused by overactive contraction with the thigh fixed or forced into extension. Strain of an iliopsoas muscle produces deep groin discomfort and tenderness that often extends into the lower abdomen. Passive external rotation of the hip in extension aggravates the pain. Several case reports in the literature have described a syndrome characterized by pain in the groin, a tender swelling in the iliac fossa, and flexion deformity of the hip associated with a femoral nerve lesion secondary to proximal avulsion of the iliacus muscle. In four of the five cases reported, hip flexor strain was secondary to hyperextension injuries of the hip in gymnastics. Green[38] suggested that early recognition of this condition, with evacuation of the hematoma, may prevent the development of a complete femoral nerve lesion.

The **rectus femoris muscle** functions as a hip flexor and an extensor of the knee. Because flexion of the hip is closely associated with extension of the knee, the muscle is active during running and walking. However, any excessive force, such as in long jumping, or repetitive activity, such as in long-distance running, can cause tendinitis of the rectus femoris tendon. Pain, often in the groin region, is caused by resistance of the extension of the knee tested while the patient is in a prone position. Also, pain can be caused by full passive flexion of the hip, which pushes the tender part, or by passive rotation, which applies local stretch. Usually the site of tenderness is approximately 8 cm below the anterior superior spine. Treatment involves local therapy measures and injections of steroids.

The **gracilis muscle** acts on both the hip and the knee, and its function is similar to that of the hip adductors. With the knee extended the gracilis is an active hip flexor, but it is inactive if the knee is allowed to flex simultaneously. The gracilis both adducts the hip joint and rotates it medially. During flexion of the hip joint the muscle is most active during the first part of the flexion of walking and bicycling. Often it can be strained when the adductors are strained, since it is part of the adductor syndrome. It is treated similarly.

Athletes may also suffer a strain of the **gluteus medius** with associated chronic tendinitis of its attachment to the trochanter. This condition is often seen in such sports as football, swimming, and ice hockey. Localized tenderness is present with discomfort on stressing the gluteus medius against resistance. Usually passive range of motion of the hip with the muscles relaxed causes no pain. Tendinitis or inflammation at the insertion of the **external rotators** of the hip attaching on the margin of the trochanter results in posterior hip pain and localized tenderness. Discomfort is accentuated by active external rotation against resistance or passive, forced internal rotation of the hip.

These various muscle-tendon injuries of the pelvis and hip are managed similarly. The degree of disability is dependent on the severity of the injury, and the functional impairment varies among sports. Prompt treatment of the acute injury is essential. If a complete muscle-tendon rupture occurs in a competitive athlete, surgical repair is usually indicated. However, most of these injuries are first- or second-degree sprains as defined by the American Medical Association nomenclature of athletic injuries.

First- or second-degree strains can be treated in four different stages. Initially the goal is to control and reduce pain, swelling, and inflammation. Treatment of an acute muscle strain involves protection, rest, ice, compression, and elevation (Table 46-3). Various physical modalities can be used in the initial stage. One is the use of cryotherapy or cold packs placed over the injured muscle for approximately 30 minutes every 2 hours. Methods of applying cold include ice wraps, evaporative cold spray, ice packs, ice slushes, and chemical gels. Cold helps raise the pain threshold, acts as a local vasoconstrictor, and decreases muscle spasm. In addition, antiinflammatory agents such as aspirin or nonsteroidal antiinflammatory drugs (NSAIDs) can be used to reduce the pain and inflammation. Swelling is often controlled and reduced by applying cold, elevating the affected part, using elastic compression wraps, and performing isometric exercise and decongestion massage. Protection and rest are facilitated by the use of crutches, orthotics, and taping. Supportive wraps, such as a hip spica wrap for groin strains (see p. 296) or an abdominal corset for oblique muscle strains over the iliac crest, help control movement and therefore reduce pain. Exercise of the uninjured joints can be started early to maintain range of motion and muscle strength.

TABLE 46-3 Treatment of muscle-tendon injuries of the hip and pelvis

Treatment	Stage I—Acute Injury Phase (First 24 to 72 hr)	Stage II—Subsidence of Acute Symptoms	Stage III—Able to Do Isometric Exercises Pain Free	Stage IV—Range of Motion 95% of Normal/Strength 75% of Normal Leg	Stage V—Strength 90% of Unaffected Leg
Rest	X				
Ice	X				
Compression	X				
Elevation	X				
Nonsteroidal antiinflammatory medication	X				
Contrast treatments		X	X		
Hydrotherapy		X	X		
Active range of motion		X	X		
Ultrasound		X	X		
Muscle stimulation		X	X		
Isometric exercise		X	X		
Well leg and upper extremity exercise		X	X	X	
Closed-chain exercises			X	X	
Isotonic and isokinetic exercises			X	X	
Stretching			X	X	
Aerobic activity			X	X	
Balance and coordination drills				X	
Agility training				X	
Sport-specific exercises				X	
Jogging				X	
Straight-ahead sprinting				X	
Return to sports					X
Maintenance flexibility and strength program					X

The second stage begins when the acute symptoms have subsided. The goals include regaining normal range of motion, reducing scar formation, relaxing any muscular spasms, reducing stiffness, and retarding muscle atrophy. Contrast treatments alternating heat and cold modalities can be used initially. An effective treatment is to apply ice for 10 minutes, followed by hot packs for 10 minutes, followed by ultrasound for 10 minutes, and ending with 10 minutes of ice therapy. Hydrotherapy using warm water (100° to 105° F [37.8° to 40.6° C]) in a whirlpool or Hubbard tank (98° to 100° F[36.7° to 37.8° C]) often reduces muscle spasms and stiffness in hip and pelvic injuries. Gentle exercises to improve range of motion and to prevent contractures can often be performed in the water. The use of heat, such as from ultrasound, radiant heat lamps, or hot moist packs can also be helpful. Exercises are always started with pain-free range of motion of the injured part, and neuromuscular reeduca-tion exercises are prescribed if there is any evidence of muscular incoordination. At times, friction or a sedative massage is used to reduce adhesion formation and congestion. High-intensity muscle stimulation and isometric strengthening exercises are initiated to reduce muscular atrophy.

The third stage involves regaining normal strength and flexibility. Once isometric exercises have been initiated and are tolerated by the patient, dynamic exercises with machine and free weights can begin. Both concentric and eccentric exercises are emphasized. Closed-chain exercises are also included in the program. Static prolonged stretching exercises to increase flexibility need to be done gently without producing pain or muscle incoordination.

In the final stage the objective is the athlete's return to previous activities with normal strength, range of motion, and mobility. Exercises should concentrate on improving flexibility, balance, and coordination. In addition, specific sports activities, such as agility and reaction exercises, are started. The use of heat before or ice after exercise can be continued. Once the patient has regained normal strength and range of motion and can perform the skill activities of the sport without any significant discomfort, he or she is allowed to return to full activity with instructions to continue proper stretching before and after participation. If active treatment of the strain is not initiated, progressive involvement of the underlying bone at the origin or insertion of the muscle may occur. **Osteitis pubis** is an irritation of the symphyseal area caused by strenuous conditioning and training of the rectus abdominis and adductor muscles. Although described in a number of athletic activities, the most common is long-distance running.[28] Radiographic evidence of the process is suggested by sclerosis of the contiguous symphyseal and pubic rami, as well as loss of definition on their medial border. Differential diagnosis includes osteomyelitis, urethritis, or chronic prostatism.

In addition, **iliac apophysitis** may occur at sites of origin of the rectus femoris or the sartorius in the long-distance, adolescent runner.[100] This continued traction injury to the origin of these muscles causes local discomfort and sometimes distortion of the architecture somewhat similar to the microavulsions that occur in Osgood-Schlatter disease of the knee.

Either osteitis pubis or iliac apophysitis responds appropriately to rest, heat, stretching of the muscles that take origin or insert into the area, and judicious use of NSAIDs.

Criteria for return to play following hip or pelvic muscle strain

- Normal strength (all muscle groups)
- Normal flexibility
- Full range of motion
- Ability to perform skill activity without discomfort
- Appropriate aerobic capacity

Pelvic Floor Myalgia

Pelvic floor myalgia is a syndrome of tension myalgia involving the muscles and fascia of the pelvic cavity. Tension myalgia of the pelvic muscles has been discussed under different names in the literature, including *levator ani syndrome, piriformis syndrome, anorectal pain,* and *coccygodynia.* All of these syndromes involve painful pelvic muscles and therefore have been grouped under one name—*pelvic floor myalgia.* The muscles that are most frequently involved are the levator ani and the coccygeus and piriformis, which form a continuous muscular sling that closes the posterior part of the pelvic outlet. Two of these muscles, the coccygeus and the levator ani, form the pelvic diaphragm that surrounds the sphincters of the excretory and reproductive structures. The pelvic diaphragm is strong enough to support the abdominal contents during running or jump-

ing, yet it is resilient enough to allow passage of a full-term infant. The third muscle, the piriformis, is the only muscle that bridges the sacroiliac joint. With the other short hip extensors, the piriformis is near the gluteal and sacral nerves in the sciatic foramen. Repetitive muscular stresses to the pelvis in athletics or in activities that involve frequent increases of inner abdominal pressure can cause pelvic floor myalgia. More frequently the condition is caused by habitual contraction of the pelvic floor muscles secondary to pain arising anywhere in the lumbosacral spinal column, sacroiliac joint, coccyx, perineum, or hips.

Clinical symptoms include back and leg pain and a heavy feeling in the pelvis. Less commonly, symptoms include dyschezia (painful bowel movements), constipation, rectal pain, and dyspareunia. These symptoms result from the relationship between the pelvic floor muscles and the various anatomic structures and their proximity to one another.

Clinical symptoms of pelvic floor myalgia

- Back pain
- Leg pain
- Heavy feeling in pelvis
- Dyschezia
- Constipation
- Rectal pain
- Dyspareunia

When the muscle tension of the pelvic floor involves the ligaments (sacrotuberous and sacrospinous), pain can be referred to either the sacroiliac or the low back region. Involvement of the piriformis muscle, through its close anatomic relation to the gluteal and sciatic nerves, can cause pain to be referred down the posterior portion of the leg and onto the hips and buttocks. The muscles can also be tender at their attachments to the sacrococcyx joint and pubic rami.

Painful pelvic floor muscles are generally found during rectal examination. In addition, many such patients have poor posture and generalized pain in the muscle attachment. If the piriformis or other short rotators of the hip are involved, resisted hip extension or rotation or excessive passive rotation of the hip in the internal location reproduces the pain.

Treatment is directed at relieving the discomfort or pain of the pelvic muscles. Deep heat or diathermy (rectal or external) or hydrotherapy in a Hubbard tank can be prescribed. Rectal massage by the technique described by Thiele[95] and general mobilization of the sacrococcygeal joint can be effective.[87] Patients can be taught to relax the pelvic floor muscles with neuromuscular reeducation by using relaxation exercises or biofeedback. Various techniques of biofeedback include the use of electrodes around the external sphincter or inside the rectum or vagina and the use of an electronic perineometer. Athletes should also be instructed to avoid activities or positions that may aggravate or precipitate

---

Treatment of pelvic floor myalgia

- Deep heat (rectal or external)
- Hydrotherapy
- Sacrococcygeal mobilization
- Biofeedback for relaxation exercises
- Patient education
- Abdominal strengthening
- Piriformis stretching
- Local injection

---

the symptoms. A home treatment program of hot tub baths, postural training, abdominal strengthening, piriformis muscle stretching, and relaxation exercises can be included in the program. Improvement usually occurs within the first week. Patients with chronic conditions occasionally are helped by injections of steroids into specific muscles (e.g., the piriformis).

Sacroiliac Joint Strain

In young athletes the sacroiliac joint is under great stress. Two forces affecting the sacroiliac joints predispose them to sprains. The first vector of forces comes from above through the lumbar spinal column and acts on the upper end of the sacrum. This force tends to push the superior portion of the sacrum downward and forward at the same time that the coccygeal portion of the sacrum is moving upward and backward. These movements are limited by the tension of the sacrotuberous, sacrospinous, and anterior sacroiliac ligaments.

The second vector of forces comes from below, acting through the femoral head and acetabulum onto the ilium and sacroiliac joint. The acetabulum is located anterior and inferior to the sacroiliac joint and tends to force the ilium into an upward and posterior rotatory motion on the sacrum. This movement is prevented by the tension of both the anterior and posterior sacroiliac ligaments. During weight bearing the downward and anterior rotating forces of the sacrum are opposed by this upward and posterior rotating force of the iliac bones. The shearing forces that result at the sacroiliac joints are considerable in athletic activity and are controlled under normal conditions by the ligamentous structures around the sacroiliac joint. A runner with short legs or with poor running mechanics increases the shearing force at the sacroiliac joint and is predisposed to ligamentous sprains.

Stressful athletic conditions that cause sudden contractions of the hamstrings or the abdominal muscles exert a posterior rotating force on the ilium and can result in sprains of the sacroiliac ligaments. Sudden, unexpected twisting motions of the trunk that occur in sports such as football, hockey, or basketball can also stress the sacroiliac joints. Vigorous pulling while bending forward, as with incorrect weightlifting techniques, or a fall on one or both buttocks can sprain the sacroiliac joint. The athlete may not be impressed with the pain initially, but on awakening the following day, he or she often experiences acute low back pain and difficulty in bending forward (e.g., to put on socks).

Unilateral pain involving the hip, buttock, low back, and the back of the upper thigh often causes the athlete to elevate the hip on the painful side to avoid weight bearing over the sacroiliac region. Physical examination reveals a poor lumbopelvic range of motion on forward flexion. With sacroiliac ligament sprains, back extension involving the long erector spinae muscles causes little discomfort, whereas pain may be elicited in dysfunction of the lumbosacral joint. Localized tenderness and a positive Lasègue's sign with pain over the joint are common findings. **Gaenslen's test** for sacroiliac involvement is performed with the patient lying on the unaffected side and hyperflexing the lower hip while hyperextending the upper hip. A positive result, in which the pain is reproduced, usually occurs. Rectal examination may reveal tenderness and swelling over the sacroiliac joint. Finally, if the strain is severe, manual compression of both iliac crests can elicit sacroiliac pain.

Treatment in the initial phase involves rest, heat, and analgesics. Gentle mobilization exercises can begin when tolerated. Often the patient can do extension exercises of the back more comfortably than flexion exercises of the back. Abdominal strengthening and postural exercises should also be prescribed. A sacroiliac belt may be helpful in stabilizing the joint motion. Injections of steroids into the sacroiliac joint are rarely necessary. The patient should be instructed in good running or lifting mechanics, and significant leg length discrepancy should be corrected to prevent recurrences.

Avulsion Injuries of the Pelvis and Hip

The same injury mechanism that results in the muscle-tendon strain in the adult athlete may avulse the cartilaginous tendon insertion from the bone in the adolescent athlete.[72] These injuries are associated with avulsions of the secondary growth center or apophysis, with traumatic separation occurring in the junction of the cartilaginous area between the apophysis and the bone. The avulsion may occur before the appearance of the secondary ossification center, which frequently is not seen until late adolescence.[15] In these circumstances, the physician must have a high index of suspicion and institute appropriate treatment. The diagnosis is subsequently confirmed by radiography several weeks later when the callus appears. Because of the thick periosteum, significant displacement is unusual in these injuries. These avulsion injuries may be mistaken radiographically for a malignancy or infection. Avulsion injuries occur most often in the apophysis of the pelvis and proximal femur and may involve various muscle insertions (Fig. 46-19).

Therapeutic efforts in avulsion injuries should decrease the risk of further displacement of the apophysis.

Gaenslen's test

- Patient lies on unaffected side
- Hyperflex uninvolved hip
- Hyperextend involved hip
- Positive test when pain is reproduced

TABLE 46-4 Rehabilitation plan for acute avulsion injuries

	Acute Injury	After Pain Subsides	When Full ROM Achieved	When 50% Strength Returned	When Full ROM and Strength Regained
Rest	X				
Limited muscle tension	X				
Analgesics	X				
Cryotherapy	X	X	X	X	X
Active ROM		X			
Passive ROM and stretching		X	X	X	X
Active-assisted ROM		X			
Isometric exercises		X	X		
Well leg exercise		X	X	X	
Upper body aerobics		X	X	X	
Isotonic exercises (injury region)			X		
Isokinetic exercises (injury region)			X		
Isotonic exercises (pelvis and lower extremity)				X	X
Isokinetic exercises (pelvis and lower extremity)				X	X
Lower extremity aerobics				X	
Sport-specific exercises					X

Modified from Metzamker JN, Pappas AM: *Am J Sports Med* 13:349, 1985.
ROM, Range of motion.

This is generally accomplished with rest, ice application, and positioning of the limb to minimize further stretch of the affected muscle. Recently, Metzamker and Pappas[67] have outlined a five-stage progressive rehabilitation program for athletes suffering from acute avulsive injuries of the hip and pelvis (Table 46-4). These include: (1) rest with positioning to relax the involved muscle, analgesics as necessary, and application of ice; (2) after the acute pain has settled, the young athlete is allowed to increase the excursion of the injured muscle involved; (3) when full range of motion has been achieved, a resistive exercise program is initiated; (4) when on dynamic objective testing it appears that the athlete has regained 50% or more of the anticipated strength of the musculotendinous unit, the incorporation of other muscles in the pelvis and lower extremity is promoted; and (5) when the athlete has achieved not only full range of motion but also full strength in the affected musculotendinous unit and the integrated muscle units of the pelvis and lower extremity, return to competitive sports is allowed. This process, however, may take several months to achieve.

Iliac Crest Injuries

The ossification center in the iliac apophysis first appears laterally and anteriorly on the iliac crest and advances posteriorly until it reaches the posterior iliac spine at maturation.[15,80] The average age of closure of the apophysis is 16 years in boys and 14 years in girls, but it may be delayed up to 4 additional years. Godshall and

Hansen[37] indicated that incomplete avulsion fracture of the iliac epiphysis or apophysis may result from a sudden severe contraction of the abdominal muscles associated with abrupt directional changes while running. They described a case in which a 14-year-old baseball player suffered a separation of the anterior portion of the left iliac apophysis during a sudden twisting maneuver. They also noted a similar injury in a 16-year-old boy who twisted his body while catching a pass in a football game. Butler and Eggert[14] described a case in which an 18-year-old football player suffered a hip pointer as a result of being hit by a helmet; when he resumed running activities, he subsequently experienced sudden severe pain and suffered an avulsion fracture of the iliac crest apophysis. Godshall and Hansen[37] and Waters and Millis[100] stressed that if an immature athlete experiences pain in the region of the iliac crest after a twisting injury, the physician should use an oblique radiograph of the iliac crest and comparison views of the opposite crest. The athletes have pain and tenderness over the iliac crest with discomfort on resisted abduction of the hip while the patient is lying on the unaffected side. Treatment is usually symptomatic; ice is applied, and excessive trunk rotations are avoided. Severe avulsion injuries may include protected weight bearing using crutches for 5 to 7 days. Radiographs confirm the separation or demonstrate a stress fracture; frequently there may be only subtle differences in contour or in physeal width.[72] In the series reported by Clancy and Foltz[16] all the patients responded after 3 to 4 weeks of rest with complete relief of symptoms within 4 to 6 weeks. There were no recurrences after the patients resumed their training program.

Iliac Spine Injuries

The **anterior superior iliac spine (ASIS)** can be avulsed by forceful contraction of the sartorius muscle in sports such as jumping and running. Hanson, Angevine, and Juhl[42] described a 16-year-old boy who suffered bilateral avulsion fractures of the ASIS during a sport. The athlete often complains of pain at the anterior aspect of the thigh in any activity that causes or produces flexion or passive extension of the hip. There may be swelling and ecchymosis at the site of the avulsion.

The **anterior inferior iliac spine (AIIS)** can be avulsed by vigorous contraction of the straight head of the rectus femoris muscle.[60] This avulsion is less common than that at the ASIS because fewer stresses are placed on the AIIS, and its ossification occurs earlier. Watson-Jones[101] reported avulsion of the AIIS associated with kicking in rugby and football. This avulsion is associated with a sudden sharp pain, an antalgic gait, and pain and weakness on hip flexion. Local tenderness and swelling are often present.

Displacement of the avulsion injury at either the superior or inferior spine is usually minimal.[104] The tensor fasciae latae and inguinal ligament prevent significant displacement of the ASIS, and the intact reflected head of the rectus femoris prevents displacement of the inferior spine. Treatment usually involves conservative measures of rest, protective weight bearing and crutches, and refraining from athletic activities for 4 to 6 weeks. Although open reduction has been recommended for a significant separation, operative intervention usually is unnecessary and the athlete can expect a complete functional recovery with conservative treatment.

Ischial Apophysis Injuries

Injuries to the ischial apophysis have received more attention in the literature than the other avulsion injuries of the pelvis, with the first case reported by Malgaigne[41,61] in 1859. This injury was called "ischial apophysiolysis" by Milch[68] in 1953 and is also known as the "hurdler's injury" (Fig. 46-18). In persons between 20 and 25 years of age the ossification center of the ischial apophysis unites with the body of the ischium.[14] The avulsion injury most commonly occurs during hurdling or gymnastics and is associated with a powerful hamstring contraction with the pelvis fixed in flexion and the knee in extension.[59] Generally, this mechanism avulses the insertion of the hamstring, whereas a dancer or cheerleader doing a split may avulse the separate attachment of the adductor magnus. Pain and disability are substantial. The patient walks with an antalgic gait and experiences discomfort on sitting. Localized tenderness is present over the tuberosity, and pain is accentuated by flexion of the thigh with the knee in extension.

There is some controversy in the literature as to whether surgical intervention is indicated. Treatment, traditionally, has been conservative. Surgical options include either excision of the fragment and reattachment of the tendons or open reduction and internal fixation of the fragment. Few authors recommend the latter. Watson-Jones[101] stated that open reduction is not indicated. Generally eventual recovery can be expected with conservative care, including rest and protective weight bearing with crutches until healing is complete. Watts[102] indicated that there is no objective loss of ability with nonoperative treatment. However, Schlonsky and Olix[85] described the cases of two patients with functional disability after nonoperative treatment. More recently Wootton, Cross, and Holt[107] have similarly reported three cases of elite athletes, including an Olympian, who were markedly disabled after a delay in diagnosis of ischial apophysis avulsion and subsequently nonunion or painful fibrous union of the fracture. In all three cases an open reduction and internal fixation was performed, and all three athletes returned to their premorbid athletic performance levels. In all three cases, objective testing of strength suggested a 30% loss in hamstring function in the displaced position. In spite of what was conceived to be adequate conservative treatment, all three patients failed to improve and continued to harbor considerable athletic disability. Even in the presence of chronicity, open reduction and internal fixation could be achieved without the need to excise the bony fragment, and reapproximation to its native ischial bed apparently was not a problem. The authors strongly supported the need for open reduction and internal fixation for all ischial apophyseal avulsions in which there is separation of at least 2 cm, and they suggested that patients with continued chronic disability in the presence of a displaced ischial apophysis be treated successfully with late open reduction and internal fixation. Healing after conservative treatment may be associated with new bone formation and enlargement, which have commonly been mistaken as a bone tumor. In a series of 39 patients with avulsion of the ischial apophysis, Barnes and Hinds[4] noted nonunion in 68%. If pain and discomfort develop with the inability to sit comfortably on the enlarged tuberosity, late excision of the fragment may be indicated.

Lesser Trochanter Injuries

An isolated avulsion fracture of the lesser trochanter is a rare injury, occurring in less than 1% of hip injuries. This injury should be suspected primarily in the adolescent athlete who has sudden anteromedial hip pain during running. The mechanism is a sudden contraction of the iliopsoas muscle with the thigh fixed. For instance, in football, if a placekicker's cleats catch in the ground, a sudden contraction of the iliopsoas muscle may avulse the lesser trochanter (Fig. 46-20). Kulund[55] also described this mechanism for avulsion of the rectus femoris. Dimon[23] collected a series of 30 patients: 25 teenagers, 4 adults, and 1 child. Of these 30 patients, 22 had participated in sports, including vigorous cheerleading, football, and track. In these cases, examination reveals an antalgic limp with tenderness anteriorly and medially on direct palpation. The patient holds the thigh in a flexed, adducted position. Painful hip flexion against resistance is demonstrated, as is an inability to straight leg

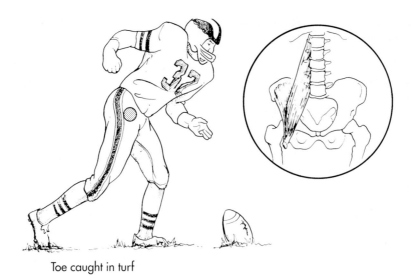

Toe caught in turf

FIG. 46-20. Mechanism of avulsion of lesser trochanter.

raise fully from a supine position. The diagnosis is confirmed by radiographs of the hip in slight external rotation, demonstrating a small metaphyseal flake of bone pulled off with the apophysis. Treatment is conservative, involving protective weight bearing with crutches for 1 to 2 weeks and restriction of sports activities. Dimon[23] found no relationship between return to activities or disability and the distance the lesser trochanter was pulled away from the femoral shaft. In his series, teenage athletes were able to begin easy running and jogging at 6 to 8 weeks after injury and had returned to full sports activities by 12 weeks.

Considerations for surgical repair of ischial apophyseal avulsion

Acute injury
- Elite athlete
- Greater than 2 cm displacement

Chronic injury
- Documented disability
- Greater than 2 cm displacement

Stress Fractures

Stress fractures of the pelvis and hip are relatively uncommon, accounting for 1.25% of injuries in joggers (Fig. 46-21). Devas[22] indicated that during running, athletes are more susceptible to femoral neck fractures than femoral shaft fractures. The literature indicates that the incidence of a stress fracture of the proximal third of the femur is approximately 2% in the general population.[57]

Pelvis. Pelvic stress fractures are seen in the anterior part of the pelvis, usually occurring in the ischial pubic ramus. These are more common in women than men. This predominant site may depend on the muscle pull

of the adductors medially and the hamstrings laterally. In a pelvic stress fracture, symptoms of perineal, groin, and adductor pain are present.

Pelvic stress fractures frequently occur in serious runners, often in individuals training for a marathon. They are particularly likely to occur during competitive racing or during interval training.[70,74] Three clinical findings, if present, in a long-distance runner with groin pain are diagnostic of a pelvic stress fracture, according to Noakes et al.[70] First, activity causes such severe discomfort in the groin that running is impossible. Second, the athlete develops discomfort in the groin when standing unsupported on the injured leg (positive standing test). Third, deep palpation reveals extreme tenderness localized to the pubic ramus and not to the overlying soft tissues.[70]

Pelvic stress fractures can be confirmed by scintigraphy or radiographs, depending on the duration of symptoms. Treatment is avoidance of running, and recovery may last as long as 12 to 16 weeks before the athlete attains preinjury level. The physician may also see a stress avulsion of the hamstring attachment to the ischium in short-distance runners.

Stress fractures of the sacrum have also been reported.[2] Like pelvic stress fractures, sacral stress fractures are seen in competitive, serious runners. Pain and tenderness are localized to the sacral region. Radiographs are usually normal, but scintigraphy or MRI can be diagnostic. A period of relative rest (nonimpact-loading sports) heals this uncommon stress fracture.[98]

Hip. Stress fractures of the lesser trochanter of the proximal femur are unusual and are suspected in patients with discomfort at the insertion at the iliopsoas muscle. When symptoms persist, this entity can be differentiated from bursitis and tendinitis by positive findings on a bone scan or serial radiographic studies. Devas[22] in 1961 and Blickenstaff and Morris[9] in 1966 indicated that early diagnosis may be difficult and that the physician must have a high index of suspicion in diag-

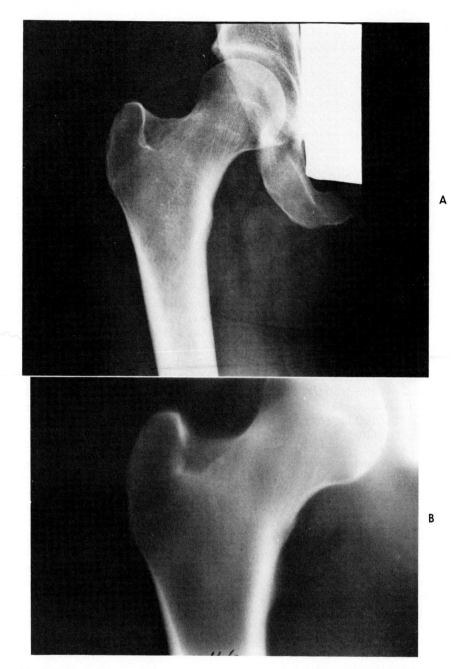

FIG. 46-21. A, Anteroposterior view and, **B,** tomogram showing compression-type stress fracture in right femoral neck of 22-year-old jogger.

nosing a **stress fracture of the proximal femur.** These authors have gone on to classify femoral neck stress fractures into Type 1 fractures that show periosteal callus without a visible fracture line, Type 2 fractures that represent a fracture in the calcar region or across the femoral neck without displacement, and Type 3 fractures that represent a displaced fracture. Similarly, Fullerton and Snowdy[30] have further classified femoral neck stress fractures as compression, tension, or displaced fractures. In most reports[35,91] the diagnosis was delayed, and the patient was treated as having a back sprain or a hip muscle strain. The predominant symptom is pain,

and the findings on physical examination may be minimal. There may be an antalgic gait, deep tenderness of the anterior aspect of the hip, and slight limitation of flexion and internal rotation with discomfort in the extremes of these movements. Attention should be given to risk factors, including excessive genu varum, tibial varum, subtalar varus, and forefoot varus. Additionally, femoral stress fractures are more commonly seen in the older athlete, whereas the younger athlete more commonly experiences tibial stress fractures. The presence of unexplained pelvic or thigh pain, even with negative findings on radiographs, should be watched closely. Radiographs of the femoral neck may not show changes for as long as 5 to 6 weeks. When a stress fracture is suspected, bone scintigraphy allows early detection and treatment.[33,34] This is particularly true of femoral neck stress fractures, which, if not treated, can lead to disastrous results with displacement and the possibility of inducing avascular necrosis.[50,64] An additional test that has been found to be helpful apart from the imaging studies above is the hop test in which the patient attempts to hop on the injured leg, inevitably reproducing the pain that these patients experience if an undisplaced stress fracture is present.

Treatment of stable femoral neck stress fractures depends on such factors as the athlete's clinical status—including pain, limp, and disability—and cooperation.[40,88] Treatment usually begins with rest and treatment of symptoms. Swimming and stationary cycling usually can begin in 2 to 3 weeks if there is no pain. If a pain-free period continues, the athlete can start light jogging on alternate days in 4 to 6 weeks. Because approximately 4 to 6 weeks are frequently needed for the stress fractures to fully heal, no vigorous physical activities should be allowed during this period. Possibly the most effective way of minimizing stress fractures is an effort to incorporate appropriate training methods among our athletes; it has been determined that major training errors were found in 22.4% of all stress fractures regardless of anatomic localization.

Once the athlete starts physical activity, it is important to watch for signs of refracturing. If pelvic or hip pain recurs, the patient should be reexamined.

In addition, the type of fracture is important in planning the treatment (Table 46-5). In the transverse type the fracture begins as a crack in the superior cortex of the femoral neck and progresses across the neck transverse to the force. Continued stress causes displacement, which progresses as the fracture line opens superiorly. Displacement of a femoral neck stress fracture may be accompanied by disastrous results, including varus deformity, nonunion, and avascular necrosis. Patients with this type of femoral neck stress fracture are best treated by percutaneous pinning because of the propensity for progressive displacement.

In contrast, compression stress fractures occur along the inferior cortex of the femoral neck and are associated with sclerosis of the cortex. Anteroposterior tomograms usually demonstrate the small fracture line. In the compression type of femoral neck stress fractures (Fig. 46-21), which is less likely to undergo displacement, conservative treatment with protective weight bearing on crutches has been effective. However, McBryde[65] has indicated that if a femoral neck fracture does not immediately become pain free on cessation of running, with or without crutches, percutaneous pinning is indicated. Bargren, Tilson, and Bridgeford[3] noted a high incidence of displacement in fatigue fractures of the femur in military trainees and developed an educational program to encourage early recognition and treatment of femoral neck stress fractures. The results of this program were very dramatic.

Femoral neck stress fractures can be devastating to the athlete as has been suggested by the study of Johansson et al.[50] These authors followed up 23 patients with stress fractures, 10 of which were Type 3, 4 of which were Type 2, and 9 of which were Type 1. Of the 23 injuries, 16 were treated with internal fixation, specifically 9 Type 3, 2 Type 2, and 5 Type 1 fractures, all of the latter representing tension injuries. Of the 23 patients, 7 developed complication of management of their underlying fractures including pseudarthrosis (one patient) avascular necrosis (three patients), and refracture (three patients). All three avascular necrosis, one pseudarthrosis, and one refracture occurred in the Type 3 injuries, suggesting a 50% complication rate in this patient population. The two remaining refractures occurred in Type 1 injuries. Both of these progressed to pseudarthrosis and were corrected by osteotomy. None of these athletes returned to elite sports. This study underscores the need

TABLE 46-5 Treatment of femoral neck stress fractures

Type	Characteristic Radiographic Appearance	Treatment	Comments
Transverse	Begins in superior cortex of neck and progresses across neck	Percutaneous pinning	Unstable, may displace
Compression	Small fracture along inferior cortex of neck; may be associated with sclerosis of fracture	Conservative non–weight-bearing ambulation	Stable

for early diagnosis and appropriate management in femoral neck stress fractures. If treated inappropriately or unrecognized, disastrous results can ensue with the ultimate need for surgical intervention to address the complications of avascular necrosis, pseudarthrosis, and refracture.

Osteitis Pubis

Osteitis pubis is a potential cause of unexplained pubic pain in athletes. Early reports indicated that this is most commonly a complication of operations on the bladder and prostate.[5] More recently there have been reports of this condition resulting from athletic activity.[42,44,106] This condition is most common in soccer players (see p. 1519), race walkers, and runners.

Radiographic features of osteitis pubis

- Symmetric bone resorption of the medial ends of the pubic bones
- Widened symphysis pubis
- Rarefaction in bones adjacent to symphysis
- Stress reaction may be present on iliac side of sacroiliac joint
- Instability of symphysis pubis is seen on films taken during weight bearing (flamingo views)

Although the cause of osteitis pubis in athletes is unclear, evidence favors repeated minor trauma from excessive or repetitive biomechanical stresses to the symphysis; with vigorous athletic activities, such as running, jumping, and kicking, shear forces are transmitted to the symphysis. Moreover, tension from the rectus abdominis or the adductors may be a factor. Hanson, Angevine, and Juhl[42] indicated that the adductor muscles originating from the inferior ischial rami may be responsible for transmitting shear forces to the pubic symphysis during kicking in soccer (Fig. 46-17).

Clinically, osteitis pubis is characterized by the gradual onset of localized pain in the region of the pubis, which may extend to the groin or lower portion of the abdomen. Such movements as pivoting on one leg, kicking a ball, sprinting, jumping, climbing stairs, or a sudden change in direction aggravate the pain.

Often the athlete thinks that he or she has strained a muscle, only to find that stretching aggravates the symptoms. The pain may become intense with pronounced localized tenderness over the pubis and the attachments at the rectus abdominis and adductor muscles and the inguinal ligament. An antalgic limp may be present, and when the condition is severe, there is adductor spasm, which results in a waddling gait. There is pain in full flexion of either leg, on passive abduction of hips, and on active resistant contractions of the abductors of the thigh. A clicking sensation may be present, indicating instability.

Harris and Murray[44] outlined the clinical and radiographic features of osteitis pubis in 37 athletes. It is characterized radiographically by symmetric bone resorption at the medial ends of the pubic bones. The symphysis is widened with rarefaction in the adjacent bone. There may not be radiographic evidence until 3 or 4 weeks after the onset of symptoms, but the signs tend to persist even after the symptoms have subsided.

Although the pathogenesis has been obscure, biopsy has shown only a nonspecific inflammation with mononuclear cell infiltrate, bone resorption, and fibrous connective tissue replacement of the symphysis of the fibrocartilage. Healing may occur gradually with sclerosis and new bone formation. Harris and Murray[44] noted that chronic stress was present in the iliac side of the sacroiliac joint of 20 of 37 athletes. Moreover, 13 had instability at the symphysis pubis on radiographs taken during weight bearing.

Osteitis pubis may be confused initially with adductor muscle strain or even a hernia. The physician must exclude other causes of apparent osteitis pubis, such as infection and ankylosing spondylitis.[47] Osteitis pubis seems to be a self-limiting disorder, usually lasting several months.

Treatment requires rest from physical exertion combined with antiinflammatory therapy. Warm, moist heat for 20 to 30 minutes and a warm (102° F [38.9° C]) whirlpool can give symptomatic pain relief. A good substitute exercise is swimming with the legs tied together using flotation devices (Fig. 46-22). Any adductor stretches or activities that stress the symphysis pubis, such as bicycling or breast-stroke swimming, should not be allowed because they aggravate the symptoms. NSAIDs and phenylbutazone have been effective.[44] Direct injection of steroids has been recommended,[105] but this should usually be avoided if possible, particularly when there is the possibility of infection. Others[21,77] have noted dramatic relief after the oral use of cortisone. Harris[45] indicated that most patients respond to conservative treatment. After about 2 months, early recalcification is usually noted on the radiograph, and light jogging can be started. Usually the athlete can return to sports in ap-

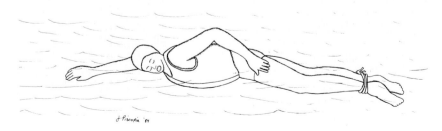

FIG. 46-22. Swimming with flotation device and legs tied together for therapy in osteitis pubis.

Radiographic examination of the hip and pelvis

by David L. Milbauer and Shashikant Patel

Avulsion fractures are common injuries in the athlete, and familiarity with the numerous musculotendinous attachments aids in the radiographic diagnosis of these injuries. For example, when an injury is related to sudden overuse of the rectus femoris muscle, an avulsion at its origin, the anterior inferior iliac spine, should be suspected (Figs. 1 and 2). Likewise, an iliopsoas injury may result in avulsion of its insertion in the lesser trochanter of the femur (Fig. 2).

In addition to acute avulsion fractures, continued strain at the origin of the gracilis and adductor musculature may result in ligamentous weakening of the symphysis pubis. This has been called "osteitis pubis."[18] Early radiographic manifestations include erosive lucencies at the origins of the adductor muscles.

In addition, frayed corners of the symphysis pubis, fluffy margins of the symphysis, periosteal reaction at the muscle attachments, osteoporosis at the symphysis, and a widened symphysis may be seen[18] (Figs. 3, *A*, and 4).

Instability at the symphysis can be demonstrated by comparison weight-bearing views. These "flamingo" views[11] are obtained with the patient standing on one leg for one view and the other leg for the comparison view. A difference in the height of the superior pubic ramus on each side of more than 2 mm may be considered abnormal (Fig. 5). In addition, if the width of the symphysis exceeds 10 mm, this may also be considered abnormal. CT may be used to demonstrate more graphically the changes seen at the symphysis pubis (Fig. 3, *B* and *C*).

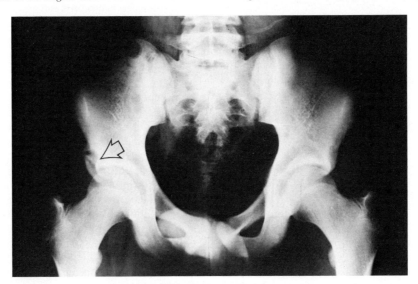

FIG. 1. Healed avulsion fracture of right anterior inferior iliac spine (*arrow*).

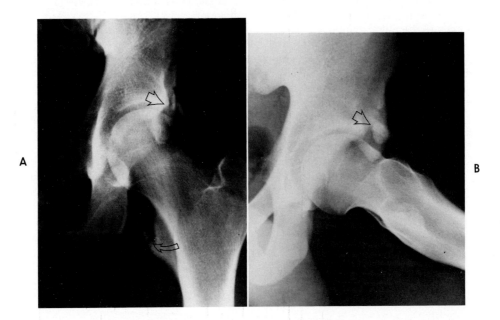

FIG. 2. A, Anteroposterior and, **B,** lateral radiographs demonstrating avulsions of anterior inferior iliac spine (*straight arrows*) and lesser trochanter of the femur (*curved arrow*).

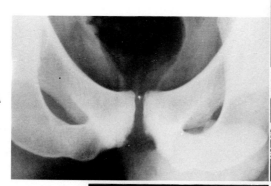

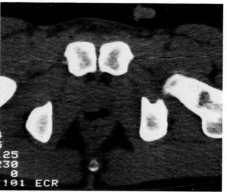

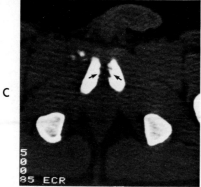

FIG. 3. Osteitis pubis. **A,** Coned-down radiograph demonstrates fluffy, irregular margins and frayed corners of symphysis pubis. Axial computed tomographic scans at **B,** superior and, **C,** inferior aspects of symphysis pubis. Note cortical irregularity and widening of the symphysis inferiorly (*arrows*).

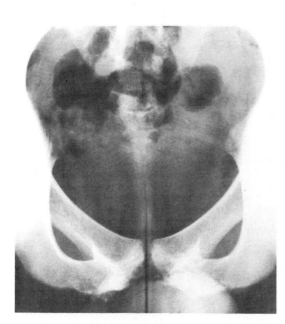

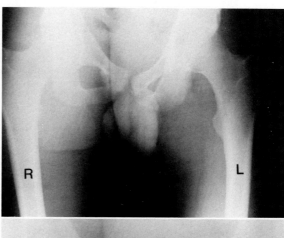

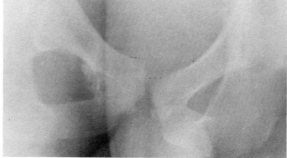

FIG. 4. Osteitis pubis, late changes. Note advanced erosion and associated sclerotic changes.

FIG. 5. Pubic symphysis diastasis. Single limb-standing anteroposterior views (flamingo views) are used to demonstrate instability at pubic symphysis.

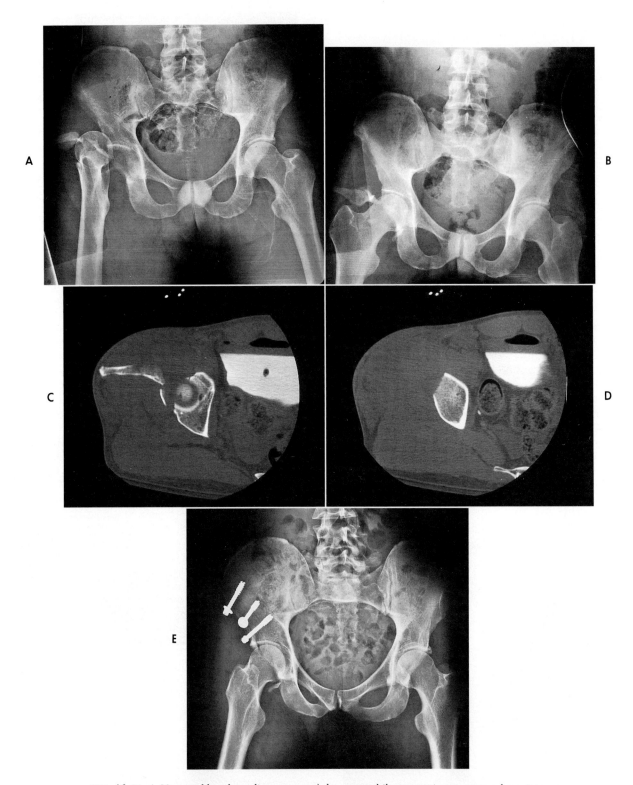

FIG. 46-23. A 22-year-old male cyclist was struck by a car while attempting to cross a busy inter-section. He was brought to the emergency room with his right leg abducted, shortened, and exter-nally rotated. He was neurologically intact. X-ray studies revealed anterior dislocation of proximal femur and large fragment of anterior hemipelvis that had been sheared off and was lying subcuta-neous with risk of skin penetration. Rapid closed reduction was accomplished. Subsequent 3-mm computed tomography cuts through pelvis revealed no intraarticular loose bodies. Open reduction of fragment was performed, reconstituting anterior column.

proximately 3 months. However, because the osteitis pubis can recur, the athlete should be given a gradual program of increased activity.[28] Only one patient in Pyle's series[77] required stabilization by arthrodesis.

Pelvic Ring Fractures

Fractures of the pelvis are usually caused by high-energy accidents and are not frequent athletic injuries. The most common type of injury is related to a vehicle accident involving passengers, pedestrians, or cyclists.[51] Cycling has become an increasingly favored sport in North America, having been a principal sport in Europe for many years. Because of the lack of sufficient cycling paths, cyclists ride on the shoulder of roads, which in large urban centers accommodate considerable traffic. As such, injuries sustained by cyclists can often be significant as a result of impact with larger cars and trucks (Fig. 46-23). Joggers may also be vulnerable to these accidents.

The mechanism of injury is usually a direct impact, but it may also be associated with rotational stresses. Fracture of the pelvis may also occur in collision sports such as football or hockey, but it is generally associated with more violent sports and recreational activities. Krissoff[54] indicated the increased popularity of hang gliding, particularly in southern California and Colorado, and discussed the severe injuries that occur in this sport, including comminuted pelvic fractures. Flynn[27] described the cases of two patients with complete disruption of the symphysis pubis as a result of horseback riding accidents (Fig. 46-24). In both cases the pubic arch was brought down violently on the anterior part of the saddle, which acts as a wedge, splitting the pubic arch and resulting

in a wide separation. Both patients were treated satisfactorily with a pelvic sling. Grossman et al[39] described the range of equestrian injuries. They indicated that most equestrian injuries result from a fall generally caused by equipment failure, particularly in polo.

Moreover, accidents during snowmobiling, the fastest growing winter sport in the northern United States, can result in forces capable of fracturing the pelvis. In the series reported by Fink and Monge,[25] most of these injuries occurred when the person was thrown from the snowmobile or when the machine overturned or struck a fixed object. These authors described a different mechanism of severe pelvic injuries associated with snowmobiling, which they refer to as the "wishbone injury," sustained when the driver's knee extends from the side of the snowmobile and the vehicle passes close to a fence post or tree. The leg then hooks around the tree while the opposite leg is fixed by the seat of the snowmobile, and the victim suffers a wide separation of the symphysis, which is often associated with severe injuries to the rectum, bladder, or pelvic organs. This type of injury also occurs when the driver uses the foot to aid in a turn and the foot catches in the snow or on a bush.

Fractures of the pelvis rarely occur in children because they have less brittleness and more pliability of the pelvis.[72] Moreover, few pelvic fractures in children are markedly displaced, and most appear to be stable because of the relatively thick periosteum. Although fractures of the pelvis may be classified in many ways, they are best considered as either stable or unstable pelvic ring fractures.

Stable fractures. Stable fractures are fractures of the individual bones in the pelvis without an associated break

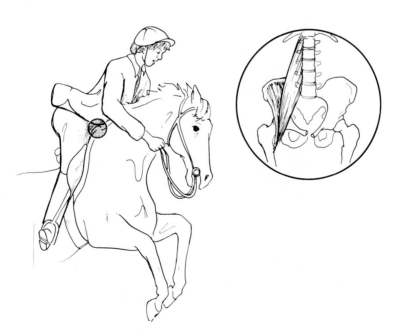

FIG. 46-24. Pelvis showing mechanism of straddle fracture of anterior pelvis. (From Berquist TH, Coventry MM: The pelvis and hips. In Berquist TH [ed]: *Orthopaedic radiology: imaging of orthopedic trauma and surgery*, Philadelphia, 1986, WB Saunders.)

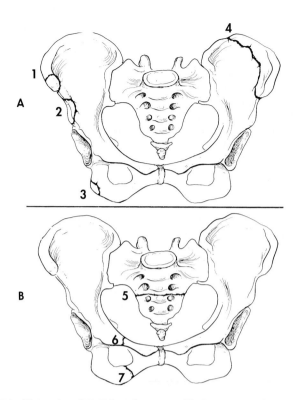

FIG. 46-25. A and **B,** Pelvis showing stable fracture of pelvis ring. Numbers 1 through 7 indicate fracture sites: *1,* anterior superior iliac spine (ASIS); *2,* anterior inferior iliac spine (AIIS); *3,* ischium; *4,* iliac wing; *5,* sacrum; *6,* superior pubic ramus; and *7,* inferior pubic ramus. (From Berquist TH, Coventry MM: The pelvis and hips. In Berquist TH [ed]: *Orthopaedic radiology: imaging of orthopedic trauma and surgery,* Philadelphia, 1986, WB Saunders.)

in the continuity of the pelvic ring. These represent approximately one third of all pelvic fractures (Fig. 46-25). Treatment is symptomatic.

A direct blow against the wing of the ilium may cause a fracture (**Duverney's fracture).**[24] The most frequent sport in which this occurs is horseback riding. Usually displacement is minimal because of the surrounding muscle attachments. These injuries are associated with pain, swelling, and tenderness over the iliac wing. Weight bearing is difficult because of the discomfort associated with the muscle contraction. This type of fracture may be overlooked on the anteroposterior radiograph, but it can easily be delineated on oblique views. Patients are treated symptomatically with bed rest initially, followed by protected weight bearing with crutches.

Pelvic trauma has also been recorded with various martial arts activities. Recently Birrer and Robinson[8] reported a case of a 27-year-old man who sustained an **anterior column fracture** of his left acetabulum after having sustained a karate kick to this area during practice. This was treated conservatively without sequelae, but it served to support the tremendous impact administered by such kicks from individuals trained in these forms of self-defense. More serious injuries such as ab-

dominal visceral rupture, cerebral contusion, and even death have been reported under these same circumstances.

Blunt trauma to the unprotected sacrum may result in isolated **transverse fractures,** but these are extremely rare in sports.[31,71] The history of a severe blow associated with pain, swelling, and tenderness over the back of the sacrum should alert the physician to the possibility of a sacral fracture. These injuries may be difficult to detect radiographically and may be missed. Fractures of the coccyx are not uncommon in sports; they result from a fall in the sitting position, such as occasionally occurs in cross-country skiing.[58] These are painful injuries. Tenderness is localized over the coccyx, and palpation externally and rectally can help in making the diagnosis. Treatment is symptomatic. Warm sitz baths may relieve the associated muscle spasms. These fractures generally heal uneventfully. When the acute symptoms subside in 2 to 3 weeks, the athlete may resume competition. Local protection with padding is advisable to prevent reinjury.

Another rare injury occasionally associated with athletic trauma is a **fracture of the ischial body.**[95] This fracture is most common in a fall from a height. Treatment is symptomatic. **Fractures of the superior or inferior pubic ramus** are uncommon in athletics.[71] These occur most frequently in the elderly age groups and are associated with a fall. In a fracture of a single ramus it is essential to search carefully for an associated injury (particularly of the sacroiliac joint) that completes the fracture of the pelvic ring. In the resilient pelvis of the child a single ramus fracture is frequent, whereas in the adult the fracture is usually a complete one through the opposite portion of the pelvic ring.[72] Generally, in stable fractures of the pelvic ring, function is minimally impaired and treatment is symptomatic with initial bed rest followed by protective weight bearing with crutches. Unilateral fractures of both pubic rami are the most common type of pelvic fractures. The mechanism is usually direct trauma and occasionally indirect forces transmitted through the femur. Symptomatic treatment and protective weight bearing until recovery is the usual treatment.

Unstable fractures. There are several patterns of unstable pelvic ring fractures.[51] Fractures that involve the pelvic ring with associated displacement are generally caused by severe forces. Although such fractures are uncommon in athletic competition, they may be seen in a number of recreational activities that cause violent forces, such as the crash of a racing car, snowmobiling,[25] or a fall from a height while hang gliding.[54] These include the **straddle fracture** (bilateral fractures of the superior and inferior pubic rami) (Fig. 46-26, *A*) or its variant with an associated symphysis separation. Dislocations and fracture-dislocations of the pelvis are referred to as **"Malgaigne fractures"**—fractures in which the anteroposterior half of the pelvic ring is disrupted (Fig. 46-26, *B*).

The anterior portion of the pelvis may be disrupted with a dislocation of the symphysis or with fracture of both superior and inferior pubic rami, and the posterior

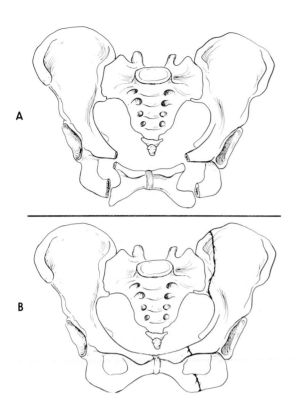

FIG. 46-26. A, Pelvis showing straddle fracture of superior and inferior pubic rami bilaterally. **B,** Pelvis showing fractures of both anterior and posterior portions of ring (Malgaigne fracture).

ring may be disrupted with a sacroiliac separation or with a fracture on either side of the joint. An epiphyseal iliac fracture may occur in children.[72] In injuries to the anterior tie arch, such as a straddle fracture, a high incidence of visceral injuries is recorded.

Because these fractures do not involve the main weight bearing arch, treatment is chiefly symptomatic and is achieved by recumbency followed by protective weight bearing. In management of unstable fractures of the pelvic ring, an attempt at accurate reduction and maintenance is important because of potential problems with persistent sacroiliac pain. If upward displacement of the hemipelvis is present, reduction is best achieved by skeletal traction applied to the involved limb with maintenance in a pelvic sling. After stability is achieved, protective weight bearing with crutches is continued. Recent experience gained with external and internal fixation devices is promising. In management of patients with an acute pelvic fracture, the physician must be alert to the possibility of associated injuries to the pelvic and abdominal viscerae. In severe pelvic fractures, the incidence of associated injuries varies from 10% to 30%.

Dislocation of the Hip

Fortunately, dislocation of the hip in an athlete is uncommon (Fig. 46-27). These injuries tend to occur in the more violent contact sports such as professional football,[19] rugby,[73] downhill skiing,[86] and cycling (Fig. 46-23). Hip dislocation represents a major injury and is a

medical emergency. The athlete is completely disabled, complains of severe pain in the hip, and resists any attempt to move the limb. In addition to having severe pain, the athlete is unable to stand or walk. Motion of the hip is painful, and there is considerable muscle spasm. In **anterior dislocations** (Fig. 46-28) the hip is held in abduction, external rotation, and slight flexion. The femoral head may be palpable anteriorly, and the greater trochanter is less prominent. **Posterior dislocations** are associated with a characteristic appearance of the athlete's holding the limb in flexion, adduction, and internal rotation. The characteristic deformity of flexion and internal rotation is caused by the marked tension in the Y ligament of Bigelow. In the posterior ischial dislocation, abduction of the limb may be present.

Clinical findings in hip dislocation

Anterior { Abduction / External rotation / Flexion }

Posterior { Adduction / Internal rotation / Flexion }

The injury usually occurs from a force transmitted along the femur with the leg in abduction, such as an impact of the knee against the dashboard in an automobile crash or a fall on the flexed knee.[95] In child athletes the pliable acetabulum allows the head to dislocate, usually without an associated acetabular fracture. However, an associated posterior acetabular ring fracture is more common in the adolescent athlete and may be difficult to demonstrate.

Left and right oblique radiographs of the pelvis, as recommended by Judet, Judet, and Letournel[51] are useful in demonstrating the posterior portion of the acetabulum. Moreover, if there is suspicion of an intraarticular injury, arthrography is helpful. CT demonstrates both acetabular and femoral head injuries and is indicated in these injuries. Central dislocation, in which there is a comminuted fracture of the central portion of the acetabulum, is fortunately a rare injury in the child and adolescent athlete. These central dislocations with comminution of the acetabulum are caused by a direct blow to the greater trochanter, such as in a fall from a height.

Dislocations of the hip are associated with considerable damage to the hip capsule and surrounding soft tissues. Anterior dislocations may be associated with an injury of the femoral nerve, whereas in posterior dislocations the sciatic nerve may be damaged. The precarious blood supply to the femoral head may also be interrupted. In a Mayo Clinic series[82] involving 24 children with traumatic hip fractures, five suffered injury to the sciatic nerve. Avascular necrosis occurs in 10% to 20% of patients.

Because the mechanism of injury involves blunt trauma to the flexed knee, careful evaluation for a con-

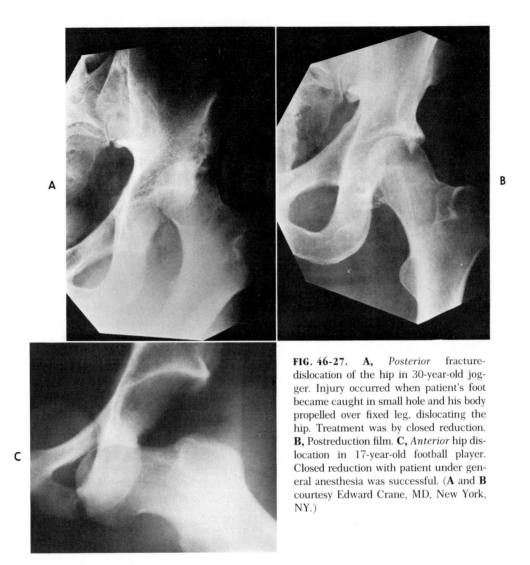

FIG. 46-27. A, *Posterior* fracture-dislocation of the hip in 30-year-old jogger. Injury occurred when patient's foot became caught in small hole and his body propelled over fixed leg, dislocating the hip. Treatment was by closed reduction. **B,** Postreduction film. **C,** *Anterior* hip dislocation in 17-year-old football player. Closed reduction with patient under general anesthesia was successful. (**A** and **B** courtesy Edward Crane, MD, New York, NY.)

comitant knee injury must be done. Early, gentle closed reduction of the traumatic dislocation of the hip is essential but should *not* be done on the athletic field.[71] A careful neurologic examination and radiographic examination is necessary *before* reduction. Adequate muscle relaxation is necessary, and this usually requires a general anesthetic, particularly in the adolescent athlete. In posterior dislocation the tight iliofemoral ligament is an obstacle to reduction. All three common methods of closed reduction[51,92,95] the Bigelow, Allis, and Stimpson techniques (see p. 1295), use the principle of hip flexion to relax the Y ligament and to bring the femoral head adjacent to the acetabulum.

In anterior dislocation, closed reduction is usually successful. Occasionally, however, a pull of the iliopsoas muscle or even a buttonhole effect of the anterior capsule may be an obstacle to reduction; this type of dislocation then requires open reduction.[51]

In posterior dislocation with a major posterior acetabular fragment, instability may be demonstrated by applying adduction and posterior pressure with the hip in moderate flexion. Posterior dislocation with instability requires open reduction and internal fixation of the posterior acetabular fracture. In a central fracture-dislocation, prognosis depends on the condition of the dome and the relationship between the femoral head and the superior acetabular dome. Satisfactory results have been achieved by conservative treatment—that is, skeletal traction for the central displacement fractures associated with an intact superior acetabular dome—and surprisingly good results have been achieved by this technique in comminuted fractures with central displacement. When the acetabular dome fragments are separated, Weber, Brunner, and Freuler[103] recommend open reduction and internal fixation with accurate repositioning of the acetabular fragments.

In the Mayo Clinic series[82] of 24 children with traumatic hip dislocations, nine had associated acetabular fractures; these were associated with other fractures about the hip. Avascular necrosis developed in five (21%) of these children. A delay in reduction beyond 24 hours increased the incidence of avascular necrosis. Avascular necrosis usually occurs within 15 months after the dislocation. The period of non–weight bearing after reduc-

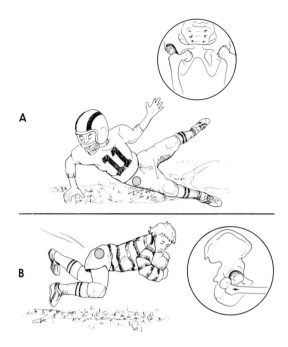

FIG. 46-28. Mechanism of **A,** anterior and, **B,** posterior dislocations of hip in athletes.

tion seems to have no effect on the outcome. After soft-tissue healing is complete in 6 weeks, the patient can resume full weight bearing and a graduated increase in athletic activities.

The result of a hip dislocation is dependent on associated injuries to the acetabulum, the amount of time between dislocation and relocation, associated nerve injuries, and associated fractures of the femoral head. If reduced promptly (within 6 to 8 hours), pure dislocations generally do well, although this is not necessarily guaranteed as is evidenced by the professional football player that experienced a traumatic subluxation of the hip resulting in aseptic necrosis and chondrolysis in the report by Cooper, Warren, and Barnes.[19]

Fractures of the Neck of the Femur

Fractures about the hip are rare in adolescent and young adult athletes.[71] They do, however, occur in the middle-aged athlete and are relatively common in elderly patients with osteoporosis and sustaining a minor torsional injury precipitating a base-of-neck fracture. Significant torsional injuries are necessary for the middle-aged athlete to sustain such an injury as reported by Frost and Bauer.[29] The authors reported 10 cases of femoral neck or intertrochanteric fractures sustained while cross-country skiing by patients whose average age was 45 years. The relative frequency with which this injury was seen in Sweden prompted the authors to call this **skier's hip.** In the young person, considerable force is required to break the strong bone of the femoral neck. The fracture may result from a direct force along the shaft of the femur, a rotational force, or occasionally a direct blow over the trochanter. Usually sufficient force

may be generated in a fall from a height or a fall from a bicycle, horse, or snowmobile.

After the injury the athlete is disabled and complains of excruciating pain in the hip. Generally the athlete cannot stand or walk, but if the fracture is of the greenstick or impacted type, the athlete may be able to bear weight with an antalgic gait. The athlete holds the limb rigid, resisting any attempt to motion. The muscle force acting across the hip creates the typical deformity with the limb held in external rotation and slight adduction. Shortening of the limb is evident. The type of fracture is delineated by anteroposterior and lateral radiographs. Ratliff's large series of children and adolescents with femoral neck fractures[79] indicated that the highest incidence occurred in the 11- to 13-year-old age group. Of the fractures, 38 were transcervical, 26 were of the basilar area of the neck, 4 were intertrochanteric, and 2 were transepiphyseal. More than half of the fractures were displaced.

Current concepts on the treatment of femoral neck fractures in the adult were reviewed by Clawson and Melcher.[17] They indicated that a gentle and accurate closed reduction followed by a rigid internal fixation using various methods is essential. We prefer multiple pins or a sliding nail plate apparatus. Femoral neck fractures in children and adolescents continue to pose a tremendous challenge. Treatment of these difficult injuries has been controversial. Although successful nonoperative treatment of undisplaced femoral neck fractures has been reported, we prefer internal fixation over closed methods, particularly because of the risk of displacement with loss of position. In displaced fractures a gentle closed reduction is done followed by internal fixation with two or three threaded pins placed just short of the epiphyseal plate; in transepiphyseal fractures, smooth pins are preferred. In intertrochanteric fractures of the hip in this age group, good results usually can be achieved by traction followed by immobilization and a spica cast on the hip.[94]

Of children with femoral neck fractures, 60% suffer a complication.[71] In femoral neck fractures, avascular necrosis is a major complication and is related to the degree of displacement and the level of the fracture. Approximately one third of children and adolescents with femoral neck fractures develop avascular necrosis. Ratliff[79] demonstrated that the pattern of avascular necrosis after femoral neck fractures in children depends on the specific pattern of the interruption of the blood supply.

Slipped Capital Femoral Epiphysis

Slipping of the capital femoral epiphysis should be suspected when the adolescent athlete complains of pain in the hip and thigh. Moreover, the pain may be referred primarily to the knee, and an athletically active youth who complains of knee pain must have the hip examined to exclude this condition.[93] In a Mayo Clinic series of 58 patients reported by Bianco,[6] this condition was more than twice as frequent in boys than girls and occurred in patients between 10 and 15 years of age.

Although the cause remains unclear, the injury has

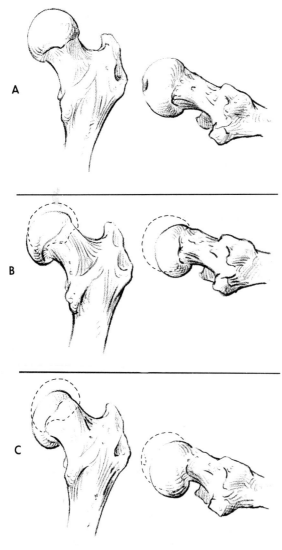

FIG. 46-29. Slipped capital femoral epiphysis. **A,** Mild. (This degree of slipping is evident only on lateral view.) **B,** Moderate slipping. **C,** Severe slipping.

been related to hormonal imbalance and a relative increase in the ratio of growth hormones to sex hormones.[45] This hormonal imbalance is reflected by the occurrence of this condition in children of two somatic types—those who are tall and thin, and those who are large and obese. The disruption in the epiphyseal plate occurs in the layer of proliferating cartilage cells adjacent to the zone of calcified cartilage. The characteristic deformity occurs as the capital epiphysis becomes displaced posteriorly and downward while there is an associated upward, anterior movement of the femoral neck on the capital epiphysis.

Slipping of the capital femoral epiphysis is classified as either acute or chronic.[93] The classification of the severity of the slip is shown in Fig. 46-29. In the preslip phase there is only subtle widening and rarefaction of the epiphyseal plate without actual displacement. In the minimal slip (Fig. 46-30) the slip may range from slight slippage that is evident on a lateral radiograph to slippage of one third of the diameter of the epiphysis. In moderate slipping there is displacement of one third to two thirds of the diameter of the epiphysis. As the slippage proceeds inferiorly and posteriorly, there is a varus deformity of the neck and adduction and external rotation of the neck in relation to the epiphysis. In severe slippage the displacement involves more than two thirds of the diameter of the epiphysis.

The usual history is groin pain that is referred to the anteromedial aspect of the thigh; the patient has an antalgic gait and an external rotation deformity of the limb. When the slipping is acute, there is usually a history of

---

Slipped capital femoral epiphysis clinical features

- Groin pain (or knee pain)
- Antalgic gait
- External rotation of hip

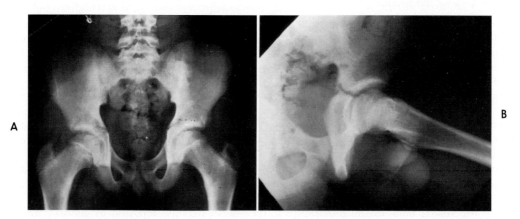

FIG. 46-30. **A,** Anteroposterior and, **B,** lateral views showing early change in epiphyseal line associated with mild slipping of right femoral epiphysis. Left hip is normal. (From Bianco AJ Jr: *J Bone Joint Surg* 47A:387, 1965.)

injury (e.g., a fall on the athletic field or a check into the boards on the ice rink).

This injury is associated with sudden pain, muscle spasm, and deformity. The acute slip is usually superimposed on a preexisting gradual slipping. These young athletes usually indicate a preexisting history of mild, aching pain and a limp for a variable period before the traumatic incident that precipitated the sudden severe slip. It is important to have a high index of suspicion when an adolescent athlete has this history because the severe slip may be precipitated by a minor injury if the preslip stage is already present. In a Mayo Clinic series,[6] all 22 patients with minimal slipping had pain and limp of gradual onset; four of the patients described an additional recent acute athletic injury.

From a diagnostic standpoint the earliest findings are related to the relative anterior displacement of the femoral neck, which causes limitation of full internal rotation of the affected hip. As the slipping progresses, a painful, lurching gait develops that is associated with an adduction deformity in external rotation. There is no internal rotation of the hip; the hip abducts as the thigh flexes. In the young athlete who complains of knee pain, external rotation of the thigh during hip flexion may indicate a slip of the capital femoral epiphysis.[55]

In the management of the patient whose epiphysis is in the preslip or minimum slip phase, Bianco[6] had uniformly good results with in situ fixation using multiple pins (Fig. 46-31). For acute, abrupt displacement of the capital femoral epiphysis, Tachdjian[94] recommended an initial attempt at closed reduction using bilateral split-Russell traction with medial rotation straps applied to the limb, and, if this is unsuccessful, gentle closed manipulative reduction with the patient under general anesthetic. If these attempts at closed reduction are unsuccessful, careful open reduction is done. Active range of motion exercises are allowed in bed as soon as the wound has healed. The patient is gradually started on non–

weight-bearing three-point crutch walking. At approximately 6 weeks, weight bearing is initiated with a gradual return to physical activities.

In patients with chronic slip of moderate or marked severity, Bianco[6] achieved good results with a cuneiform osteotomy through the femoral neck to correct the deformity. Because of the possibility of interruption of the blood supply to the femoral head, Southwick[89] recommended a biplane subtrochanteric osteotomy. Although this does not correct the abnormal relationship of the femoral head to the neck, the osteotomy seems to be effective in restoring good function. Bianco[6] preferred this approach in the older adolescent with a chronic slip in which the epiphyseal line was near closure or had closed.

Acetabular Labrum Tears

In an otherwise normal hip the acetabular labrum may be torn by a twisting motion. The physician must have a high degree of awareness when an athlete is initially seen with mechanical hip pain. Fitzgerald and Coventry[26] reported on nine patients ranging in age from 18 to 65 years who were initially seen with a sharp, catching pain localized to the groin and anterior aspect of the thigh. Besides the catching pain, these patients reported that the involved leg would give way and that this was often followed by a persistent soreness about the hip. The catching occurred with pivoting of the involved hip, especially on rising from a sitting position. On examination, an audible and palpable click may be reproduced by passively maneuvering the slightly extended hip into adduction and internal rotation. The radiographs usually are normal, but arthrography may demonstrate a filling defect in the labrum.

Relief of symptoms by the injection of bupivacaine at the time of arthrography is diagnostic and helps differentiate this group of patients from those with extraarticular disorders such as snapping of the iliopsoas tendon over the iliopectineal eminence of the superior pubic ra-

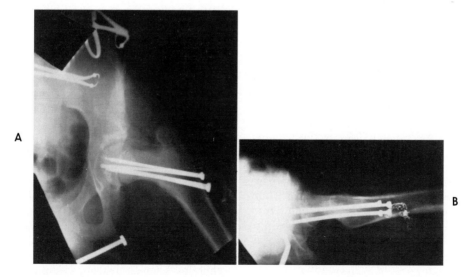

FIG. 46-31. A, Anteroposterior and, **B,** lateral views made during internal fixation with Knowles pins in patient with mild slipping. (From Bianco AJ Jr: *J Bone Joint Surg* 47A:387, 1965.)

mus. Extraarticular snapping may also be secondary to the gluteus maximus or iliotibial band. Diagnosis of a tear of the acetabular labrum requires a high index of suspicion. In Fitzgerald and Coventry's series,[26] arthrotomy with excision of the torn labrum gave excellent relief in seven of eight patients. Arthroscopy may be useful in the evaluation and treatment of this disorder. Tears can often be found on the posterosuperior portion of the labrum.

Unknown Causes

Transient Synovitis

Hip pain in the young athlete may result from acute transient synovitis of the hip, which is a nonspecific inflammatory condition. This condition often causes a painful hip in children less than 10 years of age.[94] Transient synovitis is a self-limiting condition with disappearance of the symptoms usually within several weeks. The child may report an acute or gradual onset of pain in the inguinal region, thigh, and knee and may develop an antalgic gait. Motion is usually painful and limited, and there is associated local tenderness. Although the cause remains obscure, trauma has been reported to be one factor.[94] Radiographs reveal only soft-tissue swelling with an associated effusion. Any young child who complains of pain in the hip, whether it is associated with athletic activities or not, should undergo complete evaluation to exclude rheumatoid disease, infection, or ensuing Perthes' disease (osteochondrosis of the capital femoral epiphysis). Transient synovitis precedes Perthes' disease in 1.5% to 10% of cases.[55,90] Generally, however, transient synovitis has a benign course with relief of pain and improvement in motion after a non–weight-bearing regimen with crutches is begun.

Legg-Calvé-Perthes Disease

Although Legg-Calvé-Perthes disease usually occurs predominantly in boys within a narrow age range of between 4 and 8 years, this condition also must be considered as a cause of hip pain in the young athlete between the ages of 5 and 12 years.[93] The cause of the avascularity of the femoral head remains obscure. The presenting complaints are usually pain and a limp of several months' duration. The pain is usually localized to the groin and is often referred to the anteromedial aspect of the thigh and to the knee. The discomfort is aggravated by increased activity and is improved by rest. The young athlete may report a history of an injury with an acute onset of symptoms. Approximately 25% of the patients have a history of trauma. In addition to having an antalgic limp the patient has limitation of motion, particularly abduction and internal rotation. In the acute phase there may be local tenderness and muscle spasm, and when the condition is chronic, a flexion-adduction contracture ensues. The natural history of Legg-Calvé-Perthes disease with progressive changes in the various stages was reviewed by Tachdjian.[94] In the young athlete the physician must have a high index of suspicion to recognize the incipient or synovitis stage; this stage is characterized only by swelling of the capsule and soft-tissue thick-

ening associated with widening of the articular cartilage space.

Although there are a number of treatment methods reported for Legg-Calvé-Perthes disease, conservative treatment is generally recommended. Conservative treatment uses an orthosis to maintain the femoral head in the acetabulum with the hip in abduction and internal rotation, in addition to decreasing the weight-bearing stresses from the avascular femoral head. When trilateral hip abduction orthoses designed by Tachdjian[94] and Judet, Judet, and Letournel[51] were used, these authors could recommend that the child be encouraged to pursue all normal activities as long as no weight was borne on the foot and limb. The young athlete can be taught sports activities that involve the upper extremity, such as archery or table tennis. Swimming is allowed without the orthosis if the patient does no diving or poolside weight-bearing activities. Isometric strengthening exercises using the gluteus medius, gluteus maximus, and quadriceps muscles should be done to minimize muscle deconditioning.

Once reossification of the femoral head occurs, the braces are gradually taken off and activities are slowly increased. There should be no contact sports or prolonged running or jumping until the subchondral bone of the epiphysis is formed.

SENIOR ATHLETES

People who were once athletically active and who now have disabling arthritis of the hip—often secondary to an old sports injury—present unusual problems in management. Macrotrauma and gross irregularities of the joint surface can lead to degenerative osteoarthritis. In 1976 Radin[78] discussed the theory of microtrauma leading to osteoarthritis of the hip. He suggested that the repetitive impact loading on the cartilage is a primary source of osteoarthritis and that the destruction of the cartilage is not secondary to shear stress but results from the repetitive loading of the joint. This concept of repetitive microtrauma was given support by Klünder, Rud, and Hansen,[53] who described increased osteoarthritis of the hip in soccer players. Bombelli[10] also described this concept of physiologic imbalance of the stresses across the hip and emphasized the need to decrease the forces across the hip and to increase the surface area of weight bearing.

The issue of developing premature degenerative arthritis in the hip among runners has always been somewhat contentious. To adopt the theory of microtrauma, as mentioned by numerous authors previously, the physician must anticipate such changes occurring in the hip joint and possibly even the knee joints. In a retrospective study of elite athletes, specifically long-distance runners and bobsled riders, compared with normal, healthy, untrained men, the incidence of radiologic evidence of degenerative hip disease was infinitely greater in the elite athletes.[63] These radiographic features included subchondral sclerosis, osteophyte formation, and joint space narrowing. It was interesting to note that pace was more predictive of radiographic signs of degenerative hip disease than mileage among the runners and not among the bobsled riders. However, runners that exceeded 90 km/week were more prone to develop such changes than those with less vigorous training. The authors concluded that long-term, high-intensity, high-mileage running could be a risk factor for premature degenerative arthritis among these athletes.

A selective approach to the evaluation and treatment of these patients with degenerative joint disease is essential to obtain a satisfactory result. Fortunately, only a few patients have incapacitating pain or dysfunction severe enough to consider them classic candidates for total hip replacement. A high percentage of these patients can be satisfactorily treated nonoperatively. Those with minimal pain or functional deficit may benefit from the regular use of salicylates or nonsteroidal antiinflammatory agents and a physical therapy program to maintain strength and motion. Those who have more pain or dysfunction may be satisfied with restricting their activities to nonstrenuous sports, such as golf or swimming. Generally, total hip arthroplasty has been reserved for the older, less active patient because of the predictable short prosthetic survival in the young patient who is expecting to place excessive demands on the prosthesis by strenuous working or weekend recreational activities. Age appears to relate directly to activity status and prosthetic demands.

Treatment of the athlete with degenerative joint disease of the hip

- Nonsteroidal antiinflammatory drugs
- Gentle physical therapy
- Non–impact-loading sports

Knowledge of the magnitude of the forces transmitted by the hip joint is important in setting activity guidelines and determining rehabilitation after arthroplasty. The activity guidelines after arthroplasty are not well defined. Many of these previously athletic persons have unrealistic goals, and excessive restrictions on activity often cause considerable emotional turmoil. However, the magnitude of the joint forces necessary for various activities dictates a conservative approach when recommending activity guidelines to improve the longevity of the prosthesis. Most of these patients can resume normal daily activities. Coventry (personal communication, March 1984) believes that the patient with a hip arthroplasty should avoid activities that involve repetitive impact (such as jogging) and excessive torsional strain. However, he believes that these patients can resume almost all other recreational activities in moderation, including golf, swimming, baseline tennis, and cross-country skiing. This has been further corroborated recently by Ritter and Meding,[81] who suggested that intelligent participation in such sports as walking, golf, bowling, swimming, and biking where there is no anticipated load exceeding 20 pounds on the hip replacement

---

Sports that minimize stress on total hip arthroplasty

- Walking
- Golf
- Bowling
- Swimming
- Bicycling
- Baseline tennis
- Cross-country skiing

---

is to be encouraged. In general, patients who enter the total hip arthroplasty with better overall preoperative range of motion and activity level were more likely to return to those activities postoperatively and have more favorable 6-month functional assessments than patients who either had decreased motion before surgery or who did not have or appreciate physical activity before surgery.

REFERENCES

1. Antao N: Myositis of the hip in a professional soccer player, *Am J Sports Med* 16(1):82, 1988.
2. Atwell CA, Jackson DW: Stress fractures of the sacrum in runners, *Am J Sports Med* 19(5):531, 1991.
3. Bargren JH, Tilson DH Jr, Bridgeford OE: Prevention of displaced fatigue fractures of the femur, *J Bone Joint Surg* 53A:1115, 1971.
4. Barnes ST, Hinds RB: Pseudotumor of the ischium: a late manifestation of avulsion of the ischial epiphysis, *J Bone Joint Surg* 54A:645, 1972.
5. Beer E: Periostitis and ostitis of the symphysis and rami of the pubis following suprapubic cystotomies, *J Urol* 20:233, 1928.
6. Bianco AJ Jr: Treatment of slipping of the capital femoral epiphysis, *Clin Orthop* 48:103, 1966.
7. Binck R, Levinsohn EM: Enlarged iliopsoas bursa: an unusual pain, *Clin Orthop* 224:158, 1987.
8. Birrer RB, Robinson T: Pelvic fracture following karate kick, *N Y State J Med* 11:503, 1991.
9. Blickenstaff LD, Morris JM: Fatigue fracture of the femoral neck, *J Bone Joint Surg* 48A:1031, 1966.
10. Bombelli R: *Osteoarthritis of the hip: classification and pathogenesis: the role of osteotomy as a consequent therapy,* ed 2, New York, 1983, Springer-Verlag.
11. Bowerman JW: *Radiology and injury in sport,* New York, 1977, Appleton-Century-Crofts.
12. Brignall CG, Stainsby GD: The snapping hip: treatment by Z-plasty, *J Bone Joint Surg* 73B:253, 1991.
13. Brückl R et al: Zur operativen behandlung der schnappenden hüfte, *Z Orthop* 122:308, 1984.
14. Butler JE, Eggert AW: Fracture of the iliac crest apophysis: an unusual hip pointer, *J Sports Med* 3:192, 1975.
15. Caffey JP: *Pediatric x-ray diagnosis: a textbook for students and practitioners of pediatrics, surgery, and radiology,* Chicago, 1957, Year Book Medical Publishers.
16. Clancy WG Jr, Foltz AS: Iliac apophysitis and stress fractures in adolescent runners, *Am J Sports Med* 4:214, 1976.
17. Clawson DK, Melcher PJ: Fractures and dislocations of the hip. In Rockwood CA Jr, Green DP (eds): *Fractures,* vol 2, Philadelphia, 1975, JB Lippincott.
18. Cochrane JM: Osteitis pubis in athletes, *Br J Sports Med* 5:233, 1971.
19. Cooper DE, Warren RF, Barnes R: Traumatic subluxation of the hip resulting in aseptic necrosis and chondrolysis in a professional football player, *Am J Sports Med* 19(3):322, 1991.
20. Dahlin DC: *Bone tumors: general aspects and data on 6,221 cases,* ed 3, Springfield, Ill, 1978, Charles C Thomas.
21. Daw WJ, Funke AH: Osteitis pubis treated by cortisone, *J Urol* 69:686, 1953.

22. Devas MB: Compression stress fractures in man and the grey-hound, *J Bone Joint Surg* 43B:540, 1961.

23. Dimon JH III: Isolated fractures of the lesser trochanter of the femur, *Clin Orthop* 82:144, 1972.

24. Duverney J-G: *Traité des maladies des os,* vol 1, Paris, 1751, De Bure l'Aîné.

25. Fink RA, Monge JJ: Snowmobiling injuries, *Minn Med* 54:29, 1971.

26. Fitzgerald RH, Coventry MB: Unpublished data, 1984.

27. Flynn M: Disruption of symphysis pubis while horse riding: a report of two cases, *Injury* 4:357, 1973.

28. Fricker PA, Taunton JE, Ammann W: Osteitis pubis in athletes: infection, inflammation, or injury, *Sports Med* 12(4):266, 1991.

29. Frost A, Bauer M: Skier's hip: a new clinical entity? Proximal femur fractures sustained in cross-country skiing, *J Orthop Trauma* 5(1):47, 1991.

30. Fullerton LR, Snowdy HA: Femoral neck stress fractures, *Am J Sports Med* 365, 1988.

31. Furey WW: Fractures of the pelvis with special reference to associated fractures of the sacrum, *AJR* 47:89, 1942.

32. Gardner E: The innervation of the hip joint, *Anat Rec* 101:353, 1948.

33. Garrick JG et al: Early diagnosis of stress fractures and their precursors (abstract), *J Bone Joint Surg* 58A:733, 1976.

34. Geslien GE et al: Early detection of stress fractures using ^{99m}Tc-polyphosphate, *Radiology* 121:683, 1976.

35. Gilbert RS, Johnson HA: Stress fractures in military recruits: a review of twelve years' experience, *Mil Med* 131:716, 1966.

36. Giuliani G et al: CT scan and surgical treatment of traumatic iliacus hematoma with femoral neuropathy: case report, *J Trauma* 30(2):229, 1990.

37. Godshall RW, Hansen CA: Incomplete avulsion of a portion of the iliac epiphysis: an injury of young athletes, *J Bone Joint Surg* 55A:1301, 1973.

38. Green JP: Proximal avulsion of the iliacus with paralysis of the femoral nerve: report of a case, *J Bone Joint Surg* 54B:154, 1972.

39. Grossman JAI et al: Equestrian injuries: results of a prospective study, *JAMA* 240:1881, 1978.

40. Hajek MR, Noble HB: Stress fractures of the femoral neck in joggers: case reports and review of the literature, *Am J Sports Med* 10:112, 1982.

41. Hamada G, Rida A: Ischial apophysiolysis (IAL): report of a case and review of the literature, *Clin Orthop* 31:117, 1963.

42. Hanson PG, Angevine M, Juhl JH: Osteitis pubis in sports activities, *Phys Sports Med* 6:111, 1978.

43. Harper MC, Schaberg JE, Allen WC: Primary iliopsoas bursography in the diagnosis of disorders of the hip, *Clin Orthop* 221:238, 1987.

44. Harris NH, Murray RO: Lesions of the symphysis in athletes, *BMJ* 4:211, 1974.

45. Harris WR: The endocrine basis for slipping of the upper femoral epiphysis: an experimental study, *J Bone Joint Surg* 32B:5, 1950.

46. Hedström SA, Lidgren L: Acute hematogenous pelvic osteomyelitis in athletes, *Am J Sports Med* 10:44, 1982.

47. Hollander JL, McCarty DJ Jr: *Arthritis and allied conditions: a textbook of rheumatology,* ed 8, Philadelphia, 1972, Lea & Febiger.

48. Hollinshead WH: *Anatomy for surgeons,* vol 3, *The back and limbs,* Philadelphia, 1958, Harper & Row.

49. Jacobson T, Allen W: Surgical connection of the snapping iliopsoas tendon, *Am J Sports Med* 18(5):470, 1990.

50. Johansson C et al: Stress fractures of the femoral neck in athletes: the consequence of a delay in diagnosis, *Am J Sports Med* 18(5):524, 1990.

51. Judet R, Judet J, Letournel E: Fractures of the acetabulum: classification and surgical approaches for open reduction, *J Bone Joint Surg* 46A:1615, 1964.

52. Kendall HO, Kendall FP, Wadsworth GE: *Muscles, testing, and function,* ed 2, Baltimore, 1971, Williams & Wilkins.

53. Klünder KB, Rud B, Hansen J: Osteoarthritis of the hip and knee joint in retired football players, *Acta Orthop Scand* 51:925, 1980.

54. Krissoff WB: Follow-up on hang gliding injuries in Colorado, *Am J Sports Med* 4:222, 1976.

55. Kulund DN: *The injured athlete,* Philadelphia, 1982, JB Lippincott.

56. Levinthal DH: Sports injuries in persons over 30 years of age, *Postgrad Med* 28:121, 1960.

57. Lombardo SJ, Benson DW: Stress fractures of the femur in runners, *Am J Sports Med* 10:219, 1982.

58. Lyons JW, Porter RE: Cross-country skiing: a benign sport? *JAMA* 239:334, 1978.

59. MacLeod SB, Lewin P: Avulsion of the epiphysis of the tuberosity of the ischium, *JAMA* 92:1597, 1929.

60. Mader T: Avulsion of the rectus femoris tendon: an unusual type of pelvic fracture, *Pediatr Emerg Care* 6(3):198, 1990.

61. Malgaigne JF: *A treatise on fractures (translated from the French with notes and additions by JH Packard),* Philadelphia, 1859, JB Lippincott.

62. Martens MA, Hansen L, Mulier JC: Adductor tendinitis and musculus rectus abdominis tendopathy, *Am J Sports Med* 15(4):353, 1987.

63. Marti B et al: Is excessive running predictive of degenerative hip disease? Controlled study of former elite athletes, *BMJ* 229:91, 1989.

64. Matheson GO et al: Stress fractures in athletes: a study of 320 cases, *Am J Sports Med* 15(1):46, 1987.

65. McBryde AM Jr: Stress fractures in athletes, *Am J Sports Med* 3:212, 1975.

66. Merrifield HH, Cowan RF: Groin strain injuries in ice hockey, *Am J Sports Med* 1:41, 1973.

67. Metzmaker JN, Pappas AM: Avulsion fractures of the pelvis, *Am J Sports Med* 13:349, 1985.

68. Milch H: Ischial apophysiolysis: a new syndrome, *Clin Orthop* 2:184, 1953.

69. Morrison JB: The mechanics of the knee joint in relation to normal walking, *J Biomech* 3:51, 1970.

70. Noakes TD et al: Pelvic stress fractures in long-distance runners, *Am J Sports Med* 13(2):120, 1985.

71. O'Donoghue DH: *Treatment of injuries to athletes,* ed 2, Philadelphia, 1970, WB Saunders.

72. Ogden JA: *Skeletal injury in the child,* Philadelphia, 1982, Lea & Febiger.

73. O'Leary C et al: Traumatic dislocation of the hip in rugby union football, *Ir Med J* 90(10):291, 1987.

74. Pavlor H et al: Stress fractures of pubic ramus, *J Bone Joint Surg* 64A:1020, 1982.

75. Petvik ME, Stambaugh JL, Rothman RH: Posttraumatic gluteal compartment syndrome, *Clin Orthop* 231:127, 1988.

76. Pick JW, Stack JK, Anson BJ: Measurements on human femur: lengths, diameters, and angles, *Q Bull* 15:281, 1941.

77. Pyle LA Jr: Osteitis pubis in an athlete, *J Am Coll Health* 23:238, 1975.

78. Radin EL: Aetiology of osteoarthrosis, *Clin Rheum Dis* 2:509, 1976.

79. Ratliff AHC: Fractures of the neck of the femur in children, *J Bone Joint Surg* 44B:528, 1962.

80. Risser JC: The iliac apophysis: an invaluable sign in the management of scoliosis, *Clin Orthop* 11:111, 1958.

81. Ritter MA, Meding JB: Total hip arthroplasty: can the patient play sports again? *Orthopedics* 10(10):1447, 1987.

82. Robertson RC, Peterson HA: Traumatic dislocation of the hip in children: review of Mayo Clinic series. In Harris WH (ed): *The hip,* St Louis, 1974, Mosby.

83. Rydell N: Biomechanics of the hip joint, *Clin Orthop* 92:6, 1973.

84. Sashin D: A critical analysis of the anatomy and the pathologic changes of the sacroiliac joints, *J Bone Joint Surg* 12:891, 1930.

85. Schlonsky J, Olix ML: Functional disability following avulsion fracture of the ischial epiphysis: report of two cases, *J Bone Joint Surg* 54A:641, 1972.

86. Sherry E: Hip dislocations from skiing, *Med J Austr* 146:227, 1987.

87. Sinaki M, Merritt JL, Stillwell GK: Tension myalgia of the pelvic floor, *Mayo Clin Proc* 52:717, 1977.

88. Skinner HB, Cook SD: Fatigue failure stress of the femoral neck: a case report, *Am J Sports Med* 10:245, 1982.
89. Southwick WO: Compression fixation after biplane intertrochanteric osteotomy for slipped capital femoral epiphysis: a technical improvement, *J Bone Joint Surg* 55A:1218, 1973.
90. Spock A: Transient synovitis of the hip joint in children, *Pediatrics* 24:1042, 1959.
91. Stanitski CL, McMaster JH, Scranton PE: On the nature of stress fractures, *Am J Sports Med* 6:391, 1978.
92. Stimson LA: *Fractures and dislocations,* New York, 1917, Lea & Febiger.
93. Tachdjian MO: *Pediatric orthopedics,* vol 1, Philadelphia, 1972, WB Saunders.
94. Tachdjian MO: *Pediatric orthopedics,* vol 2, Philadelphia, 1972, WB Saunders.
95. Thiele GH: Coccygodynia: cause and treatment, *Dis Colon Rectum* 6:422, 1963.
96. Trueta J, Harrison MHM: The normal vascular anatomy of the femoral head in adult man, *J Bone Joint Surg* 35B:442, 1953.
97. Vere-Hodge N: Injuries in cricket. In Armstrong JR, Tucker WE (eds): *Injury in sport: the physiology, prevention, and treatment of injuries associated with sport,* London, 1964, Staples.
98. Volpin G et al: Stress fractures of the sacrum following strenuous exercise, *Clin Orthop* 243:184, 1989.
99. Ward FO: *Human anatomy,* London, 1838, Renshaw.
100. Waters PM, Millis MB: Hip and pelvic injuries in the young athlete, *Clin Sports Med* 7(3):513, 1988.
101. Watson-Jones R: *Fractures and joint injuries,* vol 1, ed 4, Baltimore, 1957, Williams & Wilkins.
102. Watts HG: Fractures of the pelvis in children, *Orthop Clin North Am* 7:615, 1976.
103. Weber BG, Brunner C, Freuler F: *Treatment of fractures in children and adolescents,* Berlin, 1980, Springer-Verlag.
104. Weitzner I: Fracture of the anterior superior spine of the ilium in one case, and anterior inferior in another case, *AJR* 33:39, 1935.
105. Williams JGP, Sperryn PN: *Sports medicine,* ed 2, Baltimore, 1976, Williams & Wilkins.
106. Wiltse LL, Frantz CH: Nonsuppurative osteitis pubis in the female, *J Bone Joint Surg* 38A:500, 1956.
107. Wootton JR, Cross MJ, Holt KWG: Avulsion of the ischial apophysis: the case for open reduction and internal fixation, *J Bone Joint Surg* 72B:625, 1990.
108. Zoltan DJ, Clancy WG, Keene JS: A new operative approach to snapping hip and refractory trochanteric bursitis in athletes, *Am J Sports Med* 14(3):201, 1986.

ADDITIONAL READINGS

Åkermark C, Johansson C: Tenotomy of the adductor longus tendon in the treatment of chronic groin pain in athletes, *Am J Sports Med* 20(6):640, 1992.
Blasier RB, Morawa LG: Complete rupture of the hamstring origin from a water-skiing injury, *Am J Sports Med* 18(4):435, 1990.
Ikeda T et al: Torn acetabular labrum in young patients, *J Bone Joint Surg* 70B(1):13, 1988.
Kälebo P et al: Ultrasonography of chronic tendon injuries in the groin, *Am J Sports Med* 20(6):634, 1992.
Latshaw RF et al: A pelvic stress fracture in a female jogger, *Am J Sports Med* 9:54, 1981.
Martin DF et al: Osteophytic bridging of the sacroiliac joint, *Am J Sports Med* 16(6):670, 1988.
Marymont JV, Lynch MA, Henning CE: Exercise-related stress reaction of the sacroiliac joint: an unusual cause of low back pain in athletes, *Am J Sports Med* 14(4):320, 1986.
Mendez AA, Eyster RL: Displaced nonunion stress fracture of the femoral neck treated with internal fixation and bone graft, *Am J Sports Med* 20(2):230, 1992.
Puranen J, Orava S: The hamstring syndrome: a new diagnosis of gluteal sciatic pain, *Am J Sports Med* 16(5):517, 1988.
Sammarco GJ, Stephens MM: Neuropraxia of the femoral nerve in a modern dancer, *Am J Sports Med* 19(4):413, 1991.
Tehranzadeh J et al: Combined pelvic stress fracture and avulsion of adductor longus in a middle distance runner, *Am J Sports Med* 9:54, 1981.
Vingård E et al: Sports and osteoarthritis of the hip: an epidemiologic study, *Am J Sports Med* 21(2):195, 1993.
Witwity T, Uhlmann RD, Fischer J: Arthroscopic management of chondromatosis of the hip joint, *Arthroscopy* 4(1):55, 1988.

CHAPTER 47

Anatomy and Biomechanics of the Spine

Stuart Remer
Michael G. Neuwirth

The role of the vertebral column is fundamental to form and function. The spine is an articulating structure consisting of the vertebrae, intervertebral disks, and intervertebral articulations. The spine has multiple ligamentous and muscular attachments. The major portion of the axial skeleton that is located below the skull is the spine.[33] The movable segments of the spine consist of 7

Spinal segments

- Cervical   7
- Thoracic   12
- Lumbar   5
- Sacral   5
- Coccygeal 4 or 5

---

cervical, 12 thoracic, and 5 lumbar vertebrae (Fig. 47-1).[43,44] The sacrum comprises 5 fused segments, and the coccyx comprises 4 or 5 rudimentary ossicles that are fused together to form a single bone. The first coccygeal vertebra may be separate from the other vertebrae. The total number of vertebral elements is 33; however, only 24 of the vertebrae are movable in the normal spine. The spine can be considered a mechanical and *linked* structure. The vertebrae function as levers and articulate with each other in a controlled manner via the facets and disks that function as pivots. The ligaments function as passive restraints, and the muscular attachments function as activators.[55]

The spine has various essential functions. It allows motion throughout its column and between the skull and the pelvic girdle. The main movements of the spine are flexion, extension, lateral bending, and rotation. Some circumduction, which is a combination of movements, also occurs. The spine transfers weight and supports both the loads of the body and external loads. This permits upright ambulation and the ability to carry and lift objects. The structural anatomy of the spine affords protection to the delicate spinal cord. The spine also functions as a shock absorber to externally applied stresses to the trunk. The intervertebral disk is also intimately involved with this function.

Spinal motion

- Flexion
- Extension
- Lateral bending
- Rotation

BONY ANATOMY

The normal spine appears rectilinear in the coronal plane, and it has four curvatures in the sagittal plane. There is a cervical, thoracic, lumbar, and sacral curvature.[33] These curvatures give the spine increased capacity for absorbing stresses and increased flexibility. The

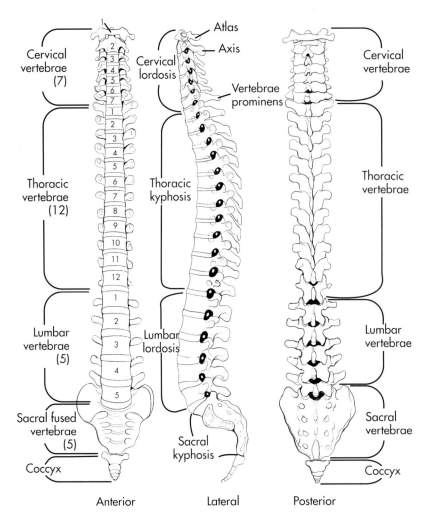

Cervical vertebrae (7)

Thoracic vertebrae (12)

Lumbar vertebrae (5)

Sacral fused vertebrae (5)

Coccyx

Atlas

Axis

Vertebrae prominens

Cervical lordosis

Thoracic kyphosis

Lumbar lordosis

Sacral kyphosis

Cervical vertebrae

Thoracic vertebrae

Lumbar vertebrae

Sacral vertebrae

Coccyx

Anterior   Lateral   Posterior

FIG. 47-1. Complete spine. Anterior, lateral, and posterior views.

vertebral bodies contribute about three fourths of the length of the presacral portion of the spine.[30] The intervertebral discs contribute about one fourth of the length of the spine. There is a gradual increase in size of the vertebral bodies as we proceed caudally from the occiput to the sacrum, and the bodies become progressively smaller toward the coccyx. The structural differences in the vertebral bodies are related to their weight-bearing capacity throughout the spine.

The typical vertebra consists of a posterior vertebral arch and an anterior body. The body is composed primarily of cancellous bone and functions primarily to support the weight of the body. The **vertebral arch** is formed by two pedicles, two laminae, two transverse processes, one spinous process, and four articulations that connect the vertebrae above and below. The vertebral body and arch enclose the vertebral foramen through which the spinal cord runs. Bony prominences, called **mamillary processes,** are found lateral to the articular facets and serve as origins and insertions of the spinal muscles. The dimensions of the pedicle from the superior to the inferior aspect are approximately half that of the corresponding vertebral body. The pedicles and the articular facets form the superior and inferior vertebral notches. The opposing inferior and superior vertebral notches form the intervertebral foramen of the intact spine.

SOFT-TISSUE ANATOMY
Ligaments

In addition to the facet articulations and the intervertebral discs, longitudinal ligaments unite the vertebral bodies. The anterior longitudinal ligament is a broad band that extends along the anterior surface of the ver-

---

Components of the vertebral arch

- Pedicles
- Laminae
- Transverse processes
- Spinous process
- Articulations

tebral body from the surface of the sacrum to the anterior tubercle of the atlas. It is most firmly attached to each vertebral body at the two ends, and it is loosely attached to the connective tissue of the annulus fibrosis of the disk where it may be elevated.[39] The posterior longitudinal ligament is a narrow band of fibers that runs along the posterior surface of the vertebral bodies from the atlas to the sacrum. It is intimately involved with the dorsum of the intervertebral disk. Two layers of fibers of the posterior longitudinal ligament span the intervertebral disk. The more superficial layer spans several segments, but the deeper layer spans only two vertebral articulations and comes up through the intervertebral foramen.[39] The fibers have thick attachments centrally and at their lateral expansions, but they leave a small segment of thinner attachments within a rhomboidal area that can permit disk protrusion. The posterior longitudinal ligament is essentially bowstrung as it crosses the vertebral bodies, which allow vascular elements to enter and leave beneath their fibers.

Neural Elements

The dermatomal and myotomal distributions of the spinal nerves will be reviewed (Fig. 47-2).[30] The relationship of the spinal nerve roots and cord segments to the vertebral level is briefly mentioned. In the cervical spine the cord segments lie at the level of the vertebrae above the root. There are eight cervical roots, and the first root emerges between the occiput and C1. The C8 root emerges between C7 and T1. No intervertebral foramina are present for the roots of C1 and C2. The spinal nerve roots for C3 to C8 form their spinal ganglia in the intervertebral foramen.

In the thoracic and lumbar regions the spinal nerve roots exit below the level of their numbered vertebral body. For example, the L1 nerve root exits below the pedicle of L1 through the intervertebral foramen composed of the posterior elements of L1 and L2. The spinal cord has been reported to terminate at the level of L1 and L2.[39] The adult spinal cord usually terminates at the inferior plate of the L1 vertebral body as the **conus medullaris.** Beyond the conus the nerve roots within the dural sac of the lumbar and sacral canals are referred to as the **cauda equina.** The nerve roots are divided into dorsal and ventral components within the region of the conus medullaris and cauda equina. The dorsal roots are

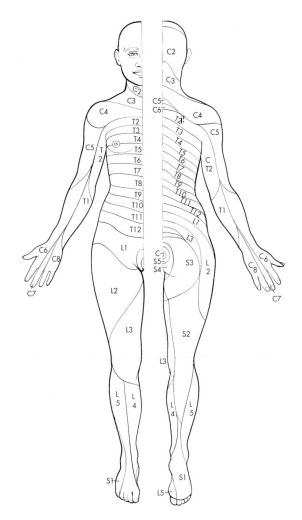

FIG. 47-2. Dermatomal distribution of the spinal nerves.

primarily sensory with their cell bodies in the dorsal root ganglion. The ventral roots are mainly motor and have their cell bodies in the gray matter of the spinal cord. The dorsal and ventral roots exit the thecal sac in separate compartments of the dura, called **root sleeves,** which come together at the dorsal root ganglion and form the mixed spinal nerve beyond that point. In the sacral region the dural sac terminates at the S2 vertebral level as the **filum terminale.** The filum terminale ends at the coccyx. The ventral rami of the sacral roots pass through the ventral sacral foramina, whereas the dorsal rami pass through the dorsal sacral foramina. The sacral hiatus is the exit point for S5 and the coccygeal roots.

The spine is innervated by three groups of rami that include the dorsal rami of the spinal nerves, the rami from the sympathetic trunk, and the sinuvertebral nerve.[30] The **dorsal rami** divide into medial and lateral branches after passing the facet joint. The medial rami innervate the facet joint, the ligamentum flavum, the supraspinous and interspinous ligaments, the medial portion of the spinal musculature, and the cutaneous regions of the neck, trunk, and buttocks. The lateral rami innervate the intertransverse ligaments, iliolumbar liga-

---

Myotomal distribution of spinal nerves

Upper extremity
- Shoulder abduction   C5
- Wrist extension   C6
- Wrist flexion and finger extension   C7
- Finger flexion   C8
- Finger abduction   T1

Lower extremity
- Knee extension   L3
- Ankle inversion   L4
- Great toe extension   L5
- Ankle eversion   S1

ments, the lateral portion of the spinal muscles, and the dorsal skin. Nerve fibers from the sympathetic trunk innervate the anterior longitudinal ligament and a superficial portion of the annulus fibrosis.

The **sinuvertebral nerve of Luschka** is formed by the confluence of the rami from the sympathetic trunk and the spinal nerve. It is formed distal to the intervertebral foramen and traverses the intervertebral foramen to come to the anterior portion of the vertebral canal, sending branches to the dura, the posterior longitudinal ligament, the superficial portion of the annulus, parts of the ligamentum flavum, and the intraspinal venous plexus. Recent work using acetylcholinesterase assays has given further support to the innervation of the outer lamina of the annulus by the sinuvertebral nerve.[5,6] Some of the fibers of the sinuvertebral nerve are efferent, but afferent fibers are thought to make up the bulk of the sinuvertebral nerve. These are thought to be involved in the pain response in diskogenic disease.

Canal Size

The anteroposterior diameter of the spinal cord varies throughout the length of the spine. In the upper cervical spine the canal diameter is widest, averaging 24 mm at C1 and 21 mm at C2. The canal narrows as we proceed down the lower cervical spine where canal diameters average about 14 mm. In the thoracic spine the average canal diameter is 14.8 mm, but the cross-sectional area is the smallest of any region of the spine. The spinal canal widens throughout the lumbar spine, and the anteroposterior diameter averages about 16 mm.

Spinal Mobility

Each mobile segment of the spine is capable of limited movements. The summation of all the mobile segments leads to overall large movements. The average total range of motion of the adult spine can be expressed in flexion-extension, axial rotation, and lateral bending. The total for flexion-extension of the spine averages 258 degrees, with 128 degrees of flexion and 130 degrees of extension possible.[30] The least amount of flexion-extension is present in the thoracic spine followed by the lumbar spine, and the largest amount of flexion-extension is present in the cervical spine. Total axial rotation of the entire spine averages 230 degrees, with 115 degrees to the left and 115 degrees to the right. The cervical spine has the largest amount of axial rotation possible followed by the thoracic spine, and the least amount of rotation possible is in the lumbar spine. Totals for lateral flexion or lateral bending of the entire spine average 147 degrees with 73.5 degrees for left lateral bend-

ing and the same amount for right lateral bending. The cervical spine has the potential for the largest amount of lateral bending, and the thoracic and lumbar spines have about the same amount of lateral bending. Overall, the cervical spine is the most mobile of the regions of the spine, followed by the lumbar and then the thoracic spines.[30]

For biomechanical analysis of the spine, several investigators have made a major effort to define instability of the various regions of the spine using various anatomic parameters. To assist in the framework of the discussion, we define stability and instability of the spine in the general sense. **Spinal stability** is defined as that quality in which vertebral structures maintain their anatomic relationships under all physiologic loads. **Spinal instability** "is the loss of the ability of the spine under physiologic conditions to maintain its pattern of displacement so that there is no initial or additional neurologic deficit, no major deformity, and no incapacitating pain."[55]

INTERVERTEBRAL DISK

The intervertebral disk comprises the nucleus pulposus and its surrounding annulus fibrosis and the cartilaginous endplates, which are between the vertebral bodies and the disk material. The intervertebral disk functions in absorbing the majority of loading on the spine. The outer annular fibers have sensory innervation, but the inner nucleus has none.[8] The matrix of the disk is principally composed of collagen fibers in a proteoglycan-water gel.[15,46,47] In the annulus the outer portion contains mostly Type I collagen. Type II collagen is present in the inner portion of the annulus.[16,17] A healthy nucleus pulposus contains only Type II collagen. The proteoglycans are macromolecules made up of a central protein core attached to side chains of glycosaminoglycans.[15]

Components of the intervertebral disk

- Nucleus pulposus
- Annulus fibrosis
- Cartilaginous endplates

Cells, water, and other noncollagenous proteins are present in the disk. The cells present in the intervertebral disk are stratified with regard to location. The cells in the annulus are cigar-shaped, whereas those in the nucleus pulposus are round.[32] The overall cell density is low. Water is the main constituent of the disk, occupying approximately 65% to 90% of the tissue volume. Most of the water is extracellular. Other noncollagenous proteins that are present in the disk have no known function.

The constituents of the disk vary with the age of the patient. The ratio of chondroitin-6-sulfate to keratan sulfate in the nucleus pulposus decreases with age.[1] The molecular weight of the proteoglycans in the nucleus de-

---

Average range of total spinal motion

- Flexion   128 degrees
- Extension   130 degrees
- Left axial rotation   115 degrees
- Right axial rotation   115 degrees
- Left lateral bending   73.5 degrees
- Right lateral bending 73.5 degrees

Disk changes with age

- ↓ Ratio of chondroitin-6-sulfate to keratan sulfate
- ↓ Molecular weight of proteoglycans
- ↓ Water content

---

creases with age. The water content of the disk decreases with age. The amount varies from about 85% in preadolescents to 70% to 75% in middle-age adults.

The disk obtains nutrition primarily through diffusion and fluid flow.[7] Solutes enter the disk via the disk-bone interface and through the annulus.[26,32,48-50] Solutes in blood vessels in the vertebral bodies diffuse into the intervertebral disk, but only a small portion of the bone endplate has blood vessels that penetrate close to the disk to form an interface with it.[23,24] The annulus, by its periphery, is vascularized and permeable and permits a greater area for diffusion of particles into the disk.[21,22] The contribution of fluid flow to the nutrition of the disk involves the behavior of the disk in response to compressive loads.[31] When a load is applied to the disk, the disk deforms and there is loss of fluid from it. Upon removal of the load the fluid that was squeezed out returns carrying solute particles.

A major role of the cells in the intervertebral disk is to form proteoglycans. The energy required for the synthesis of these molecules is primarily from glycolysis. Lactic acid levels are built up in the disk and correspond to the lower pH found in the central portion of the disk when compared with the normal pH.[39] The oxidative pathway for aerobic respiration in the disk occurs as well.

The intervertebral disk plays a major role in shock absorption of the spine. It can withstand high compressive loads far beyond that which the vertebral body can withstand. The vertebral body fractures before the disk receiving compressive loads takes on any destruction.

EMBRYOLOGY

The phylum Vertebrata in the animal kingdom comprises all animals that have a spinal column. The metamere, which has its beginning in invertebrates, is illustrated in the development of the spine. The developmental process begins in the embryologic phase, continues in the fetal phase, and completes itself postnatally, resulting in the adult spine. Following fertilization, the zygote undergoes multiple mitotic divisions resulting in an embryonic disk that exists as a bilaminar structure at the second week of intrauterine life. The primitive streak now forms in the midline with a thickening at its end known as Hensen's node. Cells from Hensen's node form the notochord, which becomes detached and forms a separate canal. The neural tube is then formed from the ectoderm over the notochord at Hensen's node. Anterior and posterior openings at the ends of the neural tube normally close on days 23 and 25, respectively.[30] The neural crest cells form from the ectodermal cells on the lateral edge of the neural tube during closure. These cells give rise to the spinal ganglia. Hensen's node on the no-

tochord is the inductor of the neural plate and of the future spinal cord. Neural tube closure constitutes an induction for the formation and closure of the posterior coverings of the spine. The mesenchyme posterior to the neural tube grows from the mesoderm to give rise to the endomeninges, which are the eventual pia mater and the arachnoid membranes. The mesenchyme also gives rise to the ectomeninges, which become the dura mater and the posterior arches of the vertebrae.

The neuroectodermal cells differentiate into three layers in the middle of the fourth week.[30] The ependymal layer is the inner layer that surrounds the lumen of the ependymal canal. The mantle layer is formed by neuroblasts and is the middle layer that forms the gray matter of the spinal cord. The marginal layer contains the nerve fibers and is the outer layer that forms the white matter of the spinal cord.

On day 18 the paraxial mesoderm begins to divide into somites, which are symmetrically paired cuboidal bodies on either side of the neural groove.[27] The somites develop in craniocaudal sequence, yielding 42 to 44 pairs. Somites divide into three-cell colonies at the end of the fourth week. The dermatome forms the dermis and subcutaneous tissue. The myotome gives rise to the musculature. The sclerotome is the initial tissue giving rise to the future vertebral column and the mesenchyme that develops on both sides of the neural tube and notochord. Eventually the sclerogenous mesenchyme undergoes chondrification and then endochondral ossification to produce the definitive skeletal columns. In contrast to previous beliefs, the sclerotome does not undergo segmentation.

The following description of the vertebrae development is from information developed by Dalgleish[9] and Verbout.[51] The notochord is surrounded by unsegmented axial mesenchyme from which the vertebrae centra and disk form. The lateral mesenchyme also shows no evidence of segmentation. The lateral mesenchyme separates into a cranial sclerotomic region, which allows for the intervertebral vessels and spinal nerves and a dense caudal sclerotomic region that forms the neural arches. With further development the notochord differentiates into the mucoid streak and the cell concentration that form the nucleus pulposus.[52,53] The future disc develops fibrocartilage. Ossification of the vertebrae is from three primary centers: the centrum and two vertebral arches.[40] Ossification is proceeding in the centra by the sixteenth week, whereas ossification is evident in the vertebral arches by the eighth week. The vertebral arch centers of ossification are well advanced of the centra in the vertebrae. The centers of ossification of the centra appear first in the lower thoracic and upper lumbar regions and proceed caudally. In the cervical region the centers of ossification of the vertebral arches appear first. The laminae of the arches unite first in the lumbar region and progress caudally. The vertebral arches eventually fuse with the centra, forming the typical vertebrae. The secondary centers of ossification appear during the fifteenth or sixteenth year at the tips of the transverse and spinous processes. These also eventually fuse in the middle of the third decade.

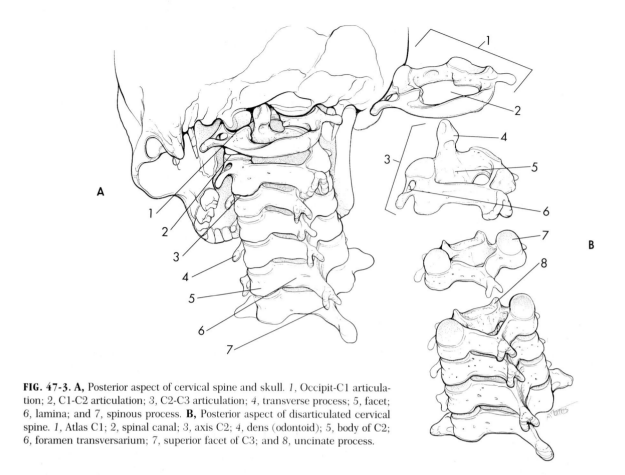

FIG. 47-3. A, Posterior aspect of cervical spine and skull. *1,* Occipit-C1 articulation; *2,* C1-C2 articulation; *3,* C2-C3 articulation; *4,* transverse process; *5,* facet; *6,* lamina; and *7,* spinous process. **B,** Posterior aspect of disarticulated cervical spine. *1,* Atlas C1; *2,* spinal canal; *3,* axis C2; *4,* dens (odontoid); *5,* body of C2; *6,* foramen transversarium; *7,* superior facet of C3; and *8,* uncinate process.

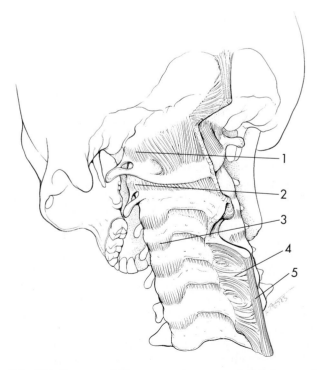

FIG. 47-4. Overview of ligamentous structure and articulations of cervical spine. *1,* Occipitoatlantal articulation; *2,* atlantoaxial articulation; *3,* synovial joint; *4,* supraspinous and interspinous ligaments; and *5,* ligamentum Nuchae.

REGIONAL ANATOMY AND BIOMECHANICS
Cervical Spine (Figs. 47-3 to 47-9)

The bony portion of the neck is formed by the cervical spine.[43] It extends from the skull to the thorax. There are seven cervical vertebrae of which the first two warrant special attention because of their unique structure. The **atlas** is the first cervical vertebra (C1), and the **axis** is the second (C2). C1 lacks a spinous process, whereas the C2 to C6 have bifid spinous processes. C7 has a prominent spinous process and is called the **vertebra prominens.**

A distinctive feature of the cervical vertebrae is the presence of the **foramen transversarium** (transverse foramen), which is an oval hole present in the transverse process of each vertebra. The transverse foramen of C7 is smaller than those of the other vertebrae and may be absent. The vertebral arteries pass through these foramina, except for C7. The diameter of the vertebral bodies of the cervical spine is smaller in the anteroposterior direction than in the transverse direction. The uncinate processes are formed by the upward turning of the lateral edges of the superior surface of each vertebral body. About 10 to 15 degrees of flexion-extension and 8 degrees of lateral flexion can occur at the occiput-C1 articulation. No axial rotation occurs at this joint.

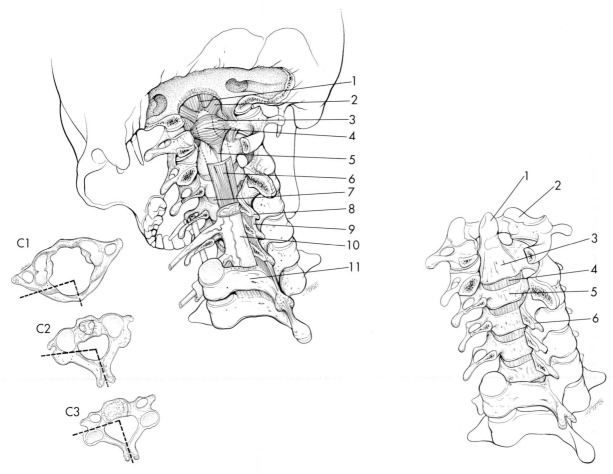

FIG. 47-5. Posterior elements and spinal cord partially removed to reveal ligamentous and neural anatomy of cervical spine. *1,* Apical ligament; *2,* atlas ligament; *3,* transverse ligament; *4,* dens of C2; *5,* body of C2; *6,* anterior longitudinal ligament; *7,* intervertebral disk; *8,* spinous process; *9,* interspinous ligament; *10,* spinal cord; and *11,* lamina.

FIG. 47-6. Posterior aspect of cervical spine with posterior elements and spinal cord removed. *1,* Dens; *2,* superior facet of C1; *3,* body of C2; *4,* intervertebral disk; *5,* vertebral body of C3; and *6,* spinous process.

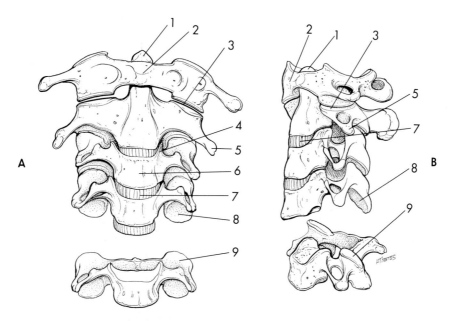

FIG. 47-7. A Anterior and, **B,** lateral views of cervical spine. *1,* Dens of C2; *2,* anterior tubercle of C1; *3,* C1-C2 articulation; *4,* uncinate process; *5,* transverse process; *6,* vertebral body; *7,* intervertebral disk; *8,* facet; and *9,* superior facet.

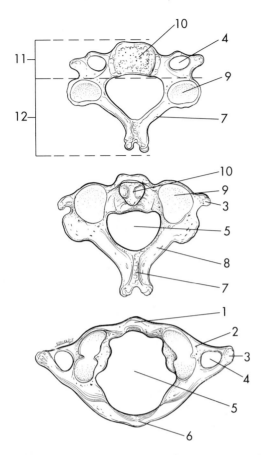

FIG. 47-8. Axial sections of cervical vertebra. *1*, Anterior tubercle of C1; *2*, lateral mass of C1; *3*, transverse process; *4*, foramen transversarium; *5*, vertebral foramen; *6*, posterior tubercle of C1; *7*, spinous process, *8*, lamina; *9*, facet articulation; *10*, vertebral body; *11*, anterior elements; and *12*, posterior elements.

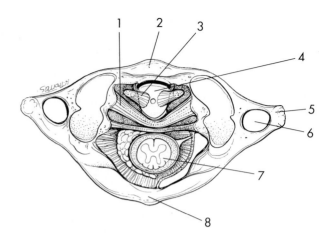

FIG. 47-9. Axial section of C1-C2 complex. *1*, Posterior tubercle of C1; *2*, spinal cord; *3*, transverse foramen; *4*, transverse process; *5*, dens of C2; *6*, anterior tubercle of C1; *7*, alar ligament; and *8*, transverse ligament.

Occipital Atlantoaxial Complex

The occipital atlantoaxial complex is formed by the articulations between the occiput, the atlas, and the axis. The atlas is a ring-shaped bone that consists of anterior and posterior arches, each of which has a tubercle and a lateral mass. It has concave superior articular facets that are kidney shaped. The atlantooccipital joints have a cup-shaped configuration and are true synovial joints. The superior articular facets of the lateral masses of the atlas articulate with the occipital condyles. The atlantooccipital membranes are anterior and posterior structures and serve as a connection between the arches of the atlas and the foramen magnum. The atlantoaxial joints are formed by the articulations between the atlas and the axis. No intervertebral disk is present between the atlas and the axis. The axis has two flat-bearing surfaces on which the atlas may rotate. The dens, or the odontoid process, is the most distinguishing feature of the axis. It is a blunt toothlike structure which projects cranially from the body of the axis to lie just posterior to the anterior tubercle of the atlas. The transverse ligament extends between the tubercles on the medial side of the lateral masses of the atlas. The dens of the axis is held up against the an-

terior arch of the atlas by the transverse ligament.[13] There is a synovial joint between them. The transverse ligament has vertically oriented upper and lower bands called the *cruciform ligament,* which passes to the occipital bone superiorly and the body of the axis inferiorly. The alar ligaments extend from the upper part of the odontoid to the lateral margins of the foramen magnum.[12] The ligaments attach the skull to the axis. The ligaments are fairly thick, and they check lateral rotation and lateral flexion movements of the head. The apical ligament is an adult derivative of the notochord. It extends from the anterior margin of the foramen magnum to the tip of the dens and provides structural support. The upward continuation of the posterior longitudinal ligament is the tectorial membrane. It extends from the body of C2 to the undersurface of the occipital bone and serves as a covering for the alar and transverse ligaments.

> Of the axial rotation of the cervical spine, 50% occurs at the C1-C2 articulation.

Range of motion. In total, the atlantoaxial articulations comprise three synovial joints. The ipsilateral joints are between the superior articular facets of the axis and the inferior articular facets of the atlas. The median joint is formed between the odontoid process, the anterior arch of the atlas, and the transverse ligament posteriorly. About 50% of the axial rotation of the cervical spine occurs at the C1-C2 articulation, which translates into about 47 degrees of axial rotation in each direction past neutral; 10 degrees of flexion-extension can occur, but little or no lateral flexion occurs at C1-C2.

Lower Cervical Spine

The typical vertebrae of the lower cervical spine comprise a vertebral body, two laminae, two pedicles, a spinous process, two transverse processes, two transverse foramina, two superior articular facets, and two inferior articular facets. The orientation of the facets of the cervical vertebrae can be demonstrated in three planes. The facets are oriented in a 30- to 50-degree angle to the horizontal or transverse plane. They are parallel to the coronal plane and are at a 90-degree angle to the sagittal plane.[28,45] The vertebral foramina have a rounded triangular shape and are relatively narrower in the lower cervical spine than in the upper cervical spine. The intervertebral foramina have average dimensions of approximately 12 mm in height by 6 mm in width by 6 to 8 mm in length.

The subaxial portion of the cervical spine has multiple ligamentous attachments. These include the anterior and posterior longitudinal ligaments that run on the anterior and posterior aspects of the vertebral body. The supraspinous and interspinous ligaments attach between and above the spinous processes. The intertransverse ligaments attach between the transverse processes of adjacent vertebral bodies. The ligamentum flavum connects the middle of the anterior surface of a lamina to the superior margin of the subadjacent lamina.[39] It extends transversely from one articular capsule to another with a small rent in the midline. The interspinous and supraspinous ligaments are reinforced in the cervical region by the nuchal ligament, which runs along the posterior border of the occiput and along the posterior border of the spinous processes to C7.

The cervical vertebrae from C2 to C7 have articulations at each level. There are two synovial joints posteriorly and the intervertebral disc anteriorly. The **oncovertebral joints of Luschka,** present between each uncinate process and the inferior lateral surface of the vertebral body, usually appear after age 30 and are believed to be associated with the degenerative changes of aging and are not true synovial joints.[43] The intervertebral disk forms a symphysis joint with the cartilage endplate of the adjacent vertebral bodies. The disks of the cervical spine are slightly thicker anteriorly than posteriorly, and their wedge shape contributes to the lordosis of the cervical spine.

Range of motion. The range of motion of the cervical spine below C2 includes flexion, extension, lateral flexion, and axial rotation between each vertebra.[30] About 90 degrees of axial rotation can occur from C3 to C7 with 45 degrees to each side of neutral; 40 degrees of flexion and 24 degrees of extension is possible. The total motion of this portion of the spine is fairly evenly distributed throughout the segments. The combined range of motion of the cervical spine is about 180 degrees of axial rotation, 90 degrees of lateral flexion, and about 145 degrees from full extension to full flexion.

Motion Segments

For biomechanical analysis, a motion segment of the cervical spine consists of two adjacent vertebrae, all the adjoining ligaments, and the intervertebral disk. The lower cervical spine has been divided into anterior and posterior columns. The posterior longitudinal ligament and all the structures anterior to it constitute the ante-

TABLE 47-1 Checklist for diagnosis of clinical instability in lower cervical spine*

Element	Point Value
Anterior elements destroyed or unable to function	2
Posterior elements destroyed or unable to function	2
Relative sagittal plane translation >3.5 mm	2
Relative sagittal plane rotation >11 degrees	2
Positive stretch test	2
Medullary (cord) damage	2
Root damage	1
Abnormal disk narrowing	1
Dangerous loading anticipated	1

From White AA, Southwick WO, Panjabi MM: *Spine* 1:15, 1976.
*Total of 5 or more = unstable.

rior column. The structures posterior to the posterior longitudinal ligament constitute the posterior column.

Stability

A checklist for clinical instability of the cervical spine has been developed by White and Panjabi[55,56] from their biomechanical analyses of the cervical spine (Table 47-1). A diagnosis of instability is made if the point value is greater than or equal to five. The various categories, which are rated by different point values, include anatomic and radiographic criteria. The criteria are as follows: the anterior and posterior elements are destroyed or are unable to function; sagittal plane translation or rotation is increased; abnormal disk space narrows; and a developmentally narrow canal, spinal cord damage, nerve root damage, or dangerous loading is anticipated.

Thoracic Spine (Figs. 47-10 to 47-13)
Structure

The thoracic spine consists of 12 vertebrae that articulate with the ribs and are denoted as T1 to T12. With the sternum and the ribs the thoracic spine forms the thorax. The contour of the thoracic spine has a normal kyphosis of approximately 20 degrees to 45 degrees (apex T7) that varies depending on the age of the person.[20] Any kyphosis at the thoracolumbar junction is considered abnormal. The upper and lower thoracic vertebrae have some characteristics of the cervical and lumbar regions. The midthoracic vertebrae are typical for that region. Throughout the thoracic spine, **costal facets** are present to articulate with the ribs. Costal facets arise from the lateral aspect of the vertebral bodies along their superior and inferior aspects. The vertebral bodies have

---

Normal thoracic kyphosis

- 20 degrees to 45 degrees
- Apex T7

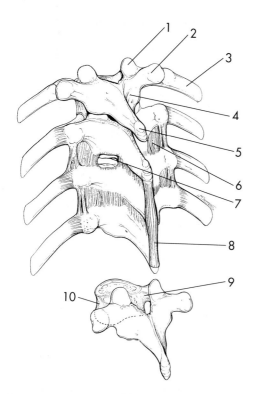

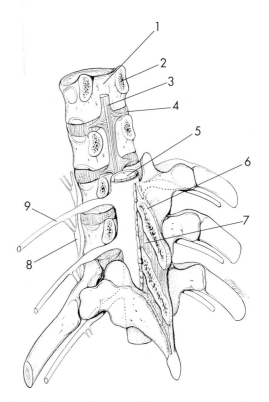

FIG. 47-10. Posterior aspect of thoracic spine. *1,* Superior facet; *2,* transverse process; *3,* rib; *4,* lamina; *5,* spinous process; *6,* synovial joint capsule; *7,* joint articulation; *8,* supraspinous ligaments; *9,* pedicle; and *10,* vertebral body.

FIG. 47-11. Posterior elements of thoracic spine removed to illustrate ligamentous and nerve anatomy. *1,* Vertebral body; *2,* pedicle; *3,* posterior longitudinal ligament; *4,* intervertebral disk; *5,* spinal cord; *6,* spinous process; *7,* interspinous ligament; *8,* sympathetic chain; and *9,* spinal nerve.

two pairs of costal demifacets on each vertebral body, except for T11 and T12, which have only one pair. The tips of the transverse process also have an anterolateral costal facet for articulation with the ribs, except for T11 and T12. The dimensions of the vertebral bodies of the thoracic spine change from T1 to T12. The anteroposterior diameter increases from T1 to T12, whereas the transverse diameter decreases from T1 to T4 and then increases to T12. From the upper thoracic spine to the thoracolumbar junction the vertebrae have a greater posterior than anterior height, resulting in the normal kyphosis of the thoracic spine.

The spinous processes throughout the thoracic spine overlay the vertebrae below them. Each vertebra is joined to the next by the intervertebral articulations. The intervertebral disk joins the adjacent vertebral bodies. The articular facets join the posterior arches of the vertebrae and form the posterior articulations. The orientation of the facets of the thoracic spine are approximately 60 degrees to the horizontal plane and 20 degrees to the coronal plane.[55]

The laminae of the thoracic spine overlap each other with the superior lamina being posterior to the inferior lamina. The overlapping of the laminae prevents hyperextension. There are no prominent interlamina spaces present until the T11-T12 level. The interlamina distance in the upper thoracic spine is less than 5 mm and

increases to T12 where the laminae are thickest. The lengths of the transverse processes are greatest at T1 and diminish progressively to T12. The pedicles have a length of approximately 15 to 25 mm in the thoracic region and decrease in the lower thoracic spine.

The structure of the typical midthoracic vertebra is as follows. The vertebral body is somewhat heart-shaped with two pairs of demifacets on each lateral aspect of the vertebral bodies for the ribs. The pedicles lie practically in the sagittal plane, slanting 10 degrees medial and approximately 10 degrees downward. The superior and inferior articular facets form the intervertebral articulations and extend out from the junction of the laminae and the pedicles. The diameter of a thoracic pedicle is approximately 5 to 6 mm. The spinous process is long and somewhat triangular in section. It is extended downward at an angle of approximately 60 degrees so that the spinous process of the next vertebra overlaps with it. The transverse process is a strong prominent structure with an anterior facet for the rib. The laminar region is small in comparison to the lumbar spine. The size of the vertebral foramen in the adult thoracic spine does not allow the passage of the distal interphalangeal joint of the index finger with an oval cross section of approximately 16 mm. The intervertebral foramina are oval in shape with dimensions of approximately 12 mm by 7 mm, but the rib head at the inferior aspect of each foramen narrows

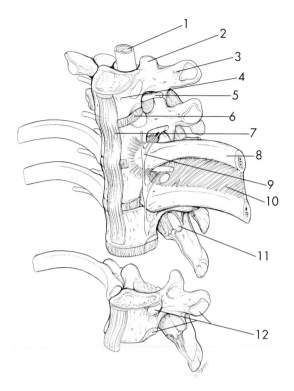

FIG. 47-12. Anterior aspect of thoracic spine. *1,* Spinal cord; *2,* superior facet; *3,* spinous process; *4,* vertebral body; *5,* spinal nerve; *6,* intervertebral disk; *7,* anterior longitudinal ligament; *8,* rib; *9,* sympathetic chain; *10,* intercostal muscles; *11,* inferior facet; and *12,* vertebral costal facets.

its size by about one third. The length of each foramen averages 6 mm. Of the total volume of the intervertebral foramina, approximately 20% is occupied by the spinal nerve.

Range of Motion

The range of motion of the thoracic spine in the adult is expressed in mean values for flexion-extension, axial rotation, and lateral flexion.[30] The total mean value for flexion-extension of the thoracic spine averages 83 degrees with full flexion of approximately 53 degrees and full extension of approximately 30 degrees. Axial rotation of the thoracic spine totals approximately 70 degrees with 35 degrees to the left and 35 degrees to the right. Axial rotation is greatest at the T12-L1 segment because of the absence of the ribs' restricting its motion. Lateral bending to the left averages 20 degrees, and lateral bending to the right averages 20 degrees in the thoracic spine.

Stability

One area of study of biomechanics of the thoracic spine that has received considerable attention is the determination of instability. In this region of the spine the structures have been grouped into three columns to form a model for spinal stability. The **anterior column** consists of the anterior longitudinal ligament, the annulus, the anterior two thirds of the disk, and the anterior two thirds of the vertebral body. The **middle column** consists of the posterior one third of the disk, the posterior one third of the vertebral body, the posterior annulus, and the posterior longitudinal ligament. The **posterior column** consists of the pedicles, laminae, spinous processes, facet capsules, and interspinous and supraspinous ligaments. Each column provides an element of stability to the spine.[10,11]

Destruction of the various columns of the spine was

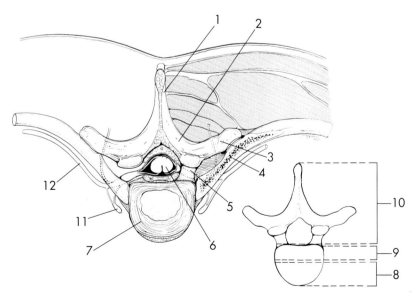

FIG. 47-13. Axial section of thoracic spine. *1,* Spinous process; *2,* lamina; *3,* transverse process; *4,* rib; *5,* pedicle; *6,* spinal cord; *7,* vertebral body; *8,* anterior column; *9,* middle column; and *10,* posterior column.

tested with respect to resultant instability.[18] Curves for load deflection were generated when the spine was subjected to physiologic loads and compression, and the same curves were generated for spines compromised for a specific column. It was found that when two columns are destroyed, the spine's ability to support the load of the head, upper extremities, and trunk decreased by 70% if the anterior and middle columns were destroyed, or 60% if the posterior and middle columns were destroyed.

The ability of the spine to resist torsion was tested by generating torsion-rotation curves under physiologic loads and then with predetermined column compromises.[19] With destruction of the anterior column the spine is unable to resist torsion at 95% loss of rigidity. Destruction of the middle and posterior columns produced only 35% loss of torsional strength. Facet joint destruction did not significantly alter the torsional resistance. The same three-column concept has also been ap-

plied to the lumbar spine with similar determinations of instability.

Lumbosacral Spine (Figs. 47-14 to 47-18)
Structure

Lumbar region. The next segment of the presacral portion of the vertebral column is the lumbar spine. There are five lumbar vertebrae, numbered L1-L5, followed by five fused sacral bodies that form the sacrum and the coccyx.[44] The alignment of the lumbar spine generally has a lordotic contour. The normal lordosis is 30 degrees to 50 degrees (apex L3) in a standing person.[20] The general anatomy of the lumbar vertebrae is similar to that of other vertebrae of the rest of the spine, having a vertebral body, two laminae, two pedicles, two transverse processes, and two superior and inferior facets, but the dimensions of the various parts of the vertebrae and the alignment of the facets differ. The lumbar vertebrae are

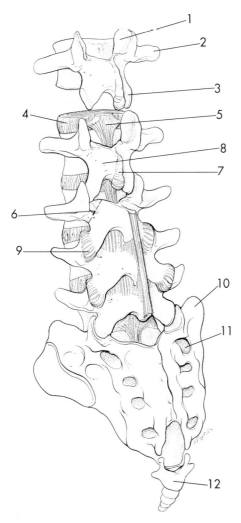

FIG. 47-14. Posterior aspect of lumbosacral spine. *1,* Superior facet; *2,* transverse process; *3,* inferior facet; *4,* intervertebral disk; *5,* posterior longitudinal ligament; *6,* pars interarticularis; *7,* spinous process; *8,* lamina; *9,* facet joint capsule; *10,* sacral ala; *11,* sacral foramina; and *12,* coccyx.

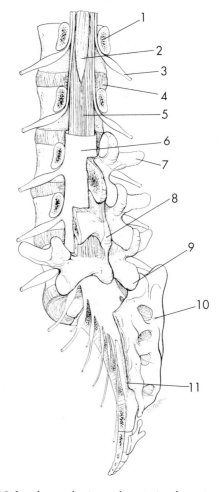

FIG. 47-15. Lumbosacral spine with posterior elements partially removed to illustrate ligamentous and neural anatomy. *1,* Pedicle; *2,* conus medullaris; *3,* spinal nerve; *4,* intervertebral disk; *5,* cauda equina; *6,* dura; *7,* transverse process; *8,* spinous process; *9,* lumbosacral facet; *10,* sacral nerve root; and *11,* coccygeal nerve root.

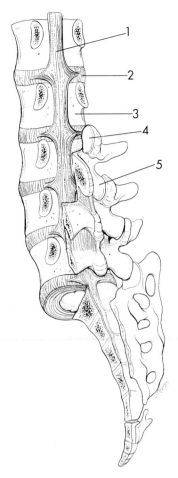

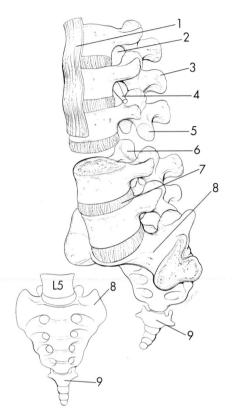

FIG. 47-16. Ligamentous structures of lumbosacral spine. *1*, Posterior longitudinal ligament; *2*, intervertebral disk; *3*, vertebral body; *4*, superior facet; and *5*, inferior facet.

FIG. 47-17. Anterior aspect of lumbosacral spine. *1*, Anterior longitudinal ligament; *2*, intervertebral foramen; *3*, spinous process; *4*, spinal nerve; *5*, inferior facet; *6*, superior facet; *7*, intervertebral disk; *8*, sacrum; and *9*, coccyx.

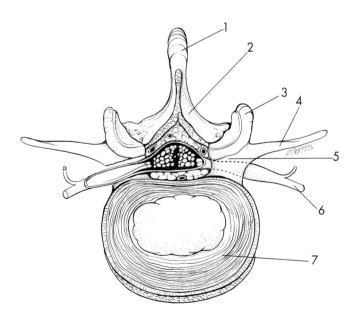

FIG. 47-18. Axial section of lumbar vertebra. *1*, Spinous process; *2*, lamina; *3*, facet; *4*, transverse process; *5*, pedicle; *6*, spinal nerve; and *7*, intervertebral disk.

larger than the thoracic or cervical vertebrae. The vertebral body has a width larger than its anterior-posterior diameter. The transverse processes from L1 to L4 come out as wings but are flattened anteriorly and posteriorly. The transverse process of L5 is much thicker and more rounded than the other transverse processes. In about 5% of the population, L5 is partially or completely incorporated into the sacrum, called *sacralization of L5.* The S1 body sometimes cannot be fused, and this is called a *lumbarized S1.*[33] The facets of the lumbar spine are oriented at a 90 degree angle to the transverse plane and at a 45 degree angle to the frontal plane.[29] The vertebral foramen can have an oval, round, or triangular shape. The intervertebral foramen comprises of the pedicles above and below, the posterior portion of the disk anteriorly, and the facet joint posteriorly. The size of the intervertebral foramina is larger than those in the cervical or thoracic portion of the spine and have mean dimensions of 18 mm by 13 mm. The length of the lumbar foramina are 8 to 15 mm. The lower lumbar foramina of L4-L5 and L5-S1 are slightly smaller than the upper lumbar foramina; however, the corresponding spinal nerve roots are somewhat larger.

The pedicles of the lumbosacral spine incline medially. The angle of inclination is usually from 5 degrees to 25 degrees. There appears to be an increase in medial inclination of the pedicles of 5 degrees per level from L1 to L5 with S1 having about 25 degrees of medial inclination.[25,54] The sagittal inclination of the pedicles parallels the vertebral endplates. The transverse diameter of the pedicle is generally smaller than the sagittal diameter. Most pedicles below L1 are generally greater than 8 mm in diameter and increase in size moving down the lumbar spine. The lower lumbar pedicles can have diameters that range from 10 to 20 mm.[30]

Sacrum. The sacrum comprises five fused vertebrae that form a triangular-shaped bone. The sacrum is part of the posterior part of the bony pelvis. It has a marked curvature with its convexity posterior and is tilted posteriorly. The lumbosacral angle is formed by the articulation of L5 with the sacrum. The sacral promontory is the anterior edge of the body of S1.

The posterior portion of the sacrum is marked by five longitudinal ridges. The median sacral crest is the central ridge and is formed by the fusion of the spinous processes of the sacral vertebrae. The intermediate crest represents the fused articular processes and is a groove with the median and the lateral crests. The lateral crests represent the fused transverse processes and form attachments for the dorsal sacroiliac ligaments. The superior ends of the crests form the superior articular facet of S1, which articulates with the inferior process of L5. The crests terminate inferiorly as the **cornua of the sacrum,** which bracket the inferior hiatus that gives ac-

cess to the sacral canal. There are four sacral foramina on each side that have their openings both anteriorly and posteriorly for egress of the nerve roots. The anterior portion of the sacrum is a flat concave surface. The anterior portion has two large lateral projections called **alae.** As we proceed inferiorly, there are fused vertebral bodies evident with anterior foramina present. The size of the foramina decreases from an average of 13 mm at S1 to approximately 4 mm at S4.

Range of Motion

For biomechanical analysis the range of motion of the adult lumbar spine is represented in mean values for flexion-extension, axial rotation, and lateral bending.[30] Flexion-extension of the lumbar spine is greatest at the L4-L5 level with a mean value of 24 degrees, and L5-S1 and L3-L4 average 18 degrees. The total flexion is 53 degrees, total extension is 30 degrees, and the total flexion-extension is 83 degrees. Total rotation of the lumbar spine averages 16 degrees with the L4-L5 and L5-S1 segments having the greatest axial rotation of the lumbar spine, which averages 4 degrees. Total lateral bending of the lumbar spine averages 20 degrees for right lateral flexion and 20 degrees for left lateral flexion.

Biomechanics

The biomechanics of the spine can be considered in terms of its kinetics, kinematics, statics, and dynamics.

Kinetics and kinematics. Motion segments are viscoelastic materials that exhibit coupled motion (motion in one direction affects motion in other directions.)[42] Motion segments have a fatigue tolerance, they absorb energy, and they move with 6 degrees of freedom (rotation about and translation along a sagittal, longitudinal, and transverse axis). The motion segment also undergoes creep (a continued deformation of the viscoelastic material with time under a constant load). The instant center of rotation of the motion segment is located in the posterior portion of the disk.

Statics and dynamics. The lumbar spine is subjected to different loads during standing, sitting, and reclining. During standing the line of the center of gravity passes anterior to L4.[4] Because the center of gravity is anterior to the center of rotation of the motion segment, a bending moment is initiated in the forward direction, which must be balanced by ligamentous and muscular forces. There are gradual increases in loads to the lumbar spine during different positions of the body. These loads translate to increased pressure on the intervertebral disks. During well-supported reclining the loads on the lumbar spine remain low. This is because the loads produced by the body weight have been eliminated, but the psoas muscle still has some pull if the hips and knees are extended. With support to flex the hips and knees in the supine position by use of pillows, the psoas muscle relaxes and the loads are further decreased.[29] During relaxed upright standing, the loads on the lumbar spine are more than twice that of reclining but are next to lowest among the various positions studied.[35-37] The compressive load on the lumbar disk is about twice that of body weight as well.

During the erect sitting position, some of the lumbar lordosis is lost even with the forward tilting of the pelvis that causes the loads on the lumbar spine to exceed those of relaxed upright standing.[35] Tight hamstrings can also reduce the forward tilting of the pelvis in the erect sitting position and can limit lumbar lordosis. The next position studied was the forward-bent standing position.[35] This produced increased loads on the lumbar spine above that of the erect sitting position because the bending moment that is produced by the weight of the upper body brings the center of gravity of the body further anterior with respect to the center of rotation of the motion segments.[29] The lumbar intervertebral disk is subjected to increased tensile and compressive stresses. Rotatory and torsional motion further increase the stresses on the disk.

Relaxed, unsupported sitting has the highest static load to the lumbar spine of the positions studied.[2,36] This occurs because there is a further decrease in lumbar lordosis, which lengthens the distance between the line of the center of gravity of the body and the center of rotation of the motion segment, thus creating a larger lever arm for the force exerted by the weight of the trunk. The larger lever arm produces an increased moment on the motion segment of the lumbar spine. Activity of the psoas musculature also contributes to the loads during sitting.[34] Supported sitting affords lower loads on the lumbar spine than unsupported sitting because a backrest supports part of the weight of the upper body. A lumbar support and a backward reclining backrest further reduce the loads. A thoracic support, which pushes the thoracic portion of the spine anteriorly, reduces the lumbar lordosis and thereby increases loads on the lumbar spine.[3]

Lifting and carrying objects can create high load to the lumbar spine. Several factors influence the loads to the lumbar spine during lifting, such as the weight of the object, the position of the spine during lifting, and the distance of the object relative to the center of rotation of the spine. In general, an object held closer to the body has a lower forward-bending moment than if the object is held further from the body. This is because the lever arm from the center of rotation of the spine is shorter if the object is held closer to the body. The loads to the lower spine are lower if the bending moment is lower.[2,38] If a person holding an object bends forward, the loads to the lumbar spine are increased. This is because the lever arm from the center of the spine is increased.[29] Objects of different sizes but of the same weight can affect the loads to the lumbar spine. A larger object has a longer lever arm produced when it is carried, thereby leading to a larger bending moment to the lumbar spine.

Lifting an object with the knees bent is generally recommended to minimize loads on the lumbar spine. If the back is kept straight and the knees are bent, the object can be held closer to the trunk when it is lifted; therefore the distance of the object from the center of rotation of the lumbar spine is less than if the object were lifted with the knees straight and the trunk bent forward. However, if the object is held far away— even with the knees bent— as it is being lifted, the loads to the lumbar spine are not reduced.[29]

Various exercises to strengthen the abdominal musculature may reduce loads on the lumbar spine. Contraction of the erector spinae muscles can be reduced by increasing intraabdominal pressure during lifting.[14] This may be particularly important when the weight of the load is to be overcome in the initial phase of lifting. Increases in intraabdominal pressure play a major role in moderating and stabilizing the forces on the lumbar spine. To strengthen the abdominal musculature, various types of sit-ups and leg lifts can be performed. However, in the process of strengthening the abdominal muscles, it is beneficial to minimize loads to the lumbar spine but still get adequate abdominal muscular development. Performing straight leg raises does little to activate the abdominal muscles but tends to produce increasing stresses on the psoas, attempting to pull the lumbar spine into hyperextension thus increasing the load. Performing sit-ups with the hips and knees flexed activates the abdominal muscles; however, if they are done through a full range of motion, lumbar disk pressure increases.[36] If the range of motion is limited so that the scapula just clears the floor, the lumbar motion is minimized, and effective motor recruitment of the muscles has been accomplished. This type of exercise is commonly known as a "trunk curl."[14] Another exercise called the "reverse curl," in which the knees and hips are flexed so that the knees can be brought to the chest, can also strengthen the abdominal muscles while limiting the stresses to the lumbar spine.[41] If this is done isometrically, the disk pressure is lower than a sit-up, and effective abdominal strengthening is accomplished. Strengthening of the erector spinae muscles can reduce loads to the lumbar spine. This can be done in the prone position as extension exercises. However, if the spine is hyperextended, increased pressures are placed on the lumbar disks. This can be minimized with abdominal support by placing a pillow under the abdomen and doing these exercises isometrically.[29]

SUMMARY

During physical activity and training, various demands are put on the human body. A significant demand is placed on the spine. The spine is required to support the body as well as act as a shock absorber throughout the activity. Stretching, range of motion, and strengthening exercises are performed to strengthen the back to reach the goal of attaining or maintaining physical fitness. A thorough understanding of the anatomy and biomechanics of the spine is essential for the following reasons: (1) to help plan general physical activity and training as well as to create an exercise program geared specifically to the development of the back musculature; (2) to comprehend the pathophysiology of sports-related spine injuries from a mild strain to a paralyzing fracture; and (3) to plan a comprehensive rehabilitation program following an injury.

REFERENCES

1. Adams P, Muir H: Qualitative changes with age of proteoglycans of human lumbar disks, *Ann Rheum Dis* 35:289, 1976.
2. Andersson GBJ, Örtengren R, Nachemson A: Quantitative studies of back loads in lifting, *Spine* 1:178, 1976.
3. Andersson GBJ et al: Lumbar disc pressure and myoelectric back muscle activity during sitting. I. Studies on an experimental chair, *Scand J Rehabil Med* 6:104, 1974.
4. Asmussen E, Klausen K: Form and function of the erect human spine, *Clin Orthop* 25:55, 1962.
5. Bogduk N, Tynan W, Wilson AS: The nerve supply to the human lumbar intervertebral discs, *J Anat* 132:39, 1981.
6. Bogduk N, Windsor M, Inglis A: The innervation of the cervical intervertebral discs, *Spine* 13:2, 1988.
7. Brown MD, Tsaltos TT: Studies on the permeability of the intervertebral disc during skeletal maturation, *Spine* 1:240, 1976.
8. Cóppes MH et al: Innervation of annulus fibrosis in low back pain, *Lancet* 336:189, 1990.
9. Dalgleish AE: A study of the development of the thoracic vertebrae of the mouse assisted by autoradiography, *Acta Anat (Basel)* 122:91, 1985.
10. Denis F: The three-column spine and its significance in the classification of acute thoracolumbar spinal injuries, *Spine* 8:817, 1983.
11. Denis F: Spinal stability as defined by the three-column spine concept in acute spinal trauma, *Clin Orthop* 189:65, 1984.
12. Dvorak J, Panjabi MM: Functional anatomy of the alar ligaments, *Spine* 12(2):183, 1987.
13. Dvorak J et al: Biomechanics of the craniocervical region: the alar and transverse ligaments, *J Orthop Res* 6(3):452, 1988.
14. Ekholm J et al: Activation of abdominal muscles during some physiotherapeutic exercises, *Scand J Rehabil Med* 11:75, 1979.
15. Emes JH, Pearce RH: The proteoglycans of human intervertebral discs, *Biochem J* 145:549, 1975.
16. Eyre DR, Muir H: Types I and II collagens in intervertebral disc, *Biochem J* 157:267, 1976.
17. Eyre DR, Muir H: Quantitative analysis of Types I and II collagens in human intervertebral discs at various ages, *Biochim Biophys Acta* 492:29, 1977.
18. Haher TR, Felmly WT, O'Brien M: Thoracic and lumbar fractures: diagnosis and management. In Bridwell KH, DeWald RL (eds): *The textbook of spinal surgery*, Philadelphia, 1991, JB Lippincott.
19. Haher TR et al: The contribution of the three columns of the spine to spinal stability: biomechanical model, *Paraplegia* 27:432, 1989.
20. Hammerberg KW: Kyphosis. In Bridwell KH, DeWald RL (eds): *The textbook of spinal surgery*, Philadelphia, 1991, JB Lippincott.
21. Holm S, Nachemson A: Cellularity of the lumbar intervertebral disc and its relevance to nutrition, *Orthop Trans* 7:457, 1983.
22. Holm S, Nachemson A: Variations in the nutrition of canine intervertebral disc induced by motion, *Spine* 8:866, 1983.
23. Holm S, Rosenqvist AL: Morphological and nutritional changes in the intervertebral disc after spinal motion, *Scand J Rheumatol Suppl* 60:A117, 1986.
24. Holm S et al: Nutrition of the intervertebral disc, *Connect Tissue Res* 8:101, 1981.
25. Johnson RM, Murhph MJ, Southwick WO: Surgical approaches to the spine. In Rothman RH, Simeone FA (eds): *The spine*, ed 3, Philadelphia, 1992, WB Saunders.
26. Katz MM, Hargens AR, Garfin SR: Intervertebral disc nutrition: diffusion versus convection, *Clin Orthop* 210:243, 1986.
27. Keynes RJ, Stern CD: Mechanisms of vertebrate segmentation, *Development* 103:413, 1988.
28. Krag MH: Biomechanics of the cervical spine. In Frymoyer JM (ed): *The adult spine: principles and practice*, New York, 1991, Raven Press.
29. Lindh M: Biomechanics of the lumbar spine. In Nordin M, Frankel VH (eds): *Basic biomechanics of the musculoskeletal system*, ed 2, Philadelphia, 1989, Lea & Febiger.
30. Louis R: *Surgery of the spine: surgical anatomy and operative approaches*, Berlin, 1983, Springer-Verlag.
31. Markolf KL, Morris JM: The structural components of the intervertebral disc, *J Bone Joint Surg* 56A:675, 1974.
32. Maroudas A et al: Factors involved in the nutrition of the human lumbar intervertebral disc: cellularity and diffusion of glycose in vitro, *J Anatomy* 120:113, 1975.
33. Moore RL: *Clinically oriented anatomy*, Baltimore, 1980, Williams & Wilkins.
34. Nachemson A: The possible importance of the psoas muscle for stabilization of the lumbar spine, *Acta Orthop Scand* 39:47, 1968.
35. Nachemson A: Towards a better understanding of back pain: a review of the mechanics of the lumbar disc, *Rheumatol Rehabil* 14:129, 1975.
36. Nachemson A, Elfström G: *Intravital dynamic pressure measurements in lumbar discs: a study of common movements, maneuvers, and exercises*, Stockholm, 1970, Almqvist & Wiksell.
37. Nachemson A, Morris JM: In vivo measurements of intradiscal pressure: discometry, a method for the determination of pressure in the lower lumbar discs, *J Bone Joint Surg* 46A:1077, 1964.
38. Németh G: On hip and lumbar biomechanics: a study of joint load and muscular activity, *Scand J Rehabil Med Suppl* 10, 1984.
39. Parke WW: Development of the spine. In Rothman RH, Simeone FA (eds): *The spine*, ed 3, Philadelphia, 1992, WB Saunders.
40. Parke WW: Applied anatomy of the spine. In Rothman RH, Simeone FA (eds): *The spine*, ed 3, Philadelphia, 1992, WB Saunders.
41. Partridge MJ, Walters CE: Participation of the abdominal muscles in various movements of the trunk in man: an electromyographic study, *Phys Ther* 39:791, 1959.
42. Pope MH, Wilder DG, Krag MH: Biomechanics of the lumbar spine. In Frymoyer JM (ed): *The adult spine: principles and practice*, New York, 1991, Raven Press.
43. Rauschning W: Anatomy and pathology of the cervical spine. In Frymoyer JM (ed): *The adult spine: principles and practice*, New York, 1991, Raven Press.
44. Rauschning W: Anatomy and pathology of the lumbar spine. In Frymoyer JM (ed): *The adult spine: principles and practice*, New York, 1991, Raven Press.
45. Shapiro I, Frankel VH: Biomechanics of the cervical spine. In Nordin M, Frankel VH (eds): *Basic biomechanics of the musculoskeletal system*, ed 2, Philadelphia, 1989, Lea & Febiger.
46. Stevens RL, Dondi P, Muir H: Proteoglycans of the intervertebral disc, *Biochem J* 179:573, 1979.
47. Stevens RL et al: Proteoglycans of the intervertebral disc, *Biochem J* 179:561, 1979.
48. Urban J, Holm S, Maroudas A: Diffusion of small solutes in the intervertebral disc: an in vivo study, *Biorheology* 15:202, 1978.
49. Urban J, Maroudas A: The chemistry of the intervertebral disc in relation to its physiological function and requirements, *Ann Rheum Dis* 6:46, 1980.
50. Urban J et al: Nutrition of the intervertebral disc: an in vivo study of solute transport, *Clin Orthop* 129:101, 1977.
51. Verbout AJ: The development of the vertebral column, *Adv Anat Embryol Cell Biol* 90:1, 1985.
52. Wamsley R: The development and growth of the intervertebral disc, *Edin Med J* 60:341, 1953.
53. Whalen JL et al: The intrinsic vasculature of the developing vertebral endplates and its nutritive significance to the intervertebral disc, *J Pediatr Orthop* 5:403, 1985.
54. Whiffen JR, Neuwirth MG: Degenerative spondylolisthesis. In Bridwell KH, DeWald RL (eds): *The textbook of spinal surgery*, Philadelphia, 1991, JB Lippincott.
55. White AA, Panjabi MM (eds): *Clinical biomechanics of the spine*, ed 2, Philadelphia, 1990, JB Lippincott.
56. White AA, Southwick WO, Panjabi MM: Clinical instability in the lower cervical spine, *Spine* 1:15, 1976.

CHAPTER 48

History, Physical Examination, and Acute Management of Spinal Injury

Henry Feuer

Active and aggressive participation in recreational and competitive sports, which has become an integral part of American life, has increased the incidence of athletic accidents. Acute spinal injuries, although uncommon during athletic events, are among the most dreaded and serious injuries that can occur. The sports medicine physician is now required to be present at competitive athletic events, and he or she must know how to both recognize spinal injury and direct initial management. This chapter deals with some of the on-the-spot evaluations and management decisions that the physician should be prepared to make in dealing with actual or suspected spine, spinal cord, and nerve root injuries.

The "downed" player on the field with obvious spinal injury is discussed first. Spine injuries with and without neurologic deficit are handled according to the well-established guidelines of the American College of Surgeons[1] with some modifications for athletes who may be wearing protective gear.

Dealing with complaints of spinal pain and paresthesias in the "walking" injured athlete during an athletic event is less straightforward. The athlete may minimize symptoms to get back into a tight game. The game clock is ticking and thousands of spectators and even television cameras may be watching the doctor's every move. The physician knows that a particular decision may be stressful and may have far-reaching consequences for both the player and the physician's reputation. Some of the guidelines that have evolved for caring for the ambulatory athlete with potentially serious symptoms are not based on scientific data; instead they are based on good judgment and the personal experiences of sports medicine physicians who deal with athletic injuries on a regular basis.

MANAGEMENT OF THE "DOWNED" PLAYER ON THE FIELD

Perhaps the most tension-producing situation for a sports medicine physician is to be called from the sidelines at a sporting event to attend to a player who is lying on the ground with a suspected spinal fracture or spinal cord injury. When the athlete complains of spinal pain, loss of strength, and numbness and tingling in the limbs, the team physician immediately suspects that a serious spinal cord injury has occurred. However, all those who may have initial contact with an injured player, such as teammates and trainers, must be taught to recognize potential spinal cord injury and must not move the injured player until proper supervision is available.[17] Failure to take precaution may aggravate an unstable spinal fracture and lead to additional neurologic injury.

For every game the team physician should assemble a team of trained paramedic personnel that responds

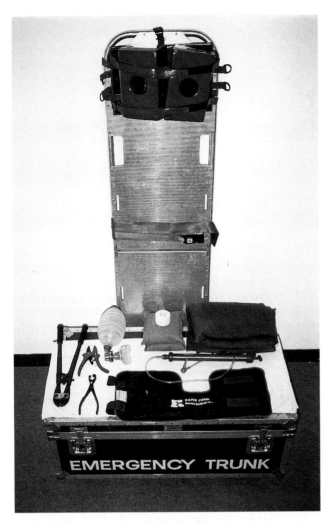

FIG. 48-1. Professional football emergency spine equipment kept on sidelines includes bolt cutters, trainer's angel, and pruning shears (for cutting mask); bag-valve mask and rapid form vacuum immobilizer with air pump (for cervical spine immobilization); sand bags, tape, rolled blanket, and spine board.

quickly when a medical emergency arises. At the beginning of each season the physician and the paramedic personnel should review and practice resuscitation, turning, and immobilization of the injured athlete. The necessary medical supplies must be inventoried and be readily available when needed. The medical equipment at a professional football game is extensive (Fig. 48-1). In contact sports the immediate availability of a spine board is advisable.

The team physician should consider the following steps in managing an athlete with a suspected acute spinal cord injury or vertebral fracture:

1. Assessment of airway, breathing, and circulation
2. Initial neurologic assessment, including the unconscious patient
3. Placing the athlete in the supine position
4. Immobilization
5. Evacuation

Airway, Breathing, and Circulation

The first responsibility of the physician is to ensure that the airway is open, breathing is adequate, and the pulse is normal. If the patient is awake, difficulty breathing or apnea should make a high spinal cord lesion suspect. **All unconscious players are presumed to have spinal fractures until proven otherwise.** (See p. 1085 for a discussion of airway management and spinal injury.)

In cervical spinal cord injury, innervation of the intercostal muscles is interrupted and breathing is performed primarily by the diaphragm and the accessory muscles of respiration supplied from the upper cervical cord. During inspiration the diaphragm descends and the abdomen expands. The resuscitation team should immediately recognize that this type of breathing is the result of a high spinal cord injury. Therefore any belt or athletic garment compressing the abdomen must be loosened. Because the diaphragm is innervated by the C3, C4, and C5 nerve roots, respiration may be seriously compromised or absent in high spinal cord injury. Ideally, all patients with spinal cord injuries should receive oxygen during resuscitation and transport, and ventilation must be carefully monitored.

Preliminary Examination on the Field

The physician should begin the initial examination by asking the awake patient a few simple questions to test his or her orientation and reliability (e.g., what period of the game is it? What is the name of the opposing team? What is the score?). The athlete should then be asked if he or she has pain in the neck or back or if he or she has had or is experiencing numbness and tingling in the extremities. If the response is affirmative, a preliminary diagnosis of spinal fracture or spinal cord injury must be considered. The player is then told to wiggle his or her hands and feet. If the legs appear to be paralyzed and there is cervical pain, careful attention must be given to examining the strength of the hand intrinsic muscles to avoid mistaking a quadriplegia for a paraplegia. **This is a common error among emergency medical personnel.** Wrist movement in a patient with a low cervical cord injury is sometimes misinterpreted by the inexperienced examiner as hand movement. Intrinsic muscles of the hand, which are supplied primarily by the C8 nerve root, can be tested by finger abduction, finger snapping, and hand grasping. Function of the intrinsic muscles *must* be tested in all cases of presumed paraplegia. Hand intrinsic weakness means injury to the cervical spinal cord and quadriplegia, not paraplegia.

If spinal cord injury is confirmed by the initial examination, a more detailed examination is repeated when the patient is placed in the supine position.

The Unconscious Athlete

The unconscious player on the field requires special consideration. All players rendered unconscious by an injury are considered to have a spinal fracture or spinal cord injury until proven otherwise. There are several physical findings that may be a clue to a spinal cord injury in an unconscious athlete:

1. Diaphragmatic breathing
2. Bradycardia
3. Warm, dry skin in the presence of hypotension
4. Grimacing to painful stimulation above the clavicle but not on the torso or lower extremities
5. Flexion of the arms but not extension to painful stimulation
6. Priapism
7. Loss of rectal tone

The unconscious athlete may have **airway problems** or even apnea if there is a high spinal cord injury. To properly care for the airway and ventilation, the athlete may have to be turned supine rapidly using the method to be described in the following section. If the airway is obstructed, the chin strap may have to be quickly cut off. In the spontaneously breathing athlete with a cervical cord injury, an obstructed airway can be opened with the classic chin lift maneuver recommended by the American College of Surgeons[1] or with the jaw thrust maneuver favored by Vegso and Torg.[24] In performing the chin lift, the assistant should place the fingers of one hand under the mandible and gently lift the chin anteriorly while being careful not to hyperextend the neck. The jaw thrust is performed by grasping the angles of the lower jaw with each hand and displacing the mandible forward.

If opening of the airway does not result in spontaneous breathing, the athlete must be ventilated. The best method at this point is to use a bag-valve face mask, which should be in the trainer's emergency kit. If this equipment is not available, mouth-to-mouth or preferably mouth–to–face mask ventilation is necessary. The athlete then requires intubation before transport. I prefer direct intubation with visualization of the vocal cords in such a situation. The American College of Surgeons[1] recommends nasotracheal intubation. Oral-tracheal intubation is accomplished with the help of an assistant who provides in-line stabilization.[26] The assistant should stand along the side of the player and place his or her own hands over the player's ears from the front. During visualization of the vocal cords the commonly used "sniffing" position, which flexes the neck at C5-C6 and extends at C1-C2, must be avoided.[26]

Turning the Athlete

The athlete with spinal cord injury must eventually be placed in the supine position for continued resuscitation, more detailed examination, and safe transportation. It is preferable to delay turning the stable athlete until the proper personnel and equipment are available. I have found the turning method described by Watkins[27] to be the most satisfactory. He suggests that at least five additional helpers be recruited to help with the turn. The physician should act as captain of the team and give all the orders. The physician should instruct the helpers on their exact duties before the turn is begun. The physician should grasp the player's shoulders so as to cradle the player's head with the forearms to maintain a neutral position during the turn (Fig. 48-2). Cervical traction at this time is not advisable because it may lead to further angulation or untoward distraction. The person

holding the head should not be responsible for any weight of the torso. Watkins[27] suggests that if the player is face down, the physician should cross his or her own arms and then cradle the player's head in the physician's arms; however, an additional person is needed to hold the player's head against the physician's arms. It is best to log roll the player onto a spine board. When a supine athlete on the ground must be lifted onto a spine board, the head and shoulders should be controlled in a similar manner to maintain alignment while the torso is lifted by three people on each side at the chest, hips, and legs (Fig. 48-3).

If the athlete is wearing a face mask, it should be removed before transport. The newer helmets have masks held in place by plastic straps that can be cut with a pocketknife or scalpel. Occasionally a bolt cutter is required to remove the face mask. In most instances, **it is advisable to leave the helmet in place until the athlete arrives at the hospital.** The chin strap also should be left on because it is helpful in immobilizing the head and helmet.

Immobilization

The athlete with a spinal cord injury must be carried off the field on a spine board. If possible the spine board should be available when turning the athlete to minimize the number of transfers. The torso is fastened to the board with straps. Sandbags or rolled blankets are placed on both sides of the head and are taped with the head to the spine board. All tape and restraints must be inspected to be sure that there is no airway obstruction or interference with abdominal breathing. If the athlete is not wearing a helmet, additional immobilization may be obtained with an extrication collar. The collar is not an alternative to proper head immobilization on the board, and it may compromise the airway of a quadriplegic. **Remember that inexperienced members of the medical team are often lulled into a false sense of security with a collar.**[10] A helmet may make it impossible to fit a cervical collar, but it should *not* be removed for the sake of the collar. When the injured player on the spine board is wearing shoulder pads but no helmet, the head needs to be elevated on padding before securing to prevent extension. If the player is wearing a helmet but no shoulder pads, there may be unwanted flexion of the neck. In this case it is necessary to place padding under the shoulders to maintain neutral alignment. An experienced emergency medical technician (EMT) on the sideline can be a great help during the immobilization process, but if one is not readily available, the sports medicine physician must be familiar with the technique.

Evacuation

Once the athlete with a spinal cord injury is carried off the playing field and before he or she is taken to the hospital, a slightly more detailed neurologic examination should be quickly performed to determine the baseline level of neurologic injury. This is extremely important because documentation of progressive neurologic deficit on sequential examinations requires urgent investigation and definitive treatment by a specialist.

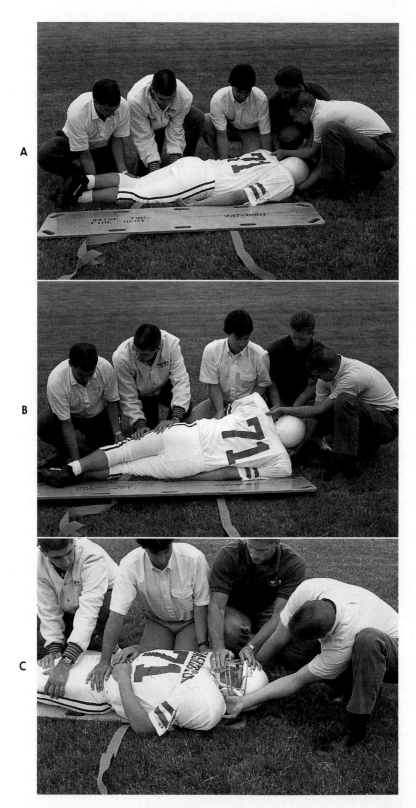

FIG. 48-2. Turning athlete from prone to supine position. **A,** Person in charge crosses his or her own arms and cradles player's head. **B,** Player is being turned with head in line with body. An assistant helps hold the head against cradled arms. **C,** Patient is ready for removal of face mask and to be secured to spine board.

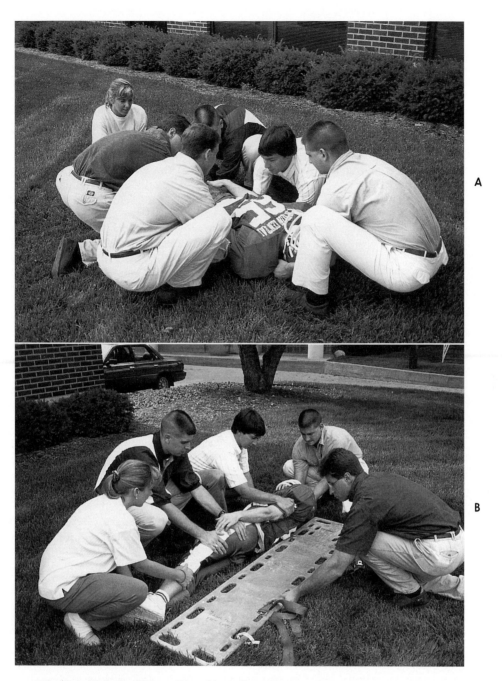

FIG. 48-3. Methods of lifting (**A**) and log rolling (**B**) an injured player onto spine board.

CASE STUDY

An 18-year-old man sustained a cervical flexion injury with severe pain. The referring hospital documented mild quadriparesis, and x-ray studies revealed a bilateral facet lock with 50% dislocation. The hospital helicopter then transported the patient. Just before landing on the roof of the hospital the resident physician on the helicopter, who had been performing serial examinations, noted that the patient had rapid deterioration to marked quadriplegia, which was confirmed by examination in the emergency department. A repeat x-ray study confirmed the marked dislocation (Fig. 48-4). Following the immediate application of skeletal traction and manipulation[2] the dislocation was reduced, and the individual improved neurologically right in front of our eyes.

We suggest that the sports medicine physician quickly check several motor functions on the sideline and record them in chart form (Fig. 48-5). A simplified on-the-scene examination can be done with the athlete fully clothed and is preliminary to the more detailed examination that is done as soon as the athlete can be undressed (Fig. 48-5 can be copied for easy reference on the field).

If hemodynamically stable, the patient should be directly transported to a designated hospital that has special capabilities for spinal injury. The sports medicine physician in attendance at a sanctioned athletic event should be familiar with the local trauma network. Before transport it is best if the baseline neurologic status is communicated by the physician on the scene directly to the consultants at the receiving hospital by a personal telephone call and a clear written report. I usually carry a portable recorder so that I can immediately dictate the neurologic examination and treatment rendered at the athletic event in case questions should arise. It is now customary to have a cellular phone on the sideline of sporting events.

In a large metropolitan area, diversion to the nearest hospital for x-ray examinations and imaging studies is unnecessary. However, in remote areas where transport distances to a trauma center are usually long, the sports medicine physician often accompanies the athlete to the local hospital and participates in the treatment. Consequently, the physician should be familiar with the next phase of management.

MANAGEMENT IN THE EMERGENCY DEPARTMENT
Evaluation and Resuscitation

When the athlete arrives in the local hospital emergency department, trauma protocols are instituted, usually in conjunction with emergency department physicians. To perform an adequate neurologic examination the athlete should be undressed completely. It is often best to cut the clothes off. If there is a helmet, its removal can be tricky in the presence of a spinal fracture. One individual should stabilize the head and helmet from a position superior to the athlete, and another person should cut the chin strap. Then the cheek pads are unsnapped with bandage scissors or a screwdriver and, after unsnapping each pad the pads are slipped out. A second individual should then initiate manual stabilization below the athlete's chin and neck, and the individual above should slip his or her fingers into the helmet ear holes, pulling laterally and easing the helmet off the head (Fig. 48-6).[12]

The vital signs are again checked, and large-bore intravenous lines are started. Because of the loss of descending sympathetic pathways in cervical and upper thoracic cord injuries, mild hypotension may be observed. This is referred to as **neurogenic shock.**[9] With sympathetic denervation there is vasodilation of visceral and lower extremity vessels with intravascular pooling of blood and hypotension. Because the individual with spinal cord injury is in the supine position, the drop in blood pressure is usually not significant. Bradycardia may re-

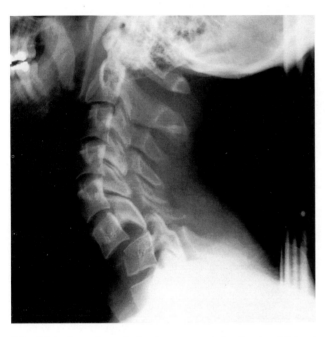

FIG. 48-4. Lateral cervical spine x-ray study showing bilateral locked facets at C6-C7.

Function	Right	Left
Shoulder abduction		
Elbow flexion		
Elbow extension		
Wrist extension		
Grasp		
Lifting thighs off board		
Knee flexion		
Knee extension		
Ankle dorsiflexion		
Ankle plantar flexion		
(+ for present; − for absent)		
Highest level of feeling pinch		

FIG. 48-5. Preliminary neurologic examination.

sult from interruption of sympathetic innervation of the heart. The term **spinal shock** refers to flaccidity and the loss of reflexes that often occurs in the acute phase of spinal cord injury.[9]

An attempt to elevate the blood pressure in neurogenic shock by overzealous use of intravenous fluids should be avoided because of the risk of inducing pulmonary edema. I prefer maintenance intravenous fluids. If the systolic blood pressure falls below 80 mm Hg in an individual with spinal cord injury and neurogenic shock, a mild vasopressor, preferably dopamine (2 to 3 µg/kg/min) is used.[19] If there is profound bradycardia, atropine (0.5 to 1.0 mg intravenously) can be used.[7] **Hypovolemic shock** should be considered with the presence of hypotension, tachycardia, pale skin, and a weak pulse, suggesting the possibility of an associated injury with blood loss. An individual with a spinal cord injury who also has hypovolemic shock is not cold and clammy because of

the "sympathectomy effect" and will not feel the pain of an intraabdominal injury.

On arrival in the emergency department, a blood count, routine blood chemistries, and a blood gas should be drawn. A Foley catheter attached to a closed drainage bag is placed in the bladder. The administration of oxygen should be continued, and oxygenation should be monitored with a pulse oximeter. Body temperature must also be monitored, particularly in extremes of climate or with air conditioning. Temperature regulation is impaired in spinal injury, and the individual may become poikilothermic. A nasogastric tube should be placed and attached to low suction. Placement of the nasogastric tube is important because the patient with a spinal injury usually has a reflex ileus. The patient may swallow large amounts of air, leading to gastric dilation with resultant reflex bradycardia and asystole.[19]

Spinal Cord Injury Medication Protocol

Based on the recommendation of the National Acute Spinal Cord Injury Studies (NASCIS), intravenous methylprednisolone is started with a dosage of 30 mg/kg in a 15-minute bolus and is followed by a 23-hour infusion of 5.4 mg/kg/hr.[5] According to this widely publicized protocol, steroids must be started within 8 hours of the injury if they are to be effective. Studies of other pharmacologic therapies in spinal cord injury are presently under way. In one study, GM-1 gangliosides, which may induce regeneration of neurons and restore neuronal function after injury in vivo, are being used following the methylprednisolone protocol.[8] Another study is evaluating the therapeutic effects of Tirilazad, a drug with especially potent lipid peroxidation inhibition properties and that lacks any corticosteroidal properties.[5]

Radiologic Assessment in the Emergency Department

Initially, a lateral cervical spine x-ray film and a chest x-ray film should be obtained at the local hospital. Additional films should not be obtained if they result in a delay in transferring the patient to a specialized hospital.

For the patient with an acute cervical spinal cord injury initial imaging study should be a lateral cervical spine x-ray with the shoulders pulled down.[26] This study should include the superior aspect of T1. In the athlete with big shoulders, a swimmer's view is frequently necessary. If the lower cervical spine cannot be visualized, computed tomography (CT) scans with lateral reconstruction are used. In the thoracic spine as well as the lumbar spine, anteroposterior and lateral views suffice. When viewing thoracolumbar spine injuries the x-ray study must be centered on the thoracolumbar junction to readily assess spinal angulation. Further radiologic assessment is extensively reviewed in Chapter 49.

Neurologic Examination in the Emergency Department

A more detailed neurologic examination is performed on the unclothed athlete as the resuscitation continues. The neurologic level of spinal injury may not correspond to the level of bone injury. It is determined by examination of both the motor and sensory systems. Motor

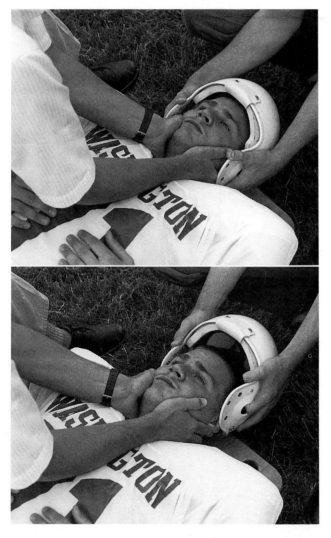

FIG. 48-6. Technique of head stabilization for removal of helmet in cervical spine injury. In general, helmet should be left in place until athlete arrives at emergency facility unless medical situation deems it necessary to remove the helmet.

TABLE 48-1 Upper extremity muscle function chart

Muscle	Root	Right	Left
Deltoid	C5	_____	_____
Biceps	C6	_____	_____
Triceps	C7	_____	_____
Intrinsics	C8	_____	_____

strength should be graded according to the following scale:

0   Zero—no muscular contraction
1   Trace—flicker of movement
2   Poor—partial arc of movement with gravity eliminated
3   Fair—complete arc of movement against gravity
4   Good—complete arc of movement against variable amounts of resistance
5   Normal

Use of this grading system allows the physician to more uniformly follow the progress of the specific injury.

It is customary to designate complete cervical cord injuries by the motor level. In cervical injuries the muscle groups should be tested in sequence, and the results should be recorded on a simple chart (Table 48-1).

A sensory level to pinprick with a clean safety pin should be sought first on the upper chest. Ordinarily there is an overlap of dermatomes, but a distinct sensory level can be discerned on the upper chest because there is an abrupt transition from the C4 to T2 dermatomes (Fig. 48-7). Pinprick sensation is then tested across the back of the hand from the medial to the lateral side. The fourth and fifth fingers are supplied by the C8 root, the second and third fingers by the C7 root, and the base of the thumb by the C6 root. The skin and the lateral aspect of the arm over the insertion of the deltoid is supplied by the C5 root.

Islands of preserved pinprick sensation should be searched for below the level of the lesion. It is important to identify whether there is preservation of pinprick sensation in the sacral dermatomes (i.e., perianal area, scrotum and penis, and vaginal labia). Sacral sparing may occur because the sacral fiber tracts within the spinal cord are the most peripheral. Preserved sensation means that the spinal cord lesion is not complete and that neurologic improvement is possible. Position sensation of the toes and touch sensation is also tested.

The level of a thoracic spinal cord injury is determined clinically by the level of sensory loss. Remember that T4 is at the nipples, T10 is at the umbilicus, and T12 just above the groin (Fig. 48-7). The T8 to T12 level supplies motor function for abdominal muscle contraction.

Testing of lower extremity strength in thoracolumbar and lumbar injuries is often difficult because of severe pain. At the thoracolumbar level there may be mixed cauda equina and spinal cord injury. Lumbar motor levels can be determined by referring to Table 48-2. (Table 48-2 may be copied for easy reference on the field.)

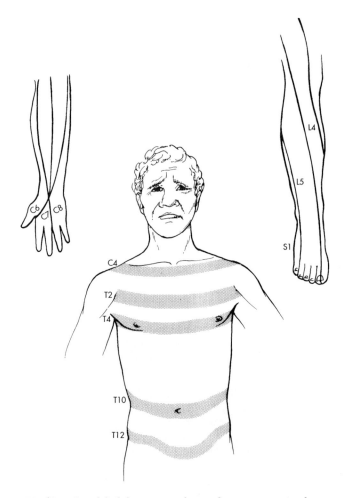

FIG. 48-7. Simplified dermatome charts of upper extremity, lower extremity, and trunk.

TABLE 48-2 Lower extremity muscle function chart

Muscle	Root	Reflex	Right	Left
Iliopsoas	L1-L3		_____	_____
Thigh adductors	L2-L3		_____	_____
Quadriceps	L3-L4	Patellar	_____	_____
Anterior tibialis	L4-L5		_____	_____
Gastrocsoleus	S1	Achilles	_____	_____

Refer to Fig. 48-7 for the sensory dermatomes in the lumbosacral area. L1 and L2 supply sensation to the inguinal region; L2 and L3 to the upper two thirds of the anterior thigh; L4 to the anterior medial leg; L5 to the big toe and the top of the foot; and S1 to the lateral foot, the sole, the back of the thigh and leg, and the sacral roots to the perineum. A tug on the Foley catheter may indicate preservation of sacral sensation.

Muscle stretch reflexes at and below the level of the injury are usually lost in acute spinal injury (spinal shock).

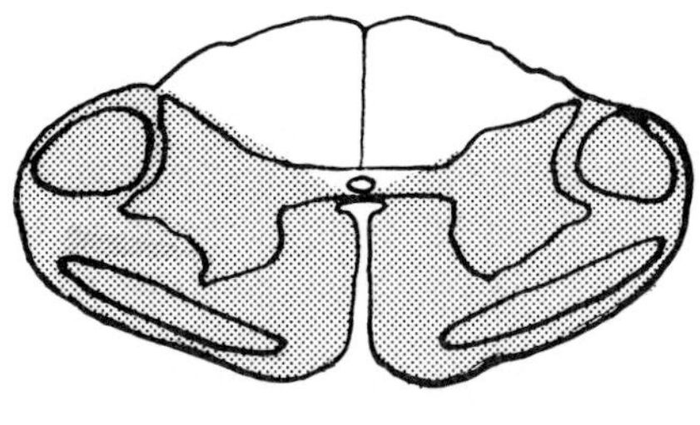

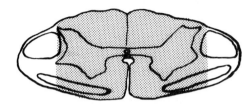

FIG. 48-8. Diagram of acute anterior spinal cord injury.

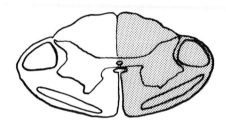

FIG. 48-9. Diagram of acute central spinal cord injury.

FIG. 48-10. Diagram of acute Brown-Séquard syndrome.

Patterns of Incomplete Lesions

Partial spinal cord injuries in the cervical area may result in classic patterns of neurologic dysfunction. In the acute anterior spinal cord lesion (Fig. 48-8), there is injury to the anterior quadrants of the cord with loss of motor function and pinprick and temperature sensation below the level of the lesion, but touch and position sense, which are transmitted in the posterior columns, are preserved.[20] This lesion usually has a poor prognosis for motor recovery.

In the central spinal cord syndrome (Fig. 48-9), most often seen in hyperextension injuries associated with acquired congenital spinal stenosis, there is characteristically greater loss of function and sensation in the upper extremities, particularly of the hands, with variable preservation of movement and sensation in the lower extremities.[21] The central spinal cord syndrome has a reasonable prognosis.

The Brown-Séquard syndrome results from a primarily unilateral spinal cord lesion (Fig. 48-10). There is an ipsilateral loss of motor power below the level of the lesion in addition to contralateral loss of pain and temperature sensation. This injury has a variable prognosis.[4] (The syndrome of spinal cord neurapraxia is discussed briefly in the next section).

Spinal Cord Injury in Young Children

Spinal cord injury in infants and children is rare except perhaps in gymnasts and divers. The important factor to remember is that spinal cord injury in the very young may occur without fracture (SCIWORA—spinal cord injury without radiographic abnormality).[16] The mechanism is believed to be subclinical subluxation secondary to wedge-shaped vertebral bodies, shallow uncinate processes, and ligamentous laxity. Even though the plain x-ray studies may be normal, studies such as CT and magnetic resonance imaging (MRI) may show a lesion in the spinal cord. Spinal cord injury may appear several days after trivial injury and may recur easily after seemingly good recovery.[15] Children with trivial symptoms should be immobilized for a long period of time and should not be allowed to return to contact sports until the spine reaches maturity.

Stroke in Sports

Extremity paralysis as a result of a stroke following a cervical injury in an athlete is rare. If there are no obvious radiologic abnormalities and the athlete develops a hemiparesis, incoordination, slurred speech, or visual difficulties, the physician should be alerted to the possibility of carotid or vertebral artery dissection or occlusion. These injuries may occur with a direct injury to the neck or following a sudden forceful rotation, hyperextension, or tilt of the neck without fracture or dislocation, in which the carotid artery is stretched across the spine. The vertebral arteries are vulnerable to compression at both the atlantoaxial level and C6 level. The onset of symptoms may be delayed for hours to days after the injury.[23] The use of crack cocaine may also be a cause of acute stroke in an athlete.[11]

ACUTE INJURIES IN THE AMBULATORY ATHLETE ON THE FIELD

The sports medicine physician is commonly called on to see an athlete who ambulates to the sidelines and complains of spine or peripheral nerve injury. Although these injuries are not as dramatic as the ones described in the first section of this chapter, management decisions can be extremely difficult for the physician. How serious is the injury? Can the athlete return to the game? Is the athlete intentionally minimizing the symptoms? Can the athlete be examined on the sidelines, or should he or she be sent to the locker room or hospital? Should x-ray studies be taken? Does the athlete need immobilization?

Neck Pain

Any athlete who has severe neck pain after an injury, who may hold his head in his hands or who may have acute torticollis and resist any movement, should be treated as having a possible unstable fracture, even though the athlete is ambulatory. The athlete should be assisted in lying down on the ground until appropriate immobilization can be obtained. If the injured athlete does not want to move the head and neck to the neutral position, he or she should be splinted as is with sandbags or rolled towels and tape. A careful baseline neurologic examination is then done, and the athlete is transported by ambulance to a hospital for x-ray studies. Most cervical spine fractures can be detected by x-ray studies and other spinal imaging studies. Most athletes will not have associated neurologic deficits. In professional football stadiums, an x-ray unit is usually available in the stadium.

An athlete who experiences neck pain after a traumatic incident on the playing field must not return to play until a full set of cervical spine radiographs, including flexion-extension views, is taken. If the x-ray studies and neurologic examination are negative, the athlete still should not be allowed to return to play any contact sport until there is full range of motion without cervical or radicular pain. Full range of motion of the neck includes touching the chin to the chest and ears to the shoulders, rotating the chin laterally to the shoulders, and fully extending the neck.[24] Motion should take place throughout all of the cervical segments including the occipitocervical junction. Flexion-extension x-ray studies to rule out ligamentous injury with instability are meaningful only if there is capability of full range of motion, which may not occur until the acute pain subsides.

When the physician is convinced that there is no fracture or ligamentous injury to explain an athlete's pain and there are no neurologic signs and symptoms, a diagnosis of cervical sprain or strain may be made. Theoretically, a sprain is a ligamentous injury, and a strain is a musculotendinous injury. Clinically it may be impossible to distinguish between the two. Athletes with ligamentous injuries should not return to play until they have full range of motion of the neck with reasonable comfort.

Numbness and Tingling in the Extremities

Numbness and tingling after an injury can be caused by lesions of the spinal cord, nerve roots, brachial plexus, or peripheral nerves. The mechanism of injury, location of any associated pain, and the neurologic examination are important in making the differential diagnosis.

Spinal Cord

If the sensory symptoms or signs are bilateral or involve the ipsilateral upper and lower extremities, the examiner should consider that a spinal cord injury has occurred even though the player may be ambulatory and has little or no back pain. The athlete must not be allowed to return to play until further diagnostic studies are performed by a neurologic specialist. As mentioned previously, a common cause of burning in both hands is the central cord injury syndrome.[13] In this injury the sensory symptoms can be severe and out of proportion to intrinsic hand muscle weakness, which may be mild.

Pinch-Stretch Neurapraxia

The most common cause of numbness and tingling in an upper extremity in contact sports is pinch-stretch neurapraxia.[25] In the old literature this disorder was referred to as burners, stingers, pinched nerves, brachial plexopathies, zingers, and brachial plexus stretch injuries.[25] Up to 50% of college and professional football players have experienced this syndrome sometime during their careers.[25] The injured athlete typically comes off the field holding his arm at his side, shaking the wrist, and rubbing the affected arm with the unaffected arm. There is a sharp, burning shoulder pain or a searing or lancinating radicular pain that may travel as far as the base of the thumb.[18] These severe sensory symptoms may last a matter of seconds to minutes. If the player is at the height of the excruciating pain, it may be hard to determine if proximal weakness is a manifestation of paralysis or a splinting secondary to severe pain. Usually the ability to flex the elbow and abduct the arm is regained within seconds at which time the pain begins to subside. If the athlete is examined a few minutes after the injury, there may be no abnormal neurologic findings. However, the athlete should be reexamined within a few days because development of weakness may be delayed.

Several mechanisms may contribute to this stereotypical painful syndrome. Lateral flexion of the cervical spine to the asymptomatic side and depression of the shoulder on the symptomatic side may stretch the upper brachial plexus. Lateral flexion with rotation and extension of the cervical spine toward the symptomatic side may compress the nerve root at the neural foramen. Shoulder depression only on the symptomatic side, hyperextension of the cervical spine, and a direct blow to the brachial plexus area may all be factors.[25] When the players are questioned about the mechanism of injury, there may be a variety of responses. Some claim their head was tilted toward the side of the injury, others state that their head was tilted away with the shoulder depressed, and still others claim that their neck was jammed or that their shoulder area received a blow. In those players who have sensory symptoms long after the pain goes away, neurologic examination with shoulder gear removed may reveal weakness of abduction and external rotation of the shoulder and flexion of the elbow. If the athlete has full, pain-free range of motion of the neck, the diagnosis of an upper brachial plexus stretch may be considered. Additionally, under no circumstances can the player with continuing paresthesias be allowed to return to the game.

Nerve Root Lesions

Nerve root syndromes are relatively uncommon following athletic injuries. Nerve roots may be injured by contiguous fractures (facet, transverse process, uncinate process, and vertebral body compression), acute soft disk herniations, or acute compression against a preexisting osteophyte. A player may hold his or her head toward the side of the affected root. Range of motion is decreased and painful. Interscapular and medial scapular pain may be prominent. Nerve root pain (radicular pain) travels from proximal to distal and is associated with paresthesias of the fingers supplied by that root (Fig. 48-7). Coughing or straining may reproduce radiating pain. Strength in the principal muscles supplied by that root are diminished, and the associated reflex is decreased or absent compared with the opposite side. Sometimes the athlete can obtain pain relief by resting the hand on his or her head. If the athlete also complains of a transient

TABLE 48-3 Peripheral nerve injuries

Nerve	Deficit
Suprascapular nerve	Diminished abduction or lateral rotation of the shoulder
Axillary nerve	Weakness of abduction of the shoulder
Long thoracic nerve	Weakness in ability of raising the arm above the shoulder (with scapular winging)
Spinal accessory nerve	Weakness of shoulder shrugging

tingling or paresthesia down the spine and into the trunk and lower extremities associated with neck flexion (Lhermitte's sign), the physician must be suspicious of a fracture or acute soft disk herniation compressing the spinal cord.

Peripheral Nerve Injury

Blows to the shoulder near the base of the neck or falling with an outstretched arm can result in numbness and weakness in the upper extremity, secondary to injury of a peripheral nerve. Vulnerable nerves are the suprascapular, axillary, long thoracic, and rarely the spinal accessory nerve.[3] Their deficits are listed in Table 48-3.

Spinal Cord Neurapraxia

Transient spinal cord injury with rapid recovery of sensory and motor systems has been referred to as the syndrome of neurapraxia of the cervical spinal cord with transient quadriplegia.[22] Other terms for this syndrome are *transient quadriparesis, transient quadriparesthesias, quadriburners, spinal cord concussion,* and *mild acute cervical spinal cord injury.*[28] Transient episodes have been associated with sensory changes only, as well as with weakness involving both arms, both legs, or all extremities. Neurapraxia usually occurs after a forced hyperextension, hyperflexion, or axial loading of the cervical spine. Mild cerebral concussions (e.g., memory loss, dizziness, and headaches), hyperventilation syndromes (e.g., dizziness and perioral numbness), and hysterical reactions (e.g., indifference and giving-way weakness) must also be considered in the differential diagnosis.

When this injury occurs, the extent of the deficit, namely whether it involves the arms, legs, or all extremities, as well as the severity of the deficit and duration of the deficit (i.e., minutes to hours), must be carefully documented. Watkins et al[28] have suggested a rating scale that is based on the extent of deficit, the duration of the deficit, and the central spinal canal diameter. This scale may be used as a guideline for return-to-play decisions.[28] However, there is no simple equation in determining who can return to play after this type of injury because frequently documentation of extent and duration of deficit and radiologic evidence of stenosis are difficult to obtain. Cantu[6] has recently made a commentary on functional cervical spinal stenosis that may well be a contra-

indication for further participation in contact sports. He defined "functional" spinal stenosis as the loss of cerebrospinal fluid (CSF) around the spinal cord that is documented either by MRI or contrasted positive CT scanning, which he believes should become the 1990s standard for defining spinal stenosis.[6] Obviously further clinical research regarding this syndrome is indicated. The great majority of physicians believe that following significant injuries of this type, athletes should curtail their careers in contact sports.

Back Pain

As with cervical spine injuries, the athlete who experiences back pain should not return to play. The athlete must be carefully reexamined as an outpatient and have lumbar spine x-ray studies done, including oblique views and flexion-extension views (if no fracture is present). If the x-ray studies and neurologic examination show no abnormalities, the athlete should not be allowed to return to play in any contact sport until pain has subsided and range of motion is back to baseline. It is helpful to have assessed lumbosacral spine motion of each player before the start of each season because there is great variation in the flexibility of spines in the young athletes.

Any athlete who has severe back pain usually has sustained at the minimum a musculoligamentous strain to the lumbosacral area. This is a nonspecific diagnosis because unless there is a fracture or disk herniation, it may be impossible to determine the specific cause of low back pain. However, the differential diagnosis should include spondylolysis with fracture of the pars interarticularis, acute disk herniation with nerve root compression, and a vertebral compression fracture[14] or fatigue fracture of the sacrum.

Spondylolysis must be suspected in any youth, most frequently 10 to 15 years of age, who develops the acute onset of low back pain and fails to improve quickly. When the patient is examined, the most typical finding is pain in the lower back reproduced by hyperextension of the lumbosacral spine or by the one-leg hyperextension test. The oblique views on the lumbar spine x-ray studies may reveal a fracture defect through the pars interarticularis, most typically at L4 or L5. However, if the pain persists and the x-ray studies are normal or equivocal, a three-phase bone scan or single photon emission computed tomographic (SPECT) scan is the most definitive study.

Acute lumbar disk herniations frequently occur or are recognized with a specific incident related to bending or lifting. The symptoms of a lumbar disk herniation present as an acute severe lower back muscle spasm followed by radiating pain to the buttocks and into a lower extremity below the knee (sciatica). The radiating pain most commonly occurs in the L5 and S1 distribution. The findings at the L4-L5 disk level with L5 root compression are weakness of the extensor hallucis longus and the anterior tibialis and sensory symptoms in the lateral leg, the dorsum of the foot, and the big toe. The findings at the L5-S1 disk level with S1 root compression are weakness of the gastrocnemius and gastrocsoleus muscles, sensory symptoms in the posterior leg and lateral foot, and a decreased or absent Achilles tendon reflex.

Occasionally a disk herniates at the L3-L4 disk level with L4 root compression. The findings there are weakness of the quadriceps muscles, sensory symptoms in the anterior thigh and medial leg, and a decreased patellar reflex.

Compression fractures are associated with severe lumbosacral muscle spasm, and the diagnosis is made from an x-ray film. A more extensive discussion of the previous differential diagnoses of lumbar spine pain is found in Chapter 52.

Thoracic Pain

Injuries to the thoracic spine are infrequent. A fall may cause a thoracic vertebral body compression fracture. Rarely an injury may lead to a thoracic disk herniation. Thoracic disk herniations may be manifested by pain radiating in the distribution of a rib (intercostal pain). Rarely they compress the spinal cord with sensory and motor findings involving the trunk and lower extremities. Thoracic disk herniations are most readily diagnosed with MRI scanning. In the differential diagnosis of thoracic pain are rib fractures, pneumothorax, and traumatic dissection of the aorta, all of which are beyond the scope of this chapter.

DEALING WITH THE PUBLIC

A serious spinal cord injury that occurs during a major high school, college, or professional athletic event makes the headlines in the local or national news media. The wise sports medicine physician has contingency plans for such an event. I would like to suggest the following:

1. Have a previously selected team spokesperson that can deal with the press. This has worked well for me with the Indianapolis Colts, Indiana Hoosiers, Purdue Boilermakers, and the Indianapolis 500.
2. Do not give an exact diagnosis until it is unequivocally established.
3. Do not talk about the prognosis soon after an injury. Wait until you can do so with some degree of certainty.
4. Discuss the case with only those athletic personnel, family, physicians, and paramedical workers directly involved with the injured athlete who have a need to know.
5. Do not tell your colleagues or friends anything you do not want the press to know.
6. Issue progress reports to your spokesperson in writing and on a predetermined time schedule.
7. Consider asking one of your partners or colleagues to see the player independently for a second opinion.
8. Think twice before trying experimental protocols and treatments.
9. Keep good records.

ACKNOWLEDGMENTS

My thanks and deepest appreciation to Julius Goodman, MD, for his energetic and invaluable assistance.

REFERENCES

1. American College of Surgeons: *Advanced trauma life support course for physicians*, Chicago, 1989, American College of Surgeons.
2. Barr JS Jr, Krag MH, Pierce DS: Cranial traction and the halo orthosis. In Cervical Spine Research Society Editorial Committee: *The cervical spine*, ed 2, Philadelphia, 1989, JB Lippincott.
3. Bateman JE: Nerve injuries about the shoulder in sports, *J Bone Joint Surg* 49A(4):785, 1967.
4. Braakman R, Penning L: *Injuries of the cervical spine*, Amsterdam, 1971, Excerpta Medica.
5. Bracken MB: Pharmacological treatment of acute spinal cord injury: current status and future prospects, *Paraplegia* 30:102, 1992.
6. Cantu RC: Functional cervical spinal stenosis: a contraindication to participation in contact sports, *Med Sci Sports Exerc* 25(3):316, 1993.
7. Chesnut RM, Marshall LF: Early assessment, transport, and management of patients with posttraumatic instability. In Cooper PR (ed): *Neurosurgical topics: management of posttraumatic spinal instability*, Park Ridge, Illinois, 1990, American Association of Neurological Surgeons.
8. Geisler FH, Dorsey FC, Coleman WP: Recovery of motor function after spinal cord injury—a randomized placebo-controlled trial with GM-1 ganglioside, *N Engl J Med* 324(26):1829, 1991.
9. Green BA, Eismont FJ: Acute spinal cord injury: a systems approach. In *Central nervous system trauma*, vol 1, 1984, Mary Ann Liebert.
10. Hadley MN: Spinal orthoses. In Cooper PR (ed): *Neurosurgical topics: management of posttraumatic spinal instability*, Park Ridge, Ill, 1990, American Association of Neurological Surgeons.
11. Levine SR et al: Cerebrovascular complications of the use of the "crack" form of alkaloidal cocaine, *N Engl J Med* 323(11):669, 1990.
12. Long SE et al: Removing football helmets safely, *Phys Sports Med* 8:119, 1980.
13. Maroon JC: "Burning hands" in football spinal cord injuries, *JAMA* 238:2049, 1977.
14. Micheli LJ: How I manage low back pain in athletes, *Phys Sports Med* 21(3):182, 1993.
15. Osenbach RK, Menezes AH: Pediatric spinal cord and vertebral column injury, *Neurosurgery* 30(3):385, 1992.
16. Pang D, Wilberger JE Jr: Spinal cord injury without radiographic abnormalities in children, *J Neurosurg* 57:114, 1982.
17. Rockett FX: *Sports injuries—the unthwarted epidemic*, Littleton, Mass, 1981, PSG Publishing.
18. Rockett FX: Observations on the "burner": traumatic cervical radiculopathy, *Clin Orthop* 164:18, 1992.
19. Rosner MJ: Medical managements of spinal cord injury. In Pitts LH, Wagner FC Jr (eds): *Craniospinal trauma*, New York, 1990, Thieme Medical.
20. Schneider RC: Syndrome of acute anterior spinal cord injury, *J Neurosurg* 12:95, 1955.
21. Schneider RC, Cherry G, Pantek H: The syndrome of acute central cervical spinal cord injury, *J Neurosurg* 11:546, 1954.
22. Torg JS, Fay CM: Cervical spinal stenosis with cord neurapraxia and transient quadriplegia. In Torg JS (ed): *Athletic injuries to the head, neck, and face*, St Louis, 1991, Mosby.
23. Tramo MJ, Hainline B: Stroke in sports. In Jordan BD, Tsairis P, Warren RF (eds): *Sports neurology*, Rockville, Md, 1989, Aspen.
24. Vegso JJ, Torg JS: Field evaluation and management of cervical spine injuries. In Torg JS (ed): *Athletic injuries to the head, neck, and face*, St Louis, 1991, Mosby.
25. Vereschagin KS et al: Burners: don't overloook or underestimate them, *Phys Sports Med* 19(9):96, 1991.
26. Wagner FC Jr: Initial assessment and management of spinal injuries. In Pitts LH, Wagner FC Jr (eds): *Craniospinal trauma*, New York, 1990, Thieme Medical.
27. Watkins RG: Neck injuries in football players, *Clin Sports Med* 5(2):223, 1986.
28. Watkins RG, Dillin WH, Maxwell J: Cervical spine injuries in football players. In Hochschuler SH (ed): *Spine: spinal injuries in sports*, Philadelphia, 1990, Hanley & Belfus.

CHAPTER 49

Radiologic Evaluation and Imaging of the Spine

Malcolm Thomas
Gordon R. Bell

Radiologic evaluation of the spine in the athlete follows the clinical assessment. The history and physical examination lead to a differential diagnosis and help determine the mechanism of injury. Radiologic studies can then be targeted to provide maximum information for the diagnostic workup, since interpretation of imaging studies is more accurate with a knowledge of the clinical data.[7,27,45,72,78] In the majority of cases the initial radiologic evaluation is the plain x-ray study. Standard x-ray views occasionally need to be supplemented by additional special views. For example, flexion-extension lateral x-ray views of the cervical spine are useful to rule out instability when standard views are normal and clinical suspicion for instability is high.[35,72] Another example is the oblique view of the lumbosacral spine to rule out a spondylolytic defect.[43] Subtle spondylolysis may be missed if such x-ray studies are not performed. In addition, more costly diagnostic studies can sometimes be avoided by appropriate use of specialized plain x-ray studies. It is therefore important for the treating physician to have a knowledge of the types of plain x-ray views that are available and their proper indications. In the majority of cases, routine radiographic views are all that is required. Nevertheless, a complete workup may require other diagnostic studies such as plain tomography, computed tomography (CT), three-dimensional computed tomography (3D-CT), myelography, postcontrast CT, and magnetic resonance imaging (MRI). Indications for these other studies are dictated by the clinical circumstances. In the professional athlete whose prompt return to play may be critical, an extensive radiologic workup may be indicated from the outset. For example, the evaluation of a professional football player with a suspected cervical spine injury, with normal plain x-ray studies and a normal, dynamic x-ray series may warrant an MRI scan to fully assess the presence of a ligamentous injury or a disk herniation.[19,32,49] In the high-school football player, on the other hand, it may be more reasonable to allow healing to occur and, if necessary, to repeat the dynamic flexion-extension lateral x-ray study at 2 weeks to assess latent instability from ligamentous disruption.[35,52,74]

This chapter outlines what is available radiologically, and suggests the type of radiologic evaluation of the injured athlete's spine.

CERVICAL SPINE EVALUATION
Plain Radiographs

Radiographic evaluation of the cervical spine begins with the plain x-ray series. This series consists of an initial lateral x-ray view followed by anteroposterior, open-mouth, and oblique views. These radiographs must be of good quality.[31,38] They must be able to demonstrate both bony architecture and soft-tissue detail. The importance of an adequate series of plain radiographs cannot be overemphasized.[31,35,52,72] To standardize for magnification the standard lateral radiograph is taken with the x-ray tube 6 feet from the film holder and is positioned against the patient's shoulder.[37] This is important when measurements are read directly from the radiograph, especially when measuring cervical canal diameter. On the lateral radiograph it is mandatory to include the entire

---

Cervical spine series

- Anteroposterior view
- Lateral view
- Open-mouth view
- Oblique views

---

cervical spine from the occiput down to the cervicothoracic junction. It may be difficult to visualize the lower cervical spine, particularly in the broad-shouldered athlete. Under such circumstances downward traction may be applied to both upper limbs.[45,72,73] If this does not help the physician to visualize the lower cervical spine, a swimmer's view with one arm fully abducted demonstrates the cervicothoracic junction.

Evaluation of the **lateral cervical radiograph** begins by looking at spinal alignment. Generally, there should be a gentle lordotic curve to the cervical spine. However, in 20% of patients in Wier's series[77] the cervical spine was straight or slightly kyphotic in the neutral position. Furthermore, depression of the chin by only 1 inch resulted in a straightened cervical spine in 70% of normal adults. In a group of 80 asymptomatic professional football players the overall sagittal cervical alignment in the neutral position was lordotic in 85% and kyphotic in 15%.[37] Therefore **lack of lordosis does not necessarily signify a pathologic condition.**[27,37,77]

Four separate radiologic lines should be visualized on the lateral cervical x-ray study.[45] The anterior and posterior borders of the vertebral bodies should form two continuous parallel gentle curves that are posteriorly concave. The spinolaminar junction is a distinct radiologic landmark that can be traced as a third continuous line. The posterior aspect of the lateral masses forms a similar continuous line. Interruption of these lines may indicate degeneration, trauma, or another pathologic condition (Fig. 49-1).

The soft tissues also must be carefully evaluated, particularly in an acute injury. From C1 to C3 the normal prevertebral soft-tissue width should be less than 5 mm.[24,77] Increase in this soft-tissue space from hematoma[32] may be the only clue to a subtle fracture and should prompt further evaluation. Below C3, this distance varies and can be as wide as the corresponding vertebral body.

The **atlantodens interval** (ADI) is the distance between the posterior aspect of the anterior arch of C1 and

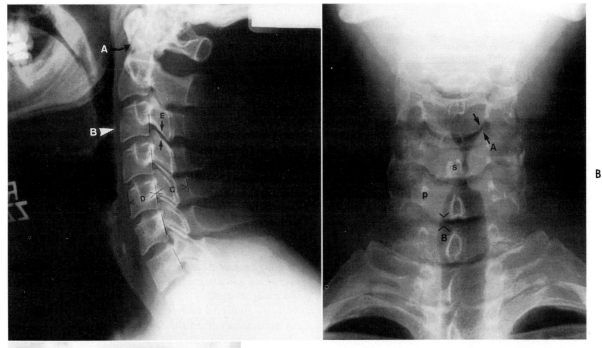

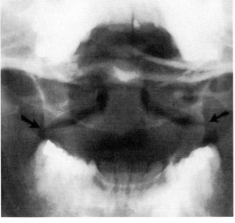

FIG. 49-1. A, Normal lateral cervical radiograph. Note gentle lordotic curve formed by posterior margins of vertebral bodies. Arrow *A* demonstrates space between odontoid and anterior arch of C1. Atlantodens interval should be less than 3 mm in adults. Arrowhead *B* demonstrates retropharyngeal soft-tissue shadow anterior to C3. This should normally be less than 5 mm. Arrowheads *C* demonstrate developmental canal diameter, measured from midpoint of posterior border of vertebral body to nearest point on corresponding spinolaminar line. Arrowheads *D* demonstrate measurement of vertebral body width. Arrows *E* demonstrates facet joints between C3 and C4. **B,** Normal anteroposterior radiograph of cervical spine. Arrows *A* demonstrate joints of Luschka. Arrowheads *B* indicate intervertebral disk space, which should be parallel to those above and below. *S* represents C5 spinous process, which should fall into vertical alignment with other spinous processes, *p* represents pedicle of C6. **C,** Normal open-mouth radiograph. This view demonstrates odontoid process, body of C2, and lateral masses of C1. Atlantoaxial joints are well visualized and should be congruent. Arrows demonstrate normal lateral margin of atlantoaxial joints.

Normal radiographic measurements

C1 to C3
Normal prevertebral soft-tissue width
- < 5 mm

C1 to C2
Atlantodens interval (ADI)
- < 3 mm in adults
- < 4 mm in children

the odontoid process. This interval should be less than 3 mm in adults and less than 4 mm in children.[24] An increase in the ADI suggests atlantoaxial instability resulting from incompetence of the transverse ligament.

White and Panjabi[76] defined a second type of instability, **subaxial instability,** by the amount of horizontal displacement and angular motion of adjoining vertebral bodies as visualized on the lateral film. Horizontal displacement of more than 3.5 mm or an angular difference 11 degrees greater than that of adjoining cervical segments indicates instability.

On the plain **anteroposterior radiograph** the cervical spine is visualized from C3 to the thoracic spine. The alignment can be assessed by looking at the spinous processes, which should line up vertically in the midline. The lateral masses should form a continuous undulating curve. Break in the continuity of this line suggests frac-

Subaxial instability

- Horizontal intersegment displacement > 3.5 mm
- Angular displacement > 11 degrees

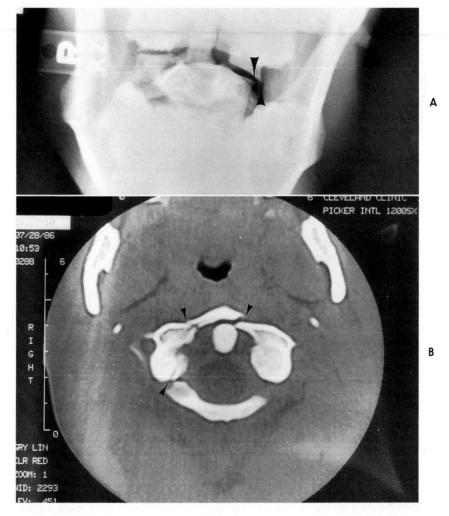

FIG. 49-2. A, Open-mouth view demonstrating Jefferson fracture in professional football player. Jefferson fracture is a bursting injury to C1 ring secondary to axial load. Arrowheads demonstrate incongruency of atlantoaxial joint with overhang of C1 lateral mass on intact axis. **B,** Computed tomography slice through atlas demonstrating anterior and posterior fractures (*arrowheads*) characteristic of Jefferson fracture.

ture or other injury. The intervertebral disk spaces and adjacent vertebral end plates should be aligned parallel to each other in a step-ladder type manner (Fig. 49-1).

The **open-mouth anteroposterior view** is used to evaluate the atlantoaxial joint. The odontoid process is well visualized and should be centered between the lat-

eral masses of C1. The atlantoaxial articulations are well demonstrated and should be congruent. The lateral edge of C1 should line up with the lateral edge of C2 (Fig. 49-1). If the lateral masses of C1 are laterally displaced in relation to C2, a Jefferson fracture should be suspected (Fig. 49-2).

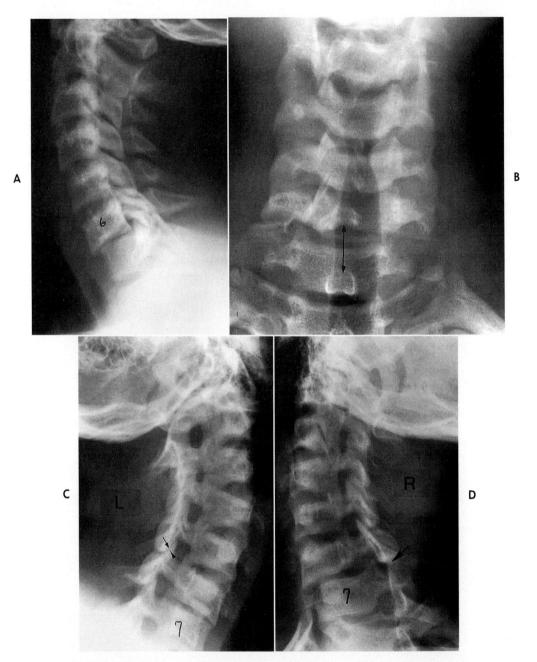

FIG. 49-3. A, Lateral cervical radiograph demonstrating unilateral facet dislocation in 15-year-old following body surfing accident. Film demonstrates anterior displacement of C6 on C7 by approximately 25% of vertebral body width. Posteriorly there is widening in distance between spinous processes of C6 and C7. **B,** Anteroposterior radiograph demonstrates widening in distance between spinous processes of C6 and C7 *(arrow)* and nonparallel C6-C7 intervertebral disk space. **C,** Left oblique view demonstrates normal alignment of facet joints in which superior articular process *(arrowhead)* is anterior to suprajacent inferior process *(arrow)*. **D,** Right oblique view demonstrates findings consistent with unilateral facet dislocation with C7 superior facet articulation *(arrow)* being displaced posterior to C6 facet.

Oblique radiographs are taken with the patient rotated 45 degrees from the frontal plane. On these x-ray films the neural foramina and pedicles are well visualized. The laminae are obliquely orientated and form a shingled appearance. The superior lamina is located posteriorly to the subjacent lamina and overlaps it slightly (Fig. 49-3).

Oblique radiographs complete the standard series for the cervical spine. Accurate interpretation, however, is aided by a careful clinical assessment. Further plain radiographic views may be necessary to elicit more information when clinical suspicion for a significant injury is high and routine radiographs are normal. **Flexion-extension lateral cervical spine radiographs** are occasionally indicated to further evaluate the stability of the cervical spine (Fig. 49-4).[35,45,72,73] Instability of the cervical spine may be assumed from the plain radiographic series if gross deformity is present. However, if the initial radiographic series is normal or has only subtle abnormalities and the clinical suspicion for a cervical injury is high, flexion and extension lateral radiographs may be helpful. These are performed by obtaining a lateral radiograph with the patient *voluntarily* flexing and extending the neck. This dynamic study may unmask anterior subluxation from hyperflexion injury.[32,35] With an acute cervical spine injury, however, muscle spasm and pain may not permit adequate flexion and extension, and the dynamic x-ray films may therefore be normal initially following injury.[72] This may potentially hide an unstable cervical spine injury.[35,52,58,74] Therefore flexion-extension films should be considered only valid if a full range of motion is possible.[73] If it is not, either flexion-extension views should be repeated when the acute pain and muscle spasm have subsided, or another study such as an MRI should be performed.

Herkowitz and Rothman[35] described the concept of subacute instability of the cervical spine. They defined this as the development of radiographic evidence of cervical instability within 3 weeks of injury following initial normal radiographs. They stressed the importance of obtaining adequate flexion-extension radiographs in cervical trauma if the standard cervical spine series is normal, and they emphasized the importance of later reevaluation, including repeat flexion-extension x-ray studies, to avoid missing an unstable cervical spine injury.[35,52,58,74]

Pillar views may also be obtained to visualize the lat-

Additional plain radiograph studies

- Lateral flexion and extension
- Pillar views

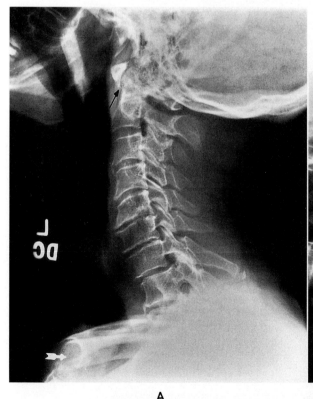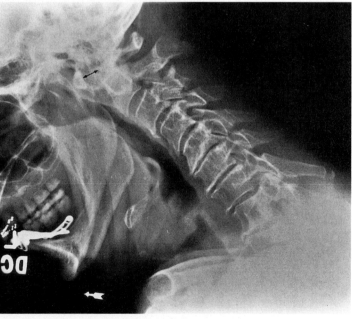

    A   **B**

FIG. 49-4. Lateral flexion and extension radiographs demonstrating C1-C2 instability. **A,** Extension view demonstrates normal atlantodental interval (*arrow*). **B,** Flexion view demonstrates increased atlantodental interval (*arrow*) of over 5 mm, indicative of C1-C2 instability.

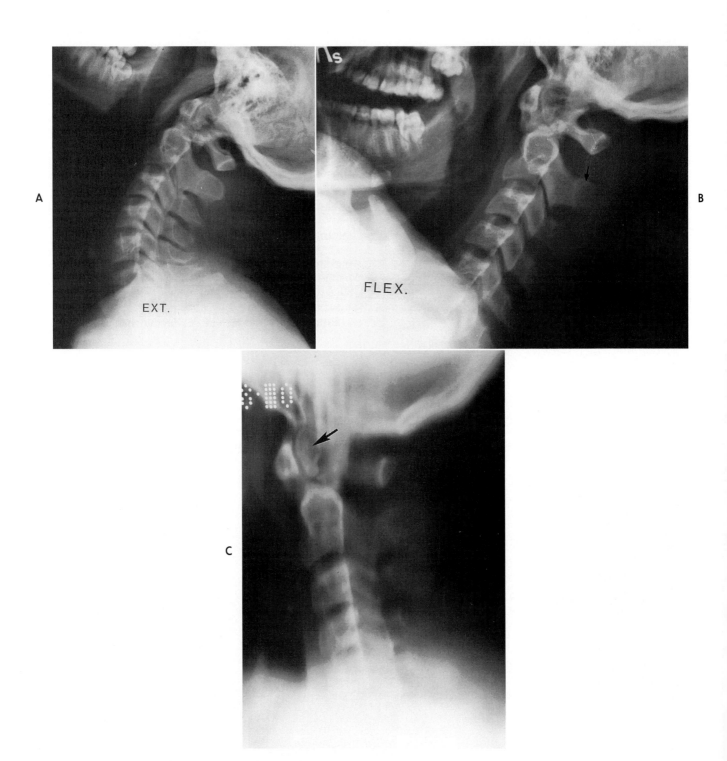

FIG. 49-5. A, Extension lateral radiograph in high-school football player demonstrating abnormality in odontoid process. This odontoid abnormality is, however, poorly defined. **B,** Flexion lateral cervical spine radiograph demonstrates anterior displacement of odontoid and atlas. There is also widening between spinous process of C2 and the arch of C1 *(arrow)*. These findings are consistent with instability from os odontoideum. **C,** Lateral tomogram confirms diagnosis of os odontoideum *(arrow)*.

eral articular masses. To obtain these radiographs, the patient must rotate the neck. Therefore pillar views should only be ordered following careful review of the other views and only if significant injury is excluded. A fracture of the lateral masses may be overlooked with the routine radiographic series, but it should be easily identified on the pillar views.[77]

Tomography

Plain, or linear, tomography still has a role in evaluation of the cervical spine. Tomography demonstrates skeletal detail in a specific plane and field. In the cervical spine the atlantoaxial region can be well visualized by tomography (Fig. 49-5). The fracture line of an undisplaced odontoid fracture is sometimes poorly defined by plain x-ray studies and can therefore be easily overlooked. Even CT of this area may miss such a fracture because the fracture is in the same plain as the CT slice.[12,57] Sagittal reconstruction from the CT may provide more information; however, this often lacks the detail of plain tomography. Tomography cannot only demonstrate the fracture anatomy, but also it is useful in evaluating eventual radiographic union. It can be used to provide detailed images of any area of suspected injury. Superimposed, nonessential anatomic detail can be eliminated, leaving a much clearer view of the area of interest (Fig. 49-6).

A particularly useful indication for plain film tomography is in providing greater detail of poorly visualized areas, such as the occipitocervical and cervicothoracic junctions. At the occipitocervical junction, tomography can provide anatomic detail of structures such as the atlantooccipital facets. Because visualization of the cervicothoracic junction is often difficult because of the presence of the shoulders, tomography may be useful to see detail of this area.

Computed Tomography

CT is an excellent imaging modality for most abnormalities of the cervical spine. CT, as it is usually performed, provides excellent anatomic detail of the spine in the axial plain. With reformatting, sagittal and coronal views are also possible. CT is the best study for providing anatomic bony detail, and in trauma it is therefore the preferred technique for providing imaging of the neural canal and for visualizing detail of the surrounding bony architecture.[10,12,57] To obtain good-quality images of the intervertebral disk, thin sections of 1.5- to 2.0-mm thickness must be obtained. It is important for the scanner gantry to be parallel to the plane of the disk to minimize image distortion.

CT is also useful in the assessment of canal size, and it can provide detailed visualization of bony changes that can occur with other conditions such as vertebral osteomyelitis or spinal tumor. CT evaluation of cervical spinal stenosis is best performed with **intrathecal contrast.**[4,49,50] This visualizes any bony injury and allows assessment of both the functional reserve around the spinal cord and the shape of the cord. Furthermore, contrast-enhanced CT provides better anatomic detail of nerve root impingement because of herniated nucleus pulposus, (Fig. 49-7) or foraminal stenosis. With CT the sagittal diameter of the spinal canal can be measured on the sagittal reformatted images, which minimizes the potential for gantry-angle distortion.[37,46] Measurement of canal dimension on axial CT images can lead to a measurement error with nonorthogonal orientation.

One of the main deficiencies of CT is its inability to visualize transverse fractures occurring in the plane of imaging such as fractures of the odontoid. In addition, dislocations may be missed on transverse CT images,[57] although this is less likely with newer generation, high-resolution CT scanning with reformatted imaging. Other potential disadvantages of CT include the time involved to perform multiple thin sections, streak artifacts as a result of the dense bone of the shoulder girdle, and changes in orientation of the spine that occur between successive motion segments.[4]

3D-CT provides an alternative way of viewing the CT information.[36] It uses the ability of computer software to

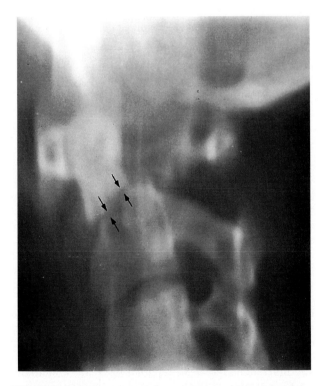

FIG. 49-6. Lateral tomogram demonstrating acute odontoid fracture with slight anterior displacement of odontoid process. Note sharp, well-defined fracture line indicative of acute injury (*arrows*), and compare this to sclerotic border seen with nonunion as in Fig. 49-5, *C.*

Limitations of computed tomography

- Difficulty defining fractures in the plane of the image
- Time factor in thin image acquisition
- Streak artifacts in individuals with dense bone in shoulder girdle
- Changes in orientation of the spine between motion segments

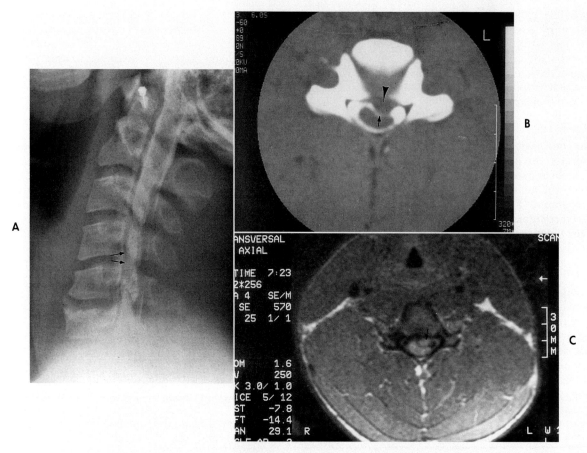

FIG. 49-7. A, Lateral cervical spine myelogram in professional football player demonstrating extradural defect in contrast column opposite C4-C5 disc space *(arrows)* consistent with herniated nucleus pulposus. **B,** Postcontrast computed tomography (CT) scan confirms presence of C4-C5 herniated nucleus pulposus *(arrowhead)* and provides excellent detail of size and shape of herniated disc and resultant cord impingement *(arrow).* **C,** Axial magnetic resonance imaging (MRI) scan at C4-C5 also demonstrates disc herniation *(arrow).* Note comparison of image quality provided by MRI to that of myelogram CT scan.

reformat the axial CT images into a three-dimensional format. The soft tissue is "removed" in the process, leaving only the skeletal detail to visualize. The images are taken in 30-degree increments about a vertical axis, and the information can be visualized on videotape by rotating around any axis in real time. The main advantage of 3D-CT is that it provides superior ability to visualize the spatial relationship of skeletal detail and bony injury (Fig. 49-8).[24]

Magnetic Resonance Imaging

MRI provides unparalleled anatomic detail of spinal anatomy, especially of soft-tissue structures.[4,49,50] The entire spinal cord, nerve roots, and axial skeleton can be visualized in any plane, most commonly in the axial and sagittal planes. MRI provides direct visualization of anatomic structures and is highly sensitive in providing information on a wide range of pathologic conditions (see Fig. 49-10). MRI can demonstrate traumatic ligament and disk disruption in a way not seen with any other mo-

dality.[19,32] As opposed to dynamic flexion-extension radiography in which disruption of ligamentous or bony structures is inferred by the presence of abnormal motion, MRI can visualize such conditions directly. In addition, the intervertebral disk can be assessed, and the spinal canal and its contents can be visualized.

Despite the excellent anatomic detail provided by MRI, it does have its drawbacks. MRI is expensive and is not recommended for patients with claustrophobia. As mentioned previously, bony detail is better visualized by CT than by MRI. Furthermore, abnormalities may be detected that may have little or no clinical significance. For example, the incidence of cervical spine intervertebral disk abnormalities demonstrated by MRI in asymptomatic individuals has been reported to be 19%, including a 10% incidence of herniated nucleus pulposus for those under 40 years of age.[7] The abnormal findings in asymptomatic subjects represent presumed clinical false-positive results, although these are not true anatomic false-positive results. The potential implications of this to

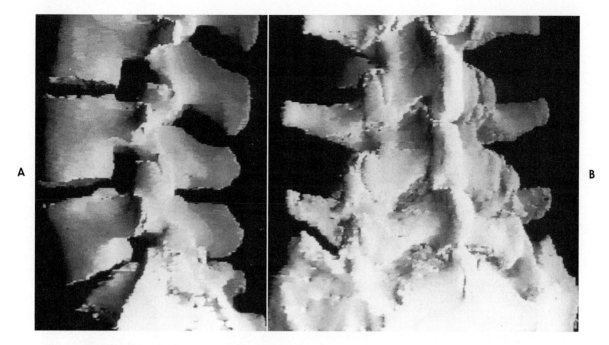

FIG. 49-8. Three-dimensional computed tomography scan of lumbar spine. **A,** Lateral view. **B,** Posterior view.

the athlete are obvious. First, it is important that MRI morphology be closely correlated with the clinical symptoms to accurately assess their significance,[7,45,72,73] and second, it is important to consider the potential clinical implications of unexpected MRI findings. For example, what, if any, is the clinical significance of a large disk herniation in an asymptomatic football player? Does this finding in the absence of symptoms portend a significant risk for potential neurologic injury? These questions have yet to be answered.

Dynamic MRI performed with the neck in neutral, flexion, and extension has been used in the evaluation of the rheumatoid cervical spine.[5] It has also been shown to be useful in evaluating other nonrheumatoid conditions, including spinal canal stenosis.[3,23,51] The advantage of dynamic MRI is its ability to demonstrate the functional relationship of the cord to bony, disk, and ligamentous components of the canal in various positions of flexion. Dynamic MRI can provide information about the dynamic nature of cord compression.[3]

In summary, MRI is an attractive imaging tool. It is noninvasive, involves no ionizing radiation, has no reported side effects, and provides unsurpassed anatomic visualization.[4,49,50] However, interpretation should be made with knowledge of both the clinical history and physical examination to minimize the potential effect of insignificant radiographic abnormalities.

ATHLETIC CONDITIONS AND INJURIES IN THE CERVICAL SPINE
Cervical Spinal Stenosis

The syndrome of transient quadriplegia from cervical spinal cord neurapraxia was described by Torg et al[68] in 1986. This syndrome is characterized by an acute transient cervical spinal cord injury following hyperextension, hyperflexion, or axial loading of the cervical spine. The symptoms and signs may be purely sensory or may have associated motor weakness of either arms, either legs, or all four extremities. Complete recovery usually occurs within 10 to 15 minutes, but it may be delayed. Neck pain may be absent initially. A full range of cervical motion is usually noted following neurologic recovery. A first priority with any patient who has sustained a neck injury with or without quadriplegia is to rule out an acute skeletal injury. After clinical assessment and stabilization, radiologic workup begins with a lateral radiograph followed by a routine plain x-ray series. In football the patient's helmet and shoulder pads are left in place because they provide some support (see Chapter 48).[72,73] Furthermore, removal of the helmet without removal of the shoulder pads may put the cervical spine in an extended position, and this could jeopardize neurologic function. These radiographs should be examined for fracture, malalignment, congenital abnormalities such as Klippel-Feil syndrome,[21] degenerative disk disease, or spinal stenosis. Flexion-extension lateral radiographs should be obtained only after the patient has fully recovered, is conscious, and has a full pain-free range of motion. These radiographs should be scrutinized for malalignment or instability. In a series by Torg et al[68] of 32 athletes who had sustained transient quadriplegia, 17 had developmental stenosis of the spinal canal. Of the other 15, 4 had radiographic evidence of ligamentous instability, 6 had identifiable intervertebral disk disease, and 5 had a congenital abnormality.

Because of the difficulty in obtaining standardized lateral cervical radiographs of known magnification, Torg et al[68] developed a ratio method to measure developmen-

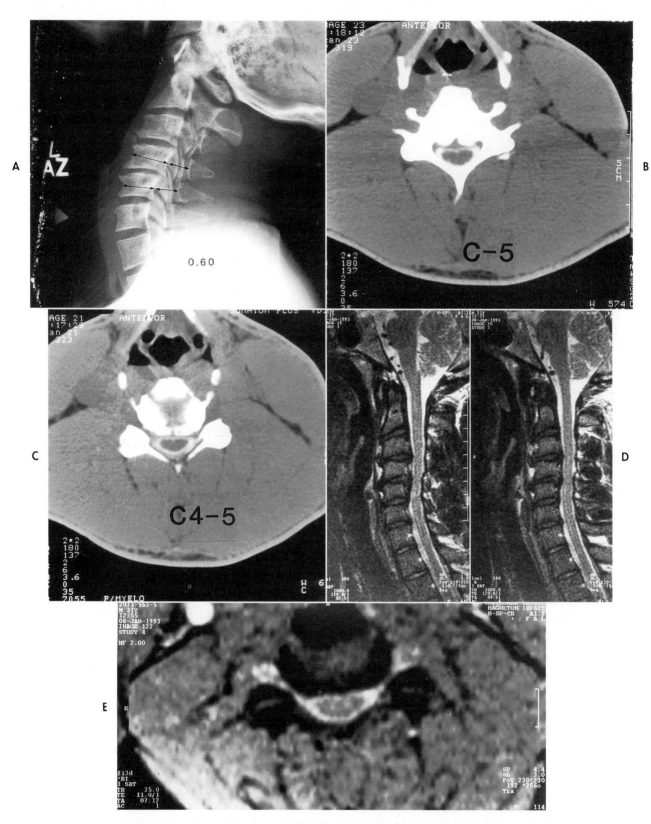

FIG. 49-9. A, Lateral cervical spine radiograph in professional football player who had sustained episodes of transient quadriplegia. Torg ratio at C4 and C5 measured 0.60, highly suggestive of cervical canal stenosis. **B,** Postcontrast computed tomography (CT) scan at C5 demonstrates flattening of cord and thinning of subarachnoid space and surrounding cerebrospinal fluid (CSF), which is consistent with canal stenosis. **C,** Postcontrast CT scan opposite C4-C5 disk space demonstrating canal stenosis with cord flattening and thinning of subarachnoid space. **D,** Sagittal T2-weighted magnetic resonance imaging (MRI) scan eloquently demonstrating extent of canal stenosis. Note that CSF should surround cord at all levels and provide reserve space; however, at C4 and C5 little or no CSF is visualized. **E,** Axial MRI scan opposite C4-C5 demonstrating flattened, bean-shaped cord with diminished surrounding CSF. This image can be directly compared with **C,** the myelogram CT at same level.

Torg ratio

Sagittal canal diameter divided by anteroposterior width of same vertebral body at midpoint
Ratio <0.80 suggests cervical stenosis

Limitations
- Abnormally small ratio may result from large vertebral body
- Up to 50% of asymptomatic individuals may have abnormal ratio
- Magnification factors can affect ratio

---

tal cervical canal diameter. This ratio is represented by the sagittal diameter of the spinal canal divided by the anteroposterior width of the midpoint of the same vertebral body (Fig. 49-9). The sagittal diameter of the spinal canal is measured from the midpoint of the posterior border of the vertebral body to the nearest point on the corresponding spinolaminar line. The sagittal diameter of the spinal canal measured from the lateral radiograph has been shown by CT correlation to accurately reflect the true midline sagittal dimension.[37]

According to the original work of Torg et al[68] a ratio of less than 0.80 indicates cervical stenosis. However, an abnormally small ratio may result from either an excessively large vertebral body or from a small spinal canal diameter. Torg et al[70] subsequently reported that professional football and elite college athletes had smaller ratios than similar age-matched controls primarily because they had a larger vertebral body rather than a smaller canal diameter. This fact was further confirmed by Herzog et al,[37] who reported a detailed radiographic analysis of 80 asymptomatic professional football players. This study was an attempt to establish normal values of cervical spine morphometry and segmental spinal motion in these athletes. A second part of their study evaluated the accuracy of radiographic screening methods for determining cervical spinal stenosis. This study detailed precise measurements of cervical spine morphometry by calculating the exact radiographic magnification factor by the use of radiopaque rulers. It was found that the magnification factor for these athletes was 21% with a range of 18% to 27%. They assessed the Torg ratio at each level of the cervical spine and found that 49% of these asymptomatic athletes had ratios of less than 0.80 at one or more levels, primarily because of the presence of excessively large vertebral body diameters rather than inordinantly small canal diameters. They concluded that although the Torg ratio was extremely sensitive in screening for cervical spinal stenosis, it was not specific.[37,53]

Herzog et al[37] further analyzed 16 athletes who were randomly selected from their population of 80 asymptomatic football players by CT and 9 of these 16 by MRI. They found that MRI was less accurate than CT in assessing bony canal size, but it was superior to CT in its ability to delineate the spinal cord and the functional reserve of the spinal canal. Herzog et al concluded that if magnification factors were unknown on the lateral cer-

vical radiograph, the Torg ratio could be used to screen for cervical stenosis provided that, if found to be abnormal, it was remeasured with plain radiographs of known magnification. The athlete who is found to have true cervical stenosis (as defined by having a sagittal diameter less than two standard deviations below the mean) should then be further examined by functional MRI to assess the spinal cord size and the functional reserve of the spinal canal. The authors stated that the significance of cervical canal stenosis could be determined only if the size of the spinal cord and the functional reserve of the canal were also known.

Work up for cervical stenosis

- Plain radiographs
- Magnetic resonance imaging (MRI)
- Postcontrast computed tomography
- Functional MRI

If MRI is unavailable, myelography and myelogram CT can be used to assess for congenital cervical stenosis.[4,42,49] When combined, these modalities accurately demonstrate canal dimensions, cord size and shape, and functional reserve. Ladd and Scranton[42] presented two cases of transient quadriplegia, one of which myelography and myelogram CT provided evidence of stenosis when the MRI was inconclusive (Fig. 49-10).

Developmental spinal canal stenosis has been recognized to be a significant factor in the development of cervical spondylitic myelopathy.* Ogino et al[54] reported a detailed clinicopathologic study of 9 patients with cervical spondylitic myelopathy. At postmortem they radiographically and histologically studied the spinal cord and neural canal. They demonstrated a direct correlation between the degree of spinal cord destruction and the ratio of the anteroposterior diameter to the transverse diameter of the spinal canal, which they called the *anteroposterior compression ratio (APCR)*.[54,55] Of the many possible factors responsible for a decrease in the APCR, they found that congenital narrowing of the spinal canal was the most significant, whereas acquired multiple spondylitic protrusions were less important. Hence congenital cervical vertebral stenosis, as demonstrated by a small developmental sagittal diameter, was an important factor leading to cervical cord damage. This factor should be considered in the radiographic evaluation of the injured athlete's cervical spine.

Eismont et al[17] investigated the relationship between cervical spine sagittal canal diameter and neurologic injury in patients sustaining cervical spinal fracture-dislocation. They studied a group of 98 patients with cervical fracture-dislocation, 15 of these injuries were sports related, and the authors demonstrated that those patients with more severe neurologic injuries had smaller canal diameters than those with less severe

---

*References 15-17, 20-22, 33, 46, 54, and 55.

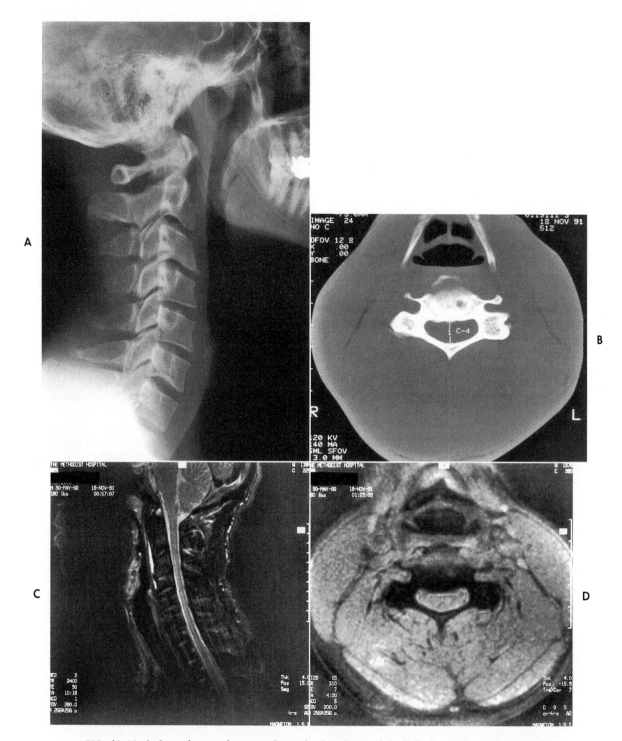

FIG. 49-10. A, Lateral cervical spine radiograph of professional football player who had sustained episodic transient quadriplegia. Torg ratio measured 0.64 at C4, suggestive of canal stenosis. **B,** Unenhanced computed tomography (CT) scan at C4 demonstrates narrowed anteroposterior canal diameter with flattening of spinal cord at C3 and C4. **C,** Sagittal magnetic resonance imaging (MRI) scan demonstrates cervical canal stenosis over several segments. Note paucity of cerebrospinal fluid (CSF) surrounding cord. **D,** Axial MRI scan at C4 demonstrates narrow anteroposterior spinal canal with flattening of cord. Image can be directly compared with CT scan at same level in **B.**

injuries. They concluded that patients with narrow midsagittal canal diameters were at increased risk for developing severe neurologic injury following a traumatic event than those with larger canals, suggesting that a large canal diameter was "protective" against spinal cord injury. The authors stated that the importance of their findings was in attempting to prevent spinal cord injury by appropriate counseling of those patients identified as being at risk.

Trauma

A detailed review of radiology as it relates to trauma is beyond the scope of this chapter. This information is readily available in most standard orthopaedic and trauma texts. It is generally accepted that the usual mechanism of injury in sports-related injuries is either hyperextension, hyperflexion, or axial compression.[26] Axial loading is thought to be the most significant mechanism of injury in serious football cervical spine injuries,[69-71] although a whole spectrum of mechanisms of injury can be seen in association with sports injuries. In their review of the epidemiologic, biomechanical, and cinematographic data compiled from the National Football Head and Neck Registry, Torg and associates[69] implicated axial loading as the primary mechanism responsible in producing severe cervical spine injuries. On this basis, high school and college football rule changes were implemented banning "spearing"; that is, with slight neck flexion, using the top of the helmet as the initial point of contact in tackling an opponent. These rule changes, effective in 1976, have been responsible for the dramatic reduction in the incidence of serious cervical spine injuries seen in football. Further work by Torg and associates[71] suggested that injuries to the cervical spine could be classified into three distinct regions: the upper (C1 to C2), middle (C3 to C4), and lower (C4 to C7) cervical segments. They reviewed 25 cases of C3 to C4 injuries sustained in athletes and found distinct differences in injury patterns when compared with cervical spine injuries at other levels. They reported that injuries to the C3 to C4 segments were unique in that bony injury was uncommon, reduction was difficult, and early aggressive treatment led to a favorable outcome.

THORACOLUMBAR SPINE

The radiographic findings in an athlete with a thoracolumbar spine injury depend on the mechanism of injury and the age of the patient. The skeletal maturity of the patient is an important factor in determining the type and frequency of injuries. In the skeletally immature athlete the spine is particularly vulnerable to injury, especially in more physically demanding sports such as football.[10,39,40] As with other injuries the risk of injury to the spine is greatest during the adolescent growth spurt.[62] However, in sports where training begins at an early age, such as gymnastics, repetitive trauma is an important factor and may result in deformity.[13,62] The most common radiographic abnormalities in the immature thoracolumbar spine include defects of the pars interarticularis, disk abnormalities (such as Schmorl's nodules,

---

> **Common radiographic abnormalities in the immature thoracolumbar spine**
>
> - Pars interarticularis defects
> - Disk abnormality
>   Schmorl's nodules
>   Scheuermann's disease
>   Apophyseal injury
> - Deformity
>   Spondylolisthesis
>   Scheuermann's disease
>   Scoliosis

Scheuermann's disease, or apophyseal injuries), and deformity.[34,62,67] Deformity may be a result of high-grade spondylolisthesis, Scheuermann's disease, or scoliosis. Although a detailed discussion of the radiologic evaluation of deformity is beyond the scope of this chapter, an association between scoliosis and some sports has been reported. Scoliosis has been reported in conjunction with sports in which the athlete sustains asymmetric loading of their trunk or shoulder girdle, such as in tennis or in javelin throwing. Sward et al[64] found a 77% incidence of scoliosis in a group of 30 top Swedish tennis players, although this was mild in degree and was asymptomatic.

In the skeletally mature athlete the incidence and type of complaint referable to the thoracolumbar spine vary with the age of the patient and with the sport. Nevertheless, the most common presenting complaint is mechanical back pain. Degenerative conditions of the spine are common in athletes as well as the general population, and they include conditions such as disk degeneration, herniated nucleus pulposus, and lumbar canal stenosis in older athletes. Although lumbar canal stenosis generally occurs in the over-50 age group, it may appear in the second or third decade of life in patients with coexisting congenital stenosis. Tumor and infection are uncommon, but they are potentially important causes of thoracolumbar spinal pain and should not be overlooked.[6,56]

> **Common radiographic abnormalities in the mature thoracolumbar spine**
>
> - Disk degeneration
> - Spinal stenosis
> - Tumor
> - Infection

Spondylolysis and Spondylolisthesis

The incidence of pars interarticularis defects in athletes has been reported for a wide variety of sports. Spondylolysis has been reported in up to 50% of football linemen,[48] 43% of divers, 30% of wrestlers, 23% of weightlifters,[60] and 16% of gymnasts.[10] The estimated incidence in the general population is between 2.3% and 6.4%.[9,79]

There is a continuum of pars interarticularis injuries that includes stress reaction, defects (spondylolysis) that may be acute or chronic, and slips (spondylolisthesis). Hyperextension has been incriminated as the predominant force in the pathogenesis of pars defects.[9] The reaction of the pars to such repetitive forces consists of microfractures with later bony remodeling (Wolfe's law), which may lead to radiographic sclerosis. When the capacity of the pars interarticularis to heal such microfractures is exceeded, a fatigue fracture occurs. This progression from stress reaction to frank fatigue fracture is well recognized.[75,79] The majority of spondylitic defects occur at the L5 level but may be seen at other levels.[6,18,43,56] Ciullo and Jackson[9] believed that the majority of pars defects seen in their population of gymnasts developed insidiously during childhood. Nevertheless, athletes of all ages are at increased risk for developing acute pars fractures, and, if diagnosed and treated at an early stage, they may heal with resolution of symptoms.[9,39,40,79] Therefore if an athletic adolescent has low back pain, the radiologic evaluation should be targeted toward diagnosis of these potentially curable conditions.

The **initial radiologic evaluation** of the adolescent athlete who has persistent low back pain is with plain x-ray studies. These include anteroposterior, standing lateral, and oblique views of the lumbar spine. With a well-centered lateral radiograph the spot lateral view of the lumbosacral junction may be unnecessary, thereby minimizing the radiation exposure to the skin, bone marrow, and gonads.[43] Flexion and extension lateral radiographs may be obtained if segmental instability is a consideration;[10] however, their use should be limited because they are unlikely to affect clinical decision making in the majority of cases. The anteroposterior x-ray study should be evaluated for alignment, presence of spina bifida occulta, and sclerosis or fracture of the pars. Indirect signs of spondylolysis include reactive sclerosis of the contralateral pedicle, pars, or lamina.[2,61]

Spondylolisthesis is demonstrated on the lateral lumbosacral radiograph as a forward slippage of one vertebra on the subjacent vertebra. Because a standing lateral film may demonstrate more slippage than a supine film,[39,44] standing lateral x-ray studies should be routinely performed. Although the lateral radiograph often demonstrates a pars defect, the oblique view is more reliable.[43] In a review of 1743 radiographs, spondylolysis was seen only on the oblique radiograph in 20% of the 165 cases in which spondylolysis was present.[43] However, if the anteroposterior or lateral radiographs demonstrate a pars defect, the oblique films may be omitted to minimize radiation exposure.[59] On the oblique radiograph the "Scottie dog" sign can be demonstrated with the pars interarticularis forming the neck of the dog. In spondylolysis, there is a break in the neck of the Scottie dog (Fig. 49-11).

The **bone scan** may be considered in the diagnostic workup of the immature athlete who has low back pain and in whom routine x-ray studies were negative. A positive scan suggests that the lesion of the pars is of recent onset. The bone scan is not normally expected to be positive in cases in which the spondylolysis is of long-standing duration, unless other associated degenerative arthritic changes are present.[6,10,18,56] Thus bone scintigraphy can help determine the age of a previously demonstrated lesion and can thereby be helpful in determining treatment. The scan can also detect a stress fracture

---

Lumbar spine series

- Anteroposterior view
- Lateral (standing) view
- Oblique view

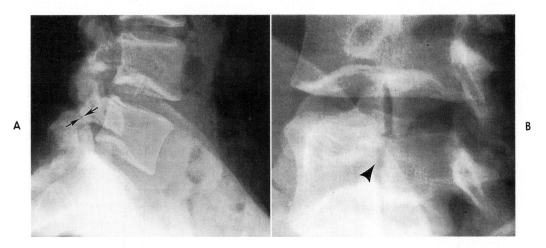

FIG. 49-11. A, Lateral lumbosacral radiograph of professional basketball player who had persistent low back pain. *Arrows* demonstrate acute fracture line in pars interarticularis of L5. **B,** Oblique lumbar spine radiographs provide greater detail of pars interarticularis and determine bilaterality of lesion. In this radiograph, acute fracture in pars interarticularis is well demonstrated as break in neck of "Scottie dog" *(arrowhead).*

to the pars interarticularis even before x-ray studies reveal the lesion.

Although bone scintigraphy is sensitive in detecting bony lesions, it is not specific. Infection, tumor, and arthritic changes may also lead to increased radionucleotide uptake. It is therefore important to correlate the findings on bone scan with both the x-ray series and the clinical setting.

The value of bone scintigraphy in the evaluation of young athletes with low back pain was assessed by Papanicolaou and associates,[56] who reviewed the bone scans and radiographs of 40 young athletes. Radiographs and bone scans were positive for spondylolysis in 14 of these athletes. In five patients the radiographs were positive, but the scans were normal, suggesting longstanding spondylolysis. Four patients had positive scans but normal x-ray studies, indicating an acute pars stress reaction. The authors concluded that bone scintigraphy was valuable in the workup of young athletes with low back pain to diagnose pars stress reactions before radiographic change and that it was useful in determining the age and activity of a lesion visualized on a plain x-ray study.

Single photon emission computed tomography (SPECT) scanning is a form of bone scintigraphy that improves the ability to localize and diagnose bony abnormalities. Like planar tomography, SPECT improves diagnostic localization by the spatial separation of overlapping bony structures. Bellar et al[6] compared planar scanning with SPECT scanning in the assessment of 162 adolescent athletes who had low back pain. In 91 patients both planar scintigraphy and SPECT were normal. In 71 patients SPECT scanning revealed a focus of increased radionucleotide uptake in the pars. In 32 of these 71 patients the planar bone scan was also abnormal; however, in 39 of the 71 patients the abnormality was demonstrated only by SPECT. The authors concluded that SPECT was more sensitive than planar scintigraphy in the assessment of a pars stress reaction (Fig. 49-12).

CT has also been used in the evaluation of the athlete with spondylolysis and spondylolisthesis. On routine CT of the lumbar spine, it may be difficult to distinguish the facet joint from a spondylolytic defect.[29] Reformatted images may provide more detail by reversing the gantry angle of the CT to allow the CT slice to pass along the pars interarticularis, thus providing direct imaging of the pars.[30]

In the majority of athletes with low back pain, CT is unnecessary. However, it is important to correlate the clinical setting with the radiologic and scintigraphic studies. Occasionally a benign tumor such as osteoid osteoma may be suspected, and CT may provide the diagnosis. If spondylolisthesis exists, CT scanning can provide information about possible neural impingement within the canal, in the neural foramen, or under the spondylolytic defect.[47]

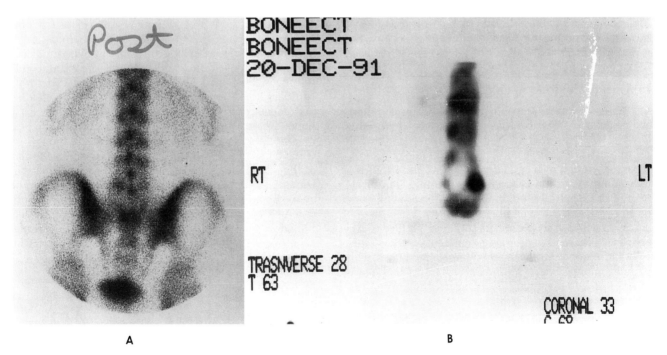

A   B

FIG. 49-12. A, Bone scan in athlete who had low back pain and whose lumbar spine radiographs were normal. Bone scan was interpreted as normal. **B,** Single photon emission computed tomography (SPECT) scan in same patient demonstrates an area of increased radionucleotide uptake in left pars interarticularis. This is consistent with acute pars fracture.

Schmorl's Nodules and Scheuermann's Disease

Schmorl's nodules are common radiographic findings on plain x ray and have a reported incidence of up to 76%.[62] They are considered to represent intervertebral disk herniations occurring through the vertebral end plates into the vertebral body and are thought to result from compression overload injury. Schmorl's nodules are reported with equal frequency among athletes and nonathletes.[62] They are well visualized on plain x-ray and MRI images.

Two types of Scheuermann's disease are recognized: thoracic and lumbar variants. Classic **thoracic Scheuermann's disease** is characterized by wedging of three or more consecutive vertebral bodies by 5 degrees or greater with associated disk space abnormalities, such as Schmorl's nodules, reduced disk height, and end plate irregularity. The apex of kyphosis in thoracic Scheuermann's disease is typically around T8. In **lumbar Scheuermann's disease** the peak incidence is at L1.[62] This form of Scheuermann's disease is reported to be more common among athletes than nonathletes, and trauma is implicated in its pathogenesis.[66] Although often asymptomatic, lumbar Scheuermann's disease may be painful.

In general, the radiologic evaluation of the athlete with suspected Scheuermann's disease is by plain x-ray study. On the lateral radiograph, vertebral wedging is the most specific finding of thoracic Scheuermann's disease and is accompanied by increased thoracic kyphosis. In the lumbar form of Scheuermann's disease, vertebral wedging and associated deformity is less common, with the radiographic findings consisting of intervertebral disk space abnormalities such as narrowing or end plate irregularities. MRI may be useful to visualize intervertebral disk abnormalities before plain x-ray changes[66]; however, its routine use is not recommended because the added information is unlikely to affect clinical decision making or to justify the added expense.

Injuries to the Ring Apophysis

Injuries to the ring apophysis, although uncommon, are a recognized cause of back pain or sciatica in the athlete.[1,8,63,67] The vertebral ring apophysis encircles the upper and lower end plates of each vertebral body and is separated from it by a cartilaginous layer. The longitudinal and intervertebral ligaments and annulus fibrosis attach to the apophysis, which fuses to the vertebral body between 12 and 25 years of age.[14] Injury is reported to occur predominantly within the anterior portion of the apophysis; however, posterior apophyseal injury is clinically more important because it can be associated with neural compression.[1,67] Most reports of injury to the posterior ring apophysis have been reported following athletic or other trauma.

The diagnosis of a fracture of the ring apophysis may be difficult, since plain radiographic changes may be subtle. Sward et al[63] documented serial radiographic changes to the ring apophysis in two adolescent gymnasts who had persistent back pain following hyperflexion and rotation injuries. Plain x-ray studies demonstrated evidence of injury to the anterior part of the T12

ring apophysis. This was manifested by excavation of the upper anterior corner of the twelfth vertebral body with progressive disk space narrowing and kyphosis at the T11-T12 intervertebral disc. There was delay in the appearance of these radiographic changes, which took up to 12 months to fully develop. The authors concluded that conventional radiography may remain unremarkable for several months following anterior apophyseal injury and that planar bone scintigraphy might also be normal because the injury is predominantly cartilaginous rather than bony. MRI, however, was able to visualize the apophyseal injury and the associated disc degeneration.

Although less common, it is important to recognize the posteriorly displaced apophyseal vertebral fracture because it may mimic the clinical presentation of a herniated nucleus pulposus.[1,8,67] Plain x-ray studies may show a small bony fragment adjacent to the posterior margin of the vertebral body that is displaced into the spinal canal. This fragment may be displaced from either the caudal or cephalad border of the posterior vertebral body, which is represented as a wedge-shaped defect in the vertebral body. CT is the method of choice in defining the degree of neural compromise, the nature and appearance of the displaced fragment, and any associated injury.[11,67]

Takata and associates[67] presented a series of 31 posterior marginal fractures of the lumbar vertebral body and proposed a classification based on CT findings. In their series only 5 of the 31 fractures could be diagnosed on the basis of the plane x-ray study. Although lateral planar tomography was useful in visualizing these injuries, CT was determined to be the method of choice. The authors concluded that injuries to the posterior ring apophysis may be more common than previously thought and may represent a common cause of sciatica in children.

Although sciatica resulting from herniated nucleus pulposus in adolescents is uncommon, athletic and other trauma is considered an important etiologic factor.[25,28,41] Kurihara and Kataoka[41] reported a series of 70 children and adolescents operated on for sciatica. Of these patients, 22 were injured during sporting pursuits, and the majority were exposed to repetitive trauma. Although the clinical presentation in this age group is similar to that of the adult, the diagnosis is often delayed because the condition is not considered.[25,28,41] The radiologic evaluation should begin with the plane x-ray series to exclude other pathologic conditions, such as disk space infection, tumor, or apophyseal injury. The next examination may be one of MRI, CT, or myelography, all of which reliably demonstrate a herniated nucleus pulposus, if present.

REFERENCES
1. Albeck MJ et al: Fracture of the vertebral ring apophysis imitating disc herniation, *Acta Neurochir (Wien)* 113:52, 1991.
2. Amato M, Totty WG, Gilula LA: Spondylolysis of the lumbar spine: demonstration of defects and laminal fragmentation, *Radiology* 153:627, 1984.
3. Ando T et al: "Dynamic" MR imaging of the cervical cord in patients with cervical spondylosis and ossification of the posterior longitudinal ligament—significance of dynamic cord compression, Rinsho Shinkeigaku-*Clin Neurol* 32:30, 1992.
4. Bell GR, Ross JS: Diagnosis of nerve root compression: myelog-

raphy, computed tomography, and MRI, *Orthop Clin North Am* 23:405, 1992.

5. Bell GR, Stearns KL: Flexion-extension MRI of the upper rheumatoid cervical spine, *Orthpaedics* 14:969, 1991.

6. Bellar RD et al: Low back pain in adolescent athletes: detection of stress injury to the pars interarticularis with SPECT, *Radiology* 180:509, 1991.

7. Boden SD et al: Abnormal magnetic resonance scans of the cervical spine in asymptomatic subjects, *J Bone Joint Surg* 72A:1178, 1990.

8. Browne TD, Yost RP, McCarron RF: Lumbar ring apophyseal fracture in an adolescent weight lifter, *Am J Sports Med* 18:533, 1990.

9. Ciullo JV, Jackson DW: Pars interarticularis stress reaction, spondylolysis, and spondylolisthesis in gymnasts, *Clin Sports Med* 4(1):95, 1985.

10. Coin CG et al: Diving-type injury of the cervical spine: contribution of computed tomography to management, *J Comput Assist Tomogr* 3:362, 1979.

11. Dake MD, Jacobs RP, Margolin FR: Computed tomography of posterior lumbar apophyseal ring fractures, *J Comput Assist Tomogr* 9:730, 1985.

12. Dorvart RH, LaMasters DL: Applications of computed tomographic scanning of the cervical spine, *Orthop Clin North Am* 16:381, 1985.

13. Dzioba RB, Gervin A: Irreversible spinal deformity in Olympic gymnasts, *Orthop Trans* 8:66, 1984.

14. Edelson JG, Nathan H: Stages in the natural history of the vertebral end plates, *Spine* 13:21, 1988.

15. Edwards WS, LaRocca SH: The developmental, segmental, sagittal diameter of the cervical spinal canal in patients with cervical spondylosis, *Spine* 8:20, 1983.

16. Edwards WS, LaRocca SH: The developmental, segmental, sagittal diameter in combined cervical and lumbar spondylosis, *Spine* 10:42, 1985.

17. Eismont F et al: Cervical sagittal spinal canal size in spine injury, *Spine* 9:663, 1984.

18. Elliott S, Hutson MA, Wastie ML: Bone scintigraphy in the assessment of spondylolysis in patients attending a sports injury clinic, *Clin Radiol* 39:269, 1988.

19. Emery SE et al: Magnetic resonance imaging of posttraumatic spinal ligament injury, *J Spinal Disorders* 2:229, 1989.

20. Epstein JA et al: Cervical myelopathy caused by developmental stenosis of the spinal canal, *J Neurosurg* 51:362, 1979.

21. Epstein N, Epstein JA, Zilkha A: Traumatic myelopathy in a seventeen-year-old child with cervical spinal stenosis (without fracture or dislocation) and a C2-C3 Klippel-Feil fusion, *Spine* 9:344, 1984.

22. Epstein N et al: Traumatic myelopathy in patients with cervical spinal stenosis without fracture or dislocation—methods of diagnosis, management, and prognosis, *Spine* 5:489, 1980.

23. Epstein N et al: Technical note: "Dynamic" MRI scanning of the cervical spine, *Spine* 13:937, 1988.

24. Fielding JW, Fietti VG, Mardam-Bey TH: Athletic injuries to the antlantoaxial articulation, *Am J Sports Med* 6:226, 1978.

25. Fisher RG, Saunders RL: Lumbar disc protrusion in children, *J Neurosurg* 54:480, 1981.

26. Funk FJ, Wells RE: Injuries of the cervical spine in football, *Clin Orthop* 109:50, 1975.

27. Gore D, Sepic S, Gardner G: Roentgenographic findings of the cervical spine in asymptomatic people, *Spine* 11:521, 1986.

28. Grobler LJ, Simmons EH, Barrington TW: Intervertebral disc herniation in the adolescent, *Spine* 4:267, 1979.

29. Grogan JP et al: Spondylolysis studied with computed tomography, *Radiology* 145:737, 1982.

30. Hardcastle P et al: Spinal abnormalities in young, fast bowlers, *J Bone Joint Surg* 74B:421, 1992.

31. Harris JH: Radiographic evaluation of spinal trauma, *Orthop Clin North Am* 17:75, 1987.

32. Harris JH, Yeakley JW: Hyperextension-dislocation of the cervical spine: ligament injuries demonstrated by magnetic resonance imaging, *J Bone Joint Surg* 74B:567, 1992.

33. Hasimoto I, Yoon-Kil T: The true sagittal diameter of the cervical spinal canal and its diagnostic significance in cervical myelopathy, *J Neurosurg* 47:912, 1977.

34. Hellstrom M et al: Radiologic abnormalities of the thoracolumbar spine in athletes, *Acta Radiol* 31:127, 1990.

35. Herkowitz H, Rothman RH: Subacute instability of the cervical spine, *Spine* 9:348, 1984.

36. Herman GT, Liu HK: Display of three-dimensional information in computed tomography, *J Comput Assist Tomogr* 1:155, 1977.

37. Herzog RJ et al: Normal cervical spine morphometry and cervical spinal stenosis in asymptomatic football players, *Spine* 16(suppl 6):178, 1991.

38. Jackson DW, Lohr FT: Cervical spine injuries, *Clin Sports Med* 5:373, 1986.

39. Jackson DW, Wiltse LL, Cirincione RJ: Spondylolysis in the female gymnast, *Clin Orthop* 117:68, 1976.

40. Kraus DR, Shapiro D: The symptomatic lumbar spine in the athlete, *Clin Sports Med* 8(1):59, 1989.

41. Kurihara A, Kataoka O: Lumbar disc herniation in children and adolescents, *Spine* 5:443, 1980.

42. Ladd A, Scranton P: Congenital cervical stenosis presenting as transient quadriplegia in athletes, *J Bone Joint Surg* 68A:1371, 1986.

43. Libson E et al: Oblique lumbar radiographs: importance in young patients, *Radiology* 151:89, 1984.

44. Lowe RW et al: Standing roentgenograms in spondylolisthesis, *Clin Orthop* 117:80, 1976.

45. Marks MR, Bell GR, Boumphrey FRS: Cervical spine fractures in athletes, *Clin Sports Med* 9:263, 1990.

46. Matsura P et al: Comparison of computerized tomography parameters of the cervical spine in normal control subjects and spinal cord–injured patients, *J Bone Joint Surg* 71A:183, 1989.

47. McAfee PC, Yuan HA: Computed tomography in spondylolisthesis, *Clin Orthop* 166:62, 1982.

48. McCarroll JR, Miller JM, Ritter MA: Lumbar spondylolysis and spondylolisthesis in college football players, *Am J Sports Med* 14:404, 1986.

49. Modic MT, Ross JS, Masaryk TJ: Imaging of degenerative disease of the cervical spine, *Clin Orthop* 239:109, 1989.

50. Modic MT et al: Cervical radiculopathy: prospective evaluation with surface coil MR imaging, CT with metrizamide, and metrizamide myelography, *Radiology* 161:753, 1986.

51. Nagele M et al: Dynamic functional MRI of the cervical spine, *Fortsch Roentgenstr* 157:222, 1992.

52. Nash CL: Acute cervical soft-tissue injury and late deformity, *J Bone Joint Surg* 61A:305, 1979.

53. Odor JM et al: Incidence of cervical spinal stenosis in professional and rookie football players, *Am J Sports Med* 18:507, 1990.

54. Ogino H et al: Canal diameter, anteroposterior compression ratio, and spondylitic myelopathy of the cervical spine, *Spine* 8:1, 1983.

55. Ono K et al: Cervical myelopathy secondary to multiple spondylitic protrusions—a clinicopathologic study, *Spine* 2:109, 1977.

56. Papanicolaou N et al: Bone scintigraphy and radiography in young athletes with low back pain, *AJR* 145:1039, 1985.

57. Post MJD et al: The value of computed tomography in spinal trauma, *Spine* 7:417, 1982.

58. Rifkinson-Mann S, Morino J, Sachdev VP: Subacute cervical spine instability, *Surg Neurol* 26:413, 1986.

59. Roberts FF, Kishore PRS, Cunningham ME: Routine oblique radiography of the pediatric lumbar spine: is it necessary? *AJR* 131:297, 1978.

60. Rossi F, Dragoni S: Lumbar spondylolysis: occurrence in competitive athletes, *J Sports Med Phys Fitness* 30:450, 1990.

61. Sherman FC, Wilkinson RH, Hall JE: Reactive sclerosis of a pedicle and spondylolysis in the lumbar spine, *J Bone Joint Surg* 59A:49, 1977.

62. Sward L: The thoracolumbar spine in young elite athletes, *Sports Med* 13:357, 1992.

63. Sward L et al: Acute injury of the vertebral ring apophysis and intervertebral disc in adolescent gymnasts, *Spine* 15:144, 1990.

64. Sward L et al: Anthropometric characteristics, passive hip flexion, and spinal mobility in relation to back pain in athletes, *Spine* 15:376, 1990.

65. Sward L et al: Back pain and radiologic changes in the thoracolumbar spine of athletes, *Spine* 15:124, 1990.
66. Sward L et al: Disc degeneration and associated abnormalities of the spine in elite athletes—a magnetic resonance imaging study, *Spine* 16:437, 1991.
67. Takata K et al: Fracture of the posterior margin of a lumbar vertebral body, *J Bone Joint Surg* 70A:589, 1988.
68. Torg JS et al: Neuropraxia of the cervical spinal cord with transient quadriplegia, *J Bone Joint Surg* 68A:1354, 1986.
69. Torg JS et al: The epidemiologic, pathologic, biomechanical, and cinematographic analysis of football-induced cervical spine trauma, *Am J Sports Med* 18:50, 1990.
70. Torg JS et al: The relationship of cervical spinal canal narrowing (stenosis) to permanent neurologic injury to the athlete: an epidemiological survey. Paper presented at the American Orthopaedic Society for Sports Medicine, Sun Valley, Idaho, July, 1990.
71. Torg JS et al: Axial loading injuries to the middle cervical spine segment, *Am J Sports Med* 196, 1991.

72. Watkins RG: Neck injuries in football players, *Clin Sports Med* 5:215, 1986.
73. Watkins RG, Dillin WH, Maxwell J: Cervical spine injuries in football players, *Spine* 4(2):347, 1990.
74. Webb JK et al: Hidden flexion injury of the cervical spine, *J Bone Joint Surg* 58B:322, 1976.
75. Weir MR, Smith DS: Stress reaction of the pars interarticularis leading to spondylolysis, *J Adolesc Health* 10:573, 1989.
76. White AA, Panjabi MM: *Clinical biomechanics of the spine*, Philadelphia, 1978, JB Lippincott.
77. Wier DC: Roentenographic signs of cervical injury, *Clin Orthop* 109:9, 1975.
78. Wiesel SW et al: A study of computed-assisted tomography. I. The incidence of positive CAT scans in an asymptomatic group of patients, *Spine* 9:549, 1988.
79. Wiltse LL, Jackson DW: Treatment of spondylolisthesis and spondylolysis in children, *Clin Orthop* 117:92, 1976.

CHAPTER 50

Diagnosis and Treatment of Cervical Spine Injuries

Louis H. Rappoport
Patrick F. O'Leary
Frank P. Cammisa, Jr.

Although cervical spine injuries are relatively uncommon in athletes, they represent a significant proportion of the most devastating injuries, those which may result in permanent disability or death. With sports participation continuing to surge, the sports medicine physician and orthopaedic surgeon should have a clear understanding of the realm of potential cervical spine injuries in the athletic population. The knowledge base begins with a fundamental comprehension of cervical spine anatomy and biomechanics. From this knowledge base, principles and guidelines of diagnostic evaluation and treatment of specific injury patterns should be mastered.

With the continuing evolution of sports medicine, the sports physician and orthopaedic surgeon have the responsibility of teaching the athletes and other involved parties a basic understanding of the cervical spine and its potential injuries. This should include continuing education concerning the prevention and recognition of serious injuries, as well as their appropriate treatment.

EPIDEMIOLOGY

The main thrust of the application of epidemiologic methods to the study of spinal injury in sports is aimed at identifying injury trends and correlating these trends with definite risk factors. During this process a directed program of training can be initiated, preparticipation screening can be made more effective, and equipment design can be modified appropriately.

To begin multifactorial analysis of the relationship between risk factors and spinal injury in athletics, data with respect to the host (age, somatotype, and conditioning of the athlete), agent (equipment and actions involved in the accident), and environment (weather and playing surface) must be accumulated in a national collection bank. After correlations have been confirmed, aggressive measures may be taken to adjust variables, and ultimately, to reduce the incidence of sports injuries, especially to the spinal cord and central nervous system. For example, in 1975 the National Football Head and Neck Injury Registry was established by Torg, Vegso, and Sennett[84] and was followed by a complete 14-year report on cervical quadriplegia in 1987. As a result of the implementation of rules changes, documented cervical spine injuries resulting in permanent quadriplegia decreased dramatically.

The application of epidemiologic methods to spinal injury in sports is difficult at best. Three primary reasons exist for these difficulties. First, most spinal injuries are self-limited and resolve without coming to the attention of health care personnel. Second, because most athletes are reluctant to document minor injuries in detail, injuries of all types are characteristically underreported. This can be easily demonstrated in preparticipation cervical radiographs showing evidence of previous injury without a given supporting history. Third, many athletic injuries in organized sports occur during practice, when health care personnel usually are not in attendance.[24]

Available epidemiologic data in most retrospective studies—the problems of which have been noted—indicate that the incidence of all spinal injuries in sports is relatively low, varying from 5% to 15%. In a prospective study analyzing head and neck injuries in college football players from 1975 to 1982, Albright et al[2] reported neck injuries occurring in 18% of players. The majority of these injuries were minor (55%); however, the remaining 45% experienced at least transient neurologic symptoms or deficits. In their review of permanent cervical cord injuries in football between 1977 and 1989, Cantu and Mueller[12] reported an incidence of 0.62/100,000 in junior high and high school players and 1.64/100,000 in college players.

Cervical spine injuries may be associated with many sporting activities, including gymnastics, football, rugby, trampoline jumping, ice hockey, racquet sports, water sports, automobile racing, motorcycle racing, snowmobiling, skiing, horseback riding, mountain climbing, skydiving, hang gliding, parachuting, and track and field events.* It is readily apparent from this list that contact sports, high-speed sports, and sports associated with unpredictable variables (e.g., skydiving) pose the greatest risk of sustaining a cervical spine injury.

Although certain trends are being established, no strict rules can be applied. Any particular mechanism with possible catastrophic sequelae may occur by chance in any sport.

BIOMECHANICAL CONSIDERATIONS IN ATHLETIC CERVICAL SPINE INJURIES

Although most investigators have attributed either hyperflexion or hyperextension forces as the major mechanism resulting in serious athletic cervical spinal injuries,* recent literature suggests that axial loading is the predominant force involved in these injuries.† Much of this literature has concerned cervical spine injuries occurring in football players, although it appears that it can be extrapolated to other high-risk sports, such as rugby, diving, and ice hockey.

The school of thought regarding axial loading as the predominant mechanism of injury has evolved from the National Football Head and Neck Registry report.[84] In this review, Torg et al[86] documented a significant decrease in the number of cervical spine injuries following the implementation of a rule change that banned "spearing," the use of the top of the helmet to make initial contact with another player. Cinematographic analysis of cervical spine injuries occurring during football games revealed axial loading to be the primary mechanism of injury.

According to Torg et al,[86] forces exerted on the cervical spine are generally dispersed via energy absorption by the paraspinal musculature and intervertebral disks through controlled spinal motion. However, with approximately 30 degrees of flexion the cervical spine becomes a straight segmented column with resultant loss of controlled spinal motion under axial loading conditions. Thus when an athlete uses the crown of the head for contact, the cervical spine assumes a straight position and axially directed forces are transmitted directly to the intervertebral disks, ligamentous tissues, and the bony structures. Axial loading of this segmented column can then result in fractures or dislocation, depending on the magnitude of the axial force and the effect of variable secondary forces such as axial rotation.

Spear Tackler's Spine

Torg et al[88] have defined an entity they have titled *spear tackler's spine* (box). Permanent neurologic injury has been documented by Torg et al in individuals with this problem, and the authors suggest that individuals who have these characteristics be precluded from participation in collision activities that expose the cervical spine to axial energy inputs.[88] In this entity the spine is always in a position to sustain an axial load.

Criteria for Spear Tackler's Spine

- Developmental narrowing (stenosis) of cervical canal
- Persistent straightening or reversal of the normal cervical lordotic curve on erect lateral radiographs obtained in the neutral position
- Concomitant preexisting posttraumatic radiographic abnormality of the cervical spine
- Documentation of having employed spear tackling techniques

Other investigators have shown the inadequacy of the helmet in protecting the cervical spine against axial compressive forces.[7] Thus it appears from this data that protective equipment may not be the answer in preventing

---

*References 2, 10-13, 22, 32, 49, 54, 56, 58, 68, 69, 75, 78, 80, 84, 85, and 89.

*References 23, 44, 49, 58, 69, and 70.
†References 68, 75, 80, 83, 84, and 86-89.

cervical spine injuries in athletes. Rather, the implementation of rules similar to those now used in football may have an effect in preventing serious cervical spine injuries in other contact sports.

HISTORY AND PHYSICAL EXAMINATION

In performing a history and physical examination of the cervical spine in sports injuries, the physician should adhere closely to well-established principles of orthopaedic clinical evaluation. Strict adherence to a set working pattern is the key to rapid and accurate diagnosis.

Several elements of the clinical evaluation are unique. First, in evaluating the history the examiner must be aware that athletes tend to underreport injuries, symptoms, or both. This phenomenon may occur on the playing field or at the preparticipation clinical evaluation. Second, the examiner should attempt to identify preexisting congenital abnormalities and their implication in preventing athletic cervical spine injuries. Third, the history of previous cervical injury and its severity should be carefully evaluated and correlated to the stresses and risks of the particular sport. Fourth, an aggressive approach to physical diagnosis and treatment is also important. The highly trained athlete cannot afford the time loss with a trial-and-error method of diagnosis or a wait-and-see attitude towards treatment. The rigorous demands of national and world-class sports make a rapid return to practice regimens and competition essential.

The preliminary history should include the origin and initiation of pain, as well as its chronologic course. The nature of the pain should be delineated along with exacerbating and ameliorating factors. The occurrence and temporal patterns of pain (e.g., night pain) should be noted. The presence of neurologic symptoms, including numbness, painful dysesthesia or paresthesia, or weakness should be noted. The specific pattern of pain or neurologic radiation should be documented. The history of deformity should include its onset of presentation, presence of progression, temporal association with pain, previous treatment, and family history of similar deformity. The history of known congenital abnormalities, such as Klippel-Feil disease or os odontoideum, should be documented because they may prove detrimental to the competitive athlete.

Previous trauma or injury to the cervical spine should be documented, and the mechanism of injury should be explained in detail. Systemic disease possibilities should also be investigated in depth, since this policy may infrequently reveal an occult tumor or infection in an athlete of any age.

Finally, the history should include an evaluation of the athlete with reference to his or her particular sport. There may be preexisting abnormalities that may not become significant until stressed in a specific manner.

Although this chapter deals specifically with the evaluation and treatment of cervical spine injuries, the physician must perform a brief, but complete, musculoskeletal examination, including evaluation of the other regions of the spine. The gait and stance of the patient should be closely observed. The patient should be eval-

uated for evidence of ligamentous laxity. Range of motion of major peripheral joints, especially of the upper extremities, should be documented. Frontal and sagittal plane spinal abnormalities should be noted. Lumbar spine range of motion should also be evaluated.

Following this general musculoskeletal examination, attention can be specifically directed to the cervical spine evaluation. An accurate examination of the cervical spine in the athlete rests on a strong foundation of applied topographic anatomy and sound neurologic examination. Palpation of bony landmarks is an essential part of the examination. For example, it is possible to palpate the transverse process of the atlas halfway between the mastoid process of the skull and the angle of the mandible. Anteriorly, it is possible to palpate the vertebral bodies. Specifically, the carotid tubercle can be palpated by pressing a finger carefully through the interval between the carotid sheath and sternocleidomastoid muscles laterally and between the trachea, esophagus, and thyroid gland medially. In cervical strains, tenderness of the longus colli muscle is common. The presence of paraspinal muscle spasm and tenderness should be noted. Percussion of the cervical spine may elicit painful areas, which can represent an occult infection of fracture. Active and passive range of motion should be evaluated for flexion, extension, rotation, and lateral bending and recorded in degrees. Pain occurring during specific cervical motions should be documented. Provocative tests, such as the Spurling's maneuver, are helpful in the diagnosis of cervical spinal disease and have been well documented elsewhere.

A thorough neurologic examination should be performed to document motor strength, sensation, deep tendon reflexes, and the presence or absence of pathologic reflexes (i.e., Babinski's or Hoffmann's). Because the athletic population is extremely well conditioned as a rule, the examiner must be sensitive to minimal muscular weakness, which is evidenced by early fatigue of the muscle group being tested. The examiner must also evaluate for muscular atrophy or fasciculations in the extremities. A detailed sensory examination that includes two-point discrimination, proprioception, light touch, pinprick, temperature discrimination, and sensitivity to pain should be performed. In addition, a rectal examination, which evaluates perianal sensation, sphincter tone, and contraction, should be performed to complete the neurologic examination.

Finally, signs of cervical fracture such as a headache, nystagmus, disorientation, and difficulty swallowing (secondary to retropharyngeal edema) may be seen with neck pain, muscle spasm, decreased motion, and possible neurologic deficit.

SPINAL CORD AND OTHER NEUROLOGIC INJURIES

Spinal cord injuries are rare in athletics, but do occur in sports such as football, diving, high-speed motor racing, boxing, karate, and gymnastics. The mechanism of injury may be a fall during play or a severe impact of the athlete's head with a stationary object (e.g., an opponent's body part) (Fig. 50-1). The clinical spectrum of

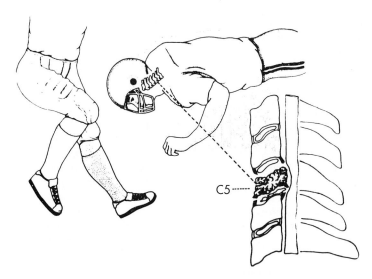

C5

FIG. 50-1. "Spearing," which involves butting opponent in midsection with one's head (illegal in American football), can result in a burst fracture and spinal cord injury.

neural element lesions ranges from complete spinal cord injuries with total loss of spinal cord function below the injury level to incomplete spinal cord injuries, which by definition preserves some degree of cord function caudal to the level of injury. Other neurologic injury patterns that may occur in athletes include isolated nerve root lesions, nerve root–brachial plexus neuropraxia, or spinal cord neuropraxia with transient quadriplegia.

The degree of spinal cord injury cannot be determined until the period of spinal shock has resolved, usually within 48 hours from injury. The return of the bulbocavernosus reflex is indicative that the patient is out of spinal shock.

The role of drug treatment for spinal cord injuries remains controversial. In a recent study, Bracken, Shepard, and Collins [9] evaluated the efficacy and safety of methylprednisolone in a prospective, randomized, double-blind, placebo-controlled, multicenter study. Methylprednisolone was administered as an initial 30-mg/kg bolus followed by a 5.4 mg/kg/hr infusion for 23 hours. The authors concluded that significant motor and sensory improvement was found in patients who were administered the steroids within 8 hours of injury. In addition, they reported no significant increase in the complication rate. Although the conclusions found in this study remain open to debate, it represents the most current controlled study on the use of steroids in the treatment of spinal cord injuries.

Recently, attention has been directed towards the use of gangliosides in the treatment of spinal cord injuries. In a small prospective, randomized, double-blind, placebo-controlled study of GM-1 ganglioside, Geisler, Dorsey, and Coleman[25] reported significant neurologic recovery 1 year following injury with the use of this experimental drug. The investigators hypothesized that gangliosides act to induce the regeneration of neural tissues. In addition, they reported no significant complications attributable to this therapy program. However, the authors clearly state that further large-scale studies are required before the routine use of GM-1 in the treatment of spinal cord injuries can be advocated.

Complete Spinal Cord Lesions

Complete spinal cord lesions define a complete transverse lesion at the level of injury, which may be a result of frank anatomic disruption of the spinal cord or may occur secondary to progressive cord hemorrhage and ischemia. At the time of diagnosis a complete loss of all motor function and sensation below the level of injury is present. The physician must carefully evaluate for the presence of sacral sparing before confirming this diagnosis. The prognosis in these patients is guarded, with recovery of significant cord function below the injury level unlikely to occur. However, nerve root function may recover one or two segmental levels below the level of injury as the edema at the traumatic cord level resolves.

Complete cord lesions in the upper cervical spine (occiput to C3) usually impair the respiratory center, resulting in death. Complete lesions of the spinal cord below C4 are seen with varying degrees of sparing of the nerve roots supplying the upper extremities. In C4-C5 lesions, there may be some late evidence of sparing of the C5 nerve root unilaterally or bilaterally, such as return of some deltoid function and shoulder motion. Injuries at the C5-C6 level may spare some or all of the C6 root function, allowing primarily elbow flexion and wrist extension. Injuries at the C6-C7 level may spare the C7 nerve root, thereby providing the patient with elbow and finger extension and wrist flexion. A C7-T1 level injury may spare the C8 nerve root, allowing for grip function.

Incomplete Spinal Cord Lesions

Incomplete spinal cord injuries can be subdivided into the (1) central cord syndrome, (2) Brown-Séquard syndrome, (3) anterior cord syndrome, and (4) posterior cord syndrome.

The **central cord syndrome** is the most common of

the incomplete cord syndromes. It occurs as the result of an insult, either hemorrhagic or ischemic, to the central portion of the spinal cord.[71] This results in a disproportionately greater neurologic deficit (motor weakness) in the upper extremities, as compared to the lower extremities, due to the somatotopic organization of the spinal cord. These patients usually present as a complete quadriplegia but with sacral sparing. They may have associated nonspecific sensory loss, as well as bowel/bladder and sexual dysfunction. Classically, this lesion occurs in older athletes with preexisting cervical spondylosis who sustain a hyperextension injury of the cervical spine.[47] However, this syndrome may occur in any age group as a result of a flexion-extension cervical spine injury. Neurologic recovery is generally greater in the lower extremities than in the upper extremities, and usually includes recovery of bowel-bladder function.

The **Brown-Séquard syndrome** represents an anatomic hemisection of the spinal cord. This results in a loss of ipsilateral motor function (corticospinal tracts) and contralateral pain and temperature sensation (spinothalamic tracts). In addition, there is loss of ipsilateral touch, vibration, and position sense (dorsal columns). Events producing this syndrome are unusual in most athletics, although penetrating injuries occurring in fencing or hunting could result in this injury pattern. More commonly, the Brown-Séquard syndrome is clinically found in association with other incomplete cord lesions.[5] There is a good prognosis for recovery of bowel-bladder function and ambulation capabilities.

The **anterior cord syndrome** represents an injury to the anterior two thirds of the spinal cord, resulting in bilateral loss of motor function and spinothalamic tract function below the level of injury. However, there is preservation of dorsal column function. In addition, bowel-bladder and sexual dysfunction are usually present. The syndrome occurs secondary to ischemic injury in the region of the spinal cord supplied by the anterior spinal artery. In general, the prognosis for recovery of functional ambulation is poor.

The **posterior cord syndrome** is exceedingly rare, resulting in loss of only dorsal column function. As the motor function is completely intact, the patient usually develops a slap-foot gait. This injury pattern occurs secondary to ischemia in the cord region supplied by the posterior spinal artery.

Selected Nerve Root Injuries

Isolated lesions of the C5 through T1 nerve roots may result following cervical spine injury. These lesions present as cervical radiculopathies with a specific dermatomal distribution on clinical examination. They must be distinguished from peripheral nerve injuries. They can occur as a result of an acute cervical disk herniation or in a setting of preexisting cervical spondylosis with osteophytic narrowing of the neuroforamen and subsequent minor trauma. A classic case occurs in the tennis player who develops radicular pain during the hyperextension movement of the cervical spine during serving (Fig. 50-2).

Avulsion injuries to the cervical nerve roots most commonly are incurred during high-velocity sports, such as

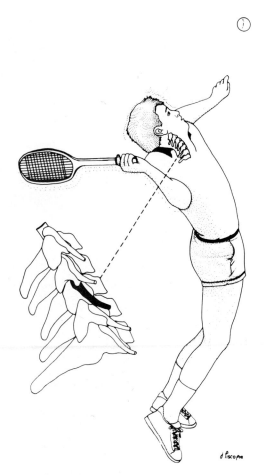

FIG. 50-2. Hyperextension injury can cause cervical radiculopathy.

automobile racing, speedboat racing, or aviation, but they can also occur in football. A postmyelogram CT scan revealing characteristic pooling of contrast around the avulsed nerve root sleeve is diagnostic (Fig. 50-3). Clinical manifestations of C5 root avulsion usually include lack of deltoid power, some diminished biceps strength, and decreased sensation and paresthesias along the proximal lateral aspect of the arm. Lesions at the C6 level primarily affect the biceps and wrist extensor motor function, as well as loss of the biceps reflex, and diminished sensation to the thumb and radial aspect of the forearm. Lesions at the C7 level affect the triceps, finger extensor, and wrist flexor motor functions, as well as loss of the triceps reflex and diminished sensation to the long finger. Injuries at the C8 level result in finger flexion weakness and decreased sensation of the little finger and ulnar aspect of the forearm. Avulsion of the T1 nerve root produces decreased intrinsic hand function and diminished sensation along the medial aspect of the elbow and arm. In addition, patients with T1 root avulsions usually have an associated unilateral Horner's syndrome.

In cases of significant functional disability, surgical procedures such as nerve grafting or reconstruction and muscle transfers may be required to improve the function of the upper extremity. In general, extensive rehabilitation is required in most cases, including the use of orthotics as necessary.

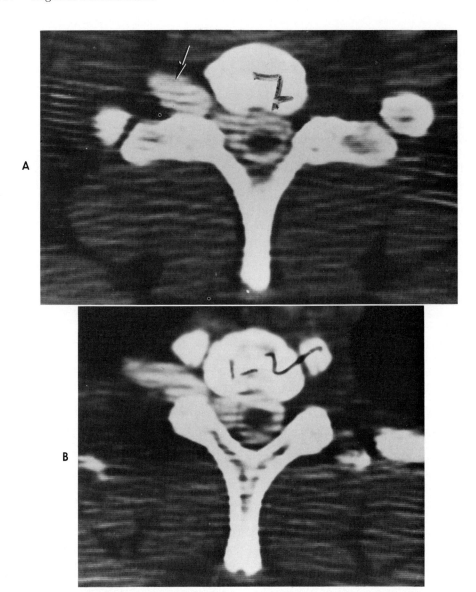

FIG. 50-3. A, Computed tomography scan taken after cervical myelogram shows dye leakage: diagnostic of nerve root avulsion at C7-T1 in patient whose brachial plexus lesion resulted from an automobile accident. **B,** Same lesion shown at level of T1-T2.

Nerve Root–Brachial Plexus Neurapraxia

Nerve root–brachial plexus neurapraxia is the most common athletic cervical neurologic injury.[77] It is more commonly known as a "stinger" or "burner."[63] It represents a traction injury to the cervical nerve roots or brachial plexus and is frequently diagnosed in football players or wrestlers. The usual mechanism of injury is shoulder depression with lateral neck flexion to the contralateral side (Fig. 50-4). Alternatively, cervical spine extension, compression, and rotation toward the affected arm can produce this injury.[47,89] The latter mechanism of injury represents the Spurling's maneuver, which is used clinically to diagnose foraminal nerve root compression. The clinical symptoms include burning (lancinating) pain, numbness, and tingling extending from the shoulder to the hand of the affected extremity. There may be associated paralysis of the extremity, usually only lasting for several minutes. On occasion the neurologic symptoms may last for days to months, especially following repetitive insults. The syndrome most commonly affects the upper trunk of the plexus (C5-C6). Athletes sustaining "burner" injuries usually have a normal cervical range of motion, distinguishing this clinical entity from a "neck" injury. Following complete resolution of symptoms an athlete with a normal neurologic examination and full painless cervical range of motion may return to his or her normal level of activity.

Athletes who experience multiple clinical episodes or have persistent symptoms 3 weeks following the injury should have routine radiographic evaluation of the cer-

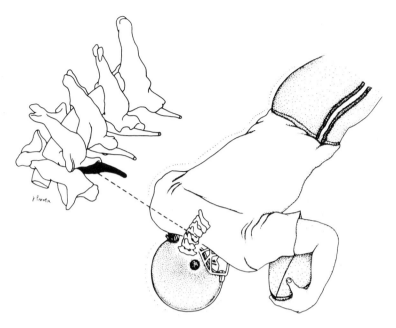

FIG. 50-4. Acute lateral flexion of cervical spine causes brachial neurapraxia, known in football as a "burner."

vical spine, as well as a complete neurologic evaluation, including an electromyographic (EMG) and nerve conduction study.[33,77] If the neurophysiologic evaluation is negative, the patient should begin a physical therapy program, including stretching and strengthening exercises of the neck musculature. Return to athletic competition is allowed as previously described. In addition, football players should wear well-fitted shoulder pads and a cervical roll to limit the neck range of motion at impact.[33,77,89] The lesion should be considered an axonotmesis if the EMG is abnormal. In these cases, return to contact sports should be delayed until the symptoms have resolved, full cervical muscle strength has been achieved, and a repeat EMG shows evidence of axonal regeneration, usually 4 to 6 weeks following injury.[77]

Spinal Cord Neurapraxia with Transient Quadriplegia

The clinical entity of cervical spinal cord neurapraxia has been well described in the literature.[38,77,79,82,85] The syndrome consists of transient sensory and motor abnormalities occurring after a forced hyperextension, hyperflexion, or axial loading injury of the cervical spine. Specific sensory changes include burning pain, numbness, tingling, or complete anesthesia, whereas motor symptoms can range from weakness to complete paralysis. As defined by Torg et al[85] the episodes are distinctly transient with complete recovery of neurologic function generally occurring after a 10- to 15-minute period, although a gradual recovery over 48 hours may occur in some individuals. In the diagnosis of this specific entity, neck pain should not be present at the initial clinical evaluation. Although the majority of cases have been reported in football players, the injury has also been reported to occur in ice hockey, basketball, and boxing.[85]

In the review by Torg et al,[85] radiographic findings included developmental stenosis, congenital fusion, cervical instability, or intervertebral disk disease. There were no cases of radiographic evidence of cervical spine fracture or dislocation. Ladd and Scranton[38] reported two cases of transient quadriplegia in football players, both of whom had radiographic evidence of congenital cervical stenosis.

Although most investigators have agreed that the sagittal diameter of the spinal canal is the key radiographic measurement in the correlation of cervical canal size and spinal cord injury, there appear to be inconsistencies in the methods of determination.[16,48,61,85] To establish normal values for the sagittal diameter of the spinal canal, consistent spinal landmarks and imaging techniques (magnification factors) must be used. Because of inconsistencies in the literature a ratio method was developed to compensate for the various evaluation techniques.[61] The ratio method consists of a comparison of the anteroposterior width of the spinal canal to the anteroposterior width of the corresponding vertebral body at its midpoint. These measurements can be determined on a routine lateral radiograph of the cervical spine from the third to the sixth vertebral bodies. In using this method a ratio of less than 0.80 has been defined as indicating significant cervical stenosis because of its association with a transient quadriplegic event in athletes.[61,79,82,85] In other words, it is inferred that in patients who have preexisting spinal canal stenosis, a sustained injury that results in a further decrease in the sagittal dimension of the canal can lead to a transient quadriplegic event. However, in a study by Odor et al,[57] approximately one third of football players evaluated had a ratio of less than 0.80 at one or more cervical levels. Thus while a relationship between cervical stenosis (Torg criteria) and a transient quadriplegic event appears to exist, a ratio of less than 0.80 does not necessarily predispose an athlete to a transient quadriplegic event. In addition, athletes who sustain an episode of transient quadriplegia do not appear to be at increased risk for an additional transient quadriplegic event, or more importantly, for the development of a permanent neurologic injury. Although these patients can generally be treated nonoperatively, surgery may become necessary in select cases, such as in the athlete with an associated central disk herniation.

The question of restriction of activities in athletes who have sustained an episode of transient quadriplegia remains unclear. Advice regarding return to play or risk of future injury should be based on the following factors: (1) severity and frequency of symptoms, (2) nature of the sporting activity, (3) duration of signs, (4) radiographic evaluation (i.e., severity of stenosis), (5) neurologic evaluation, (6) age of the athlete, (7) anticipated duration of the athlete's career, and (8) medicolegal considerations.[59,81]

RADIOGRAPHIC EVALUATION

The athlete with a presumptive diagnosis of a cervical spine injury should undergo a routine radiographic evaluation of the cervical spine for definitive diagnosis.[76] Plain radiographs should be used for the initial evaluation. A cross-table lateral radiograph should be the first study obtained.[36,46,47,60] This should be performed with the patient remaining on the spine board or stretcher so as not to incur neurologic injury with movement of the patient. All seven cervical vertebrae must be easily identified on the radiograph, including the C7-T1 disk space. In athletes with large shoulders it may be necessary to place gentle traction on the arms to depress the shoulders. Alternatively, a swimmer's view can be obtained. If there remains difficulty in visualization of the cervicothoracic junction, lateral tomograms or a CT scan may be necessary. An open-mouth odontoid view and anteroposterior view should then be obtained.

The lateral radiograph should reveal a gentle lordotic curve. Continuous lines along the anterior and posterior borders of the vertebral bodies, the posterior cortices of the lateral masses, and the spinolaminar line should be identified. The prevertebral soft tissues should be evaluated because they represent an indirect sign of cervical injury. The atlantodens interval (ADI) should be no greater than 3 mm in adults[20] or 4 mm in children. On the open-mouth odontoid view, the C1-C2 lateral masses should be aligned and the odontoid should be centered between the C1 lateral masses. In addition, a fracture of the odontoid process may be visualized on this view. On the anteroposterior view the spinous processes should be well aligned, the vertebral endplates parallel to each other, and the tracheal air shadow in the midline. The uncovertebral joints and lateral masses should be symmetric.

In the event these standard views show an essentially normal spine and there is a high index of suspicion of a cervical injury, additional views can then be obtained. Further studies include oblique views to evaluate the intervertebral foramina, pedicles, and facet joints, pillar

views to rule out lateral mass fractures, and lateral flexion-extension radiographs to rule out instability. The latter views should be performed actively by the patient because passive neck motion could result in neurologic injury. White, Southwick, and Panjabi[90] have developed radiographic criteria for segmental instability in the cervical spine. Translational instability is defined as ≥3.5 mm of displacement in the sagittal plane, whereas angular instability is defined as a minimal difference of 11 degrees between adjacent spinal segments.

Conventional tomography is useful in evaluating areas of the cervical spine that are difficult to visualize on routine radiographs (e.g., the cervicothoracic junction). In addition, fractures oriented in the axial plane, which can be difficult to evaluate with routine axial CT, can often be well visualized with conventional tomography. Facet and lateral mass fractures can also be clearly delineated with conventional tomography.[15]

In the evaluation of most cervical spine fractures, CT provides the best delineation of the fracture pattern and bony anatomy. Bony fragmentation within the spinal canal and spinal canal size can be clearly assessed with axial CT images. Reformatted sagittal plane images can be useful in evaluating axial plane fractures. CT can also be used to critically assess "suspicious" plain radiographs and may detect occult fractures not visualized with conventional radiography.[8,14] When combined with intrathecal contrast, CT evaluates for neural element compression, although this is largely being replaced with magnetic resonance imaging (MRI). If used, intrathecal contrast should be administered through a lateral C1-C2 puncture without turning the patient to the prone position. There are distinct differences in the CT appearance of the spine of children compared with those of adults because of the presence of incomplete ossification.[64]

MRI is being increasingly used in the diagnostic evaluation of cervical spine injuries. It is most useful in the evaluation of the cervical neural elements and soft-tissue structures.[51] Parenchymal spinal cord injury, extradural compression of the spinal cord, and nerve roots can be well visualized with MRI. MRI may be quite useful in the evaluation of the athlete with a neurologic deficit that does not appear to be associated with a bony injury on routine radiographs and CT images. In this setting, MRI may detect intrinsic spinal cord injury or extradural neural element compression resulting from a cervical disk herniation or hematoma. For example, in the evaluation of older individuals with preexisting cervical spondylosis who sustain a hyperextension injury associated with a central cord syndrome, MRI can distinguish intrinsic cord damage, such as intramedullary hematoma or edema, from extradural compression.[27] This diagnostic information is quite critical in that the presence of significant extradural neural element compression usually requires acute surgical management. Posterior ligamentous injuries can be well visualized with MRI, and this information can be used by the surgeon in planning an appropriate management plan. In the diagnostic evaluation of cervical facet dislocations or fracture-dislocations, MRI is quite useful in evaluating for a concomitant disk herniation, which may accompany these injuries.

Some investigators have attempted to correlate the

MRI findings in acute cervical spine trauma with both the severity of clinical neurologic injury and the prognosis for recovery.[21,65,66] Significant spinal cord intramedullary hematoma has been associated with the most severe neurologic deficits and the worst prognosis for recovery. On the other hand, the MRI appearance of a normal spinal cord or one showing only small focal areas of cord edema has been associated with the least severe neurologic deficits and the best prognosis for recovery.

Therefore the complete radiographic evaluation of the athlete who has sustained a cervical spine injury may consist of a series of imaging techniques designed to provide valuable and complementary information.

SPECIFIC CERVICAL SPINE INJURIES
Upper Cervical Spine Injuries
Atlantooccipital Dislocation

Injuries at the atlantooccipital level are rare (Fig. 50-5). They generally occur secondary to high-speed trauma. The majority of atlantooccipital dislocations are fatal, resulting from devastating neurologic injury at this level with resultant respiratory arrest. Should the patient survive, careful early realignment and halo-vest immobilization should be performed, followed by posterior occipitocervical fusion, generally to the C1 or C2 level. Cervical traction must be avoided in these injuries because

significant distraction of neurologic tissues can occur secondary to the severe ligamentous disruption between the occiput and C1.

C1 Fractures

Fractures of the atlas (C1) usually occur secondary to an axial compressive load, which forces the occipital condyles into the lateral masses of C1. The four major types of atlas fractures described in the literature are (1) anterior arch fracture or avulsion, (2) posterior arch fracture, (3) lateral mass fracture, and (4) burst (Jefferson's) fracture (Fig. 50-6). In contrast to injuries at the occiput-C1 level, fractures of the ring of C1 rarely produce a neurologic injury because they are decompressive lesions. They generally result in symptoms of severe neck pain and headaches.

Fractures of the atlas may be difficult to evaluate with routine radiographs, and as such, plain tomography and CT may be required for complete evaluation. An open-mouth odontoid view should be performed to evaluate for the presence of lateral mass displacement of C1.

Although the major mechanism of injury in fractures of the atlas is axial loading, these injuries also involve secondary forces, such as shear, flexion, extension, or rotation. As a result, contiguous or noncontiguous cervical spine injuries must be ruled out. Levine and Edwards[42] have shown that approximately 50% of patients with posterior arch fractures have an associated cervical spine injury, with the most common being posteriorly displaced odontoid fractures or traumatic spondylolisthesis of the axis.

Isolated anterior or posterior arch fractures can be treated in a rigid orthosis or halo vest for 3 months because they are stable injuries. However, the presence of associated cervical injuries may alter the treatment plan.

Unilateral fractures of the lateral mass of C1 generally occur only on one side of the neural arch, although an additional posterior arch fracture on the opposite side has been reported.[42] Characteristically, the open-mouth radiograph reveals variable asymmetric displacement of the lateral mass.

Jefferson's, or burst, fracture of the atlas involves combined anterior and posterior arch fractures on both sides of the neural arch. There is usually a symmetric displacement of the lateral masses on the open-mouth radiograph. In a cadaveric study, Spence, Dedser, and Sell[73] have shown that a total lateral mass displacement greater than 6.9 mm implies rupture of the transverse ligament.

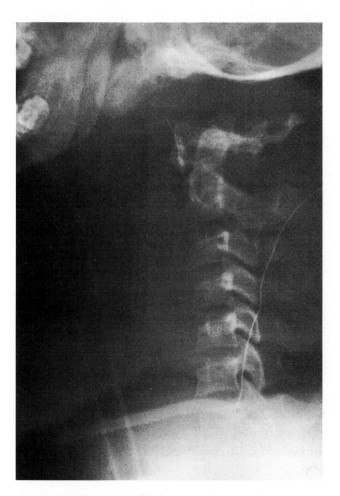

FIG. 50-5. Atlantooccipital dislocation with severe displacement.

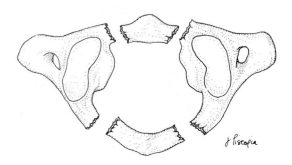

FIG. 50-6. Jefferson's fracture of first cervical vertebra.

However, the clinical significance of this associated transverse ligament insufficiency with respect to C1-C2 instability is controversial. Levine and Edwards[42] have shown that late C1-C2 instability does not seem to occur in this subset of patients, whether or not reduction of the lateral masses was performed. In their review, no patient had an ADI greater than 5 mm on review of flexion-extension radiographs following fracture healing. The authors theorized that isolated transverse ligament disruption occurring with atlas fractures leaves the remaining stabilizing soft-tissue structures intact (i.e., the alar ligaments), thereby preventing gross instability.

The role of reduction of lateral mass displacement remains controversial. The development of posttraumatic arthrosis of the C1-C2 articular facets with resultant chronic neck pain has not been definitively correlated to the presence or absence of residual lateral mass displacement, although painful nonunions and malunions of atlas fractures appear to occur.[72]

Although still somewhat controversial, it appears that the majority of lateral mass and Jefferson's fractures can be treated by halo-vest immobilization until fracture healing has occurred, usually in 3 months. Tomography can be used to assess fracture healing during the course of treatment. Flexion-extension lateral radiographs should be obtained following fracture healing to rule out significant C1-C2 instability. Although there are not definitive guidelines at present, patients with significant lateral mass displacement (>7 mm) can be treated with skeletal traction to achieve lateral mass reduction. Prolonged axial traction (a minimum of 6 weeks) is required to maintain reduction because a halo vest cannot provide adequate cervical spine distraction for fracture reduction.

Following early fracture healing the patient should be immobilized in a halo vest until fracture union. Alternatively, fractures with significant displacement can be reconstructed by an anterior reduction and plate fixation technique via a transoral approach.[30] Although the latter is a technically demanding procedure, it allows for the preservation of significant rotation at the C1-C2 motion segment.

In patients with associated chronic C1-C2 instability, assessment of union of the posterior arch fracture is important. If the posterior fracture has healed after halo-vest immobilization, a posterior C1-C2 fusion can be performed. If the posterior arch fracture has not healed, options for treatment include posterior occiput-C2 fusion, anterior C1-C2 reduction and plate fixation,[30] or posterior C1-C2 transarticular screw fixation.[28] Alternatively, the latter two procedures can be performed as the initial treatment if significant instability is present with resultant preservation of the occipitocervical motion segment. However, these latter procedures do require proper technical training before their clinical use.

Atlantoaxial Instability without Fracture

Rupture of the atlantoaxial ligamentous complex (transverse, apical, and alar ligaments) can occur without an associated fracture, resulting in atlantoaxial instability. These ligamentous injuries can occur following severe flexion loads and can lead to a significant increase in the ADI (Fig. 50-7). Patients with preexisting rheumatoid arthritis or connective tissue disease may require less force to produce this injury. The resultant instability may result in spinal cord injury because the odontoid process compresses the spinal cord against the posterior

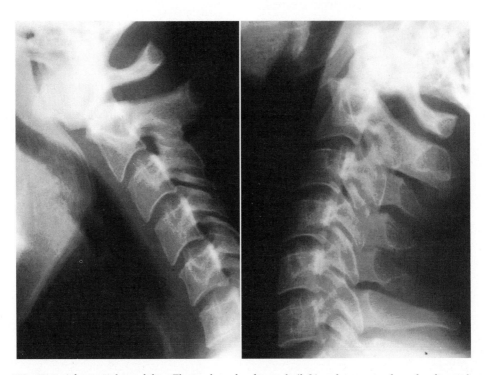

FIG. 50-7. Atlantoaxial instability. Flexion lateral radiograph (*left*) and extension lateral radiograph (*right*) revealing dynamic C1-C2 instability.

arch of C1. However, damage to the spinal cord is rare unless significant displacement occurs because the space available for the cord is large in this region.

Fielding et al[20] have shown that the normal anterior ADI in adults is ≤3 mm. The transverse ligament was found to rupture in the ADI range of 3 to 5 mm, with an ADI >5 mm indicative of incompetency of the remaining atlantoaxial ligamentous complex.

Because atlantoaxial instability is a pure ligamentous injury, stabilization can only be achieved via a surgical approach. Treatment of this injury consists of a posterior C1-C2 fusion, most commonly with a wire construct.

C1-C2 Rotatory Subluxation

Atlantoaxial rotatory subluxation is a condition that primarily affects children, but it may also occur in adults. This condition may occur spontaneously, such as following an upper respiratory infection in children, or it may result from trauma. The patient has a painful torticollis associated with significant apprehension to cervical range of motion. The injury rarely results in a neurologic deficit. The mechanism of injury is believed to be primarily a combination of distraction and axial rotation, resulting in subluxation of the lateral C1-C2 articulation. In long-standing cases the subluxation often becomes fixed in the abnormal position. Atlantoaxial rotatory subluxation has been classified into four types, depending on the severity and direction of C1 displacement and the presence and degree of associated increase in the ADI.[19]

Critical radiographic analysis is essential in establishing the diagnosis. The anteroposterior open-mouth radiograph demonstrates overriding of the C1-C2 articulation on the side of subluxation ("wink sign"), and the contralateral joint appears normal. The lateral radiograph is critical in determining the ADI and should be obtained in flexion and extension if there is a suspicion of instability. Dynamic CT scans in left and right axial rotation positions can be helpful in demonstrating the fixed relationship at the C1-C2 articulations.

Children with acute injuries usually respond to a brief period of cervical traction followed by symptomatic collar immobilization. Acute deformities in adults may be reduced with skeletal traction followed by halo-vest immobilization for 8 to 12 weeks. Acute deformities that do not reduce with traction obligate surgical reduction and

posterior C1-C2 arthrodesis. Recurrent deformities and those that are associated with significant C1-C2 instability (>5 mm) or neurologic deficit require posterior C1-C2 stabilization and fusion. Alternatively, direct anterior reduction and C1-C2 plate fixation can be performed for unstable or irreducible (closed) deformities.[30] Chronic subluxations (>3 months) may not reduce with traction, and often require posterior fusion for pain relief.

Odontoid Fractures

Anderson and D'Alonzo[3] have classified fractures of the odontoid into three types according to the fracture location (Fig. 50-8). Type 1 fractures represent a ligamentous avulsion of the tip of the odontoid process; Type 2 fractures occur at the neck of the odontoid process; and Type 3 fractures occur at the base of the odontoid process and extend into the body of C2. Odontoid fractures should also be evaluated based on the degree of displacement and angulation at the fracture site. These fractures may be diagnosed on plain radiographs, including open-mouth odontoid views. In addition, the physician should evaluate the prevertebral soft tissues on the lateral radiograph at the C2 level, since abnormal widening represents an indirect sign of injury. If necessary, tomography may be performed to aid in diagnosis to define the extent of the fracture, and to rule out an associated fracture of the posterior arch of C1, which may alter the treatment plan.

Type 1 fractures are considered stable because the fracture occurs cephalad to the intact transverse ligament. Type 1 fractures are rare and can be treated symptomatically in a cervical collar.

Type 2 fractures can result from hyperextension, flexion, rotation, or lateral forces in various combinations. The treatment of Type 2 fractures remains controversial. These fractures have a poor prognosis for healing and a nonunion rate of 15% to 85%, despite adequate immobilization. In a multicenter study, Clark and White[14] reported a 68% union rate for Type 2 fractures treated by halo-vest immobilization. Risk factors for nonunion included (1) age >50, (2) displacement >5 mm, (3) posterior (vs anterior) displacement, and (4) improper treatment (i.e., overdistraction in a halo).[29,53,67] Initial treatment of a young patient without risk factors for nonunion consists of halo-vest immobilization for 12 weeks in a re-

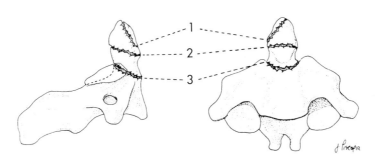

FIG. 50-8. Anderson and D'Alonzo's classification of odontoid fractures. Type 1 fractures represent ligamentous avulsion of tip of odontoid process. Type 2 fractures occur at neck of odontoid process. Type 3 fractures occur at base of odontoid process and extend into body of C2.

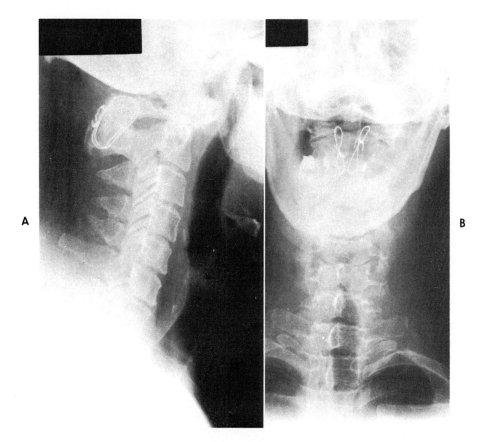

FIG. 50-9. Posterior C1-C2 fusion for Type 2 odontoid fracture. **A,** Lateral view. **B,** Anteroposterior view.

duced position. Follow-up tomography and flexion-extension radiographs can then be performed to assess fracture healing and stability. Nonunions of odontoid fractures are generally treated with a posterior C1-C2 fusion. Patients with significant risk factors for nonunion can initially be treated by a posterior C1-C2 fusion (Fig. 50-9). Alternatively, several investigators have recommended direct anterior odontoid screw fixation[18,53] or transoral reduction and plate fixation[43] to preserve C1-C2 axial rotation. These techniques are useful in cases of a concomitant posterior arch fracture of C1. In addition, the transarticular C1-C2 fusion technique of Magerl has been recommended in specific injury patterns.[28,34]

Type 3 fractures, which extend into the cancellous bone of the C2 body, have a high rate of union. These fractures are generally treated with halo-vest immobilization for 3 months. Although impacted, nondisplaced fractures can alternatively be treated in a rigid cervical orthosis. Follow-up assessment of fracture union and stability should be routinely performed.

Traumatic Spondylolisthesis of C2

Traumatic spondylolisthesis of C2, also called *hangman's fracture*, most commonly occurs in automobile accidents, but it also occurs with increased frequency in athletes of football, ice hockey, gymnastics, aquatic, and equestrian sports. Neurologic injury directly attributable to the fracture is uncommon. Diagnosis can usually be made on the routine lateral radiograph. Supervised flexion-extension lateral radiographs can be performed in the awake, intact patient to assess the degree of instability. Tomography can be used to assess complex injury patterns. These bipedicular fractures can be associated with significant anterior translation of C2 on C3, including complete facet dislocation. Modification of the Effendi classification by Levine and Edwards[40] identifies four fracture patterns.

Type 1 fractures are either nondisplaced or have <3 mm of translation without concomitant angulation. These fractures are believed to occur secondary to a hyperextension–axial loading force.[40] These fractures are stable because there is no associated significant ligamentous injury, and union should be anticipated in most patients. Treatment consists of immobilization in a cervical orthosis for approximately 3 months.

Type 2 fractures are associated with both significant translation (>3 mm) and angulation (Fig. 50-10). The mechanism of injury appears to be an initial hyperextension-loading force, resulting in a longitudinal fracture through the neural arch followed by secondary flexion and compression forces.[40] The latter forces result in disruption of the posterior longitudinal ligament and C2-C3 disk space with preservation of the anterior lon-

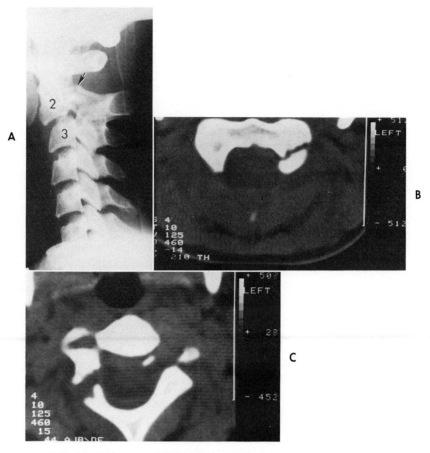

FIG. 50-10. Type II traumatic spondylolisthesis of C2. **A,** Lateral radiograph revealing C2-C3 subluxation and angulation. **B,** Computed tomography (CT) scan showing fracture of left pedicle of C2. **C,** CT scan illustrating fracture of right pedicle of C2.

gitudinal ligament. Radiographically, an area of compression of the anterosuperior portion of the body of C3 is noted in many patients, in addition to the anterior translation and angulation at the C2-C3 segment. Treatment consists of initial fracture reduction via halo traction (10 to 20 pounds) in a slightly extended neck position with the intact anterior longitudinal ligament preventing excessive distraction. Patients with moderately displaced fractures (3 to 6 mm of initial translation) can then be placed into a halo vest for 2 to 3 months. Satisfactory results occur in the majority of these cases. In patients with severely displaced fractures (>6 mm of initial translation), consideration should be given to prolonged traction (4 to 6 weeks) to allow for early fracture healing in the reduced position followed by halo-vest immobilization until fracture union (3 months total).[41] Early mobilization in a halo vest in the latter group of patients often leads to a significant loss of fracture reduction with a resultant higher nonunion rate.

Type 2A fractures are associated with significant angulation, but they have minimal translational displacement. They represent a variant of the Type 2 fracture with the mechanism of injury being flexion and distraction.[40] In comparison to the Type 2 fracture pattern the fracture line of the Type 2A fracture is more oblique and

posterior, lying just anterior to the facet joints. The identification of this injury pattern is critical in that applied traction can cause a significant increase in angulation with widening of the posterior portion of the disk space. Treatment consists of immediate halo-vest immobilization and mild axial compression performed for fracture reduction. These fractures generally heal after 3 months of halo-vest immobilization.

Type 3 fractures are associated with severe angulation, translation, and an additional unilateral or bilateral C2-C3 facet dislocation. The mechanism of injury is thought to be flexion-compression. Neurologic injuries are more common with this fracture type because of the potential for severe deformity and instability. Because the facets are often "free-floating," closed reduction may not be possible and if obtained may not be stable. Intraoperative reduction and stabilization is required in most cases. In the past, C1-C3 fusion was performed for this injury; however, this includes fusing the normal C1-C2 motion segment. Currently, open reduction and stabilization of the bipedicular fracture with C2 screw compression osteosynthesis (Judet) in combination with a posterior plate device for stabilization of the C2-C3 segment[4,35,55] may be the best approach. This technique uses lateral mass screw fixation in C3. Alternatively,

C2-C3 oblique wiring in combination with halo-vest immobilization may be performed.[41]

Middle Cervical Spine Segment Injuries

Although athletic cervical spine injuries at the C3-C4 segment are rare, they appear to be distinctly different from fractures occurring in the other cervical regions. Torg et al[87] analyzed 25 cases of C3-C4 traumatic injuries in football players and identified axial loading as the predominant mechanism of injury. Traumatic bony injuries occur relatively infrequently at this level. Rather, intervertebral disk and ligamentous injuries are predominant. In addition, acute disk herniations at this level are often associated with an episode of transient quadriplegia. Unilateral or bilateral facet dislocations at the C3-C4 level may be difficult to reduce with skeletal traction, and therefore they often require closed or open reduction under anesthesia followed by stabilization.

Lower Cervical Spine Injuries

Lower cervical spine injuries differ from those in the upper cervical spine in that there is a decreasing ratio of canal diameter/cord diameter, thereby increasing the likelihood of a neurologic injury. The injury spectrum may range from avulsion and minor compression fractures to complex ligamentous and osteoligamentous injuries. Complete evaluation of these patients must include a careful assessment for the presence of spinal deformity, instability, or neural element compression, especially in cases with an associated neurologic injury.

Avulsion Injuries

Fractures of the spinous processes of the mid-lower cervical spine, also known as "clay shoveler's" fractures

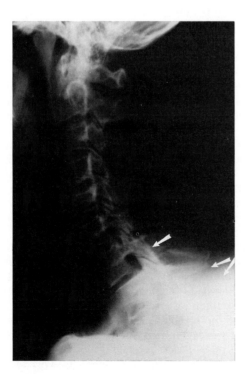

FIG. 50-11. Spinous process or "clay shoveler's" fracture.

(Fig. 50-11), have been reported in powerlifters and football players.[32,56] The fracture is most commonly seen at the C7 level. Several mechanisms have been postulated for this fracture. Most likely it occurs secondary to a sudden contraction of the trapezius and rhomboid muscles, which originate in the lower cervical spine, resulting in avulsion of the spinous process. Alternatively, a severe flexion force may result in a spinous process avulsion via force transmission through the supraspinous and interspinous ligaments. Fractures at the C7 level may be misdiagnosed on initial radiographs because of poor visualization of this area. Isolated fractures of the spinous processes are stable injuries, and they respond well to symptomatic treatment with a cervical orthosis, such as a Philadelphia collar or a sternal occipital mandibular immobilization (SOMI) brace in more significant injuries.

The extension "teardrop" fracture represents an avulsion of the anteroinferior corner of a vertebral body. The fracture occurs secondary to a hyperextension force, which results in an avulsion of the anterior longitudinal ligament at its insertion point. Although most commonly occurring at C2, this injury can also occur in the lower cervical spine. These injuries can be associated with late segmental disk degeneration. Treatment consists of a brief period of cervical collar immobilization for symptomatic relief.

Compression Fractures

Anterior column wedge compression fractures are associated with a variable loss of anterior vertebral height. In isolated injuries the middle column must be intact, and there should be no associated posterior ligamentous disruption. Careful radiographic assessment, including dynamic lateral radiographs, CT scan, or MRI, may be necessary to rule out associated injuries. Established radiographic parameters for assessment of cervical instability should be used (see p. 1120).[89]

Isolated fractures with less than 25% anterior compression are considered to be stable injuries and can be treated with orthotic immobilization. Fractures with greater than 50% loss of anterior vertebral height are often associated with posterior ligamentous injury because the posterior ligamentous structures (i.e., supraspinous and interspinous ligaments and facet joint capsules) fail in tension with resultant segmental instability. If there is associated segmental instability, surgical stabilization is mandatory. This can generally be accomplished by posterior segmental interspinous wiring and fusion. However, in the presence of an additional posterior element fracture (spinous process, lamina, or facet), interspinous wiring stabilization usually requires fusion of an adjacent normal motion segment. Although other posterior wiring techniques are available, posterior cervical arthrodesis with lateral mass screws and plate fixation appears to be the current procedure of choice with resultant fusion limited to the involved spinal segment.[4,55]

Facet Joint Injuries

Injuries to the articular facets can be divided into subluxations or dislocations, fractures, or a combination of the two. In turn, these injuries can be either unilateral or bilateral. All facet injury patterns can be associated with neurologic deficits.

Unilateral and bilateral facet dislocations represent pure ligamentous injuries with disruption of the supraspinous ligament, interspinous ligament, ligamentum flavum, and facet capsule. Although unilateral and bilateral facet dislocations can be well visualized on lateral radiographs, tomography, CT scans, and MRI are useful in the evaluation of associated fractures or soft-tissue injuries. Most important, a concomitant cervical disk herniation may occur with facet subluxations or dislocations.[17] Although disk herniations appear to occur more commonly with bilateral facet dislocations, they may also be found in association with unilateral facet injuries. The treating physician must be cognizant of the possibility of an associated disk herniation because reduction maneuvers may result in further disk extrusion and resultant neurologic injury.

Unilateral facet dislocation occurs secondary to a flexion-rotation force with an associated axial compressive load. Anatomically, this may result in a unilateral-"perched" facet (Fig. 50-12) or complete facet dislocation with the cephalad inferior facet lying anterior to the caudal superior facet of the involved segment. On the lateral radiograph, there is an approximate 25% vertebral body subluxation, and the dislocated facets have the appearance of a "bow-tie."[36]

Bilateral facet dislocations occur secondary to severe flexion-axial loading forces. As in unilateral facet injuries, "perched" facets or complete facet dislocations may be apparent. Because of the bilaterality of these in-

juries, there is an approximate 50% vertebral body subluxation present at the involved segment. As a result, neurologic deficits are more commonly found in association with these injuries.

The optimal treatment approach for facet dislocations remains controversial. Because of the risk of concomitant disk herniation, the question arises as to whether all of these patients should have routine myelographic or MRI evaluation before attempted reduction. Although this appears to be ideal, there are some technical, logistical, and financial disadvantages to this approach. A generalized treatment approach, such as that outlined by Eismont, Arena, and Green[17] appears to be the most reasonable. All patients should initially be placed in Gardner-Wells tong traction. In patients without neurologic deficits, skeletal traction up to 50 pounds may be used for attempted closed reduction. Careful radiographic and neurologic monitoring should be performed during the reduction maneuvers. If closed reduction is successful and the patient remains neurologically intact, temporary halo-vest immobilization is used and an MRI obtained to rule out disk herniation before elective surgical stabilization. In cases without associated disk herniation, segmental posterior spinal fusion should then be performed because these are ligamentous injuries and spontaneous healing or fusion is unpredictable. Interspinous process wiring for stabilization appears to be adequate in most cases. In cases with a concomitant disk herniation, anterior cervical diskectomy and fusion should be the initial procedure followed by posterior stabilization (Fig. 50-13). Alternatively, some investigators recommend surgical treatment solely via an anterior approach in these patients, adding plate fixation for stabilization,[1,62] although this remains controversial.

If closed reduction is difficult, MRI evaluation should be urgently performed, since these cases may have an associated concomitant disk herniation. Pending the results of MRI, further treatment can then proceed along the previous guidelines, although in these cases posterior open reduction is required before posterior stabilization. In addition, as recommended by Eismont, Arena, and Green,[17] patients who have a significant neurologic deficit or who develop worsening symptoms or progressive neurologic deficit during attempted closed reduction should undergo immediate MRI evaluation before continuing with the treatment plan.

The spectrum of facet injuries also includes facet fractures, which may be isolated or more commonly occur in association with facet dislocations or other injuries. In turn, facet fractures may be either unilateral or bilateral in location. Facet fractures can often be visualized on lateral and oblique radiographs, although CT scans (with sagittal reconstruction) can be helpful in diagnostic evaluation and treatment planning (Fig. 50-14).

Unilateral facet fractures can be associated with significant neurologic deficits, ranging from isolated root deficits to spinal cord syndromes. Although reduction can generally be achieved with traction, significant residual rotational instability warrants surgical stabilization and fusion. Oblique segmental wiring has been recommended over standard spinous process wiring tech-

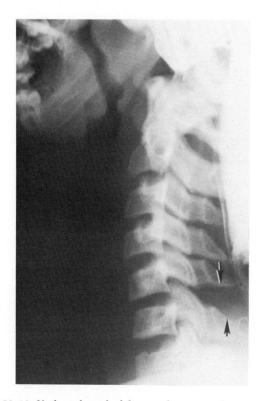

FIG. 50-12. Unilateral-perched facet with associated posterior ligamentous disruption.

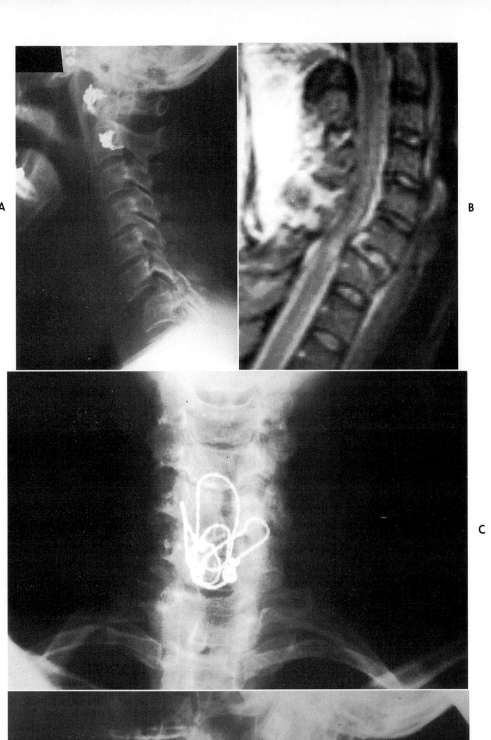

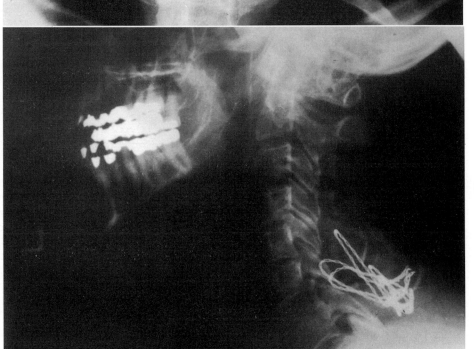

FIG. 50-13. Bilateral facet dislocation with concomitant disk herniation. **A,** Lateral radiograph reveals bilateral C6-C7 facet dislocation. **B,** Magnetic resonance image showing associated C6-C7 disc herniation. Patient underwent initial anterior cervical decompression and fusion, followed by posterior fusion with wire stabilization. Anteroposterior (**C**) and lateral (**D**) postoperative radiographs illustrating combined anterior and posterior stabilization and fusion.

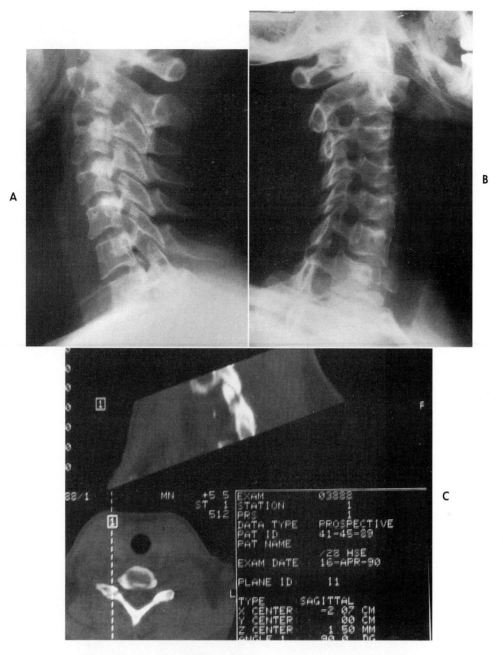

FIG. 50-14. Lateral (**A**) and oblique (**B**) raidographs reveal unilateral facet fracture at C6-C7 with foraminal encroachment. **C,** Axial computed tomography scan with sagittal reconstruction helps to visualize fractured facet.

niques because the latter does not provide adequate resistance to the rotational forces. However, posterior stabilization techniques using lateral mass fixation appear to have a role in the treatment of these injuries, since excellent stability is achieved with these fixation constructs.[4,35,55] Clearly, the experienced spinal surgeon must carefully weigh the advantages of these latter fixation techniques with the increased potential risk.

Isolated **bilateral facet fractures** are rare. They are usually found in association with dislocations or other complex injury patterns. In fractures occurring at the base of the superior facets there is loss of the posterior bony buttress, allowing significant segmental translation. As a result the incidence of neurologic deficits in association with these injuries is high. Fractures that are limited to the extreme apical portion of the superior facets may preserve some stability via the remaining bony facet buttress. Fractures of the inferior facets usually occur at the base and are less likely to be associated with a neurologic deficit. Treatment is similar to that for unilateral facet fractures.

Vertebral Body Burst Fractures

Vertebral body burst fractures represent one of the most devastating injuries to the cervical spine. The predominant mechanism of injury is severe axial loading associated with secondary hyperflexion. By definition these fractures involve the middle vertebral column (posterior vertebral body). Generally, there is significant vertebral body comminution and variable bony retropulsion into the spinal canal (Fig. 50-15). In addition, posterior ligamentous disruption or posterior element fractures are often associated with these injuries. As a result of these injury components, significant segmental kyphosis may be present. Because of the canal encroachment and spi-

nal column deformity, spinal cord injury is generally present, ranging from complete to incomplete deficits.

Although these fractures are readily apparent on plain radiographs, additional radiographic evaluation is necessary to fully delineate the pathologic anatomy. CT scans provide visualization of the bony elements and assess the severity of spinal canal compromise. MRI evaluation assesses neural element compression and can be used to assess the severity of posterior ligamentous disruption.

Following initial evaluation, including complete neurologic assessment, the patient should be placed into skeletal traction. This not only aids in spinal realignment, but also may result in significant spinal canal decompres-

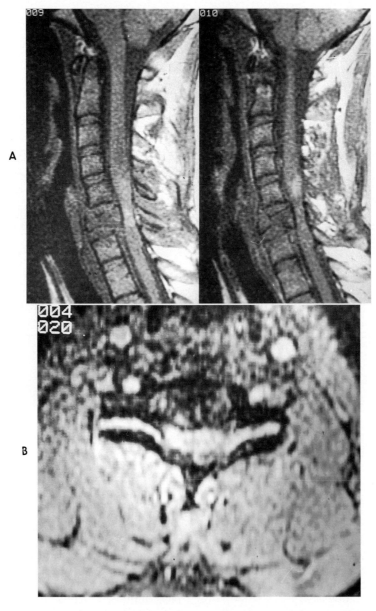

FIG. 50-15. C6 burst fracture. Sagittal (**A**) and axial (**B**) magnetic resonance images reveal vertebral body comminution and bony retropulsion into spinal canal with resultant spinal cord compression. Increased signal intensity within spinal cord (sagittal view) is indicative of intrinsic spinal cord injury.

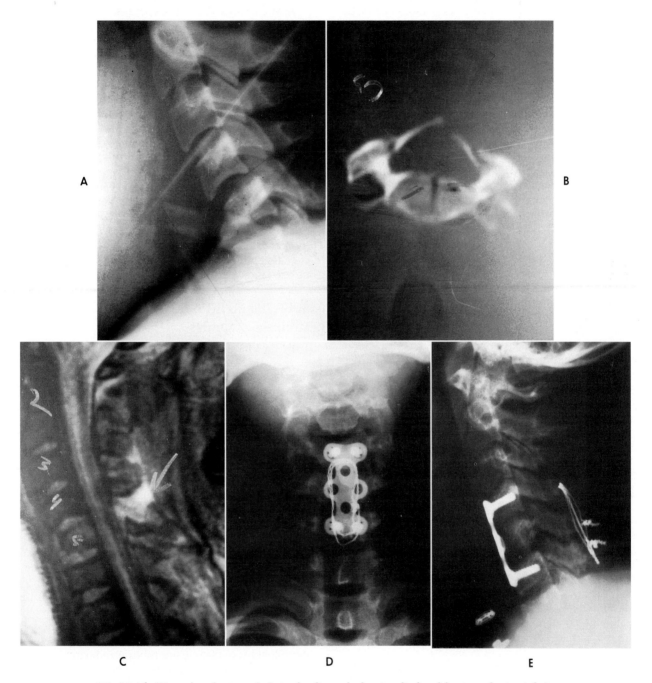

FIG. 50-16. C5 teardrop fracture. **A,** Lateral radiograph showing displaced fracture of anteroinferior portion of C5 vertebral body with mild retrolisthesis of posteroinferior portion of C5. Widening of C4-C5 interspinous process distance is apparent. **B,** Axial computed tomography scan reveals sagitally oriented fracture of vertebral body and posterior element fractures. **C,** Sagittal magnetic resonance image reveals C4-C5 posterior ligamentous disruption. Patient underwent anterior cervical decompression and fusion with unicortical plate fixation, followed by posterior fusion with wire stabilization. Anteroposterior (**D**) and lateral (**E**) postoperative radiographs showing combined anterior and posterior stabilization and fusion.

sion via ligamentotaxis of the retropulsed bony fragments. MRI evaluation can be performed in traction to assess for residual canal compromise. In patients with persistent spinal cord compression associated with an incomplete neurologic deficit, anterior surgical decompression should be performed on an urgent basis. If there is no evidence of residual neural element compression and spinal alignment has been restored, the patient can temporarily be maintained in traction or halo vest, and surgical stabilization can be performed when feasible.

As these injuries generally represent unstable three-column lesions, combined anterior and posterior surgical stabilization and fusion is recommended. Anterior corpectomy with spinal canal decompression as necessary should be performed with the patient stabilized in traction. Tricortical iliac crest or fibula can be used as grafting material for reconstruction of the anterior and middle spinal columns. In addition, in these severe destabilizing injuries, adjuvant anterior plate fixation can be used to augment the fixation construct.[1,62] Although investigators have used anterior reconstruction and plate stabilization as the sole procedure in cases with associated posterior ligamentous disruption, this practice remains controversial. Montesano et al,[52] in a biomechanical analysis, have shown that anterior plate fixation does not appear to be adequate stabilization in flexion-type injuries associated with posterior ligamentous disruption. Therefore despite the use of anterior cervical plate fixation, concomitant posterior stabilization is recommended. If the posterior osseous structures are intact, interspinous process wiring provides secure stabilization. However, in the presence of associated spinous process or lamina fractures, lateral mass plate fixation is an excellent alternative, allowing for limitation of the fusion to the involved levels and providing ideal spinal stability.[4,26,55]

Teardrop Fractures

A severe flexion–axial loading mechanism may also result in a teardrop fracture. This three-column injury is characterized by a displaced fracture of the anteroinferior portion of the superior vertebral body, segmental disk disruption, and posterior ligamentous injury or fracture. As a result, there is often associated retrolisthesis of the posteroinferior portion of the involved vertebral body with variable neural element compression (Fig. 50-16). Thus there is a high incidence of neurologic deficit, either partial or complete, with this injury pattern.[39]

In general, the clinical evaluation and treatment of this injury is the same as for burst fractures. Because these injuries represent grossly unstable lesions, combined anterior and posterior stabilization and fusion is required.

Other Fractures

Lamina fractures generally occur in association with other major cervical spine injuries (e.g., burst fractures). Occasionally, lamina fractures can occur as isolated injuries, resulting from extension–axial loading forces. These patients must be carefully evaluated for concomitant injuries with appropriate radiographic analysis. If there is no evidence of neural element compression, instability, or associated injury, these patients can usually be managed in a rigid orthosis for 6 to 8 weeks to allow for fracture healing. Follow-up flexion-extension radiographs should be performed to document stability.

Fractures of the lateral mass result in a complete separation of the lateral mass from the involved vertebral body (Fig. 50-17).[37] As in lamina fractures, these injuries usually occur in association with other major cervical spine injuries (e.g., facet dislocation), but they can be diagnosed as isolated entities. In addition, the treating physician must be cognizant of the possibility of associated vertebral artery injury because the fracture may course through the transverse foramen. Anatomically, these injuries disrupt the facet articulation of the motion segments directly above and below the involved vertebra. Because these injuries result in significant instability, surgical stabilization and fusion is required. At surgery the involved lateral mass can be reduced under direction before stabilization. Although traditionally interspinous process wiring of the adjacent segments has been used for stabilization, lateral mass plating appears to offer an excellent alternative because the intermediate screw can be used for stabilization of the fractured lateral mass.[55]

SOFT-TISSUE INJURIES
Strains and Sprains

By far the most common neck injuries in athletes are strains and sprains. Strains are defined as injuries to the muscle-tendon unit, whereas sprains are defined as ligamentous or capsular injuries. The clinical differentiation between these two entities may be difficult; however, the treatment plan is generally similar.

Strains and sprains may be associated with the whiplash injury pattern. A whiplash injury is produced by an extension-flexion mechanism, such as occurs when a vehicle comes to an abrupt stop. This injury can also occur in gymnastics, football, rugby, and diving. Muscles, ligaments, soft tissues, and supporting skeletal structures of the entire cervical spine can be affected. This may include injuries to the trachea, esophagus, anterior and posterior longitudinal ligaments, cervical intervertebral disks, facet joints, and all muscles supporting the neck.

Strains and sprains can range in severity from minor muscle pulls to more severe tears and disruption of ligamentous structures. More extensive ligamentous and capsular disruptions may lead to instability and possible neurologic sequelae. Thus routine radiographic evaluation is required in more serious cervical sprains to rule out spinal instability.[33]

Most strains and sprains respond well to conservative management, including immobilization in a soft cervical collar and use of antiinflammatory drugs and physical therapy modalities. Some of these injuries have a protracted course and may require extensive therapy before the patient can return to athletic competition (see Chapter 51). In general, return to sports is allowed when full, painless range of motion has been reestablished.

Cervical Disk Injuries

Cervical disk herniations are relatively common and affect participants in many sports, ranging from noncon-

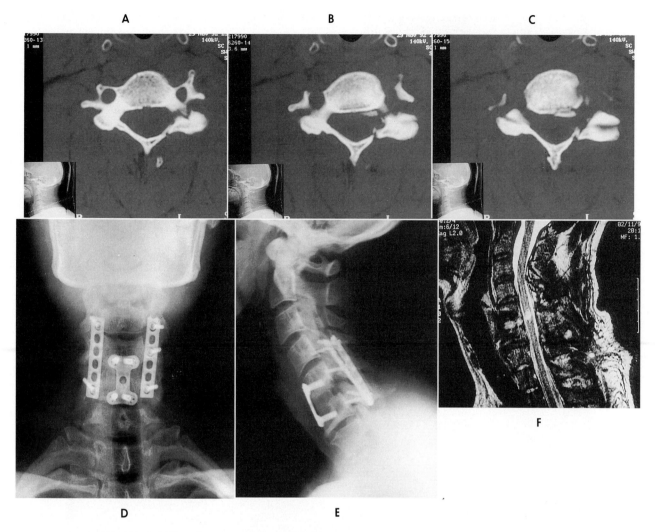

FIG. 50-17. C5 lateral mass separation fracture with concomitant complete C5-C6 transdiskal injury and associated anterior cord syndrome in a football player. **A,** Axial computed tomography (CT) image reveals left lateral mass separation fracture. Pedicle fracture line courses just posterior to intertransverse foramen. **B** and **C,** Axial CT images showing C5 inferior end plate fractures associated with severe C5-C6 transdiskal injury. Injury pattern resulted in severe instability at C5-C6 level and left C4-C5 facet disruption secondary to displaced C5 lateral mass fracture. Because of the presence of severe instability, patient underwent combined anteroposterior stabilization procedure. First phase consisted of C5-C6 anterior cervical decompression and fusion with unicortical plate fixation. Second phase consisted of C4 to C6 posterior fusion with lateral mass plate fixation. Extension of posterior fusion to include C4-C5 level was required because of C4-C5 facet disruption. Anteroposterior (**D**) and lateral (**E**) postoperative radiographs showing combined anterior and posterior stabilization and fusion. **F,** Sagittal magnetic resonance image 11 weeks after injury showing persistent increased signal within spinal cord despite patient's improving neurologic status.

tact activities, such as swimming and tennis, to contact sports, such as football and rugby (Fig. 50-18). Most are unisegmental and unilateral, although bilateral symptoms can occasionally be found at one or more levels. The spectrum of symptoms may include restricted cervical motion; neck pain; and radicular upper extremity pain, weakness, or sensory changes. A careful history and physical examination, including complete neurologic evaluation, can often localize the injury.

The symptoms and signs of disk herniation may result from either compression of the nerve root by a soft ex-

truded posterolateral disk fragment or from a combination of disk degeneration, osteophyte production, and fragment extrusion. The latter constellation of injury is more likely to occur in middle-aged and older athletes; however, it may also be found in younger athletes who have sustained repetitive cervical loading in contact sports.

Following appropriate diagnostic evaluation, nonoperative treatment in the form of rest, immobilization, medication, physical therapy, and occasionally epidural steroid injections is successful in the majority of cases. If

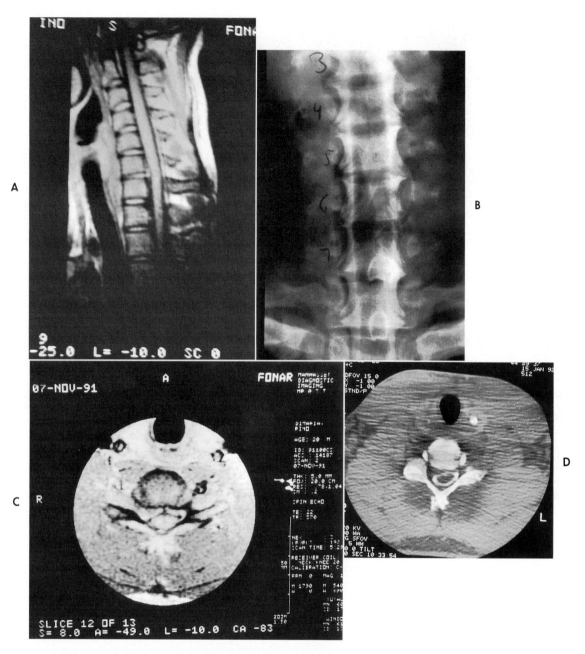

FIG. 50-18. C6-C7 disk herniation. Sagittal (**A**) and axial (**B**) magnetic resonance images reveal right-sided disk herniation. **C,** Preoperative anteroposterior myelogram reveals right C7 root compression. **D,** Postmyelogram computed tomography confirms diagnosis.

conservative treatment fails or if a significant or progressive neurologic deficit is present, surgical decompression is generally recommended. Anterior cervical decompression and fusion is the procedure of choice, although in some cases of soft posterolateral herniations, posterior foraminotomy and disk excision can be performed alternatively.

Although a large central disk herniation with or without associated cervical spondylosis or stenosis is a rare occurrence, it can cause variable spinal cord compression and associated long-tract findings. The latter cases

must be approached expediently with surgical decompression following complete diagnostic evaluation.

Major Ligamentous Injuries

Disruption of the posterior ligamentous complex can occur following severe axial compression-flexion injuries to the cervical spine, resulting in segmental instability. On the lateral radiograph, widening of the spinous processes with a variable amount of angulation and translation at the involved interspace is evident (Fig. 50-19). In some cases dynamic flexion-extension radiographs are

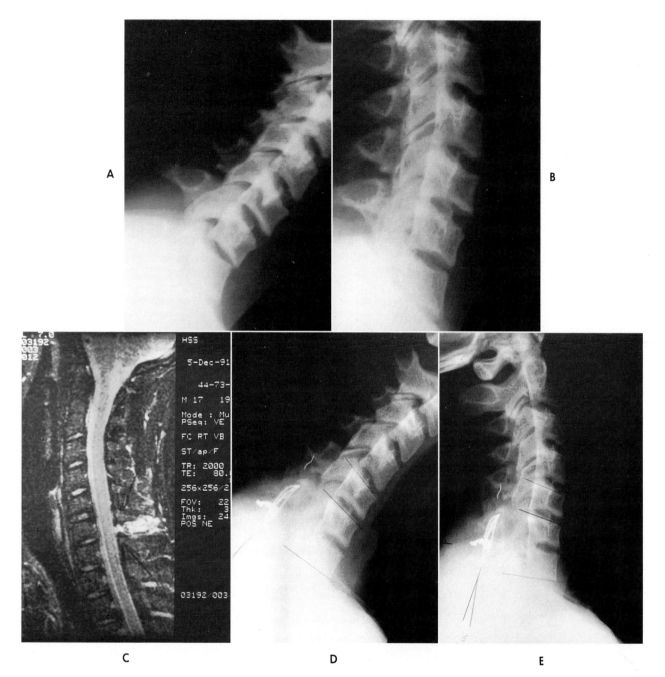

FIG. 50-19. C6-C7 traumatic instability secondary to posterior ligamentous complex disruption. Lateral flexion (**A**) and extension (**B**) radiographs showing dynamic segmental instability. **C,** T2-weighted sagittal magnetic resonance image showing posterior ligamentous injury. Patient underwent posterior fusion with spinous process wire stabilization. Flexion (**D**) and extension (**E**) postoperative lateral radiographs reveal solid fusion.

necessary to demonstrate these radiographic findings. The criteria proposed by White, Southwick, and Panjabi[90] may be used in the determination of clinical instability on flexion-extension radiographs. In addition, MRI may be useful in delineating the extent of segmental soft-tissue involvement.

If significant segmental instability is present, segmental posterior fusion is recommended because sufficient

healing is unlikely to occur in these pure, soft-tissue lesions. Stabilization can be achieved using spinous process wiring.[74]

Although not reported in athletes, subacute instability of the cervical spine has been reported in traumatic settings.[31] Subacute instability is defined as the development of radiographic instability within 3 weeks of cervical injury in association with a normal initial radiographic evaluation. It has been attributed to elastic and plastic deformation of the ligamentous structures and intervertebral disk. Despite initial normal radiographic and neurologic evaluation, these patients have radiographic instability, usually associated with a neurologic deficit, at follow-up examination. Therefore follow-up radiographic evaluation, including flexion-extension views, should be considered in all patients who sustain a cervical spine injury, albeit in the presence of a normal initial evaluation.

Hyperextension Injuries

In athletes with preexisting cervical spondylosis (Fig. 50-20), a hyperextension injury may result in a significant neurologic deficit, most commonly the central cord syndrome,[71] despite the absence of a fracture. In this clinical setting the hyperextension force results in spinal cord compression between the vertebral body osteophytes anteriorly and the buckled ligamentum flavum posteriorly. In some cases the lateral radiograph may reveal slight posterior displacement of the superior vertebrae, indicating variable disruption of the longitudinal ligaments and intervertebral disk.[45] MRI can be used to assess the presence and severity of soft-tissue disruption, extradural neural element compression, and intrinsic cord injury.[27]

In most cases patients can be treated nonoperatively with orthotic immobilization and neurologic monitoring. In cases with significant soft-tissue disruption, instability, or extradural neural element compression, surgical decompression or stabilization may be necessary.

DIAGNOSIS, EVALUATION, AND GENERAL TREATMENT PRINCIPLES
Clinical Manifestations

The clinical manifestations of injuries to the cervical spine can vary tremendously. The severity of injury can range from mild to life threatening. Whether or not neurologic symptoms are present, the most common presenting complaint from the patient's point of view is cervical pain.

Acute "On-the-Spot" Assessment and Care

Until the exact extent of any cervical spinal injury can be ascertained, every effort should be made to evaluate the patient's clinical status without disturbing the longitudinal alignment of the neck and spine. The basic principles of the acute evaluation are to perform as complete an assessment as possible and to prevent further injury.

The acute assessment of the injured athlete begins with the standard cardiopulmonary evaluation: airway, breathing, and circulation. The physician must ensure that there is no airway compromise secondary to obstruction or neuromuscular malfunction. If the patient is unconscious, he or she should be presumed to have a cervical spine injury until proven otherwise. If the patient is conscious, an attempt should be made to establish a presumptive diagnosis through careful history and physical examination. Patients who complain of neck pain, numbness, weakness, or paralysis should be presumed to have a cervical spine injury. If an injury is suspected, the physician should perform as detailed an assessment of neuromuscular function as possible to differentiate between a spinal cord injury and a brachial plexus lesion.

Patient Transportation

If a cervical spine injury is suspected, great care must be taken to prevent independent movement of the head and neck before the en block movement of the patient. This is especially true when a patient must be removed from the water after a diving injury. It is imperative that the head and neck are supported via manual traction by a designated individual until the cervical spine has been properly immobilized. At no time should a patient be lifted carelessly after a suspected spinal injury no matter how insignificant the injury might seem at initial assessment. During transportation the same guidelines should be followed. The head and neck can be supported by hand traction, manual halter traction, or with other neck immobilization devices. Techniques for transfer and immobilization have been previously established (see Chapter 48).[33,88] If a cervical collar is to be used, it should be applied in a manner that neither causes any neck deformity nor increases the risk of neck injury during its application. Vital signs should be monitored during transportation whenever there is a significant possibility of compromise.

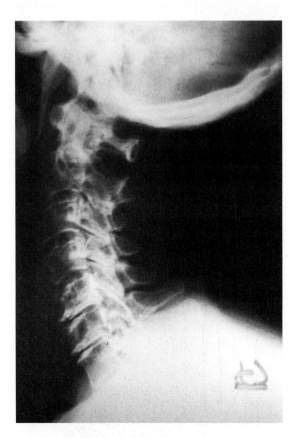

FIG. 50-20. Cervical spondylosis.

Primary Emergency Room Care

Once the patient arrives in the emergency room, cardiopulmonary evaluation should be performed rapidly followed by a complete neurologic examination, as previously outlined. The patient is observed for spontaneous movement of the upper and lower extremities. The physician should evaluate for evidence of previous injury, such as isolated or extensive muscle atrophy from previous neurologic injury.

In serious injuries to the cervical spine the bulbocavernosus and anal wink reflexes should be evaluated. Thereby, the presence or absence of spinal shock should be recorded as well as the duration and cessation of spinal shock. If a complete spinal cord lesion remains following the conclusion of spinal shock, further spinal cord recovery is extremely unlikely.

In the athlete with a less severe injury to the cervical spine a detailed neurologic examination is still necessary. It should include tests not only of power, sensation, and reflexes, but also of function and endurance. In some minor nerve root lesions results of initial motor strength evaluation may appear normal, but repeated testing may uncover fatigability or weakness.

If a cervical spine injury is suspected the physician should then proceed to a thorough diagnostic radiographic assessment to document the level and extent of injury.

General Treatment Principles

The two essential principles in the treatment of cervical spinal injury are to ensure that further neurologic injury does not occur and to relieve any spinal cord compression as soon as possible. Initially, neural element decompression can be achieved by careful realignment of an existing spinal deformity. After obtaining appropriate spinal alignment, persistent, extradural, mechanical compression of the spinal cord should be treated by urgent surgical decompression of the involved segment. This can be performed via an anterior, posterior, or combined approach, depending on the pathologic location determined by radiographic evaluation.

If satisfactory spinal alignment can be obtained after a significant cervical spine injury and further diagnostic evaluation reveals no evidence of persistent neural element compression, the patient can be initially managed in cervical traction, such as Gardner-Wells tong traction. Further treatment in the form of orthotic immobilization or surgical stabilization depends on the specific pathologic lesion. The recommended management of specific pathologic entities is discussed in detail on pp. 1121-1136.

Most cervical spine injuries respond to nonoperative treatment regimens. Operative intervention is indicated in cases of significant spinal deformity, instability, or neural element mechanical compression.

PREVENTION

The most important aspect of prevention of injury to the cervical spine or to any spinal region is proper education of the athlete and other involved parties, including the coach and the trainer. This educational process must begin as early as possible and must be reinforced frequently. The individual prospective participant should be advised in detail of the nature of the sport and the various mechanisms of injury. For example, the importance of proper blocking techniques in football must be carefully outlined to the player. "Spearing," which may result in a significant spinal cord injury, must be prevented at all levels of sport. The proper use of athletic gear may prevent injuries, such as "burners."

The significance of being in good physical condition must be emphasized. For most sports, muscle tone and function should be optimal and the athlete should have no underlying bony abnormalities. There is no doubt that an athlete who is in peak physical condition is less likely to be injured in sporting activities. A complete preseason physical examination for players of all ages should be performed. From this evaluation a detailed program of physical fitness training can be outlined for athletes in various sports at different skill levels so that the involved muscles can be developed to the appropriate level of function. In football, for example, neck-strengthening exercises play a critical role in the prevention of cervical spine injuries. Should a significant underlying orthopaedic condition be detected in the routine physical examination, the orthopaedic surgeon can direct the potential athlete to a sport that poses less risk to the cervical spine.

RETURN TO PLAY

A major question that arises in the management of athletes who have sustained a cervical spine injury is whether or not the athlete can return to normal activity level. Although investigators have developed classification systems in an attempt to predict the risk for further injury with continued athletic participation, their recommendations have been based primarily on clinical experience, given the limited availability of objective data concerning athletic cervical spine injuries.[6,46,89]

In general, athletes who have sustained cervical strains or sprains, intervertebral disk injury, or minor fractures and avulsions can return to contact activities when the clinical evaluation reveals (1) no reported cervical spine symptoms, (2) full, painless cervical spine range of motion, (3) full muscle strength, (4) no evidence of radiographic instability, and (5) a normal neurologic evaluation.[50,77,81] Athletes who do not meet the above criteria should be restricted from contact activities. In addition, Torg and Glasgow[81] have established criteria for return to contact activities for specific bony or ligamentous injury patterns.

Patients who have undergone a single-level anterior cervical fusion for disk herniation can be allowed to return to contact activities provided the above criteria are met and a solid fusion has been achieved. Similarly, a patient who has a solid posterior single-level fusion may be allowed to return to contact activities. Athletes who have undergone two- or three-level cervical fusions should not be allowed to return to contact activities because of the altered biomechanics of the cervical spine. In these cases forces are distributed over fewer motion segments, leading to increased risk for the development of degenerative changes of the facets and intervertebral disk.[81]

Although this discussion has presented useful guidelines, each case must be evaluated on an individual basis. Although the specific injury pattern plays a major role in the decision-making process, the specific sport and level of activity should also be seriously considered.

SUMMARY

It is impossible to do justice to all the ramifications of cervical spine injuries in sports in a short chapter such as this. This chapter should serve as a guide and a knowledge base for the diagnosis and treatment of athletic cervical spine injuries. The reader is referred to the publications listed in the references for more detailed information concerning cervical spine injuries in athletes.

REFERENCES

1. Aebi M, Zuber K, Marchesi D: Treatment of cervical spine injuries with anterior plating: indications, techniques, and results, *Spine* 16:S38, 1991.
2. Albright JP et al: Head and neck injuries in college football: an eight-year analysis, *Am J Sports Med* 13:147, 1985.
3. Anderson L, D'Alonzo R: Fractures of the odontoid process of the axis, *J Bone Joint Surg* 56A:1663, 1974.
4. Anderson PA et al: Posterior cervical arthrodesis with AO reconstruction plates and bone graft, *Spine* 16:S72, 1991.
5. Bailes JE, Maroon JC: Management of cervical spine injuries in athletes, *Clin Sports Med* 8:43, 1989.
6. Bailes JE et al: Management of athletic injuries of the cervical spine and spinal cord, *Neurosurgery* 29:491, 1991.
7. Bishop PJ, Wells RP: The inappropriateness of helmet drop tests in assessing neck protection in head-first impacts, *Am J Sports Med* 18:201, 1990.
8. Borock EC et al: A prospective analysis of a two-year experience using computed tomography as an adjunct for cervical spine clearance, *J Trauma* 31:1001, 1991.
9. Bracken MB, Shepard MJ, Collins WF: A randomized, controlled trial of methylprednisolone or naloxone in the treatment of acute spinal cord injury, *N Engl J Med* 322:1405, 1990.
10. Brady TA, Cahill BR, Bodnar LM: Weight training–related injuries in the high school athlete, *Am J Sports Med* 10:1, 1982.
11. Bruce DA, Schut L, Sutton LN: Brain and cervical spine injuries occurring during organized sports activities in children and adolescents, *Clin Sports Med* 1:495, 1983.
12. Cantu RC, Mueller FO: Catastrophic spine injuries in football (1977-1989), *J Spinal Disord* 3:227, 1990.
13. Cheng CL et al: Bodysurfing accidents resulting in cervical spinal injuries, *Spine* 17:257, 1991.
14. Clark CR, White AA: Fractures of the dens: a multicenter study, *J Bone Joint Surg* 67A:1340, 1985.
15. Clark CR et al: Radiographic evaluation of cervical spine injuries, *Spine* 13:742, 1988.
16. Eismont FJ: Cervical sagittal spinal canal size in spine injury, *Spine* 9:663, 1984.
17. Eismont FJ, Arena MJ, Green BA: Extrusion of an intervertebral disc associated with traumatic subluxation or dislocation of cervical facets, *J Bone Joint Surg* 73A:1555, 1991.
18. Etter C et al: Fixation of dens fractures with a cannulated screw system, *Spine* 3:S25, 1991.
19. Fielding JW, Hawkins RJ: Atlantoaxial rotatory fixation, *J Bone Joint Surg* 59A:37, 1977.
20. Fielding JW et al: Tears of the transverse ligament of the atlas, *J Bone Joint Surg* 56A:1683, 1974.
21. Flanders AE et al: Acute cervical spine trauma: correlation of MR imaging findings with degree of neurologic deficit, *Neuroradiology* 177:25, 1990.

22. Frymoyer JW, Pope MH, Kristiansen T: Skiing and spinal trauma, *Clin Sports Med* 1:309, 1982.
23. Funk FJ, Wells RE: Injuries of the cervical spine in football, *Clin Orthop* 109:50, 1975.
24. Garrick JG, Requa RK: Injuries in high-school sports, *Pediatrics* 61:465, 1978.
25. Geisler FH, Dorsey FC, Coleman WP: Recovery of motor function after spinal cord injury—a randomized, placebo-controlled trial with GM-1 ganglioside, *N Engl J Med* 324:1829, 1991.
26. Gill K et al: Posterior plating of the cervical spine: a biomechanical comparison of different posterior fusion techniques, *Spine* 13:813, 1988.
27. Goldberg AL et al: Hyperextension injuries of the cervical spine: magnetic resonance findings, *Skeletal Radiol* 18:283, 1989.
28. Grob D, Magerl F: Operative stabiliserung bei frakturen von C1 und C2, *Orthopade* 16:46, 1987.
29. Hadley MN, Browner C, Sonntag VKH: Axis fractures: a comprehensive review of management and treatment in 107 cases, *Neurosurgery* 17:281, 1985.
30. Harms J: Orthopaedics—traumatology I, rehabilitationskrankenhaus. Personal communication, Karlsbad-Langensteinbach, Germand, 1993.
31. Herkowitz HN, Rothman RH: Subacute instability of the cervical spine, *Spine* 9:348, 1984.
32. Herrick RT: Clay shoveler's fracture in power lifting: a case report, *Am J Sports Med* 9:29, 1981.
33. Jackson DW, Lohr FT: Cervical spine injuries, *Clin Sports Med* 5:373, 1986.
34. Jeanneret B, Magerl F: Primary posterior fusion C1/2 in odontoid fractures: indications, technique, and results of transarticular screw fixation, *J Spinal Disord* 5:464, 1992.
35. Jeanneret B et al: Posterior stabilization of the cervical spine with hook plates, *Spine* 16:S56, 1991.
36. Kaye JJ, Nance EP Jr: Cervical spine trauma, *Orthop Clin North Am* 21:449, 1990.
37. Krag MH: Cervical spine: trauma. In *Orthopaedic knowledge update 4*, Park Ridge, Ill, 1993, American Academy of Orthopaedic Surgeons.
38. Ladd AL, Scranton PE: Congenital cervical stenosis presenting as transient quadriplegia in athletes, *J Bone Joint Surg* 68A:1371, 1986.
39. Levine AM: Cervical spine and cord: trauma. In *Orthopaedic knowledge update 3*, Park Ridge, Ill, 1990, American Academy of Orthopaedic Surgeons.
40. Levine AM, Edwards CC: The management of traumatic spondylolisthesis of the axis, *J Bone Joint Surg* 67A:217, 1985.
41. Levine AM, Edwards CC: Treatment of injuries in the C1-C2 complex, *Orthop Clin North Am* 17:31, 1986.
42. Levine AM, Edwards CC: Fractures of the atlas, *J Bone Joint Surg* 73A:680, 1991.
43. Louis R: Department of orthopaedics and spinal surgery: Hopital de la Conception. Personal communication, Marseille, France, 1993.
44. MacNab I: Acceleration injuries of the cervical spine, *J Bone Joint Surg* 46A:1797, 1964.
45. Marar BC: Hyperextension injuries of the cervical spine, *J Bone Joint Surg* 56A:1655, 1974.
46. Marks MR, Bell GR, Boumphrey FR: Cervical spine fractures in athletes, *Clin Sports Med* 9:13, 1990.
47. Marks MR, Bell GR, Boumphrey FR: Cervical spine injuries and their neurologic implications, *Clin Sports Med* 9:263, 1990.
48. Matsuura P et al: Comparison of computerized tomography parameters of the cervical spine in normal control subjects and spinal cord–injured patients, *J Bone Joint Surg* 71A:183, 1989.
49. McCoy GF et al: Injuries of the cervical spine in schoolboy rugby football, *J Bone Joint Surg* 66B:500, 1984.
50. Micheli LJ: Sports following spinal surgery in the young athlete, *Clin Orthop* 198:152, 1985.
51. Mirvis SE et al: Acute cervical spine trauma: evaluation with 1.5-T MR imaging, *Raidology* 166:807, 1988.
52. Montesano PX et al: Biomechanics of cervical spine internal fixation, *Spine* 16:S10, 1991.
53. Montesano P et al: Odontoid fractures treated by anterior odontoid screw fixation, *Spine* 3:S33, 1991.

54. Mueller FO, Blyth CS: Fatalities from head and cervical spine injuries occurring in tackle football: 40 years' experience, *Clin Sports Med* 6:185, 1987.
55. Nazarian SM, Louis RP: Posterior internal fixation with screw plates in traumatic lesions of the cervical spine, *Spine* 16:S64, 1991.
56. Nuber GW, Schafer MF: Clay shoveler's injuries: a report of two injuries sustained from football, *Am J Sports Med* 15:182, 1987.
57. Odor JM et al: Incidence of cervical spinal stenosis in professional and rookie football players, *Am J Sports Med* 18:507, 1990.
58. Paley D, Gillespie R: Chronic repetitive unrecognized flexion injury of the cervical spine (high jumper's neck), *Am J Sports Med* 14:92, 1986.
59. Patterson D: Legal aspects of athletic injuries to the head and cervical spine, *Clin Sports Med* 6:197, 1987.
60. Pavlov H, Torg JS: Roentgen examination of cervical spine injuries in the athlete, *Clin Sports Med* 6:751, 1987.
61. Pavlov H et al: Cervical spinal stenosis: determination with vertebral body ratio method, *Radiology* 164:771, 1987.
62. Ripa DR et al: Series of ninety-two traumatic cervical spine injuries stabilized with anterior ASIF plate fusion technique, *Spine* 16:S46, 1991.
63. Rockett FX: Observations on the "burner": traumatic cervical radiculopathy, *Clin Orthop* 164:18, 1982.
64. Rothman SL: Computed tomography of the spine in older children and teenagers, *Clin Sports Med* 5:247, 1986.
65. Schaefer DM et al: Magnetic resonance imaging of acute cervical spine trauma: correlation with severity of neurologic injury, *Spine* 14:1090, 1989.
66. Schaefer DM et al: Prognostic significance of magnetic resonance imaging in the acute phase of cervical spine injury, *J Neurosurg* 76:218, 1992.
67. Schatzker J, Rorabeck CH, Waddell JP: Nonunion of the odontoid process, *Clin Orthop* 108:127, 1975.
68. Scher AT: Diving injuries to the cervical spinal cord, *South Afr Med J* 59:603, 1981.
69. Scher AT: Rugby injuries of the spine and spinal cord, *Clin Sports Med* 6:87, 1987.
70. Schneider RC: Serious and fatal neurosurgical football injuries, *Clin Neurosurg* 12:226, 1966.
71. Schneider RC, Cherry GR, Pantek H: Syndrome of acute central cervical spinal cord injury with special reference to mechanisms involved in hyperextension injuries of the cervical spine, *J Neurosurg* 11:363, 1954.
72. Segal LS, Grimm JO, Stauffer ES: Nonunion of fractures of the atlas, *J Bone Joint Surg* 69A:1423, 1987.
73. Spence K, Dedser D, Sell K: Bursting atlantal fracture associated with rupture of the transverse ligament, *J Bone Joint Surg* 52A:543, 1970.
74. Stauffer ES: Management of spine fractures C3 to C7, *Orthop Clin North Am* 17:45, 1986.
75. Tator CH: Neck injuries in ice hockey: a recent, unsolved problem with many recent contributing factors, *Clin Sports Med* 6:101, 1987.
76. Thomas JC: Plain roentgenograms of the spine in the injured athlete, *Clin Sports Med* 5:353, 1986.
77. Torg JS: Management guidelines for athletic injuries to the cervical spine, *Clin Sports Med* 6:60, 1987.
78. Torg JS: Trampoline-induced quadriplegia, *Clin Sports Med* 6:73, 1987.
79. Torg JS: Cervical spinal stenosis with cord neuropraxia and transient quadriplegia, *Clin Sports Med* 9:279, 1990.
80. Torg JS, Das M: Trampoline-related quadriplegia: review of the literature and reflections on the American Academy of Pediatrics position statement, *Pediatrics* 74:804, 1984.
81. Torg JS, Glasgow SG: Criteria for return to contact activity following cervical spine injury, *Clin J Sport Med* 1:12, 1991.
82. Torg JS, Pavlov H: Cervical spinal stenosis with cord neuropraxia and transient quadriplegia, *Clin Sports Med* 6:115, 1987.
83. Torg JS, Sennett B, Vegso JJ: Spinal injury at the level of the third and fourth cervical vertebrae resulting from the axial loading mechanism: an analysis and classification, *Clin Sports Med* 6:159, 1987.
84. Torg JS, Vegso JJ, Sennett B: The national football head and neck injury registry: 14-year report on cervical quadriplegia (1971-1984), *Clin Sports Med* 6:61, 1987.
85. Torg JS et al: Neuropraxia of the cervical spinal cord with transient quadriplegia, *J Bone Joint Surg* 68A:1354, 1986.
86. Torg JS et al: The epidemiologic, pathologic, biomechanical, and cinematographic analysis of football-induced cervical spine trauma, *Am J Sports Med* 18:50, 1990.
87. Torg JS et al: Axial loading injuries to the middle cervical spine segment: an analysis and classification of twenty-five cases, *Am J Sports Med* 19:6, 1991.
88. Torg JS et al: Spear tackler's spine: an entity precluding participation in tackle football and collision activities that expose the cervical spine to axial energy inputs, *Am J Sports Med* 21(5):640, 1993.
89. Watkins RG: Neck injuries in football players, *Clin Sports Med* 5:215, 1986.
90. White AA, Southwick WO, Panjabi MM: Clinical instability in the lower cervical spine: a review of past and current concepts, *Spine* 1:15, 1976.

CHAPTER 51

Nonoperative Treatment and Rehabilitation of Disk, Facet, and Soft-Tissue Injuries

Jeffrey A. Saal
Michael F. Dillingham

The majority of cervical spine athletic injuries can be successfully treated without surgical intervention. This chapter outlines an approach to rehabilitation that encompasses a comprehensive exercise training approach to treatment. X-ray–guided cortisone injections into inflamed facet joints or the epidural space are discussed as a means to shorten the pain control phase of treatment. Additionally, nonpharmacologic methods, such as acupuncture and physical therapy modalities, are discussed as facilitators of the rehabilitation process.

ANATOMY AND BIOMECHANICS

The cervical spine serves to protect the spinal cord while allowing combined motions in three dimensions.

The bone structures surround and protect the spinal cord and its enveloping membranes. Supporting ligaments are also important structural elements. The C1-C2 complex is designated as the upper cervical segment with the C3 to C7 levels forming the middle and lower cervical segments. The occipitoatlantal complex forms a combination of bony structures that enables unique motions to occur. Nodding motion of the head occurs primarily at the atlantooccipital joints. The atlas-axis complex with the odontoid process allows for approximately 50% of the cervical spine rotation. Available rotation totals approximately 80 degrees in each direction. Total cervical flexion and extension approximates 100 degrees. Flexion increases foraminal size but stretches nerve roots. Flexion also stretches the anterior aspect of the cord across the posterior aspect of the vertebral body. Extension decreases foraminal size and causes ligamentum flavum buckling. C3 is the first vertebra to have a true vertebral body and an intervertebral disk.

The shape of the vertebral bodies positions the uncovertebral joint, or joints of Luschka, in a posterolateral position. With the development of degenerative changes, uncal osteophytes can narrow the nerve root canal. The vertebral bodies are thought to act as shock absorbers during axial loading via a hydraulic-type mechanism. The intervertebral disk with its annulus fibrosis and nucleus pulposus transmits forces to the vertebral bodies

---

Cervical biomechanics: motion and canal size

Flexion
- Increases foraminal size
- Stretches nerve roots
- Stretches anterior cord over posterior vertebral bodies

Extension
- Decreases foraminal size
- Causes ligamentum flavum bucking

of the cervical spine. The disks resist torsional and flexion loads on the cervical spine. They play a particularly important role in potential injury to the neural axis when spondylotic changes narrow the canal or when acute annular rupture with nuclear extrusion occurs. The planar orientation of the facet joints allows for flexion, extension, and rotational motions. To a lesser extent, lateral bending motions are allowed, although this is a combined motion pattern that includes rotation occurring in the midcervical segments.

The spinal segments form a complex network of supporting structures and restraints. From the base of the skull the tectorial membrane extends inferiorly to form the posterior longitudinal ligament. This ligament runs along the posterior aspect of the vertebral bodies, providing longitudinal supports and an element of protection from posterocentral disk herniations encroaching on the spinal canal and theca. The anterior longitudinal ligament runs along the anterior aspect of the vertebral bodies, providing resistance to hyperextension movements. The ligamentum flavum lies posteriorly in the neural arches and adds stability when the cervical spine is hyperflexed. The facet joint and neural arch combined with the ligamentous supporting tissue provide posterior stability.

Deep muscles of the cervical spine including the interspinalis, semispinalis, splenius, and erector spinae along with the suboccipital muscles are postural support muscles. The levator scapulae, rhomboids, and trapezius muscles ensure the coupling effect of the scapulothoracic mechanism and the cervical spine. The cervical nerve root may be injured by disk or osteophytes as it traverses toward the intervertebral foramen. The nerve root complex is clearly adherent to the periosteum of the transverse process. This renders the neural complex relatively fixated and prone to both compressive and traction forces.[39]

MECHANISMS OF INJURY

The biomechanics and classification of cervical spine injury and recovery have been well studied by a multitude of authors.* Important injury mechanisms include axial loading or compression, flexion, extension, lateral bending, horizontal shear forces, rotational forces, or a combination of any of these. The cervical spine is relatively stable in each plane of motion mentioned unless a rotational force component is present. This can

---

*References 4, 7, 14-16, 20-24, 36, and 38.

Mechanisms of injury
■ Axial loading
■ Flexion
■ Extension
■ Lateral shear
■ Rotation
■ Combination

TABLE 51-1 Head and cervical spine fatalities (1945-1984)

Body Part	No. of Fatalities	Percentage of Total
Head	433	67.3
Cervical spine	111	17.3
Other	99	15.4
TOTALS	643	100

lead to a variety of subluxations, dislocations, fractures, and fracture-dislocations.[2] The treatment of fractures and spinal cord injuries is discussed in Chapter 50. Epidemiologic, cinematographic, and other experimental studies have demonstrated that **axial loading** or **compression injury** is responsible for a significant percentage of cervical spine and spinal cord injuries in sports.[6] This is especially so if the head is positioned in a slightly forward flexed posture forming a column with absence of the normal cervical lordosis.

Flexion injuries occur in most collision sports, including football, rugby, and ice hockey.[34] If the forces cause hyperflexion without compression, segmental distraction with or without disruption of the supraspinous and interspinous ligaments and facet capsule ligaments can occur with acute disk rupture. **Flexion with compression forces** lead to compression wedge fractures or comminuted vertebral body fractures. **Extension injuries** potentially lead to disruption of the anterior ligamentous complex, and if they are combined with compressive forces, dislocations as well as dislocations and fractures may ensue.[10]

EPIDEMIOLOGY

Cervical spine injuries have the potential to be catastrophic. Table 51-1 shows a total of 544 head and cervical spine fatalities from 1945 through 1984. The decade of 1975 through 1984 had a precipitous drop in frequency of cervical spine fatalities (Table 51-2). Fig. 51-1, A, from the National Football Head and Neck Injury Registry, shows the incidence of cervical spine fractures, subluxations, and dislocations for high school and college football. Fig. 51-1, B, presents the annual incidence of quadriplegia secondary to cervical injury. It demonstrates a significant decline in 1977. This drop in catastrophic injuries and fatalities was a result of a combination of factors.

Upon analysis of the epidemiologic and biomechanical data the mechanism of these injuries has been more clearly demonstrated. The majority of these injuries were a result of axial load applied to a flexed cervical spine. Shortly after this fact came to light, rule changes were instituted. The helmet could not longer be used as a weapon. The player could not make initial contact with the head while tackling or blocking. This rule change was implemented in 1976.

Improved on-site medical care is probably an additional factor in catastrophic injury reduction. School districts are encouraging attendance of properly trained personnel during practice and at games. In 1958 a California appellate court reviewed the case of a high school

TABLE 51-2 Head and cervical spine fatalities by decades

Years	Head		Cervical Spine	
	No. of Fatalities	Percentage of Total	No. of Fatalities	Percentage of Total
1945-1954	87	20.1	32	28.8
1955-1964	115	26.6	23	20.7
1965-1974	162	37.4	42	37.9
1975-1984	69	15.9	14	12.6
TOTALS	433	100	111	100

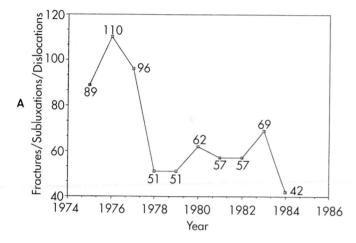

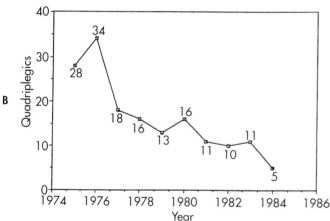

FIG. 51-1. Incidence of **A,** cervical spine fractures, subluxations, and dislocations, and **B,** quadriplegia secondary to cervical injury in high school and college football.

football player who was unable to get up off the turf after being tackled. His coach instructed team members to carry the athlete off the field. This instruction resulted in the injured player's permanent quadriplegia. Medical experts testified that the improper transport of the injured player caused the neurologic damage.

In 1968 the National Operating Committee on Standards in Athletic Equipment (NOCSAE) was founded in an effort to establish safety standards. Helmet and shoulder pad characteristics were analyzed. It was concluded that proper fit and maintenance were the critical factors in ensuring that equipment would prevent injury.

SOFT-TISSUE INJURY
Disk

The disk can be either the source of athletic disability by virtue of its intrinsic innvervation, or the cause of injury and inflammation to a traversing nerve root. The natural history of a cervical spine degenerative process from repetitive injuries (not necessarily related to sporting activities) leads to a degenerative cascade, as elucidated by Kirkaldy-Willis.[17] With an accumulation of disruptive forces to the annulus fibrosis over a period of time, radial fissures and nuclear desiccation occur. This then leads to the biomechanical changes that create degenerative changes in the facet joints, leading to capsule laxity with further instability and progressive disk disruption. With eventual progression of the degenerative process and enlargement of the articular processes, osteophytes form initially at the uncovertebral joints leading to foraminal and central canal stenosis.

As evidenced by the remarkable degenerative process noted in the relatively young population of professional athletes involved in collision sports, the physician assumes that the repetitive trauma to the cervical spine may play a significant role in the advancement of the degenerative process. It is also thought that repetitive trauma with resultant accumulation of redundant fibrous tissue and ligamentous hypertrophy may also lead to soft-tissue stenosis and a predisposition for neurologic injury. This mechanism could eventually contribute to a radiculopathy. Acute cervical disk herniation can occur with or without myelopathy or radiculopathy.

Cervical Facet Joint and Capsule

The athlete typically will have experienced an extension injury to the cervical spine, such as when a football lineman blocks an oncoming defender. The athlete complains of a "jammed neck." An overstressed facet joint or strained facet joint ligamentous capsule elicits these symptoms. Pain typically is referred to the interscapular region or head dependent on which facets have been injured.[1] The evaluator should be able to localize which facet joints are involved and thereby guide the treatment program to the precise localization of the injury.

Musculotendinous Unit

Occasionally an athlete primarily injures a musculotendinous segment. This usually occurs as a result of forceful overstretching of the muscle group past its capable length. However, most often the injury involves the facet joints and ligamentous complex. Primary soft tissue

TABLE 51-3 Medication check list

Medication	Indications and Use
Nonsteroidal antiinflam-matory drugs	Useful for antiinflamma-tory action and analge-sics
Narcotic analgesics	To be avoided because of endorphine blockade and addictive potential
Muscle relaxants	To be avoided because of their central nervous system anxiolytic ef-fects
Sleep hypnotics	To be avoided because of their central nervous system depressive ef-fects
Tricyclic antidepressants	Useful to promote sleep and decrease seritoner-gic pain stimuli

TABLE 51-4 Noninvasive treatment modalities

Clinical Presentation	Treatment Modality
Radicular pain associated with disk herniation	Traction techniques
Soft-tissue restriction	Ultrasound Electrotherapy Soft-tissue mobilization Deep massage
Joint hypomobility	Joint mobilization Manipulation

injury can lead to secondary and tertiary problems. These problems may include substitution patterns for pre-viously established engrams, interference of normal joint kinetics, muscle strength imbalance, sclerotomal-referred pain, and trigger point sensitivity. Predisposing factors for development of these injury types include poor flexibility, strength, endurance and power, improper training techniques, and soft-tissue contractures.

REHABILITATION

The ultimate goal of rehabilitation is to return the ath-lete to competition as rapidly and as efficiently as possi-ble. The principles of physiatric rehabilitation of the in-jured athlete have been detailed elsewhere, and the reader who wishes more information should consult these comprehensive works.[11,25-27] The rehabilitation program has two major subsections: the pain control phase[26] and the training phase.

Pain Control Phase

It is imperative that the pain control phase be short-ened as much as possible. The judicious use of nonste-roidal inflammatory medications is beneficial during this phase. Central nervous system (CNS)–acting medica-tions should be avoided. This caveat applies not only to narcotic analgesics, but also to muscle relaxant medica-tions that act as CNS anxiolytics (Table 51-3).[25] Passive treatment with manual techniques,[8] traction,[19] and deep-heating modalities[25] can improve motion and re-duce pain in a great many cases, but if they fail to do so after four to six treatment sessions, more aggressive steps are appropriate (Table 51-4).[28]

Traction

Traction is useful for the treatment of disk herniation associated with radicular pain. Initially, manual traction should be tried before institution of mechanical traction devices. The angle of pull usually requires slight spinal flexion. Intermittent mechanical traction has additional benefits by allowing maximum spinal lengthening. Ver-

tebral space gapping persists for approximately 20 min-utes following traction. In cases of spinal stenosis the fix-ated neural complex may be irritated by the lengthening effects of the traction, and therefore traction must be used with caution.

Soft-tissue muscular syndromes are usually exacer-bated by traction. Modalities and stretching techniques should be used to increase soft-tissue length before us-ing traction on the patient with disk herniation. Tem-poromandibular joint (TMJ) pain may be provoked by traction especially in the patient with a previous history. Home traction devices are usually not as effective as the intermittent mechanical devices; however, some of the newer devices hold promise.

Injection Therapy

Recent advances have allowed for the rapid control of pain and postinjury inflammation by the use of precisely applied injection techniques (Table 51-5). The establish-ment of a precise diagnosis is the initial key element to the success of the rehabilitation program. If the athlete has a facet joint injury that remains painful and is not responding to mobilization techniques[8] and nonsteroidal antiinflammatory drugs (NSAIDs), a facet joint injection with cortisone is beneficial. The pain referral zones as-sociated with facet joint injury has been elucidated and can help the evaluator determine the spinal level that is likely to be responsible for the pain syndrome.[1] Facet joint injection with corticosteroid reduces the inflamma-tory response and thereby facilitates the early institution to the exercise training program. The athlete who has experienced an intervertebral disk herniation with result-ant radicular pain referral is probably benefited by an epi-dural cortisone injection.[40] Recent biochemical evidence has demonstrated an inflammatory enzyme (phospho-lipase A_2) that is liberated at the time of disk herniation, resulting in an intense neural inflammatory reaction that can cause pain and axonal damage to the spinal nerve root.[30,32,33] Cortisone inhibits the enzymatic action of PLA_2, thereby aborting the inflammatory response asso-ciated with disk herniation.

Acupuncture

Acupuncture can be successfully used to control pain nonpharmacologically.[35] This technique can be a major contributor to the rehabilitation program when used in conjunction with the other tools of rehabilitation as dis-kussed previously. Acupuncture can reduce muscle hy-

TABLE 51-5 Advanced pain control methods

Clinical Presentation	Treatment Techniques
Persistent radicular pain	Selective epidural cortisone injection
	Epidural cortisone injection
	Acupuncture
Facet joint synovitis and capsular pain	Facet joint cortisone injection
Muscle hypertonicity and trigger point sensitivity	Acupuncture
	Trigger point injection with local anesthetic
Cervicogenic headaches	Acupuncture
	Facet joint injection to symptomatic and relevant joints

pertonicity and trigger point sensitivity. Additionally, acupuncture can control radicular pain by CNS endorphin increase and dorsal column gate control. We have been using acupuncture as part of our treatment regimen for over 20 years.

Training Phase

The most important phase of rehabilitation is the training phase. The training program we use is called **cervicothoracic stabilization** (CTS).[37]

Physical and Functional Capacity Assessment

Before the commencement of the training program, accurate assessment of the patient's physical and functional capacity is required. An accurate diagnosis and complete functional examination provide the guidelines for program progression.[29] Localization and clinical reproduction of symptoms in specific posture patterns are essential when designing the initial training parameters. Consistent reproduction of symptoms with postural positioning and relief through posture alteration are the keys to identifying the initial functional range. The determinants often encompass a variable equation between the underlying pathologic condition and the secondary bony restrictions, muscular restrictions, irregularity of force coupling patterns of movement, and inflammation. Therefore careful correlation of the patient's history, mechanism of injury, and physical and functional examination is important in recognizing abnormal movement patterns.

Biomechanical and Kinesiologic Principles

The cervical spine must permit support of the head while allowing great degrees of movement to optimize function of the sensory organs housed within the cranium. Cervical spine mobility should allow an individual to look quickly behind him, over his shoulders, up at the stars, and down at a newspaper. The cervical spine moves in flexion, extension, lateral flexion, and rotation. Lateral flexion and rotation are considered combined movements.[3,9,12]

Total movement of the cervical spine is the composite of segmental motion of all the cervical vertebrae. The major portion of rotational movement occurs in the upper

cervical portion between the occiput, the atlas, and the axis.[3] The remaining motion occurs at the lower cervical segments, C4 to C7.[3]

Poor posture and irregular movement patterns alter the normal segmental use of cervical vertebrae. All postures that are considered poor or undesirable are those aggravating dorsal thoracic kyphosis, resulting in a rounding of the shoulders. The faulty posture thrusts the head forward from the lower cervical spine and increases the upper cervical lordosis with compensatory occipital-atlas extension.[5,13] Poor posture during lifting, carrying, pushing, and pulling activities may contribute to additional forward translation and compression stresses on cervical structures.

Movement patterns on a poor postural base contribute to repetitive microtrauma of cervical structures including facets, disks, ligaments, articular capsules, and muscles. These patterns of movement contribute to habitual overuse of isolated motion segments while minimizing normal movement of others. Habitual dysfunction of isolated segments may generate bony hypertrophy, ligamentous laxity, and breakdown of disk and facet articulations.[29] The underlying combination can perpetuate itself in pain, spasm, and the dysfunction cycle.[18,29]

Correct dispersal of segmental movement depends on the balanced relationship between the head (occiput), the cervical spine, and the thoracic cage. This balanced relationship may be termed the **position of optimal function** (POF). POF is the functional range of the cervical spine in which each segment operates in its safest, most balanced, and pain-free position. It is a position that optimizes the biomechanical balance between the thoracic "base" and the flexible, balanced cervical spine. POF does not mean eliminating all lordosis by forcing a dorsal glide into a military posture. Rather, **POF is a balanced position with slight occipital-atlas flexion, and a comfortable or small degree of cervical lordosis is available to each individual.**

Alteration of this cervical position may not be attempted without consideration of the entire spine. All spinal curves transect a plumb line to remain in balance with gravity.[3] An increase in any one curve must be compensated by a proportionate increase or decrease in the other curves. For example, lumbar flexion associated with slump sitting contributes to collapsing of the thoracic cage or increased thoracic kyphosis. The increased thoracic kyphosis and rounded shoulder provide a poor base of support for the cervical spine. This poor base thrusts the head forward at the cervicothoracic junction with a resultant compensatory occipital-atlas extension position.

Cervicothoracic Stabilization Training

Training the balanced cervical spine must include postural stabilization retraining of the entire spine. Lumbar spine stabilization offers a properly aligned base of support for the thoracic cage. If the thoracic cage is conceptualized as the platform on which the cervical spine rests, the thoracic cage position is the key to postural control of the balanced cervical spine.

The critical components of a balanced spine are muscular strength and symmetry. The anterior and posterior muscles of the thoracic cage may be thought of as cables that effectively influence the articular interaction of the thoracic spine, scapulothoracic articulation, and glenohumeral joints.

A shortening of the anterior musculature that includes the pectoralis major, pectoralis minor, and anterior deltoid muscles contributes to a shortened, narrow, and collapsed thoracic cage. Pectoralis minor muscle fibers run inferiorly, obliquely, and medially, forming the tip of the coracoid process to the anterior third through fifth ribs. The fibers pull the anteroscapulae laterally and anteriorly, resulting in a rounded shoulder postural position.

A lengthened, widened, and opened thoracic cage requires equivalent soft-tissue extensibility between these muscle groups. Additionally, the posterior interscapular musculature that includes the middle and lower fibers of the trapezius, rhomboids, and serratus anterior muscles must be both flexible and strong enough to support the "shoulders back–chest out" posture.

The muscles with force vectors that lie anteriorly and posteriorly to the cervical spine also act as cables that influence the joint alignment and symmetry of the head and cervical spine in relation to the thoracic cage. A shortening of the suboccipital, sternocleidomastoid, upper trapezius, levator scapulae, splenius capitis, longissimus capitis, spinalis capitis, and semispinalis capitis musculature contributes to a flattened lower cervical spine with a compensatory occipitalatlas extension position. Lengthening of these muscles in balance with the anterior flexors frees up the motion segments to attain a balanced position of the occiput resting on the atlas. The balanced neutral cervical position offers an appropriate starting base for segmental mobility and stabilization training.

The stability of the cervical column depends on dynamic muscular control. The musculature must be strong and symmetric for position maintenance during cervicothoracic stabilization training (CTST). This re-

duces compression forces, chronic soft-tissue strain, and excessive forces on the cervical intervertebral disks.

CTST requires specialized training and coordination using body mechanics, posture, movement principles, and active exercise. The principles of stabilization training include retraining the musculature to control and use cervical mobility and stability of the diseased (painful) spinal segment. CTST promotes the necessary strength, coordination, and endurance to maintain the cervical spine in a stable and safe position during loading, mobility, and weight-bearing activities. CTST optimizes the cervicothoracic spine's capacity to absorb loads in all directions while minimizing direct stress and strain in relation to individual cervical tissues. It eliminates repetitive microtrauma to the cervical segments and limits progression of injury, thereby allowing healing to take place.[29]

CTST focuses on the balance of neutral spine, restoration of segmental mobility, dynamic muscular control, and the appropriate use of stabilization principles. The components of training must therefore encompass mobility and stability within a functional range. The emphasis of the mobility phase is restoration of segmental movement from a balanced position. It is important to enhance dynamic stability while avoiding cervical joint fixation and soft-tissue rigidity. Additionally, restoration of motion may be limited by pain and pathologic changes.[31] A fine line exists between a tolerable range of movement and its end range that exacerbates the patient's symptoms. Proper flexibility and mobility exercise applied to area of restriction gives the patient a valuable tool for controlling pain and improving function.[31] Flexibility training geared at restoring lost movement is discussed later in the chapter.

Although mobility provides an important function in daily living, stabilization in the balanced position is essential when lifting, carrying, pushing, and pulling objects. Muscle control helps maintain the balanced position while performing daily tasks that use the upper and lower extremities independent of the trunk or spine. Spinal stabilization training focuses on cocontraction of axial musculature while allowing isolated movement at the peripheral joints.

Dynamic stabilization encounters a larger range of muscular activity depending on the task. For example, an activity such as backing a car out of a driveway requires mobility in conjunction with contraction of muscles to place the head in a position to increase the visual field.

An activity such as lifting an object requires muscular stabilization of the cervical spine in a safe position while transmitting the forces away from the spine to the upper and lower extremities. CTST must encompass the range of mobility to stability by altering the type of exercise, the position of exercise, the resistance of exercise, and the related functional activities.

During an acute phase of pain, rest to the injured areas and use of cervical supports may be indicated. The cervical supports should hold the neck in a comfortable, balanced position. Initial patient education entails neck

---

Soft-tissue flexibility training: major areas of concern

Anterior muscles
- Sternocleidomastoid
- Scaleni
- Pectoralis major
- Pectoralis minor
- Biceps (long head)

Posterior muscles
- Rectus capitis posterior major
- Rectus capitis posterior minor
- Obliquus capitis inferior
- Obliquus capitis superior
- Levator scapulae
- Superior trapezius
- Latissimus dorsi
- Teres major
- Subscapularis
- Rhomboids
- Middle trapezius
- Lower trapezius
- Serratus anterior

first aid, positions of comfort, time contingent activity and rest, application of ice, and body mechanics. The patient learns hands-on knowledge to control symptoms while performing activities of daily living.

Patient education. The training phase begins with educating the patient in neck and back basics. The purpose of back basics is to instruct an individual who has either a low back or cervicothoracic injury in spine care, spinal anatomy, neutral spine concepts, and stabilization.

Postural reeducation. Following neck and back basic principles, postural reeducation begins. A balanced posture is the "state of muscular and skeletal balance that protects supporting structures of the body against injury or progressive deformity regardless of the attitude."[3]

The cervical spine is a flexible structure than can be tilted, rotated, and lowered by contracting the muscles attached to it. Balanced on top of the cervical spine is the head with its center of gravity anterior to its base, the atlas.[3] It is the ligaments and muscles of the neck with their insertion points at the base of the skull that play a key role in maintaining a balanced position of the head in relationship to the cervical and thoracic spines.[3]

The therapist begins by having the patient sit with front and side mirror views. This positioning enables the patient to see any postural deviations of the spine. It is important for the patient to see his or her habitual posture so that change may be facilitated.

Next, the therapist helps the patient find a **neutral balanced position of the lumbar and cervicothoracic spine.** Instruction includes both verbal and subtle hands-on cueing. With the patient's feet on the floor in front of him or her, the patient sits balanced on the ischial tuberosities in a stabilized lumbar spine position. The therapist then demonstrates to the patient where the thoracic cage and cervical spine neutral positions are in relationship to the lumbar spine. Generally, this involves lengthening the anterior and posterior soft tissues with special attention given to releasing the posterior neck muscles, thereby allowing the head to assume a slightly forward and balanced position on the cervical spine. If the patient is in a more acute stage, this training may need to begin in the supine position.

The next phase of postural reeducation is to use the balanced neutral position in a basic movement sequence such as a transition from sitting to standing. In this sequence the patient has a tendency to extend the head back and down and tighten the posterior and posterolateral muscles of the neck. The therapist instructs and directs the patient to move forward from the hips while maintaining a neutral spine and allowing the chin to drop slightly as the patient leaves the chair. Most patients do not realize that they are pulling their heads back and tightening their neck muscles in this habitual movement pattern. A hand on the back of the neck helps demonstrate this pattern and provides kinesthetic feedback.

Flexibility. If the patient is unable to attain a balanced cervical position because of soft-tissue or joint restrictions, the next step must include flexibility training before proceeding. Flexibility is an integral component of CTST. Adequate flexibility of the anterior chest wall, in-

terscapular region, and cervical musculature is essential to assume a balanced posture.

Isolation of upper extremity movement without compensatory cervicothoracic motion requires adequate flexibility of the shoulder girdle musculature and the internal rotators. Additionally, restoration of normal scapulothoracic movement must be accomplished.[13,18]

The two components of cervical flexibility are joint mobility and soft-tissue extensibility. Joint mobility is accomplished through mobilization techniques. Mobilization describes the application of a force along the rotational or translational planes of motion of a joint.[29] Specific joint mobilization may be accomplished through a gentle active range of motion. Clearly defined beginning and ending positions with careful attention to movement of the segment in question are essential to correct execution of the exercise. An appropriate exercise applied improperly does not achieve the desired effect.[31]

Stretching techniques provide increased soft-tissue extensibility. Stretching defines an activity that applies a deforming force along a linear plane of motion.[29] The shortened musculature in the cervical, scapulothoracic, and shoulder girdle areas is the chief target for stretching. The specific muscle groups can be divided into anterior and posterior groups. The anterior muscle groups include the sternocleidomastoid, scaleni, pectoralis major, pectoralis minor, and the long head of the biceps muscles. The posterior muscle groups contain the deep occipital muscles (i.e., rectus capitis posterior major and minor, obliquus capitis inferior and superior, levator scapulae, superior trapezius, latissimus dorsi, teres major, subscapularis, rhomboids, middle and lower trapezius, and serratus anterior.

Techniques proven effective in promoting musculotendinous flexibility include ballistic stretching, passive stretching, static stretching, and neuromuscular facilitation. Ballistic stretching is not recommended because repeated bouncing stretches contracting muscle and may lead to further injury. Early passive stretching by the treating practitioner should be performed with caution. A sustained stretch beyond the patient's safe available excursion may contribute to prolonged duration of symptoms or additional injury. It is advisable to instruct the patient to initiate static stretching between or at the end of the tolerable range of motion. Static stretching requires spine-safe techniques. The stretch is initiated from the balanced position. Prevention of collapsed thoracic cage and forward head positioning minimize abnormal stretching patterns. A position that applies a gradual stretch to the cervical musculature and upper extremity musculature is achieved and maintained for a 15- to 60-second period.

An improved range of shortened soft-tissue musculature restores capacity for normal movement patterns. Full range is desired for tissue health and function. It minimizes or prevents abnormal excursion, which contributes to adaptive shortening and functional disability. Finally, full range establishes adequate extensibility of tissues for dynamic stability vs. protective rigid stability.

It is important to stabilize the shoulder girdle before

TABLE 51-6 The progression of cervicothoracic stabilization exercises

	Cervicothoracic Stabilization Levels		
	I (Basic)	**II (Intermediate)**	**III (Advanced)**
Direct cervical stabiliza- tion exercises	Cervical active range of motion Cervical isometrics	Cervical gravity Resisted isometrics	Cervical active Range gravity resisted
Indirect cervical stabiliza- tion exercises			
Supine, head supported	Theraband chest press Bilateral arm raise Supported dying bug	Unsupported dying bug	Chest flyes Bench press Incline dumbbell press
Sit	Reciprocal arm raise Unilateral arm raise Bilateral arm raise Seated row Latissimus pulldown	Swiss ball reciprocal Arm raises Chest press	Swiss ball bilateral Shoulder shrugs Supraspinatus raises
Stand	Theraband reciprocal Chest press Theraband straight Arm latissimus Pulldown Theraband Chest press Latissimus pulldown Standing rowing Crossovers Triceps press	Standing rowing Biceps pulldown	Upright row Shoulder shrugs Supraspinatus raises
Flexed hip-hinge position	0 to 30 degrees Reciprocal arm raise Unilateral arm raise Bilateral arm raise Interscapular flyes	30 to 60 degrees Incline prone flyes Reciprocal deltoid raise Cable crossovers	60 to 90 degrees Bilateral anterior Deltoid raises Interscapular flyes
Prone	Reciprocal arm raise Unilateral arm raise Bilateral arm raise	Quadriped Head unsupported Swiss ball bilateral Anterior deltoid raises Swiss ball prone Rowing Swiss ball prone flyes	Head supported Prone flyes Latissimus flyes
Supine, head unsupported	Not advised for Level I	Partial sit-ups Arm raises	Swiss ball chest flyes Swiss ball reciprocal

stretching the cervical musculature. This stabilization may be accomplished by grabbing the base of a chair to depress and stabilize the shoulder girdle from moving. Once the shoulder girdle is stabilized, the head is directed away from the shoulder in rotation, lateral flexion, or combined patterns. As the available excursion improves, a steady application of additional force may be added by the use of proper hand placement. If deficits in range of motion remain after patient instruction, passive stretching and neuromuscular facilitation techniques are appropriate. These methods require a skilled practitioner to perform hold-relax and contract-relax methods to the appropriate shortened musculature. As normal range of both joint and soft tissue is achieved, muscle strength, endurance, and coordination can be addressed through stabilization routines.

Lumbar stabilization. A good cervicothoracic program begins with a lumbar stabilization program. Lumbar stabilization programs include exercises such as partial sit-ups, diagonal sit-ups, prone reciprocal arm and leg sit-

ups, and superman (prone with both legs and arms extended). Necessary precautions in monitoring and supporting the spine during this initial phase are important so as not to exacerbate cervical symptoms. The lumbar stabilization exercise program strengthens and aligns the lumbopelvic base of support for a neutral cervicothoracic posture (Table 51-6). (See Figs. 53-16 to 53-20.)

Cervicothoracic stabilization training regional exercises. CTST may be divided into regional exercises for the cervical, interscapular, chest, and upper extremity musculatures. The patient must learn to use the muscle groups in an isolated fashion and in cocontraction patterns, performing increasingly difficult tasks and demands applied to the body.

Cervical spine. The cervical spine regional musculature includes cervical spinal extensors and anterior musculature (i.e., rectus capitis anterior, rectus capitis lateralis, longissimus cervicis, and longus capitis). The anterior musculature stabilizes the cervical spine in the neutral position during muscular contraction of the ster-

---

Treatment phases of a stabilization program

Find neutral position
- Standing
- Sitting
- Jumping
- Prone

Prone gluteal squeezes
- With arm raises
- With alternate arm raises
- With leg raises
- With alternate leg raises
- With arm and leg raises
- With alternate arm and leg raises

Supine pelvic bracing

Bridging progression
- Basic position
- One leg raised
- With ankle weights stepping
- With ankle weights balanced on gym ball

Quadriped
- With alternate arm and leg movements
- With ankle and wrist weights

Kneeling stabilization
- Double knee
- Single knee
- Lunges with and without weight

Wall slide quadriceps strengthening

Position transition with postural control
- Abdominal program
   Curl ups supported and unsupported
   Dying bug supported and unsupported
   Diagonal curl ups
   Diagonal curl ups on incline board
   Straight leg lowering
- Gym program
   Latissimus pulldowns
   Angled leg press
   Lunges
   Hyperextension bench
   General upper weight exercises
   Pulley exercises to stress postural control

---

tion, and resistance of the exercise provides a progression of CTST. Cervicothoracic exercises presented here are arranged according to these principles of program progression (Table 51-7). The types of exercise selected challenge the individual's stabilization skills by altering the activity from static positioning to dynamic balancing. Each exercise incorporates varying degrees of upper extremity movement progressing from unilateral arm raises, to reciprocal arm raises, to bilateral arm raises. The patient's stabilization skills may continue to be challenged with transitional movements. Transitional movements include a change of position such as sitting to standing or entire body movement in space such as pivoting and turning. The movement from the supine position to the sitting position may be a difficult stabilization skill for the patient to achieve. Once stabilization skills are mastered in the transitional movement phase of the program, predictable loading and unexpected loading may be added. The patient's balance may be challenged with the use of the Swiss gymnastic ball. Power drills involving speed, strength, falls, and contact require the highest level of stabilization skills.

Varying the exercise position determines the required amount of trunk stabilization. Initially, exercises can be performed in the supine position with the head supported in the balanced position. Exercises progress to the sitting, kneeling, and standing positions. Finally, the prone and the flexed hip-hinge stance positions may be introduced into the program. The flexed hip-hinge stance is a standing position with varying degrees of knee and hip flexion. The type of resistance advances from isometric to isotonic contractions. During isometric contractions the muscle remains at a constant length. Isometrics vary the patient's positioning and direction relative to gravity resulting in direct stabilization of the cervical spine. Initially, the patient may begin isometric contractions in the supine position with the head supported. The patient then progresses to isometrics in the seated position or off the edge of a table against gravity. Exercises are performed with the cervical spine in the neutral position. An active range of resistance results in dynamic stabilization of the cervical spine. The dynamic cervical stabilization requires great segmental control from a neutral spine position. It is restricted to the tolerable range available to each patient. Avoidance of end range movement can minimize the exacerbation of symptoms.

Training the interscapular, shoulder, and upper extremity musculatures provides indirect stabilization support for the cervical muscles. The training must couple cocontraction of cervicothoracic stabilizers with isotonic contractions of interscapular, shoulder, and upper extremity musculatures against resistance. Method of resistance during isotonic contractions progress from rubber tubing or Theraband to pulley systems and free weights, and finally, to free body weight such as boxes. Rubber tubing, Theraband, a Swiss gym ball, and 3- to 6-pound dumbbells can provide the diversity necessary for a successful home program.

Shoulder girdle. Before gym training the patient must demonstrate consistent postural control and stabilization skill. Gym training challenges the stabilization ability of

nocleidomastoid as when a patient raises his or her head off the table while in the supine position. Emphasis is placed on the cervical extensors to balance shear stress on the intervertebral segments.

Thoracic region. The primary thoracic stabilizers are the abdominal, spinal extensor, and latissimus dorsi muscles. In the scapulothoracic area the major muscles of concern include the middle and lower trapezius, serratus anterior, and rhomboid muscles. The chest wall musculature to concentrate on includes the clavicular head of the pectoralis major and pectoralis minor muscles. The upper extremity musculature also requires training, using the supraspinatus, biceps, triceps, and deltoid muscles.

As the program advances, the patient is instructed in cocontraction techniques, which consist of active use of the trunk stabilizing muscles to balance the spine while an extremity performs a task. Advancing the type, posi-

TABLE 51-7 Variables for cervicothoracic stabilization progression

Training Level	Trunk Position	Exercise Pattern	Resistance Type
I (Basic)	Supine Sit Kneel Stand Flexed hip-hinge position (0 to 30 degrees) Prone	Reciprocal arm movement Unilateral arm movement	Theraband (elastic resistance)

II (Intermediate)	Supine
	Sit
	Kneel
	Stand
	Flexed hip-hinge position
	  (30 to 60 degrees)
	Prone
	Transition positions
	  Sit-stand
	  Supine-sit
		Reciprocal arm movement
		Unilateral arm movement
			Weight machine
			Pulleys
			Free weights

III (Advanced)	Supine
	Sit
	Kneel
	Stand
	Flexed hip-hinge position
	  (60 to 90 degrees)
	Prone
	Balance challenged with
	  Swiss ball
	Transition position
	  Sit-stand
	  Supine-sit
		Reciprocal arm movement
		Unilateral arm movement
		Bilateral arm movement
		Predictable loading*
			Weight machine
			Pulleys
			Free weights
			Free-form objects

	Free form	Specialized sports drills Unexpected loading† Falls Contact (football tackling and blocking) Power drills‡	Live sports activity

*Tasks that involve cervicothoracic load placement accomplished in definable postural positions (e.g., lifting a box from a high shelf).
†Loads placed on the cervicothoracic spine that occur without warning and in various postural positions (e.g., catching a falling object or bracing for a sudden fall).
‡High-speed movement patterns using near-maximum loads.

the patient; thus skill level assessment is necessary before advancement. The training goals include increasing muscular strength and endurance of trunk stabilizing and extremity musculature in a spine-safe technique. The targeted exercises for the shoulder girdle are listed in Table 51-8, and targeted exercises for the upper trunk or interscapular region are listed in Table 51-9. Table 51-10 provides the targeted groups for the upper extremity.

Resistance exercises additionally train strength, power, and endurance. The type of resistance and the number of sets and repetitions determine whether strength, power, or endurance are trained. Specificity of training with sets and repetitions must match with the individual's activities of daily living, occupation, and sports.

Exercises must be constantly matched with the patient's strength, endurance, and stabilization ability. Pain is one guide for exercise progression. An increase in axial or radicular pain requires a reevaluation of the exercise program. The pain increase may result from either poor technique or inadequate coordination of available strength and endurance. Additionally, the degree of in-

jury may present a limitation to progression in the exercise program.

EQUIPMENT CONSIDERATIONS AND PREVENTION OF INJURIES

Technique training in football, rugby, and other collision sports is imperative. Learning proper tackling techniques and proper equipment fit and design are absolute necessities. Proper fitting of football shoulder pads, for example, should allow for appropriate shock absorption and protection of the shoulders. They should be fitted snugly to the chest and fit the midcervical spine to the trunk. These features can be accomplished by having a long and rigid front and back panel fitted securely around the entire chest. Lateral build-ups can play an important role in prevention of cervical spinal root and plexus injuries.

RETURN TO PLAY

An injured athlete should return to play only when specific criteria are met. A great number of catastrophic

TABLE 51-8 Shoulder girdle muscle strengthening exercises useful in cervicothoracic stabilization training

Exercise Routines	Primary Muscle Groups
Theraband-resisted reciprocal chest press	
Theraband-resisted chest press while standing	
Initial and final positions Theraband-resisted diagonally	Pectoralis major muscles
Symmetric-internal rotation	
Chest press	Pectoralis major, pectoralis minor, and anterior deltoid muscles
Bench press	Pectoralis major, pectoralis minor, and anterior deltoid muscles
Incline dumbbell press	Anterior deltoid, pectoralis major, pectoralis minor, and serratus anterior muscles
Chest flyes and chest flyes while on a Swiss gym ball	Pectoralis major, pectoralis minor muscles
Supine reciprocal arm raises while on a Swiss gym ball	Anterior deltoid, pectoralis major, pectoralis minor, and serratus anterior muscles
Initial and final positions Upright rowing	Deltoid, pectoralis major, pectoralis minor muscles
Reciprocal arm and anterior deltoid arm raises	Anterior deltoid muscles
Lateral deltoid raises	Middle deltoid muscles
Prone reciprocal arm raises	Posterior deltoid muscles
Supraspinatus raises in standing position	Supraspinatus muscles
Theraband-resisted diagonal-internal rotations	Pectoralis major and subscapularis muscles
Theraband-resisted diagonal-external rotations	Infraspinatus muscles

NOTE: Cocontraction of direct cervical and thoracolumbar stabilizers must accompany these exercise routines.

TABLE 51-9 Interscapular muscle strengthening exercises useful in cervicothoracic stabilization training

Interscapular Muscle Strengthening Exercises	Primary Muscle Groups
Seated rowing	Latissimus dorsi, rhomboid, middle trapezius, and posterior deltoid muscles
Theraband-resisted rowing while standing and rowing from a low pulley while standing	Trapezius muscles
Theraband-resisted pulldown and closed-hand pulldown	Serratus anterior and latissimus dorsi muscles
Theraband-resisted pulldown	Serratus anterior and latissimus dorsi muscles
Open-hand pulldown	Latissimus dorsi, rhomboid, middle trapezius, and posterior deltoid muscles
Incline prone flyes final position	Rhomboid, middle trapezius, and thoracolumbar paraspinal muscles
Prone flyes, bilateral arm raises while on a Swiss gym ball and prone flyes while on a Swiss gym ball	Rhomboid, middle trapezius, and thoracolumbar paraspinal muscles
Prone reciprocal arm raises while on a Swiss gym ball	Rhomboid, middle trapezius, and thoracolumbar paraspinal muscles
Reverse flyes while standing in a flexed hip-hinge position	Rhomboid, middle trapezius, and thoracolumbar paraspinal muscles

NOTE: Cocontraction of direct cervical and thoracolumbar stabilizers must accompany these exercise routines.

TABLE 51-10 Upper extremity muscle strengthening exercises useful for cervicothoracic stabilization training

Upper Extremity Muscle Strengthening Exercises	Primary Muscle Groups
Biceps pulldown	Biceps brachii muscles
Standing biceps curl	Biceps muscles
Standing triceps press	Triceps brachii muscles

NOTE: Cocontraction of direct cervical and thoracolumbar stabilizers must accompany these exercise routines.

cervical spine injuries can be prevented. Appropriate training in the techniques of blocking and tackling are most important. Furthermore, guidelines presented for return to play following an injury must be observed. Allowing players to return to competition without full range of motion and with neurologic deficit courts disaster.

Even the most persuasive athlete, coach, agent, or parent should not alter return-to-play guidelines. Also, the guidelines should not afford special consideration to the team's star halfback vs. the team's platoon player. Individual players should decide how much pain they can endure. Obviously the timing within a given season and the importance of a particular contest may allow an athlete to push himself or herself through the pain more easily. Nevertheless, structural injury that has led to neurologic loss, joint instability, or significant loss of motion should restrict the player from returning to action prematurely.

SUMMARY

Rehabilitation of cervical spine injuries in athletes requires a comprehensive approach. A precise diagnosis permits the institution of an equally precise rehabilitation program. The training phase of the program must

---

Return to play criteria

- Full range of motion
- Normal strength with less than 20% side-to-side differential
- Normal neurologic examination
- No persistent swelling
- No unchecked joint instability
- Ability to run without pain
- No intake of pain medication
- Has received instruction about proper warm-up, flexibility and strength programs, proper use of ice and heat, proper use of taping and bracing to protect the injured area, and reporting increases in pain and postexercise swelling
- Has been informed about the risks of future injury and disability given the previously sustained injury

be emphasized. The passive aspects of the pain control phase should be kept to a minimum. Proper equipment, coaching, and injury prevention counseling are all integral portions of the rehabilitation process.

ACKNOWLEDGMENTS

The authors want to acknowledge the assistance of Tara Sweeney, PT, and Carol Prentice in the preparation of the cervicothoracic muscular stabilization techniques portion of this chapter.

REFERENCES

1. Aprill C, Dwyer A, Bogduk N: Cervical zygoapophyseal joint pain patterns. II. A clinical evaluation, *Spine* 15(6):458, 1990.
2. Babcock J: Cervical spine injuries, *Arch Surg* 111:646, 1976.
3. Bland JH: *Disorders of the cervical spine*, Philadelphia, 1987, WB Saunders.
4. Burke DC, Tiong TS: Stability of the cervical spine after conservative treatment, *Paraplegia* 3(3):191, 1975.
5. Capian D: *Back trouble: a new approach to prevention and recovery*, Gainesville, Fla, 1987, Triad Publishing.
6. Clancy WG Jr, Brand RL, Bergfeld A: Upper-trunk brachial plexus injuries in contact sports, *Am J Sports Med* 5:209, 1977.
7. Daffner R, Deeb Z, Rothfus W: "Fingerprints" of vertebral trauma: a unifying concept based on mechanisms, *Skeletal Radiol* 15:518, 1986.
8. Farrell JP: Cervical passive mobilization techniques: the Australian approach. In Saal JA (ed): *Physical medicine and rehabilitation: state of art reviews: neck and back pain*, vol 4, Philadelphia, 1990, Hanley & Belfus.
9. Foreman SM, Croft AC: *Whiplash injuries: the cervical spine acceleration-deceleration syndrome*. Baltimore, 1988, Williams & Wilkins.
10. Forsyth H: Extension injuries of the cervical spine, *J Bone Joint Surg* 46A:1792, 1964.
11. Franson RC, Saal JS, Saal JA: Human disc phospholipase A_2 is inflammatory, *Spine* 17(6S):S129, 1992.
12. Gracovetsky S: *The spinal engine*, New York, 1988, Springer-Verlag.
13. Gustavson R: *Training therapy: prophylaxis and rehabilitation*, New York, 1985, Thieme Medical.
14. Harris J, Edeiken-Monroe B, Kopaniky D: A practical classification of acute cervical spine injuries, *Orthop Clin North Am* 17:15, 1986.
15. Heulke D, Nusholtz G: Cervical spine biomechanics: a review of the literature, *J Orthop Res* 4:232, 1986.
16. Holdsworth F: Review article: fractures, dislocations, and fracture dislocations of the spine, *J Bone Joint Surg* 52A:1534, 1970.
17. Kirkaldy-Willis WH: *Managing low back pain*, New York, 1983, Churchill-Livingstone.
18. Knott M, Voss D: *Proprioceptive neuromuscular facilitation: patterns and techniques*, New York, 1956, McGraw-Hill.
19. LaBan MM, Macy JA, Meerschaert JR: Intermittent cervical traction: a progenitor of lumbar radicular pain, *Arch Phys Med Rehabil* 73(3):295, 1992.
20. Lysell E: Motion in the cervical spine: an experimental study on autopsy specimens, *Acta Orthop Scand Suppl* 123:1, 1969.
21. Paley D, Gillespie R: Chronic, repetitive, unrecognized flexion injury of the cervical spine (high jumper's neck), *Am J Sports Med* 14:92, 1986.
22. Panjabi M, White A III, Johnson R: Cervical spine mechanics are a function of transection of components, *J Biomech* 8:327, 1975.
23. Panjabi M et al: Three-dimensional load-displacement curves due to forces on the cervical spine, *J Orthop Res* 4:152, 1986.
24. Roaf R: A study of the mechanics of spinal injuries, *J Bone Joint Surg* 42B:810, 1960.
25. Saal JA: General principles and guidelines for rehabilitation of the injured athlete. In Saal JA (ed): *Physical medicine and rehabilitation, sports injuries: state of the arts reviews*, vol 1, Philadelphia, 1987, Hanley & Belfus.
26. Saal JA: Rehabilitation of sports-related lumbar spine injuries. In Saal JA (ed): *Physical medicine and rehabilitation: state of the art reviews: sports injuries*, vol 1, Philadelphia, 1987, Hanley & Belfus.
27. Saal J: Rehabilitation of the injured athlete. In DeLisa J (ed): *Principles and practice of rehabilitation medicine*, ed 2, Philadelphia, JB Lippincott (in press).
28. Saal JA, Saal JS: Initial stage management of lumbar spine problems. In Herring SA (ed): *Physical medicine and rehabilitation clinics of North America*, vol 2, Philadelphia, 1991, WB Saunders.
29. Saal JS: Flexibility training. In Saal JA (ed): *Physical medicine and rehabilitation: state of the art reviews*, vol 1, Philadelphia, 1987, Hanley & Belfus.
30. Saal JS: The role of inflammation in lumbar pain. In Saal JA (ed): *Physical medicine and rehabilitation: state of the art reviews: neck and back pain*, vol 4, Philadelphia, 1990, Hanley & Belfus.
31. Saal JS: Nonoperative treatment of lumbar pain syndromes. In White AH, Anderson R (eds): *Conservative care of lumbar spine*, Baltimore, 1991, Williams & Wilkins.
32. Saal JS et al: High levels of inflammatory phospholipase A_2 activity in lumbar disc herniations, *Spine* 15(7):674, 1990.
33. Saal JS et al: Human disk PLA_2 induces neural injury: a histomorphometric study. Poster presented at the annual meeting of Orthopaedic Research Society, San Francisco, February 1993.
34. Schneider R: The treatment of the athlete with neck, cervical spine, and spinal cord trauma. In Schneider RC (ed): *Sports injuries: mechanisms, prevention, and treatment*. Baltimore, 1985, Williams & Wilkins.
35. Sjolund BH, Terenius L, Eriksson M: Increased cerebrospinal fluid levels of endorphins after electroacupuncture, *Acta Physiol Scand* 100:382, 1977.
36. Sunderland S: *Nerves and nerve injuries*, ed 2, New York, 1978, Churchill-Livingstone.
37. Sweeney T et al: Cervicothoracic muscular stabilization techniques. In Seal JA (ed): *Physical medicine and rehabilitation: state of the art reviews: neck and back pain*, vol 4, Philadelphia, 1990, Hanley & Belfus.
38. Thompson R: Current concepts in management of cervical spine fractures and dislocations, *J Sports Med* 3:159, 1975.
39. Wiens JJ, Saal JA: Rehabilitation of cervical spine and brachial plexus injuries. In Saal JA (ed): *Physical medicine and rehabilitation: state of the art reviews*, vol 1, Philadelphia, 1987, Hanley & Belfus.
40. Wilson SP et al: Cervical epidural steroid injection (CESI): clinical classification as a predictor of therapeutic outcome. Paper presented at the seventeenth annual meeting of the Cervical Spine Research Society, New Orleans, Dec 5-8, 1989.

CHAPTER 52

Diagnosis and Treatment of Lumbar and Thoracic Spine Injuries

Gordon W. Nuber
Mark K. Bowen
Michael F. Schafer

Back pain is a universal malady that affects 80% of the population at one time or another.[45] Associated conditions in the general population include lack of proper physical conditioning, sedentary life-style, smoking, and workmen's compensation.[9,24] The incentives to recover are frequently less tangible for the general population compared with an athletic population. Athletes are frequently well motivated, well conditioned, more active, and younger than the symptomatic population at large. Back pain in an athlete frequently results from trauma, either of a repetitive, microscopic nature or from a major traumatic event.

Although athletes, like the general population, most frequently sustain injuries to the lumbar spine, the thoracic spine is often injured as well.[*] Numerous traumatic and nontraumatic causes are considered. Athletic endeavors that predispose an individual to injury are identified. It is our goal to identify the causes and natural history of back problems in the athletic population and to formulate a succinct approach to the work-up, diagnosis, and treatment of these disorders. Because this is not a text of surgical methodology, the surgical procedures are not discussed in detail. We have elaborated on those techniques that we have found helpful in assessing and treating the athlete's injured spine.

As in all areas of sports medicine, knowledge of the anatomy and biomechanics of the spine is essential to our understanding of both the normal and pathologic condition. These areas were covered in Chapter 47 and should be reviewed. Simply, the spinal column is a series of

---

*References 7, 15, 21, 26, 28, 86, and 98.

stacked vertebral blocks that are held together by cartilage cushions, or disks. These blocks support the entire weight of the body and still allow for rotational and bending motions, uniplanar and complex. In the thoracic region the rib cage adds rigid support to this bony column. In the lumbar area the paraspinal and abdominal muscles support the spine, acting as "guy wires." The most common injury, musculoligamentous strain, is directly related to the strength of the column and its supporting structures and to the workload it must sustain.[36] Even in the well-conditioned athlete many athletic endeavors overload the column and cause minor or serious breakdown. The effect of aging on disk composition and spine kinematics is as important in the athlete as it is in the population at large.[65,89,90]

The inability to compete, even temporarily, affects the entire life-style of the athlete. The goal of the treating sports medicine physician is to minimize the length of disability and return the athlete to safe participation as soon as possible. This goal can only be met with a sound understanding and knowledge of the pathophysiology and treatment of these problems.

PATHOPHYSIOLOGY

Spine injuries in athletes occur from repetitive stress (microtrauma) or major (macrotrauma) traumatic injury. Most of these injuries are self-limited and respond to rest and restriction of activity in 1 to 2 weeks. Only recently have the intrinsic and environmental factors that predispose an athlete to injury come into focus. The effects of overtraining must be studied, and through the use of the preparticipation examination, athletes prone to injury must be identified and counseled regarding sport selection and training methods.[8,53,93]

Fractures

Injuries to the thoracic spine are relatively rare (Table 52-1). Because of the unique thoracic spine anatomy and the stability provided by the rib cage, fractures are unusual except in the case of high-impact sports.[46,68,73] These sports include alpine skiing, tobogganing, snowmobiling, automobile racing, skydiving, and hang gliding.

Compression-type fractures are seen most commonly, involve only the anterior column, and are gener-

Sports in which thoracic vertebral fractures are reported

- Alpine skiing
- Tobogganing
- Snowmobiling
- Automobile racing
- Sky diving
- Hang gliding

ally stable. Vertebral compression greater than 50% or angulation of 20 degrees at the thoracolumbar junction suggests a condition of chronic instability and possible further kyphotic deformity.[88]

Burst-type fractures involve both the anterior and middle columns in the three-column model of Denis[16] and Denis et al.[17] The injury usually involves an axial load of significant force with failure of both the anterior and posterior portions of the vertebral body. Typically, the posterior column is uninvolved, but severe injuries with significant compression and angulation of the vertebral body may lead to posterior ligamentous damage and instability. The spinal cord at the thoracolumbar junction takes up approximately 50% of the cross-sectional diameter of the canal and usually is not specifically involved in the typical burst fracture. Denis et al[17] classified burst injuries into five subgroups, depending on endplate involvement, rotation, and lateral wedging.

A flexion-distraction force causes a "seat belt" injury that typically involves all three columns of the spine. These injuries often result from motor vehicle accidents in which passengers wear a lap harness without a shoulder restraint. A distractive force at point of impact causes failure of the three columns from posterior to anterior with a focus near the anterior column acting as a hinge.[88] Vertebral column failure may occur either through the bony or ligamentous anatomy or through a combination of both. The classic **Chance fracture** involves failure of bone only.

Fracture-dislocations are the most severe of the injuries to the spine. All three columns of the spine are involved, and injury occurs as a result of a combination of tension, compression, rotation, or shear forces. These are the most unstable of the spine injuries and are fre-

TABLE 52-1 Thoracolumbar injuries

Pattern	Involvement	Features
Compression fracture (flexion load)	Anterior column	Unstable if compression > 50% or angulation > 20 degrees at thoracolumbar junction
Burst fracture (axial load)	Anterior and middle columns (occasionally posterior)	Usually unstable
"Seat belt" injury (flexion-distraction load)	Anterior, middle, and posterior columns	May be bony (Chance fracture) or ligamentous
Fracture-dislocation (combination of tension, compression, rotation, or shear force)	Anterior, middle, and posterior columns	Very unstable, often associated with neurologic or abdominal injury

quently associated with neurologic and intraabdominal injuries.

Musculoligamentous Injuries

Soft-tissue **sprains, strains,** and **contusions** are probably the most frequent injuries sustained by athletes. In most cases the injury is self-limited, and healing occurs without long-term disability, frequently before the athlete consults the physician. A clear understanding of the injury is limited, since many cases of back pain are dumped into this category after only a cursory examination. Certainly, pain that lasts more than a few weeks should arouse suspicion on the part of a more specific diagnosis.

Micheli[62] described an **"overgrowth syndrome"** that occurs in the adolescent athlete during a growth spurt as a result of overgrowth of the bony elements compared with the soft-tissue elements. This overgrowth may lead to muscular spasm, tight lumbodorsal fasciae and hamstrings, and combined with weak abdominal muscles, a functional lumbar lordosis and compensatory roundback posture. This syndrome usually responds to stretching of the tight posterior structures.

Vertebral Growth Plate Injury

Scheuermann's disease is defined as a dorsal kyphosis of more than 50 degrees with wedging of at least three vertebral bodies by at least 5 degrees, disk space narrowing, and irregularity of the end plates.[7,81] A similar lesion has been described at the dorsolumbar junction.[95] Schmorl[83] described the herniation of the intervertebral disk through the vertebral end plate in 1927

Diagnostic criteria of Scheuermann's disease

- Kyphosis > 50 degrees
- Wedging of at least three vertebral bodies by at least 5 degrees
- Disk space narrowing
- Irregularity of end plates

(Schmorl's nodules). The herniation that was thought to be traumatic has a predilection for young men and is located at the level of the lower thoracic and upper lumbar vertebrae.[6] Micheli[62] found similar changes in the growth plate of young athletes at the thoracolumbar junction, but the findings did not meet the strict criteria for Scheuermann's disease. The changes have been classified as vertebral growth plate fractures in athletes but may be a continuum of the same entity.

The radiographic findings of **dorsolumbar kyphosis** are similar to Scheuermann's disease and include wedging of adjacent vertebrae, Schmorl's nodules, diminished disk space height, fragmentation of epiphyseal rings, and vertebral margin sclerosis.[30,95] If the disk herniates from below the apophyseal ring, a typical **"limbus vertebra"** is created that should not be confused with a fracture or disk space infection.[27] These findings are more common in athletes involved in weightlifting and repetitive

flexion-extension activities, such as swimming, rowing, gymnastics, and diving.

Diskogenic Pain

The lumbar disk motion segment is defined as the two lumbar vertebrae, the intervening annulus-disk complex, and the interspinous soft-tissue elements. As humans age, the disk "degenerates," losing water content from the nucleus pulposus and elastic recoil from the annular fibers.[10] The intervertebral disk and the facet joints are subjected to significant compressive forces. Besides these compressive loads the disk withstands tensile and shear stresses that occur with rotation and bending movements. Intervertebral disk injuries occur primarily in the fourth decade of life and are uncommon in adolescents. Miller, Schmatz, and Schultz[65] found that disk degeneration begins in males during the second decade of life and in females a decade later. They also found that by the age of 50, 97% of all lumbar disks are degenerated. The disk usually fails because of some combination of bending torsion and tension.[72] Disc protrusion most commonly occurs at the posterolateral corner of the disk, where coverage by the posterior longitudinal ligament is deficient.

Lumbar disk motion segment

- Two lumbar vertebrae
- Intervening annulus-disk complex
- Interspinous soft-tissue elements

Pain usually occurs because of nerve root impingement, which leads to ischemia of the root and subsequent inflammation.

Nachemson and Morris[67] have demonstrated increases in intradiskal pressure related to activities such as lifting weights, sitting, or bending—all of which are activities important to most athletic activity. Continued degeneration and injury of the intervertebral disk motion segment lead to microinstability, facet arthrosis, spur formation, and disk space narrowing—all of which are signs of degenerative disk disease. These changes in the older athlete can lead to further neural encroachment and central or lateral recess stenosis.[9]

Scoliosis

Curvature of the spine in the coronal plane is termed *scoliosis.* The cause of scoliosis may be either functional or structural. **Functional scoliosis** usually results from such extraspinous factors as limb length discrepancy or pelvic obliquity and corrects with the elimination of the underlying problem.[64] **Structural scoliosis,** on the other hand, is a fixed deformity that may result from congenital, paralytic, or idiopathic conditions. Most cases of structural scoliosis result from idiopathic conditions and are found during childhood and adolescence. The presence of a fixed deformity of the spine does not preclude the individual from participation in athletic activity. The

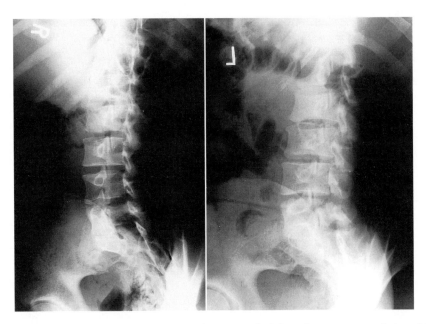

FIG. 52-1. Radiographs of high school football lineman with defect of pars interarticularis at L5 bilaterally on oblique views of lumbar spine.

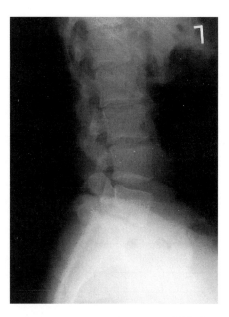

FIG. 52-2. Lateral radiograph displaying spondylolisthesis of L5 on S1 in professional football defensive lineman.

preparticipation physical examination is an excellent opportunity to check the athlete for any spinal deformity.

Spondylolysis and Spondylolisthesis

Athletic activities such as football, gymnastics, weightlifting, and rowing have been associated with either symptomatic or asymptomatic defects in the posterior bony elements of the spine.[20,41,55,85] **Spondylolysis** is a defect in the pars interarticularis portion of the vertebra (Fig. 52-1). **Spondylolisthesis** is the slipping of one ver-

tebra on another because of the bony defect in the pars interarticularis (Fig. 52-2). It is believed that athletic activity that demands repetitive hyperextension of the lumbar spine places the posterior bony elements at risk. Jackson[39] reported that 40% of athletes who had back pain that lasted longer than 3 months had pars defects or stress reactions of the posterior spine. Spondylolysis and spondylolisthesis are classified into five categories by

---

Classification of spondylolysis and spondylolisthesis

- Dysplastic type
- Isthmic type
  Lytic type
  Elongated type
  Acute fracture type
- Degenerative type
- Traumatic type
- Pathologic type

Wiltse, Newman, and MacNab.[96] The categories include the dysplastic, isthmic, degenerative, traumatic, and pathologic types. The type most commonly encountered in athletes is the isthmic type, which can be further subdivided into lytic, elongated, and acute fracture types. When spondylolisthesis occurs, the degree of slippage is graded by the classification of Meyerding.[61] The superior border of the inferior vertebra is divided into equal quadrants, and the slip is graded by the displacement of the superior vertebra on the inferior vertebra. Grade 1 slips are into the first quadrant, Grade 2 into the second, and so on. **Spondyloptosis** is a complete slippage of the superior vertebra off the inferior vertebra.

Frederickson et al[23] have demonstrated that the natural history of spondylolysis and spondylolisthesis is usually benign. In the general population, spondylolysis is rarely disabling or progressive to spondylolisthesis. There appears to be some hereditary predisposition to spondylolysis that plays a role in the development of the pars defect. Athletic participation accentuates the forces, both bending and torsional, on the lower spine. Therefore it seems plausible that rather than just exacerbating the symptoms of a previous defect, participation in sports may actually be instrumental in the creation of the defect. There seems to be two groups of affected athletes: those with a long-standing defect made worse by activity and those who acquire the defect through activities that load the posterior spine on a repetitive basis.

Other Anatomic Abnormalities

The presence of a **transitional vertebra, sacralized lumbar vertebra** or **lumbarized sacral vertebra** has been implicated in the cause of back pain, particularly in the middle-aged athlete.[87] These anomalies are quite common and may only play a pathologic role in the individual who stresses the spine through athletic or heavy labor types of activity. It is not certain whether asymmetry of the lumbar spine and subsequent stress give rise to pain and disability that would otherwise not occur.

Neoplasms

The incidence of benign and malignant neoplasms of the thoracic and lumbar spine is no greater in athletes than in the general population. Certainly, for any athlete who has persistent back pain and no particular inciting event, neoplasm should be considered in the clinical and diagnostic workup. A history of malignancy is an obvious warning sign because the spine is an obvious site of bony metastasis via Batson's plexus.[32]

Infections/Diskitis

Spine infections may involve the vertebral body, the disk space, or, rarely, the spinal canal and its contents. **Vertebral osteomyelitis** is an entity most commonly seen in the older- or younger-aged population.[31] Back pain, particularly in a child, should arouse the suspicion of inflammatory or infectious cause, rather than simply ascribing the pain to a musculoligamentous cause. Spinal infections in children usually present as **disk space infections,** whereas in the adult pyogenic infections occur in the vertebral body from seeding of the nutrient end arteries.[52]

Inflammatory conditions of the spine, particularly of the **spondyloarthropathies,** frequently present in males in their middle to late twenties, who are typically a very athletic population. Ankylosing spondylitis, Reiter's syndrome, and the enteropathic spondyloarthropathies must all be considered in the workup of the athlete with back pain.

Other Causes

Less frequent causes of back pain in the athletic population include **metabolic derangements** and **referred pain** from structures such as the kidney, abdomen, or gynecologic areas. Athletes who are involved in such impact sports as football and who have flank or back pain must be evaluated for a kidney injury.

Intervertebral disk calcifications are usually found in the cervical spine rather than the thoracolumbar area, but they may be symptomatic and lead to disk herniation.

Metabolic diseases, such as cystic fibrosis, and storage diseases, such as Gaucher's disease, have been associated with back pain. Gaucher's disease weakens the bone and leads to compression fractures.

Infarction of the vertebral body secondary to sickle-cell disease may also occur and needs to be differentiated from osteomyelitis.[48]

DIAGNOSIS

History

As with any physiologic or anatomic abnormality, the diagnostic workup of back pain is dependent on a good history and physical examination.

The athlete who sustains an acute traumatic injury should be immobilized, and a complete neurologic evaluation should be obtained before transport to the nearest emergency facility.

The most common presenting symptoms of an acute traumatic injury is pain. The injury's onset and related events are the initial, most important diagnostic clues. Many athletes, particularly those involved in high-impact sports, live with constant aches and pains and may minimize the significance of pain. *When did the pain begin? Was the pain associated with a traumatic event, or did it start insidiously and progress? What types of activities was the athlete involved in? High force or repetitive?* Obviously, fractures, muscles strains, and ligamentous sprains are frequently associated with some inciting event. The mechanism of injury also clues the examiner to the type and location of the injured segment. *Was the original injury caused by a hyperextension force such as that seen in football linemen, or was the mechanism one of rotation and twisting?* Hyperextension injuries clue the examiner to consider the posterior spinal elements. Rotation and flexion injuries may predispose the anterior spinal elements to injury.

Pain of an insidious nature may be related to chronic repetitive trauma or to nontrauma-related injuries. *Is the pain associated with any other symptoms?* Fever or chills may suggest an infectious cause. *Is there a previous history of the same or similar symptoms or treatment for the same?* The age of the patient may clue the examiner to the possible cause. Juvenile and adolescent athletes are more likely to have spondylolisthesis or spondylolysis, tumors, or infections. The adult athlete is more likely to have pain of a diskogenic nature.

Where is the pain located, and does it radiate? Pain located in the midline implies injury to the central bony ligamentous structures, whereas pain along the paraspinal area implies muscle spasm. Severe flank pain with blood in the urine indicates a primary urologic injury. *Does the pain radiate in a true dermatomal pattern? Does the pain radiate below the knee, implying true radiculopathy, or is the pain more of a referred nature, radiating only to the thigh, hip, and buttocks, such as what is referred to as sclerotomal pain?* The athlete should be questioned about the distribution of the radiating pain and any associated numbness or weakness of the lower extremity. L4 nerve root pain typically radiates along the anterior thigh and medial aspect of the knee. L5 nerve root compression may cause pain and numbness along the lateral aspect of the leg and the dorsum of the foot. S1 nerve root pain radiates into the posterior calf and into the lateral and plantar aspect of the foot. Athletes describing pain in a nonanatomic pattern should be questioned about other neurologic or psychosomatic conditions. Incontinence or urinary retention are symptomatic of cauda equina syndrome, a surgical emergency.

What motions or activities make the pain worse? What motions or activities relieve it? Pain at rest unrelated to trauma may be the result of infection or tumor and should be diligently pursued. *What effect do activities such as walking, sitting, bending, or lying down have on the production or exacerbation of the pain?* Pain related to walking and standing in the older athlete suggests the possibility of spinal stenosis. Leg pain with walking that is relieved by stopping but that is not positional should arouse the suspicion of a vascular cause.

Are there associated conditions such as metabolic or systemic disease that cause or impact the athlete's pain? In what sport does the athlete participate? Certain high-impact sports such as football, gymnastics, weightlifting, and rowing have a high predisposition to back problems and are associated with specific diagnoses (e.g., football linemen and gymnasts with spondylolisthesis). Although most athletes are dedicated to their recovery, other factors such as associated trauma, active litigation, and workmen's compensation should be ascertained, since they may also have an impact on recovery.

Physical Examination
Inspection and Palpation

The physical examination requires inspection of the entire spine. Observation of the spine requires that the patient wear a gown that opens in the back and exposes the entire length of the spine. This generally allows the female or young athlete the required amount of modesty while allowing the examiner a satisfactory inspection. The physician should look for skin abnormalities, including cafe au lait spots and hairy patches in the young athlete.[47] Angular deformity in the sagittal (kyphosis) or coronal (scoliosis) planes should be sought. A rib hump or shoulder height asymmetry may indicate scoliosis or Sprengel's deformity. The physician should palpate the midline for bony prominences, palpating for pain or deformity. The paraspinal and flank areas should also be palpated.

Range of Motion

Spine motion, including forward flexion-extension, side bending, and lateral rotation, is observed next. Any limitation of motion or production of pain, including the location of pain, should be noted. Motion of the hips should also be recorded to distinguish this area from a source of referred pain. Restricted motion of the spine and hip and chest expansion should alert the physician to the possibility of spondyloarthropathy.

Neurologic Evaluation

A complete neurologic examination should be performed. The athlete should be observed during normal walking, then on the toes, and then on the heels. Toe walking measures S1 nerve root function, whereas heel walking measures L4 and L5 motor function. Extensor hallucis weakness is associated with L5 nerve root function. Quadriceps weakness is a function of the L3 and L4 nerve roots and may be elicited by having the athlete step up repetitively on a low platform. Hip flexion strength should also be tested; it determines L1 and L2 nerve root function. The Trendelenburg test determines hip abductor weakness.

A complete sensory examination checks both light touch and pin prick over all dermatomes in the lower extremity. The L4 nerve root sensory distribution is along the medial aspect of the knee, the L5 along the lateral calf and dorsum of the foot, and the S1 along the lateral border of the foot and its plantar surface. The sacral dermatomes, S2, S3, and S4, innervate the perineal and genital areas. Decrease in sphincter tone or loss of sensation in this area may indicate an impending cauda equina syndrome. Reflexes should be checked for symmetry. Evidence of hyperreflexia, clonus, or a positive Babinski's test may be significant for an upper motor neuron lesion.

Special Testing

The **straight leg raising test** is considered positive if it produces sciatic pain radiating below the knee. The test should be performed with the patient both lying and sitting and is a measure of neural irritability. A more specific test for measuring neural irritability is the **contralateral straight leg raise test.** In this test the asymptomatic leg is elevated; results are positive if it recreates sciatic pain radiating down the contralateral leg. The reverse prone straight leg raise, or **femoral stretch test,** is performed by extending the straight leg at the hip and recreating symptoms. This tests L3 and L4 nerve root irritation.

The **Lasègue test** is performed with the hip bent at 90 degrees of flexion and the patient supine. The knee is slowly extended until radicular pain is produced.

The **Bowstring sign** is produced by applying pressure to the popliteal space while the sciatic nerve is under stretch. An increase in pain is considered positive.

Special tests

- Straight leg raising test
- Contralateral (reverse) straight leg raising test
- Femoral stretch (reverse prone straight leg raising) test
- Hamstring tightness test
- One-legged hyperextension test
- Lasègue test
- Bowstring sign

Hamstring tightness is often associated with spondylolysis of a painful nature. A test to provoke pain at the site of the spondylolysis is the **one-legged hyperextension test** described by Ciullo and Jackson.[11] In this test the athlete is asked to stand on one leg and arch the back backwards. If the test is positive, the athlete points to the area of pain, localizing the site of the lesion.

Vascular Evaluation

A complete examination, particularly in the older athlete, should include palpation of the peripheral pulses. The symptoms of spinal stenosis and arterial claudication may be difficult to distinguish.

DIAGNOSTIC STUDIES
Radiography

Plain radiographs are the most frequently ordered diagnostic study performed during workup of the athlete with back pain. There is concern that this examination rarely gives pertinent information and that the abnormalities depicted rarely correlate with symptoms.[25,97] We believe that an athlete who has not responded to activity restriction and physical modalities over 2 to 3 weeks should have radiographs performed. The athlete suspected of an acute major trauma should have a radiograph performed immediately. A clinical suspicion of infectious, neoplastic, or metabolic abnormalities also warrants immediate radiography. An anteroposterior and a lateral view of the thoracic or lumbar spine while the patient is standing is standard (Fig. 52-3). The standing position accentuates any bony deformity such as a spondylolisthesis or disk space narrowing. The use of lateral flexion-extension views to check for instability may be obtained, but they seldom contribute to our understanding of the symptoms.

Computed Tomography

Computed tomography (CT) is an imaging technique that allows visualization of bony and soft-tissue neural compression. The advantage over myelography is that it

is noninvasive and affords better visualization of lateral pathologic conditions, such as foraminal stenosis and lateral disk herniations.[33,42,77] Three-dimensional surface reformations may allow for unimpaired visualization of the bony architecture and its impact on neural compression.[2,76] One potential drawback of standard CT vs. magnetic resonance imaging (MRI) and myelography is the convention of visualizing only the lower three lumbar vertebrae. This creates the possibility of missing unsuspected higher lesions. CT of a disk herniation relies on the demonstration of an asymmetric soft-tissue bulge in the spinal canal (Fig. 52-4). If this bulge causes significant neural encroachment, there is loss of the normal neural anatomy and loss of the epidural fat that normally surrounds the nerve roots. The addition of a water-soluble contrast agent in conjunction with CT enhances the accuracy of the study.[42,43]

CT may have its greatest advantage in the evaluation of the posttraumatic burst fracture and canal encroachment by retropulsed bony fragments. Subtle fractures of the spine may also be best visualized using CT. These fractures include fractures of the facets or other posterior spinal elements.

Myelography

The current use of water-soluble agents during myelography has provided for better visualization of nerve roots, the conus, and the thoracic cord than with oil-soluble agents (Fig. 52-5). The incidence of arachnoiditis and symptoms of headaches, nausea, vomiting, and seizures have also substantially lessened. Although these changes have enhanced the reliability of the test and have made it less toxic, it remains an invasive test, and controversy remains as to which test (myelography, CT, or MRI) is the most reliable to evaluate the neural elements (Fig. 52-6).[3,5,34,82] To date, no clear-cut advantage

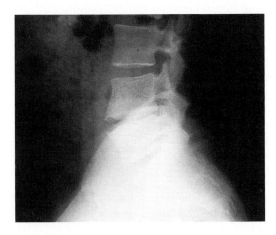

FIG. 52-3. Lateral radiograph displaying narrowing of disk space and anterior osteophyte formation in professional football offensive lineman.

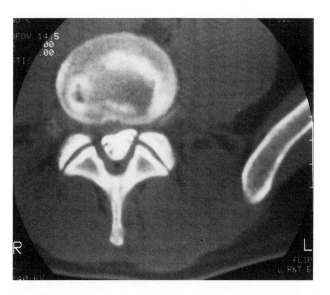

FIG. 52-4. Computed tomography of lumbar spine of baseball pitcher performed immediately following water-soluble myelography. Right lateral disk herniation at L4-L5 with ventral compression of thecal sac.

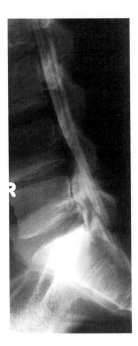

FIG. 52-5. Lumbar myelogram in professional baseball player. Lateral view demonstrates symmetric ventral compression of contrast-filled dural tube at L4-L5 disk level, suggesting disk herniation.

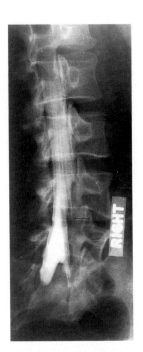

FIG. 52-6. Lumbar myelogram of professional baseball pitcher showing amputation of right inferiorly coursing L5 nerve root (*arrow*). Same patient as in Fig. 52-4.

of one over the other has been shown. In instances in which a complete blockage of myelographic dye is shown, it is imperative that a CT scan distal to the blockage be performed. In one study of cases of complete blockage, CT showed abnormalities distal to the blockage in 59% of the cases.[34]

Magnetic Resonance Imaging

In recent years MRI has served as a useful tool in the diagnosis of soft-tissue abnormalities in athletes. The advantage of MRI is that it is noninvasive, unlike myelography, and it does not expose the athlete to radiation, unlike CT.[56,66,74,75] It is an excellent technique to determine early degenerative changes in the disk space, but it may be too sensitive, leading to overdiagnosis and treatment (Figs. 52-7 and 52-8). As with any imaging modality the patient must not be treated on the basis of a diagnostic test to the exclusion of clinical findings.

MRI also has the capacity to identify intraspinal abnormalities above and below the primary area of interest. One disadvantage of MRI may be its ability to demonstrate lateral recess nerve root compression compared with that which is possible with myelography. MRI also lags behind myelography and CT in the diagnosis of spinal stenosis.

An important advantage of MRI is its use of an intravenous paramagnetic contrast medium, such as gadolinium, when evaluating the postoperative patient. The enhanced imaging is superior to both myelography and contrast-enhanced CT in the differentiation of postoperative scarring from retained disk fragments.[35]

Diskography

The current role of diskography in the diagnostic workup of the athlete, or any patient with back pain, is controversial. The concept behind the use of the test is twofold. First, proponents of diskography believe that the injection of a contrast medium into a disk space, coupled with CT, allows for a morphologic assessment of the intervertebral disk space. Classification systems of the normal and pathologic space have been proposed. Second, symptoms elicited during the injection are thought to correlate with localization of the offending pathologic condition.[13] Some physicians have recommended diskectomy and fusion based on this correlation. MRI, because of its noninvasive nature and ability to determine early disk degeneration, may hold more promise in the future.[84,100]

Bone Scintigraphy

Bone scanning (technetium-99 phosphate) uses radiation from radiopharmaceuticals to detect abnormalities in the skeletal system.[69] It is particularly useful in the evaluation of infectious, neoplastic, metabolic, ischemic, and traumatic disorders of the spine. Unfortunately, it is not very specific. In most cases it is used as an adjunctive diagnostic modality and is combined with some other imaging study (radiography, CT, or MRI) to enhance the diagnosis. A "hot spot" on a bone scan correlates with an area of increased bone metabolic activity, and a "cold spot" correlates with alteration in vascularity. A bone scan may be useful in athletes to determine the presence of a spondylolytic defect caused by trauma.

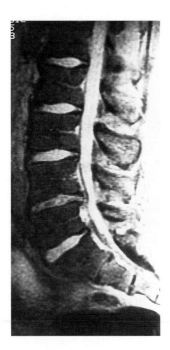

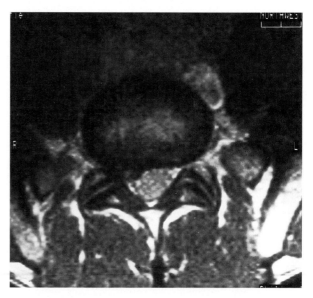

FIG. 52-7. Magnetic resonance image displays degeneration of disk and bulging at L4-L5 disk space level.

FIG. 52-8. Magnetic resonance image showing laterally herniated L5-S1 disk fragment in professional basketball player who subsequently underwent laminectomy and excision.

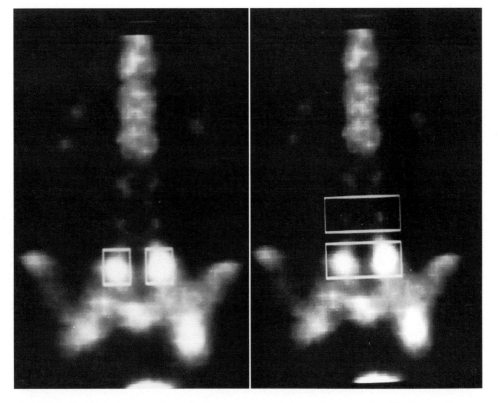

FIG. 52-9. Bone scintigram with single photon emission computed tomography of lumbosacral spine indicates increased localization of radionuclide in pars interarticularis of L5 vertebra bilaterally in high school football player. Findings are compatible with spondylolysis in this region.

Single Photon Emission Computed Tomography

Single photon emission computed tomography (SPECT) scanning is a recent advance in our diagnostic armamentarium. It combines the advantages of bone scanning with those derived from tomogaphic imaging (Fig. 52-9).[14,94] This allows an evaluation of bony structures that normally overlap. It can be particularly useful in the evaluation of spondylolysis, spondylolisthesis, and pseudoarthrosis of the spine. We have also found it to be useful in evaluating an athlete with low back pain when the bone scan is negative.

Thermography

The thermogram records changes in skin temperature, allegedly mapping areas of physiologic change. To date, there has been no conclusive studies to validate its usefulness as a diagnostic adjunct in the evaluation of the athlete with low back pain. We neither currently use it, nor recommend its use in the workup of back injuries.

Electrodiagnostic Studies

The role of electrodiagnostic testing in the evaluation of the athlete with radiculopathy or low back pain is uncertain. Although this type of testing may be quite accurate in the detection of radiculopathy, we tend to rely on an extensive physical examination and diagnostic workup and use the previously mentioned tests to localize the lesion. Electrodiagnostic studies may be useful in distinguishing peripheral neuropathy secondary to a metabolic disorder, such as diabetes mellitus, or a demyelinating disorder.

TREATMENT

The goals of any treatment program should be to minimize disability secondary to injury and return the athlete to sport activity in as short a time as possible. In keeping with this concept, exercise is the most commonly prescribed treatment for athletes with back pain. We have found that a well-structured exercise program not only assists in the rehabilitation of back injuries, but also serves as an excellent means of prevention. Numerous studies have proposed a relationship between trunk muscle strength, endurance, and low back disorders.[4,22,50,54] Patients with back problems frequently lack strength, flexibility, and endurance of the musculature about the thoracolumbar spine, abdomen, and pelvic girdle. Many athletes emphasize strengthening the thoracic, upper, and lower extremity musculature at the expense of the less glamorous spine and pelvic girdle. Recently, attention has been focused on the importance of not only strength, but also general physical fitness in the prevention of back injuries.[12] In a study of firefighters the incidence of back injuries was 10 times higher in the least-conditioned group compared with the most-conditioned group. Even in an athletic population an assessment of the athletes' physical capacity before participation is important to identify those who are at risk for injury. Thus before discussing specific injuries and their treatment, it would be prudent to discuss injury prevention.

Preparticipation Examination

The preparticipation examination is an integral part of the evaluation of athletes at risk for injury, whether it be back injuries or cardiovascular disease. According to Van Handel[93] the examination aids the physician in evaluating for the potential adverse effects of exercise and athletic participation in four specific areas. First, it aids in the diagnosis of disease or injury in the symptomatic or asymptomatic individual. Second, it assesses the cardiovascular, pulmonary, and muscular endurance levels of the athlete. Third, it assesses the safety of exercise and athletic participation and the safety and efficacy of interventions. Last, it provides a comparison for adaptation and the basis for exercise prescription. Where the preparticipation screening breaks down is in the scope of the examination and the resources that are available to provide such screening to the athlete. Although most athletic programs require a preseason physical examination, few examinations, unless at the college, professional, or elite level provide sufficient information or depth to form the basis for exercise prescription.

Ideally, the preparticipation examination should identify structural abnormalities of the spine and previous spine injuries that warrant attention. The examination should identify structural abnormalities of the spine and previous spine injuries that warrant attention. The examination should assess muscular strength, flexibility, and endurance.[49,71] Armed with this information the team physician can outline a program of fitness and exercise that lessens the risk of injury.

Preparticipation spinal evaluation

- Identify structural abnormalities
- Elucidate previous spinal injury
- Assess muscle strength, flexibility, and endurance

Exercise Prescription
Strengthening

As previously mentioned, strengthening exercises are currently thought to be important in the treatment and prevention of back injuries.[37,38,91] The rationale behind such an approach is multifactorial. The abdominal, paraspinal, and pelvic musculature support the thoracic and lumbar spine by acting as "guy wires." Individuals with low levels of muscular strength for a given endeavor are at greater risk for back injuries.[12] Even a well-conditioned athlete can have a relatively weak abdominal, paraspinal, and pelvic musculature. Which exercises are most beneficial for a healthy back and athletic performance is still unclear. For years the Williams' exercises, which emphasized flexion, were most popular. Recently there has been a trend emphasizing extension exercises and restoring the normal extension/flexion strength ratio of $1.3:1.0$.[1,50] Patients with low back pain are found to have this ratio significantly reduced. The purpose of therapeutic exercise then is to reduce pain,

Normal spinal muscle balance
Extension/flexion
1.3:1.0

restore range of motion, and strengthen the musculature to restore functional capacity.[50]

Swiss Ball Exercise Program

Our approach to an exercise program is to emphasize all areas, both flexion and extension, and torsional muscular strength and endurance. A unique and new method of developing this strength and endurance is to use the **Swiss ball exercise program** (Figs. 52-10 to 52-14).

The underlying concept of the Swiss ball exercise program is to attain adequate musculoligamentous control of the lumbar spine forces. When this control is obtained, repetitive injuries to the intervertebral disks, facet joints, and related structures can be minimized.

The Swiss ball exercise program has a series of basic exercises that must be mastered before progressing to more advanced exercises. The basic level emphasizes postural control, starting from the most primitive postural positions of supine and prone lying with advancement to kneeling, standing, and position transition movements. The precise observation of meticulous technique is imperative in these exercise. Each of the exercises is designed to develop isolated and co-contraction muscle patterns to stabilize the lumbar spine in the neutral position.[78]

Basic stabilization routines
■ Hamstring stretching
■ Quadriceps stretching
■ Hip flexor stretching
■ Hip rotator stretching
■ Gastrocsoleus stretching
■ Abdominal curls—basic program
■ Pelvic bracing
■ Prone neutral spine positioning
■ Prone leg raises
■ Sidelying leg raises
■ Bridging
■ Advanced bridging
■ Bridging with stepping
■ Ball-balanced bridging
■ Quadriped
■ Kneeling stabilization
■ Squat strengthening—wall slides and counter squats
■ Position transition with and without weight

When the athlete has mastered the basic exercises, he or she is started on the Swiss ball exercise program. This program helps develop lumbopelvic kinesthetic awareness in as many positions as possible. The ultimate goal is to design the program so that it can be tailored to the injured athlete in his or her individual sport.

Flexibility

Flexibility and mobility of the lumbar spine and pelvis are also essential to the treatment and prevention of low back pain. Patients with low back pain have been shown to have significant motion limitations in lumbar flexion and extension.[54] Limitations of rotation and lateral bend-

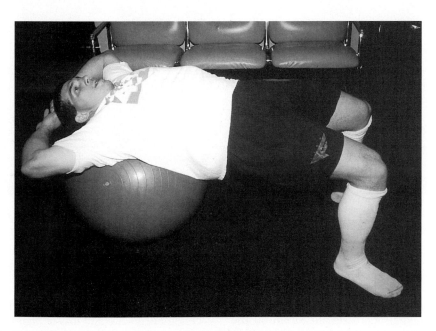

FIG. 52-10. Neutral position emphasizes flat lumbar spine with hips at neutral position and knees flexed at 90 degrees. While maintaining this position athlete may march in place or alternate extending the leg.

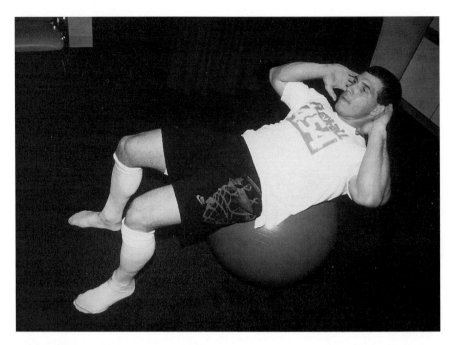

FIG. 52-11. While in neutral position, partial sit-ups can be performed on the ball. This strengthens abdominals, spine extensors, quadriceps, and gluteal muscles.

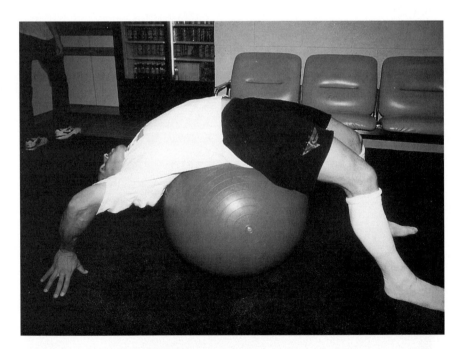

FIG. 52-12. Supine lumbar and thoracic extension exercises stretch out abdominal and hip flexor muscles. It also strengthens entire trunk musculature.

ing are also common.[57,59] It stands to reason that limitation of motion in one of the mobile segments, such as pelvic extension or flexion, increases the strain on the other segments. Thus maintenance of muscular flexibility and joint mobility should be a goal of any exercise and rehabilitation program.

Aerobic Fitness

Injury to the spine associated with pain leads to a deconditioned state and loss of physical fitness. One of the goals of the exercise program should be to maintain aerobic fitness. Deficits in aerobic capacity do not have a direct correlation with spine injury or pain, but it stands

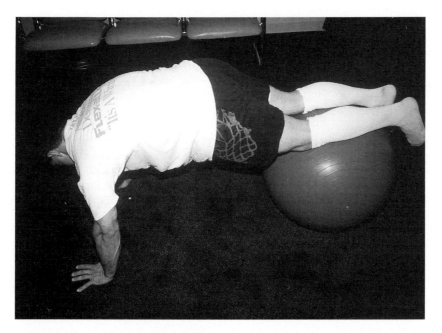

FIG. 52-13. Prone push-ups from the ball strengthen arms, shoulders, and spinal extensor musculature. It is imperative that athlete maintains a neutral lumbar lordosis during this exercise to derive maximum benefit.

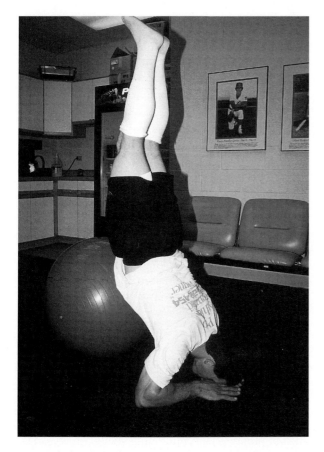

FIG. 52-14. An advanced exercise is the handstand. This incorporates the entire trunk musculature and demands high degree of kinesthetic awareness.

to reason that overall aerobic fitness is important to injury prevention. The preferred exercise program should emphasize activities that avoid high-impact and ballistic-type spinal movements.

Approach to Specific Injury

Unlike back injuries in the general population the athlete frequently responds to injury in an exaggerated manner. The desire to compete and continue with the chosen activity frequently makes it difficult for the athlete to comply with prescribed treatment. Thus one of the goals of the treating physician should be to educate the athlete about the pathogenesis of his or her pain. A second goal should be to outline as specific a treatment plan as possible and formulate a timetable of desired goals and objectives for the injured athlete. A third goal should be to involve the athlete in the formulation of the treatment plan and provide activities that keep the athlete active and minimize the psychologic stress resulting from inactivity.[9] The athlete accepts his or her potential disability only when he or she is involved with the treatment protocol and is educated regarding the pathogenesis of the problem.

Treatment goals

- Educate athlete about problem
- Outline specific treatment program
- Formulate a timetable
- Involve athlete in treatment plan
- Provide athlete with activities to minimize inactivity stresses

General Measures

Fortunately, most of the thoracic and lumbar injuries treated by sports medicine physicians are self-limited musculoligamentous sprains that improve spontaneously. Despite this, a number of therapeutic modalities have been promoted to influence the clinical outcome and return the athlete to activity as soon as possible. Most of these modalities have little scientific foundation and have not been shown to be of significant clinical benefit.

Medication. Nonsteroidal antiinflammatory drugs (NSAIDs) are frequently used in the initial treatment of back pain, although they have not been shown to have any significant benefit over the use of aspirin or acetaminophen. They generally are well tolerated and help provide analgesia without the addictive or depressant effects of narcotics. **Narcotics** are used only in extreme cases of trauma and severe pain. We have found the use of **antispasmodics** to be of limited value, and we prescribe them infrequently.

The use of **oral steroids** in a tapered dose may also be contemplated in the initial treatment of low-back pain, particularly in those athletes with radicular symptoms.

Modalities. Therapeutic modalities such as **cryotherapy** and **heat** are also frequently used in the treatment of musculoligamentous injuries. Ice has been used in the management of soft-tissue injuries for decades. Local application of ice causes lower cell metabolism, vasoconstriction, reduced nerve conduction velocity, decreased muscle contractility, and increased pain threshold.[58,80,99] Application of ice for a duration of 15 to 30 minutes is generally accepted to have the most beneficial effect on subcutaneous tissue. The therapeutic effect of heat on the back has been empiric in nature. Modalities that produce heat include warm compresses and other modalities such as diathermy and ultrasound. The physiologic effects of heat application include increased cellular metabolic rate, vasodilatation, increase in the inflammatory process, increase in the elastic properties of collagen, and psychologic relaxation.[51,80,92] The desired depth of penetration of the heating modality determines which should be selected. Diathermy and ultrasound are selected when the desired treatment area lies deep to the skin. Muscle spasm, soft-tissue contracture, and edema are generally treated with heat modalities.

Electrical stimulation, either galvanic (direct current) or faradic (alternating current), has been used by physical therapists in the management of soft-tissue injuries about the spine. The physiologic effects of these modalities are believed to be similar to those of the other modalities and include vasoconstriction, decrease in nerve irritability, and local analgesia. To date, these therapeutic effects have not been well documented.

Phonophoresis is a method of driving a drug through a membrane using ultrasound. A medication such as hydrocortisone or xylocaine with a coupling gel is worked into the skin over the target tissues. Ten percent hydrocortisone cream either alone or in combination with xylocaine is commonly used in acute or chronic inflammatory conditions of the spine. Depth of penetration of the agent allegedly is from 5 to 10 cm, depending on the vibrational frequency of the ultrasound.[29,79]

Transcutaneous electric nerve stimulation (TENS) is a modality that produces an intermittent or pulsed electric signal transmitted via surface electrodes. TENS units are used for the control of both acute and chronic low back pain. The basis for their use lies in the work of Melzack and Wall,[60] who theorized that stimulation of cutaneous afferents blocks pain stimuli in the substantia gelatinosa. Another theory suggests that its benefit may be obtained by elevating endorphins, the body's endogenous opiate system. Electroacupuncture is a modality similar to TENS but is rooted in the theory of acupuncture. To date, we have had no experience with this modality to disprove or validate its use.

Manipulation. Spinal manipulative therapy is a controversial modality that is accepted by a large group of athletes. Manipulation of the spine has been practiced since the time of Hippocrates, and its use has promoted significant debate over its clinical efficacy and purpose. The goal of manipulative therapy is to relieve pain and increase function. Theoretically, these goals are achieved via mechanical, neurophysiologic, and psychologic effects.[70] On a mechanical level, manipulation provides freer motion in spinal segments that have lost their extensibility as a result of immobilization and adhesion formation. The neurophysiologic effects, like many of the other modalities, are rooted in the gate control theory of Melzack and Wall.[60] In this case the manipulation provides the sensory input that closes the gate to painful stimuli. Psychologic effects of manipulation are provided by the "laying on of the hands," a modality frequently overlooked in importance by today's practitioner. Short-term benefits of spinal manipulation are modest, but its recurrent use and its use in chronic back pain has not been substantiated.[44] Even its greatest supporters con-

---

Contraindications to spinal manipulation

- Spinal instability
- Spondylolysis
- Fractures
- Acute herniated disks

---

sider spinal instability, spondylolysis, fractures, and acute herniated disks as contraindications to its use.

Bed rest and traction. Prolonged bed rest and traction are also unproven modalities in the treatment of back pain. Mechanical low back pain responds as well to 2 days of bed rest as it does to 1 week.[18]

Dorsolumbar Kyphosis (Scheuermann's Disease)

Conservative treatment consisting of activity limitation with occasional bracing is usually sufficient to return the athlete to activity. An initial period of restriction from strenuous activity combined with the previously mentioned physical therapy modalities frequently relieves the pain. Once the athlete is pain free an exercise program aimed at progressive conditioning should be undertaken with a gradual return to athletic activity.[95] Bracing with a Milwaukee brace is undertaken only if the deformity is severe and the athlete is skeletally immature. Surgery is only rarely indicated.

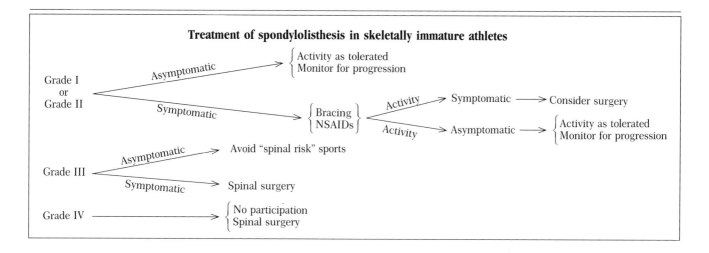

Spondylolysis and Spondylolisthesis

Various approaches to the treatment of the athletically active individual with spondylolysis have been proposed. These range from restriction of activity to surgical fusion. Most patients with spondylolysis and spondylolisthesis respond to activity restriction, bracing, and antiinflammatory medication. The brace we use is a Boston type, anterior opening, antilordotic brace that is worn by the athlete full-time for at least 4 months. Once the patient becomes asymptomatic, he or she can return to athletic activity. Frederickson et al[23] allows athletic activity in the brace if the patient is asymptomatic. The incidence of spondylolysis is approximately 4.4% in children and 6% in adults.[23] Slippage (spondylolisthesis) is believed to occur at the same time as the pars interarticularis defect is discovered, and the likelihood of further slippage with activity is remote.

The skeletally immature athlete with a Grade I (25%) or Grade II (25% to 50%) slip is allowed to be active as long as he or she remains asymptomatic. The likelihood of further slippage is low, but the skeletally immature athlete should be monitored for progression. The child with a symptomatic Grade I or Grade II slip who does not respond to conservative care over the course of 1 year may require surgical stabilization. A Grade III (50% to 75%) slip is probably at higher risk to ultimately progress further. Asymptomatic athletes may be advised to avoid sports that put the spine at further risk, such as contact sports, pole vaulting, gymnastics, and weightlifting. The symptomatic athlete requires a fusion. If the patient has significant radicular symptoms, a decompression and fusion is warranted. (There is considerable controversy about the role of reduction of the slippage and fusion vs. decompression and fusion alone. A full discussion of this

controversy is beyond the scope of this chapter.) In the mature athlete with radicular symptoms a decompression is combined with an in situ fusion. The Grade IV (75% to 100%) slip probably precludes participation in athletic activity. This group usually experiences radicular symptoms and has severe hamstring tightness and marked cosmetic deformity. Because of severe symptoms, this group usually requires a surgical fusion approached from both back and front. In the skeletally immature athlete an attempt at reduction and fusion is warranted.

Herniated Nucleus Pulposus

A herniated disk may occur at either the thoracic or the lumbar area. Disk herniation at the thoracic area is rare. Lumbar disk herniation, on the other hand, is not uncommon in the active athlete. A number of athletes, many in the professional ranks, have returned to play after both conservative and operative treatment for disk herniations. These athletes have returned to sports such as baseball, golf, football, and basketball (all activities that place significant stress on the spine). Herniated disks in children and adolescents can be extremely disabling and difficult to diagnose because of the paucity of neurologic abnormalities. Frequently the only positive sign is the straight leg raise with crossover.[19]

The initial treatment of the individual with a ruptured lumbar disk is conservative. The only true surgical emergencies are the cauda equina syndrome (bowel or bladder dysfunction) or ascending motor weakness. Medication should be directed at pain relief without the depressant effects of narcotics. We usually prescribe a nonsteroidal medication. Bed rest should not be prolonged, and the various physical therapy modalities may help in mo-

---

"Spinal risk" sports

- Contact sports
- Pole vaulting
- Gymnastics
- Weightlifting

Initial treatment of lumbar disk herniation

- NSAIDs
- Bed rest (2 to 3 days)
- Mobilization with modalities
- Epidural steroid injection

bilizing the patient. We have found the use of epidural cortisone injections administered by our anesthesiology staff to be particularly useful in the early treatment.[40] Depending on the response of the patient, we repeat injections up to three times, spaced at 2-week intervals.

Only 5% to 10% of patients with a lumbar-herniated disk and radicular symptoms require surgical intervention. Those athletes who do not respond in 6 to 12 weeks of conservative treatment undergo diagnostic workup and disk fragment excision. With an adequate postoperative exercise and conditioning program, we have been successful in returning both the amateur and professional athlete to their desired sport.

Surgical indications in lumbar disk herniation

- Cauda equina syndrome (emergency)
- Ascending motor weakness
- Failure of 6 to 12 weeks of conservative treatment for radicular symptoms
- Documented disk herniation

Spinal Stenosis

Spinal stenosis is the most common cause of neurologic leg pain in the older athlete. The pathologic condition invloves neural compression secondary to degenerative disk collapse, facet arthritis, and narrowing of the neural foramen. Bony impingement and soft-tissue compression by either the disk anteriorly or the ligamentum flavum posteriorly may occur. Initial treatment is symptomatic and includes the use of oral anti-inflammatory drugs, and restriction of those activities that elicit the pain. Aerobic conditioning is promoted. Epidural steroid injections have met with mixed results in our hands.

Surgical decompression is warranted in documented cases of compression when symptomatic modalities provide incomplete relief. Preservation of the facet joint on at least one side is important to provide lumbar stability. Extensive decompression may lead to segmental instability. Return to athletic activity after such extensive laminectomy should be predicted on the physician's knowledge of the remaining spinal stability.

Athletics After Spine Surgery

The decision to return an athlete to athletic activity after injury or surgery must be individualized. The two most common scenarios are patients following laminectomy and patients following arthrodesis. As previously mentioned, laminectomy in a stable spine poses little threat to the return to activity. Fusion, on the other hand, places increased mechanical stress on the mobile segments above and below the fusion. Extensive fusion, as performed in scoliosis surgery, generally should preclude the individual from participation in contact sports and gymnastics. Shorter fusions in patients without neurologic deficit, such as in spondylolisthesis, may increase the risk of long-term deterioration of segments above and below the fusion, but they were not proven to potentiate greater risk than that to the general population.[63] Be-

cause of this, we believe that athletes may return to contact sports after short fusions for spondylolysis.

SUMMARY

Spine injuries make up approximately 10% of all athletic injuries. The basis for treatment of injuries to the spine should be anchored in an understanding of basic science, pathology, prevention, diagnosis, treatment, and rehabilitation. The sports medicine physician who understands these fundamentals best serves the athletic patient population through a logical and organized approach to their individual problems. Most athletes are well motivated and seek prompt return to athletic endeavors. We hope that this chapter stimulates a greater degree of interest and understanding of thoracolumbar spine injuries.

REFERENCES

1. Beimborn DJ, Morrisey MC: A review of the literature related to trunk muscle performance, *Spine* 13:655, 1988.
2. Bell GR, Modic MT: Radiology of the lumbar spine. In Rothman RA, Sinecone FA (eds): *The spine*, ed 3, Philadelphia, 1992, WB Saunders.
3. Bell GR et al: A study of computer-assisted tomography. II. Comparison of metrizamide myelography and computed tomography in the diagnosis of herniated lumbar disc and spinal stenosis, *Spine* 9:552, 1984.
4. Berkman M et al: Voluntary strength of male adults with acute low back syndrome, *Clin Orthop* 129:84, 1977.
5. Bolander NF, Shonstrom NS, Spengler DM: Role of computed tomography and myelography in the diagnosis of central spinal stenosis, *J Bone Joint Surg* 67A:240, 1985.
6. Boukris R, Becker KL: Schmorl's nodes and osteoporosis, *Clin Orthop* 104:275, 1974.
7. Bradford DS et al: Scheuermann's kyphosis and roundback deformity, *J Bone Joint Surg* 56A:740, 1974.
8. Brady TA, Bernard RC, Bodner LM: Weight training: related injuries in the high school athlete, *Am J Sports Med* 10:1, 1982.
9. Brigham CD, Schafer MF: Low back pain in athletes, *Adv Sports Med Fitness* 1:145, 1988.
10. Brown AD, Tsaltis T: Studies on the permeability of intervertebral disc during skeletal maturation, *Spine* 1:240, 1982.
11. Ciullo JV, Jackson DW: Pars interarticularis stress reaction, spondylolysis, and spondylolisthesis in gymnasts, *Clin Sports Med* 4:95, 1985.
12. Cody LB et al: Strength and fitness and subsequent back injuries in firefighters, *J Occup Med* 21:269, 1979.
13. Colhound E et al: Provocation discography as a guide to planning operations on the spine, *J Bone Joint Surg* 70B:267, 1988.
14. Collier BD et al: Painful spondylolysis or spondylolisthesis studied by radiography and single photon emission computed tomography, *Radiology* 154:207, 1985.
15. Dehaven KE, Lintner DM: Athletic injuries: comparison by age, sport, and gender, *Am J Sports Med* 14:218, 1986.
16. Denis F: The three-column spine and its significance in the classification of acute thoracolumbar spinal injuries, *Spine* 8:817, 1983.
17. Denis F et al: Acute thoracolumbar burst fractures in the absence of neurologic deficit, *Clin Orthop* 189:142, 1984.
18. Deyo RA, Diehl PK, Rosenthal M: How many days of bed rest for acute low back pain: a randomized clinical trial, *N Engl J Med* 315(17):1064, 1987.
19. Epstein JA et al: Lumbar intervertebral disk herniation in teenage children: recognition and management of associated anomalies, *Spine* 9:427, 1984.
20. Ferguson PJ, McMaster MC, Stanitski CL: Low back pain in college football linemen, *J Bone Joint Surg* 56A(6):1300, 1979.

21. Ferrera MS et al: The injury experience and training history of the competitive skier with a disability, *Am J Sports Med* 20(1):55, 1992.
22. Foster DN, Fulton MN: Back pain and the exercise prescription, *Clin Sports Med* 10(1):197, 1991.
23. Frederickson BC et al: The natural history of spondylolysis and spondylolisthesis, *J Bone Joint Surg* 66A(5):699, 1984.
24. Frymoyer JW et al: Spine radiographs in patients with low back pain: an epidemiological study in men, *J Bone Joint Surg* 66A:1048, 1984.
25. Frymoyer JW et al: Epidemiologic studies of low back pain, *Spine* 5:419, 1980.
26. Gaine D et al: An epidemiologic investigation of injuries affecting young competitive female gymnasts, *Am J Sports Med* 17(6):811, 1989.
27. Ghelman B, Freiberger RH: The limbus vertebra: an anterior disc herniation demonstrated by discography, *AJR* 127:854, 1976.
28. Goldstein JD et al: Spine injuries in gymnasts and swimmers, *Am J Sports Med* 19(5):463, 1991.
29. Griffin JE, Touchstone JC: Effects of ultrasonic frequency on phonophoresis of cortisol into swine tissue, *Am J Phys Med* 51:62, 1972.
30. Hafner RHV: Localized osteochondritis (Scheuermann's disease), *J Bone Joint Surg* 34B:38, 1952.
31. Hanley EN, Phillips ED: Profiles of patients who get spine infections and the type of infections that have a predilection for the spine. In Wiesel SW (ed): *Seminars in spine surgery,* vol 2, Philadelphia, 1990, WB Saunders.
32. Harrington KD: Metastatic disease of the spine, *J Bone Joint Surg* 68A:1110, 1986.
33. Haughton VM et al: A prospective comparison of computed tomography and myelography in the diagnosis of herniated lumbar disc, *Radiology* 142:103, 1982.
34. Herkowitz HN et al: The use of computerized tomography in evaluating nonvisualized vertebral levels caudad to a complete block on a lumbar myelogram: a review of thirty-two cases, *J Bone Joint Surg* 69A:218, 1987.
35. Hueffle MG et al: Lumbar spine postoperative MR imaging with GD-OTRA, *Radiology* 167:817, 1988.
36. Ishmael WK, Shorbe HB: *Care of the back,* ed 3, Philadelphia, 1985, JB Lippincott.
37. Jackson CD, Brown MD: Analysis of current approaches and a practical guide to prescription of exercise, *Clin Orthop* 179:46, 1983.
38. Jackson CP, Brown MD: Is there a role for exercise in the treatment of patients with low back pain? *Clin Orthop* 179:39, 1983.
39. Jackson DW: Low back pain in young athletes: evaluation of stress reaction and discogenic problems, *Am J Sports Med* 7:364, 1979.
40. Jackson DW, Rettig A, Wiltse RL: Epidural cortisone injections in the young athletic adult, *Am J Sports Med* 8(4):239, 1980.
41. Jackson DW, Wiltse LL, Cirincione RJ: Spondylolysis in the female gymnast, *Clin Orthop* 117:68, 1981.
42. Jackson RP et al: The neuroradiographic diagnosis of lumbar-herniated nucleus pulposus I, *Spine* 14:1356, 1989.
43. Jackson RP et al: The neuroradiographic diagnosis of lumbar-herniated nucleus pulposus II, *Spine* 14:1362, 1989.
44. Kahnovitz N: Lumbar spine. In Poss R: *Orthopaedic knowledge update III,* Rosemont, Ill, 1990, American Academy of Orthopaedic Surgeons.
45. Kelsey JL, White AA: Epidemiology and impact of low back pain, *Spine* 5:133, 1980.
46. Kien JS: Thoracolumbar fractures in winter sports, *Clin Orthop* 216:38, 1987.
47. King HA: Back pain in children, *Pediatr Clin North Am* 31:1083, 1984.
48. Koren A, Garty I, Katzuni E: Bone infarction in children with sickle cell disease: early diagnosis and differentiation from osteomyelitis, *Eur J Pediatr* 142:93, 1984.
49. Lagrana NA et al: Quantitative assessment of back strength using isokinetic testing, *Spine* 9:287, 1984.
50. Lee CK: The use of exercise and muscle testing in the rehabilitation of spinal disorders, *Clin Sports Med* 10(1):197, 1991.
51. Lehman JF, Warren CG, Schom SM: Therapeutic heat and cold, *Clin Orthop* 99:207, 1974.
52. Lestini WF, Bell GR: Spinal infections: patient evaluation. In *Seminars in spine surgery,* vol 2, Philadelphia, 1990, WB Saunders.
53. Linder CW et al: Preparticipation health screening of young athletes: results of 1268 examinations, *Am J Sports Med* 19(3):187, 1981.
54. Longrana NA, Lee CK: Isokinetic evaluation of trunk muscles, *Spine* 9:171, 1984.
55. Mandelbaum BR, Cross MC: Spondylolysis and spondylolisthesis. In Reider B (ed): *Sports medicine: the school-age athlete,* Philadelphia, 1991, WB Saunders.
56. Masaryk TJ et al: High resolution MR imaging of sequestered lumbar intervertebral discs, *AJNR* 9:351, 1988.
57. Mayer TG et al: Quantification of lumbar function. II. Preliminary data on isokinetic torso rotation testing with myoelectric spectral analysis in normal and low back pain subjects, *Spine* 10:912, 1985.
58. McMaster WC: A literary review on ice therapy in injuries, *Am J Sports Med* 5(3):124, 1977.
59. McNeill T et al: Trunk strengths in flexion, extension, and lateral bending in healthy subjects and patients with low back disorders, *Spine* 5:529, 1980.
60. Melzack R, Wall PD: Pain mechanisms: a new theory, *Science* 50:971, 1965.
61. Meyerding HW: Spondylolisthesis, *Surg Gynecol Obstet* 54:371, 1932.
62. Micheli LJ: Low back pain in the adolescent: differential diagnosis, *Am J Sports Med* 7(6):362, 1979.
63. Micheli LJ: Sports following spinal surgery in the young athlete, *Clin Orthop* 198:152, 1985.
64. Micheli LJ, Trapman E: Spinal deformities. In Torg S, Welsh RP, Shephard RJ (eds): *Current therapy in sports medicine,* ed 2, St Louis, 1990, Mosby.
65. Miller JAA, Schmatz C, Schultz AB: Lumbar disc degeneration: correlation with age, sex, and spine level in 600 autopsy specimens, *Spine* 13(2):173, 1988.
66. Modi MT et al: Degenerative disc disease: assessment of changes in vertebral body marrow with MR imagery, *Radiology* 166:193, 1988.
67. Nachemson A, Morris JM: In vivo measurements of intradiscal pressure, *J Bone Joint Surg* 46A:1077, 1964.
68. O'Leary P, Boiardi R: The diagnosis and treatment of injuries of the spine in athletes. In Nicholas JA, Hershman EB (eds): *Lower extremity and spine in sports medicine,* ed 1, St Louis, 1986, Mosby.
69. Papanicolaou N et al: Bone scintigraphy in young athletes with low back pain: observations and indications, *AJR* 145:1039, 1985.
70. Paris SV: Spinal manipulative therapy, *Clin Orthop* 179:24, 1983.
71. Paulsen E: Back muscle strength and limits in lifting burdens, *Spine* 6:73, 1981.
72. Punjabi MM, White AA III: Physical properties and functional biomechanics of the spine. In White AA III, Punjabi MM (eds): *Clinical biomechanics of the spine,* ed 2, Philadelphia, 1990, JB Lippincott.
73. Reid DC, Saboe L: Spine fractures in winter sports, *Sports Med* 7:393, 1989.
74. Ross JJ et al: Thoracic disk herniation: MR imaging, *Radiology* 165:511, 1987.
75. Ross JS et al: Assessment of extradural degenerative disease with gadolinium-DTPA–enhanced MR imagery: correlation with surgical and pathological findings, *AJNR* 10:1243, 1989.
76. Rothman SLG: Computed tomography of the spine in older children and teenagers, *Clin Sports Med* 5(2):247, 1986.
77. Ruskin S, Kentry J: Recognition of lumbar disc disease: comparison of myelography and computed tomography, *AJNR* 3:215, 1982.
78. Saal JA: Rehabilitation of sports-related lumbar spine injuries. In Saal JA (ed): *Physical medicine and rehabilitation state of the art reviws: sports injuries,* Vol 1, No 4, Philadelphia, 1987, Hanley and Belfus, Inc.
79. Santiesteban AJ: The role of physical agents in the treatment of spine pain, *Clin Orthop* 179:24, 1983.

80. Sawyer M, Zbieranek CK: The treatment of soft tissue after spinal injury, *Clin Sports Med* 5(2):387, 1986.

81. Scheuermann HW: Kyphosis dorsalis juvenilis, *Z Orthop* 41:35, 1921.

82. Schipper J et al: Lumbar disk herniation: diagnosis with CT or myelography, *Radiology* 165:227, 1987.

83. Schmorl G: Die pathologische anatomie der wirbelsunk, *Verh Dtsch Orthop Gr* 21:3, 1927.

84. Schneidermer G et al: Magnetic resonance imaging in the diagnosis of disc degeneration: correlation with discography, *Spine* 12:276, 1987.

85. Semon RL, Spengler D: Significance of lumbar spondylolysis in college football players, *Spine* 6:172, 1981.

86. Spencer CW, Jackson DW: Back injuries in the athlete, *Clin Sports Med* 2:191, 1983.

87. Stanish W: Low back pain in middle-aged athletes, *Am J Sports Med* 7:367, 1969.

88. Stauffer ES et al: Fractures and dislocations of the spine. Part II. The thoracolumbar spine. In Rockwood CA, Green DP, Bucholz RW (eds): *Fractures in adults,* ed 3, Philadelphia, 1991, JB Lippincott.

89. Tanz SS: Motion of the lumbar spine: a roentgenologic study, *AJR* 69:399, 1953.

90. Thurston AJ, Harris JO: Normal kinematics of the lumbar spine and pelvis, *Spine* 8:199, 1983.

91. Tollison CB, Kriegal ML: Physical exercise in the treatment of low back pain. I. A review, *Orthop Rev* 17:724, 1988.

92. Topperman PS, Devlin M: Therapeutic hot and cold, *Postgrad Med* 73(1):69, 1983.

93. Van Handel PJ: The preparticipation fitness test, *Clin Sports Med* 10(1):1, 1991.

94. Webb S et al: Three-dimensional display of data obtained by single photon emission computed tomography, *Br J Radiol* 60:557, 1987.

95. Wilcox PG, Spencer CW: Dorsolumbar kyphosis or Scheuermann's disease, *Clin Sports Med* 5(2):343, 1986.

96. Wiltse LL, Newman PH, MacNab I: Classification of spondylolysis and spondylolisthesis, *Clin Orthop* 117:23, 1976.

97. Witt I, Vestergaard A, Rosen KA: A comparative analysis of x-ray findings of the lumbar spine, *Spine* 9:298, 1984.

98. Wroble RR, Albright JP: Neck and low back injuries in wrestling, *Clin Sports Med* 5:255, 1986.

99. Yackzan L, Adams C, Francis KT: The effects of ice massage on delayed muscle soreness, *Am J Sports Med* 12(2):159, 1984.

100. Yasama T, Ohno R, Yamauchi Y: False negative lumbar discograms: correlation of discographic and histologic findings in postmortem and surgical specimens, *J Bone Joint Surg* 70A:1279, 1988.

CHAPTER 53

Assessment and Nonsurgical Management of Athletic Low Back Injury

Stanley A. Herring
Stuart M. Weinstein

Low back pain probably began with the development of bipedal ambulation and has spanned the ages, often precipitated by physically demanding activities such as sports. The treatment of low back pain also predates recorded history. Manual therapy techniques such as spinal mobilization were practiced by North and South American Indian tribes. The Old Testament mentions laying on of hands. Hippocrates (460-370 BC) recorded the first history of low back pain treatment, describing and illustrating joint manipulation and traction. His successor, Galen (131-202 AD), taught manual medicine techniques for the spine and extremities. By the Middle Ages Chinese, German, English, French, Dutch, and Arabic physicians described hands-on treatment for spinal and peripheral joint problems. Starting with this era and into the nineteenth century, "bone setters" treated the spine and extremities with techniques often handed down through generations. Bone setting received great attention at the 1882 annual meeting of the British Medical Society and later in a 1925 edition of *The Lancet*.[20,76,133,168]

The use of exercise to prevent and treat such diseases as low back pain dates back to at least ancient Greece. Hippocrates not only taught manual therapy and traction, but also recognized the necessity and value of sufficient exercise for healthy living and treatment of disease. Galen too incorporated exercise into preventive and therapeutic medicine. He also developed a system of resistance training using dumbbells, heavy weightlifting, and isometric contraction exercises.[17,183] During the Renaissance the leading European medical schools taught hygiene and exercise as part of the general curriculum. Also, as early as the fifteenth century, publications promoting self-help in the form of exercise for disease and health were available.[17,171] Beginning with the latter part of the sixteenth century and throughout the seventeenth century a gradual rekindling of the interest in strength training occurred.[183] By the nineteenth century the term *physical education,* including discussions of strengthening, was described in the literature regarding the importance of exercise in the prevention and treatment of diseases.[17,189] In the late twentieth century functional restoration following lumbar spine injury has again become the focus of most rehabilitation programs. This chapter focuses on the assessment and rehabilitation of lumbar spine problems in the athletic population. Based on concepts originating in antiquity, a comprehensive and state-of-the-art approach to rehabilitation is presented.

EPIDEMIOLOGY

Perhaps the most often repeated statistics regarding low back pain are the 60% to 90% lifetime incidence and 5% annual incidence.[18,60,151,178] Males and females are equally affected, with the peak incidence at approximately 40 years of age.[59,79,151] However, 12% to 26% of children and adolescents have been reported to experience lumbosacral pain as well.[52,167] The natural history of lumbosacral pain appears to be favorable. Up to 90% of cases of low back pain apparently resolve without medical attention in 6 to 12 weeks; 40% to 50% are symptom free within 1 week.[3,16,44,58,198] Even 75% of the patients with sciatica report relief of pain at 6 months.[187,191] However, these statistics, which at first glance appear reassuring, should be tempered by the knowledge that as

---

Low back pain

- Up to 90% resolve *without* medical treatment in 6 to 12 weeks
- 40% to 50% are symptom free in 1 week
- 70% to 90% have recurrent episodes

---

many as 70% to 90% of patients have recurrent episodes of low back pain.[34,83,86] Although there may be *symptomatic* improvement, anatomic and functional changes may persist that increase the chance for reinjury.

Given the pervasiveness of low back pain in the general population, it can be intuitively determined to be universally present in the physically active population. Although physical fitness may maintain the health of the lumbar spine,[29,151] excessive physical activity, including acute dynamic overload and chronic repetitive exertion, can be detrimental. Most sporting activities can result in injury to the lumbosacral spine, but low back pain is most frequently reported in gymnastics, football, weightlifting, wrestling, dance, and rowing.[87,91,134,135,172] Injuries in gymnastics frequently involve the lumbosacral spine.[42,66,135] Pars interarticularis injuries are the most well-recognized injuries and have approximately a 10% incidence in female gymnasts, almost four times the frequency of the general population.[92,93,135] Other athletic

---

Sports in which low back pain is common

- Gymnastics
- Football
- Weightlifting
- Wrestling
- Dance
- Rowing

---

activities requiring repetitive flexion, extension, and rotation such as football also result in spondylitic injury and other lumbosacral problems. Of high school football players, 6% have some type of low back problem, and 30% of college players are affected.[55,123,170,201] Low back pain, including pars interarticularis injuries, is the most frequent injury in weightlifting.[26,108,175] Retired wrestlers commonly report lumbosacral problems as well.[71]

Similar to the industrially injured patient, significant time loss from athletic participation secondary to low back injury does occur. One National Football League survey noted a 12% incidence of spine injuries necessitating time loss.[162] Low back pain is the fourth most frequent injury in the general dance population and is often severe enough to cause the participant to miss several weeks or an entire season of performance.[134] Ballet dancers appear to be experiencing lumbosacral injuries at a growing rate. During the 1990-1991 season a San Francisco Ballet injury survey revealed 24% of all injuries were to the spine.[64] This made the spine the leading site of injury, and one half of all the spine injuries were to the lumbosacral region. The low back has been noted to be the second most common site of injury in aerobic dance.[159] Crew participation also places the lumbosacral spine at risk.[88]

Although the previously listed sports are most often associated with low back pain, other athletic activities are not spared. Low back injuries have been reported as the second or third most frequent anatomic site of injury in basketball.[7,80,138,203] The athlete playing the center position was the most frequently injured, and lumbosacral spine pain accounted for approximately 15% of missed playing time. Pain in the low back region accounts for approximately one third of all figure skating injuries.[56] Almost 40% of men's professional tennis tour players missed at least one tournament because of back pain.[54] Low back pain ranks second in frequency among injuries to professional golfers and first among amateur golfers.[47,48] Baseball, jogging, cycling, and almost all sports are mentioned in the literature as having some spine-related problems.[85] Even such activities, such as swimming, that are often prescribed as therapy for lumbosacral problems are associated with lumbosacral injury. This may not be surprising when one realizes that a competitive swimmer undergoes approximately 600,000 lumbar rotatory movements per year.[49] The anatomic structures and functional deficits that develop with sports-related injuries of the lumbar spine are the same as for the general population. However, the demands of the sport may precipitate more significant symptoms, and comprehensive rehabilitation necessitates a thorough understanding of the interplay between the lumbar spine and the specific biomechanical demands of the individual sport.

FUNCTIONAL ANATOMY AND BIOMECHANICS

A working knowledge of the functional anatomy and biomechanics of the lumbar spine provides a basis for understanding the rehabilitative concepts that are presented later in this chapter. The optimum lumbar spine mechanism is an intrinsically stable yet physiologically mobile structure. The lumbar spine comprises a series of five articulated motion segments plus the thoracolumbar junction (i.e., T12-L1). The **motion segment,** or three-joint complex, which is the basic kinematic unit of the spine, consists of one intervertebral disc situated anteriorly between the endplates of two adjacent vertebral bodies and two posterior synovial facet joints formed by the articular processes of the superior and inferior vertebrae. The caudal vertebrae are larger in proportion to their greater load-bearing capacity. The intervertebral disc comprises the central nucleus pulposus—a fibrogelatinous mass containing 80% to 90% water, collagen, and a mucopolysaccharide matrix—and the peripheral annulus fibrosis, which is formed by the concentric lamellae of obliquely oriented cartilaginous fibers. Individual lumbar nerve roots exist bilaterally below the pedicle of each respective vertebra and travel laterally in the intervertebral foramen. The lateral recess is a semidistinct region within the spinal canal that is medial to the intervertebral foramen.

Pain Generators

Given the multiplicity of potential pain generators in the lumbar spine, determination of a clinically relevant pain generator remains difficult. Kuslich, Ulstrom, and Michael[112] present an interesting study in which lumbar spine surgery was performed with local anesthesia to allow selective stimulation of distinct anatomic structures. The various pain provocation patterns were recorded. As expected, inflamed or compressed nerve roots always produced pain with mechanical stimulation, and this typically followed a dermatomal pattern. The diskovertebral joint was the next most common pain producer. This included the outer annular fibers, the posterior longitudinal ligament, and the peripheral aspect of the vertebral endplate. Centralized low back pain and occasional buttock pain were reported with stimulation of these structures.

In 1940 the innervation of the annulus fibrosis was studied[158] and the scientific premise that the disk could be a source of pain was investigated.[82] It is now widely accepted that the outer one third of the intervertebral disk is innervated, whereas the remainder of the annulus and the nucleus pulposus is not. Both encapsulated and free nerve endings have been demonstrated,[119] implying both proprioceptive and nociceptive functions. The greatest concentration of nerve receptors occurs in the lateral margin of the disk, less so posteriorly, and few-

---

Potential pain generators in the lumbar spine
■ Vertebral body—periosteum
■ Intervertebral disk—outer one third of annulus fibrosis
■ Facet joint—capsule and ligaments
■ Spinal nerve root—dorsal root ganglion, dura, and radicular arteries and veins
■ Ligaments—anterior and posterior longitudinal ligaments and supraspinous and interspinous ligaments
■ Muscles

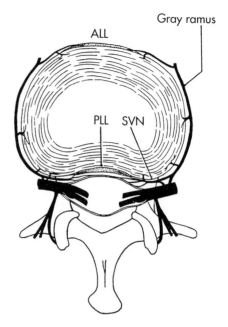

FIG. 53-1. Nerve supply of lumbar intervertebral disk depicted in transverse view of lumbar spine. Branches of gray rami communicans and sinuvertebral nerves *(SVN)* are shown entering disk and anterior longitudinal ligaments *(ALL)* and posterior longitudinal ligaments *(PLL)*. Branches from sinuvertebral nerves also supply anterior aspect of dural sac and dural sleeve. (From Bogduk N, Twomey LT: *Clinical anatomy of the lumbar spine*, ed 2, New York, 1991, Churchill Livingstone.)

est are found anteriorly. The posterior margin of the annulus and the posterior longitudinal ligament is supplied by the sinuvertebral nerve, which is formed by a branch of the ventral rami (somatic) and from a branch of the gray ramus communicans (autonomic).[22] Anteriorly, including the anterior longitudinal ligament, and laterally the disk is innervated by gray ramus communicans and ventral rami (Fig. 53-1). The actual significance of the sympathetic innervation of the disc is not clear beyond a vasomotor function, which is minimal, because the vascular supply to the disc is relatively sparse.

In general, the role of the facet joint as a pain producer has received much negative attention.[30] The conclusion of Kuslich, Ulstrom, and Michael[112] regarding the pain-producing capacity of the facet joint was that the capsule was rarely a source of pain, and when present, it never radiated pain beyond the buttock. The facet joint synovium and articular cartilage were not thought to be pain originators. From a strictly anatomic perspective the lumbar facet joints are richly innervated, receiving branches from up to three different segmental levels via the medial branches of the primary dorsal rami. In an animal model the lumbar facet joints have been shown to contain both high threshold mechanosensitive afferents that serve primarily as nociceptors and low threshold afferent fibers that modulate proprioceptive feedback.[8,202] These nerve endings are located in the facet joint capsule and in the border regions within the ligamentum flavum, muscles, and tendons. This implies that

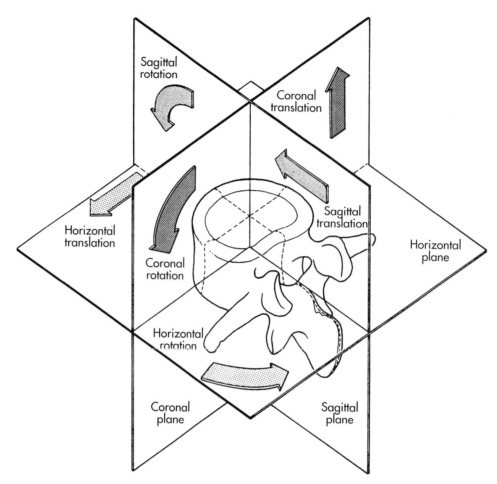

FIG. 53-2. Cardinal planes of segmental motion. (From Bogduk N, Twomey LT: *Clinical anatomy of the lumbar spine*, ed 2, New York, 1991, Churchill Livingstone.)

excessive tensile loading of the facet joint capsule may be the mechanism whereby facet-mediated nociception occurs. Finally, the musculoligamentous supporting structures of the lumbar spine are innervated by lateral, intermediate, and medial branches of the primary dorsal rami. The pain-producing areas of these muscles may be primarily at the muscle-tendon junction, tendon-bone junction, and neurovascular bundle sites.[21,112]

Kinematics and Injury

Movement of the trunk on the lower extremities is accomplished by the additive effect of each motion segment and lumbopelvic motion occurring at the hip joints. The cardinal planes of segmental motion include flexion and extension (i.e., sagittal translation and rotation), torsion (i.e., axial or horizontal rotation and translation), and side bending (i.e., coronal rotation and translation) (Fig. 53-2). The inherent efficiency of lumbar segmental motion allows functional range of motion while protecting the three-joint complex from excessive forces.

Flexion and extension occur predominantly at the lower two lumbar segments (i.e., L4-L5 and L5-S1) with up to 20 degrees occurring at each segment. This motion is defined by an **instantaneous axis of rotation**

(IAR) (Fig. 53-3). Similar to the glenohumeral joint, maintenance of this axis of rotation is critical for proper joint stability. Through lumbar flexion and extension of a normal three-joint complex a finite distribution of IAR points exist that are known as a **centrode** (Fig. 53-4), but this centrode becomes more dispersed and random in an injured or degenerative segment.

Pure lumbar flexion is tolerated well. Pain produced following a flexion injury can potentially result from a sprain of the interspinous ligaments or facet joint capsule, a strain to the thoracolumbar fascia or spinal extensor muscles, and possibly a facet joint meniscoid structure or a fibroadipose tissue flap (or a redundant synovial fold) that becomes trapped in the superior or inferior capsular recess. Annular tears are unlikely with flexion because the IAR, which is located near the endplate of the lower vertebra, lies close to the annulus; thus the lever arm is short, and the tensile force that is generated within the annular collagen fibers is not excessive. However, if the nucleus pulposus fragments and impinges the annular fibers, pain may potentially result. Both a trapped facet meniscoid and nuclear fragmentation may result in the acute "locked" back syndrome following pure forward flexion.

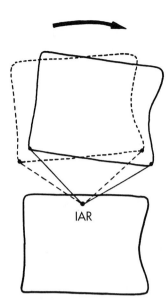

FIG. 53-3. During flexion-extension, each lumbar vertebra exhibits an arcuate motion in relation to vertebra below. Center of this arc lies below moving vertebra and is known as instantaneous axis of rotation *(IAR)*. (From Bogduk N, Twomey LT: *Clinical anatomy of the lumbar spine,* ed 2, New York, 1991, Churchill Livingstone.)

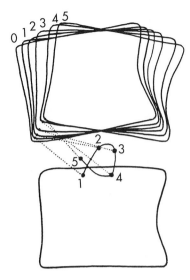

FIG. 53-4. As vertebra moves from extension to flexion, its motion can be reduced to small sequential increments. Five such phases are illustrated. Each phase of motion has a unique instantaneous axis of rotation (IAR). In moving from position *0* to position *1*, vertebra moves about IAR number *1*. In moving from position *1* to position *2*, it moves about IAR number *2*, and so on. Dotted lines connect vertebra in each of its five positions to location of IAR about which it moved. When IARs are connected in sequence, they describe a locus, or path, known as centrode. (From Bogduk N, Twomey LT: *Clinical anatomy of the lumbar spine,* ed 2, New York, 1991, Churchill Livingstone.)

Compressive load to the normal lumbar spinal column is borne predominantly by the anterior vertebral endplates and the annulus fibrosis and less so by the posterior facet joints. Axial compression does not result in annular disruption because pressure generated within the nucleus is evenly distributed to the annular fibers. When bearing excessive loads, as occurs when lifting heavy objects or after falling onto the buttocks or rigid lower extremities, the patient is at risk for vertebral endplate fracture. The force vectors associated with lumbar extensor muscle contraction that parallel the lumbar spine longitudinal axis can result in compressive loads on the order of 4000 N,[131] which can result in endplate fractures when lifting heavy objects, despite proper lifting technique. Power weightlifters, for example, develop compensatory hypertrophy of the vertebrae, which adds protection against this compressive load. Endplate herniations, per se, may not be painful given the relative lack of nociceptive receptors at this site, but a secondary inflammatory cascade within the nucleus with subsequent nuclear "degradation" and internal disc disruption can develop (Fig. 53-5). Ultimately, annular disruption and herniation may occur, although not acutely following compressive overload.

Although extension forces are not common in most activities of the general population, they are present in a vast number of athletic events. Extension injury may theoretically result in spinous process impingement and periostitis, although this is not often clinically evident. More likely to occur are injuries to the facet joints, for example, impingement of the inferior facet joint capsule on the lamina of the vertebra below. If the extension moment is strong enough, bony limitation on the ipsilateral side can result in a rotational component (spinous pro-

cess rotating ipsilaterally) with subsequent tensile damage to the contralateral facet joint and capsular avulsion (Fig. 53-6).

Torsional stress is relatively poorly tolerated by the three-joint complex. The annulus fibrosis does not readily tolerate torsion. Between 3 and 12 degrees of rotation, microtears to the outer annulus can occur with frank failure beyond 12 degrees. Farfan et al[53] have studied torsional injury and have found that the relative contribution to the resistance of torsion is 65% from the ipsilateral (impacted) facet joint and 35% from the annulus. The 90-degree orientation of the lumbar facet joints allows only 2 to 3 degrees of pure rotation, thus protecting the annulus in a "safe" range. However, with rotation greater than 3 degrees, ipsilateral facet joint impaction can lead to facet fracture or pars interarticularis injury, including fracture (spondylolysis) or pars stress reaction.[92] Further, the IAR moves posteriorly, placing the outer annulus at risk for circumferential tears and the contralateral facet joint at risk for capsular tear or avulsion (Fig. 53-7).

Combined movements through the lumbar spine carry the highest injury potential. As just demonstrated, pars interarticularis injury can occur with rotation and is probably more common with repetitive loading in extension and rotation. It is the forward flexed and rotated spine that is at the greatest risk for disk injury.[127] Flexion results in preferential loading of the disk anteriorly, which may displace the nucleus posteriorly.[109] Increased tensile force in the posterior annular collagen fibers is

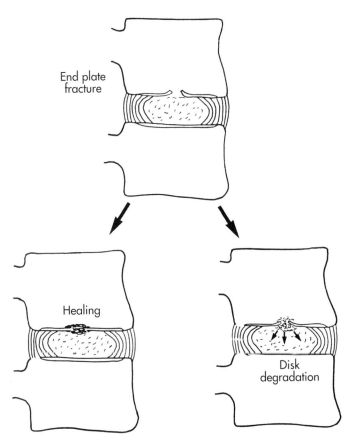

FIG. 53-5. Compression injury of intervertebral joint. Excessive compression force may result in fracture of vertebral endplate. This lesion may heal and be of no consequence, but may initiate process of disk degradation affecting nucleus pulposus near fracture site but gradually extending into rest of nucleus. (From Bogduk N, Twomey LT: *Clinical anatomy of the lumbar spine,* ed 2, New York, 1991, Churchill Livingstone.)

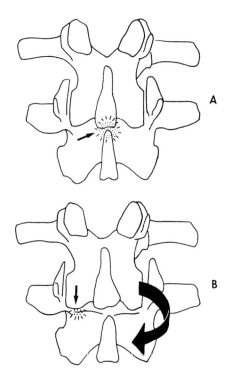

FIG. 53-6. Extension injuries of lumbar spine. **A,** If extension is limited by impaction of spinous processes, periosteal irritation of tips of spinous processes might become source of pain. **B,** If extension is limited by impaction of inferior articular process, irritation of periosteum of lamina might become painful. Otherwise, if extension is limited by bony contact, any remaining extension force is accommodated by segment rotating backwards about impacted articular processes, causing injury of contralateral zygapophyseal joint. (From Bogduk N, Twomey LT: *Clinical anatomy of the lumbar spine,* ed 2, New York, 1991, Churchill Livingstone.)

poorly tolerated, and with forward bending and rotation the posterolateral margin of the disk is at risk. Further, compressive loading of the disk in a flexed position may also risk disk herniation in a posterolateral direction where the posterior longitudinal ligament is thinnest and least protective.

Supporting and Stabilizing Systems

Support and stability of the lumbar spine is maintained by both passive and active restraints. The midline ligamentous system, which comprises the supraspinous ligaments, interspinous ligaments, posterior longitudinal ligaments, the ligamentum flavum, and the facet joint capsule, are passively stretched as the lumbar spine flexes. Because the lever arm of the ligaments, especially the supraspinous ligament, is relatively longer than the intrinsic musculature, more force is generated within these ligaments to counterbalance the anterior shear of forward bending.[70] This is supported by the absence of electric activity in the hip extensors and erector spinae muscles as the "flat back" posture is attained. Absolute lumbar kyphosis is not necessary to maintain adequate

counterpressure. There is recent suggestion that despite electric silence the passive tension generated in these back muscles with flexion may be fivefold greater than the ligamentous tension, contributing further to the antiflexion moment.[21]

Various muscular mechanisms have been proposed, which when activated, can directly and indirectly reduce shear to the three-joint complex resulting from excessive translation during flexion, extension, rotation, and side bending. The muscular stabilizers of the spine include the intersegmental muscles (i.e., multifidi, rotatores, and interspinales), abdominal muscles (i.e., particularly the transversus abdominis and obliquus internus), latissimus dorsi, erector spinae, iliopsoas, and quadratus lumborum. The "abdominal mechanism," acting via the thoracolumbar fascia (TLF) as described by Gracovetsky, Farfan, and Heleur,[69] can provide counterbalancing shear forces during the lifting of excessive loads. The TLF has bony attachments to the spinous processes in the midline, ribs, and pelvis superiorly and inferiorly, and the lateral free margin blends with the obliquus internus, transversus abdominis, and latissimus dorsi (Fig. 53-8). Contraction of these abdominal and trunk muscles results in the development of tension in the TLF,

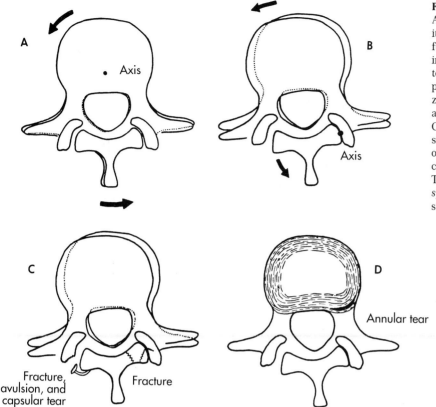

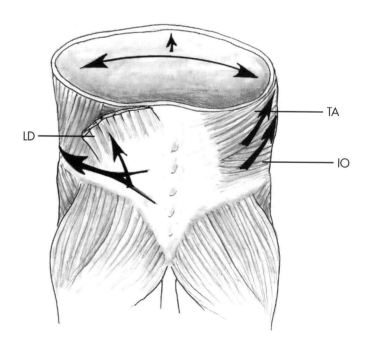

FIG. 53-7. Rotation injuries of lumbar spine. Axial rotation of lumbar segment is initially limited by impaction of zygapophyseal joint, but further rotation may occur about new axis in impacted joint, resulting in disk being exposed to lateral shear force and contralateral zygapophyseal joint swinging backwards. Impacted zygapophyseal joint may sustain fractures of its articular processes or of pars interarticularis. Contralateral joint may sustain fracture, avulsions, or tears of its capsule. Annulus fibrosus of intervertebral disk may sustain peripheral, circumferential tears. (From Bogduk N, Twomey LT: *Clinical anatomy of the lumbar spine*, ed 2, New York, 1991, Churchill Livingstone.)

resisting flexion of the lumbar spine without generating excessive shear. Given the relatively long lever arms of these abdominal muscles, this mechanism is effective and active independent of the degree of lumbar flexion. Similarly, contraction of the erector spinae and transversospinalis musculature contained within the TLF, which is known as the *hydraulic amplifier mechanism*,[69] generates internal tension and leads to protection against shear. The gluteus maximus and hamstrings, acting in a closed kinetic chain, generate 15,000 inch-pounds of torque, maintain the pelvis in a posteriorly rotated position and thereby generate passive tension in the TLF. These muscles contribute little to directly counterbalancing the anterior shear produced with bending and lifting.

Protection against torsional injury may be afforded by the short intersegmental muscles. There is, however, some controversy regarding the role of these muscles in stabilizing the lumbar spine.[21,31,147] The multifidi span only two to four segments and lie close to the midline and center of rotation of the motion segment. This implies poor mechanical advantage as a prime mover, and indeed these muscles are not effective prime movers. The force vectors of the multifidi indicate that they can generate posterior rotation in a sagittal plane (Fig. 53-9). Contraction of the abdominal oblique muscles results in combined motion into flexion and rotation, previously demonstrated to be an "at risk" postural attitude. The multifidi, however, are recruited to cocontract with the obliquus internus counterbalancing the forward shear force, stabilizing the segment, and allowing the internal

FIG. 53-8. Thoracolumbar fascia (TLF) and intraabdominal pressure (IAP) mechanisms. Intraabdominal pressure represented by triradiate arrows within abdominal cavity increases tension along transversus abdominis (*TA*) and obliquus internus (*IO*) muscles. TA and IO muscles insert onto TLF mechanism and, with latissimus dorsi (*LD*), produce tension within TLF. (From Sullivan MS, Jantzen W: Enhancing back support mechanisms through rehabilitation, *Crit Rev Phys Med Rehabil* 2:40, 1990.)

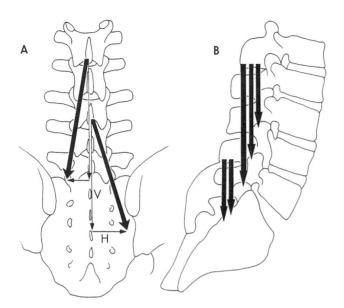

FIG. 53-9. Force vectors of multifidus. **A,** Posteroanterior view. Oblique line of action of multifidus at each level (*bold arrow*) can be resolved into major vertical vector (*V*) and smaller horizontal vector (*II*). **B,** Lateral view. Vertical vectors of multifidus are seen to be aligned at right angles to spinous processes. (From Bogduk N, Twomey LT: *Clinical anatomy of the lumbar spine,* ed 2, New York, 1991, Churchill Livingstone.)

oblique to produce pure axial rotation with less risk to the annulus and facet joints. Thus the multifidi are effective stabilizers and can balance shear forces and seemingly produce rotation, although not as primary rotators. The multifidi also secondarily maintain the lumbar lordosis by the nature of their force vectors posterior to the vertebral bodies. The multisegmental muscles of the spine (i.e., erector spinae) have been shown to be more effective prime movers with the greatest efficiency occurring with the fibers that originate from the pelvis, span the most segments, and are located most laterally from the midline.[31] The psoas may act as both a stabilizer and a prime mover.[21]

NATURAL HISTORY OF DISK HERNIATION

The classic paper by Mixter and Barr[136] popularized the role of surgery for the management of the herniated disk with radiculopathy in the midtwentieth century. The natural clinical course of this problem, however, has been shown to be self-limited in a large majority of cases, even in the presence of motor impairment.[2,28,164,191] Within the past decade a number of studies have demonstrated the presumed pathoanatomic correlate of this observed clinical improvement.* A brief review of these studies in total may allow for a better appreciation of the principles on which a comprehensive nonsurgical treatment program is developed. The success of nonsurgical management was predicated on a combination of epidural corticosteroid management and exercise. Although

---

*References 25, 28, 35, 41, 51, 117, 165, 179, and 180.

one of these studies[179] stated that minimal treatment (i.e., bed rest and education) may be necessary to accomplish clinical improvement, this approach may be both realistically and intuitively unsound in an athletic population in which time loss and "light" duty do not lend themselves to maximal performance. All but two of the studies compared initial computed tomography (CT) with follow-up CT[25,165]; the former compared initial CT imaging to follow-up magnetic resonance imaging (MRI), and the latter compared initial MRI to follow-up MRI. As expected the majority of herniated disks occurred at the lower two lumbar motion segments, namely L4-L5 and L5-S1. In general, clinical improvement paralleled radiographic improvement or resolution of herniated disks. The length of time for follow-up imaging examination ranged from 9 to 25 months. One study examined at least one portion of the cohort group every 3 months, finding that within 1 month, regression of disk material can be seen.[117]

Of the follow-up scans, 50% to 80% demonstrated a 50% or greater reduction in the size of the intervertebral disk herniation. Interestingly, the largest disk herniations, including free fragments that would have previously been considered surgically "desirable," demonstrated the greatest resolution in size in most studies,[28,35,117,165] including complete resolution. Postulated mechanisms for this observation include a foreign body reaction triggered by nuclear material that enters the epidural space, aggressive granulation into the disk fragment with subsequent phagocytosis, and fluid shifts (i.e., an increased ability of the fragment to imbibe water and subsequently dehydrate completely).

Although the correlation of spontaneous regression of herniated disk material and clinical signs and symptoms may seem logical, what remains unclear is why clinical improvement can occur in the absence of any morphologic change in the size or shape of disk herniations. Additionally, the persistence of symptoms and possibly signs occurs in some people despite resolution of the disk herniation. The presence of disk herniations in asymptomatic people has also been demonstrated by CT,[199] MRI,[19] and myelography,[84] implying a mechanism beyond simple mechanical pressure on a nerve root as the cause of all radiculopathies. The biochemical mechanisms that may explain these findings follow.

BIOCHEMISTRY AND BIOPHYSIOLOGY

Mechanical, vascular, biochemical, and neurochemical factors may all contribute to the clinical syndromes of low back pain and radiculopathy. Of all the peripheral nerves the nerve root is the least tolerant to compressive force, most likely because of the relative lack of epineurial tissue.[177] Although compression can lead to focal demyelination and edema with resultant impairment of axoplasmic transport, ischemic changes also contribute to nerve root dysfunction.[161] Jayson[96] has reviewed the vascular role in the pathogenesis of nerve root damage. Even in the absence of significant mechanical pressure, compression of epidural, radicular veins results in a cascading effect of dilation of noncompressed veins, venous hypertension with obstruction to normal capillary flow, and perineurial fibrosis and atrophy. Olmarker, Rydevik, and Holm[146] have demonstrated the susceptibility of the lumbar nerve root, in an animal model, to rapid compression resulting in hypoxic changes. The sensory nerve root was shown to be more affected than the motor nerve root, and recovery also occurred earlier in the motor root. This finding supports the more common clinical observation of residual sensory dysfunction (e.g., numbness or paresthesias) following radiculopathy. Epidural veins have also been shown to have a lower compressive threshold than other neurovascular structures,[145] again supporting the concept that low compressive forces can result in vascular-induced hypoxic injury.

Proposed mechanisms of herniated disk resolution

- Foreign body reaction
- Aggressive granulation with phagocytosis
- Fluid shifts (dehydration)

The biochemical and neurochemical contributions to low back pain and sciatica have received much attention within the past two decades. In 1979 Marshall, Trethewie, and Curtain[120] postulated that chemical radiculitis might explain nonmechanical radicular pain. Nuclear material was found to be antigenic and capable of producing an autoimmune reaction in vitro. In clinical studies serum titers of antibodies to glycoproteins in patients with acute sciatica and severe back pain without sciatica were found to rise over a period of several weeks following the onset of symptoms. McCarron and colleagues[124] found that an inflammatory reaction occurred as early as 5 days after injection of a nucleus pulposus preparation in the epidural space of dogs.

The inflammatory response to injury, including sensitization of the sensory nerve fibers to painful stimuli, is ultimately a protective mechanism. The mechanical and biochemical processes that occur during the course of disk injury or degradation may be complimentary. Chemical, cellular, and humoral responses may also play a role. Normally, an enzymatic homeostasis exists within a lumbar disk, which prevents the unintended breakdown of the outer annular fibers by collagenase and elastase.[143] The acidic environment accompanying disk injury that is presumed to be secondary to ischemic changes may result in the altered enzymatic expression of the nuclear chondrocytes. Recent studies have shown that phospholipase A_2 (PLA_2), is released from the disk following injury,[166] and PLA_2 has also been shown to be a strong inflammatory mediator.[57,166] PLA_2 may act directly on neural membranes[139] or increase the production of prostaglandins and leukotrienes. These strong nonneurogenic chemical pain mediators that also include serotonin, histamine, and bradykinin may sensitize nociceptive receptors directly, alter nerve impulse transmission, sensitize neurons to mechanical stimulation, cause vascular congestion and neural ischemia, and attract polymorphonuclear cells and monocytes.

Neurogenic pain mediators such as substance P, vasoactive intestinal polypeptide (VIP), and calcitonin gene-related peptide (CGRP) occur in primary afferent neurons and the dorsal root ganglion. They are released in response to noxious stimuli, including mechanical compression (i.e., stenosis or disk herniation) and vibration.[9,150,192,193,195] Transport of substance P to the pain transmission pathways of the spinal cord (i.e., substantia gelatinosa) has been demonstrated,[150] implicating its role in pain modulation. Neurotransmitter delay could account for the sometimes observed latency of onset of radiculopathy following disk herniation. Immunohistochemical studies have revealed substance P nociceptors in the posterior longitudinal ligament,[111] lumbar facet joints,[13] and outer annulus.[194] Substance P release may sensitize these nociceptors and lower their threshold for pain impulse transmission. These neuropeptides may also stimulate release of histamine from mast cells and leukotrienes, interconnecting the neurogenic and nonneurogenic mediators of spinal pain (Fig. 53-10).

DIAGNOSIS

Specificity of diagnosis in the acutely or subacutely injured athlete is the principle by which early aggressive, nonsurgical, or even surgical intervention is instituted to resolve symptoms and restore function. The assessment of lumbar spine syndromes requires a working knowledge of spinal biomechanics and the degenerative spinal cascade,[103] a high index of suspicion for previously undiagnosed conditions, proper clinical correlation of supplemental diagnostic imaging and electrophysiologic tests, and a concern for the athlete's development of disability and chronic pain syndromes.

Motion Segment Injury

A comprehensive pathomechanical schema of low back pain and three-joint complex deterioration has been described by Kirkaldy-Willis et al.[103] The degenerative cascade of the motion segment is subdivided into three distinct stages: segmental dysfunction, instability, and stability (Fig. 53-11). The main principle in this degenerative cascade is that pathologic changes that occur in one part of the three-joint complex (e.g., diskovertebral or facet joint) typically cause pathologic changes in the other joint or even in adjacent segments. The different biomechanical manifestation of these changes (e.g., hypomobility or hypermobility) can occur in adjacent segments in the same individual. Secondary soft-tissue changes, including spasm and shortening of ligaments, fasciae, and musculotendinous structures, also contribute to pain and impaired function. The various phases of this cascade are clinically correlatable. Because initial presentation of symptoms can occur anywhere along this continuum, the implication is that subpain threshold degenerative changes occur throughout life.

Phase I

Phase I, or **segmental dysfunction,** is a state of **segmental hypomobility.** In this stage the restricted motion of the three-joint complex typically results from

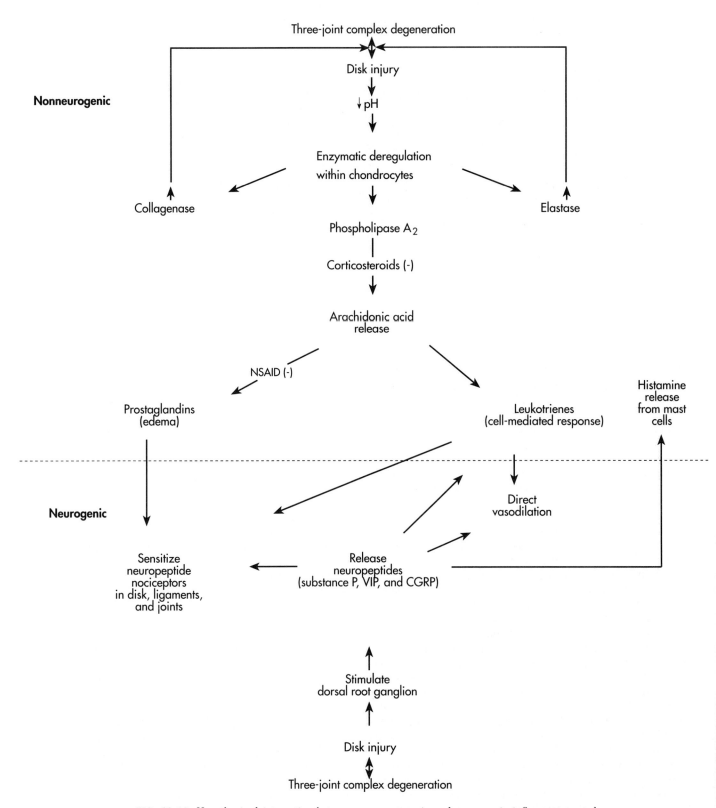

FIG. 53-10. Hypothesized interaction between nonneurogenic and neurogenic inflammatory and pain mediators.

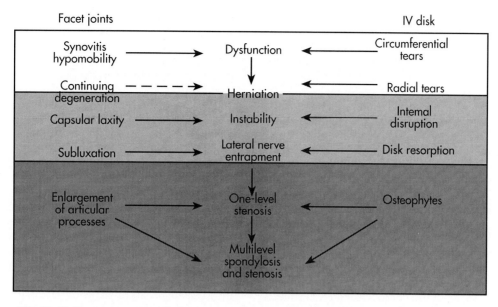

FIG. 53-11. Degenerative cascade. Interaction of facet joint and disk changes. Changes in facet joints appear on left and changes in disk on right. Lesions that occur as a result of interaction of these changes are seen in center. (From Kirkaldy-Willis WH, Burton CV: *Managing low back pain,* ed 3, New York, 1992, Churchill Livingstone.)

facet joint overload as opposed to disk herniation. This represents the pathomechanical correlate of the common clinical diagnosis of "sprain-strain" syndrome. Abnormalities of the facet joint can include synovitis; capsular fibrosis, or shortening; and later articular cartilage degeneration, resulting in pain, inflammation, and restricted motion or glide. Secondary muscle spasm and muscle contraction and shortening, especially of the short polysegmental muscles, contribute further to joint hypomobility. Symptomatically, nonradiating low back pain may be worse with static standing, walking, lumbar extension, or extension combined with rotation. Theoretically, flexion relieves this joint-induced discomfort, but even forward bending may aggravate a restricted joint capsule or musculotendinous unit. Physical signs include local tenderness; muscle spasm; limited active and passive range of motion with compensatory changes at the sacroiliac or thoracolumbar junction joints; excessive anterior pelvic tilt (i.e., increased lordosis); hamstring inflexibility; and typically a normal neurologic examination. Referred pain patterns are common in Phase I and are usually described as sclerotomal referral patterns in contrast to radicular pain. Usually pain can be referred to the buttock or proximal thigh. Pain radiating below the knee is negatively correlated with facet syndrome.[78] Although Mooney and Robertson[137] suggested that facet syndrome can be associated with distal referral patterns, volumes of injected materials (e.g., 3 to 8 ml) may have exceeded the capacity of the facet joint capsule (e.g., 1 to 2 ml)[155] and the distal radiation of pain may have represented extravasation of irritative substances over nerve roots. Other syndromes have been postulated to explain the referred pain patterns that are nonradicular. The lumbar dorsal ramus syndrome is mediated solely

through the posterior primary rami, which were previously shown to innervate the facet joint, posterior neural arch, and some musculoligamentous structures in the dorsal aspect of the three-joint complex.[20]

Diskogenic low back pain is less commonly acknowledged in this early phase, but logically, annular disruption and tears can occur as a result of the decreased load-bearing capacity of a dysfunctional facet joint. Both circumferential and radial tears can be painful; the latter is more likely to result in disk protrusion or herniation in the later part of Phase I. However, the onset of disk degeneration is frequently painless. Gibson et al[65] evaluated disk herniations in adolescents and found that 10% of asymptomatic teenagers had at least one abnormal level as shown by MRI. The typical clinical presentation of diskogenic low back pain is pain exacerbated by activities that cause anterior shear or translation (i.e., flexion), torsional shear (i.e., twisting), and the Valsalva maneuver. The tissue injury complex includes the richly innervated outer annular fibers and the posterior longitudinal ligament (PLL). If a disk protrusion or herniation is present, it is typically in a posterolateral direction where the annular fibers are least well protected by the PLL and shear force is greatest with combined forward bending and twisting. Chemical or mechanical irritation of the nerve roots can result in lower extremity radiating pain or paresthesias. Experience suggests that with disk herniation and radiculopathy, the ratio of back to lower extremity pain varies, but with an extruded fragment resulting in radiculopathy, low back pain may be minimal or absent. Central disk herniations can result in back pain without radiating signs or symptoms. Often the athlete with a central disk protrusion may have atypical symptoms that are more suggestive of posterior element pain.

As previously discussed the presence of a disk herniation, even with radiculopathy, is not an absolute indication for surgery. However, there are certain physical signs that may assist with prognosticating the outcome of a disk herniation, thus allowing early recognition of a herniation refractory to nonsurgical treatment. Schnebel, Watkins, and Dillin[169] have demonstrated, in vitro, that compressive forces on the L5 nerve root from an L4-L5 disk herniation increases with flexion of the L4-L5 motion segment and are compounded by increasing tension in the nerve root. Extension decreases the compressive force. The persistent peripheralization of pain[45] despite properly performed McKenzie extension exercises[128] or a positive crossed straight leg raise[102] (i.e., pain in the symptomatic leg worsened by raising the contralateral lower extremity) may be a poor prognostic indication for successful nonsurgical outcome.

Proper interpretation of the straight leg raise test is important.[107] A positive response indicates dural tension and probable tethering of the nerve root over a herniated disk. However, the test is only considered positive if symptoms are elicited within the range of 30 to 70 degrees. Care must be taken to prevent posterior pelvic rotation in the seated position, which can result in false-positive findings. Further, a positive response does not predict the size or location (e.g., lateral recess, central) of a disk herniation.[181] Also, a negative response does not rule out the presence of a disk herniation. Beyond 70 degrees, passive stretch of musculoligamentous structures may increase pain, but neural tension is not increased. Last, straight leg raising cannot identify tension on any nerve root rostral to L5; therefore the reverse straight leg raise or femoral stretch test is necessary to identify radicular pain from an upper lumbar disk herniation. This can be performed in a prone position by passively extending the hip or in a supine position by passively lowering the affected limb below the plane of the examination table.

A subset of disk herniation, the far lateral disk herniation,[94,106] also has a typical presentation. The location of the nerve root impingement is at the foraminal exit zone or extraforaminally. The radiculopathy therefore involves the nerve root from the level above (i.e., a far lateral disk herniation at L5-S1 affects the L5 nerve root). Clinically, the herniation does not usually cause lower back pain but rather lower extremity pain, sensory disturbance, and/or weakness usually in an L3, L4, or L5 distribution. Radiculopathy of the S1 nerve root cannot occur from a true far lateral disk herniation unless an S1-S2 disk is congenitally present or there is an extra lumbar vertebra (i.e., L6). Symptoms are frequently worse with standing or walking, and they occasionally are reduced with sitting. Straight leg raises or reverse straight leg raises are typically negative or minimally positive despite potentially severe symptoms. Overall, this condition acts similarly to spinal stenosis (see p. 1183).

Phase II

In Phase II, **segmental hypermobility** and occasional frank instability exist. Clinically, this phase is more difficult to conceptualize. The hypermobility may result from facet joint capsular laxity and loss of the instantaneous axis of rotation of the three-joint complex.[176] Compensatory hypermobility often exists adjacent to a hypomobile or dysfunctional segment. These sites of secondary hypermobility are frequently the painful areas of the lumbar spine. Standard flexion-extension radiographs may not reveal excessive translation. Further, flexion-extension x-ray studies may be abnormal in asymptomatic people,[77] implying that a chemical mediator may be necessary to initiate symptoms in this phase. This relates to our clinical impression that the quality of motion is more representative of injury than is quantity. Observing dysrhythmia, a catching sensation or painful arc with recovery phase from forward bending, can be indicative of hypermobility. Passive mobility testing through a skilled manual examination can elicit excessive segmental motion, pain, and reactive paravertebral spasm with torsional loading across a specific segment.

Disk-related abnormalities in Phase II include internal disk disruption and narrowing of the intervertebral disk space. The additive effect of multiple annular tears allows random distribution of nuclear material throughout the disk.[27] The pain-generating potential of an internally disrupted disk may result from a combination of sensitized annular nociceptive nerve endings or neurobiochemical mediators. Relative instability of the three-joint complex is enhanced by the decreased resistance to torsional load following annular incompetence and facet joint laxity following reduction in disk space height. Radiculopathy can occur as a result of direct mechanical impingement, dynamic lateral entrapment from narrowing of the lateral recess, and primary radiculitis from PLA_2 and neuropeptides. Dynamic lateral entrapment occurs as the lax facet joint capsule allows excessive glide of the superior facet in the sagittal plane. This can also occur following diskectomy and chemonucleolysis before fixed bony or degenerative changes ensue.

Clinically, many athletes experience symptoms relating to Phase II. Back pain with rotation and limited tolerance for rotational activities are common. Often MRI may reveal only degenerative changes of the intervertebral disk or small central disk protrusions. *Radiologist-generated reports of "not clinically significant" when referring to these findings should be interpreted with caution.* Comprehensive review of T2-weighted axial and sagittal MRI images may also reveal an increased quantity of fluid in the facet joints, suggestive of facet joint inflammation.

Phase III

For the majority of younger athletes, there is little clinical relevance of Phase III (stenosis); however, congenital spinal stenosis with a superimposed disk protrusion or herniation can result in typical stenotic symptoms (see the next pargraph) in the young athlete. With greater numbers of people 50 years and older participating in athletics, it is important to recognize the degenerative processes of the facet and diskovertebral joints and the role of spinal stenosis in this phase. The prevalence of disk herniations diminishes in people older than 55,[187] and these are typically far lateral herniations reflecting degenerative bony constraints, reduction in elasticity, and biochemical alterations of the disk.

Spinal nerve entrapment is a relatively common result of fixed lateral recess stenosis, degenerative spondylolisthesis, and less so, central stenosis. Fixed lateral stenosis can occur because medial facet joint osteophytes narrow the lateral recess or forward subluxation of the superior facet persists. Degenerative spondylolisthesis occurs because erosion of the superior articular facet allows forward displacement of the upper vertebral body on the lower body, trapping the nerve root that exists one level below between the inferior facet and the back of the vertebral body.[103] Such slips are usually isolated to one segment, typically L4-L5, impinging on the L5 nerve root. When present, symptomatic central stenosis can result in bilateral, multilevel radiculopathy.

Clinically, lumbar radiculopathy evidences as neurogenic claudication in Phase III. Symptoms of pain, paresthesia, or muscle cramps can develop with erect posture during extension and exercise (i.e., walking and running). Venous compression and ischemia may explain the pathophysiology of these symptoms. Occasionally, the radicular symptoms are manifest by buttock pain, which may be mistaken for hip joint injury in this population. Unlike true vascular claudication, exercising in a flexed posture (e.g., while bicycle riding) is typically well tolerated, and this may be an effective form of exercise for the spinal stenotic population.

Selective Injection

Selective spinal injections, such as epidural steroid, nerve root sheath, and intraarticular facet joint, have diagnostic and therapeutic value. The goal of diagnostic injections is to differentiate the qualitative and quantitative contribution of posterior element, diskogenic, and radicular pain. Given the multiplicity of pain generators in the lumbar spine, selective injection of an anesthetic into a potential source may prove the origin of pain. Generally, selective injections are valuable in the setting of multilevel disease, as demonstrated by imaging studies or electrophysiologic testing, in situations with no correlatable anatomic abnormalities such as with suspected chemically mediated symptoms or in postoperative cases in which anatomic boundaries are disrupted and imaging studies are more difficult to interpret. Corticosteroid administration accounts for the therapeutic benefit of these injections. **Epidural steroid injections** may be useful for disk-related conditions, including annular tears, disk herniations and radiculopathy, and for spinal stenosis. **Selective epidural injections** (or selective nerve root blocks) are indicated for radiculopathy resulting from either a herniated disk or spinal stenosis not responsive to epidural injection or a far lateral disk herniation and for noncompressive inflammatory radiculopa-

thies. **Facet joint injections** may have a role with persistent posterior element symptomatology. Experience suggests that a positive response to facet joint injection is more likely if a bone scan with single photon emission computed tomography (SPECT) imaging is positive for facet joint arthropathy. As shown, however, the interplay between the components of the three-joint complex often implies that pain production may be multifactorial. Unfortunately, a precise diagnosis is not always obtainable despite thorough investigation with diagnostic imaging and selective injection. Good clinical judgment and clinical correlation is always necessary in determining proper diagnosis and appropriate rehabilitation. Selective injections are never the sole treatment modality.

Of paramount importance in identifying a specific pain generator or maximizing the therapeutic role of corticosteroid administration is precise needle localization. This can be obtained only by the use of fluoroscopy and contrast dye.* An epidurogram, radiculogram, or arthrogram is desired. Although epidural injections are not frequently performed under fluoroscopic guidance, incorrect needle placement has been reported from 15% to 40% of the time including intravenous, intraligamentous, and subcutaneous infiltrations.[156,196,197] Without the use of a contrast agent, intravenous injection may not be identified even with correct needle placement in the epidural space. This is particularly true with a caudal approach in the older population when the epidural venous plexus may be more pronounced. The low pressure venous system may collapse with "drawback" testing, thus giving a false assurance of proper localization. The caudal epidural via the sacral hiatus is frequently used for abnormalities at L4-L5 or L5-S1, and the translumbar route is used for more rostral segmental abnormalities or if previous surgery, especially fusion, has been performed at L5-S1.

Typically, the anesthetic and corticosteroid preparations are administered simultaneously. The desired anesthetic effect is always partial without a profound sensory, motor, or sympathetic blockade. A short-acting anesthetic (e.g., 0.5% lidocaine in volumes of 8 to 10 ml via the caudal approach and 3 to 5 ml via the translumbar approach) is used for epidural injections. The shorter acting anesthetic reduces the risk of a prolonged sympathetic block should this unintentionally develop. A longer acting anesthetic such as 0.5% bupivacaine is used for facet joint and nerve root sheath infiltration. The total volume injected is approximately 1 ml or less to prevent facet capsule rupture or spillover into the epidural space,

---

*References 36, 38, 46, 50, 61, 97, 98, 110, 156, and 196.

Injection agents

- Epidural—Short-acting anesthetic (0.5% lidocaine) plus corticosteroid
- Facet joint—Long-acting anesthetic (0.5% bupivacaine) plus corticosteroid
- Nerve root sheath—Long-acting anesthetic (0.5% bupivacaine) plus corticosteroid

---

Selective injections

- Epidural steroid injection
- Selective epidural injection (selective nerve root block)
- Facet joint injection

thereby reducing the diagnostic value of the procedure. Pain reproduction during the needle placement and contrast instillation may also help to identify a painful structure. Typically, nonaffected nerve roots are not hypersensitive to mechanical irritation by the spinal needle or contrast dye.[46,61] Comparison of preinjection and postinjection pain levels by verbal report or visual analog scale is extremely helpful in gauging the response to the anesthetic. Provocative testing such as evaluating spinal range of motion and straight leg raising may also add to the diagnostic process. Placebo responses can occur both immediately and with weekly follow-up assessment.

The corticosteroids act by disrupting the inflammatory cascade via arachidonic acid, decreasing prostaglandin synthesis and cytokine action, and by impeding cell-mediated inflammatory reactions. Possibly, corticosteroids act to decrease substance P and VIP and to reduce ectopic neuronal discharge and conduction block. Fibroblast and capillary proliferation is decreased and collagen deposition reduced, thereby implying a reduction in scar tissue formation. Last, corticosteroids may stabilize PLA_2, thus limiting the inflammatory cascade of cellular and noncellular responses (Fig. 53-10). Interestingly, anesthetic agents alone may also stabilize PLA_2 leading to a therapeutic response via a "diagnostic" block.

The decision to administer any injection is based on a number of factors including the acuteness of pain, the response to other treatments including oral antiinflammatory medications, and the risks of the procedures. The presence of nonprogressive neurologic deficits does not rule out the use of an epidural steroid injection. As shown earlier, nonsurgical recovery from radiculopathy may in fact be facilitated by epidural corticosteroids. Usually, a maximum of four injections per year typically performed in a series over a 2- or 3-month period may be administered, depending on outcome and a favorable diagnostic or therapeutic response. *Persistent crossed straight leg raise immediately following a technically well-performed epidural injection is a poor prognostic sign for nonsurgical success.* In this setting, sometimes epidural injection and selective nerve root block are combined. The duration of response to the selective nerve root block has also been shown to have some predictive value regarding a positive outcome following surgical decompression.[37] Epidural injections can be performed without a preinjection imaging study if the clinical presentation is classical for diskogenic or lumbar radiculopathy, but lack of response to a single injection demands a more thorough diagnostic workup.

As with any invasive procedure, a thorough review of relative risks[75] and informed consent are absolutely required. Although rare, risks include allergic reaction; infection, including epidural abscess;[160] spinal headache (greater risk with translumbar approach); temporary partial paralysis, or the remote possibility of permanent paralysis from direct mechanical trauma or infection; vasovagal reactions; neurotoxicity (including meningitis or arachnoiditis possibly resulting from preservatives in some steroid or anesthetic preparations);[142] transient hyperglycemia in diabetics; and adrenal suppression.[185]

REHABILITATION

Rehabilitation principles can be applied to all spinal disorders in the acute, subacute, and chronic settings and in both nonoperative and surgical patients. As noted earlier in this chapter, disk herniations, including large extruded fragments, have sometimes been demonstrated to resolve without surgery, and resolution of signs and symptoms can occur even if the disk material remains in the spinal canal. Invariably, changes in soft-tissue and articular mobility and loss of strength and overall fitness occur in cases of disk herniation and with other nonsurgical spinal problems. Indeed, after 6 months of lumbosacral discomfort, up to 70% loss in trunk musculature strength has been reported.[122] Therefore addressing these spinal problems with a comprehensive rehabilitation program is beneficial especially in the athletic patient where physical demands remain high. Further, improvements in quality of life in those patients choosing to avoid surgery can be enhanced by educational programs and physical therapy despite the degree of injury present.[125] Postoperatively, soft-tissue and articular adaptive changes are also dramatic. One year status after lumbar diskectomy trunk strength loss of at least 30% for almost every parameter tested has been reported.[100]

In both surgical and nonsurgical patients absence of symptoms does not imply normal function. Correction of soft-tissue inflexibility and reestablishment of proper spinal segmental motion are necessary. Normal trunk and lower extremity strength, endurance, and power should be combined with education and training for posture, body mechanics, proprioception, and supervised return to sporting activity. This constitutes a comprehensive rehabilitation program. The acute phase goals of such a spinal rehabilitation program include: (1) education and protection of the injured tissue; (2) control of pain and reduction of inflammation; (3) early mobilization of joint and soft-tissue structures; and (4) implementation of therapeutic exercise.

The subacute phase goals of a spinal rehabilitation program include (1) full, pain-free range of motion of the injured and adjacent segments and other spinal and lower quadrant structures that influence the lumbar spine; (2) optimal strength, endurance, and coordination of the neuromuscular system affecting the lumbar spine; and (3) prevention of further injury and recurrences.

Acute Phase

The goals of the acute phase can be accomplished with the use of (1) education, (2) physical modalities, (3) appropriate medication, (4) manual therapy, (5) mechanical therapy, and (6) therapeutic exercise.

Education

Education is perhaps the most important component of any back care program including acute injury.[90] Instructions regarding proper body mechanics and review of activities of daily living allow the patient to sit, stand, bathe, and perform other tasks in a fashion that will not cause further injury to the spine. Education also teaches patients about the natural history of their spine injury and provides an opportunity to discuss a framework for comprehensive treatment. Different back school programs are available and useful; however, spine education alone should not be equated with a total treatment program.[173]

Physical Modalities

The use of physical modalities is another way to help meet the goals of the acute phase of rehabilitation. Pain and inflammation can be controlled while the spinal injury is provided with a period of relative rest. Cold treatment (cryotherapy) decreases spasm, pain, and capillary blood flow. The skin is cooled quickly, but the rate of muscle cooling is directly proportionate to the thickness of overlying fat and ranges from 10 to 30 minutes.[114,115] Heat (thermotherapy) also decreases spasm and pain, but it increases arterial and capillary blood flow. Superficial heating modalities such as heating pads, hydrocollator packs, and use of a whirlpool only penetrate to a depth of 2 cm or less. If a deeper response to these heating modalities is obtained, it is attributable to reflex pathways.[115] Cryotherapy is preferable following acute spine injury. Both superficial heat and cold control pain and spasm, but cryotherapy also helps decrease acute inflammation. Diathermy, or deep heat, (e.g., ultrasound, microwave, or shortwave) is usually reserved for the subacute or chronic injury if these modalities are used for their thermal effects. Therapeutic electricity, another physical modality, has the physiologic effects of reducing acute muscle spasm, decreasing edema, and relieving pain. It usually is delivered as high-voltage pulse galvanic stimulation (HVGS). Transcutaneous electric nerve stimulation (TENS) was initially used for chronic pain, but it may also have some beneficial effect on acute pain.[62,157] Therapeutic electricity therefore can be beneficial in the acute phase of rehabilitation, but treatment provides little benefit if used in isolation.[39,101]

Physical modalities useful in back treatment

- Cryotherapy (acute)
- Heat (subacute/chronic problems)
- High-voltage pulse galvanic stimulation
- Transcutaneous electric nerve stimulation

Medications

Medications are frequently prescribed for acute lumbar spine pain.

Nonsteroidal antiinflammatory drugs. Nonsteroidal antiinflammatory drugs (NSAIDs) provide both an analgesic and antiinflammatory effect. The analgesic effect is often present at a lower medication dose than the antiinflammatory effect, and the duration of the analgesic effect of the NSAID may be different from its antiinflammatory effect.[89] The NSAIDs interfere with prostaglandin production via arachidonic acid, but they do not modulate cell-mediated responses (Fig. 53-10). Patients respond differently to nonsteroidal antiinflammatory medications. A physician cannot predict response based

on pharmacokinetics or the chemical classification of the drug,[33] but changing to a different chemical classification if one NSAID is not effective may be reasonable. Potential side effects should be remembered, and reasonable patient warnings should be issued before using the NSAIDs or any medication. Studies evaluating the true effectiveness of NSAIDs in acute spine pain have not clearly shown efficacy, reflecting the complex nature of the problem and study design issues.[39,101,154]

Analgesics. As with NSAIDs, nonnarcotic analgesia can also be obtained with acetaminophen. Patients who cannot tolerate NSAIDs may still get analgesia from acetaminophen, and in addition, there is no cross tolerance between the NSAIDs and acetaminophen.[23] The combination of acetaminophen and NSAIDs may enhance pain relief. Stronger analgesics (narcotics) also can be used short term in cases of more severe back pain. If the narcotics are used, they should be prescribed at an adequate dose for pain relief and on a time-contingent basis. If the narcotics are used for a short time in this fashion, there is little chance of addiction.[174]

Muscle relaxants. The use of muscle relaxants for acute spinal pain is controversial; again, few studies demonstrate efficacy.[39] The site of action of these medications has been variously described as the muscle spindle or the central nervous system.[23] The latter may explain why muscle relaxants can often cause lethargy, thus impairing the patient's ability to participate in the other aspects of his or her rehabilitation program.

Corticosteroids. The NSAIDs, acetaminophen, narcotics, and muscle relaxants are used at least partly for their analgesic properties. In contrast, corticosteroids do not have any direct analgesic effect; pain relief results from the drug's antiinflammatory action. Oral corticosteroid treatment has been reported for the treatment of acute spinal pain.[72] Also, corticosteroids can be delivered via the epidural route as discussed earlier in this chapter. Conflicting reports of efficacy of epidural steroid injection exist.[14,15,32,75,197] Research design, patient selection, and other factors must be assessed when reviewing this literature. Medication prescription in the acute phase of spine rehabilitation should be based on sound principles and should be used as part of an overall treatment plan.

Manual Therapy

A variety of different manual therapy techniques can be used to modulate pain and introduce controlled motion to the lumbar spine during the acute phase of rehabilitation. Stimulation of mechanoreceptors and other pain-sensitive structures may produce input into the central nervous system, resulting in pain modulation and alteration of the state of muscle contraction. Soft-tissue and mild articular mobilization can initially provide pain control and still provide relative protection of the injured tissue. At the same time, early mobilization can provide controlled stresses to healing tissue.

Mechanical Therapy

To help meet the goals of the acute phase of spinal rehabilitation, mechanical therapies can also be employed. Lumbar traction has been used for over 2000 years in the treatment of low back 0ain. To achieve true distraction of the vertebral bodies with the body in the horizontal position, a traction force of at least 25% of body weight must be exerted.[23] The reduction of the disk protrusion, if obtained, is temporary.[74,121] There also appears to be only a small decrease in intradiskal pressure with horizontal traction.[141] Traction can also be used via a special frame anchoring the lower extremities and providing handles for the patient to pull. This so-called *auto-traction* allows the patient to control the amount of traction. Favorable results have been reported, but some studies have shown an actual increase in intradiskal pressure with auto-traction, perhaps because of the contraction of thoracic musculature when the patient is placed in the auto-traction device.[4,144] Inversion gravity traction may cause actual distraction of the vertebral bodies by 0.3 to 4.0 mm. The effects on disk protrusion are unknown, and potential side effects from inversion traction include hypertension, tachycardia, gastrointestinal reflux, and berry aneurysm rupture.[63] These types of traction may provide pain relief not only by intervertebral distraction, but also by stretching muscle or other soft-tissue structures and providing a period of relative rest. If symptoms are predominantly diskogenic, traction may be applied in a prone lying position, which helps to maintain neutral or extended lumbar postures. If symptoms appear to be mostly posterior element in nature, lumbar traction applied in flexion may be employed. Once again, this mechanical modality should be used as a component of a comprehensive rehabilitation program.

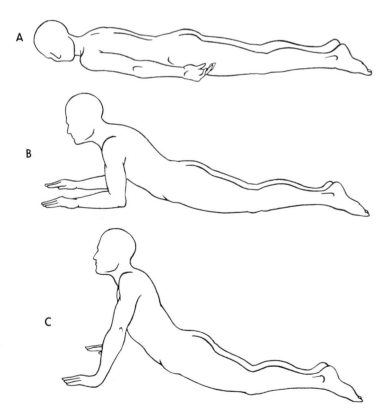

FIG. 53-12. Extension exercises. **A,** Prone—unsupported. **B,** Prone—on elbows. **C,** Press-up.

Therapeutic Exercise

During the acute phase of rehabilitation of the lumbar spine, active treatment is instituted, since simply resting the injured spine may actually have deleterious effects. Long-term bed rest has generalized debilitating effects on muscle strength and flexibility, cardiovascular fitness, and bone density,[24] as well as specific negative effects of increased spinal segmental stiffness and decreased disk nutrition.[186] Absolute bed rest of longer than 3 days has not been shown to reduce disability or dysfunction in cases of lumbosacral spine problems.[40] Initial exercise may involve movement into extension or flexion based on whether the patient's predominant symptoms are diskogenic or posterior element. Also, the exercise activity that causes centralization of the pain (i.e., less radicular discomfort) and does not significantly exacerbate low back pain is the appropriate initial exercise.

In the majority of acute diskogenic injuries, **extension exercises** are the initial exercise of choice. Exercises begin with the patient lying in the prone position with support under the abdomen to maintain a neutral position. The patient may progress as tolerated to prone lying without support, prone lying with support under the chest, prone on elbows, and press-ups (Fig. 53-12).[45,128,129,152,173] Lateral trunk shifts need to be corrected before initiating extension exercises. Care must also be taken to prevent irritation of segments that already have compensatory hypermobility as a result of segmental stiffness. Therefore some of the manual therapy techniques discussed above may be helpful with the introduction of extension exercises in acute diskogenic patients. It has been suggested that extension exercises may reduce pain by decreasing intradiskal pressure and allowing anterior migration of the nucleus pulposus.[129,141] Whether or not there is an actual decrease of the disk protrusion is unclear, but there may be increased mechanoreceptor input activating the pain gate mechanism[132] or decreased tension on the nerve root with extension positioning.[169] As the patient progresses, instruction on extension posturing in standing could be helpful, particularly after prolonged sitting or activities requiring forward bending. Large central disk herniations, which can cause functional spinal stenosis or other causes of spinal stenosis, may result in increased symptoms with extension positioning. An internally deranged disk occasionally increases pain with extension as a result of associated segmental hypermobility. If there is increase in radicular discomfort, presence of instability, or increase in low back pain, unless associated with concomitant reduction in radicular pain, extension exercises should be avoided.

Williams' flexion exercises[20] were historically described for diskogenic symptoms (Fig. 53-13). The concept was that the compressive load on the posterior disk margin decreased, and the intervertebral foramen opened. However, flexion exercises also increase intradiskal pressure[140] and may exacerbate symptoms in patients with an acute disk protrusion.

Depending on the severity of the patient's acute discogenic symptoms, maintenance of some **cardiovascu-**

lar fitness may also be possible and desirable. No exercise should be done that significantly intensifies the patient's symptoms; however, many patients with acute diskogenic symptoms may tolerate such activities as swimming, the use of a cross-country ski machine, or other aerobic activities that place the spine in more of a neutral or extended position.

If the acute episode of lumbosacral discomfort suggests a predominantly posterior element component, flexion exercises may be chosen initially. These exercises may decrease facet joint compressive forces while providing stretch to the lumbar musculature, ligaments, and myofascial structures. Strengthening the abdominal muscles may also occur with the partial sit-up position. Single knee-to-chest exercises help stretch the contralateral hip flexor and ipsilateral hip extensors, and double knee-to-chest exercises promote stretching of the lumbar and hip extensors. Pelvic tilts can be performed in the supine position and while standing. If there is increase in radicular discomfort or significant increase in lumbosacral pain, these flexion exercises should be discontinued.

Patients with posterior element symptoms can also attempt to maintain a baseline level of cardiovascular fitness if such attempts do not cause a significant increase in their symptoms. These patients may best tolerate stationary bicycle riding in slight lumbar flexion, stair

climbing, or other such activities that challenge the cardiovascular system while unloading the posterior elements of the lumbar spine.

With a proper mixture of education, physical modalities, mechanical modalities, medication, manual therapy, and the introduction of appropriate initial exercise, the acute phase goals of rehabilitation of lumbar spine problems should be met. Rehabilitative efforts are not complete as the patient's discomfort resolves. As the reactivation program continues, the goals of the subacute phase of rehabilitation must be addressed.

Subacute Phase
Connective Tissue Changes

Initially, the goal of full, pain-free range of motion of the injured and adjacent motion segments of the lumbar spine and lower quadrant must be met. Whether the surrounding soft tissue was injured primarily or immobility and stiffness occurred secondary to injury to the three-joint complex or both depends on the initial injury. Injured connective tissue structures that restrain motion include ligaments, tendons, joint capsules, and fasciae. These structures are composed of cells, fibers, and ground substance, and the arrangement and proportion of these basic constituents determine the mechanical properties of the individual soft tissue. The collagen fibers in these structures have varying degrees of waviness, which is reduced by tensile loading. At a point just slightly *beyond* the limit of physiologic tensile loading, there is some individual collagen fiber failure. Such progressive loading of collagen does cause plastic deformation (i.e., some collagen fiber microfailure with resultant permanent lengthening of the remaining collagen fibers). Plastic deformation should not be confused with creep, which occurs with tensile loading *within* the elastic limits of the tissue. Thus with creep phenomenon, removal of the tensile load results in the collagen returning to its original length. Manual therapy techniques applied to connective tissue affect both of these biophysical properties. Initial gentle manual therapy may temporarily elongate connective tissue and provide pain relief. Basic science research suggests that more aggressive manual therapy produces enough internal force to cause plastic deformation of collagen-containing connective tissue.[113,182]

A variety of hands-on therapy techniques are available to provide graded tensile or compressive loads to connective tissue. These techniques include massage, fascial-tendon stretching, traction, and joint mobilization, which can also affect the connective tissue. Changes following a ligamentous injury include edema, cellular and vascular granulation proliferation, increased synthesis of col-

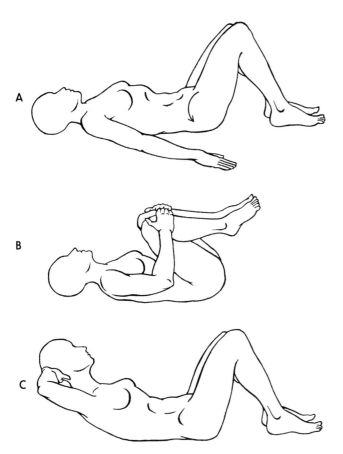

FIG. 53-13. Flexion exercises. **A,** Posterior pelvic tilt—"flat back." **B,** Double knee to chest. **C,** Partial sit-up.

"Hands-on" therapy techniques

- Massage
- Fascial-tendon stretching
- Traction
- Joint mobilization

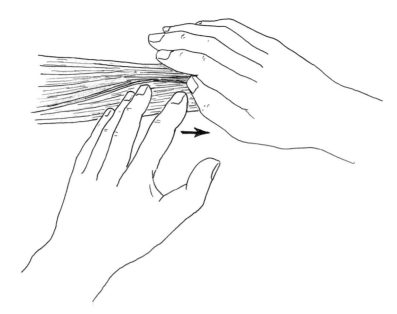

FIG. 53-14. Diagram of myofascial release. (From White AH, Anderson R: *Conservative care of low back pain*, Baltimore, 1991, Williams & Wilkins.)

lagen, remodeling of collagen fibers into a longitudinal pattern, and maturation of fiber cross-linking.[6] Immobilization causes weakening of the ligamentous insertion sites as well.[81] It has also been shown that early mobilization and tensile loading of damaged ligaments may promote proper alignment of collagen fibers during remodeling.[101] Since tissue is optimally healed along lines of physiologic stress, directed physical therapy with manual soft-tissue techniques may be helpful as a component of a comprehensive rehabilitation program.

Myofascial System

The same concepts apply to other collagen-containing tissue such as the myofascial system. Like ligaments, the fascia is connective tissue consisting of layers of collagen and elastin in a ground substance matrix. The fascial sheaths are continuous and interwoven. All structures from the dermis to the periosteum are enveloped with fasciae. The superficial fascia is thinner and allows for more freedom of movement, whereas the deeper fascia is thicker and stronger and is designed for structure and support. The fascia functions to separate and support muscles, allowing for independent muscle function, but at the same time joining them into a functional unit. The fascia also works to absorb shock, transmit mechanical force, and exchange metabolites from fibrous elements to the circulatory and lymphatic systems. Injury to the myofascial system with resultant pain, swelling, and immobility can cause desiccation of the fascia with loss of elasticity and failure to maintain critical fiber distance. Layers of the fascia lose their normal gliding function, and increased cross-linking of fibers may occur. If the myofascial system loses it mobility, there can be secondary loss of spinal articular mobility and lower extremity flexibility. Myofascial releasing techniques are designed to apply pressure and shear to the layers of the fascia, promoting improved elasticity and freedom of movement (Fig. 53-14).[12,73] Reestablishment of normal mobility in connective tissue structures provides relief of discomfort and contributes to the reestablishment of normal flexibility and biomechanics.

Mobilization

Both connective tissue changes and intrinsic changes in the three-joint complex can produce segmental dysfunction. Mobilization of soft-tissue structures alone often does not achieve the goal of full, pain-free range of motion of the spine and lower quadrant. Optimal joint mobility is also required. Assessment of segmental spinal motion and treatment to restore proper mobility demand expert manual techniques.[12,118,149,188] Standard grades of mobilization can be used for pain control or stretching. Grades I and II are gentle movements within resistance-free range of motion. These are often referred to as *oscillations* and are used for pain control. Grades III and IV are larger amplitude forces that move the joint into its restricted range of motion and are used for actual stretching. Grade V, often referred to as a *manipulation*, is a brief thrust that takes the joint beyond its physiologic range of motion. The presence of soft-tissue or articular disease can decrease the available excursion of movement in each grade of mobilization (Fig. 53-15). Mobilization and manipulation in a healthy spinal segment does not cause any true facet gapping; however, there is some gliding of the synovial facet joints.[126] *There is no convincing evidence of actual realignment of vertebral bodies or reduction of disk herniations with mobilization or manipulation techniques.*[59,95] Applying force through a motion segment can produce pain relief and with a stronger movement can produce tissue stretching.

The key to mobilization is to direct energy only at a specific level. The hypomobile segments can be mobilized while protecting the hypermobile segments. Gross

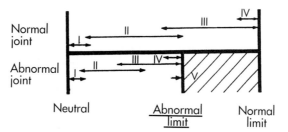

Movements of <u>abnormal</u> joints are usually, but not invariably, limited, and since the <u>available</u> excursion of movement is reduced, the grades of treatment are proportionately reduced.

FIG. 53-15. Grades of mobilization for normal and abnormal joints. (From Grieve GP: *Mobilization of the spine*, ed 3, New York, 1979, Churchill Livingstone.)

rotatory manipulation most likely causes movement at the segment of least resistance (i.e., the segment that is already hypermobile). Also, the use of manipulative treatment in the presence of acute radiculopathy is controversial and has been associated with complications.[23] MacDonald and Bell[116] have demonstrated positive effects from manipulative treatment in a small population of patients with lumbosacral pain without radicular symptoms. The symptoms were of 2 to 4 weeks' duration, and symptoms present for more than 4 weeks showed no preferential response to manipulative treatment. Studies by Koes et al[104,105] have demonstrated that manual therapy is superior to treatment provided by the general practitioner or placebo treatment for cases of low back pain. DiFablo[43] has critically reviewed the literature on manual therapy and demonstrated that there appears to be a role for this type of treatment in some patients with low back pain. *No data exist to support the role of long-term soft-tissue or articular mobilization or manipulation in the treatment of spine pain.* Such protracted passive treatment places the patient in a dependent role and can be counterproductive in attempts to move toward participatory function-oriented care.

Exercise

To meet the goal of optimal strength, endurance, and coordination of the neuromuscular systems as it affects the lumbar spine and to meet the goal of prevention of further injury and recurrences, rehabilitation beyond the absence of symptoms is necessary. As shown, an early exercise program is usually appropriate. Exercises can control pain, possibly via endorphin release, optimize soft-tissue repair and regeneration, and improve muscular performance. Exercises that improve the function of the spinal muscles are generally known as spinal stabilization.[153,163] Stability of the lumbar spine is provided by bony architecture; disk mechanics; ligamentous support; and muscular strength, endurance, and coordination. Optimal muscle strength can protect the spinal motion segment from chronic repetitive stress or acute dynamic overload. The concept of spinal stabilization implies a muscle "fusion." The specific muscular stabilizers

---

> **Muscular stabilizers of the lumbar spine**
>
> - Abdominal muscles (particularly the transversus abdominis and obliquus internus)
> - Latissimus dorsi
> - Spinal intersegmental muscles (multifidi, rotators, and interspinals)
> - Iliopsoas
> - Erector spinae
> - Quadratus lumborum

---

of the lumbar spine include (1) abdominal muscles, particularly the transversus abdominis and obliquus internus; (2) latissimus dorsi; (3) spinal intersegmental muscles (i.e., multifidi, rotators, and interspinalis); (4) iliopsoas; (5) erector spinae; and (6) quadratus lumborum.

Any spinal exercise must address stability before movement and endurance before strength. Training begins with exercises designed to help locate the neutral spine position, which allows for increased awareness of lumbosacral motion and pelvic control. **Neutral spine** is defined as the midpoint of available range of motion between anterior and posterior pelvic tilt, not the absence of lordosis (Fig. 53-16). Neutral positioning is advantageous because it is a loose-packed position that decreases tension on ligaments and joints, it allows more balanced segmental force distribution between the disk and facet joints, it is close to the center of reaction and allows movement into flexion and extension quickly, it provides the greatest functional stability with axial loading, and it is usually the position of greatest comfort. Cocontraction of the abdominal and extensor musculature, especially the gluteals, is required to maintain this braced position. The patient can perform this exercise initially in a standing position and later advance to sitting and jumping activities. Ultimately the patient can progress to more challenging antigravity positions such as supine lying with and without alternating arm and leg raises (Fig. 53-17), bridging (Fig. 53-18), prone lying, and quadriped (i.e., hands and knees position) with and without alternating

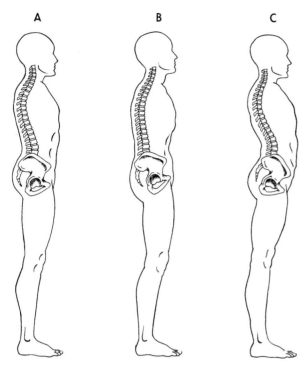

FIG. 53-16. Neutral spine posture. **A,** Neutral pelvis—"pelvic bracing." **B,** Excessive posterior pelvic tilt—hypolordosis. **C,** Excessive anterior pelvic tilt—hyperlordosis.

arm and leg raises (Fig. 53-19). The latter exercises also emphasize the short intersegmental muscles such as the multifidi. These tonic or postural stabilizers of the spine tend to fatigue first and atrophy first following spinal injury. Initially, resisted exercises of the trunk limited to short arcs performed in rotation, flexion, extension, and side bending also preferentially strengthen these short segmental stabilizers. Once neutral spine stabilization is mastered, position transition exercises while maintaining precise pelvic control and exercises of the extremities with and without resistance are added. These facilitate neuromuscular coordination and enhance endurance and strength gains. The use of a gymnastic ball enhances these rehabilitation techniques (Fig. 53-20).

Torque to the lumbar spine is intrinsic to most activities, and most sporting activities have demands that force the lumbar spine and pelvis out of a neutral position. Therefore strengthening of the prime movers, including the abdominal and erector spinae muscles, is required, but protection against shear and torsion must be maintained usually through the TLF mechanism. Specific strengthening of the obliquus and latissimus dorsi muscles is required. Abdominal exercises have been universally regarded as a treatment for low back pain. Sagittal plane sit-ups are used in the stabilization routine, but they are limited to partial curl-ups, since lifting the head and upper torso only activates the obliquus and rectus abdominis. When performing a pull-down weight routine

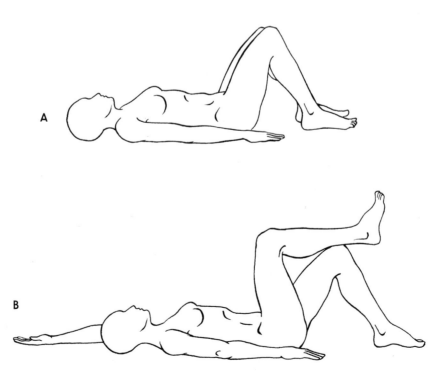

FIG. 53-17. Stabilization exercises. **A,** Supine pelvic bracing. **B,** Supine pelvic bracing with alternating arm and leg raises ("dead bug").

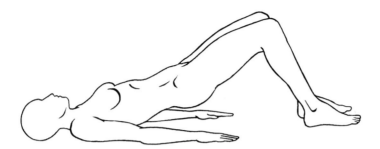

FIG. 53-18. Stabilization exercises. Basic position of bridging.

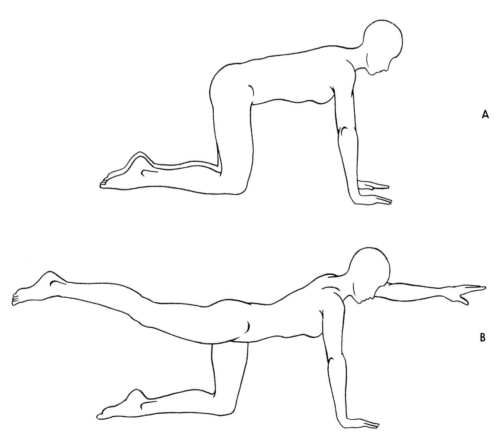

FIG. 53-19. Stabilization exercises. **A,** Quadruped position with pelvic bracing. **B,** Quadruped position with pelvic bracing and alternating arm and leg raises.

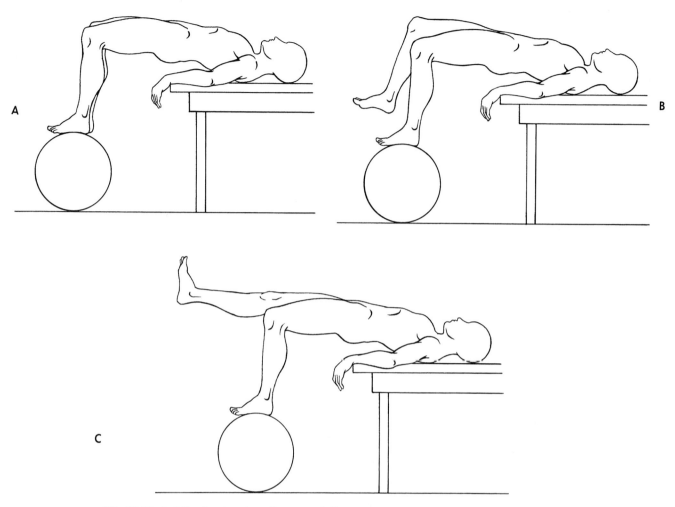

FIG. 53-20. Stabilization exercises. Gymnastic ball exercises. Degree of difficulty increases from **A** to **C.**

for the latissimus dorsi muscles, it is critical to maintain neutral spine positioning and avoid the tendency toward lumbar hyperextension with the arms overhead. Lower extremity strengthening is necessary because these muscles work in a coordinated manner with the trunk, especially during lifting, when the gluteal and hamstring muscles are the prime posterior rotators of the pelvis and trunk. Quadriceps muscle strengthening is important for support of body weight during squatting.

Cardiovascular Fitness

Cardiovascular fitness should also be continued in the subacute phase of rehabilitation. In addition to the general aerobic benefits of exercise, nutrition to injured tissues may be enhanced. Cardiovascular fitness provides the necessary aerobic base for sports training. Along with aerobic training, anaerobic fitness should be developed and maintained based on the demands of the particular sporting activity. Training for total body muscle strength, endurance, and power, specific for the demands of the sport, should also be combined with the spine stabilization-strengthening program. The program content varies from sport to sport, but helps ensure that

sports-specific rehabilitation and training occur in preparation for successful return to activity. This comprehensive approach also helps prevent further injury and recurrences. The practitioner must be familiar with both the spine and the sport to prescribe full rehabilitation and meet the goals of the subacute phase of treatment.

SPINE AND PELVIC ROLE IN LINKAGE SYSTEM

The spine and pelvis contribute significantly to the body's overall ability to perform physically. They are critical links in the total kinetic chain and have been referred to as the "engine" or "motor" for sports performance.[68] The trunk and pelvis act as a functional unit connecting the lower extremities to the upper extremities. The trunk and pelvis funnel much of the ground reactive force into the upper extremity and are capable of generating additional forces.

This linkage system is particularly relevant in overhead throwing and racquet sports. The shoulder girdle itself is incapable of generating the necessary force (i.e., 60 Nm of internal rotation torque) to produce the tremendous angular velocities (i.e., greater than 7000 de-

---

Exercise training for the lumbar spine

Soft-tissue flexibility
- Hamstring musculotendinous unit
- Quadriceps musculotendinous unit
- Iliopsoas musculotendinous unit
- Gastrocsoleus musculotendinous unit
- External and internal hip rotators

Joint mobility
- Lumbar spine segmental mobility
- Hip range of motion
- Thoracic segmental mobility

Stabilization program
- Finding neutral spine position while in the standing, sitting, jumping, and prone positions
- Prone gluteal squeezes with arm raises, alternate arm raises, leg raises, alternate leg raises, arm and leg raises, and alternate arm and leg raises
- Supine pelvic bracing
- Bridging progression (basic position, one leg raised with ankle weights, stepping, and balancing on a gym ball)
- Quadruped with alternating arm and leg movements using ankle and wrist weights)
- Kneeling stabilization (double knee, single knee, and lunges with and without weight)

- Wall slide quadriceps strengthening
- Position transition with postural control

Abdominal program
- Curl-ups
- Dead bugs (supported, nonsupported)
- Diagonal curl-ups
- Diagonal curl-ups on incline board
- Straight leg lowering

Gym program
- Latissimus pull-downs
- Angled leg press
- Lunges
- Hyperextension bench
- General upper-body weight exercises
- Pulley exercises to stress postural control

Aerobic program
- Progressive walking
- Swimming
- Stationary bicycle riding
- Cross-country ski machine
- Running (initially supervised on a treadmill)

From Saal JA: *Orthop Rev* 19:698, 1990.

---

grees/sec) of the shoulder during the acceleration phase of throwing.[5,148] Although the rotator cuff and scapula act as stabilizers to protect the integrity of the glenohumeral joint and shoulder girdle, it is the much greater mass of the trunk and pelvis that generates a significant degree of the kinetic energy necessary for overhead athletic performance and transfers that energy into the upper extremity.[1] If motion of the axial skeleton is limited, a significant decrease in the velocity of a thrown ball has been reported.[184] Also, if the ground reactive force is lessened, the transfer of energy to the upper extremity is also reduced. Peak ball velocities of a thrown water polo ball are approximately one half that of a thrown baseball where ground reactive force can be generated.[130]

If the trunk and pelvis do not act as a rigid cylinder, there is loss of control, dissipation of energy, and alteration of shoulder biomechanics. Lumbosacral spine fatigue may result in the assumption of a more lordotic posture. Watkins et al[190] suggested that this excessive lordosis results in a lagging of the shoulder and upper extremity behind the torso during throwing (i.e., the so-called slow arm). This results in control problems and in compensatory change in the shoulder girdle biomechanics leading to possible injury. It is of interest that the most highly skilled pitchers consistently demonstrated trunk muscle firing patterns that produce the most trunk flexion and rotation. Also, professional pitchers show more efficient rotator cuff firing patterns when throwing as compared with less skilled amateurs.[67] In addition, isokinetic shoulder muscle strength appears to have little bearing on throwing velocity.[11] The lower extremities, pelvis, and trunk provide the necessary kinetic energy for throwing in these athletes.

These same structures also function as force attenuators during the follow-through phase of throwing. Greater than 500 N of force is necessary to slow down the upper extremity,[5] which is far greater than the force-generating capacity in the rotator cuff and scapular stabilizers. During the acceleration phase of throwing the trunk decelerates, transferring its kinetic energy to the upper extremity. During the follow-through phase of throwing the trunk rotates again, reacquiring some of its energy and theoretically decreasing the burden on the rotator cuff and scapular stabilizers to decelerate the upper extremity.[99]

The thoracolumbar fascia, its muscular attachments, and the midline ligament structures help maintain the trunk as a rigid cylinder. These structures also help dissipate the shear forces imparted to the three-joint complex. Any breakdown in the pelvis and trunk function affects the entire kinetic chain. Fatigue, inflexibility, and strength imbalance can lead to less efficient energy transfer, a breakdown in proper mechanics, and alteration of technique. This can result in a drop in performance or injury.

This information suggests that training and conditioning programs for many sports could benefit by including measures to specifically obtain and maintain proper trunk, pelvis, and lower extremity flexibility, strength, power, and endurance combined with work on biomechanics and technique.

SUMMARY

The comprehensive rehabilitation of athletic low back injury requires a fundamental understanding of the demands of the sport, the mechanisms of injury, the functional anatomy and biochemistry of normal and aberrant segmental motion, and the potential pain generators. If possible, a precise diagnosis may aid in the rehabilitation process. The rehabilitation principles that apply to the spine are essentially the same that apply to all musculoskeletal injuries—control pain and inflammation, restore joint and soft-tissue mobility, maximize strength and endurance, and progressively return the athlete to sport-specific activities. The dynamic muscular control of the lumbar spine mechanism demands exhaustive physical reconditioning for the athlete to maintain high performance levels.

Lack of response to such a treatment program demands a reevaluation of the diagnosis including a high index of suspicion for a missed diagnosis and even evaluation of any potential psychosocial barriers to recovery. It can be said that the injured athlete may in fact be the "ultimate" worker's compensation patient. Theoretically, disability can be fueled by many factors including poor communication from the health care provider, fear of the severity of injury and reinjury, peer pressure, lack of management support, and financial and legal issues. Even with athletes, disability may be the path of least resistance and failure to rehabilitate successfully should alert the physician to this possibility. Ultimately, education and *pre*habilitation may be the most effective *re*habilitation.

ACKNOWLEDGMENT

Figs. 53-12, 53-13, and 53-16 through 53-20 were prepared by Steve Kechley.

REFERENCES

1. Abrams JS: Special shoulder problems in the throwing athlete: pathology, diagnosis, and nonoperative management, *Clin Sports Med* 10:839, 1991.
2. Alaranta H et al: A prospective study of patients with sciatica: a comparison between conservatively treated patients and patients who have undergone operation. III. Results after one year follow-up, *Spine* 15:1345, 1990.
3. Anderson GBJ: Epidemiologic aspects of low back pain in industry, *Spine* 6:53, 1981.
4. Andersson G, Schultz H, Nachemson A: Intervertebral disc pressures during traction, *Scand J Rehabil Med Suppl* 9:88, 1983.
5. Andrews JR: Forces about the shoulder. Proceedings of the thirty-ninth annual meeting of the American College of Sports Medicine, Dallas, May, 1992.
6. Andriacchi T et al: Ligament injury and repair. In Woo SL-Y, Buckwalter JA (eds): *Injury and repair of the musculoskeletal soft tissues*, Park Ridge, Ill, 1988, American Academy of Orthopaedic Surgeons.
7. Apple DF, O'Toole J, Annis C: Professional basketball injuries, *Phys Sports Med* 10:81, 1982.
8. Avramov AI et al: The effects of controlled mechanical loading on group II, III, and IV afferent units from the lumbar facet joint and surrounding tissue: an in vitro study, *J Bone Joint Surg* 74A:1465, 1992.
9. Badalamente MA et al: Mechanical stimulation of dorsal root ganglion induces increased production of substance P: a mechanism for pain following nerve root compromise? *Spine* 12:552, 1987.
10. Barker H: *Leaves from my life*, London, 1928, Heineann.
11. Bartlet LR, Storey MD, Simons BD: Measurement of upper extremity torque production and its relationship to throwing speed in the competitive athlete, *Am J Sports Med* 17:89, 1991.
12. Basmajian JV, Nyberg R (eds): *Rational manual therapies*, Baltimore, 1993, Williams & Wilkins.
13. Beaman D et al: Substance P innervation of lumbar facet joints. Proceedings of the seventh annual meeting of North American Spine Society, Boston, July 9-11, 1991.
14. Benzon HT: Epidural steroid injection for low back pain and lumbosacral radiculopathy, *Pain* 24:277, 1986.
15. Berman AT et al: The effects of epidural injection of local anesthetics and corticosteroids on patients with lumbosciatic pain, *Clin Orthop* 188:144, 1984.
16. Berqguist-Ullman M, Larsson U: Acute low back pain in industry: a controlled prospective study with special reference to therapy and confounding factors, *Acta Orthop Scand Suppl* 170:1, 1977.
17. Berryman JW: Exercise and the medical tradition from Hippocrates through antebellum America: a review essay. In Berryman JW, Park RJ (eds): *Sport and exercise science: essays in the history of sports medicine*, Chicago, 1992, University of Illinois Press.
18. Biering-Sorenson F: Physical measurements as risk factors for low back trouble over a one-year period, *Spine* 9:106, 1984.
19. Boden S et al: Abnormal magnetic resonance scans of the spine in asymptomatic patients, *J Bone Joint Surg* 72A:403, 1990.
20. Bogduk N: Lumbar dorsal ramus syndrome, *Med J Aust* 2:537, 1980.
21. Bogduk N, Twomey LT: The lumbar muscles and their fascia. In *Clinical anatomy of the lumbar spine*, ed 2, Melbourne, 1991, Churchill Livingstone.
22. Bogduk N, Twomey LT: Nerves of the lumbar spine. In *Clinical anatomy of the lumbar spine*, ed 2, Melbourne, 1991, Churchill Livingstone.
23. Borenstein D, Wiesel S: *Low back pain: medical diagnosis and comprehensive management*, Philadelphia, 1989, WB Saunders.
24. Bortz W: The disuse syndrome, *West J Med* 141:169, 1984.
25. Bozzao A et al: Lumbar disc herniation: MR imaging assessment of natural history in patients treated without surgery, *Radiology* 185:135, 1992.
26. Brady TA, Cahill BR, Bodner LM: Weight training–related lumbar spine injuries, *Am J Sports Med* 10:1, 1982.
27. Buirski G: Magnetic resonance signal pattern of lumbar discs in patients with low back pain: a prospective study with discographic correlation, *Spine* 17:1199, 1992.
28. Bush K et al: The natural history of sciatica associated with disc pathology, *Spine* 17:1205, 1992.
29. Cady LD, Thomas PC, Karwasky RJ: Program for increasing health and fitness of firefighters, *J Occup Med* 27:110, 1985.
30. Carrette S et al: A controlled trial of corticosteroid injection into facet joints for chronic low back pain, *N Engl J Med* 325:1002, 1991.
31. Crisco JJ, Panjabi MM: The intersegmental and multisegmental muscles of the lumbar spine: a biomechanical model comparing lateral stabilizing potential, *Spine* 16:793, 1991.
32. Cuckler JM et al: The use of epidural steroids in the treatment of lumbar radicular pain: a prospective, randomized, double-blind study, *J Bone Joint Surg* 67A:63, 1985.
33. Dahl S: Nonsteroidal antiinflammatory agents: clinical pharmacology/adverse effects/usage guidelines. In Wilkens RF, Dahl SL (eds): *Therapeutic controversies in the rheumatic diseases*, Orlando, Fla, 1987, Grune & Stratton.
34. Dehlin O, Hendenrund B, Horal J: Back symptoms in nursing aides in a geriatric hospital, *Scan J Rehabil Med* 8:47, 1976.
35. Delauche-Cavallier M-C et al: Lumbar disc herniation: computed tomography scan changes after conservative treatment of nerve root compression, *Spine* 17:927, 1992.
36. Derby R: Diagnostic block procedures: use in pain localization, *Spine* 1:47, 1986.
37. Derby R et al: Response to steroid and duration of radicular pain as predictors of surgical outcome, *Spine* 17(suppl):176, 1992.

38. Destouet JM: Lumbar facet syndrome: diagnosis and treatment, *Surg Rounds Orthop* 2:22, 1988.

39. Deyo R: Conservative therapy for low back pain: distinguishing useful from useless therapy, *JAMA* 250:1057, 1983.

40. Deyo R, Diehl A, Rosenthal M: How many days of bed rest for acute low back pain? a randomized clinical trial, *N Engl J Med* 315:1064, 1986.

41. Didry C et al: Medically treated lumbar disc herniation: clinical and computed tomographic follow-up, *Presse Med* 20:299, 1991.

42. Dietrich M, Kurowski P: The importance of mechanical factors in the etiology of spondylolysis: a model analysis of loads and stresses in human lumbar spine, *Spine* 6:532, 1985.

43. DiFablo RP: Efficacy of manual therapy, *Phys Ther* 72:853, 1992.

44. Dixon ASJ: Diagnosis of low back pain—sorting the complainers. In Jayson M (ed): *The lumbar spine and back pain,* New York, 1976, Grune & Stratton.

45. Donelson R, Silva G, Murphy K: The centralization phenomenon: its usefulness in evaluating and treating referred pain, *Spine* 15:21, 1990.

46. Dooley JF et al: Nerve root infiltration in the diagnosis of radicular pain, *Spine* 13:79, 1988.

47. Duda M: Golf injuries: they really do happen, *Phys Sports Med* 15:191, 1987.

48. Duda M: Golfers use exercise to get back in the swing, *Phys Sports Med* 17:109, 1989.

49. Eagleston RE: Personal communication, 1993.

50. El-Khoury GY et al: Epidural steroid injection: a procedure ideally performed with fluoroscopic control, *Radiology* 168:554, 1988.

51. Ellenberg ME et al: Prospective evaluation of the course of disc herniation in patients with radiculopathy, *Arch Phys Med Rehabil* 74:3, 1993.

52. Fairbank JCT et al: Influence of anthropometric factors and joint laxity in the incidence of adolescent back pain, *Spine* 9:461, 1984.

53. Farfan HF et al: The effects of torsion on the lumbar intervertebral joints: the role of torsion in the production of disc degeneration, *J Bone Joint Surg* 52A:468, 1970.

54. Feeler LC: Racquet sports, *Spine* 4:337, 1990.

55. Ferguson RJ, McMaster HS, Stanitski CL: Low back pain in college football linemen, *Phys Sports Med* 2:63, 1974.

56. Fortin JP, Roberts D: Competitive figure skating injuries, *Arch Phys Med Rehabil* 68:642, 1987.

57. Franson RC, Saal JS, Saal JA: Human phospholipase A_2 is inflammatory, *Spine* 17(suppl):129, 1992.

58. Fry J: *Back pain and soft tissue rheumatism: advisory services colloquium proceedings,* London, 1972, Clinical & General.

59. Frymoyer JW: Back pain and sciatica, *N Engl J Med* 318:291, 1988.

60. Frymoyer JW et al: Risk factors in low back pain: an epidemiological survey, *J Bone Joint Surg* 65A:213, 1983.

61. Gamburd R: Use of selective injections for the diagnosis and management of lumbar spine problems, *Clin Phys Med Rehabil* 2:79, 1991.

62. Gersh M: Postoperative pain and transcutaneous electrical nerve stimulation, *Phys Ther* 58:1463, 1978.

63. Gianakopoulos G et al: Inversion devices: their role in producing lumbar distraction, *Arch Phys Med Rehabil* 66:100, 1985.

64. Gibbs R: Personal communication, 1993.

65. Gibson MJ et al: Magnetic resonance imaging of adolescent disc herniation, *J Bone Joint Surg* 69B:699, 1987.

66. Goldstein JD et al: Spine injuries in gymnasts and swimmers: an epidemiologic investigation, *Am J Sports Med* 19:463, 1991.

67. Gowan ID et al: A comparative electromyographic analysis of the shoulder during pitching, *Am J Sports Med* 15:586, 1987.

68. Gracovetsky S: The spine as a motor in sports: application to running and lifting. In Hochschuler SH (ed): Spinal injuries in sports, *Spine* 4:267, 1990.

69. Gracovetsky S, Farfan H, Heleur C: The abdominal mechanism, *Spine* 10:317, 1985.

70. Gracovetsky S et al: Analysis of spinal and muscular activity during flexion-extension and free lifts, *Spine* 15:1333, 1990.

71. Granhed H, Morelli B: Low back pain among wrestlers and retired weightlifters, *Am J Sports Med* 16:530, 1988.

72. Green L: Dexamethasone in the management of symptoms due to herniated lumbar disc, *J Neurol Neurosurg Psychiatry* 38:1211, 1975.

73. Greenman PE: *Principles of manual medicine,* Baltimore, 1989, Williams & Wilkins.

74. Gupta R, Ramarao S: Epidurography in reduction of lumbar disc prolapse by traction, *Arch Phys Med Rehabil* 59:372, 1978.

75. Haddox JD: Lumbar and cervical epidural steroid therapy, *Anesth Clin North Am* 10:179, 1992.

76. Harris JD: History and development of manipulation and mobilization. In Basmajian JV, Nyberg R (eds): *Rational manual therapies,* Baltimore, 1993, Williams & Wilkins.

77. Hayes MA et al: Roentgenographic evaluation of lumbar spine flexion-extension in asymptomatic individuals, *Spine* 14:327, 1989.

78. Helbig T, Lee CK: The lumbar facet syndrome, *Spine* 13:61, 1988.

79. Helliüvaara M: Risk factors for low back pain and sciatica, *Ann Med* 21:257, 1989.

80. Henry JH, Lareau B, Neigut D: The injury rate in professional basketball, *Am J Sports Med* 10:16, 1982.

81. Herring SA: Rehabilitation of muscle injuries, *Med Sci Sports Exerc* 22:453, 1990.

82. Hirsch C: An attempt to diagnose the level of a disc lesion clinically by disc puncture, *Acta Orthop Scand* 18:132, 1949.

83. Hirsch C, Jonsson R, Lewin T: Low back symptoms in a Swedish female population, *Clin Orthop* 63:171, 1969.

84. Hitselberger WE, Witten PM: Abnormal myelogram in asymptomatic patients, *J Neurosurg* 28:204, 1986.

85. Hochschuler SH (ed): Spinal injuries in sports, *Spine: State Art Rev* 4:1990.

86. Horal J: The clinical appearance of low back disorders in the city of Gothenburg, Sweden, *Acta Orthop Scand Suppl* 118:8, 1969.

87. Hoshina H: Spondylolysis in athletes, *Phys Sports Med* 8:75, 1980.

88. Howell DW: Musculoskeletal profile and incidence of musculoskeletal injuries in light-weight women rowers, *Am J Sports Med* 12:278, 1984.

89. Huskisson E: Nonnarcotic analgesics. In Wall PD, Melzack R (eds): *Textbook of pain,* New York, 1989, Churchill Livingstone.

90. Jackson CP: Historic perspectives on patient education and its place in acute spinal disorders. In Mayer TG, Mooney V, Gatchel RJ (eds): *Contemporary conservative care for painful spinal disorders,* Philadelphia, 1991, Lea & Febiger.

91. Jackson DW: Low back pain in young athletes: evaluation of stress reactions and discogenic problems, *Am J Sports Med* 7:364, 1979.

92. Jackson DW, Wiltse LL, Cirincione RJ: Spondylolysis in the female gymnast, *Clin Orthop* 117:68, 1976.

93. Jackson DW et al: Stress reactions involving the pars interarticularis in young athletes, *Am J Sports Med* 9:304, 1981.

94. Jackson RP, Glah JJ: Foraminal and extraforaminal lumbar disc herniation: diagnosis and treatment, *Spine* 12:577, 1987.

95. Jayson M IV et al: Mobilization and manipulation for low back pain, *Spine* 6:409, 1981.

96. Jayson MIV: The role of vascular damage and fibrosis in the pathogenesis of nerve root damage, *Clin Orthop* 279:40, 1992.

97. Jeffries B: Epidural steroid injections, *Spine* 2:419, 1988.

98. Jeffries B: Facet steroid injections, *Spine* 2:409, 1988.

99. Jobe FW et al: The shoulder in sports. In Rockwood CA Jr, Matsen FA III (eds): *The shoulder,* Philadelphia, 1990, WB Saunders.

100. Kahanovitz W, Viola K, Gallager M: Long-term strength assessment of postoperative diskectomy patients, *Spine* 14:402, 1989.

101. Kellet J: Acute soft tissue injuries—a review of the literature, *Med Sci Sports Exerc* 18:489, 1986.

102. Khuffash B, Porter RW: Cross leg pain and trunk list, *Spine* 14:602, 1989.
103. Kirkaldy-Willis WH et al: Pathology and pathogenesis of lumbar spondylosis and stenosis, *Spine* 3:319, 1978.
104. Koes BW et al: The effectiveness of manual therapy, physiotherapy, and treatment by the general practitioner for nonspecific back and neck complaints: a randomized clinical trial, *Spine* 17:28, 1992.
105. Koes BW et al: Randomized clinical trial of manipulative therapy and physiotherapy for persistent back and neck complaints: results of one-year follow-up, *BMJ* 304:601, 1992.
106. Kornberg M: Extreme lateral lumbar disc herniation: clinical syndrome and computed tomography recognition, *Spine* 12:586, 1987.
107. Kosteljanetz M, Bank F, Schmidt-Olsen S: The clinical significance of straight-leg raising (Lasègue's sign) in the diagnosis of prolapsed lumbar disc: interobserver variation and correlation with surgical findings, *Spine* 13:393, 1988.
108. Kotani T, Ichikova N, Wakabeyosh W: Studies of spondylolysis found amount weight lifters, *Br J Sports Med* 6:4, 1971.
109. Krag MH et al: Internal displacement distribution from in vitro loading of human thoracic and lumbar spinal motion segments: experimental results and theoretical predictions, *Spine* 12:1001, 1987.
110. Krempen JF, Smith BS, DeFreest LJ: Selective nerve root infiltration for the evaluation of sciatica, *Orthop Clin North Am* 6:311, 1975.
111. Kurkala et al: Immunohistochemical demonstration of nociceptors in the ligamentous structures of the lumbar spine, *Spine* 10:156, 1985.
112. Kuslich SD, Ulstrom CL, Michael CJ: The tissue origin of low back pain and sciatica: a report of pain response to tissue stimulation during operations on the lumbar spine using local anesthesia, *Orthop Clin North Am* 22:181, 1991.
113. Lee M: Mechanics of spinal joint manipulation in the thoracic and lumbar spine: a theoretical study of posteroanterior force techniques, *Clin Biomech* 4:249, 1989.
114. Lehmann J: Therapeutic heat and cold, *Clin Orthop* 99:207, 1974.
115. Lehmann J, DeLateur B: Diathermy and superficial heat and cold therapy. In Kottke FJ, Stillwell GK, Lehmann JK (eds): *Krusen's handbook of physical medicine and rehabilitation*, ed 3, Philadelphia, 1982, WB Saunders.
116. MacDonald RS, Bell CMJ: An open controlled assessment of osteopathic manipulation in nonspecific low back pain, *Spine* 15:364, 1990.
117. Maigne J-Y, Rime B, Deligne B: Computed tomography follow-up study of forty-eight cases of nonoperatively treated lumbar intervertebral disc herniation, *Spine* 17:1071, 1992.
118. Maitland GD: *Vertebral manipulation*, ed 5, London, 1986, Butterworth.
119. Malinsky J: The ontogenetic development of nerve terminations in the intervertebral discs of man, *Acta Anat (Basel)* 38:96, 1959.
120. Marshall LL, Trethewie ER, Curtain CC: Chemical radiculitis: a clinical, physiological, and immunological study, *Clin Orthop* 129:61, 1979.
121. Matthews J: Dynamic discography: a study of lumbar traction, *Ann Phys Med* 9:275, 1968.
122. Mayer T et al: Quantification of lumbar function. II. Sagittal plane trunk strength in chronic low back pain patients, *Spine* 10:765, 1985.
123. McCarrol JR, Miller JM, Ritter M: Lumbar spondylolysis and spondylolisthesis in college football players, *Am J Sports Med* 14:404, 1986.
124. McCarron RF et al: The inflammatory effect of nucleus pulposus: a possible element in the pathogenesis of low back pain, *Spine* 12:760, 1987.
125. McCoy CE et al: Patients avoiding surgery: pathology and one-year life status follow-up, *Spine* 16(suppl):198, 1991.
126. McFadden KD, Taylor JR: Axial rotation in the lumbar spine and gapping of the zygapophyseal joints, *Spine* 15:295, 1990.
127. McGill SM: The influence of lordosis on axial trunk torque and trunk muscle myoelectric activity, *Spine* 17:1187, 1992.
128. McKenzie RA: Prophylaxis in recurrent low back pain, *N Z Med J* 89:22, 1979.
129. McKenzie RA: *The lumbar spine, mechanical diagnosis, and therapy*, Walkance, New Zealand, 1981, Spinal Publications.
130. McMaster WC, Long SC, Caiozzo V: Isokinetic torque imbalances in the rotator cuff of the elite water polo player, *Am J Sports Med* 19:72, 1991.
131. McNeil T et al: Trunk strengths in attempted flexion, extension, and lateral bending in healthy subjects and patients with low back disorders, *Spine* 5:529, 1980.
132. Melzack R, Wall PD: Pain mechanisms: a new theory, *Science* 150:971, 1965.
133. Mennell J: *Back pain: diagnosis and treatment using manipulative technique*, Boston, 1960, Little, Brown.
134. Micheli LJ: Back injuries in dancers, *Clin Sports Med* 2:473, 1983.
135. Micheli LJ: Back injuries in gymnastics, *Clin Sports Med* 4:85, 1985.
136. Mixter WJ, Barr JS: Rupture of the intervertebral disc with involvement of the spinal canal, *N Engl J Med* 211:210, 1934.
137. Mooney V, Robertson J: The facet syndrome, *Clin Orthop* 115:149, 1976.
138. Moritz A, Grana WA: High school basketball injuries, *Phys Sports Med* 6:91, 1978.
139. Myers R et al: Human disc PLA_2 induces neural injury: a histomorphometric study. Proceedings of the seventh annual meeting of NASS, Boston, July 9-11, 1991.
140. Nachemson A: Disc pressure measurements, *Spine* 6:93, 1981.
141. Nachemson A, Elfstrom G: Intravital dynamic pressure measurements in lumbar discs: a study of common movements, maneuvers, and exercises, *Scand J Rehabil Med (suppl)* 1:1, 1970.
142. Nelson DA: Dangers from methylprednisolone acetate therapy by intraspinal injection, *Arch Neurol* 45:804, 1988.
143. Ng SCS et al: Abnormal connective tissue degrading enzyme patterns in prolapsed intervertebral discs, *Spine* 11:695, 1986.
144. Ohnmesis D et al: Treatment of acute back pain, *Spine* 3:65, 1989.
145. Olmarker K, Rydevik B: Pathophysiology of sciatica, *Orthop Clin North Am* 22:223, 1991.
146. Olmarker K, Rydevik B, Holm S: Edema formation in spinal nerve roots induced by experimental, graded compression: an experimental study on pig cauda equina with special reference to differences in effects between rapid and slow onset of compression, *Spine* 14:569, 1989.
147. Panjabi MM et al: Spinal stability and intersegmental muscle forces: a biomechanical model, *Spine* 14:194, 1989.
148. Pappas AM, Zawacki RM, Sullivan TJ: Biomechanics of baseball pitching: a preliminary report, *Am J Sports Med* 13:216, 1985.
149. Paris SV: Manipulation of the lumbar spine. In Weinstein JN, Wiesel SW (eds): *The lumbar spine*, Philadelphia, 1990, WB Saunders.
150. Pedrini-Mille A et al: Stimulation of the dorsal root ganglion and degradation of rabbit annulus fibrosus, *Spine* 15:1252, 1990.
151. Plowman SA: Physical activity, physical fitness, and low back pain. In Holloszy JO (ed): *Exercise and sport sciences review*, vol 20, Philadelphia, 1992, Williams & Wilkins.
152. Ponte JT, Jensen GJ, Kent BE: A preliminary report on the use of the McKenzie protocol versus William's protocol in the treatment of low back pain, *J Orthop Sports Phys Ther* 6:130, 1984.
153. Porterfield JA: Dynamic stabilization of the trunk, *J Orthop Sports Phys Ther* 6:271, 1985.
154. Quintet R, Hadler M: Diagnoses and treatment of backache, *Semin Rheum* 8:261, 1979.
155. Raymond J, Dumas JM: Intraarticular facet block: diagnostic test or therapeutic procedure? *Radiology* 151:333, 1984.
156. Renfrew DL et al: Correct placement of epidural steroid injections: fluoroscopic guidance and contrast administration, *Am J Neuroradiol* 12:1003, 1991.
157. Roeser W et al: The use of transcutaneous nerve stimulation

for pain control in athletic medicine: a preliminary report, *Am J Sports Med* 4:210, 1976.

158. Roofe PG: Innervation of the annulus fibrosus and posterior longitudinal ligament, *Arch Neurol Psychiat* 44:100, 1940.

159. Rothenberger LA: Prevalence and types of injuries in aerobic dancers, *Am J Sports Med* 16:403, 1988.

160. Rustin MHA, Flynn MD, Coomes EN: Acute sacral epidural abscess following local anesthesia injection, *Postgrad Med J* 59:399, 1983.

161. Rydevik BL, Myers RR, Powell HC: Pressure increase in the dorsal root ganglion following mechanical compression: closed compartment syndrome in nerve roots, *Spine* 14:574, 1989.

162. Saal JA: Rehabilitation of sports-related lumbar spine injuries. In Saal JA (ed): *Physical medicine in Rehabilitation: state of the art reviews: Spine,* Philadelphia, 1987, Henley and Belfus.

163. Saal JA: Dynamic muscular stabilization in the nonoperative treatment of lumbar pain syndromes, *Orthop Rev* 19:691, 1990.

164. Saal JA, Saal JS: Nonoperative treatment of herniated lumbar intervertebral disc with radiculopathy: an outcome study, *Spine* 14:431, 1989.

165. Saal JA, Saal JS, Herzog RJ: The natural history of lumbar intervertebral disc extrusions treated nonoperatively, *Spine* 15:683, 1990.

166. Saal JS et al: High levels of inflammatory phospholipase A_2 activity in lumbar spine disc herniation, *Spine* 15:674, 1990.

167. Salminen JJ: The adolescent back: a field survey of 370 Finnish school children, *Acta Paediatr Scand Suppl* 315:1, 1989.

168. Schiotz E, Cyriax J: *Manipulation: past and present,* London, 1975, Heinemann.

169. Schnebel BE, Watkins RG, Dillin W: The role of spinal flexion and extension in changing nerve root compression in disc herniations, *Spine* 14:835, 1989.

170. Semon RL, Spengler D: Significance of lumbar spondylolysis in college football players, *Spine* 6:172, 1981.

171. Smith G: Prescribing the rules of health: self-help and advice in the late eighteenth century. In Porter R (ed): *Patients and practitioners: lay perceptions of medicine in preindustrial society,* Cambridge, 1985, Cambridge University Press.

172. Stanitski CL: Low back pain in young athletes, *Phys Sports Med* 10:77, 1982.

173. Stankovic R, Johnell O: Conservative treatment of acute low-back pain: a prospective randomized trial: McKenzie method of treatment versus patient education in "mini back school," *Spine* 15:120, 1990.

174. Stimmel B: Pain, analgesia, and addiction: an approach to the pharmacologic management of pain, *Clin J Pain* 1:14, 1985.

175. Stith WJ: Exercise and the intervertebral disc, *Spine* 4:259, 1990.

176. Stokes IAF, Frymoyer JW: Segmental motion and instability, *Spine* 12:688, 1987.

177. Sunderland S: *Nerves and nerve injuries,* ed 2, New York, 1978, Churchill Livingstone.

178. Svensson HO et al: Low back pain in relation to other diseases and cardiovascular risk factors, *Spine* 8:277, 1983.

179. Tchang SPK, Kirkaldy-Willis WH: Spontaneous regression of herniated nucleus pulposus, *AJR* 146:882, 1986.

180. Teplick JG, Haskin ME: Spontaneous regression of herniated nucleus pulposus, *AJR* 145:337, 1985.

181. Thelander U et al: Straight leg raising test versus radiologic size, shape, and position of lumbar disc hernias, *Spine* 17:395, 1992.

182. Threlkeld AJ: The effects of manual therapy on connective tissue, *Phys Ther* 72:893, 1992.

183. Todd T: A brief history of resistance exercise. In Pearl W, Moran G (eds): *Getting stronger,* Bolinas, Calif, 1986, Shelter Publishing.

184. Toyoshima S et al: Contribution of the body parts to throwing performance, *Biomechanics IV,* Baltimore, 1974, University Park Press.

185. Tuel SM, Meythaler JM, Cross LL: Cushing's syndrome from epidural methylprednisolone, *Pain* 40:81, 1990.

186. Urban J, McMullin J: Swelling pressure of lumbar intervertebral discs: influence of age, spinal level, composition, and degeneration, *Spine* 13:179, 1988.

187. Vanharanta H: Etiology, epidemiology, and natural history of lumbar disc disease, *Spine* 3:1, 1989.

188. Van Hoesen L: Mobilization and manipulation techniques for the lumbar spine. In Grieve GP (ed): *Modern manual therapy of the vertebral column,* New York, 1986, Churchill Livingstone.

189. Warner JH: *The therapeutic perspective: medical practice, knowledge, and identity in America 1820-1885,* Cambridge, 1986, Harvard University Press.

190. Watkins RG et al: Dynamic EMG analysis of torque transfer in professional baseball pitchers, *Spine* 14:404, 1989.

191. Weber H: Lumbar disc herniation: a controlled, prospective study with ten years of observation, *Spine* 8:131, 1983.

192. Weinstein JN: Recent advances in the neurophysiology of pain, *Physical medicine in rehabilitation: state of the art reviews: Spine,* Philadelphia, 1990, Henley and Belfus.

193. Weinstein JN: Neurogenic and nonneurogenic pain and inflammatory mediators, *Orthop Clin North Am* 22:235, 1991.

194. Weinstein JN, Claveric W, Gibson S: The pain of discography, *Spine* 13:1344, 1988.

195. Weinstein JN et al: Neuropharmacologic effects of vibration on the dorsal root ganglion: an animal model, *Spine* 13:521, 1988.

196. White AH: Injection technique for the diagnosis and treatment of low back pain, *Orthop Clin North Am* 14:553, 1983.

197. White AH, Derby R, Wynne G: Epidural injection for the diagnosis and treatment of low-back pain, *Spine* 5:78, 1980.

198. White AWM: Low back pain in men receiving workmen's compensation, *Can Med Assoc J* 95:50, 1966.

199. Wiesel SW et al: A study of computer-assisted tomography. I. The incidence of positive CAT scans in an asymptomatic group of patients, *Spine* 9:549, 1984.

200. Williams P: *Low back and neck pain: causes and conservative treatment,* ed 3, Springfield, Ill, 1974, Charles C Thomas.

201. Wooden MJ: Preseason screening of the lumbar spine, *J Orthop Sports Phys Ther* 3:6, 1981.

202. Yamashita J et al: Mechanosensitive afferent units in the lumbar facet joint, *J Bone Joint Surg* 72A:865, 1990.

203. Yost JG Jr, Elfieldt HJ: Basketball injuries. In Nicholas JA, Hershman EB (eds): *The lower extremity and spine in sports medicine,* St Louis, 1986, Mosby.

PART V The Skeletally Immature Athlete

CHAPTER 54

Sports Medicine Musculoskeletal Considerations for Children and Adolescents

Angela D. Smith

GENERAL CONSIDERATIONS
Physical and Psychologic Differences

Children participate in many of the same sports as their parents, but the injuries that they sustain often differ. Children's bone absorbs more energy before breaking.[25] The long bones have cartilaginous growth plates near the ends for longitudinal growth, apophyses with their own growth plates for attachment of musculotendinous structures to the long bone shaft, and growing articular cartilage. The porosity of the bone, the presence of growth plates, and other biomechanical differences lead to a different spectrum of injuries in children and growing adolescents compared with those in adults. In addition, the psychologic development and the motivating forces of young sport and fitness activity participants differ from adults, which lead to variations in level of participation, injury patterns, and rehabilitation methods.

Epidemiology of Children's Sports Injuries

Satisfactory epidemiologic data are difficult to gather because soft-tissue injury and overuse injury data are often missed by those who examine only records from emergency rooms[30,36] or orthopaedic surgeons.[22,31] Despite these limitations, useful information is available. In a prospective study of Massachusetts emergency department records, 1 of every 14 teenagers in monitored communities required hospital treatment for a sports injury.[30] Adolescent participants in football, wrestling, and girls' gymnastics had injury rates as high as 81%, 75%, and 40%, respectively, over a 2-year period.[31] Similarly high rates were noted by McLain and Reynolds[47] in a 1-year study: 61%, 40%, and 46%, respectively. A study of top collegiate women's gymnastic injuries found that a new injury could be expected during 9% of exposure periods, and reinjury could be expected during 71% of exposure periods.[68] DeLee and Farney[26] studied Texas high school football athletes over one season and found .003 injuries per hour of exposure (an injury caused the athlete to miss at least a part of a game or practice or to be treated by a physician). Of 4399 athletes sustaining 2228 injuries, 137 required hospitalization. Younger football players (8 to 15 years of age) have significantly fewer injuries than high school football athletes presumably because of the older athletes' greater mass, speed, and skill.[34,65] The lower incidence of injuries of youth sport participants compared with high school athletes in organized sports is also noted for basketball, soccer, wrestling, baseball, and ice hockey.[33]

Catastrophic injuries that lead to quadriplegia or death (directly from neurologic trauma or indirectly from medical causes) may occur.[52] Rule changes that prohibit "spearing" with the head in football[52,79] and body checking in PeeWee hockey in some Canadian provinces[66] have resulted in a decrease in the incidence of serious injuries. However, in both girls' and boys' gymnastics an increase in injuries is noted between the Garrick and Requa[31] and McLain and Reynolds[47] studies, possibly reflecting differences in difficulty level of gymnastics skills performed, since the more skilled gymnasts generally were not training on the school teams surveyed in the Garrick and Requa study (Garrick, personal communication, 1994). The skill level of gymnasts also advanced between the periods studied.

Despite concerns about sports injuries, participation in organized sport activity has been shown to be safer than free play at home or on the playground.[22] In a classic 1966 study of emergency room visits for trauma, only 4.3% of the injuries were caused by sports; bicycling injuries added another 4.5% of injuries.[36] Of all injuries in that report, 71.3% occurred in either the home or the yard. In a more recent report that monitored school-related injuries sustained by children from elementary school through high school, sports accounted for only 53% of the injuries sustained by children either on the school grounds or during a school-sponsored activity.[42] Among elementary school students, only 40% of school-related injuries were associated with sports; the percentage rose to 54% for middle school students and 69% for senior high school students. During two major soccer tournaments that involved 25,000 players, only half of the consultations with medical personnel were a result of injuries that occurred during matches.[55] The incidence of injury during tournament soccer play was .014 injuries per exposure hour for boys and .032 for girls. The increased injury rate for girls compared with boys was also found in a community-based epidemiologic study from Sweden; the study found that in all age groups from 8 to 16 years the incidence of injuries from soccer was at least twice as great among girls as boys.[27]

Although concern has been raised regarding possibly increasing the incidence of injury among young sports participants, Tenvergert and colleagues found no change in the number of sports injuries treated in the Netherlands from 1982 to 1988.[78]

Residual Disability

Some injuries from childhood and adolescent sports continue to cause problems in adulthood. Female collegiate gymnasts, who were interviewed 10 to 70 months following completion of their gymnastic careers, were found to have a 45% incidence of residual problems from gymnastic injuries. Twenty-nine percent believed that their current level of sport activity was limited by these injuries.[82]

Positive Influences of Sport and Fitness Activities on Youth

Although injuries sustained by young athletes are always of concern, it seems that sport injuries are no more frequent or more serious than the injuries from activities around the home, at the playground, or on urban streets. In addition, children who participate in organized sport and fitness activities have opportunities to develop self-discipline, self-confidence, independence, and interpersonal skills. Participants in organized sport and fitness activities may be instructed in physical and psychologic skills, appropriate strengthening and flexibility exercises, and training methods that can decrease their chances of suffering an injury.[5]

The introduction of an active life-style in youth, especially when coupled with instruction in lifelong activity skills and injury prevention methods, may influence a child's desire and ability to maintain a high level of activity for subsequent decades. Many reports have linked decreased mortality from numerous causes to participation in aerobic activities.[13,29,61,69] Recent reports indicate that the bone stock built up in youth is influenced by activity[54,60] and that greater bone mass and better balance prevent fractures later in life.[23] This chapter addresses the basic principles and methods that can be used in the prevention and treatment of injuries that result from sport and fitness activity in children.

DIFFERENCES BETWEEN MATURE AND IMMATURE MUSCULOSKELETAL SYSTEMS
Longitudinal Growth Plate Injury

Cartilaginous growth plates provide longitudinal and appositional growth to the skeleton. Longitudinal growth

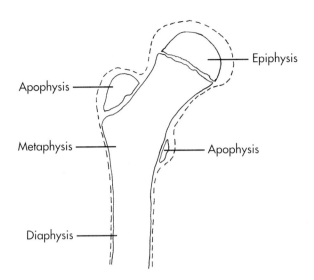

FIG. 54-1. Longitudinal, latitudinal, and appositional growth in proximal femur.

occurs between the epiphysis and the metaphysis of a long bone and at the joint surface. A long bone increases in breadth by appositional and latitudinal growth (Fig. 54-1). The loads on these growth regions are primarily compressive, although shear and torsional loads are also prominent. Growth plates have decreased strength during puberty.[16] Some physes that contribute to longitudinal growth, such as the distal femoral, distal tibial, and distal radial physes, seem particularly susceptible to failure from sport activity, especially during adolescence.

Injury to a physis may mimic the signs and symptoms that typically indicate a sprain or a strain in an adult. Therefore before performing range of motion and stress tests on an injured child's joint, the possibility of physeal injury should be ruled out. The initial physical examination should include careful palpation of the growth plates of the injured region, and radiographs should generally be obtained before manipulating or stressing the region. For any child with knee or anteromedial thigh pain, slipped capital femoral epiphysis or other hip injury should be considered in the differential diagnosis.

Apophyseal Injury

The apophyseal growth plates, which are present at sites of insertion of musculotendinous structures into the skeleton, are subjected to traction forces and may fail with sport activity. This is especially likely if the muscle-tendon unit that inserts on the apophysis is relatively inflexible compared with the length of the adjacent skeletal structure. It appears that these relative imbalances are most likely to occur during rapid growth spurts. A young athlete whose muscles are too tight relative to the adjacent long bones and joints sustains repeated microtraumatic tensile load injuries to the apophysis through which the muscle attaches to the long bone. If the individual ignores the resulting pain from the inflammation, a single rapid and forceful contraction of the inserting muscle-tendon unit may avulse the apophysis.[8,43]

Chronic, repetitive avulsion may lead to marked enlargement of the apophysis or spur formation, as can be seen in "break dancer's hip"[85] and chronic Osgood-Schlatter disease at the tibial tubercle.

Physis vs. Ligament Injury

The strength of the physis compared with the strength of the ligaments supporting a joint is important in the consideration of growth plate injuries. At certain ages the physis may be more likely to fail than the ligament. In general, the physis seems more likely to fail during times of rapid growth, such as the period of **peak height velocity** near puberty.[7] For girls the peak age for physeal injury is age 11 years, and for boys it is 12 to 14 years.[49] Whether the physis or the ligament fails may depend on the insertion sites of the ligamentous structures[12]: if the ligament inserts into the metaphyseal region, then a Salter II fracture (beginning with a metaphyseal fracture on the tension side of the bone) or a ligament sprain may occur. If the ligament inserts into the epiphyseal region, a fracture may be initiated through the physis on the tension side of the bone. However, in some circumstances, even in young children, the ligament may fail before the physis.[16,23,70,76]

Diaphysis and Metaphysis

Immature bone has greater porosity than adult bone.[37] In children and adolescents, porosity is greatest at the regions undergoing the most rapid remodeling, particularly at the metaphysis. Because of the increased porosity, metaphyseal buckle (torus) fractures may result from relatively minor trauma.[44] Torus fractures often leave one cortex completely intact and the opposite cortex minimally buckled or overlapped. There is some evidence that children who sustain metaphyseal distal radius fractures have decreased bone density compared with their peers, particularly if the fracture was caused by low-energy trauma.[41]

Plastic Deformation

The biomechanical properties of a child's bone allow plastic deformation of the bone so that a long bone may bend rather than break (Fig. 54-2). Deformed bone may return nearly to its original shape because of elastic recoil of the surrounding soft tissues.[57] If it does, the limb may have significantly injured structures but no obvious radiographic abnormality of the adjacent bone or it may be plastically deformed with no radiographically apparent, discrete fracture line. Correction of marked plastic deformity may require manipulation to complete the fracture and allow the injured bone to be reduced to a more anatomic position.

Periosteum

The bones of children have thicker, stronger, and more vascular periosteal envelopes. When a child's bone fractures, the thick periosteum may not tear completely (Fig. 54-3). A distal radius torus fracture is often initially thought by the injured child and parents to be a simple bruise or a sprain because the intact periosteum provides such stability with this fracture pattern. Intact perios-

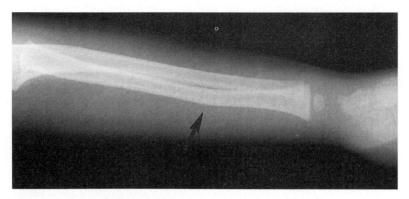

FIG. 54-2. Radius shows plastic deformation.

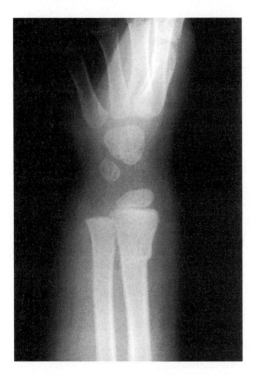

FIG. 54-3. Buckle or torus fracture of distal radius is one of the most frequently occurring fractures of children.

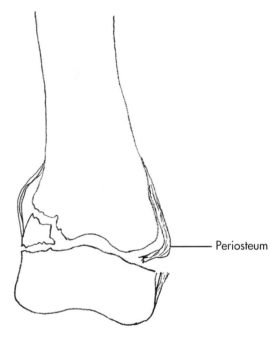

FIG. 54-4. Periosteal hinge may aid in fracture stabilization, but enfolded periosteal flap may block reduction.

teum limits the motion of the free bone fragments and can be used as a hinge in fracture immobilization and stabilization. However, a flap of periosteum may become entrapped in the fracture gap and prevent closed reduction (Fig. 54-4).

Because of the vascularity of a child's periosteum and the presence of growth-enhancing hormones and other circulating growth factors, new bone may be formed rapidly within an empty periosteal sleeve, so bone with an apparently anatomic form grows as the protruding fracture fragments remodel. The reformation of a normally shaped clavicle following what may have appeared to be a severe acromioclavicular separation (but is generally a fracture of the distal clavicle in a child) is an example of the remarkable regenerative power of periosteal bone formation.

Articular Cartilage

The articular cartilage of a skeletally immature individual is thicker than in an adult and contains growth cartilage. Regions that are injured relatively frequently from recurrent trauma to growing articular cartilage and the underlying supporting bone are the proximal humerus, the distal femur, and the radiocapitellar joint.

Osteochondritis Dissecans

Berndt and Harty[11] showed that a single injury to the articular cartilage may result in partial or complete separation of the articular fragment, from the remainder of the epiphysis, sometimes with an epiphyseal bone wafer. Consistent with this theory, patients with chondral or osteochondral injury of the talus most frequently have sustained one or more ankle sprains in the past. There-

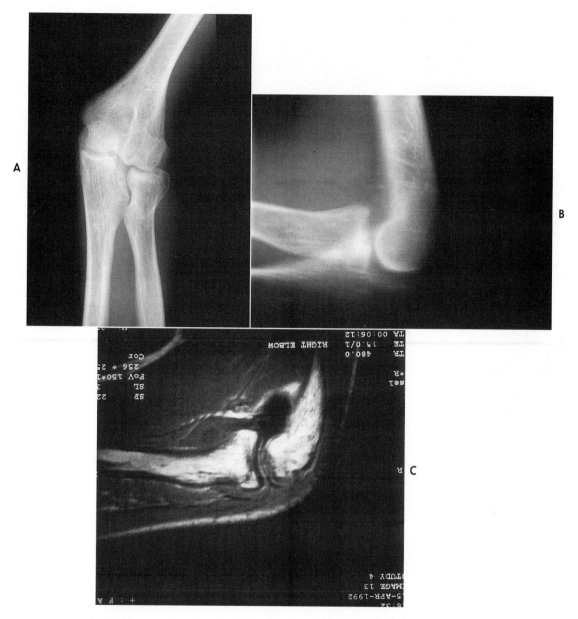

FIG. 54-5. A, Plain radiograph shows enlargement and irregularity of radial head in basketball player. **B,** Lateral tomogram confirms lack of congruence between radial head and capitellum and loss of normal contour of subchondral bone. **C,** Magnetic resonance imaging scan indicates injury to capitellum found at surgery to have severe fragmentation of articular cartilage and sclerotic subchondral bone.

fore the name more frequently given to this talar dome lesion now is osteochondral fracture of the talus.

Osteochondritis dissecans (OCD) of the distal femur of a skeletally immature individual probably does not occur from a single injury. Mubarak and Carroll[50,51] noted that no researcher has produced a typical OCD lesion in the distal femur from a single injury unless the articular cartilage was breached, and many OCD lesions of the knee are found to have intact overlying articular cartilage at the time of surgery. The authors proposed a strong likelihood of endogenous factors (such as generalized tissue laxity, family history, other epiphyseal abnormalities, or possible endocrine dysfunction) that predispose an individual to developing OCD. They found no

difference between the activity levels of OCD patients and control groups. Bearing this hypothesis in mind, OCD of the distal femur, often found bilaterally, may already be present because of the endogenous factors and the symptoms brought on by such activities as jumping.

Child and adolescent pitchers who exceed reasonable pitching limits but recall no single significant traumatic event may sustain permanent chondral and osteochondral injury, most frequently affecting the radiocapitellar joint (Fig. 54-5). The humeral head may be involved, although less frequently. Small articular fragments may become completely separated from the joint surface and grow in size (nourished by synovial fluid) until they are large enough to become symptomatic.

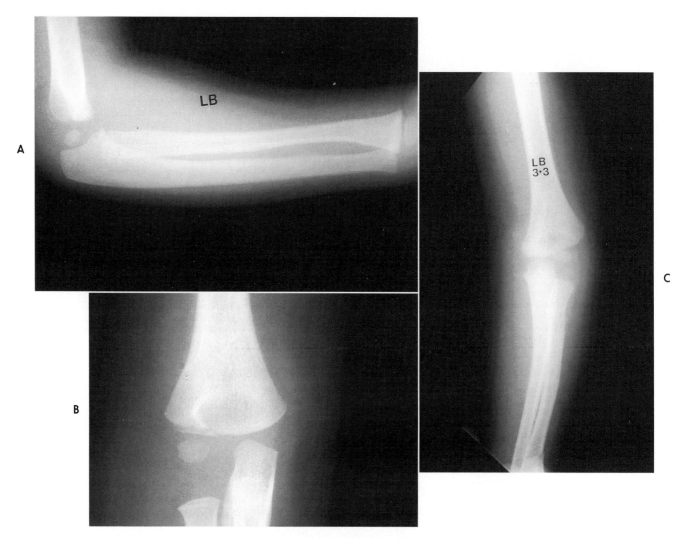

FIG. 54-6. A, Flake of bone from distal humeral metaphysis may be difficult to see on radiograph of this lateral condyle fracture. Three-year-old child fell on her outstretched hand. Distal radius fracture was treated initially, but lateral humeral condyle fracture was not noted. **B,** Close-up of anteroposterior view. **C,** Marked displacement of nonimmobilized humerus fracture occurred.

Fractures Through Nonossified Cartilage

As the cartilaginous model of a bone undergoes endochondral ossification, the skeletal contours become apparent radiographically. Before ossification occurs, some injuries must be suspected by the clinical setting and radiographic findings of soft-tissue swelling and abnormal alignment rather than relying on visible fracture lines. Injuries to a child's elbow require close attention to the physical examination and subtle radiographic findings because of the higher frequency of bone injury relative to ligamentous injury in the 5- to 13-year age group and the difficulty of visualizing fracture lines through the unossified regions of the elbow joint (Fig. 54-6). These principles are particularly important in diving accidents or other cervical spine injuries in which a child may have complete transection of the spinal cord despite normal radiographic appearance and alignment of the vertebrae.[14] Sleeve fractures of the patella, which generally occur on take-off for a jump, must also be suspected based on the clinical picture, since only a tiny fleck of displaced bone may be seen on radiographs despite displacement of most of the articular cartilage (Fig. 54-7).[86]

Menisci

The final major difference in biomechanical properties between the musculoskeletal structures of children and adults involves the vascularity of the menisci of the knee. Adult menisci generally have vessels in only the outer (peripheral) one third. In the menisci of young children the vascular channels frequently extend inward to or even beyond the halfway mark.[24] This property has implications for meniscal healing and may have implications for the types of injuries sustained at different ages, since children younger than 10 years rarely tear menisci that are otherwise normal (Fig. 54-8). Discoid menisci may rarely become symptomatic at young ages, however.

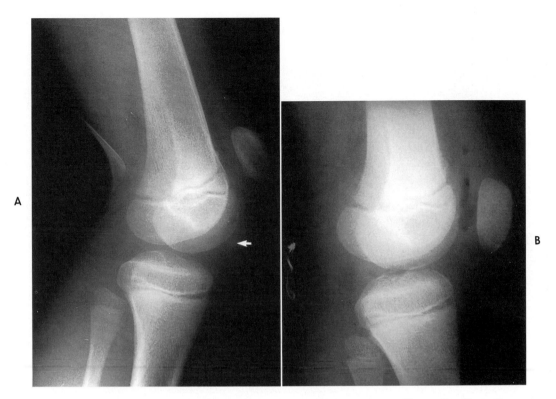

FIG. 54-7. A, Tiny flake of bone from inferior pole of patella is nearly invisible on plain films. Abnormally proximal position of patella and age of child suggested diagnosis of sleeve fracture of patella. **B,** Sleeve fracture of patella following open reduction.

The incidence of symptomatic meniscal lesions of all types was approximately 2/10,000 children under 19 years in one report.[1] Another study found that 7 of 15 children ages 7 to 12 years who had diagnostic arthroscopy for acute knee hemarthrosis had meniscal tears.[76]

ACUTE INJURIES
Age-Related Fracture Variation

There is an increased incidence of fractures at the periods of most rapid growth of a child or adolescent known as *peak height velocity*.[7] The typical patterns and locations for fractures vary somewhat by age, however. For instance, the metaphyseal torus fracture of the distal radius generally occurs among children ages 7 to 11 years, but the torus fracture of the distal tibia is sometimes called the *toddler's fracture* because of the typical age group. Distal femoral growth plate fractures are not very unusual among adolescents participating in sports activities; however, much more force than the typical sport injury (e.g., injury from a motor vehicle accident) is required to cause similar injuries among prepubertal children.

Fractures of the distal tibial growth plate vary in their anatomy according to how much of the physis has fused. With the understanding of this principle, ankle radiographs of pubescent children and adolescents should be examined carefully for the often subtle signs of a distal tibial triplane fracture or a Tillaux fracture. Intraarticu-

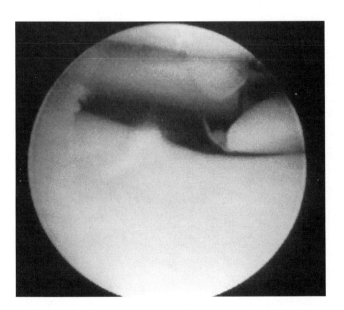

FIG. 54-8. Tear in central portion of lateral meniscus. One of three separate acute meniscal tears sustained by 10-year-old gymnast when she also ruptured anterior cruciate ligament.

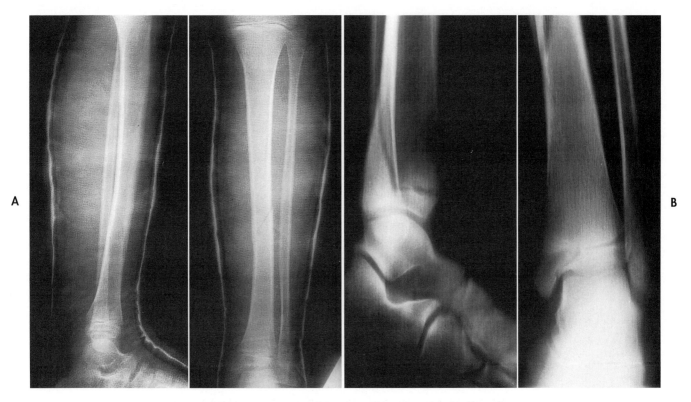

FIG. 54-9. Roller skater sustained long spiral fracture of tibia. Intraarticular physeal injury was suggested on plain films (**A**), but only fully appreciated with tomograms (**B**).

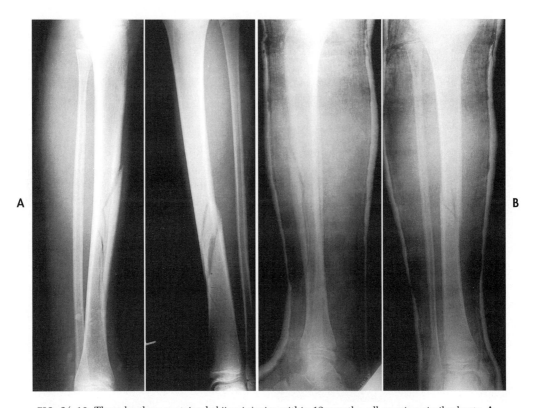

FIG. 54-10. Three brothers sustained skiing injuries within 12 months, all wearing similar boots. **A,** Fractured tibia and apparent plastic deformation of fibula of 7-year-old boy. **B,** Fracture of tibia and possible plastic deformation of fibula of 12-year-old boy. The 16-year-old sustained complete rupture of anterior cruciate ligament.

lar fractures may be difficult to visualize on the initial radiographs, but they often displace if they are not immobilized appropriately (Fig. 54-9).

Children are more likely to sustain fractures and less likely to sustain ligamentous sprains than adults. A study of recreational alpine skiers found that children under 10 years had nine times the incidence of lower leg fractures compared with skiers over 20 years, who were more likely to sustain knee sprains (Fig. 54-10).[28]

Classification of Physeal Fractures

Fractures through the growth plates at the ends of long bones are generally classified as described by Salter and Harris,[67] using a nomenclature that has prognostic value regarding potentially abnormal growth subsequent to the fracture (Fig. 54-11). Growth abnormalities caused by damage to physeal cells may lead to shortening or angular deformity of the injured limb. The Type 1 fracture involves only the physis. A Type 1 fracture may be innocuous, such as a nondisplaced fracture of the distal fibula in a 14-year-old boy. However, a completely displaced Type I fracture of a proximal femur of a 6-year-old child often leads to marked deformity as a result of arrest of growth, with or without avascular necrosis. The Type II fracture line courses through a portion of the physis and then exits the opposite side of the bone through the metaphysis. Even with accurate reduction of the fracture displacement, growth may slow or stop in the injured region of the physis (Fig. 54-12). The Type 3 fracture line

traverses the physis, crosses the epiphysis, and enters the joint (Fig. 54-13). If displacement persists, the articular surface is malaligned. With significant articular surface malalignment, premature development of osteoarthritis is likely. As in the Type III fracture, the Salter-Harris Type 4 fracture line crosses the articular surface. However, it also crosses the metaphysis so that persistent displacement of fracture fragments may cause the bone of the epiphysis on one side to unite with the bone of the metaphysis on the other side of the fracture line, leading to bony deformity that increases with growth. The articular surface concerns for the Type III fracture are also present for the Type IV fracture. In the Type V fracture, cells of the growth plate are crushed, even though no radiographic evidence of fracture may be present, since this fracture involves only the physis itself.

The existence of the Type V fracture has been called into question by Peterson and Burkhart,[62] who have neither seen a pure Type V fracture in their files nor found satisfactory documentation of one in the literature. Ogden[56] believes that an injury to the physis that is initially invisible on radiographs but causes growth arrest is actually an injury to the vascularity of the physis itself or of the perichondrial ring, rather than a compressive injury that mechanically injures the growth chondrocytes of the physis. He has described additional fracture types: Type VI involves only the zone of Ranvier; Type VII is completely intraepiphyseal; Type VIII is a metaphyseal

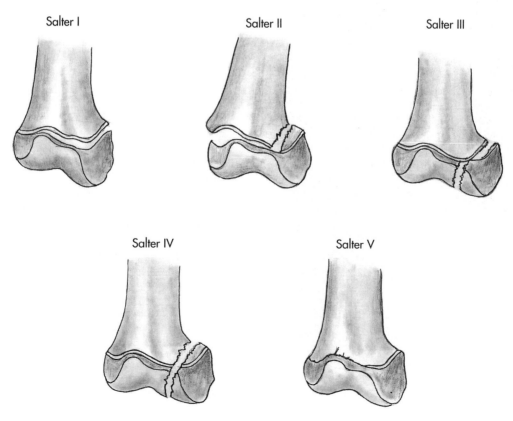

FIG. 54-11. Salter-Harris classification of physeal fractures.

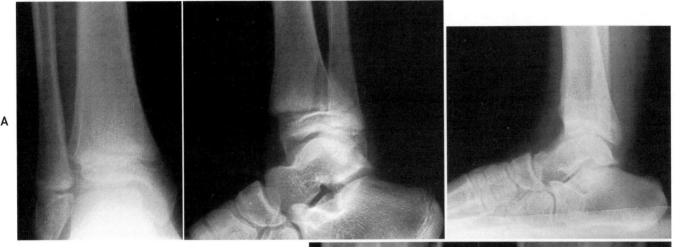

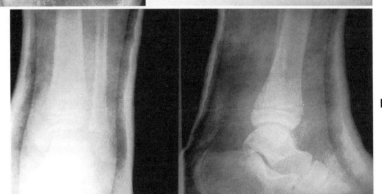

FIG. 54-12. A, Displaced Salter 2 fracture of distal tibia. **B,** Postreduction radiographs showed satisfactory position. **C,** Years later, patient complained of ankle pain during high school gymnastics. Observation of Harris lines in distal tibia shows that growth of anterior portion of physis continued following injury but at a slower rate than posterior portion, causing deformity that led to decreased plantarflexion at maturity.

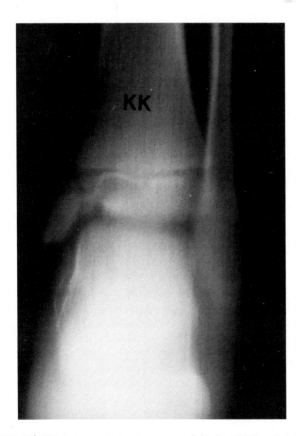

FIG. 54-13. Anteroposterior tomogram of displaced Salter 3 fracture of distal tibia.

fracture that significantly injures the peripheral vascular supply; and Type IX involves only the diaphyseal appositional new bone formation.

The resumption of normal growth can be monitored by observing the Harris lines in the metaphysis. Once any residual angulation has corrected, visible transverse lines in the metaphysis should remain parallel to the physis (Fig. 54-14).

Sprains

Children and adolescents may sustain most of the sprains seen among adult athletes. (Sprains involving the acromioclavicular or sternoclavicular joints are rare because the clavicle almost always fractures instead.) However, the same force that might cause a sprained ligament may cause a fracture in or near the joint. Both a sprain and a fracture may be present, as in the combination of a tibial eminence fracture and medial collateral ligament sprain (Fig. 54-15).[15,23] Accurate diagnosis is critical. Once a sprain has been diagnosed definitively, treatment usually follows the same recommendations given to adults. The time course to healing, however, is generally more rapid in growing individuals than in adults.

Meniscal Injury

Because of the increased vascularity of the child's meniscus, the prognosis for healing of a torn meniscus is

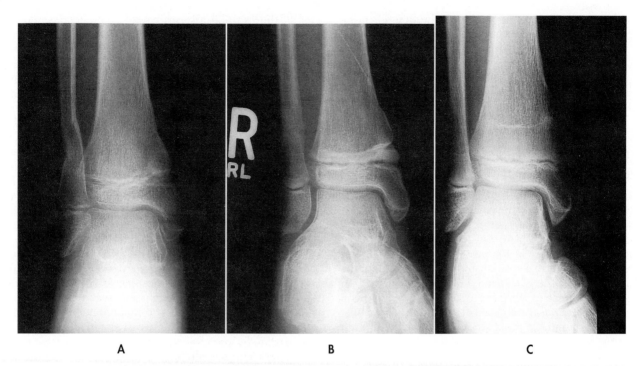

FIG. 54-14. A, Appearance of displaced Salter 2 fracture of distal tibia and metaphyseal fracture of fibula after closed reduction. Most medial portion of physis remains widened. **B,** Six months after injury Harris lines appear parallel to physis. **C,** Eighteen months after injury fibula has completely remodeled, and normal growth continues.

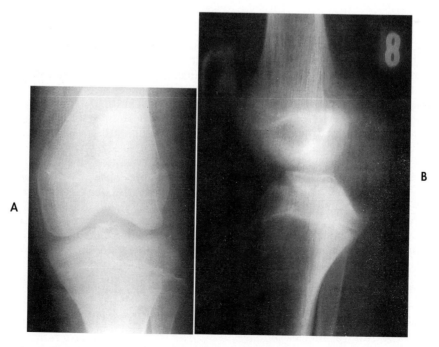

FIG. 54-15. A, Fourteen-year-old girl with tibial eminence fracture and partial avulsion of medial collateral ligament from femur. **B,** Lateral tomogram of tibial eminence fracture before open reduction and internal fixation.

probably better than for an adult and the time for healing is shorter. It is recommended for adults that unstable, avascular portions of a torn meniscus should generally be excised and any region that has reasonable potential for healing should be repaired or allowed to heal in situ if stable. Discoid menisci are resected back to a stable rim that resembles as closely as possible a normal meniscus.

OVERUSE INJURIES
Inflexibility and Injury

Fractures of the growth plate resulting from sudden, acute traumatic injuries represent an obvious difference in the injury patterns of mature and immature athletes. Injuries to the growth plate also occur from repetitive microtrauma, especially in the presence of a predisposing injury or an abnormal relationship between the lengths of a muscle and the adjacent long bone. The elongation of adjacent muscles appears to follow the long bone growth as the adjacent muscles respond to the stimulus of stretch. If a muscle is not stretched routinely through its entire range of motion (for example, the gastrocnemius muscles of a child with spastic diplegia), the muscle length becomes short relative to the adjacent bones and joints. The problem is particularly apparent in the muscles that cross two joints, for example, the gastrocnemius, hamstrings, and rectus femoris. Relatively tight muscles lead to bone injury by several mechanisms: (1) by traction from muscle contraction or excessive stretch, (2) by compression causing mechanical abnormality within the joint or on the opposite side of the joint, or (3) by rubbing or snapping over a bony prominence.

Injury-Prone Profile

It appears that individuals with marked laxity of the joint ligaments and capsular structures require particularly strong surrounding muscles to support the joint and satisfactory balance of both the strength and the flexibility of the adjacent muscles. Among male college freshman physical education students, Lysens and colleagues[45] found that the combination of traits most likely to be associated with overuse injuries included being tall, endomorphic habitus, little static strength but high explosive strength, and poor muscle flexibility with high ligamentous laxity. Overuse injury–prone females were also tall and had little static strength and upper body strength but high explosive strength and limb speed. The athletes also had poor muscle flexibility combined with high ligamentous laxity.[45] Graded relationships have been noted between gastrocnemius inflexibility and calcaneal apophysitis[48] and rectus femoris inflexibility, Osgood-Schlatter disease, and jumper's knee.[74]

Locations of Overuse Injury

Among Finnish children the knee, low back, and foot and ankle predominate as locations of overuse injuries.[39] In the study of Orava and Puranen[59] of athletes younger than 16 years the two most common overuse injuries were calcaneal apophysitis and Osgood-Schlatter disease, each occurring in 16% of the injured athletes. Half of all the exertion injuries were located at musculotendinous insertion sites. Other studies have found sport-specific patterns of overuse injury that include upper extremity injuries, including wrist pain in gymnasts,[46] pain in adolescent pitchers' shoulders,[80] and exertional compartment syndrome in the forearms of a female field hockey player and gymnast.[84] These findings are not surprising given the sport-specific adaptations found among adolescent athletes by Kibler and colleagues,[40] such as decreased flexibility in the lower body among athletes in sports that primarily exercise the lower body and extra external rotation but decreased internal rotation of the dominant shoulder compared with the nondominant shoulder among athletes in sports that primarily exercise the upper body.

Apophysitis

When a muscle is relatively tight, the traction force on its bony attachments becomes excessive. The skeletally immature athlete with a tight iliopsoas muscle, for instance, may develop pain and inflammation at its insertion into the lesser trochanter. This apophysitis, if ignored, predisposes the athlete to an avulsion fracture in the event of a sudden strong contraction of the muscle (Fig. 54-16, A). Other regions of frequently occurring apophysitis include the tibial tubercle (Osgood-Schlatter disease), the calcaneus, the ilium and ischium, and the medial epicondyle of the distal humerus (Fig. 54-16, B to D).

Pain on Opposite Side of Joint

Tight or inflexible muscles may also lead to pain syndromes on the opposite side of the joint, particularly if the muscles on the opposite side of the joint are relatively weak. Patellofemoral pain syndrome often is associated with tight hamstring and gastrocnemius muscles (e.g., inflexible muscles on the posterior aspect of the lower extremity associated with pain at the anterior aspect of the extremity).[17] Similarly, tight calf muscles may cause anterior ankle pain as the talus is forced against the anterior rim of the tibia near the end of the stance phase of gait or when dorsiflexing in landing after a jump.

Inflexible calf muscles may also cause excessive eversion of the hindfoot late in the stance phase of gait, producing excessive traction on the posterior tibial muscle and its insertion into the navicular. This is a frequent cause of a previously asymptomatic accessory navicular becoming painful in a growing child. (Therefore the first and usually the only treatment recommendation in this case is stretching exercises, not expensive orthotic devices that might be included in the initial treatment plan for an adult with this problem.) Another frequently noted association correlates inflexibility of the posterior shoulder muscles to the anterior pain of impingement syndrome.

Excessive Pressure

The third type of problem that can be directly caused by inflexible muscles is excessive pressure on a bony prominence. This may result in an inflammation of the muscle-tendon unit (as in iliotibial band tendinitis or

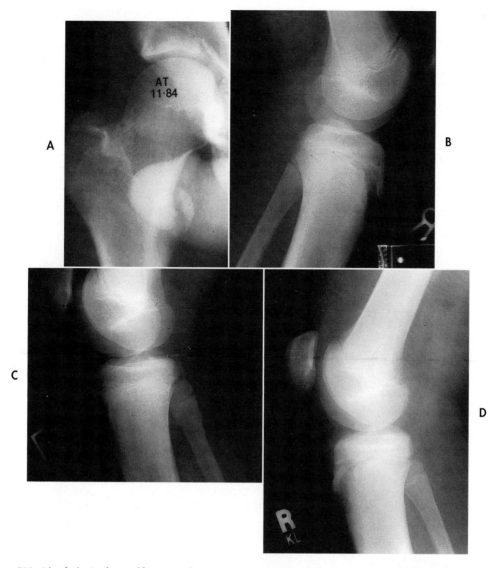

FIG. 54-16. A, Avulsion of lesser trochanter occurred less than 10 meters from finish of a 100-meter race. Athlete had noted some aching in his groin for previous 2 weeks. **B,** Basketball player had painful, swollen, tibial tubercle for 2 weeks. His proximal tibial physis is at risk for acute, complete fracture. **C,** Unaffected left knee. **D,** Right knee after 3 weeks of relative rest, using knee immobilizer. New bone has formed in gap between metaphysis and apophysis.

"friction syndrome" at the level of the lateral femoral condyle) or in inflammation of a bursa between the muscle-tendon unit and the bony prominence (as in greater trochanteric bursitis).

Inflexibility and Soft-Tissue Injury

Tight muscles predispose a growing individual to soft-tissue injuries of the muscle-tendon unit. Traction injury from a sudden, forceful muscle contraction generally occurs along the entire musculotendinous junction.[75] Injury in the substance of the tendon may occur in the presence of preexisting inflammation or previous injury. Muscle strains generally occur among older children and adolescents, although they may rarely occur among even

preschool children without apparent flexibility deficits (unpublished data).

Overuse Injuries of Skeletal Tissues

Overuse injuries of bone in the skeletally immature athlete may be caused by repetitive compressive forces. Gymnasts have been reported to develop stress reaction of the distal radial growth plate, which may cause permanent growth disturbance and deformity of the distal radius, apparently from repetitive weightbearing on their hands (Fig. 54-17).[20,21,46,81] A similar injury to both the distal radius and ulna was found in a break dancer.[32] When found in the early phase of epiphyseolysis, relative rest (allowing only those activities that do not cause

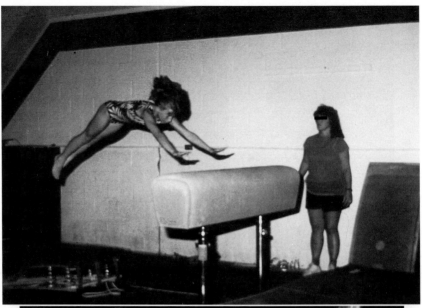

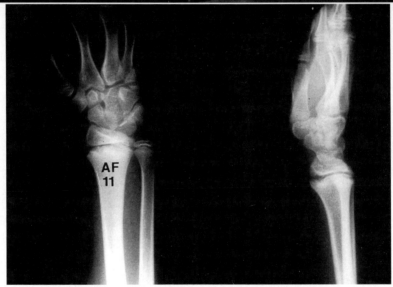

FIG. 54-17. Recurrent loading of dorsiflexed wrists in gymnasts has been associated with stress reaction and even growth arrest of distal radius. Radiograph shows widening and irregularity of physis.

pain or swelling at the site of injury) and the use of a brace that prevents full dorsiflexion generally leads to full recovery. If overgrowth of the ulna occurs because of growth arrest of the distal radius, lengthening of the radius or shortening of the ulna may be required to correct wrist deformity. Epiphyseolysis has been observed in the proximal humerus of adolescent pitchers.[9] Rest should lead to healing.

Osteochondritis dissecans (OCD) of the capitellum and radial head may be noted in the dominant upper extremity of throwing athletes, particularly those who play in multiple leagues or practice sidearm throwing excessively (Fig. 54-5). OCD of the knee may be related to repetitive microtrauma in some athletes, particularly those

involved in repetitive jumping activities such as gymnastics and basketball. OCD lesions may be treated with simple relative rest if symptoms resolve completely. However, if locking, recurrent effusion, or persistent pain is noted, surgical intervention (pinning or excision of fragments) is recommended.

Symptomatic spondylolysis has been found to occur more frequently in sports that require repetitive hyperextension of the lumbar spine, such as diving, swimming, gymnastics, football, and ice hockey (Fig. 54-18). For elite gymnasts there is evidence that practicing more than 15 hours/week is a predisposing factor for the development of spinal abnormalities.[35] Spondylolysis symptoms generally resolve with relative rest, but bracing may

---

Common combinations of adolescent injuries that may be preventable

Shin splints and posterior tibial tendinitis
- Foot: pronated
- Weak muscle: posterior tibial (may be secondary)
- Tight muscle: gastrocnemius
- Malalignment: genu valgum, none

Plantar fasciitis and Achilles tendinitis
- Foot: cavus
- Weak muscle: none
- Tight muscle: gastrocnemius and plantar fascia
- Malalignment: none

Recurrent ankle sprains
- Foot: cavus
- Weak muscle: peroneal
- Tight muscle: gastrocnemius
- Malalignment: none

Patellofemoral pain syndrome
- Foot: any, often pronated
- Weak muscle: vastus medialis
- Tight muscle: hamstrings, gastrocnemius, and quadriceps
- Malalignment: torsional or angular

Osgood-Schlatter disease
- Foot: any
- Weak muscle: quadriceps (secondary)
- Tight muscle: quadriceps
- Malalignment: none

Iliotibial band friction syndrome
- Foot: any
- Weak muscle: quadriceps (secondary)
- Tight muscle: tensor fasciae latae
- Malalignment: genu varum

Low back pain
- Foot: any
- Weak muscle: abdominals and spinal extensors
- Tight muscle: hamstrings and hip flexors
- Malalignment: femoral torsion, none

Female athlete's triad

- Disordered eating
- Amenorrhea
- Osteoporosis

---

be recommended if symptoms persist or if a radionuclide bone scan shows increased uptake at the pars interarticularis.

Unusual stress fractures have been reported in adolescent and preadolescent athletes, including a scaphoid waist fracture in a weightlifter,[64] a first rib fracture in a gymnast,[63] a second metacarpal fracture in a tennis player,[83] and a supracondylar femur fracture in a rugby player doing squat lifts.[87] Another supracondylar femur fracture was reported in a 9-year-old runner,[2] and a proximal tibial stress fracture was reported in a 15-year-old male distance runner.[18] Young athletes who have sustained unusual or multiple stress fractures should be questioned regarding their nutritional practices and (for females) their menstrual status (Figs. 54-18, *D*, and 54-19). Females, especially athletes in "appearance" sports such as gymnastics, figure skating, diving, and dance, are most likely to develop eating disorders at puberty or around the time of entrance into college. Athletes who have disordered eating patterns and who train excessively may develop serious menstrual irregularity. This combination can lead to the female athlete triad of dis-

ordered eating, amenorrhea, and osteoporosis, markedly increasing the athlete's susceptibility to fractures.[5] Kadel, Teitz, and Kronmal[38] found that young ballet dancers who danced more than 5 hours/day and who had been amenorrheic for longer than 6 months were more likely to sustain stress fractures than those who danced less and had more regular menstrual periods. A similar study of female ballet dancers of an average age of 18.7 years found an increased number of bone injuries among the dancers with abnormal menses.[10] Those with body mass index (BMI [body weight in kilograms divided by height in meters^2]) less than 19 had more days of chronic low-grade injury than those with a greater BMI. Male athletes who participate in sports where the competitive class is determined by weight, such as wrestling, are also at risk for developing disordered eating patterns and the subsequent associated nutritional risks.[58]

Strength Training for Prevention of Overuse Injury

Strong muscles in a limb provide protection from stress fractures to the adjacent bones by reducing joint reaction forces and by sharing load with the adjacent bones. Therefore strength training should be considered an important part of any training program in adolescence. Extremely few stress fractures are reported among normal preadolescents, so the necessity of strength training by prepubescents for fracture prevention is probably low. However, stress fractures may occur among children when marked changes occur in training patterns; thus strength training may help prevent overuse injuries of bone as well as injuries of soft tissue. (Fig. 54-20).

SPECIAL DIAGNOSTIC CONSIDERATIONS

Additional diagnoses must be considered when evaluating an immature athlete with an injury compared with a skeletally mature athlete. For example, a positive stress test of the knee may be the result of a fracture rather than a ligament injury. Knee pain may not reflect any local injury at all but an injury of the hip such as an anterior dislocation or a slipped capital femoral epiphysis (Fig. 54-21). The on-field examination must be modified, taking these alternative diagnoses into account.

For the immature athlete, strong consideration should be given to obtaining plain radiographs before performing stress maneuvers to avoid possible displacement of a nondisplaced fracture. In an athlete with an obvious knee injury, excessive motion when a valgus stress is applied could be caused by a medial collateral ligament sprain or by displacement of a distal femoral physeal fracture. Similarly, excessive motion with Lachman testing

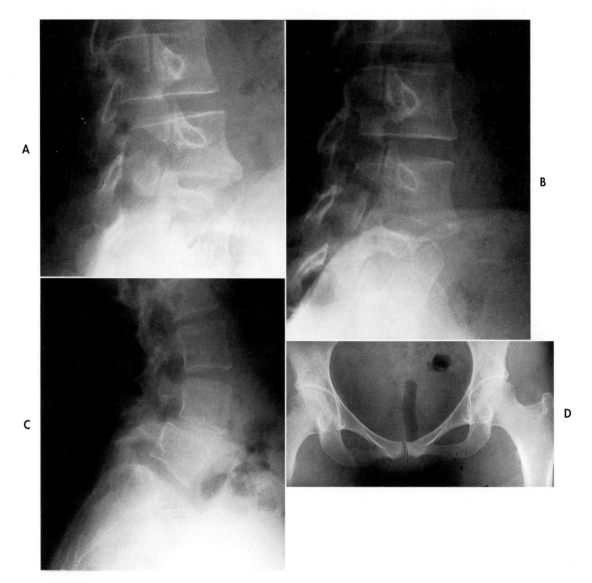

FIG. 54-18. A, This female swimmer had back pain, normal plain radiographs, and radionuclide bone scan that showed unilateral increased uptake at L4 pars interarticularis. Six months later unilateral defect was visible radiographically. Twelve months after onset of pain, she had bilateral L4 defects. Another year later, during which she had only negligible symptoms, she also had unilateral defect of L3 **(B)** and mild spondylolisthesis at level L4-L5 **(C). D,** Three years after initial presentation, her back was asymptomatic but she had activity-related pain deep in right buttock. Stress fracture of inferior pubic ramus presumably occurred because she now had no visible flexion of lumbar spine, yet performed better than average on a sit-and-reach test. To do sport activities that required good mobility of this region, she apparently overstressed origin of hamstrings from ischium. Menses were normal, but she later admitted to being bulimic. Stress fracture healed with relative rest.

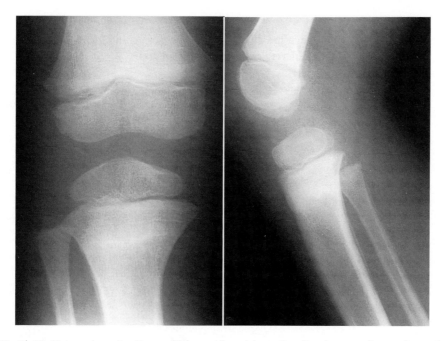

FIG. 54-19. Extremely active 5-year-old boy with malabsorption disorder was of normal size, but developed an activity-related limp. Radiographs showed stress fractures of proximal tibia and fibula.

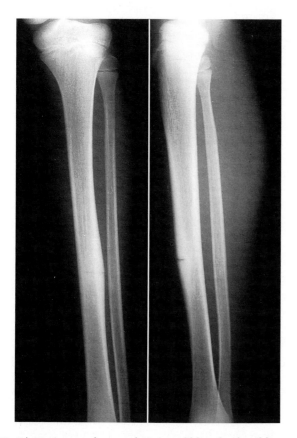

FIG. 54-20. Apparently normal 10-year-old boy developed limp on fifth day of basketball camp, playing 5 hours a day. He denied any pain. By its radiographic appearance, stress fracture of tibia had been present for at least several weeks. Treated with patellar-tendon bearing cast, it healed uneventfully. Boy was allowed to walk, bearing full weight in cast.

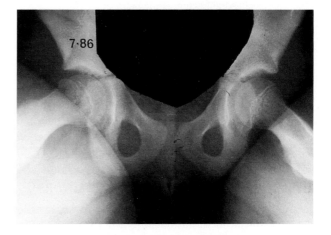

FIG. 54-21. Mild slipped capital femoral epiphysis may appear normal on anteroposterior radiograph, and findings can be subtle even on frog lateral. Right femoral head is no longer aligned with femoral metaphysis, and growth plate looks irregular and widened.

Frequently diagnosed conditions to consider in the differential diagnosis of a child or adolescent (in addition to usual differential diagnoses for adults)

Acute injury
- All joints
  Physeal injury
  Sprain (ligament or capsule)
  Strain (muscle)
  Congenital anomaly
  Neoplasm
  Infection
- Cervical spine
  Subluxation or dislocation
  Spinal cord injury despite normal vertebral alignment
- Chest
  Sternoclavicular dislocation is generally a medial clavicle physeal injury until late adolescence or adulthood
- Shoulder
  Acromioclavicular separation is usually a distal clavicle physeal injury in children and young adolescents
  In proximal humerus fractures, look for such injury as bone cyst
- Elbow
  Serious distal humerus fractures may not be visible on routine x-ray films
  Avulsion of medial epicondyle
  Consider elbow injury if only fracture of the radius or ulna can be seen, rather than both
- Wrist
  Large majority are distal radius and ulna fractures
  Sprain rare in childhood and early adolescence
  Rule out carpal fracture or dislocation
- Finger
  Flexor or extensor tendon may avulse with a fleck of bone or only a cartilaginous fragment
- Hip
  Slipped capital femoral epiphysis
  Dislocation with or without fracture
  Avulsion of anterior superior iliac spine, anterior inferior iliac spine, ischial tuberosity, or lesser trochanter
- Knee
  Tibial eminence fracture
  Distal femoral or proximal tibial physeal fracture
  Tibial tubercle avulsion
  Sleeve fracture of the patella
  Slipped capital femoral epiphysis
- Ankle
  Triplane fracture or Tillaux fracture
  Osteochondral fracture of the talus
  Disruption of fibrocartilaginous junction of secondary ossification center to epiphysis (at medial or lateral malleolus or posterior process of talus)
  Tarsal coalition
- Foot
  Disruption of fibrocartilaginous junction of secondary ossification center to epiphysis at base of fifth metatarsal
  Tarsal coalition

Overuse injury
- All joints
  Inflammatory process
  Metabolic disease
  Neoplasm
  Infection
- Shoulder
  Epiphyseolysis (stress fracture) of proximal humeral physis
- Elbow
  Medial or lateral epicondylitis
  Osteochondritis dissecans of capitellum or radial head
- Wrist
  Stress fracture of distal radius or ulna physis
- Lumbar spine region
  Spondylolysis
  Spondylolisthesis
  Posterior iliac crest apophysitis
- Hip
  Apophysitis of anterior superior iliac spine, anterior inferior iliac spine, iliac crest, ischial tuberosity, lesser trochanter, greater trochanter
  Snapping hip syndrome (usually iliopsoas or iliotibial band)
  Osteoid osteoma of proximal femur
- Knee
  Osgood-Schlatter disease
  Patellofemoral pain syndrome
  Prepatellar bursitis
- Tibia
  Osteoid osteoma
- Ankle
  Achilles tendinitis
  Tarsal coalition
  Osteochondritis dissecans of talus
  Painful os trigonum (older adolescents)
- Foot
  Calcaneal apophysitis (Sever's disease)
  Plantar fasciitis

could result from either a torn anterior cruciate ligament or from the avulsion of the ligament and its osteochondral insertion from the remainder of the tibia.

DIFFERENCES IN OTHER ETIOLOGIC FACTORS

Among older participants in sport and fitness activities factors involved in the development of overuse injuries include training errors, changes in training techniques, and problems with equipment and playing surface. All of these may contribute to the development of an overuse injury in a child or adolescent as well.

Training Error

Young participants may be even more likely than adults to make errors in training because they often have less patience in following a plan of gradually increasing distance, speed, intensity, and complexity of activity. Training errors are especially likely as an injured young athlete returns to activity. Most teenagers want to resume a full, normal training regimen with their peers as soon as they are allowed back into practices with the group. Prevention of recurrent injury then requires careful counseling and monitoring of the athlete who is returning to sports participation.

Equipment

Because of the expense of playing equipment and appropriate footgear, many young athletes wear "hand-me-downs" that fit poorly or that are worn to the point that protection is inadequate. Footgear is often suboptimal—fashionable, poorly cushioned, nonsupportive sneakers may be worn for all activities, including distance running. Few families can afford to buy court shoes, running shoes, and aerobic dance shoes each year for their children's rapidly growing feet. Many young athletes therefore participate in sports for many hours each week with insufficient cushioning or stability. If the previous owner of the gear wore it unevenly, problems may be compounded. More expensive equipment items such as helmets, skates, and ski boots are likely to have had previous owners. They may not fit properly and may lead to acute or overuse injury.

Congenital Abnormality

Underlying congenital abnormalities should be considered when evaluating the young individual for either a preparticipation physical examination or for an injury. The physician who treats a child or adolescent for a sports injury may be the first to diagnose a congenital or developmental abnormality such as mild spastic hemiplegia, tarsal coalition, vertebral anomaly, or discoid meniscus.

ADDITIONAL FACTORS INDIRECTLY RELATED TO THE MUSCULOSKELETAL SYSTEM
Coordination Changes

Growing individuals are subject to temporary changes in coordination during growth spurts and weight gains. These changes, combined with the frequent changes in relative muscle flexibility, increase the chance of sport injury during the periods of rapid growth. Problems with coordination are particularly noted by individuals involved in activities that require extreme body awareness, such as ballet, gymnastics, figure skating, diving, and ski jumping.

Matching

Unlike adults, who tend to be matched relatively well by ability and by size in organized sports, the matching for children and adolescents is inadequate. In most organized sports activities the children are matched simply by age. Matching by height, weight, or Tanner sexual maturity stage is more appropriate for most contact and collision sports (Fig. 54-22). However, given the differences in rates of growth, maturation, and emotional development,[72] the best methods for matching have not been defined and their usefulness has not been proven.

Motivation

Immature athletes may have motivational differences compared with older athletes. A young athlete may be pushed by a parent or coach, or he or she may be self-motivated to the point that the athlete is afraid to let someone know when he or she has pain. This situation

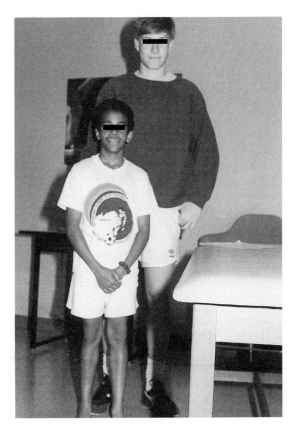

FIG. 54-22. Two 14-year-old boys who played on same soccer team.

may lead to either increased incidence of injury or increased severity of an injury. Athletes should be encouraged to report the presence of pain or significant discomfort. Coaches and parents should be alert for a decrement in performance or favoring of an extremity, both of which may be signs of injury.

Other psychologic considerations are important in relation to child and adolescent athletes. Young people who perceive that the only way to be valued by or to retain attention from their coaches and parents is through athletic success may develop psychologic problems such as depression or disordered eating. Depression or disordered eating may in turn cause increased injury as a result of physical or mental fatigue, weakness, or osteoporosis.[95] Adolescent girls who exercise excessively and feel extreme pressure to excel may develop the female athlete triad of disordered eating, amenorrhea, and osteoporosis. These individuals may first consult a physician for a stress fracture, and issues other than just training error and anatomic malalignment must be explored.

An athlete may perceive (sometimes correctly) that his or her worth to a parent is more as a successful athlete than as a unique individual. These young people may be afraid to admit an injury until it is so severe that either major treatment or prolonged treatment is required. Some young athletes use an injury as a reason to discontinue an activity. If pain and apparently slow healing (gauged by continued subjective complaints by the injured athlete) seem out of proportion to the injury, the athlete's health care professionals should be sensitive to possible underlying psychologic causes or emotional needs and should refer the patient for counseling, if appropriate.

Coaches

Younger athletes are more likely than adults to have less qualified coaches. The coaches in many organized sports are either volunteer coaches or school coaches who have little education in the principles of good coaching techniques. The coaches may lack knowledge in appropriate training methods, equipment maintenance and safety rules, and child and adolescent psychology. Astonishingly, many such coaches still promote training practices that have been deemed unsafe for a decade. Sports medicine professionals can provide much needed service to their communities by helping to establish coaching education guidelines and actively participating in coaching education programs.

"PREHABILITATION" TIPS

Given the relationships already noted between flexibility deficits and certain injuries, it is logical to consider resolving deficits *before* beginning a sport or fitness activity. This has become known as "prehabilitation." Adolescents without obvious strength or flexibility deficits may also benefit from preseason conditioning, as indicated by a 63% reduction in knee injuries of high school football players who participated in a total body conditioning program.[19] Marked reductions in overuse injuries of the upper and lower extremities were found in a longitudinal study of elite figure skaters after preseason evaluation, and required strengthening and flexibility exercises were added to the training program.[73]

Flexibility Deficits

Growing children and adolescents can be checked for flexibility problems quickly, easily, and reliably. A complete or directed flexibility examination should be included in preparticipation examinations, in examinations for injury, and before allowing return to unrestricted activity. Tests such as the sit-and-reach field test allow rapid assessment of several areas of flexibility, but they are not specific enough to determine the site of the flexibility deficit that needs to be addressed. The flexibility tests shown on pp. 1221 and 1222 are highly reproducible and have small interobserver and intraobserver error (unpublished data). In general, the muscle groups that are most likely to lack normal flexibility are those that cross two joints, and these are most useful to test for prehabilitation purposes. When measures of flexibility are to be followed longitudinally, the athlete should be instructed not to perform any stretching exercises within a few hours of the test.

Strength Deficits

Identification of strength deficits of major muscle groups is another important component of prehabilitation. The musculoskeletal injuries of children and ado-

lescents are often treated only to the point of healing with the idea that "children are so active that they complete their own rehabilitation naturally." A significant number of the children who "rehabilitate naturally" without any instruction or supervision return to the doctor with a recurrent ankle sprain from weak peroneal muscles or patellofemoral pain related to residual quadriceps atrophy. Any strength deficits identified during the preparticipation physical examination should certainly be corrected before unlimited sport activity is allowed.

Strength Training

Some children, and many adolescents, may wish to include resistance training in their routines to improve performance. Few give injury reduction as a reason for pursuing strength training, but some evidence for a role in injury reduction exists.[19] Both the American Academy of Pediatrics and the National Strength and Conditioning Association support the participation of children and adolescents in carefully supervised, appropriate, strength training activities.[4,53] Several authors have shown that strength gains can be made, even by prepubescent athletes, although no major changes are found in muscle bulk.[71] The equipment should be adjusted to fit the youth, maximal lifts should not be attempted, the amount of resistance should be low enough that 6 to 15 repetitions of the exercise can be completed in good form, and muscle flexibility exercises should be incorporated into the program.[5,53,71]

REHABILITATION TIPS
Why Not Rehabilitate?

Young athletes often fail to completely rehabilitate an injury for many reasons. One frequently noted reason is the failure of physicians to prescribe a rehabilitation program, believing that children either rehabilitate sufficiently through their usual daily activities or that they do not comply with a prescribed program. As a result, asymptomatic children who were immobilized over 2 years earlier for a fracture may have residual atrophy noted when examined for another reason (unpublished data). Other young athletes may train and compete with injuries[68] because they are afraid to lose training time and competitive experience or ranking. Taylor and colleagues[77] have shown that strained muscles generate less contractile force than uninjured muscles. Training with an unhealed or unrehabilitated injury therefore probably predisposes the athlete to further injury because of lack of strength and neuromuscular coordination.

Improving Compliance

It is difficult enough for adults to adhere to a prescribed exercise program for training or rehabilitation. For children and adolescents the difficulties may be increased because of shorter attention spans and greater perceived demands on their time. Therefore when a young athlete is prescribed a rehabilitation program, it is important to follow several additional principles that may be dealt with more superficially when working with

Text continued on p. 1225.

Flexibility deficit test

Scientific evidence for relationship

- Quadriceps inflexibility and anterior knee pain
- Hamstrings inflexibility and patellofemoral pain
- Triceps surae inflexibility and calcaneal apophysitis

Specific flexibility deficits related to frequently occurring injuries

- Muscles that cross two joints are more likely to cause injury from muscle and long bone disproportion
- Triceps surae
  - Plantar fasciitis
  - Calcaneal apophysitis
  - Achilles tendinitis
- Hamstrings
  - Patellofemoral pain
  - Low back pain and abnormal posture (increased sway-back and roundback)
  - Muscle strain
  - Avulsion fracture from origin or insertion
- Quadriceps
  - Osgood-Schlatter disease and other traction disorders of knee extensor mechanism
  - Patellofemoral pain
  - Anterior inferior iliac spine avulsion
- Rectus femoris inflexibility
  - Avulsion fracture of anterior inferior iliac spine
  - Muscle strain
- Sartorius inflexibility
  - Avulsion fracture of anterior superior iliac spine
- Adductors
  - Muscle strain

- Iliopsoas
  - Avulsion fracture of lesser trochanter
  - Poor posture (increased lumbar lordosis) and back pain
- Lumbodorsal muscular and fascial structures
  - Lumbar strain
  - Thoracic kyphosis
- Lateral rotators of the shoulder and posterior capsule (patient lacks internal rotation or horizontal flexion)
  - Shoulder subluxation may contribute to osteochondritis dissecans of the humeral head
  - Shoulder impingement or overlap syndrome
- Biceps and triceps
  - May contribute to osteochondritis dissecans of the capitellum
- Wrist flexors and pronator
  - May contribute to medial epicondylitis

Reproducible flexibility tests

- Hip flexors
  - Thomas test. Adolescents should have no contracture
- Iliotibial band (tensor fasciae latae)
  - Ober or modified Ober test (Fig. 54-23). Abduct hip, extend hip, and flex ipsilateral knee, then observe how close to midline the knee returns as the hip adducts (by gravity in the Ober test and by gently swinging the knee toward midline in the modified test).
  - The extended hip should adduct to neutral (knee at midline).
- Rectus femoris (quadriceps) (Fig. 54-24).
  - Patient lies prone with anterior superior iliac spine on firm surface and knees together. Examiner records angle

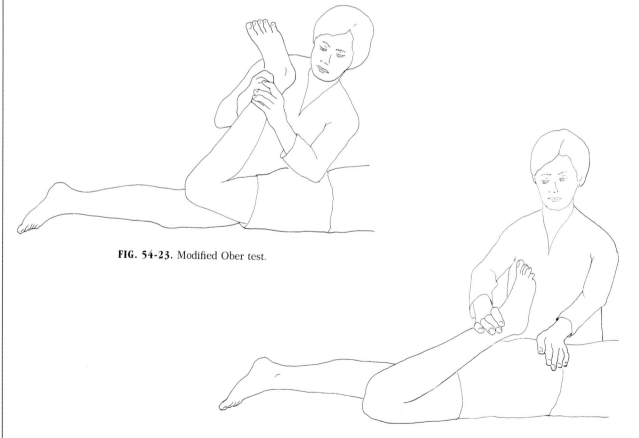

FIG. 54-23. Modified Ober test.

FIG. 54-24. Rectus femoris flexibility test.

Continued.

Flexibility deficit test—cont'd

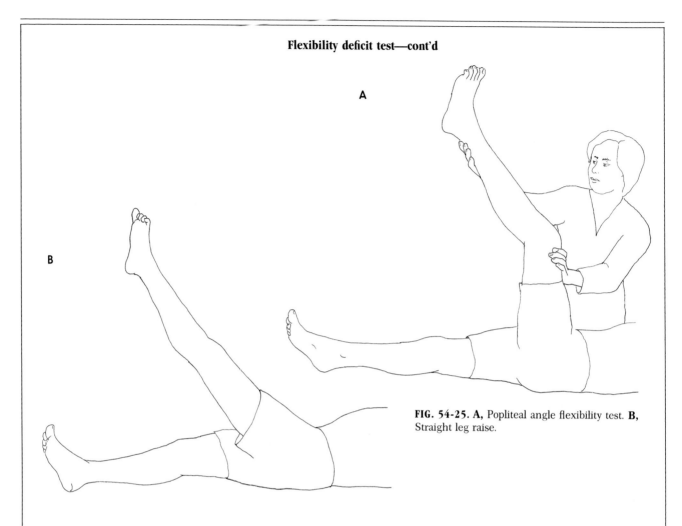

FIG. 54-25. **A,** Popliteal angle flexibility test. **B,** Straight leg raise.

gle of maximal knee flexion. (Maximal knee flexion with hip extended − Maximal knee flexion with hip flexed = Amount of contracture of rectus femoris. Adolescents should be able to touch heel to buttock unless they are unusually mature males.

■ Hamstrings
Straight leg raise is less reliable than popliteal angle.
For popliteal angle, examiner passively flexes the patient's hip and ipsilateral knee each 90 degrees, then (maintaining the hip flexion at 90 degrees) extends the knee until tension is noted in the hamstrings; the angle between the tibia and true vertical is recorded (Fig. 54-25, *A*).
Adolescents should be able to straight leg raise to 85 degrees and have popliteal angle of 10 degrees or less (Fig. 54-25, *B*)

■ Gastrocnemius
Align the heel with the tibia by supinating the foot. Fully extend the knee.
Passively dorsiflex the ankle as far as possible with the examiner's body weight leaning against the patient's foot; do not allow the patient to "help" by contracting the ankle dorsiflexors (this often pulls the hindfoot out of alignment with the tibia and gives inflated measurements) (Fig. 54-26). Adolescents should have 10 degrees or more of ankle dorsiflexion with the knee extended.

■ Shoulder medial rotators
Here, comparison with the opposite side is important.
With the scapula firmly on the examination table and the shoulder abducted 90 degrees, flex elbow 90 degrees to be able to use forearm as a goniometer arm. For most average adolescents, medial and lateral rotation are about 90 degrees each; dominant arm of throwers and tennis players and both shoulders of swimmers often have excessive lateral rotation and diminished medial rotation.

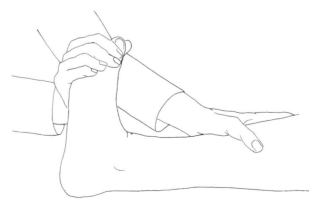

FIG. 54-26. Gastrocnemius flexibility test.

Simple stretches that work

- Triceps surae (Fig. 54-27)

  Wall stretch: both feet should be perpendicular to the wall

  To stretch the right gastrocnemius, put the right foot back and hold the right knee straight. Lean forward as if doing a push-up against the wall.

  To stretch the right soleus, do not change the position of the feet, but simply sit back a bit, flexing the right knee slightly; the athlete should feel a deeper muscle stretch than gastrocnemius stretch.

- Hamstrings (Fig. 54-28)

  Sit on a firm surface with the chest on the thighs, knees bent, and hands gently grasping lateral borders of the feet.

  "Walk" the heels away from the buttocks until a slight stretch is felt.

  Hold this position for 30 seconds, then lift the chest up to release the stretch, walk heels further away, lean chest down onto thighs again, keeping shoulders and upper back relaxed.

  Repeat several times. This can also be done standing up if no place is available to sit, but it is impossible to relax into the stretch as well when standing. For additional exercise, see *Adductors* below.

- Quadriceps (Fig. 54-29)

  Lie prone with anterior superior iliac spine firmly on table or floor and knees together.

  Bend one knee and grasp that foot or ankle with the opposite hand. Bring the foot toward the buttock, and try to touch the buttock with foot.

  To increase the stretch, extend the hip further.

  If this exercise is done while standing, make certain that hip remains extended and adducted to neutral position.

- Adductors

  Straddle stretch. Easy way for teenagers to do this (while talking on the telephone, reading, etc.) is to lie supine, perpendicular to a wall, with the feet on the wall and buttocks as close to the wall as possible. Allow feet to slide outward on the wall (abducting hips). As flexibility increases, move buttocks closer to the wall and let the feet slide farther apart.

  This exercise may also be done seated on the floor. Add to stretch by leaning trunk towards one leg or straight between the legs.

  These exercises stretch the adductors and hamstrings.

  The specific muscle stretched is dependent on relative positions of the trunk and hips.

- Iliopsoas or rectus femoris (hip flexors)

  Perform Thomas test. Increase stretch by letting the limb that is to be stretched hang off the edge of the table.

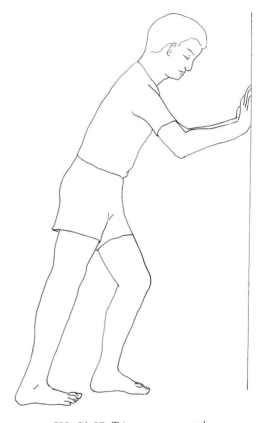

FIG. 54-27. Triceps surae stretches.

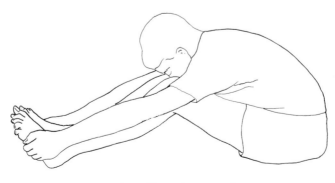

FIG. 54-28. Hamstrings stretches.

Continued.

Simple stretches that work—cont'd

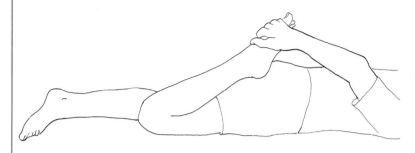

FIG. 54-29. Quadricep stretches.

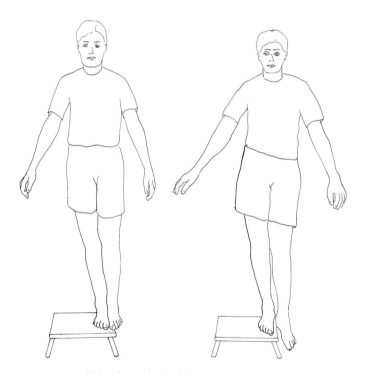

FIG. 54-30. Iliotibial band stretches.

- Iliotibial band (Fig. 54-30)
    The hip is in the neutral position, feet are pointing forward with no trunk rotation. Adduct the hip that is to be stretched.
    To stretch the right iliotibial band, cross the left foot in front of the right foot and push the right greater trochanter into the iliotibial band.
    An alternative is to stand on a platform on the right foot, let the left hip drop a few inches lower than the right hip, not twisting or rotating at all.

- Lumbodorsal muscular and fascial structures
    Seated hamstring stretch as on p. 1223.
    Curl up, as in partial sit-up.
- Posterior shoulder muscles and capsule
    Lie supine with the shoulder abducted approximately 90 degrees and the elbow flexed 90 degrees. The upper arm is supported on the table, and weight is in the hand or on the wrist. Allow passive medial rotation of the shoulder.
    Standing or sitting, lift the arm to a position parallel to the floor and reach across the body. The opposite hand pushes against the elbow to bring the upper arm close to the chest.

adults. The first goal is to convince the athlete that the rehabilitation program is important. Most adolescents feel invulnerable. They rarely believe that they can be injured again, even if they are incompletely rehabilitated. Adolescents do not wish to be perceived as being different from their friends, and they are less likely than adults to understand why a rehabilitation program is necessary. Therefore it is important to spend time explaining the relationship of the rehabilitation program to the resolution of the injury, to the return of normal performance, and to the athlete's ability to participate in the sport both safely and successfully.

Keep it Short

The rehabilitation program should be as short as possible to improve the chances for compliance. Keeping the length of the rehabilitation exercise period to 15 minutes, 6 days a week is a reasonable goal. The most critical exercises should be emphasized because the individual otherwise tends to do the simplest exercises, which are generally the least useful for the rehabilitation process. The exercise program should incorporate the use of equipment that is fun, enticing, and readily available. Finally, the athlete should receive advice on integrating the rehabilitation program into his or her daily schedule. Ideas such as doing the program during the first television show watched or the first telephone call are generally received positively. A program of small rewards, such as a special treat each seventh day, can also help the young athlete remain compliant.

Keep it Simple

Unless instructed otherwise, children and adolescents perform required exercises in the easiest and least uncomfortable manner possible. Therefore when instructing them in strengthening exercises, specific instructions concerning the speed of motion, the muscles for concentrated focus, and the expected amount of discomfort or difficulty should be provided. Similarly specific instructions are necessary for stretching exercises. Many adolescent athletes who stretch every day that their team practices have no idea (either by name or by the general location of the body) which muscles they are supposed to be stretching with *any* of the exercises they do. My impression, based on questioning of office patients, is that most participants in school sports do not even understand whether a particular exercise is designed to stretch muscles or strengthen them. Misconceptions and lack of understanding frequently extend even to young people who have been rehabilitating under the supervision of a physical therapist or a certified athletic trainer, underscoring the need for frequent explanation and questioning of their understanding of therapeutic exercise programs.

Four Rules of Participating while Injured

The principles of relative rest and protected mobilization apply well to injuries of children and adolescents. With most injuries the individual remains able to participate at some level of either usual, limited, or rehabilita-

---

> **Four rules of participation while injured**
>
> - Pain absent or minimal
> - No limping or favoring
> - No pain the next morning
> - No ice or pain medication *before* sport activity

---

tive fitness activity. Treatment of injuries such as Osgood-Schlatter disease may not require any absolute prohibition against sport participation. Instead, the athlete may participate within the limits set by four rules. The child or adolescent may participate as long as (1) pain is either absent or slight so that the prescribed therapeutic exercise program can be completed effectively and correctly, and the expected rate of progress is seen; (2) the athlete is not limping or favoring the injured limb; (3) there is no pain the following morning; and (4) neither local ice application nor recent NSAID administration that could mask pain are allowed *before* sport activity, since masking of symptoms may exacerbate the index injury or cause a new injury because of the lack of the normal protective mechanisms in the injured limb. (Ice or NSAIDs may be used before performing the controlled, therapeutic exercises.) Recovering injured sport participants must learn to listen to their bodies' signals to avoid further tissue damage to injured and uninjured parts.

SUMMARY

Through appropriately directed preparticipation examinations, coaching education, careful selection and preparation of equipment and playing surfaces, and any indicated prehabilitation, sports injuries of children and adolescents can probably be reduced by up to 50%.[4] Throughout prehabilitation, injury treatment, and rehabilitation, attention to muscle flexibility and strength is especially important for the child and adolescent population. During injury evaluation, age-appropriate diagnoses must first be considered from data provided by inspection and palpation alone, bearing in mind the possibility of displacing or further displacing a fracture or a slipped capital femoral epiphysis with manipulative examination. Even after reviewing the radiographs the entire clinical picture provided by the history, physical examination, and other studies must be integrated to ensure the correct diagnosis and to lead to appropriate treatment. The injured individual can then be cared for in a holistic manner including discussions with parents, coaches, therapists, and certified athletic trainers as indicated to ensure the best physical and psychologic preparedness for returning to full activity as soon as is safely possible.

REFERENCES

1. Abdon P, Mats B: Incidence of meniscal lesions in children: increase associated with diagnostic arthroscopy, *Acta Orthop Scand* 60:710, 1989.
2. Adams JE: Bone injuries in very young athletes, *Clin Orthop* 58:129, 1968.

3. American Academy of Orthopaedic Surgeons: Position statement on prevention of hip fractures, July, 1993.

4. American Academy of Pediatrics Committee on Sports Medicine and Fitness: Strength training, weight and power lifting, and body building by children and adolescents, *Pediatrics* 86:801, 1990.

5. American College of Sports Medicine: Current comment: prevention of sport injuries of children and adolescents, *Med Sci Sports Exerc* 1993.

6. American College of Sports Medicine: The female athlete triad: disordered eating, amenorrhea, and osteoporosis, *Sports Med Bull* 28(1):6, 1993.

7. Bailey DH et al: Epidemiology of fractures of the distal end of the radius in children as associated with growth, *J Bone Joint Surg* 71A:1225, 1989.

8. Bak K: Separation of the proximal tibial epiphysis in a gymnast, *Acta Orthop Scand* 62:293, 1991.

9. Barnett LS: Little League shoulder syndrome: proximal humeral epiphyseolysis in adolescent baseball pitchers: a case report, *J Bone Joint Surg* 67A:495, 1985.

10. Benson JE et al: Relationship between nutrient intake, body mass index, menstrual function, and ballet injury, *J Am Diet Assoc* 89:58, 1989.

11. Berndt AL, Harty M: Transchondral fractures (osteochondritis dissecans) of the talus, *J Bone Joint Surg* 41A:988, 1959.

12. Birch JG, Herring JA, Wenger DR: Surgical anatomy of selected physes, *J Pediatr Orthop* 4:224, 1984.

13. Blair SN et al: Physical fitness and all-cause mortality: a prospective study of healthy men and women, *JAMA* 262:2395, 1989.

14. Bohlman HH: Acute fractures and dislocations of the cervical spine: an analysis of three hundred hospitalized patients and review of the literature, *J Bone Joint Surg* 61A:1119, 1979.

15. Bradley GW, Shives TC, Samuelson KM: Ligament injuries in the knees of children, *J Bone Joint Surg* 61:588, 1979.

16. Bright RW, Burstein AH, Elmore SM: Epiphyseal-plate cartilage: a biomechanical and histological analysis of failure modes, *J Bone Joint Surg* 56A:688, 1974.

17. Brukner P, Khan K: *Clinical sports medicine,* Sydney, Australia, 1993, McGraw-Hill.

18. Cahill BR: Stress fracture of the proximal tibial epiphysis: a case report, *Am J Sports Med* 5:186, 1977.

19. Cahill BR, Griffith EH: Effect of preseason conditioning on the incidence and severity of high school football knee injuries, *Am J Sports Med* 6:180, 1978.

20. Caine D et al: Stress changes of the distal radial growth plate: a radiographic survey and review of the literature, *Am J Sports Med* 20:290, 1992.

21. Carter SR et al: Stress changes of the wrist in adolescent gymnasts, *Br J Radiol* 61:109, 1988.

22. Chambers RB: Orthopaedic injuries in athletes (ages 6 to 17), *Am J Sports Med* 7:195, 1979.

23. Clanton TO et al: Knee ligament injuries in children, *J Bone Joint Surg* 61:1195, 1979.

24. Clark CA, Ogden JA: Development of the menisci of the human knee joint, *J Bone Joint Surg* 65B:538, 1983.

25. Currey JD, Butler G: The mechanical properties of bone tissue in children, *J Bone Joint Surg* 57:810, 1975.

26. DeLee JC, Farney WC: Incidence of injury in Texas high school football, *Am J Sports Med* 20:575, 1992.

27. DeLoes M, Goldie I: Incidence rate of injuries during sport activity and physical exercise in a rural Swedish municipality: incidence rates in 17 sports, *Int J Sports Med* 6:461, 1988.

28. Ekeland A, Holtmoen A, Lystad H: Lower extremity equipment-related injuries in alpine recreational skiers, *Am J Sports Med* 21:201, 1993.

29. Frisch RE et al: Lower prevalence of breast cancer and cancers of the reproductive system among former college athletes compared to nonathletes, *Br J Cancer* 52:885, 1985.

30. Gallagher SS et al: The incidence of injuries among 87,000 Massachusetts children and adolescents: results of the 1980-81 statewide childhood injury prevention program surveillance system, *Am J Public Health* 74:1340, 1984.

31. Garrick JG, Requa RK: Injuries in high school sports, *Pediatrics* 61:465, 1978.

32. Gerber SD, Griffin PP, Simmons BP: Break dancer's wrist: a case report, *J Pediatr Orthop* 6:98, 1986.

33. Goldberg B: Injury patterns in youth sports, *Phys Sports Med* 17:175, 1989.

34. Goldberg B et al: Injuries in youth football, *Pediatrics* 81:255, 1988.

35. Goldstein JD et al: Spine injuries in gymnasts and swimmers: an epidemiologic investigation, *Am J Sports Med* 19:463, 1991.

36. Izant RJ, Hubay CA: The annual injury of 15,000,000 children: a limited study of childhood accidental injury and death, *J Trauma* 6:56, 1966.

37. Jowsey J: Age changes in human bone, *Clin Orthop* 17:210, 1960.

38. Kadel NJ, Teitz CC, Kronmal RA: Stress fractures in ballet dancers, *Am J Sports Med* 20:445, 1992.

39. Kannus P, Nittymaki S, Jarvinen M: Athletic overuse injuries in children: a 30-month prospective follow-up study at an outpatient sports clinic, *Clin Pediatr* 7:333, 1988.

40. Kibler WB et al: A musculoskeletal approach to the preparticipation physical examination: preventing injury and improving performance, *Am J Sports Med* 17:525, 1989.

41. Landin L, Nilsson BE: Bone mineral content in children with fractures, *Clin Orthop* 178:292, 1983.

42. Lenaway DD, Ambler AG, Beaudoin DE: The epidemiology of school-related injuries: new perspectives, *Am J Prev Med* 8:193, 1992.

43. Lepse PS, McCarthy RE, McCullough FL: Simultaneous bilateral avulsion fracture of the tibial tuberosity, *Clin Orthop* 229:232, 1988.

44. Light TR, Ogden DA, Ogden JA: The anatomy of metaphyseal torus fractures, *Clin Orthop* 188:103, 1984.

45. Lysens RJ et al: The accident-prone and overuse-prone profiles of the young athlete, *Am J Sports Med* 17:612, 1989.

46. Mandelbaum BR et al: Wrist pain syndrome in the gymnast: pathogenetic, diagnostic, and therapeutic considerations, *Am J Sports Med* 17:305, 1989.

47. McLain LG, Reynolds S: Sports injuries in a high school, *Pediatrics* 84:446, 1989.

48. Micheli LJ, Ireland ML: Prevention and management of calcaneal apophysitis in children: an overuse syndrome, *J Pediatr Orthop* 7:34, 1987.

49. Mizuta T et al: Statistical analysis of the incidence of physeal injuries, *J Pediatr Orthop* 7:518, 1987.

50. Mubarak SJ, Carroll NC: Familial osteochondritis dissecans of the knee, *Clin Orthop* 140:131, 1979.

51. Mubarak SJ, Carroll NC: Juvenile osteochondritis dissecans of the knee: etiology, *Clin Orthop* 157:200, 1981.

52. Mueller FO, Cantu RC: Catastrophic injuries and fatalities in high school and college sports, fall 1982–spring 1988, *Med Sci Sports Exerc* 22:737, 1990.

53. National Strength and Conditioning Association: Position paper on prepubescent strength training, Lincoln, Neb, 1985.

54. Nilsson BE. Westlin NE: Bone density in athletes, *Clin Orthop* 77:179, 1971.

55. Nilsson S: Soccer injuries in adolescents, *Am J Sports Med* 6:358, 1978.

56. Ogden JA: Skeletal growth mechanism injury patterns, *J Pediatr Orthop* 2:371, 1982.

57. Ogden JA: The uniqueness of growing bones. In King RE, Wilkins KE, Rockwood CA (eds): *Fractures in children*, ed 3, Philadelphia, 1991, JB Lippincott.

58. Oppliger RA et al: Bulimic behaviors among interscholastic wrestlers: a statewide survey, *Pediatrics* 91:826, 1993.

59. Orava S, Puranen J: Exertion injuries in adolescent athletes, *Br J Sports Med* 12:4, 1978.

60. Ott SM: Bone density in adolescents, *N Engl J Med* 325:1646, 1991.

61. Paffenbarger RS Jr et al: The association of changes in physical activity level and other lifestyle characteristics with mortality among men, *N Engl J Med* 328:538, 1993.

62. Peterson HA, Burkhart SS: Compression injury of the epiphyseal growth plate: fact or fiction? *J Pediatr Orthop* 1:377, 1981.

63. Proffer DS, Patton JJ, Jackson DW: Nonunion of a first rib fracture in a gymnast, *Am J Sports Med* 19:198, 1991.

64. Reider B, Yurkofsky J, Mass D: Scaphoid waist fracture in a weight lifter: a case report, *Am J Sports Med* 21:329, 1993.

65. Roser LA, Clawson DK: Football injuries in the very young athlete, *Clin Orthop* 69:219, 1970.

66. Roy MA et al: Body checking in pee wee hockey, *Phys Sports Med* 17:119, 1989.

67. Salter RB, Harris WR: Injuries involving the epiphyseal plate, *J Bone Joint Surg* 45A:587, 1963.

68. Sands WA, Shultz BB, Newman AP: Women's gymnastics injuries: a 5-year study, *Am J Sports Med* 21:271, 1993.

69. Sandvik L et al: Physical fitness as a predictor of mortality among healthy, middle-aged Norwegian men, *N Engl J Med* 328:533, 1993.

70. Schaefer RA, Eilert RE, Gillogly SD: Disruption of the anterior cruciate ligament in a 4-year-old child, *Orthop Rev* 725, 1993.

71. Sewall L, Micheli LJ: Strength training for children, *J Pediatr Orthop* 6:143, 1986.

72. Shaffer TE: Schering symposium on sports medicine: the uniqueness of the young athlete: introductory remarks, *Am J Sports Med* 8:370, 1980.

73. Smith AD: A four-year longitudinal study of injuries of elite figure skaters, *Med Sci Sports Exerc* 23:S151, 1991.

74. Smith AD, Stroud L, McQueen C: Flexibility and anterior knee pain in adolescent elite figure skaters, *J Pediatr Orthop* 11:77, 1991.

75. Speer KP, Lohnes J, Garrett WE: Radiographic imaging of muscle strain injury, *Am J Sports Med* 21:89, 1993.

76. Stanitski CL, Harvell JC, Fu F: Observations on acute knee hemarthrosis in children and adolescents, *J Pediatr Orthop* 13:506, 1993.

77. Taylor DC et al: Experimental muscle strain injury: early functional and structural deficits and the increased risk for reinjury, *Am J Sports Med* 21:190, 1993.

78. Tenvergert EM, Ten Duis HJ, Lkasen HJ. Trends in sports injuries, 1982-1988: an in-depth study on four types of sport, *J Sports Med Phys Fitness* 32:214, 1992.

79. Torg JS et al: The National Football Head and Neck Injury Registry, 14-yr report on cervical quadriplegia, 1971-1984, *JAMA* 254:3439, 1985.

80. Tullos HS, King JW: Lesions of the pitching arm in adolescents, *JAMA* 220:264, 1972.

81. Vender MI, Watson K: Acquired Madelung-like deformity in a gymnast, *J Hand Surg* 13:19, 1988.

82. Wadley GH, Albright JP: Women's intercollegiate gymnastics: injury patterns and "permanent" medical disability, *Am J Sports Med* 21:314, 1993.

83. Waninger KN, Lombardo JA: Stress fracture of index metacarpal in a tennis player, *Med Sci Sports Exerc* 25:S21, 1993.

84. Wasilewski SA, Asdouian PL: Bilateral chronic exertional compartment syndromes of forearm in an adolescent athlete: case report and review of literature, *Am J Sports Med* 19:665, 1991.

85. Winkler AR, Barnes JC, Ogden JA: Break dance hip: chronic avulsion of the anterior superior iliac spine, *Pediatr Radiol* 17:501, 1987.

86. Wu CD, Huang SC, Liu TK: Sleeve fracture of the patella in children: a report of five cases, *Am J Sports Med* 19:525, 1991.

87. Yasuda T et al: Stress fracture of the right distal femur following bilateral fractures of the proximal fibulas: a case study, *Am J Sports Med* 20:771, 1992.

CHAPTER 55 Injuries to the Foot and Ankle

Vincent J. Turco

Injuries to the foot and ankle are among the most frequently encountered entities in the treatment of sports-related injuries. This chapter includes discussions of the diagnosis and treatment of ankle and foot injuries in adolescents and the recognition of some less common entities that are frequently overlooked. Most of the problems in the skeletally immature athlete have adult counterparts. The major difference is that in the younger athlete the foot and ankle are predisposed to additional trauma associated with the epiphyses, apophyses, and congenital anomalies.

The importance of an early, accurate diagnosis based on a knowledge of the normal anatomy, biomechanics, and the mechanism of injury is emphasized. An accurate diagnosis is the basis for good treatment and results. In the care of sports injuries prognosis is especially important; the common question is "How soon can I get back to sports?" Early recognition of the problem provides a realistic prognosis for the athlete. The following factors help the physician make an accurate diagnosis and prognosis in the initial assessment:

1. A good history, which should include the mechanism of injury.
2. Clinical assessment, including inspection and careful palpation for areas of maximal localized point tenderness and stability.
3. Proper radiographic assessment, including comparable views of the uninjured side, if necessary. In selected cases other imaging studies such as computed tomography (CT) scans, magnetic resonance imaging (MRI) scans, or bone scans may be necessary.
4. Correlation of the mechanism of injury, complaints, and clinical and radiographic evaluations with the normal anatomy and biomechanics.

NORMAL ANATOMY AND BIOMECHANICS

An accurate diagnosis, rational treatment, and rehabilitation demand a comprehension of the normal anatomy and biomechanics. There is an anatomic and functional interplay between the foot and ankle because the tibiotalar, subtalar, and midtarsal joints are interrelated. Anatomic and biomechanical abnormalities in any of these articulations are reflected by changes in range of motion and function and subsequent adaptive changes according to Wolff's law of form and function. Fick[9] recognized this functional interrelationship between the foot and ankle when he described the upper ankle joint as "articulation crurotalarias" and the lower ankle joint "articulation talocalcaneal navicularias."

The stability of the ankle joint is provided both by bones and ligaments. The tibiotalar articulation is one of a tenon and mortise. The talar body is the tenon, and the mortise comprises the medial malleolus, the undersurface of the tibia, and the lateral malleolus. The tibia is joined to the fibula by a rather complex and somewhat elastic syndesmosis that includes the distal anterior and posterior tibiofibular ligaments and the interosseous ligament, which is the distal continuation of the interosseous membrane. The medial malleolus projects about halfway down the medial surface of the talus and is broader and stronger than its lateral counterpart. The thick, strong deltoid ligament complex affords additional

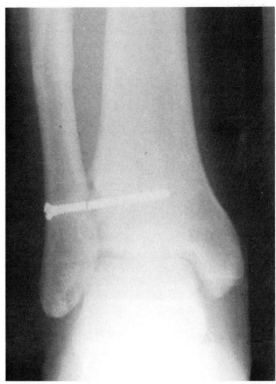

FIG. 55-1. Normal mechanics. Diastasis of tibiofibular syndesmosis with concomitant fracture of fibula and torn deltoid ligament incurred while playing football. Tibiofibular separation was reduced and stabilized with transfixion screw. Stress fracture of screw occurred because rigid fixation to tibia prevented normal axial and rotatory motion of fibula. It is interesting to note that patient was relieved of ankle pain after screw fractured. This hardware should be removed after ligament heals to permit mobility of fibula. Bone absorption around screw usually occurs in absence of metal fatigue.

support medially. Laterally, the fibula is longer and extends more distally to the level of the subtalar joint. The fibula is slightly constricted at the level of the ankle joint (a common area for fracture) and expands distally to form the lateral malleolus. The lateral malleolus has a greater surface contact with the adjacent talus than the medial malleolus. Additional lateral support is provided by the three lateral ligaments: the anterior talofibular, the calcaneofibular, and the posterior talofibular ligaments. The anterior and posterior tibiotalar capsules are lax to permit dorsiflexion and plantar flexion. The inherent stability of the ankle mortise is enhanced because the dome-shaped surface of the trochlea fits snugly in the slightly concave surface of the tibia. The anterior surface of the dome or trochlea of the talus has been described by Inman[13] as a frustum of a cone. The dome is wider anteriorly and laterally. The anteroposterior measurement of the superior surface of the talus is greater than the reciprocal articular surface of the tibia. Therefore a portion of the dome of the talus is always out of the mortise and not in contact with the tibia. At any time in any position, only about 50% of the dome of the trochlea is in contact with the tibia.

The ankle is often inaccurately described as a hinged joint. It is actually a *hingelike* joint. In vertical motion of the foot the trochlea of the talus glides in and out of the mortise as the talus moves up and down. In plantar flexion the anterior portion of the dome of the talus is out of the mortise, and the narrower posterior portion of the trochlea is in the mortise; therefore there is more lateral laxity in the mortise in the position of plantar flexion. In dorsiflexion the wider anterior part of the trochlea is in the mortise, and for this reason twisting motions with the foot in dorsiflexion exert a more forceful stress on the

malleoli, particularly the lateral malleolus because of the large articular facet between the body of the talus and the fibula. A slight amount of rotatory and axial motion occurs in the fibula with normal plantar flexion and dorsiflexion of the ankle (Fig. 55-1).[2] This motion can be appreciated by palpation of the proximal tibiofibular joint as the ankle is dorsiflexed and plantar flexed.[12] Forceful inversion and eversion, particularly eversion, transmit greater stress to the fibula and the syndesmosis. It is important to remember that vertical movement in the ankle joint is accompanied by simultaneous motion in the subtalar and midtarsal joints. As the talus moves vertically in the mortise, the foot moves vertically and horizontally. In dorsiflexion the foot pronates (eversion). In plantar flexion the foot supinates (inversion). In horizontal motions the calcaneus and navicular rotate around the talus medially in varus and laterally in valgus. Most of the mobility occurs in the talonavicular and anterior talocalcaneal articulations. Little motion occurs at the stable, S-shaped calcaneocuboid joint. The navicular and calcaneus move simultaneously, in unison, around the head of the talus in both horizontal and vertical motions of the foot (talocalcaneonavicular complex). The forefoot follows the hindfoot.

Knowledge of the mechanics of the talocalcaneonavicular complex is basic to an understanding of the symptoms and clinical findings in peroneal spasm, congenital anomalies, and traumatic problems involving the ankle, subtalar, and midtarsal joints. Movement in the talocalcaneonavicular complex accounts for the apparent vertical motion in a fused ankle. After ankle fusion, mobility in the midtarsal, anterior subtalar, and tarsometatarsal joints increases because of added stress secondary to a stiff ankle. In calcaneonavicular coalitions subtalar motion is limited because the calcaneus and navicular are not mobile and therefore cannot invert and evert around the talus. The degenerative changes at the talonavicular and calcaneocuboid joints often associated with talocalcaneal coalition and subtalar fusion, as in a Grice procedure, are the result of added stress to these joints. The lack of mobility caused by coalitions or trauma of the talocalcaneonavicular complex is the reason patients have difficulty walking on uneven terrain. It is interesting to note that patients with peroneal spasm are usually more comfortable walking at an incline because plantar flexion is limited in the foot as a result of its fixed valgus position and the foot is incapable of the inversion that is necessary for plantar flexion. If motion is decreased in any one of the joints of the upper and lower ankle the overall motion is affected.

Little motion occurs at the tarsometatarsal (Lisfranc) joints. The first metatarsal articulates with the medial or first cuneiform; it is slightly adducted and is the most mobile of the metatarsals. The second metatarsal base is lodged in a mortise formed by all three cuneiforms and is very stable. This anatomic relationship of the second metatarsal base provides the major stability of the Lisfranc region. Further stability of the second metatarsal base is afforded by the first cuneiform–second metatarsal ligament (Lisfranc ligament). The clinical application of the anatomy of this area is discussed in Chapter 25. We have noted that the perimeter of the foot—the medial and lateral exposed areas—is a common site for injury. The first and fifth tarsometatarsal articulations are the most mobile metatarsals.

During the important push-off phase of running and walking the five metatarsal heads bear considerable weight and are subjected to high forces. Although there is controversy about the exact percentage of weight carried by each metatarsal, there is no doubt that, clinically, the first metatarsal bears the higher load. This is in part because the sesamoid bones of the great toe enhance weight bearing. During the push-off phase the metatarsophalangeal joints are in dorsiflexion and the sesamoid bones of the great toe are pulled distally beneath the large first metatarsal head. These sesamoids are therefore susceptible to overuse injuries and fractures. Indiscriminate removal of these bones can result in transfer metatarsalgia and further problems caused by the resulting biomechanical disadvantage of sesamoid removal.

The two heads of the gastrocnemius muscle and the soleus muscle are collectively known as the triceps surae. The tendon of insertion of this muscle group has been called by various synonyms: "Achilles tendon," "tendocalcaneus," "tendo Achillis," and "tendon of the triceps surae." The Achilles tendon is the thickest and strongest tendon in the body, which reflects its functional importance. The gastrocnemius muscle is superficial and has two bellies of which the medial is larger. Both heads of the gastrocnemius originate on the distal femur, and they synchronize motion of the foot and knee. The deeper soleus originates from the tibia and fibula. The Achilles tendon is the conjoint tendon of the gastrocnemius and soleus, and because of a gentle spiral in its downward descent into the calcaneus, the gastrocnemius inserts primarily laterally and the soleus inserts medially. Because the insertion at the calcaneal tuberosity is medial to the midline, the heel is pulled into equinus and inversion by contraction of the triceps surae. Difficulties during the push-off phase of running and walking are a consequence of deficiency in this muscle group and detract from performance in walking, running, and jumping.

MECHANISM OF INJURY

A careful history of the mechanism of injury is most helpful in arriving at an accurate diagnosis, especially in difficult cases of obscure trauma in which the subjective complaints appear to be out of proportion to the gross clinical assessment. A good history should be taken before the clinical and radiographic evaluations. The examiner should listen to the patient, let the patient talk, and ask the pertinent questions. Equal time should be devoted to the history and the clinical examination. The mechanism of injury is as important as the clinical examination and often provides the diagnosis if the examiner applies his or her knowledge of the normal anatomy and mechanics of the foot and ankle. The mechanism of injury does not refer to the general type of accident, such as "motor vehicle accident," or "a fall down stairs." The mechanism of injury is determined by the specific position of the foot and the direction and magnitude of the injuring force. The position of the foot and the direction of the stress at the instant of injury indicate the ligaments, joints, or bones most likely to be injured based on knowledge of normal anatomy and mechanics. Each mechanism usually causes specific injuries. We do not mean to imply that the exact mechanism of injury is always readily determined. However, a patient and an understanding physician can often elicit a meaningful history. When possible the patient should be asked to reconstruct the exact mechanism, or the physician can demonstrate to the patient the various positions of the foot and mechanisms of force. The common types of injuries are (1) **direct injuries** and (2) **indirect injuries.**

Mechanism of injury

- Specific position of the foot
- Direction and magnitude of injuring force

Direct Injuries

Direct injuries are incurred by, for example, being stepped on or being hit by an object such as a high-flying hockey puck. This type of mechanism, when accurately described, readily rules out sprains and dislocations. Direct injuries are usually obvious on careful examination because of the telltale bruise they leave. The depth of the injury varies with the force applied, which frequently is a factor of the velocity of the injuring object. Direct injury can cause an abrasion of the skin, myositis of the muscle, periostitis, or fracture of the bone. Injury to the tendons can cause tendinitis. Neuritis and phlebitis can result from injuries to the superficial nerves and blood vessels. It is possible to incur infractions by a direct injury, particularly by being hit by a puck in the more competitive levels of hockey or by a ball. A fall directly on the heel can result in a fracture of the plantar surface of the os calcis or a periostitis—so-called stone bruise of the heel. One should bear in mind that it is possible to incur an injury by a combination of both direct and indirect mechanisms. This can occur, for example, when the foot is stepped on with the foot anchored and the weight of the body falling sideways, providing a torsion strain in either pronation or supination on the foot. In these cases the direct blow can be misleading because the damage is caused primarily by the twisting of the anchored forefoot. In this type of injury the entire extremity or linkage system from the spine to the foot must be examined to evaluate possible injury at other sites.

Indirect Injuries

Indirect injuries are the more difficult category from which to elicit the precise mechanism of injury. Ligament sprains of the ankle and foot are common, and they directly reflect the direction of the excessive motion that results in injury. Occasionally, the physician is fortunate enough to be a direct witness to the mechanism of injury. However, more often the history must be elicited from the player, coach, trainer, or parents. In some instances a review of game films may be helpful.

The important factors to consider and the questions to ask are as follows. Was the foot in the position of dorsiflexion, plantar flexion, inversion, eversion, or hyperflexion of the toes in a ballet position? There may be a combination of both direct and indirect trauma. Was the foot anchored? When the patient fell, was the fall backwards, forwards, to the right, or to the left? The examiner should ask questions of the mechanisms that produce predictable injuries. Did the patient hear a pop, snap, or tear? Was the onset of disability, pain, swelling, or discoloration immediate or delayed? Was the athlete able to finish the game? Could the athlete bear weight? Where is the area of most pain?

A good history takes time and patience. By letting the patient talk and asking the pertinent questions the chances of reconstructing the mechanism of injury are increased. **The correlation of the mechanism of injury with the knowledge of normal anatomy and biomechanics enables the examiner to detect unrecognized injuries that often cause prolonged, unexplained morbidity.** Unrecognized trauma with improper treatment may also result in more problems that could have been avoided with a proper diagnosis and treatment.

Straight hyperdorsiflexion in the neutral position causes injuries to the anterior tibiotalar joint, which may result in occult fractures of the anterior lip of the tibia or the neck of the talus. If the pain is predominantly posterior, the physician should look for injuries to the Achilles tendon or posterior tibial tendon. With the foot in dorsiflexion the mortise is fully occupied by the widest part of the talus. Hence with a valgus stress the talus pushes the fibula laterally, causing a sprain, avulsion, or even separation of the tibiofibular syndesmosis.

Hyperplantar flexion of the forefoot so that it is pointing straight down can cause infractions in the region of

the posterior tibiotalar joint with strain of the anterior tibiotalar capsule.

An inversion stress with the foot plantar flexed may cause stretching of the lateral ligaments and result in separation of the distal fibular epiphysis.

Some physicians minimize the importance of eliciting the mechanism of injury because they believe that either surgical or nonsurgical treatment can be rendered regardless of this exact knowledge. However, our experience overwhelmingly supports the necessity of determining the true mechanism to fully understand the extent of injury. The physician should never fail to review the injuring force intraoperatively to expand understanding of the problem at hand. From this understanding, realistic treatment, rehabilitation, and ultimately prevention can follow.

INJURIES AND CONDITIONS OF OSSEOUS STRUCTURES
Coalitions

Tarsal coalitions occur initially as cartilaginous bars that calcify and may become completely osseous or remain osteocartilaginous (Fig 55-2). Diagnosis is particularly difficult during the pure cartilaginous stages. Many cases undoubtedly remain asymptomatic throughout life and may be fortuitously diagnosed on radiographs taken for ankle sprains or fractures. The symptomatic cases are usually seen as episodes of recurrent peroneal spastic flatfoot, or they may become symptomatic after injury. These cartilaginous bars are one of the causes of painful flatfeet. A common complaint is difficulty walking on uneven terrain.

Occasionally, the pain may be so disabling that a short period of plaster immobilization is necessary to reduce the peroneal spasm that is seen clinically. Such cases may remain entirely asymptomatic after such treatment. However, there are instances in which the symptomatic episodes are so frequent or disabling that surgical intervention is necessary.

Clinically, recurrent episodes of peroneal spasm and decreased foot mobility secondary to loss of normal motion in the talocalcaneonavicular complex associated with flatfoot should alert the examiner to this entity. Radiographic studies confirm the diagnosis, but special views are frequently required. Anteroposterior, lateral, oblique, and posterior subtalar (Harris) views are indicated. If these radiographs fail to confirm or adequately

---

Evaluation of coalitions

Subtalar coalition
- Anteroposterior, lateral, and oblique views
- Harris heel view
- Computed tomography scans

Calcaneonavicular coalition
- Oblique foot film

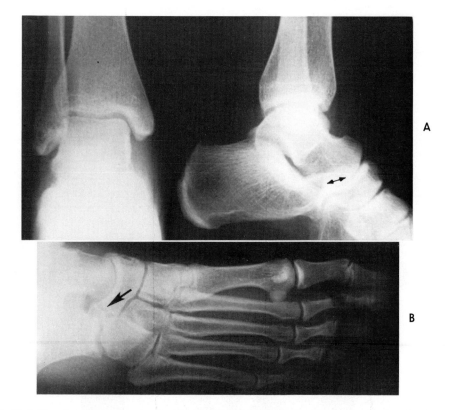

FIG. 55-2. Tarsal coalition associated with ankle injuries. This patient had been diagnosed as having chronic "recurrent lateral ligament sprain." She incurred recurrent acute episodes with minimal trauma. In addition to tenderness over lateral ligaments, she had peroneal spastic flatfoot and heel valgus with painful limited horizontal mobility of foot. Limited subtalar motion increased stress on ankle. **A,** Anteroposterior and lateral views of ankle were normal. Calcaneonavicular bar was suspected from lateral view of foot. **B,** Oblique view of foot clearly demonstrates calcaneonavicular bar.

delineate the suspected injury, tomograms or CT scans should be considered.

The most common coalition is at the calcaneonavicular site. The talocalcaneal coalition is usually in the region of the sustentaculum tali but may be in the region of the posterior subtalar compartment (Fig. 55-3). The solid bony coalitions are more likely to cause symptoms because they cause a greater restriction in motion than a cartilaginous synostosis. Because the navicular normally accompanies the anterior calcaneus in motions at the talocalcaneonavicular joint, the common coalition between the anterior end of the calcaneus and the lateral aspect of the navicular has a less deleterious effect on foot mechanics than the subtalar coalitions. This biomechanical fact explains why symptoms and degenerative changes are more prominent in the subtalar synostosis. Although the great majority of coalitions occur with flatfeet, this entity has also been described in the region of the sustentaculum tali in clubfeet.[28]

Once diagnosis is confirmed, the decision whether to resect the bar or perform triple arthrodesis is based on the presence or absence of degenerative changes.[6] Talonavicular beaking caused by increased stress at this articulation is a common adaptive attritional change (Fig. 55-4). Excision is performed with the hope of retaining talocalcaneonavicular-mobility and preventing attritional changes. Interposition of fat or the extensor

digitorum brevis muscle is commonly performed to discourage reformation of the coalition, and early motion after a short period of casting for comfort and wound care is in order (Fig. 55-5).

If a triple arthrodesis is indicated because of early arthrosis, it is best to perform this procedure after the foot has attained radiographic evidence of skeletal maturity. Technically, the surgery should be performed by denuding the articular surface only to subchondral bone. This is done to maintain foot size and avoid discrepancy in shoe size and for cosmesis. The procedure is best performed through lateral and medial incisions centered over the sinus tarsi and talonavicular joints, respectively. If the presenting flatfoot deformity is unacceptable, all three joints must be mobilized to allow correction before fusion, which necessitates removal of the bar. Internal fixation is used routinely and may allow only a short leg cast postoperatively.

Effects of tarsal coalition

Tarsal coalition	→	Limited talocalcaneonavicular motion	→	Increased ankle stress

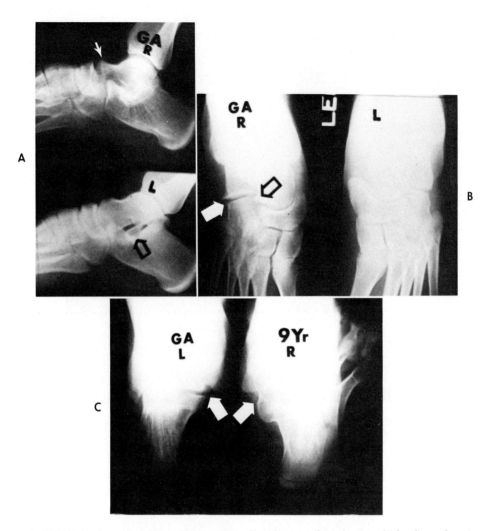

FIG. 55-3. Talocalcaneal coalition. This condition disturbs normal mechanics of talocalcaneal navicular complex. Loss of subtalar motion increases stress on midtarsal joints, causing degenerative changes of talonavicular and calcaneocuboid joints. **A,** Lateral radiograph. Comparison lateral views show talonavicular beaking on involved right side. Notice sinus tarsi is closed on right and open on normal left side, consistent with valgus angulation of heel. **B,** Anteroposterior view demonstrates arthritic changes at calcaneocuboid joint. **C,** Harris axial view. Bony subtalar fusion in region of sustentaculum tali. This patient underwent triple arthrodesis through medial and lateral approach with percutaneous Kirschner wire transfixion. Operation relieved pain and had excellent cosmetic and functional results.

Tarsal coalition may be unrecognized until an ankle sprain or fracture occurs. It is important to note that coalitions limit motion of the talocalcaneonavicular complex and therefore increase stress at the ankle joint. Coalition should be suspected when pain and peroneal spasm persist beyond the usual disability time following a simple sprain or fracture. An ankle injury per se should not cause peroneal spasm. A spastic flatfoot with limited subtalar motion is evidence of subtalar or midtarsal injury. In cases of ankle instability that require lateral ligament reconstruction, the physician should take proper radiographs of the foot to make certain an occult coalition is not present. The associated coalition may become more symptomatic after reconstruction.

Navicular
Accessory Navicular or Overgrown Navicular Tuberosity

A prominence in the medial midfoot in the region of the navicular can be either an accessory tarsal navicular or a prominent overgrown navicular tuberosity. The prominence in itself predisposes to painful bursa, callosities, and pressure from shoes but is usually asymptomatic. We have noted a tendency for the localized prominence to become less accentuated in the growing child because of the slower growth of the accessory ossicle in comparison to the major bones of the foot.

An accessory tarsal navicular has become noted as a cause of painful flatfeet. We believe that the accessory bone occurs concomitantly with flexible flatfeet but that it is a minor factor in the etiology of the deformity. Extensive experience with congenital foot deformities has pointed out to us that the main anatomic finding in flexible pes planus is a voluminous calcaneonavicular socket associated with relaxed collagen structures. In such instances close inspection often reveals an oblique talus, talonavicular sag, or lateral subluxation of the navicular on the talar head. It is easy to understand anatomically that plication or advancement of the posterior tibial ten-

don and spring ligament is a partial and simplistic solution to a complex entity that involves all the collagen structures, including bone. To further complicate the anatomic injury of pes planus, we have personal operative experience with cavus feet that had congenital complete absence of the posterior tibial tendon.[30]

The persistently painful overlying bursa and localized arthrosis of the accessory joint may necessitate excision. If surgery is necessary, the accessory ossicle is found in the tendon of the posterior tibialis at its insertion. The posterior tibial tendon normally attaches to the sustentaculum tali, the navicular tuberosity, the spring ligament, and the plantar aspect of the forefoot. In accessory tarsal navicular the posterior tibial tendon often lacks its multiplicity of insertions in favor of a single insertion to only one of the many normal areas, usually the accessory ossicle or the plantar aspect of the foot. During surgery an attempt should be made to preserve the insertion of the posterior tibial tendon, resect the ossicle, and remove the overgrown navicular tuberosity while sparing the main talonavicular joint. The posterior tibial tendon should be transplanted distally and plantarward to enhance support of the spring ligament for the talar head (Fig. 55-6).

Fracture of Tarsal Navicular

The tarsal navicular can be injured in jumps or falls by a mechanism of injury similar to that described for calcaneal fractures. Stress fractures can also occur. Avulsion fractures usually involve the talonavicular capsule; they usually are minimally displaced and heal with routine fracture care. Avulsion fractures of the navicular may accompany tarsometatarsal injuries but are usually not a factor in the care of these problems. Vertical fractures of the navicular, however, can occur in basketball, gymnastics, and other jumping sports and demand ag-

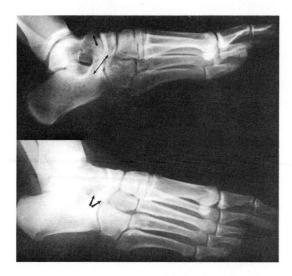

FIG. 55-4. Calcaneonavicular coalition. Distomedial aspect of calcaneus is joined to lateral aspect of navicular. This is the most common coalition. Lateral view demonstrates adaptive attritional changes of talonavicular joint. Oblique view is best for visualization of this bar. In this case, excision of coalition is contraindicated because of preexisting degenerative changes at talonavicular joint.

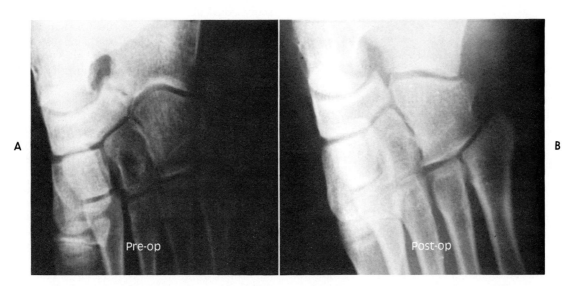

FIG. 55-5. Calcaneonavicular synchondrosis in 12-year-old boy. Cartilaginous coalition was excised to relieve pain and recurrent peroneal spastic flatfoot. **A,** Preoperative. Typical calcaneonavicular cartilaginous bar. **B,** Postoperative. Bar excised using Cowell's technique. Talonavicular joint is not violated. Good result with supple foot.

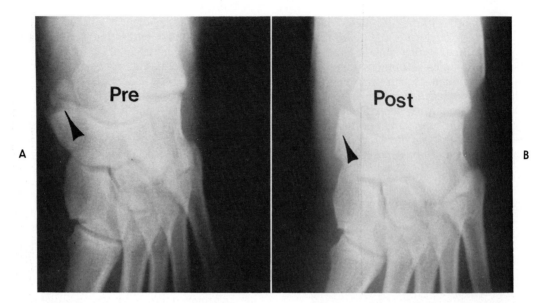

FIG. 55-6. Accessory navicular. Preoperative and postoperative views. This runner complained of localized pain and bursal swelling over region of navicular tuberosity. **A,** Preoperative radiographs show cystic changes and irregularity at accessory joint. Arthritic changes were more prominent at surgery. Pain is usually caused by attritional changes of accessory joint or painful callus with bursal thickening over an accessory ossicle or overdeveloped tuberosity of navicular. **B,** Postoperative radiographs, show that accessory navicular and overdeveloped navicular tuberosity have been excised. It is important to spare articular surfaces of talonavicular joint. Surgery is extraarticular.

gressive treatment because of the possibility for delayed union and nonunion. Initial care of vertical undisplaced fractures consists of non–weight-bearing cast immobilization. Displaced fractures require reduction and fixation. Accessory tarsal navicular can be mistaken for an acute fracture. We have seen instances in which a previously asymptomatic accessory navicular became symptomatic because of an injury to the articulation between the accessory bone and the main body of the navicular or the talar head.

Calcaneus
Pump Bumps

We are aware that many entities in the area of the posterior calcaneal tuberosity may cause problems secondary to a local irritation by the heel counter of the shoe or mechanical interference with the Achilles tendon. There is, however, a specific entity that we call "pump bump," which is caused by a broad-based lateral exostosis, usually bilateral, in the region of the calcaneal tuberosity.[14] Pump bumps are not to be confused with osteophytes projecting from the posterior midline under the Achilles tendon or with a prominent calcaneal tuberosity. In some cases the lateral broad-based exostosis can be visualized in a Harris calcaneal radiographic projection. This bony irregularity is more commonly symptomatic in females, perhaps because of the differences of women's shoes. Local padding, heel elevation, application of ice, use of antiinflammatory medications, and restricted activity may control symptoms. A small group of cases, however, requires local surgical excision.

A transverse skin incision is centered over the exosto-

sis, and any fibers of the Achilles tendon that interfere with exposure are detached. The exostosis is removed and rasped smooth. The Achilles tendon is reconstituted, and a cast is used postoperatively for comfort and to protect the insertion of the tendon. Results of this procedure are good (Fig. 55-7).

Achilles Tendinitis

Achilles tendinitis is a common problem in running sports. Basically, the mechanism of injury is repetitive contraction leading to an overuse phenomenon. The clinical diagnosis is based on local pain, usually near the Achilles tendon insertion, which can be exacerbated by forceful dorsiflexion of the foot with the knee in extension. Dorsiflexion may be limited.

The pathologic process can involve local bursae, the tendon sheath, or the tendon substance. The tendon sheath of the Achilles tendon is unusual in that there is no tenosynovium. There is instead peritendon, which includes the epitenon and paratenon. Therefore inflammation of the sheath of the Achilles tendon is properly termed "peritendinitis."[27] There are two bursae at the calcaneal insertion of the Achilles tendon; one between the skin and tendon and another between the tendon and bone. Initial treatment includes judicious use of antiinflammatory medications, application of ice, rest, heel elevation, and stretching exercises. The devoted, high-performance athlete may require surgery for bursectomy, peritendon removal, excision of areas of degenerated tendon, or partial ostectomy.[19] Degenerative changes occur only in the older athlete. Often the integrity of the tendon-bone complex is violated during this type of sur-

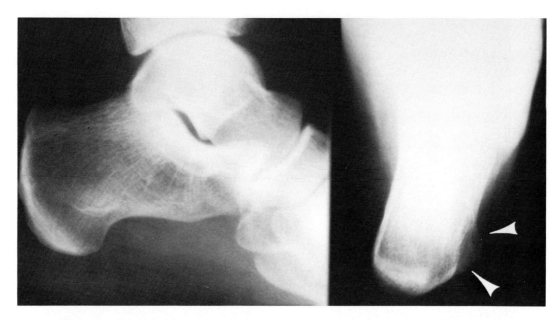

FIG. 55-7. "Pump bump." This young woman had localized discomfort over lateral posterior bony prominence of calcaneus that caused difficulties with athletic shoewear. On lateral view calcaneus is normal. Axial view of calcaneus demonstrates a broad-based exostosis, which was subsequently removed, giving complete relief of symptoms.

gery, and postoperative plaster immobilization is determined on an individual basis. Vigorous stretching and strengthening exercises are indicated postoperatively.

In young, active adolescents the clinical entity of **calcaneal apophysitis** can occur. This diagnosis is presumptive because these young athletes do not require surgery. Radiographic findings are controversial but may consist of fragmentation and irregular ossification of the calcaneal apophysis. Rest, salicylates, and shoe inserts are usually successful in alleviating the symptoms of pain.*

Fracture of the Calcaneus

Fractures of the calcaneus, although uncommon in the young, do occur and present the same problems as in adults. Intraarticular fractures usually cause attritional changes of the subtalar or calcaneocuboid joints; the loss of mobility in these joints causes difficulty walking on uneven terrain. Extraarticular injuries of the calcaneus can occur in the anterior process, posterior tuberosity, or body.

Fractures of the anterior end of the calcaneus are caused by indirect trauma. These are osteochondral fractures, really avulsions of the bifurcated Y ligament, which joins the anterior end of the calcaneus to the navicular and the medial aspect of the cuboid. These are usually undisplaced or minimally displaced osteochondral fractures, often an unrecognized cause of foot pain. This injury should be suspected in cases of chronic pain

in the midfoot and with normal ankle examination with painful limited subtalar motion (Fig. 55-8). Most osteochondral fractures can be treated closed with plaster immobilization. Surgery is necessary for large displaced fragments or persistent disability after closed treatment.

Localized pain laterally in the region of the calcaneocuboid joint is usually caused by an avulsion fracture associated with the calcaneocuboid ligament. Fractures of the anterior tuberosity of the calcaneus that involve the calcaneocuboid joint are notorious for causing disabling pain and limited horizontal motion in spite of anatomic reduction. This area is injured by indirect injury and is prone to occur in motorcycle injuries.

Comminuted fractures of the calcaneus are uncommon in adolescents. These injuries occur in a fall, jump, or collision. The usual mechanism is a direct axial compression, which drives the posterior facet of the talus through the body of the calcaneus, disrupting the articular surface of the calcaneus. An axial Harris view is necessary to accurately assess the damage. In undisplaced fractures plaster immobilization and early motion are recommended as soon as acute pain and swelling subside and motion is tolerable. The sources of disability in terms of pain and function are (1) piling-up of bone fragments below the lateral malleolus associated with tenosynovitis of the peroneals; (2) upward displacement of the posterior tuberosity and relative shortening of the Achilles tendon, causing difficulty with push-off because of the mechanical disadvantage; (3) subtalar and calcaneocuboid arthritis limiting horizontal mobility of the foot; and (4) peroneal spastic flatfoot.

The objectives of treatment are to avoid, if possible, or at least minimize the sequelae of comminuted fractures of the calcaneus. When closed reduction is unsuccess-

---

*Editors' note: Recovery may take months to a year of compliance combined with a maintenance program of stretching, strength, and endurance exercises. Changing from jumping sports to bicycling or swimming may help. Students may require an elevator pass to avoid stairs.

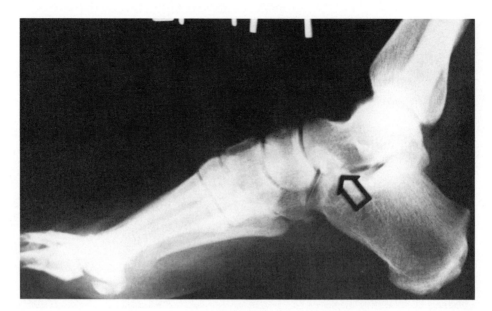

FIG. 55-8. This patient had chronic pain in midfoot and believed she had a sprained ankle. Radiographs show fracture of anterior process of calcaneus. These injuries are often unrecognized and diagnosed as ankle injuries. Often, radiographs of foot are omitted. History, physical examination, and proper radiographs are key to accurate diagnosis of this injury. Most fractures are undisplaced and do well with closed treatment in plaster. Surgical excision is recommended for grossly displaced osteochondral fragments or when persistent disability is present following closed treatment. Open reduction and internal fixation is indicated rarely for large, displaced fragments.

ful, surgical intervention may be indicated, especially in the adolescent. Impingement on the lateral malleolus after the fracture is healed can be treated with surgical excision of the bony prominence and lysis of the peroneal tendons. The fracture pattern is variable, and the treatment for each case should be tailored to the specific injury.

Discussion of the various techniques is beyond the scope of this chapter. Our purpose is to call attention to this injury in the young athlete and to stress the importance of restoring anatomic alignment and mechanics, especially the tuber angle of Böhler (Fig. 55-9).

Talus

Posterior Talar Injuries

Posterior process compression injury. Injuries to the posterior process of the talus are uncommon, often missed athletic injuries. These injuries are usually misdiagnosed as chronic ankle sprains. Posterior impingement symptoms are usually caused by trigone injuries or posteromedial talocalcaneal coalition.

Anatomy. The posterior aspect of the body or trochlea of the talus has two bony tubercles separated by a groove that contains the flexor hallucis longus tendon. The posterior talofibular ligament is attached to the longer lateral tubercle, which projects more posterially. The posterior portion of the deep deltoid ligament inserts on the smaller medial tubercle. The size of the lateral tubercle varies; it may be long or short. A long lateral tubercle is called **Stieda's process.** In about 10% of feet the lateral tubercle is a separate ossicle attached to the bone

by fibrous tissue known as the **os trigonum** (Fig. 55-10).[25] The size of Stidea's process may vary in the same patient. It is not usual to have an os trigonum and Stieda's process contralaterally. In dorsiflexion and plantar flexion the trochlea of the talus glides in and out of the ankle mortise. In plantar flexion the posterior portion of the talus is in the mortise, articulating with the tibia. This knowledge of anatomy and biomechanics of the ankle is essential for an understanding of the mechanism of injury.

Mechanism of injury. The typical mechanism of injury is forceful, extreme plantar flexion of the ankle. In extreme equinus the more prominent lateral tubercle is compressed between the posterior lip of the tibia and the underlying calcaneus. The injury may result from one severe equinus incident or from repetitive overuse as in athletes or ballet dancers en pointe. Compression of the lateral tubercle can cause a fracture, or "trigonitis" of an os trigonum.

Clinical examination. Patients with posterior talar process injuries complain of posterior ankle pain. Point tenderness is noted in the posterolateral aspect of the ankle

---

Posterior talar process compression injury

- Occurs with extreme forceful ankle plantar flexion
- Pain in posterior ankle region
- Tenderness in region between Achilles tendon and lateral malleolus
- Symptoms reproduced by ankle plantar flexion

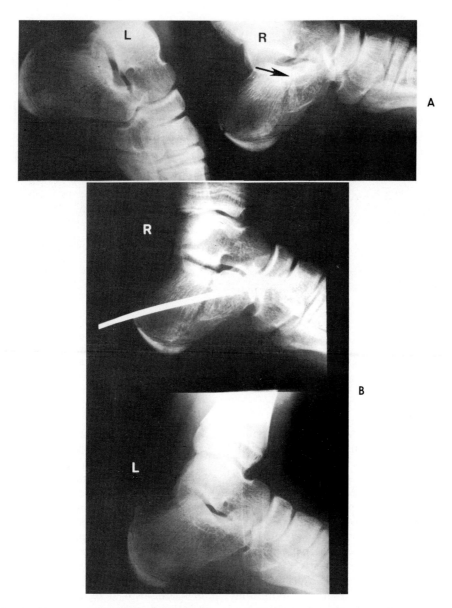

FIG. 55-9. Fourteen-year-old boy injured his right foot playing ice hockey. He jammed his skate into boards with forceful direct impact but without twisting his ankle. He developed immediate, severe pain and was unable to stand. Examination revealed pain, swelling, and tenderness over heel with bony prominence below lateral malleolus. **A,** Fracture of right os calcis with comparative view of uninjured left foot. Note depressed fracture of calcaneus with loss of Böhler's, or tuber, angle. Harris axial view showed involvement of sustentaculum tali and fragment below lateral malleolus. **B,** Intraoperative radiograph with comparison view of normal side. Reduction using Essex-Lopresti technique of reduction and fixation. Heavy Steinman pin extends into cuboid anteriorly; posteriorly, pin is incorporated in short leg cast. Pin is removed in 6 weeks. Note restoration of subtalar anatomy and Böhler's angle.

deep in the interval between the Achilles tendon and the lateral malleolus. Symptoms are consistently reproduced by plantar flexion. These patients have difficulty walking on the tips of toes, downhill, and in high heels. Symptoms are relieved by activities and shoe wear that require dorsiflexion. Swelling and findings of collateral ligament instability are notably absent. In my experience, few patients had symptoms or clinical findings of flexor hallucis tendinitis. Impingement from posteromedial talocal-

caneal coalition is readily excluded by the absence of peroneal spasm and limited subtalar motion typical of coalition. Posterior impingement from coalition usually becomes symptomatic after an ankle sprain or fracture; also a history of chronic recurrent ankle sprains is common. The differential diagnosis includes tendinitis of the Achilles, tibialis posterior, and peroneal tendons. Unlike posterior impingement, these patients feel better in equinus; also palpation over these tendons is asymptomatic.

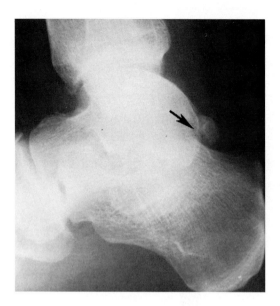

FIG. 55-10. Os trigonum. Posterior process of talus is unfused with talus in fewer than 10% of individuals. This radiograph is an example of asymptomatic prominent os trigonum. Smooth, round surfaces differentiate accessory ossicle from fracture of trigonal process. With right mechanism of injury, this ossicle can be separated and can become temporarily symptomatic.

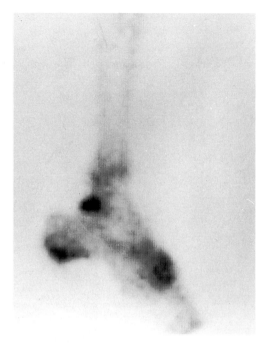

FIG. 55-11. Technetium scan from acute fracture of trigone process. (From the NISMAT collection.)

We have already noted normal ankle stability and asymptomatic palpation over bony landmarks. Comparison examination of the normal side should be routine. A good history of the patient's complaints, mechanism of injury, and clinical and radiographic studies should readily distinguish posterior tibiotalar problems.

Imaging studies. In addition to routine anteroposterior, lateral, and oblique views of the foot and ankle, we take comparison lateral views of the ankle in dorsiflexion and plantar flexion. Often the fracture is best visualized in the dorsiflexion lateral view of the ankle. An incidental, asymptomatic os trigonum is usually smooth and round compared with the irregularly fractured Stieda's process. A technetium bone scan distinguishes trauma from an incidental normal os trigonum (Fig. 55-11).

Treatment. For acute undisplaced fractures of the trigone process the recommended treatment is 6 weeks of cast immobilization with the ankle in neutral position. Initial treatment for chronic injuries is rest, use of anti-inflammatory medications, restriction of activities, and use of an orthosis to prevent plantar flexion. Surgical excision is recommended for the patients who have persistent, disabling pain after nonoperative treatment (Fig. 55-12). The trigone fragment can be removed by either a posteromedial or posterolateral approach. We personally prefer a medial approach. The medial approach affords easy access to the posterior neurovascular bundle, flexor hallucis, and flexor digitorum. The major advantage of the medial approach is that the danger of sural nerve entrapment is avoided. No functional problems with the ankle, lateral collateral instability, or flexor hallucis have been noted following excision of the trigone fragment. We have had great success with athletes who

have undergone excision of a symptomatic os trigonum, and we advocate this procedure for patients with persistent disabling complaints following nonoperative management. Following surgery, convalescence and return to full sports activity averages 4 to 6 months. Results have been gratifying after surgical treatment.

Fractures of the posterior process of the talus are uncommon injuries and probably occur more often than has been reported. Posterior impingement is one of the unrecognized causes of ankle pain in athletes. Recognition and diagnosis depend on an awareness, a good history of mechanism of injury, complaints, clinical examinations, and appropriate imaging studies.

Osteochondritis Dissecans—Dome of Talus

Osteochondral lesions may involve any part of the talus. This discussion is limited to osteochondral defects located in either the medial or lateral border of the talar dome. There is controversy concerning the etiology of these defects in the superior articular surface of the talus. In the past this condition was believed to be caused by a local ischemic necrosis secondary to circulatory impairment. Currently, it is believed that this condition is traumatic in origin.[1,4,22] The lesion is commonly called "osteochondritis dissecans" when there is no history of isolated incidence of trauma. When a specific incident of trauma is elicited, the condition has been called "osteochondral fracture," "transchondral fracture," or "flake" or "dome fracture." We believe the defect is the result of trauma to the superomedial or superolateral border of the trochlea. The trauma may be a single isolated injury associated with concomitant fracture or sprain of the ankle. It is also conceivable that repetitive episodes of an-

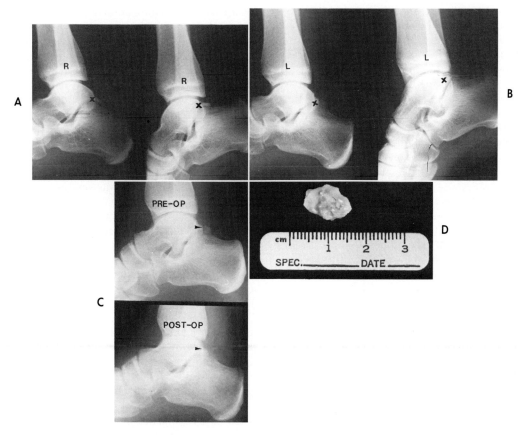

FIG. 55-12. Fifteen-year-old boy was seen with history of pain following hyperplantar-flexion injury of right foot incurred 1 year previously while playing basketball. Diagnosis was "sprained ankle ligaments." His complaints were inability to run, especially downhill, because of posterior ankle pain. Plantar flexion, resisted and passive flexion, and extension of big toe reproduced posterior ankle pain. Localized tenderness was noted over posterior aspect of ankle. Local steroid injection gave temporary relief. **A,** Normal right side in dorsiflexion and plantar flexion. Posterior process of talus is best visualized in plantar flexion. Sudden forceful hyperplantar flexion can result in fracture as posterior process impinges on posterior edge of tibia. **B,** Injured left foot in dorsiflexion and plantar flexion shows fracture of posterior process with impingement and slight irregularity of adjacent tibiotalar articular surfaces. **C,** Preoperative and postoperative views. Findings at surgery were nonunion of posterior process of talus and attritional changes in talus and tibia at site of injury. Patient was relieved of his complaints and resumed sports. **D,** Excised posterior process of talus. Nonunited osteocartilaginous fragment was removed through posteromedial approach.

kle sprain may traumatize this vulnerable part of the talar dome. The defect may be evident in the initial radiographs following an injury. In some cases the defect may not be seen in the initial radiographic study but becomes evident in studies made after healing of the associated ankle injury. The lesion is an osteochondral defect located along the superomedial or superolateral border of the dome, adjacent to the respective malleolus. In our experience the lateral side is involved more often. In anteroposterior orientation the lateral lesion is usually located anterior to the middle part of the lateral border of the trochlea. The medial defect is either in the middle or posterior to the midline of the medial border of the trochlea. The significance of localization in the anteroposterior plane is relevant to an understanding of the mechanism of injury. Accurate anteroposterior localization is also necessary to plan the surgical approach for excision of an osteochondral fragment.

Mechanism of injury. A brief review of the normal anatomy and mechanics of the ankle is necessary to understand the mechanism of injury. The talus functions like a ball bearing between the tibia and the foot, and its dome is susceptible to trauma by compression. Because no ligaments or tendons insert on the dome, this part of the talus is not susceptible to traction-avulsion fractures. There are no muscle attachments on the talus; it moves passively by virtue of articulations and ligament attachments with the other tarsal bones. The wedge-shaped talar dome is wider anteriorly. In dorsiflexion and plantar flexion the dome (trochlea) glides in and out of the ankle mortise. In plantar flexion the posterior half of the dome is in contact with the tibia. Because the talar dome is narrower, it fits more loosely in the mortise—there is more "play." In dorsiflexion the wide anterior portion of the dome occupies the mortise. In dorsiflexion the mortise is fully occupied, and the talus fits more snugly because there is less "play" in the mortise. The mechanism of injury is inversion. An inversion force produces a medial or lateral dome fracture, depending on whether the ankle is plantar flexed or dorsiflexed.

Medial osteochondral fracture of the dome is the result of an inversion injury sustained when the ankle is in plantar flexion. In equinus the narrow posterior part of the dome is in the mortise. Hence the talus can tilt into slight varus, especially when the lateral ligaments are stretched or torn. In equinus a sudden inversion force compresses the tibia against the talus, shearing the posteromedial border of the dome, which is in contact with the tibia. This is the typical mechanism that occurs in running and jumping sports. For example, if a basketball player twists an ankle when landing from a jump and the foot is in equinovarus, a sudden inversion force compresses the tibia against the medial border of the talar dome, causing an osteochondral fracture of the posteromedial border. This mechanism is often associated with lateral ligament injury.

Lateral osteochondral fractures of the dome result from an inversion force exerted when the ankle is dorsiflexed. In dorsiflexion the widest anterior part of the dome is in the mortise. The mortise is fully occupied by the talus, resulting in a snug contact between the talus and the fibula. With a sudden inversion force in this position, the superolateral border of the talus impinges on the adjacent fibula, causing an infraction of the lateral dome of the talus. Because the anterior portion of the talus is in the mortise, the defect is usually located more anteriorly than in the medial fracture. The same mechanism can also cause concomitant chip fractures of the medial surface of the fibula when the talus is forced against the adjacent fibula.

In cadaver experiments Berndt and Harty[4] produced lateral lesions by exerting an inversion stress with the ankle dorsiflexed. When the same inversion force was applied in plantar flexion, they produced osteochondral fractures of the medial border of the talar dome.

Diagnosis. It should be emphasized that the symptoms and clinical findings may be acute or chronic, and the diagnosis in acute injuries may be difficult. The lesion may be unrecognized or diagnosed as a ligament sprain. It is easy to overlook this fracture because many patients with chronic cases have lax ankles, and the patients with acute cases may have associated lateral ligament injuries. In acute cases the osteochondral defect of the talus may be obscured by associated ankle fractures.

The dome fracture may not be evident on the first radiographs and is detected at the time of open reduction of a fracture or becomes evident in subsequent radiographs. In all open reductions for ankle fracture the joint should be inspected for osteochondral fractures. In the chronic cases the athlete may or may not recall a specific incident of trauma, and the lesion may conceivably result from repeated sprains of overuse. In chronic cases the patient complains of pain and tenderness localized

over either the anterolateral or anteromedial aspect of the ankle. Patients may have mechanical complaints with recurrent exacerbations of symptoms associated with sports. The swelling over the medial or lateral compartments is usually minimal, except in acute exacerbations. These patients usually complain of a dull, aching pain after the acute episode subsides. In a review of 49 osteochondral fractures Alexander and Lichtman[1] found that 92% had a prior severe ankle sprain or an ankle fracture. These patients complained of chronic symptoms before the definitive diagnosis was made.

Radiographic examination. The diagnosis can usually be made with standard anteroposterior, lateral, and oblique mortise views of the ankle. On occasion the lesion may be best visualized in views of the foot. As previously noted, on occasion the fracture may not be evident in the initial radiographs. Occasionally, a healed defect may be an incidental finding, and the history and clinical findings must be correlated with the radiograph. The osteochondral defect may be overlooked in radiographs of poor quality.

Supplemental radiographic studies may be necessary in suspected cases. These studies include tomography, arthrotomograms, bone scanning, and high-resolution CT scanning (Fig. 55-13). In selected cases, CT scanning provides accurate visualization of the extent and location of the defect. Osteochondral defects should be differentiated from sprains of lateral ligaments and syndesmosis, posttraumatic osteophytes of the ankle, osteoid osteoma, and subchondral cysts. Normal subtalar motion readily excludes problems involving the subtalar and midtarsal joints.

Treatment. Incomplete and undisplaced osteochondral fractures can be treated with plaster immobilization,

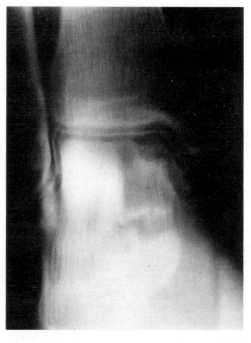

FIG. 55-13. Arthrotomogram of medial dome fracture. (From the NISMAT collection.)

early motion, and delayed weight bearing until radiographs show evidence of healing.

Early surgical excision is recommended for displaced fragments. Open reduction with internal fixation has been advised.[1] We prefer to excise the fragment to avoid the risk of nonunion and arthritic changes and the necessity of prolonged non–weight bearing postoperatively.

The surgical procedure consists of an arthrotomy with excision of the loose fragment. The fragment is usually removed in one piece. The edges of the crater are smoothed, and the nidus is perforated with multiple drill holes made with a fine Kirschner wire. After surgical excision we prefer protected weight bearing as soon as the wound is well healed and the patient can tolerate it. The rationales for early weight bearing are to stimulate better healing of the articular defect with physiologic stress and to avoid disuse atrophy and stiffness. Alexander and Lichtman[1] reported 88% excellent long-term results after early and delayed excision of osteochondral fragments.

Lateral lesions can be exposed and excised through an anterolateral arthrotomy of the ankle. Exposure and excision of the lateral lesion is easier than the medial because the defect is usually located in the anterolateral border of the dome. The lesion is visualized by plantar flexing the ankle, and the lateral laxity facilitates exposure. Exposure and excision of medial fragments is more difficult because the site of injury is more posterior and the medial compartment is tighter. Excision of a medial fragment may require a limited partial incision of the deltoid. Because exact location in the anteroposterior plane is more important for the medial lesion, CT scanning may be necessary. Before surgery the patient should be warned that osteotomy of the malleolus may be necessary to expose and remove a medial dome defect; we routinely expose medial lesions through an anteromedial arthrotomy so that we are prepared to do an osteotomy of the medial malleolus, if necessary. In doing a medial malleolar osteotomy, it should be remembered that the posterior tibial tendon lies in a fibroosseous tunnel located in the malleolus and not posterior to the bony prominence. Before the osteotomy is performed, a screw hole is predrilled in the malleolus in preparation for rigid anatomic fixation of the malleolar fragment. As another precaution the malleolus should be osteotomized below the "shoulder" of the tibia, distal to the top of the talus. The malleolar fragment, with the attached deltoid, is reflected distally to expose the medial aspect of the ankle. If there is any question regarding postoperative stability, a Kirschner wire can be inserted in addition to the screw to prevent rotation. Because the site of osteotomy is below the weight-bearing part of the mortise, earlier mobilization and weight bearing can be allowed. The risks of osteotomy include the danger of nonunion and iatrogenic injury to the articular surfaces. Arthroscopic surgery by an experienced arthroscopist with proper equipment also has a place in selected cases, particularly for lateral lesions (see Chapter 21).

Summary. Osteochondritis dissecans is considered an osteochondral fracture. This condition should be included among the causes of occult ankle pain. It is often associated with ankle fractures and sprains. An osteochondral fracture may be located in the superomedial or superolateral border of the talar dome. The lateral osteochondral fracture is incurred by an inversion injury with the ankle dorsiflexed. An acute inversion injury with the foot in plantar flexion results in a posteromedial fracture of the dome. The diagnosis can usually be made on routine radiographs or occasionally a bone scan, or CT scanning may be necessary. Accurate location in the anteroposterior plane is essential to planning surgical approach, especially for the defects in the medial border of the talar dome. The method of treatment is tailored for each patient. Nonoperative treatment is indicated for nondisplaced fractures. Surgical excision is recommended for displaced fragments and for cases of persistent disability after conservative treatment. Postponing surgical treatment does not deleteriously affect the long-term result; therefore there is no harm in temporizing. Early surgery may be considered in the high-performance or professional athlete who is anxious to return to sports as soon as possible. The diagnosis demands a good history of the mechanism of injury, record of the complaints, physical examinations, and radiographic studies.

Forefoot
Fifth Metatarsal Problems

The fifth metatarsal is a common site of foot problems in the athlete. There are several entities that may develop at the base of the fifth metatarsal, and they should be considered separately because of their clinical significance.

Fifth metatarsal problems

- Iselin's disease
- Os vesalianum
- Avulsion fracture of base
- Fractures of the distal one third
- Jones fracture of the proximal one third

Traction apophysitis of the fifth metatarsal base— Iselin's disease. Traction apophysitis of the proximal end of the fifth metatarsal was first described by Iselin, a German, in 1912.[20] This uncommon entity is caused by the peroneus brevis attachment. This entity occurs during the period of rapid growth. It is an overuse syndrome that occurs in running, jumping, and inversion stress. This apophysis can also be irritated by a snug-fitting shoe, especially skates. These patients have painful swelling and localized point tenderness over the peroneal insertion on the tuberosity; resisted contraction of the peroneal brevis reproduces symptoms. Radiographs may show soft-tissue swelling over the apophysis or slight separation of the apophysis. We have seen unilateral and bilateral involvement. Usually the parents are concerned about a fracture or "bone disease." The apophyseal line is longitudinal and is readily differentiated from the transverse line seen with an avulsion fracture. This physeal line is

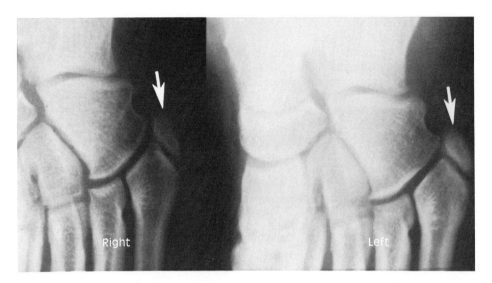

FIG. 55-14. Os vesalianum. Major League baseball player had bilateral prominences at bases of fifth metatarsals. Overlying bursa and callus were noted. Oblique views show bilateral os vesalianum. This ossicle should not be mistaken for avulsion fracture or os peroneum. Os peroneum is an accessory ossicle located more proximally in peroneus longus, juxtaposed to calcaneocuboid joint. Symptoms in this case were relieved with proper footwear. In selected cases, surgical excision may be indicated.

present and is an incidental finding in children without complaints and negative clinical findings.[8] A technetium bone scan shows increased uptake, but it is rarely necessary. Treatment is symptomatic rest and avoidance of the aggravating activity. When pain and tenderness are completely gone, rehabilitation, stretching, and strengthing exercises may be instituted to tolerance. This condition is comparable to Osgood-Schlatter disease; symptoms always subside with skeletal maturity.

Os vesalianum. Os vesalianum should not be mistaken for an avulsion fracture (Fig. 55-14). The os vesalianum is actually an accessory bone that lies within the insertion of the peroneus brevis tendon. The os peroneum is within the peroneus longus in juxtaposition to the cuboid at which point the peroneus longus enters the sole of the foot. There may be a symptomatic bursa overlying the prominent base of the fifth metatarsal in a splayfoot or an os vesalianum that should be treated with appropriately padded footwear and possibly excision at maturity for recalcitrant symptomatic cases. In the skeletally immature athlete an apophysitis of the growth center may cause localized pain and swelling as a result of overuse or improper footwear (Iselin's disease).

Fractures of the proximal fifth metatarsal. Of all the metatarsals the fifth is the most vulnerable and susceptible to fracture. The characteristic features and the management of fractures of the base, proximal one third, and distal diaphysis are discussed here.

The most common fracture occurs at the base. The base of the fifth metatarsal tuberosity is conical and extends more proximally. It is weaker and more cancellous; the peroneus brevis inserts on this bony prominence. A sudden inversion stress results in an avulsion fracture of the tendon insertion. In children, fracture must be dif-

ferentiated from a normal apophysis. A normal apophyseal line is longitudinal, whereas fracture lines are in the transverse plane (Fig. 55-15). Two accessory ossicles, the os vesalianum and os peroneum, are readily recognized and differentiated by their round, smooth surfaces and extraosseous location proximal and lateral to the base of the metatarsal. Treatment for most cases is protective strapping, surgical wooden shoe with cane or crutches during the initial acute phase, and activity and weight bearing as tolerated. In selected cases a walking cast is required for 4 to 6 weeks to relieve pain and allow more normal activities while avoiding the inconvenience of crutches or a cane. These fractures usually heal in a few weeks without residual disability.[8]

Fractures of the distal third. Fractures of the distal one third of the fifth metatarsal usually result from a fall. As the foot hits the ground, there is a combination of a direct and indirect twisting force. This is an oblique or spiral fracture in the distal one third; usually there is minimal displacement. The treatment is essentially the same as outlined for avulsion fractures of the base (Fig. 55-16). These fractures are characterized by swelling and discoloration over the dorsolateral aspect with point tenderness over the distal one third.

Jones fracture. Transverse fracture in the proximal one third of the diaphysis of the fifth metatarsal, unlike the previously described fractures, is not a "simple" fracture to be taken lightly. This injury is notorious for delayed union, nonunion, and refracture after apparent healing. This fracture has been given the eponym "Jones fracture." Sir Robert Jones[15] himself suffered this injury while dancing. He described his own injury and five other cases in 1902. The mechanism of injury described by Jones was almost identical to that reported by Ka-

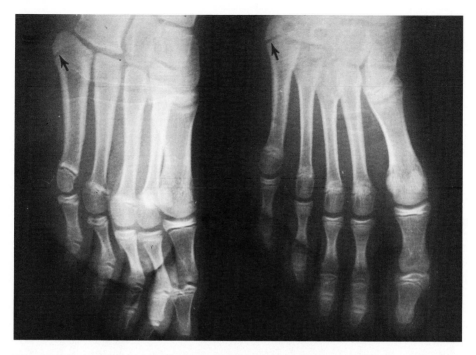

FIG. 55-15. Fractured base of fifth metatarsal. This 11-year-old boy twisted his foot while running and felt a "pull" with immediate pain on lateral aspect of foot. Radiographs show simple fracture of fifth metatarsal. These heal with symptomatic treatment, usually short leg weight-bearing cast for few weeks. Notice fracture line is oblique and readily distinguished from epiphyseal line, which is longitudinal and parallel to metatarsal.

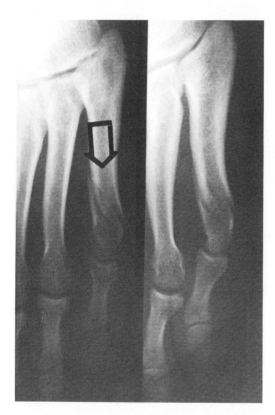

FIG. 55-16. Fracture of distal third of fifth metatarsal. Notice fracture is spiral or oblique in distal diaphysis. Fracture line is not smooth or wide. This injury rarely causes problems. This is a "nuisance" injury that heals with routine symptomatic treatment.

vanaugh, Brower, and Mann[16] in 1978—the inverted foot is loaded in weight bearing "with the heel off the ground." This is the mechanism often reported in basketball injuries. Typically, this is a transverse fracture in the proximal one third of the diaphysis distal to the cuboid metatarsal and the intermetatarsal ligaments. In some cases the initial radiographs may be negative or show a partial incomplete fracture; after several weeks, repeat radiographs show a complete, wide fracture line with smooth edges, unlike the thin fracture line usually seen in other fractures. The radiographic appearance of the fracture line along with the following characteristics suggest a stress fracture: (1) patients may not seek immediate medical attention, (2) history of minimal trauma, (3) minimal swelling, (4) absence of the usual hematoma discoloration, and (5) prolonged healing time. Some patients have reported vague discomfort in the foot before the minimal trauma that produced the fracture, again suggesting the possibility of a stress fracture. The absence of external periosteal callus and obliteration of the medullary canal in the healing phase distinguishes this fracture from the usual metatarsal fracture. There is varying opinion regarding treatment.

Torg et al[30] suggest that a short leg non–weight-bearing cast helps healing. In cases of delayed union, nonunion, and refracture the advantages of open reduction must be considered. Torg et al[30] and Dameron[8] recommended open reduction and bone grafting. Kavanaugh, Brower, and Mann[16] have reported good results with intramedullary screw fixation without bone graft for cases of delayed union, nonunion, and selected fresh injuries.

For initial treatment of a new injury, we use a below-knee, non–weight-bearing cast for 3 weeks followed by a walking cast until radiographs and clinical examination show solid union. Even after union the patient is forewarned regarding the probability of refracture, delayed healing, and nonunion.

In cases of delayed union and nonunion we have used intramedullary screw fixation with good results (Fig. 55-17). In selected cases, such as professional or high-performance athletes, we consider initial open reduction to minimize disability time and avoid refracture. We have treated one case of refracture successfully with a walking cast.

Sesamoiditis of the Great Toe

The sesamoid bones of the great toe lie within the conjoint tendons of (1) the abductor hallucis and medial head of the flexor hallucis brevis, and (2) the adductor

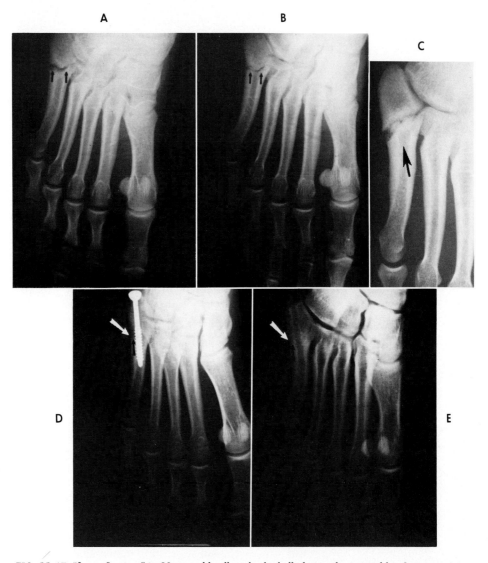

FIG. 55-17. "Jones fracture" in 22-year-old college basketball player who twisted his foot, sustaining fracture in proximal third of fifth metatarsal. Treated with plaster cast for 6 weeks. At follow-up visit 11 weeks after injury, patient complained of pain, tenderness, and slight swelling over fracture. Options were (1) more plaster immobilization, (2) restriction of activities and rest, and (3) surgery. Patient returned 3 weeks later with increased pain. He elected to have surgery 3 months after injury to minimize disability time, resume sports sooner, and avoid danger of refracture. Three years previously a similar fracture in other foot eventually healed without surgery. **A,** Initial radiograph. Typical transverse fracture in proximal third of fifth metatarsal. **B,** After 6 weeks. No callus. Note widening of fracture line with smooth edges. **C,** Spot preoperative radiograph shows wide fracture line, sclerosis, and obliteration of intramedullary canal. This establishes nonunion. **D,** Compression screw was used with no bone graft. Plaster immobilization was used for 6 weeks. **E,** Screw was removed 6 months postoperatively. Solid union was achieved. Return to athletics was asymptomatic.

hallucis and the lateral head of the flexor hallucis brevis. Partition of the sesamoids is common.

The function of these bones is to transmit weight from the ground to the first metatarsal head. The sesamoids are pulled distally when the metatarsophalangeal joint is dorsiflexed, and this functionally extends the weight-bearing surface of the first metatarsal plantarward, below the lesser metatarsals. Hence the sesamoids bear considerable weight. Overuse syndromes can cause inflammation in this area that is consistent with a diagnosis of sesamoiditis. Aseptic necrosis and chondromalacia can also occur. All of these problems may respond to treatment with arch supports, metatarsal pads, or a metatarsal bar, along with decreased activity. The initial treatment should be nonoperative.*

Differentiating between bipartite sesamoid and sesamoid fracture is a common clinical problem. Fracture is associated with pain localized at the sesamoid, sharp radiographic margins, and unilateral involvement. A bipartite sesamoid has smooth radiographic margins, is not painful in the absence of injury, and is frequently bilateral. Jahss[14] reported that bipartite sesamoids are larger than uninjured, normal sesamoids. Occasionally,

---

*Editors' note: Steadfast attention to making the supports and bars take weight behind the sesamoid is extremely important and requires careful attention to placement, height, and width of the bars or inserts. (See Chapter 27 for technique.)

because of repetitive overloading, stress fractures of the sesamoids occur. These are best seen radiographically on sesamoid views. A technetium bone scan is often necessary to confirm the diagnosis of fracture vs. a normal bipartite sesamoid. Sesamoid studies demand comparable views. Stress-fractured sesamoids respond to rest and metatarsal unloading with pads or a bar (Fig. 55-18).

In our experience the fibular sesamoid of the great toe is usually the one to be fractured, although some authors have reported fracture of the tibial sesamoid to be more common.[11,14] Considered risks of surgical removal of the lateral sesamoid should include the possibility of a postoperative hallux varus caused by weakening of the valgus forces of the adductor hallucis and the lateral head of the flexor hallucis brevis and painful plantar scar. Metatarsalgia may be a persistent problem regardless of the mode of treatment. A localized form of Sudeck's atrophy, which is an extremely challenging therapeutic problem, can occur from combinations of patient disposition, delay in diagnosis, and impaired function.

Fractures and Dislocations of the Toes

Fractures and dislocations of the toes occasionally occur in athletes. Younger athletes with open physes are more likely to sustain a fracture through the physis rather than simple dislocation. This is a reflection of the comparative weakness of the growth area at the hyper-

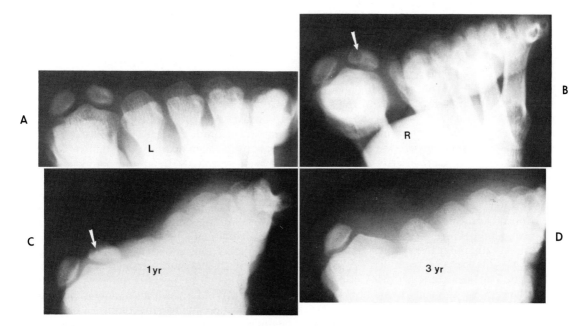

FIG. 55-18. Young runner complained of persistent pain beneath first metatarsal head of her right foot. **A,** Normal left foot sesamoid view. Note how sesamoids extend weight-bearing surface further plantarward than first metatarsal in comparison with other four metatarsals. **B,** Sesamoid view of right foot clearly shows fracture of lateral sesamoid of great toe. **C,** Patient was treated with restricted activities and metatarsal bar. Her fracture was healing, but some pain persisted. We advised further conservative care. **D,** Patient returned 3 years after injury and after excision of fibular sesamoid elsewhere. Pain was now increased, and symptoms of metatarsalgia were prominent. These cases have a guarded prognosis after surgical excision. We prefer nonoperative treatment, plaster immobilization, and shoe correction or orthosis.

trophic cell zone between the calcified and uncalcified areas and has been attributed to the minimal amount of collagenous matrix in this layer.[24] Because of the superior strength of the ligaments in adolescents, avulsion fractures rather than sprains are the rule. Growth aberrations caused by physeal damage and bony bridging can occur.

Knowledge of the orientation, location, and time of appearance of the physes of the foot is important to avoid confusion in the diagnosis of fracture. Congenital anomalies, accessory ossicles, irregular epiphyseal centers, and bipartite bones can also present problems in diagnosis. In such circumstances the examiner should rely on the mechanism of injury, local physical findings, and comparison radiographs for help. Most fractures of the foot and ankle do not cause difficulties in diagnosis or treatment; however, certain fractures require special consideration.

Subungual Exostosis

Subungual exostosis is a bony projection that may be confused with an ingrown toenail. An exostosis can be caused by repetitive trauma or represented by a small bone tumor.[3,23,33] The common site of occurrence is the dorsomedial aspect of the distal phalanx of the great toe, but it can be present in the lesser toes or the fingers.[25] We have seen several adolescent runners who complained of discomfort from local irritation caused by shoe pressure. In fact, the patient commonly trims the toenail to alleviate the painful pressure over the mass. Deformities of the nail are common, and on occasion the athlete may have been treated unsuccessfully for an ingrown toenail.

Radiographically, the mass is osteocartilaginous and almost always located on the dorsomedial aspect of the distal phalanx of the great toe. The stalk may be narrow or broad, and the medullary canal of the phalanx and the stalk are confluent. Overlying irregularities of the nail may be noticeable.

Zimmerman[33] suggested excising the mass through the lateral or distal aspect of the toe, leaving the toenail in place, or partially removing the nail plate to improve exposure. We perform the procedure using local tourniquet hemostasis, and we remove the entire nail for best visualization. It is important to remove the entire mass; otherwise, recurrence is probable.[23] The defect remaining in the nail bed should be dressed open, and it rapidly heals by secondary intention. The patient should be forewarned about possible toenail deformities.

Although the mass has been compared with an osteochondroma, it differs in that the stalk is not always directed away from the physis and occurs at the end of the bone, opposite from the growth center. It is also reported histologically that the cartilaginous cap is composed of fibrocartilage and not the typical hyaline cartilage of the true osteochondroma.

Soft-Tissue Injuries
Posterior Tibial Tendon

The posterior tibial tendon is a prime supinator of the foot and assists in plantar flexion. The tendon reinforces the medial aspect of the calcaneonavicular socket and normally inserts into the navicular tuberosity, sustentaculum tali, spring ligament, cuneiforms, and plantar metatarsal bases. By reinforcing the spring ligament, this tendon aids in support of the talar head and prevents pes planus. Many cases of rupture of the tibialis posterior have been reported to occur in previous flatfeet, and excessive strain has been proposed as the mechanism.[5,7,17] Cases of rupture after multiple steroid injections have also been noted.[27] After rupture of the posterior tibial tendon, there is a tendency for increased heel valgus and pronation that is a consequence of the loss of a medial restraint on the tarsal navicular, and this leads to lateral subluxation of the navicular. Attenuation of the spring ligament as part of the degenerative process leading to the tendon rupture may be an additional factor in promoting the progressive flatfoot.

Tendinitis and tenosynovitis of the posterior tibial tendon can be caused by a direct blow, irritation by a shoe or equipment, and overuse. Occasionally there may be a history of one isolated incident of overstretching, and the tendon may be torn partially or completely. We have encountered ganglions around the posterior tibial tendon, which cause a soft cystic swelling in the region of the malleolus. These patients have a typical history of swelling that varies in size commensurate with activity. It should be remembered that the posterior tibial tendon is not posterior to the medial malleolus but is located in a fibroosseous tunnel within the substance of the malleolus. For this reason the tendon is prone to be irritated by irregular osteophytes in the region of the medial malleolus. Posterior tibial tendon irritation is treated by rest, heel elevation, and antiinflammatory medications. Surgical lysis with excision of the bony osteophyte may be necessary in chronically symptomatic cases. In the young, healthy athlete, we have seen only partial ruptures of the posterior tibial tendon.

Peroneal Tendons

Problems involving the peroneal tendons in athletes may result from a direct blow or a combination of a direct injury accompanied by sudden dorsiflexion with eversion. Subluxation of the peroneal tendons occurs when the retinaculum that maintains the tendons posterior to the fibula is torn. Thus the retinaculum can be torn as a consequence of acute injury, stretching by repetitive trauma, or overuse. This condition should be differentiated from a ligamentous injury or tenosynovitis of the tendons. One or both of the tendons may be involved. A careful history and examination readily differentiate a subluxation of the peroneal tendons from an ankle ligament injury. Many of these patients have an associated tenosynovitis. The patient complains of a "clicking," slipping sensation over the lateral malleolus. Localized tenderness is present over the peroneal tendons. The examiner may see or even feel subluxation of these tendons as the patient contracts the peroneal tendons against resistance. Forceful, repetitive equinus position—as in ballet—can predispose to pathologic conditions of the peroneal tendons. In chronic disabling cases satisfactory results have been recorded with a surgical correction as advocated by O'Donoghue[21] and Savastano.[26]

Partial tear of the peroneus brevis tendon occurs with

a severe inversion sprain. We have also seen this partial rupture associated with ankle dislocation. This tear is usually a longitudinal splitting of the peroneus brevis that is in close contact with the fibula. Clinically, these patients have a soft swelling over the peroneal tendon just proximal to the lateral malleolus. Excision of the torn portion of the tendon and retinaculum repair, if necessary, has produced good results with relief of complaints.

Flexor Hallucis Longus Muscle

The flexor hallucis longus muscle arises from the posterolateral aspect of the lower leg and runs medially to enter the foot in a groove in the posterior surface of the talus. This groove is formed by the larger, lateral tubercle, which serves as an attachment for the posterior talofibular ligament and a smaller tubercle, medially. Distally, the flexor hallucis longus tendon passes under the sustentaculum tali, which serves as a pulley. In the sole of the foot it is located above the flexor digitorum longus to which it is connected by a tendinous slip. After it crosses the common toe flexor, the tendon runs forward between the two sesamoids of the great toe and inserts onto the base of the distal phalanx. Because of its anatomic relationships and function, tenosynovitis, partial ruptures, and nodules of this muscle are reflected in problems with the great toe that may include pain, triggering, and difficulties with push-off. This has been most often discussed in relation to ballet dancers and has been responsive to antiinflammatory medications and, on occasion, surgery.

Laceration of the flexor hallucis longus commonly occurs in the region of the medial arch of the foot near the first metatarsophalangeal joint. In our experience many of these injuries are secondary to puncture wounds from stepping on glass or other sharp objects and may involve the metatarsophalangeal joint capsule. We have had extensive operative experience with congenital foot deformities in which prior operative procedures have included transection without repair of the flexor hallucis longus, and there have been few significant functional problems related to the great toe in children. There is a connecting slip of tendon between the flexor digitorum longus and the flexor hallucis longus in the sole of the foot that can provide active interphalangeal flexion of the great toe if the tendon is interrupted proximal to this decussation. Nonoperative treatment can give good results if deformities of the interphalangeal joint do not result. Operative treatment with direct repair is an attractive option because of the possibility of restoring active interphalangeal joint flexion. However, because the flexor hallucis longus tendon is anatomically wedged between the two sesamoids, the two heads of the flexor hallucis brevis, the plantar plate of the metatarsophalangeal and interphalangeal joints, and the sensory branches of the medial plantar nerve, the possibility of independent interphalangeal joint flexion may not be realized. Loss of function in this joint is rarely a clinical problem despite loss of flexion, even in the athlete. However, neuritic symptoms caused by laceration are common complaints after such an injury. There have been isolated reports of deformity of the great toe interphalangeal joint after the occurrence of flexor hallucis longus laceration.[10] It has been our observation that the younger patients have fewer complaints and problems with this injury.

Abductor Hallucis Problems

The abductor hallucis arises from the medial plantar surface of the os calcis and runs forward and medially to the medial sesamoid of the great toe. The posterior neurovascular bundle enters the sole of the foot beneath this muscle belly. This structure is prone to strain from overuse, contusion, or shoe pressure. Injury to the abductor hallucis can be mistaken for symptomatic pes planus or even a tarsal tunnel syndrome because of its proximity to the posterior tibial nerve. Improper footwear is often the cause of symptoms in this area. The symptoms usually subside with rest, proper footwear, and antiinflammatory medication.*

---

*Editors' note: In sprinters who do not strike on the heel as much as on the midfoot and toes, abductor hallucis strain can be severe and associated with cramps. Stretching and orthotics, as well as gait analysis, may be necessary in the serious runner. It is important to check the entire leg for weakness when symptoms have been present for more than 6 weeks. Proximal weakness, if not rehabilitated, may lead to recurrence.

REFERENCES

1. Alexander AH, Lichtman DM: Surgical treatment of transchondral talar-dome fractures, *J Bone Joint Surg* 62A:646, 1980.
2. Barnett CH, Napier JR: The axis of rotation at the ankle joint in man, its influence upon the form of the talus, and the mobility of the fibula, *J Anat* 86:1, 1952.
3. Bendl BJ: Subungual exostosis, *Cutis* 26:260, 1980.
4. Brahms MA: Common foot problems, *J Bone Joint Surg* 49A:1653, 1967.
5. Berndt AL, Harty M: Transchondral fractures (osteochondritis dissecans) of the talus, *J Bone Joint Surg* 41A:988, 1959.
6. Cowell HR, Elener V: Rigid painful flatfoot secondary to tarsal coalition, *Clin Orthop* 177:54, 1983.
7. Cozen L: Posterior tibial tenosynovitis secondary to foot strain, *Clin Orthop* 42:101, 1965.
8. Dameron TB: Fractures and anatomical variations of the proximal portion of the fifth metatarsal, *J Bone Joint Surg* 57A:788, 1975.
9. Fick R: *Handbuch der anatomie und mechanik der gelenke: Handbuch der anatomie des menchen*, vol 2, sec 1, part 3, Jena, Germany, 1911, Gustav Fischer Verlag.
10. Frenette JP, Jackson DW: Lacerations of the flexor hallucis longus in the young athlete, *J Bone Joint Surg* 59A:673, 1977.
11. Helal B: The great toe sesamoid bones: the lus or lost souls of Ushaia, *Clin Orthop* 157:82, 1981.
12. Helfet AJ: *The management of internal derangements of the knee*, London, 1963, JB Lippincott.
13. Inman VT: *The joints of the ankle*, Baltimore, 1976, Williams & Wilkins.
14. Jahss MH: The sesamoids of the hallux, *Clin Orthop* 157:88, 1981.
15. Jones R: Fracture of the base of the fifth metatarsal bone by indirect violence, *Ann Surg* 35:697, 1902.
16. Kavanaugh JH, Brower TD, Mann RV: The Jones fracture revisited, *J Bone Joint Surg* 60A:776, 1978.
17. Kettlekamp DB, Alexander HH: Spontaneous rupture of the posterior tibial tendon, *J Bone Joint Surg* 51A:759, 1969.
18. Reference deleted in proofs.
19. Leach RE, James S, Wasilewski S: Achilles tendonitis, *Am J Sports Med* 9:93, 1981.
20. Lehman RC et al: Iselin's disease, *Am J Sports Med* 14(6):494, 1986.
21. O'Donoghue D: *Treatment of injuries to athletes*, Philadelphia, 1962, WB Saunders.
22. O'Farrell TA, Costello BG: Osteochondritis dissecans of the talus, *J Bone Joint Surg* 64B:494, 1982.

23. Oliveira AD et al: Subungual exostosis: treatment as an office procedure, *J Dermatol Surg Oncol* 6:555, 1980.
24. Salter RB, Harris WR: Injuries involving the epiphyseal plate, *J Bone Joint Surg* 38A:587, 1956.
25. Sarrafian SK: *Anatomy of the foot and ankle*, Philadelphia, 1983, JB Lippincott.
26. Savastano AA: Surgical treatment of recurrent dislocation peroneal tendons. dic Surgeons, Chicago, personal communication.
27. Simpson RR, Gudas CJ: Posterior tibial tendon rupture in a world-class runner, *J Foot Surg* 22:74, 1983.
28. Tachdjian MO: *Pediatric orthopedics*, vol 2, Philadelphia, 1972, WB Saunders.
29. Reference deleted in proofs.
30. Torg JS et al: Fractures of the base of the fifth metatarsal distal to the tuberosity, *J Bone Joint Surg* 66A:209, 1984.
31. Turco VJ: Injuries to the ankle and foot in athletics, *Orthop Clin North Am* 8:669, 1977.
32. Reference deleted in proofs.
33. Zimmerman EH: Subungual exostosis, *Cutis* 19:185, 1977.

ADDITIONAL READINGS

Dezwart DF, Davidson JS: Rupture of posterior tibial tendon associated with fracture of the ankle, *J Bone Joint Surg* 65A:260, 1983.

Inman VT (ed): *DuVries' surgery of the foot*, ed 3, St Louis, 1973, Mosby.

Johnson KA: Tibialis posterior tendon rupture, *Clin Orthop* 177:140, 1983.

Kumar SJ et al: Osseous and non-osseous coalition of the middle-facet of the talocalcaneal joint, *J Bone Joint Surg* 74A(4):529, 1992.

Leach RE et al: Pathologic hindfoot conditions in the athlete, *Clin Orthop* 177:116, 1983.

Macnicol MF, Voutsinas S: Surgical treatment of the symptomatic accessory navicular, *J Bone Joint Surg* 66B:218, 1984.

Mann RA (ed): *DuVries' surgery of the foot*, ed 4, St Louis, 1978, Mosby.

Moorman CT, Monto RR, Bassett FH: So-called trigger ankle due to an aberrant flexor hallucis longus muscle in a tennis player, J Bone Joint Surg 74A(2):294, 1992.

Parra G: Stress fractures of the sesamoids of the foot, *Clin Orthop* 18:281, 1960.

Peiro A et al: Triplane distal tibial epiphyseal fracture, *Clin Orthop* 160:196, 1981.

Powell HDW, Cantab MA: Pes planovalgus in children, *Clin Orthop* 177:133, 1983.

Schmidt TL, Weiner DS: Calcaneal fractures in children: an evaluation of the nature of the injury in 56 children, *Clin Orthop* 171:150, 1982.

Smith AD, Carter JR, Marcus RE: The os vesalianum: an unusual case of lateral foot pain, *Orthopedics* 7:86, 1984.

Ward WG, Bergfeld JA: Fluoroscopic demonstration of acute disruption of the fifth metatorsophalangeal sesamoid bones, Am J Sports Med 21(6):895, 1993.

Williams R: Chronic nonspecific tendovaginitis of tibialis posterior, *J Bone Joint Surg* 45B:542, 1963.

CHAPTER 56 Knee Injuries

Alan M. Strizak

Epidemiologists report yearly increases in sports injuries of youngsters. This may reflect an actual increase in incidence or merely an increased awareness of the problem among primary care physicians, or some combination of the two. While many of these injuries are similar to those occurring in adults, knee injuries in the pediatric population present special problems, both in diagnosis and treatment. This chapter is devoted to the unique problem of the injured knee in the pediatric athlete.

The pediatric knee is generally protected by its softer cartilage, more pliable bone, and ligamentous attachments that are stronger than the periosteum supporting a wide-open growth plate. The child is lighter than the adult and has a lower center of gravity, shorter lever arms, and decreased muscle strength, thereby considerably reducing the magnitude of forces that can be generated across the lower extremities. As any builder knows, this combination of lower center of mass and more pliable materials protects buttressing structures from stress and strain. Thus clinically detectable injuries to ligaments and menisci of the knee are unusual occurrences in children.

EXTENSOR MECHANISM

The extensor mechanism is the most common location for a symptomatic pathologic condition in the skeletally immature athlete's knee. It is also indirectly involved in almost every other abnormality that upsets knee mechanics. Its health and strength are the barometer most often used to gauge overall knee function.

Larson[52] reported that 9.2% of knee injuries that were incurred at age 15 or younger were subluxations or dislocations of the patella. This reinforces Hughston's work[40] that showed that 65% of subluxations or dislocations of the patella occur before the age of 18 years in athletes.

Certainly, a large percentage of undiagnosed or misdiagnosed "internal derangements of the knee" in the prearthroscopic era can be attributed to undetected pathologic conditions of the extensor mechanism. Although the patellofemoral pain syndromes are most often ascribed to the loose-ligamented young female, Hughston[40] found that of 35 athletes with recurrent dislocations and subluxations of the patella, 77% were male and only 23% were female. Furthermore, recurrences after the initial patellar dislocation were relatively frequent. Cofield and Bryan[22] found that 44% of patients suffered at least one recurrence following their acute patellar dislocation. The average follow-up time was 11.8 years, but 13 of the 48 cases came to reconstructive surgery between 5 months and 5 years after the initial dislocation. Crosby and Insall[23] confirmed Hughston's observation of a decrease in tendency for redislocation with age.

Mechanics of the Patellofemoral Joint

The bony patella protects the anterior aspect of the knee and provides a mechanical advantage for the quadriceps in tibiofemoral extension. As a sesamoid bone it glides in a helical fashion over a 5- to 7-cm course in and out of the femoral sulcus with flexion and extension of the knee.[24] The exact course and stability of the patella are determined by both bony and soft-tissue relationships. The articular surface of the patella pays a large biomechanical price, with patellofemoral compression forces minimal in standing, less than body weight during walking, up to 2.5 times body weight with stair climbing, and increasing up to 8 times body weight in performing a full squat (Fig. 56-1).[48] The extensor mechanism provides the dynamic stability needed by the knee joint to support weight and yet remain mobile in the anteroposterior plane. The normal motion of the patella on the

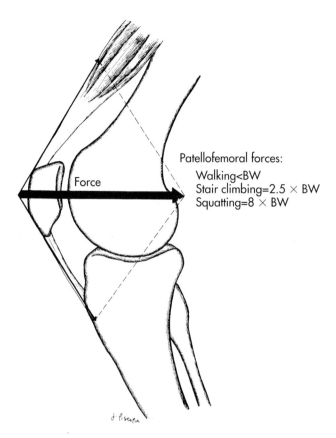

FIG. 56-1. Patellofemoral forces vary with knee flexion.

Patellofemoral forces:

Walking<BW
Stair climbing=2.5 × BW
Squatting=8 × BW

femur is guided passively by bony contour and patellofemoral ligaments.[24] It is also fine-tuned dynamically by the vastus medialis obliquus part of the quadriceps muscle (Fig. 56-2).[54,55]

The cartilaginous anlage of the patella begins to ossify at approximately 2 to 3 years of age, usually beginning in multiple small foci and expanding outward to "coalesce" by adolescence. In some adolescents the superolateral ossification center fails to fuse, being attached only by fibrous or fibrocartilaginous tissue to the remainder of the ossified patella. This so-called bipartite patella often occurs bilaterally and may be completely asymptomatic or, alternatively, a nidus for chondromalacic degeneration. Ogden, McCarthy, and Jokl[78] postulated that at least some cases of bipartite patella are the result of "traumatically induced chondroosseous disruption of the superolateral pole of the incompletely ossified patella" and offer an analogy to Sinding-Larsen-Johansson disease at the inferior pole. Rarely, this condition may be confused with fracture after acute trauma.[76,78]

Radiographic fragmentation of the proximal pole of the patella has also been reported in 10- to 11-year-old asymptomatic boys.[9]

The pyramid-shaped patella is wider proximally than distally, and its articular surface is angulated into medial and lateral facets by a longitudinal ridge. At the most medial portion of the medial facet is the "odd facet," which was described by Goodfellow, Hungerford, and Zindel[33] as the portion that makes no contact with the

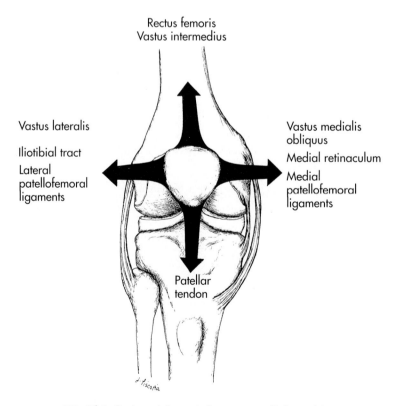

FIG. 56-2. Static and dynamic forces on patellofemoral joint.

articular surface of the femur from 0 to 90 degrees of flexion. However, between 90 and 135 degrees the patella rotates on a vertical axis, and the ridge between the medial and odd facet engages the lateral aspect of the medial femoral condyle. As the knee approaches full flexion, the patella slips into the intercondylar notch and rotates and shifts laterally, thus engaging the odd facet with the articular surface of the medial femoral condyle. These patellofemoral relationships have been described on tangential radiographs and in special cases can now be visualized on CT scans of the patellofemoral articulation (Fig. 56-3). This is particularly applicable to cases of patellofemoral incongruency, either congenital or traumatic.

A frontal view of the knee discloses a lack of symmetry between the mechanical and anatomic axes of the fe-

mur. With reference to the extensor mechanism, this translates as an angle between the direction of the quadriceps pull and patellar tendon alignment. This quadriceps angle, or **Q angle,** is measured at the angle of intersection between a line from the middle of the patella to the anterior superior iliac spine and a line from the center of the patella to the tibial tubercle with the foot pointing directly forward. A Q angle greater than 15 degrees may be associated with a propensity for patellar subluxation and is a gross indication of the lateral vector force on the patella as the knee is extended. From the lateral view the extensor mechanism also demonstrates some important geometric relationships. According to Insall and Salvati[42] the ratio of the length of the patellar tendon to the length of the patella itself is roughly 1:1 on lateral radiographs in the normal adult population. A

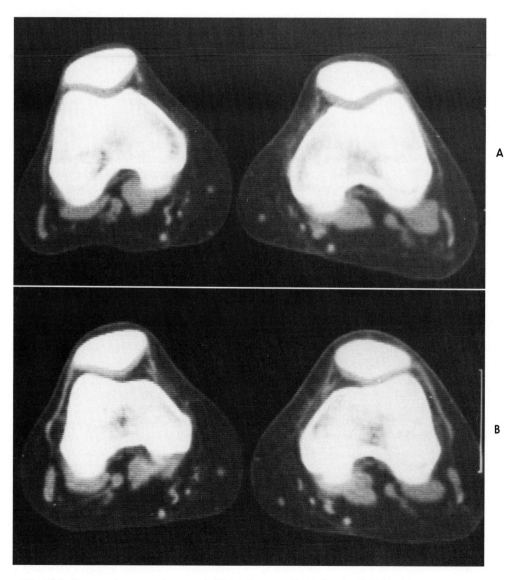

FIG. 56-3. Computed tomography scan. **A,** Thirty degrees of knee flexion. **B,** Fifteen degrees of knee flexion. Note subluxation.

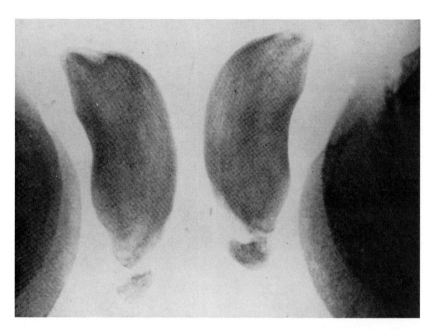

FIG. 56-4. Patellae with inferior ossicle.

deviation of greater than 20% from this value is arbitrarily cited as abnormal, but this ratio can be markedly distorted in children without associated patellofemoral symptomatology.[42]

A ratio of much less than one is called "patella baja" or "patella infera" and is almost always iatrogenic. In the past this phenomenon occurred almost exclusively as the result of excessive distal patellar realignment. More recently it has been reported with increasing frequency as a complication of anterior cruciate ligament (ACL) reconstruction. The opposite situation, "patella alta," is an extremely common naturally occurring phenomenon. It has been associated with patellar hypermobility, chondromalacia, and growth-related syndromes such as Osgood-Schlatter disease.[42]

The dynamic and changing nature of the patellofemoral articulation in the growing child does not allow the clinician to rely heavily on the Insall-Salvati ratio. Young athletes who participate in jumping sports, in a way similar to children with cerebral palsy and spastic quadriceps, often develop an elongated inferior pole of the patella resembling a consolidation of the inferior ossicle of Sinding-Larsen-Johansson disease (Fig. 56-4).[47,67,89,98] This effectively returns the Insall-Salvati ratio toward normal by prolonging the bony region of the patellar tendon despite a patella with an articular surface riding high above its groove. Osgood-Schlatter disease can then be thought of as a similar normalization process of the insertion of the patellar tendon itself.

These disorders seem to represent pathologic tightness in the extensor mechanism as a result of quadriceps overdevelopment from spasticity, strengthening, or jumping activities — or merely as a result of bony growth around the knee that outstrips muscular growth with as-

sociated patella alta. Paradoxically, these rapidly growing youths with patella alta and Osgood-Schlatter disease often excel in the jumping sports that further add to the burdens imposed on the extensor mechanism.[72]

Micheli[71] stated that growth is one of the major risk factors in overuse injuries in skeletally immature athletes. The key tissue in growth is cartilage, and growing cartilage is seen in the immature skeleton in three locations: the epiphyses, apophyses, and articular surfaces (Fig. 56-5). That chronic, repetitive microtrauma can adversely affect the epiphyseal plate is well manifested in the syndrome of slipped capital femoral epiphysis.

Not so commonly appreciated, however, are the subtle but significant effects that rapid growth has on soft-tissue relationships spanning and neighboring the epiphyseal plate. At the knee joint the periarticular epiphyseal plates are the fastest growing in the body and may distort the soft-tissue balance of the extensor mechanism (Fig. 56-6). The relatively thick and taut tensor fasciae latae and iliotibial tract may contribute to a progressive lateral and proximal migration of the quadriceps expansion, perhaps adding to an already present tendency toward lateral patellar subluxation. The cause of this growth factor in the common patellofemoral stress syndrome remains to be defined.[71]

In one study Micheli and associates[72] demonstrated some positive correlations between patella alta and growth rate during the adolescent growth spurt in girls. The correlation in males was not so clear, and the authors concluded that "there is not a simple one-to-one relationship of patellar height to femoral growth rate in all patients."

Growth cartilage in the traction apophyses has also been implicated in pathologic states, the most familiar of

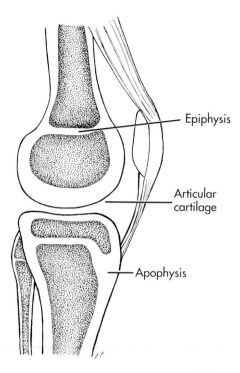

FIG. 56-5. Growth areas in immature skeleton.

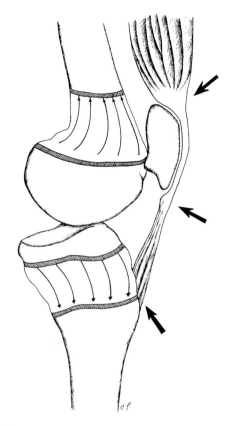

FIG. 56-6. Rapid longitudinal skeletal growth may lead to "tightness" of soft tissues. Problems *may arise at a number* of places (*arrows*). (Modified from Mitcheli LJ: *Orthop Clin North Am* 14:353, 1983.)

which is Osgood-Schlatter disease of the tibial tubercle. As in the patellofemoral stress syndrome, rapid cartilaginous growth leads to relative tightening of periarticular soft-tissue structures. Thus it is possible that a young athlete entering a growth spurt may suddenly require a rigorous stretching program not previously necessary and may just as suddenly "outgrow" the musculoskeletal tightness as the growth rate slows.

The third place that growing cartilage is seen is in the articular surface itself. It may be the growing skeleton's increased sensitivity to shear effects that is a contributing factor in osteochondritis dissecans. This growth phenomenon may also add to the deformation of the surface of the patella that may start with proximal and lateral migration of the quadriceps mechanism. Again, the role of these growth factors in the cause of some of the more common pathologic states in and around the knee in skeletally immature athletes remains to be clearly defined.

Pathomechanics of the Extensor Mechanism

Symptomatic difficulties in the patellofemoral articulation can be related to these factors: (1) local pathologic conditions, such as low profile of the femoral sulcus or deficiencies of the local supporting musculature; (2) distant abnormalities, such as angular and rotatory malalignment of the involved extremity; or (3) generalized conditions, such as hyperlaxity syndromes or obesity.[23,24,33,40,52]

Most frequently, patellar subluxations become symptomatic during adolescence. The symptom complex itself is often nondescript and poorly localized, and the athlete reports mostly a lack of confidence about the stability of

---

Factors contributing to patellofemoral malalignment

Local pathologic conditions
- Hypoplastic trochlea
- Hypoplastic patella
- Patellar configuration
- Hypoplastic or aplastic vastus medialis obliquus
- Tight lateral retinaculum
- Patella alta

Distant abnormalities
- Q angle
- Genu valgum
- Tibia vara
- Femoral anteversion
- Abnormal tibial torsion

Generalized conditions
- Hyperlaxity syndrome
- Obesity

---

the knee and unpredictable episodes of giving way. The key to diagnosis is a high index of suspicion in complaints associated with the knee in the young athlete. Physical examination should then be centered on the local and distant abnormalities that can predispose the young athlete to pathologic conditions of the patellofemoral joint. (Details of the physical examination can be found in Chapter 32.)

Nonsurgical management, with emphasis in five areas, is the appropriate treatment in young athletes. Management includes (1) patient education and activity modification; (2) musculoskeletal rehabilitation; (3) weight reduction, when appropriate; (4) nonsteroidal antiinflammatory medications, when necessary; and (5) bracing. This approach has proved useful in the majority of cases.

The keystone to treatment is rehabilitation. Initially, isometric quadriceps setting exercises are prescribed and are augmented by appropriate hamstring stretching. If a tight iliotibial tract is present, denoted by a positive result to the Ober test, iliotibial band tract stretching is performed. When the athlete is relatively comfortable, progressive resistance exercises are instituted. These include straight leg raising, hip adductor strengthening, hip abductor strengthening, and hip flexor strengthening. Free weights are used initially to provide minimal resistance in the early stages of this form of isotonic training. As the young athlete develops strength, isotonic training on Universal or Nautilus equipment can be added. Finally, terminal 10-degree flexion-extension exercises are added.

When the athlete has made documented strength gains, straight-ahead running is performed. If this can be performed pain free, agility drills and figure-8 running may be added. Finally, sport-specific drills are done before the athlete resumes competition.

In a small number of patients tightness of the extensor mechanism is found (positive Ely test). These athletes probably have a high-pressure patellofemoral compression syndrome, and quadriceps stretching is included in the rehabilitation program.

A patella-restraining brace is used during therapy and when the athlete returns to participation. Any of the standard patellar-restraining braces, such as the Marshall or Palumbo types, are useful in the treatment of these problems.

An alternative technique that combines both active exercise and supportive bracing is **McConnell[63] taping**. An Australian physiotherapist, Ms. Jenny McConnell, reasoning that pain inhibits muscle function, proposed a technique of taping that corrects abnormal glide, tilt, and rotation components of patellar tracking. With patellofemoral pain relieved, quadriceps muscle training becomes more effective. Rapid results can be achieved, even while the athlete continues with modified activity.

For athletes who fail to respond satisfactorily to these measures or who are unable or unwilling to live with the limitations imposed on their activities by their symptomatology, surgical correction may be necessary. To return the skeletally immature athlete to sports activities, the surgical approach should be guided by two principles: (1) the purpose of surgery is to restore the abnormal structure or function to as normal a state as possible, and (2) the simplest, safest, and least invasive procedures should be attempted first.

With young athletes the principle of "less is more"

should govern management. Arthroscopic evaluation with lateral retinacular release and thorough joint inspection and lavage is the usual first step in surgical management and proves a therapeutic success in most well-selected cases.[14,65]

Rarely is more extensive surgical intervention required. In the skeletally immature athlete, bony procedures, particularly in the area of the tibial tubercle, must be avoided. Iatrogenic damage to the proximal tibial physis can lead to premature closure and deformity. Dynamic balancing of the patella in its groove most often is satisfactorily accomplished with proximally directed soft-tissue reconstructive procedures. Distally based procedures are rarely necessary.

Chondromalacia Patellae

All too often the phrase "chondromalacia of the patella" is used as a catch-all term for any vague anterior knee discomfort. Chondromalacia is specifically a softening of articular cartilage and is diagnosed visually and histologically. There is some relationship, as yet undefined, between patellar instability and malalignment in chondromalacia of the patella. The etiologic histories of malalignment and chondromalacia are generally similar, although direct trauma to the patella can precipitate chondromalacia in some cases without obvious malalignment. In fact, symptomatic or asymptomatic chondromalacia may exist in athletes with no detectable (known) etiologic factors.

Arthroscopy has proved a useful tool in making the visual diagnosis necessary in chondromalacia patellae.[74] It has also expanded the list of differential diagnoses in the young athlete with vague anterior knee pain, including meniscal lesions, osteochondral and chondral fractures, and the plica syndrome. The multifactorial cause of patellofemoral pain syndrome in young athletes necessitates thorough history-taking and physical examination to rule out an associated pathologic condition in the rest of the lower extremity and the general body habitus, including posture and even athletic technique. Conservative management is the watchword; often the most important treatment is patient education and "tincture of time."[86]

When the proper criteria have been met, however, arthroscopic surgery under local anesthesia can be extremely useful. Although it may increase operating times slightly, arthroscopy under local anesthesia permits tactile confirmation of intraarticular injury that may or may not mimic the patient's preoperative complaints. This helps restrict the tendency toward overdiagnosis and thus "overtreatment."[73]

Furthermore, it would seem eminently logical that the best assessment of patella tracking and thus the need for lateral release is achieved with the patient awake and actively contracting the muscles involved. Overenthusiastic lateral release may cause more problems than it solves, particularly in the pediatric population, which is more flexible and whose muscle balance is in a constant state of flux.

When properly prepared preoperatively, adolescent and preadolescent patients tolerate the local anesthetic experience surprisingly well. The few who do not are easily converted to general anesthesia and are essentially no worse off for the attempt. Any information gained in the process could only be to the diagnostic and therapeutic benefit of the patient and the physician.

Plica Syndrome

In discussing the adolescent athlete with a chronically painful, snapping knee and a mild effusion but no arthrographic abnormalities, the extensor mechanism is most often the instigating source of injury. However, the various meniscosynovial plications must also be considered.

Painful snapping is produced on active knee flexion or extension as the pathologically tough fibrous band slips back and forth over the femoral condyle, usually the medial one. Tenderness is found over the anterior portion of the medial femoral condyle. Most plicae are not symptomatic, particularly in youngsters, but for those that are, arthroscopy is a powerful diagnostic and therapeutic tool. There remains some dispute about whether mere division of the plica is sufficient for cure or whether total open excision is necessary for optimal treatment of these lesions. The usual prognosis is favorable with minimal surgery, however.*

Reflex Sympathetic Dystrophy

In preadolescent females the differential diagnosis of "vague knee pain" is made more complicated by the syndrome of reflex sympathetic dystrophy (RSD). Like the plica syndrome there is great controversy about the frequency of this problem in this population, and the proper diagnosis is entirely dependent on a high index of suspicion on the part of the examiners.

Although RSD in adults seems to occur with equal frequency in males and females, a study of 80 cases of childhood RSD found a male/female ratio of 1:6 (mean age 11 years; range 3 to 17 years).[27] Interestingly, there was also a higher incidence of lower extremity involvement than in adult series.[62] Although RSD is less common in children than adults, it is not as rare as one might think, and the prognosis with proper treatment is much better.

Awareness of the possibility of RSD may prevent an ill-advised surgical intervention. Histories and clinical presentations may vary—some cases seem to arise after trauma, some insidiously or spontaneously. Dietz, Mathews, and Montgomery[27] described the signs of vasomotor instability, discoloration, temperature difference, and tache cérébrale. The tache cérébrale is manifested by an erythematous streak in the skin that appears 15 to 30 seconds after stroking with a blunt object like the head of a safety pin. The authors found the line to persist for as long as 15 minutes. Along with dysesthesia to light touch, this tache cérébrale is one of the most consistent signs of childhood RSD.

Radiographic evaluation is not as consistently reliable in the pediatric population as in adult population with RSD. Perhaps because of the high metabolic rate of pediatric bone, radiographs and bone scans are not reliably abnormal in children with RSD, another distinction from the adult form of the syndrome.

Diagnosis should be followed by treatment with mobilization and massage. Immobilization, so frequently and fearlessly employed in the treatment of childhood musculoskeletal pain, is to be avoided in RSD patients, and surgery is to be condemned. Because the prognosis with nonsurgical management is much better in children than adults, sympathetic blocks and sympathectomy are usually unnecessary.

Fractures and Dislocations of the Extensor Mechanism

Lateral dislocation of the patella is a common injury in the skeletally immature athlete. It can result from a direct blow or, more commonly, from active quadriceps muscular response to valgus, external rotation loading. Spontaneous reduction is the rule, so much so that it is often impossible to differentiate true dislocation from the usual lateral subluxation of the patella. This makes radiographic evaluation of a knee with such a history extremely important. When possible, a series of tangential views of the patellofemoral joint are particularly valuable in revealing osteochondral fractures or dysplastic patellofemoral indices that might dispose the athlete to a future of chronic patellar instability.*

The management of acute patellar dislocation in the young athlete is almost always nonsurgical. Many physicians prefer immobilization of the knee in full extension for 3 to 6 weeks.[51] However, there is really nothing to mitigate against simple, immediate symptomatic treatment followed by early rehabilitation to strengthen the quadriceps, as dictated by patient comfort. This drastically decreases the length of disability and unnecessary "down time" for the competitive athlete.† Of course, well leg exercise and cardiovascular training can continue during the rehabilitation process.

Adolescents are also susceptible to the extremely rare "intraarticular" dislocation of the patella (Fig. 56-7). This is a much more severe injury than the common lateral dislocation that is often associated with concomitant ligament or quadriceps tendon rupture.[75] Also, in contrast to lateral dislocation, intraarticular dislocation of the patella usually requires open reduction and surgical repair of the extensive soft-tissue damage incurred.

Fracture of the patella itself is an uncommon injury in the young athlete. The mechanism of injury is similar to that in the adult: sudden acute flexion against a forceful, eccentric quadriceps contraction with or without a direct blow to the bony patella.

Equally rare in children are stress fractures of the patella. One reported case occurred from participation in soccer and basketball (Fig. 56-8).[25] Like other stress fractures those in the patella may be seen initially as pain on activity. Scintigraphy may aid in the early diagnosis before radiographic changes are present. Rest is usually all that is required for treatment, except for those frac-

---

*See Chapter 41 for further discussion.

*Techniques are described in Chapter 33.
†McConnell taping techniques can also be employed.

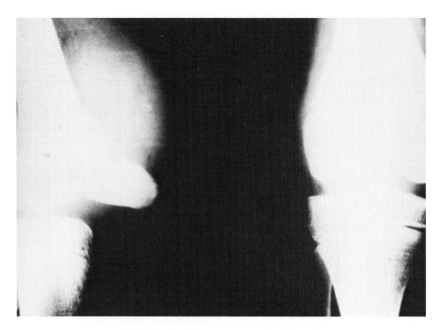

FIG. 56-7. Intraarticular dislocation of patella.

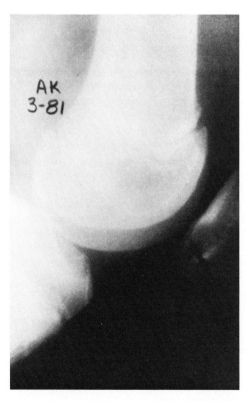

FIG. 56-8. Stress fracture of patella in 12-year-old soccer and basketball player. (From Dickason JM, Fox JM: *Am J Sports Med* 10:248, 1982.)

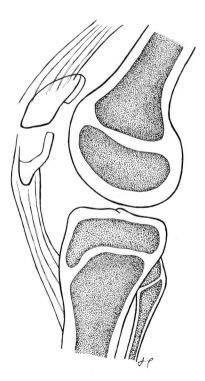

FIG. 56-9. Sleeve fracture of patella.

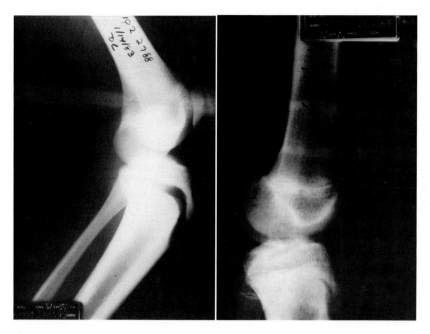

FIG. 56-10. Lateral radiographs of "lay-up" fracture of proximal tibia (before and after reduction).

tures prone to displacement. If displacement occurs, anatomic reduction and internal fixation is indicated.

Houghton and Ackroyd[39] coined the term "sleeve fracture" of the patella for disruption of the patellar tendon origin attached to a considerable sleeve of osseocartilaginous tissue, often including much of the articular surface of the patella itself. The osseous component of the fragment may be extremely slight, rendering simple radiographic identification of the injury extremely treacherous (Fig. 56-9).

Again, the key to diagnosis is a high index of suspicion in young athletes participating in jumping sports. The usual history is a sudden episode of giving way in a knee during a vigorous quadriceps contraction (e.g., the takeoff for a basketball lay-up shot). There is immediate pain and effusion, and complete inability to extend the knee against resistance. The patella may be seen to retract proximally.

The severity of this fracture must not be underestimated by its benign radiographic appearance. Anatomic restoration of the avulsed articular surface is essential to the continued good function of the involved knee.[101] These young athletes must get a lifetime of performance from this damaged patellofemoral articulation, even if their athletic pursuits are curtailed. A return to competition is rarely possible without surgical intervention.

Fractures of the Proximal Tibial Physis

Another interesting fracture arises in the young athlete engaged in jumping sports. It also typically occurs during a basketball player's drive to the basket or a high-jumper's takeoff. In fact, it almost always involves the take-off leg with or without contact. This "lay-up" fracture involves avulsion of the proximal tibial physis, including the tibial tubercle (Fig. 56-10). Anatomic resto-

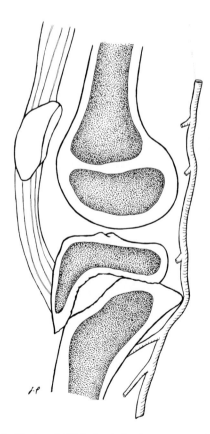

FIG. 56-11. Displaced tibial physis fractures may cause vascular injury from posterior displacement of distal fragment.

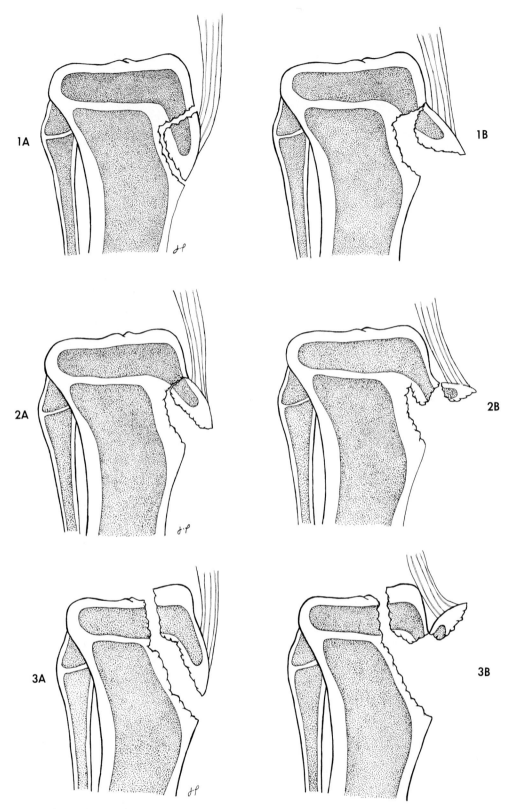

FIG. 56-12. Classification of tibial tuberosity fractures. Types of injury to tibial tuberosity. **Type 1A,** Fracture is distal to normal junction of ossification centers of proximal end of tibia and tuberosity. Displacement is minimal. **Type 1B,** Fragment is hinged (displaced) anteriorly and proximally. **Type 2A,** Primary fracture failures is at junction of ossification of proximal end of tibia and tuberosity, essentially in line with a transverse continuation of proximal tibial epiphysis. In **Type 2B** tuberosity fragment is comminuted, and more distal fragment may end up being more proximally displaced. In **Type 3** fracture extends to joint and is associated with displacement of anterior fragment or fragments, leading to discontinuity of joint surface. In **Type 3A** tuberosity and anterior aspect of proximal tibial epiphysis are a composite unit. In **Type 3B** unit is comminuted, major site of fragmentation being juncture of ossification centers of tuberosity and proximal end of tibia. (Modified from Ogden JA, Tross RB, Murphy MJ: *J Bone Joint Surg* 62A:205, 1980.)

ration of the proximal tibial physis is of primary importance in treating these injuries.[6,19] Simple closed reduction is often successful with fractures of the Salter-Harris Type I or II. Intraarticular fractures of the Salter-Harris Type III or IV require open reduction and internal fixation to achieve an anatomic reduction. Occasionally, with complete displacement of the epiphysis, there may be associated vascular damage as a result of displacement of the distal metaphysis, particularly in hyperextension injuries (Fig. 56-11). Other potential complications of these fractures include late angulation, compartment syndrome, and peroneal palsy.[19,88]

Of course, fractures of the proximal tibial epiphysis may also occur after trauma-producing varus or valgus stress at the knee. They are less frequent than other epiphyseal fractures about the knee, but they are often hazardous. The proximal tibial epiphysis is relatively protected by the irregularity of its metaphyseal-physeal interface and collateral ligaments, which span the epiphy-

sis to insert distal to the growth plate itself. Thus when a fracture occurs at this location, it is often the result of a high-energy mechanism.

Fractures of the Tibial Tuberosity

Although relatively uncommon, fractures of the tibial tuberosity have received some attention in the literature (Table 56-1). Watson-Jones[95] originally characterized these fractures in three types. Ogden, Tross, and Murphy[80] modified Watson-Jones's classification, placing greater emphasis on the intraarticular extension of the fracture and comminution of the tuberosity (Fig. 56-12). Watson-Jones believed that the mechanism of injury was violent flexion of the knee against a tightly contracting quadriceps muscle. Bowers[16] agreed with this mechanism but thought, as did Ogden, Tross, and Murphy,[80] that an alternative mechanism of injury was a strong contraction of the quadriceps with the knee flexed and the foot fixed (Fig. 56-13). Most cases reported in the

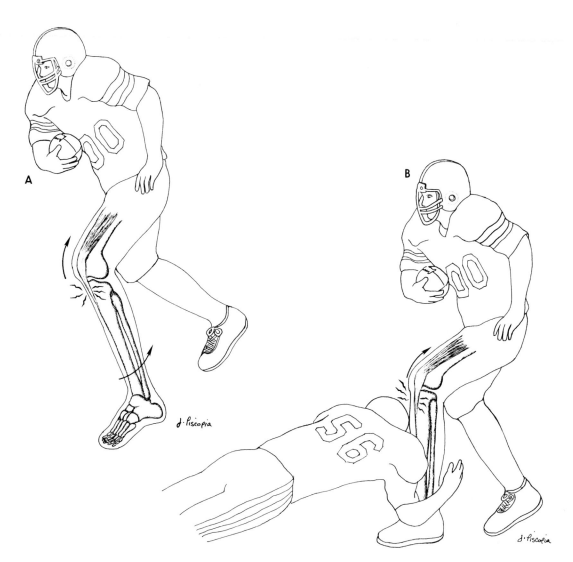

FIG. 56-13. Mechanisms of injury in tibial tuberosity fractures. **A,** Violent flexion of knee against tightly contracting quadriceps. **B,** Strong contraction of quadriceps with knee flexed and foot fixed.

TABLE 56-1 Sports in which tibial tuberosity fractures have been reported

Series Reported	Jumping	Football	Running	Other	Total
Hand et al.	3	4	—	—	7
Ogden et al.	7	1	2	4	14
Bowers	1	—	—	—	1
TOTAL	11	5	2	4	22

Data from Hand WL et al: *J Bone Joint Surg* 53A:1579, 1971; Ogden JA et al: *J Bone Joint Surg* 62A:205, 1980; and Bowers KD: *Am J Sports Med* 9:356, 1981.

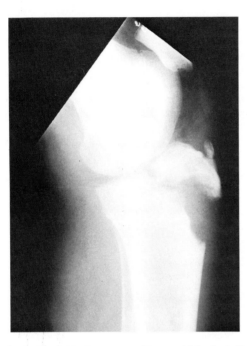

FIG. 56-14. Type 3A fracture in 16-year-old basketball player. Treatment was by open reduction and internal fixation. Note Osgood-Schlatter lesion. (From the NISMAT Collection.)

literature were associated with jumping and other sports movements. Many authors believe that a strong association exists between these fractures and Osgood-Schlatter disease. Ogden et al[79] believed that Osgood-Schlatter disease altered the biochemical response of tissue in the physis of the tuberosity, affecting the amount of columnar cartilage compared with fibrocartilage. If there is more columnar cartilage (which is weak when subjected to tensile stress) than fibrocartilage (which specifically resists such stress) before there is adequate maturation of the secondary ossification center, the physis might be predisposed to tensile failure.

The goal of treatment in these injuries is anatomic restoration of the fragment. Nondisplaced fractures may be treated by a cylinder cast with the knee in full extension. Displaced fractures (Fig. 56-14) must be anatomically reduced and internally fixed.[36,38,53] Screw fixation is most commonly used, although fragmentation may make staples and wire fixation more appropriate. If closed treatment is used, radiographs should be taken within the first 10 days to ensure that displacement of the distal

fragment has not occurred as the result of isometric quadriceps contraction. At 6 weeks, union across the physeal fracture should be present (trauma-induced epiphyseodesis). Without evidence of solid union, premature efforts at rehabilitation may lead to recurrent avulsion. Appropriate treatment with anatomic restoration of the distal fragment, allows these young athletes to return to sports without sequelae, although a theoretic complication of genu recurvatum exists. At the time of surgery the patellar tendon should be visualized, since Maybar[60] reported a case of avulsion of the patellar tendon from the displaced tibial tubercle fragment.

Ligamentous and meniscal injury may also accompany Type III and even some Type II fractures of the tibial tuberosity.[29] These structures should be visualized by arthrotomy or arthroscopy at the time of open reduction or by MRI if nonsurgical management is being considered. An aggressive approach to these injuries should be applied with repair of any ligamentous or meniscal injury to achieve a satisfactory result.

Osgood-Schlatter Disease

A common condition seen in adolescent athletes is Osgood-Schlatter disease. Independently described in 1903 by Osgood[81] and Schlatter,[87] this condition is a disturbance in the tibial tuberosity. The patients are generally between 11 and 15 years of age. Onset of symptoms often begins with the beginning of the growth spurt. Males are much more commonly affected.[91] Involvement is often bilateral. Pain is generally localized to the area of the tibial tubercle. Invariably, sports activities aggravate the symptoms, and the adolescents often give up sports before they seek treatment. When the affected adolescent is examined, a prominence of the proximal tibia in the area of the tibial tubercle is noted. This area is formed by enlargement of the tibial tubercle and associated soft-tissue swelling. Swelling may be apparent in the distal portion of the patellar tendon, over the tibial tubercle, and in some cases in the local subcutaneous tissue.[91,97] Intraarticular effusion is absent. Active flexion and extension may be limited by pain or swelling. Extension of the knee against resistance is also painful. Generally, contracture of the ipsilateral quadriceps muscle group is found, as represented by a positive result to the Ely test.

Radiographically, soft-tissue swelling may be visible anteriorly in acute cases. The tibial tubercle may take on a number of patterns. Irregular, multiple areas of ossification are commonly seen. Ossification may be com-

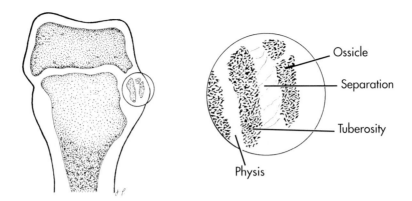

FIG. 56-15. Possible mechanism of formation of Osgood-Schlatter lesion. Primary lesion is avulsion of small areas (ossicles) of anterior portions of developing ossification center of tibial tuberosity with callus formation in intervening area thus building up anterior portion of tuberosity. Growth plate of tuberosity remains intact. (Modified from Ogden JA, Southwick WO: *Clin Orthop* 116:180, 1976.)

pletely absent, however. Classification of the radiographic appearance is difficult because of variability in normal ossification of the tibial tuberosity. It should, however, be stressed that ossification in the patellar tendon is not seen in Osgood-Schlatter disease. Ossification in the patellar tendon is more common in skeletally mature patients and does not represent Osgood-Schlatter disease, whereas irregular ossification in the tibial tuberosity in the appropriate clinical setting confirms the diagnosis of Osgood-Schlatter disease.[79]

Ogden and Southwick[79] noted that the tibial tubercle develops from three imperceptibly merging areas with cytoarchitecture varying in both the arrangement of hyaline cartilage cells and in the amount of interposed fibrocartilage and fibrous tissue. Ossification occurs by membranous ossification. The lesion in Osgood-Schlatter disease appears to be, according to Ogden et al,[80] an avulsion of small regions (ossicles) of the anterior portions of the developing ossification center of the tibial tuberosity with formation of callus in the intervening areas building up the anterior portion of the tuberosity (Fig. 56-15).[79] Thus histologically, only lesions occurring in the tuberosity should be considered to be Osgood-Schlatter disease. Others have reported the lesion to be multiple "microtears" in the patella tendon insertion on the tibial tuberosity.[29]

Treatment of this lesion is generally conservative.[10,91] Because histologically Osgood-Schlatter disease is the result of small avulsions and these avulsions are seen in growing athletes with tight muscles, treatment is di-

rected at relieving the tensile force on the tubercle exerted by the quadriceps. In the acute state, ice and a compressive wrap is applied. Analgesics may be required in severe cases. A period of rest from sports is suggested. When the athlete is comfortable, stretching of the quadriceps is instituted on a three-times-daily basis. Stretching is followed by a 20-minute application of ice to the area of the tibial tubercle. When the patient can easily touch the heel of the affected leg to the buttock in the prone position, quadriceps strengthening is added. Also at this point, slow resumption of athletic participation is allowed. At no point in the treatment program is cast immobilization used. Young athletes are told at the time of treatment that a residual deformity will probably be present in the tuberosity.

A small percentage of adolescents do not improve with conservative therapy. Before embarking on any more invasive therapy, compliance with the stretching program must be determined. Often patients who have not improved have not been stretching adequately or frequently. Another important factor in treatment is the amount of growth remaining in the tuberosity. Completion of growth in the tuberosity is associated with amelioration of symptoms in most cases. In fact, surgical treatment of Osgood-Schlatter disease is simply epiphyseodesis. In patients close to closure of the physis, patience is indicated.[99] However, in the younger athlete with a wide open physis and 2 to 3 years of athletic participation lost during the turbulent adolescent years if conservative therapy is continued beyond 6 months, surgery should be considered. Any number of procedures may be used, and generally results are excellent.[15,49,50,91] Following surgical epiphyseodesis, athletic resumption may occur when bony union has occurred.

Bipartite Patella

A bipartite patella is normally classified as a developmental anomaly and is generally asymptomatic (Fig. 56-16). It is often bilateral and is more common in males by nine to one.[78] Normally, bipartite patella is an incidental finding, but in some instances the lesion can be-

---

Conservative treatment of Osgood-Schlatter disease

- Quadriceps stretching
- Ice
- Compressive wrap
- Analgesics if necessary
- Quadriceps strengthening (straight leg raising) later
- *No* cast immobilization

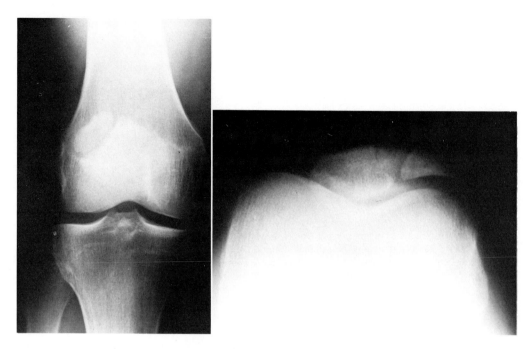

FIG. 56-16. Bipartite patella.

come a source of problems.[35,78,96] Most often pain in the superolateral aspect of the patella has its onset after direct or indirect trauma. In young athletes, participation in sports is limited by the localized pain and tenderness. Following examination of routine radiographs, a bone scan should be obtained. If the involved patella has an abnormally increased uptake in the superolateral area identical to the location of the accessory ossification center, an acute traumatic disruption of the cartilage between the ossification centers should be considered.[78] These patients should be placed in a cylinder cast for 3 weeks. Following cast removal, symptoms should be relieved and the patient may begin on a progressive muscle rehabilitation program. Other patients may have chronic pain in the region of the bipartite patella and remain symptomatic despite a trial of cast immobilization. In these adolescents excision of the accessory ossification center provides satisfactory relief of symptoms.

During excision of the accessory ossification center the articular surface of the patella is clearly exposed to allow a clean line of excision. A lateral release should accompany the resection. Resumption of heavy demand sports after rehabilitation generally takes 4 to 6 months because the leg requires extensive rehabilitation of weakened muscle groups from preoperative and postoperative atrophy.

LIGAMENTOUS INJURIES

Although uncommon, ligament disruptions do occur in childhood.[17,21,28] Considering the frequency of pediatric knee trauma, ligament injury is extremely rare before 14 years of age. These injuries generally do not appear in the knee until about the time of physeal closure.

Physeal closure is a gradual and irregular phenomenon, and it may be that in early adolescence some physes, although apparently "open" radiographically have begun to develop areas of bony consolidation, protecting them from growth plate injuries.

In the assessment of such injuries in the pediatric population the physician is hampered by the inability to rely on one of the most reliable tools—a good clinical history. These injuries are usually acute in presentation, and the acutely injured child is a notoriously poor historian. Coaches, teachers, or parents may provide helpful information, but often the trauma occurs during unsupervised play with no skilled observers. Nevertheless, the physician must persist with a careful history of the exact nature and duration of symptoms, remembering that many neoplasms of the musculoskeletal system in childhood present after traumatic episodes.

This puts even more importance on a good physical examination, again a tricky business in a child who is frightened or in pain. Because the mechanisms of injury to the pediatric knee are similar to that of the adult, many of the principles of the usual adult knee evaluation prove useful.

The physician must begin with observation—ambulatory gait, running, jumping, and hopping, when possible. This act of testing establishes the seriousness of the injury immediately. Does the child stand with full extension and good alignment, or is there flexion contracture or genu recurvatum? Can the child squat fully and "duck walk," or is there a painful or painless block to full flexion? Are there any clicks or pops elicited by these maneuvers? Does the child's neuromuscular coordination and balance seem appropriate for his or her age? The physician must suspect something other than a ligament injury in the child who is always falling or who has pain that is only minimally activity related or interferes with sleep patterns. In fact, persistent musculoskeletal pain of any kind is a red flag in trauma to active young children, who get over the pain of long bone fractures in a matter of days.

The physician may now focus his or her observations on the knee itself. Is it swollen, warm, or erythematous? Are there bruises or abrasions on the extremities and where are they located? This may be an important clue to the mechanism of injury, and the anticipation of what might be injured is often crucial to the success of the physical evaluation.

With observations duly recorded the examiner may now begin the hands-on evaluation of the knee. With children it is especially important to begin with the uninjured knee and glean all the information the physician can before proceeding from areas of least discomfort to those that are blatantly painful. Children have a natural flexibility that is often lost in late adolescence, and the uninvolved knee is important for baseline measurements, lest the unwary examiner mistake physiologic laxity for ligamentous injury. The spine and upper extremities should be examined to help determine the degree of laxity.

Although the mechanisms of acute trauma to the knee remain fairly constant as we age, the nature of the damage sustained is somewhat different in the pediatric population. For example, valgus or external rotation, hyperextension, and hyperflexion injuries occur in children, just as they do in adults. However, the precise combination of epiphyseal and ligament injuries is much harder to predict, despite knowing the mechanism and forces involved. In the pediatric population the usual tests for anterior-posterior and valgus-varus instability remain useful, but radiographic documentation of the positive findings becomes crucial. In the acute injury it has been shown that gross anterior laxity in a child with avulsion of the tibial spine is strongly suggestive of concomitant collateral ligament injury.[32] Stress radiographs are the simplest way to determine whether the abnormal motion is occurring through the knee joint or a neighboring physis. It also helps in the differentiation of anterior from posterior laxity when there is question of cruciate ligament incompetence. Aspiration of the knee may help secure the diagnosis both by confirming hemarthrosis and by easing capsular pain on examination stress. Fat globules in the aspirate suggest osteochondral fracture. Local anesthesia can also be instilled to decrease pain and guarding. If there remains further doubt about the intraarticular status of the knee, arthrographic evaluation is urged to make the precise anatomic diagnosis. If some question still exists of the extent of injury, examination with the patient under anesthesia with stress radiographs and arthroscopy is indicated. The dictum of "diagnose aggressively, treat conservatively" holds in this population.[37]

The ACL has come under increasing scrutiny in the pediatric age group, and these injuries are being reported with increasing frequency. Although far less frequent before the physes close, the ACL injury in childhood occurs because of the requirements for high levels of activity and athletic participation in this population.

Libscomb and Anderson[56] reported on their technique of ACL reconstruction in 24 adolescents ages 12 to 15 years. Their technique used the gracilis and semitendinosis passed through a proximal tibial tunnel crossing the epiphyseal plate. The femoral tunnel was created entirely within the epiphysis, distal to the growth plate, and only one patient demonstrated a significant growth disturbance. Although the results of the series were otherwise similar to those of midsubstance ACL tears in adults, personal experience has suggested better results with simple arthroscopic ACL repair when enough ligament remains to repair. Just as patients who undergo ACL reconstruction immediately after acute disruption often experience ankylosis secondary to exuberant fibrous tissue response so, too, that same fibrous response can help to heal and hypertrophy the repaired ACL (L. Johnson, personal communication, 1992).

The skeletally immature knee ACL tear is an excellent indication for Dr. Lanny Johnson's technique of arthroscopic ACL repair using an intraarticular staple. Using a relatively short staple does not violate the epiphyseal plate, and excellent results have been achieved in cases that meet the appropriate criteria. The staple is routinely left in place unless secondary procedures are necessary.

Even more unusual is a **congenital absence of the ACL.** It should be suspected in cases where the adolescent complains of sensations of instability and even pivot shift but no pain, swelling, and often no history of classical injury mechanisms. It may present as an isolated finding or as part of a combination of lower limb anomalies. Because femoral lengthening may produce posterior subluxation of the knee, some have argued that the cruciate ligaments should be evaluated arthroscopically before the correction of leg length inequalities. Hamstring lengthening may be considered to alleviate some of this tendency toward posterior subluxation if congenital absence of the cruciate ligaments is discovered. These patients are also prone to suffer meniscus lesions and patellofemoral pain,[43] and there is some evidence that congenital absence of the ACL is probably more common than previously suspected, particularly as one part of a combination of a wide variety of congenital anomalies.[93] Radiographs can confirm the diagnosis with hypoplasia or total aplasia of the tibial spines. These patients must be differentiated from the familiar population of hyperlax adolescents with naturally symmetric and physiologic knee ligament laxity.

Posterior cruciate ligament (PCL) injury is uncommon in the skeletally immature population and is usually the result of hyperextension, an avulsion fracture of the ligament origin from the femur.[85] However, there has been at least one report in the literature of childhood PCL disruption after a fall on a flexed knee.[84] Nonsurgical management resulted in unsatisfactory residual instability and therefore open reduction and internal fixation was recommended for the avulsion fracture.

The situation for ACL tears remains more controversial. In 1988 McCarroll, Rettig, and Shelbourne[61] reported on a study of 40 patients with midsubstance tears of the ACL, acute or chronic, under 14 years of age with open physes. Of 24 patients who were treated surgically, 10 underwent extraarticular procedures, tenodesing the iliotibial band with one or two techniques. The remaining 14 had intraarticular reconstructions using ipsilateral patellar tendon autografts. Each of these had extraarticular augmentation; six with dynamic biceps transfer and eight with iliotibial band tenodesis. Interestingly enough the authors did not alter their intraarticular "over-the-top" approach in these reconstructions, drilling osseous tunnels without regard for the open proximal tibial physis. Nevertheless, no growth anomalies were encountered, confirming the experience of other investigators that growth plate disturbances are relatively infrequent even when the growth plate is surgically violated in these procedures.

Similarly, Graf et al[34] studied 12 skeletally immature patients who had acute ACL tears between January 1984 and September 1987 (average age 14.5 years; range 11.7 to 16.3 years). Four patients underwent arthroscopic meniscus repair and an ACL-stabilizing procedure. Eight were treated nonsurgically with rehabilitation and protective bracing. All eight managed nonsurgically developed instability within an average time of 7 months. Seven of these patients went on to develop new meniscal tears an average of 15 months after the initial ACL injury. The authors concluded that "brace management appears unsuccessful in preventing instability and further meniscal damage in athletic adolescents who are unwilling to curtail sports activities." The incidence of unsatisfactory clinical outcomes was significantly greater in patients managed conservatively, and so a more aggressive approach to ACL reconstruction in this "growing" population was recommended.[34,44] Youngsters who wish to continue in athletic pursuits are counseled for intraarticular ACL reconstruction; the failure of nonsurgical management outweighs the risk of growth plate injury.

In contrast, a 1989 study from Australia comes to a different conclusion.[8] Between November 1980 and June 1986 212 arthroscopies of all kinds were performed at Adelaide Children's Hospital, and ACL tear was the most common arthroscopic finding. More than half of the ACL injuries were partial tears, but six of the seven complete midsubstance ACL tears demonstrated additional injury. All ACL injuries were routinely managed by correcting associated intraarticular injury but not repairing or reconstructing the ACL itself. Apparently, of 31 ACL injuries, only four underwent any kind of repair. During the study period only four patients developed subsequent intraarticular injury and three of these were after the tears were reported as partial tears. Their statistics showed that in children and adolescents the chance of making a correct diagnosis on clinical grounds alone is 56%. Arthroscopy can improve this to a 99% accuracy with minimal risk of morbidity.

Collateral stability of the knee in full extension is crucial for successful nonsurgical management. If complete complex ligamentous disruptions are discovered, these should usually be acutely repaired for best results. During repair, it is best to try not to cross the open physis with large drill holes or reattached ligamentous complexes. There must be an extended period (2 to 3 years) of observation for growth anomalies and undetected physeal injuries. Partial ligament injuries can be treated conservatively, but they also require continued follow-up and reexamination. It has been noted that such ligamentous injuries in the skeletally immature athlete often result in long-term knee laxity, although no consistent short-term disability.[21]

FRACTURES OF THE TIBIAL EMINENCE

Fractures of the tibial eminence in children result from a forceful avulsion of the ACL. Although the anterior intercondylar region does not correspond exactly with the described insertion of the ACL, in practice the fracture fragment of cartilage and bone includes the ACL and a variable-sized portion of the anterior intermeniscal area. The anterior horn of the lateral meniscus and the intermeniscal ligament are slightly behind the eminence avulsion and do not interfere with reduction. The anterior horn of the medial meniscus is more anterior and has been described as blocking the reduction of the tilted or elevated fragment. The area of the ACL and tibial eminence corresponds to the intercondylar notch of the femur and so does not have an articular match, although contact is apparently made in full extension.[48]

The mechanism of injury is similar to that seen in mature individuals sustaining ACL tears: hyperextension, bending, and twisting forces. It is also conjectured that the relative laxity of the immature knee may allow the femoral condyle to "knock off" the tibial eminence in some injuries. Boys, particularly in latency or adolescent periods (7 to 15 years), are the usual recipients of these injuries, and most series note bicycle accidents as a common cause. Here the patient usually has an immediate, painful, bloody effusion with decreased range of motion. Clinical instability of the knee joint, even with a dangling ACL is uncommon. This is thought to be because this injury is truly isolated and other supporting structures are spared, unlike the adult injury.

Meyers and McKeever[69,70] described a large series of eminence fractures and used radiographic displacement criteria to grade the severity and guide the therapy (Fig. 56-17). Grade I fractures were visible but essentially undisplaced. Grade II fractures were angulated anteriorly, appearing to be pried up from the tibia, but were in continuity posteriorly. In Grade III fractures the eminence was completely displaced from the tibia and could be seen floating either horizontally or at right angles to the plateau.

After aspiration of the hemarthrosis and, perhaps, local anesthesia, treatment of the fractures depends on the grade of displacement. Minimally displaced fractures can be casted without further reduction. Meyers and McKeever[69,70] suggested casting the knee at 20 degrees of flexion based on a report of a case in which a Grade II fracture was converted to a Grade III fracture because of the pull of a taut cruciate in full extension. On the other hand, Roberts described anatomic studies using

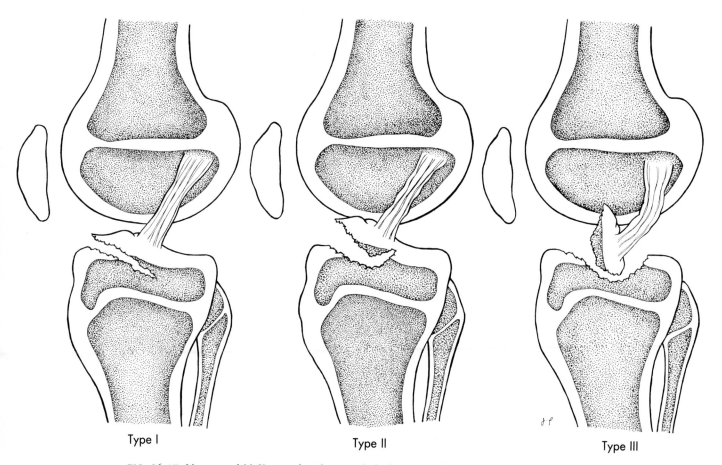

FIG. 56-17. Meyers and McKeever classification of tibial eminence fractures. **Type I,** Minimal displacement. **Type II,** Displacement of anterior portion, producing beaklike appearance. **Type III,** Complete displacement of fragment. (Modified from Meyers M, McKeever F: *J Bone Joint Surg* 52A:1677, 1970.)

the femoral intercondylar area of contact to push the displaced fragment back into place and suggested immobilization in full extension for 6 to 8 weeks.[48] Grade III fractures are significantly displaced and must be reduced.[103] Closed reduction may be attempted with the patient under local or general anesthesia, depending on patient compliance. Reduction is effected by fully extending the knee with the position confirmed by radiograph. If displacement remains, an open reduction is indicated. Reduction may be blocked by the anterior horn of the medial meniscus, although the actual occurrence of this is disputed. Exploration and open reduction–internal fixation of this fragment is best done through a medial incision no larger than the fracture fragment itself because once reduction is made, fixation is relatively simple.[7] The fragment is secured with sutures to the meniscus or to the bone. An alternative procedure is arthroscopic reduction and pin fixation or transosseous suturing. This technique is most useful in Type III fractures and is associated with decreased hospital time and morbidity.[66]

Although most patients are asymptomatic, other studies have suggested less consistent success in the clinical outcome of these injuries.[97] Computed instrument

testing has suggested a minor, but nevertheless permanent alteration of cruciate ligament stability in these knees, even in the absence of any subjective complaints or other objective physical findings. These changes cannot be attributed to changes in the architecture of the tibial eminence because even nondisplaced fractures can show permanent radiographic changes.[83]

Rehabilitation after healing is important because stiffness and thigh wasting are significant and usually take months to resolve. The problem with the late-presenting Grade III eminence fracture is one of mechanical blocking, occasionally with effusions and atrophy, but usually not instability. Surprisingly, stable knees have been reported several years after treatment of the late presentation of mechanical blocking with excision of the shortened, neglected ACL avulsion.

MENISCAL INJURIES AND DISCOID LATERAL MENISCUS

Although rare in the preadolescent group, meniscal injuries are being noted with increasing frequency in adolescents. The role of the menisci in stabilization of the knee joint and transmission of forces across it is now well documented. The loss of stability and load-sharing function of the meniscus does lead to further instability and often early degenerative changes within the knee.

In the series by Medlar, Mandiberg, and Lyne [68] of 26 patients who underwent total meniscectomy while their growth plates were open, ligamentous laxity, early degenerative arthritis, and symptomatic knee pain was common at the time of follow-up (average 8.3 years postoperatively). In fact, the authors found only 42% excellent or good results. Manzione et al [59] found that 60% of their 20 patients who underwent meniscectomy while still with open physes had unsatisfactory results an average of 5.5 years after surgery. However, these studies suffer from relatively small numbers and relatively brief follow-up time. In 1992 Wroble et al [100] studied 39 patients from 10 to 35 years old who had undergone total meniscectomy at ages less than 16 years old. Although of all patients who worked fulltime, only four had changed to less physically demanding jobs, only 38% could participate in sports without limitations. Radiologic abnormalities were observed in 90%, and only 27% of the patients were asymptomatic. Although unsatisfactory radiographic ratings occurred more often with medial meniscectomy, lateral meniscectomy led to a higher percentage of unsatisfactory subjective and objective ratings. The authors concluded that meniscus repair was the treatment of choice with peripheral meniscal lesions and that in nonreparable lesions partial excision is preferable to total meniscectomy. Similarly, Abdon et al [1] found that only 74% of 89 children who underwent single meniscectomy were pleased with the outcome. Objective ratings were even lower (52% to 58% satisfactory), and significantly poorer results were found after lateral as opposed to medial meniscectomy. The presence of a meniscal tear causing mechanical block also causes damage and altered joint mechanics, accelerating local cartilage wear and promoting atrophy of the extremity. Presentation of these problems is not unlike that in the mature knee in which pain, swelling, "locking," and atrophy may be noticed. In Fowler's series [30] the most common configuration of symptomatic meniscal tears was the "bucket handle," which he thought was most likely a continuation of lesser tears. Some authors have pointed out the usefulness of arthroscopy in the diagnosis of children's knee complaints. [82,104] Not only was the procedure believed to be technically easier and freer of complications in the more mobile adolescent knee, but there was significant information gained in the somewhat difficult differential diagnosis of adolescent knee pain. Again, excision of only symptomatic and clearly damaged menisci is indicated, as in adults. Many menisci that might have been damaged and removed at arthrotomy can be explored arthroscopically without iatrogenic damage and thus preserved.

The **discoid lateral meniscus** must also be considered in a differential diagnosis of adolescent knee pain, especially when associated with clicking. Although somewhat unusual in the United States, the incidence is higher in Japan. [26,31] Kaplan [45,46] and subsequently others have demonstrated that at no time in normal embryologic development does either meniscus assume a discoid shape before achieving its familiar semilunar configuration. Kaplan concluded that the primary problem was one of hypermobility, the result of inadequate posterior fixation that caused the snapping of the meniscus to and fro within the joint with secondary hypertrophy. Because of this mechanism, discoid menisci are not always discoid, and in fact, they may make various configurations, depending on the response to the instability.

Two types of discoid lateral menisci have been described — the complete type and the Wrisberg type. The complete type, which is attached peripherally, presents with symptoms in late adolescence or early adulthood. In this type, a saucerization style of resection often produces good results. [12] The Wrisberg type has no peripheral attachment of the posterior horn except for the ligament of Wrisberg, which is more significantly hypertrophied. This more unstable meniscus snaps back and forth, occasionally blocking full extension, and must be resected by cutting the hypertrophied ligament of Wrisberg. The entire unstable portion of the meniscus must be removed, resulting essentially in a total meniscectomy with results often unsatisfactory as in other total meniscectomies in the skeletally immature population.

Plain radiographs may occasionally suggest the discoid configuration by widening of the lateral joint space and hypoplasia of the lateral tibial spine, but this is not reliable for making the diagnosis. Arthrograms may be helpful, but they often miss the symptomatic, hypertrophied, Type II discoid meniscus. Even magnetic resonance imaging (MRI) may produce some confusion by overreading the discoid shape of the meniscus, leading to an unsettling number of false positives. This reinforces the value of arthroscopy in accurate diagnosis and effective treatment of the discoid meniscus.

OSTEOCHONDRAL FRACTURES AND OSTEOCHONDRITIS DISSECANS

Osteochondral fractures of the articular surface of the knee and the clinical entity of osteochondritis dissecans (OCD) are considered together because of the likelihood of shared etiologic factors, variations in presentation, and pathologic conditions differing only in the size, location, and age of the defect. The cause of OCD has been the subject of ongoing conjecture in the orthopaedic literature. Postulated mechanisms have included localized avascular necrosis, possibly secondary to vascular changes peculiar to the epiphyseal area, trauma, and a tertiary center of ossification in the growing skeleton. Kettlekamp and DeRosa [48] remained unconvinced that OCD and osteochondral fractures are at all related. Carroll and Mubarak [20] pointed out the lack of consistent occurrence with trauma, joint hypermobility, tibial spine prominence, and other local anatomic features. An association with a short or tall obese body habitus was noted, and a relationship with an undefined "constitutional defect" was therefore suggested.

Berndt and Harty [11] nicely demonstrated the traumatic cause of OCD of the talus by using anatomic correlation, histologic descriptions, individual case presentations, and laboratory-produced lesions in the talar dome. There was no need to use a vascular etiologic source to explain something that appeared so clearly related to trauma. Similar parallels may be drawn to the lesion called OCD of the knee. Aicroth,[3-5] in discussing OCD of the knee, believed that the radiographic and clinical picture could largely be explained by trauma and used anatomic correlations to demonstrate this point.

The clinical presentations of acute subchondral fracture and subacute or chronic OCD may be rather different. The osteochondral fracture clearly occurs with trauma, often dramatically so, typically resulting from torque to the knee. It is rapidly followed by a bloody effusion, pain, and mechanical block. This clinical picture is typical enough to reliably make the diagnosis in any adolescent. The radiographs may reveal a minimal defect or no obvious changes at all, depending on the amount of bone taken with the cartilaginous fragment and on the position of the defect.

In skeletally immature patients the presentation of OCD is much less dramatic. A history of trauma may or may not be elicited, or the trauma occurred many weeks or months before the patient was initially seen. The complaint is usually of ache and pain, especially with activity, occasionally accompanied by swelling. "Locking" is rather unusual, but "catching" is common. The affected extremity may show thigh muscle atrophy, occasional effusion, and sometimes tenderness in the intercondylar notch when the knee is flexed. Occasionally pain can be elicited with internal rotation of the leg on the thigh as the knee is put through a range of motion. Radiographs demonstrate a demarcated, disk-shaped, nondisplaced area of lucency in the subchondral bone usually on the medial femoral condylar border of the intercondylar notch. It appears less often on the lateral condyle and only occasionally on the patella (Fig. 56-18).

Smillie[90] described the usual areas of involvement of these osteochondral injuries, relating external or internal injury mechanisms to the site of trauma.

- *Lateral femoral condyle exogenous.* Usually the result of a direct blow, such as a kick to the lateral aspect of the knee. An osteochondral fracture of the anterior and inferior weight-bearing surface of the femoral condyle is produced.
- *Lateral femoral condyle endogenous.* Seen with dislocation of the patella, which produces a relatively small fragment at the superior lateral aspect of the femoral condyle.
- *Medial aspect of the medial femoral condyle exogenous.* Again, from a direct blow to the knee, typically a dashboard injury. An osteochondral fracture of the medial femoral articular surface is produced.
- *Lateral aspect of the medial femoral condyle endogenous.* Associated with a twist or direct blow to the leg that produces a lesion in the site typical of OCD. There may be a slight variation in the location of this lesion, depending on the prominence of the tibial spine.

Treatment depends on the acuteness, magnitude, and presentation of the osteochondral fracture defect. Recent injury with involvement of the weight-bearing articular surface and "locking" must be repaired promptly. A de-

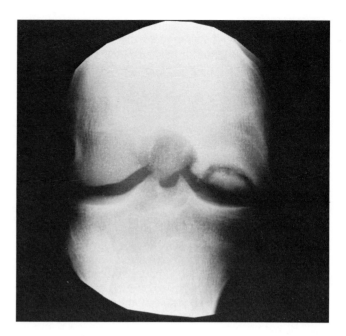

FIG. 56-18. Osteochondritis dissecans in its "classic" location on lateral aspect of medial femoral condyle in 12-year-old boy.

lay may cause further injury secondary to mechanical damage to the remaining articular cartilage, difficulty in replacing the fragment anatomically because of partial healing of the defect, and muscular deconditioning. A delay in treatment dictates a shift in treatment strategy. A large chondral defect is unlikely to remain, but an irregular chondral surface may have developed. Specific treatment with resection and drilling may be unwise unless arthrotomy is indicated for other reasons. Locking, as evidence of a loose body or other mechanical impingements, warrants debridement of the fracture. An exercise rehabilitation program may be indicated in the adolescent and is preferable to allowing him or her to "run it out." Thus the basis of treatment is symptomatic and preventive. This usually involves modification of activity, possibly with immobilization in a plaster cast until the pain and swelling resolve. Activities are then gradually increased unless recrudescence of symptoms appears. Again, rehabilitation of the muscles involved may be necessary if this problem has been long standing and there is significant atrophy.

An aggressive approach can be justified in athletes nearing skeletal maturity because the prognosis becomes far worse after epiphyseal closure. At this time, persistent symptoms despite 6 months of conservative care may be considered justification for surgical intervention. This may involve arthroscopy or arthrotomy with drilling of the lesion either inside-out or, according to some, preferably outside-in so as not to violate the articular surface of the lesion when intact.

Bradley and Dandy[18] have reported no apparent ill effects from drilling through the articular surface. The authors believe that this technique avoids additional incisions and allows more accurate drill hole placement. The lesions were not in weight-bearing areas and no internal fixation was used. Because rapid relief of pain was reported after drilling and a normal radiographic appearance was restored in 10 of 11 knees over 1 to 5 years, the authors suggested that when fragments are fixed internally, the effective part of the operation may be the hole and not the fixation.

It is far more common, however, to find the symptomatic lesion as a completely or partially loose body. Thus the most frequent surgical choice is limited to whether to excise the osteochondral fragment and drill the bed of the lesion or to replace and internally fix the fragment. Although a recent study suggests better results with open reduction–internal fixation, it is technically more demanding and not often feasible.[41] The osteochondral fragment is often smaller than its bed and may need to be further smoothed with a rongeur. Cancellous bone graft from the ipsilateral tibial metaphysis has been used to fill the defect until the articular surfaces are flush.[57]

The prognosis with excision of the fragment is poor enough that some advocate various autografts and allografts.[2,64,102]

Unlike the prognosis for the young adult, the outlook in adolescent OCD is good. Few adolescents require surgery for excision or replacement of the defect, although operation may be required when symptoms of locking or pain and swelling persist. The long-term prognosis remains favorable, and normal knee function is expected in adulthood.

INJURIES CAUSING GROWTH DISTURBANCE ABOUT THE KNEE

As opposed to meniscal, ligamentous, and osteochondral injuries, fractures involving the physis that produce growth disturbances are unique to the immature skeleton. Growth injuries about the knee are especially important because of the potential magnitude of the leg length discrepancy and the possibility of significant angular deformity, resulting in abnormal knee mechanics. Approximately 70% of the longitudinal growth of the femur and 55% of the longitudinal growth of the tibia is produced by the physes about the knee. Significant fractures of the knee are more common in the distal femur than the proximal tibia. The proximal tibia has a more irregular metaphyseal-physeal interface and appears to be more resistant to displacement from trauma. The growth plate itself is a composition of transitional forms of chondrocytes and their surrounding matrix. Because of alterations in the collagen orientation of this matrix, the mechanically weakest strata occur through a band at the interface of the zone of cell hypertrophy with its zone of provisional calcification. However, because of the normal irregularities of the metaphyseal-physeal interface, the actual fracture line usually wanders about this boundary zone.

Growth can also be altered by damage to the vascular supply to the area. The metaphyses and epiphyses of the tibia and femur about the knee have separate blood supply systems. Injury to either the epiphyseal or metaphyseal blood supply may cause a growth disturbance even without a radiographic "bridging."

The Salter-Harris classification of epiphyseal fractures has been thoroughly accepted by orthopaedists. The five classes of fractures are relatively easy to use and appear to have clinical significance. Ogden[76] pointed out that this system does not recognize other determinants of bone growth injuries, such as damage to the metaphysis, diaphysis, periosteum, localized vascular supply, and germinal centers of chondrocytes. He has therefore de-

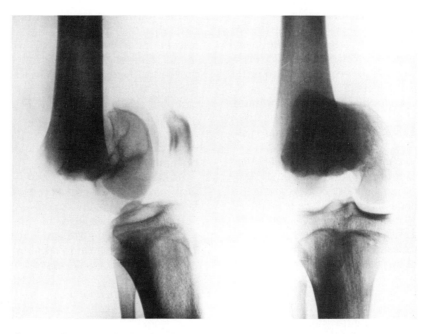

FIG. 56-19. Displacement of Salter-Harris fractures, Types I and II, requires reduction and possible fixation. This injury occurred during a football blocking drill. (From the NISMAT Collection.)

scribed an alternative system with nine major classifications and subclassifications of growth-altering injuries. Its main usefulness is in increasing awareness of those other possible traumatic causes of growth disturbance.

The most common and significant growth injury about the adolescent knee is fracture in and about the distal femoral growth plate.

In distal femoral epiphyseal fractures the use of the familiar Salter-Harris classification scheme to recommend appropriate treatment is particularly treacherous. Experience has shown that in more than 20% of cases, secondary growth disturbances necessitated late reconstructive procedures. In distal femoral epiphyseal fractures, it seems that the degree of initial displacement is a better predictor of subsequent growth disturbance than the Salter-Harris classification. Perhaps total energy absorption plays a role or perhaps it is a vascular effect, but in 1977 Lombardo and Harvey[58] showed that distal femoral epiphyseal fractures initially displaced more than 50% have the poorest prognosis despite the Salter-Harris classification.[92]

In all such injuries the end result appears to depend to some extent on the adequacy of reduction.[58] Salter I and II fractures of the distal femur may be adequately treated with closed reduction and casting, occasionally using percutaneous fixation (Fig. 56-19). As the patient approaches maturity, the importance of anatomic reduction of nonarticular fractures becomes less important. Fractures involving the articular surface, Salter-Harris Type III (Fig. 56-20) and Type IV require anatomic re-

duction. Fixation may be across the epiphysis, the metaphysis, or the physis itself as is dictated by the fracture configuration. Secure reconstruction of the joint surface is crucial to early rehabilitation and complete return of normal knee function.

The unstable knee in an adolescent demands stress radiographs to demonstrate whether the site of injury is in the joint or at the physis. This is especially true in Salter I injuries (Fig. 56-21), which may be occult, or in Salter II fractures (Fig. 56-22), where there is a small Thurston-Holland fragment. Treatment of these fractures has two goals: anatomic restoration of the articular surface and normal growth potential. Conversely, with all fractures involving the distal femoral epiphysis, a complete examination of the ligamentous integrity of the joint is essential. Bertin and Goble[13] concluded that physeal fracture does not preclude ligament damage. Six of their 16 patients with distal femoral epiphyseal fractures were found to have late ligamentous insufficiency (ACL and medial collateral ligament [MCL]). They believed that the initial associated ligamentous injury was overlooked because attention was directed toward fracture management without consideration of possible ligament injury.

Torg, Pavlov, and Morris[94] found late ACL laxity in two of their six athletes with Salter-Harris Type III fractures of the medial femoral condyle. They believed that the usual mechanism of injury was a valgus force applied to the distal femur and hypothesized that the medial femoral condylar fragment was held in a normal relationship

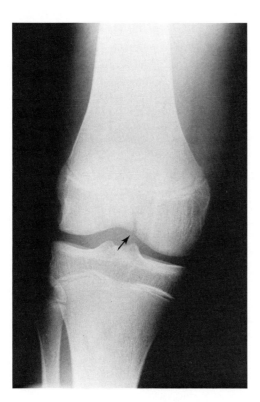

FIG. 56-20. Salter-Harris Type III fracture of distal femoral physis. In some cases stress views may be required to demonstrate fracture. (From the NISMAT Collection.)

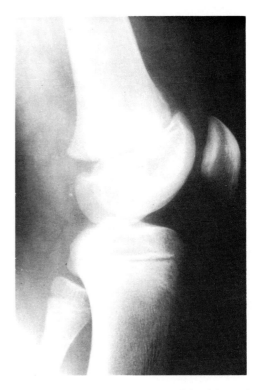

FIG. 56-21. Salter-Harris Type I fracture of distal femoral physis. (From the NISMAT Collection.)

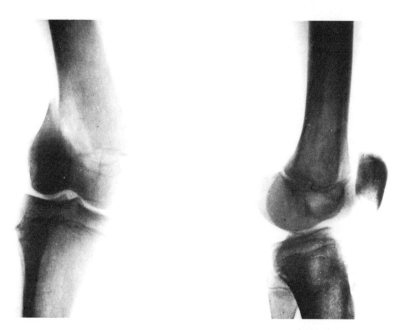

FIG. 56-22. Salter-Harris Type II fracture. (From the NISMAT Collection.)

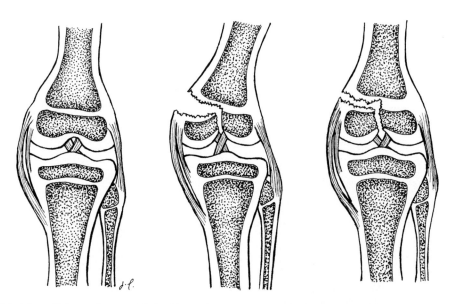

FIG. 56-23. Pathomechanics of Salter-Harris Type III fracture of medial femoral condyle involve valgus force applied to distal part of femur and knee, resulting in fracture across medial aspect of distal femoral physis, extending through epiphysis into intercondylar notch. Medial condylar fragment is held in relationship to proximal part of tibia by medial collateral and posterior cruciate ligaments. Femoral lateral condylar fragment rotates on lateral tibial condyle either laterally or posteriorly, or both. Because of restraining effect of anterior cruciate and lateral capsular ligaments, spontaneous reduction occurs. With excessive rotation of femoral lateral condylar fragment anterior cruciate ligament becomes vulnerable to injury. (Modified from Torg JS, Pavlov H, Morris VB: *J Bone Joint Surg* 63A:586, 1981.)

to the proximal part of the tibia by the MCL and posterior cruciate ligament (PCL) (Fig. 56-23). However, with excessive rotation of the lateral femoral condylar fragment, the ACL becomes vulnerable to injury. Because of ligamentous restraint imposed by the MCL and the PCL on the medial fragment, they thought that treatment should be manipulative reduction followed by non–weight-bearing immobilization in a cylinder cast.

As a result of these published cases of late instability, a strong case can be made for careful arthroscopic evaluation of the cruciate ligaments after closed reduction of these fractures. This is particularly true in cases in which at the time of acute injury, stability testing of the knee is difficult. If a concomitant ligament injury is found, repair can be undertaken at the time of fracture treatment, hopefully obviating the need for a late reconstruction. If reconstruction is not carried out, identification of the ligament injury at least permits a thorough discussion with the young athlete's parents of the need for continuing long-term follow-up to avoid unpleasant late accusations.

Among the rarest of epiphyseal injuries about the knee are those of the proximal fibula.[77] A case report by Abrams et al[2] presented a Salter-Harris Type III fracture of the proximal fibula in a 15-year-old female high school gymnast. The mechanism of injury was reported as a fall from the balance beam with varus stress, and the fracture healed without apparent sequelae after 3 weeks in a cylinder cast at 15 degrees of flexion with partial weight bearing.

SUMMARY

The great majority of knee problems that arise in the skeletally immature athlete are similar to those of the adult, as described elsewhere in this text. However, a thorough understanding of those few characteristics that are unique to the pediatric population is absolutely crucial to the proper management of these injuries.

REFERENCES

1. Abdon P et al: A long-term follow-up study of total meniscectomy in children, *Clin Orthop* 257:166, 1990.
2. Abrams J et al: Salter-Harris type III fracture of the proximal fibula: *Am J Sports Med* 14(6):514, 1986.
3. Aicroth P: Osteochondral fractures and their relationship to osteochondritis dissecans of the knee, *J Bone Joint Surg* 53B:448, 1971.
4. Aicroth P: Osteochondritis dissecans of the knee: a clinical survey, *J Bone Joint Surg* 52B:440, 1971.
5. Aicroth P: Osteochondral fractures and osteochondritis dissecans in sportsmen's knee injuries, *J Bone Joint Surg* 59B:108, 1977.
6. Aitken AP: Fractures of the proximal tibial epiphyseal cartilage, *Clin Orthop* 41:92, 1965.
7. Almgard L, Wikstadt I: Late results of surgery for osteochondritis dissecans of the knee joint, *Acta Chir Scand* 127:588, 1964.
8. Angel KR, Hall DJ: The role of arthroscopy in children and adolescents, *Arthroscopy* 5(3):192, 1989.
9. Batten J, Menelaus MD: Fragmentation of the proximal pole of the patella, *J Bone Joint Surg* 67B:249, 1985.
10. Beddow FH: Treatment of 103 patients with Osgood-Schlatter's disease, *J Bone Joint Surg* 48A:384, 1960.
11. Berndt A, Harty M: Transchondral fractures of the talus, *J Bone Joint Surg* 41A:988, 1959.
12. Berson B, Herman G: Torn discoid menisci of the knee in adults, *J Bone Joint Surg* 61A:303, 1979.
13. Bertin KC, Goble EM: Ligament injury associated with epiphyseal fractures about the knee, *Clin Orthop* 177:183, 1983.
14. Bigos SJ, McBride GG: The isolated lateral retinacular release in the treatment of patellofemoral disorders, *Clin Orthop* 186:75, 1984.
15. Bosworth DM: Autogenous bone pegging for epiphysitis of the tibial tubercle, *J Bone Joint Surg* 16:829, 1934.
16. Bowers KD: Patellar tendon avulsion as a complication of Osgood-Schlatter's disease, *Am J Sports Med* 9:356, 1981.
17. Bradley GW, Shives TC, Samuelson KM: Ligament injuries in the knees of children, *J Bone Joint Surg* 61A:558, 1979.
18. Bradley J, Dandy DJ: Results of drilling osteochondritis dissecans before skeletal maturity, *J Bone Joint Surg* 71B:642, 1989.
19. Burkhort SS, Peterson HA: Fractures of the proximal tibial epiphysis, *J Bone Joint Surg* 61A:996, 1979.
20. Carroll ND, Mubarak SJ: Juvenile osteochondritis dissecans of the knee, *J Bone Joint Surg* 59B:506, 1977.
21. Clanton TO et al: Knee ligament injuries in children, *J Bone Joint Surg* 61A:1195, 1979.
22. Cofield RH, Bryan RS: Acute dislocation of the patella: results of conservative treatment, *J Trauma* 17:526, 1977.
23. Crosby EB, Insall J: Recurrent dislocation of the patella, *J Bone Joint Surg* 58A:9, 1976.
24. DaSilva GL, Bratt JF: Stress trajectories in the patella: study by the photoelastic method, *Acta Orthop Scand* 41:608, 1970.
25. Dickason JM, Fox JM: Fracture of the patella due to overuse syndrome in a child: a case report, *Am J Sports Med* 10:248, 1982.
26. Dickhout S, Delee J: The discoid lateral meniscus syndrome, *J Bone Joint Surg* 64A:1068, 1982.
27. Dietz FR, Mathews KD, Montgomery WJ: Reflex sympathetic dystrophy in children, *Clin Orthop* 258:225, 1990.
28. Fairbank HAT: Internal derangement of the knee in children and adolescents, *Proc R Soc Med* 30:427, 1936.
29. Falster O, Hesselbalch H: Avulsion fracture of the tibial tuberosity with combined ligament and meniscal tear, *Am J Sports Med* 20(1):82, 1992.
30. Fowler PJ: Meniscal lesions in the adolescent: the role of arthroscopy in the management of adolescent knee problems. In Kennedy JC (ed): *The injured adolescent knee*, Baltimore, 1979, Williams & Wilkins.
31. Fujikawa K, Isoki F, Mikura Y: Partial resection of the discoid meniscus in the child's knees, *J Bone Joint Surg* 63B:391, 1989.
32. Garcia A, Neer CS II: Isolated fractures of the intercondylar eminence of the tibia, *Am J Surg* 95:593, 1958.
33. Goodfellow J, Hungerford DS, Zindel M: Patellofemoral joint mechanics and pathology: functional anatomy of the patellofemoral joint, *J Bone Joint Surg* 58B:287, 1976.
34. Graf BK et al: Anterior cruciate ligament tears in skeletally immature patients: meniscal pathology at presentation and after attempted conservative treatment, *Arthroscopy* 8(2):229, 1992.
35. Green WT: Painful bipartite patella, *Clin Orthop* 110:197, 1975.
36. Hand WL, Hand CR, Dunn AW: Avulsion fractures of the tibial tubercle, *J Bone Joint Surg* 53A:1579, 1971.
37. Hayes AG, Nageswar M: The adolescent painful knee: the value of arthroscopy in diagnosis, *J Bone Joint Surg* 59B:499, 1977.
38. Henard DC, Bobo RT: Avulsion fractures of the tibial tubercle in adolescents, *Clin Orthop* 177:182, 1983.
39. Houghton GR, Ackroyd CE: Sleeve fractures of the patella in children, *J Bone Joint Surg* 61B:165, 1979.
40. Hughston JD: Subluxation of the patella, *J Bone Joint Surg* 50A:1003, 1968.
41. Hughston J, Hergenroeder P, Cournenay B: Osteochondritis dissecans of the femoral condyles, *J Bone Joint Surg* 66A:1340, 1984.
42. Insall J, Salvati E: Patella position in the normal knee joint, *Radiology* 101:101, 1971.
43. Kaelin A, Hulin PH, Carlioz H: Congenital aplasia of the cruciate ligaments, *J Bone Joint Surg* 68B:827, 1986.

44. Kannus P, Jarvinen M: Knee ligament injuries in adolescents, *J Bone Joint Surg* 70B:772, 1988.

45. Kaplan EB: Discoid lateral meniscus of the knee joint, *J Bone Joint Surg* 39A:77, 1957.

46. Kaplan EB: Some aspects of functional anatomy of the human knee joint, *Clin Orthop* 23:18, 1962.

47. Kaye JJ, Freiberger RH: Fragmentation of the lower pole of the patella in spastic lower extremities, *Radiology* 101:97, 1971.

48. Kettlekamp DB, DeRosa GP: Biomechanics and functional role of the patellofemoral joint. In *American Academy of Orthopaedic Surgeons instructional course lectures,* vol 25, St Louis, 1976, Mosby.

49. King AC, Blundell-Jones G: A surgical procedure for the Osgood-Schlatter lesion, *Am J Sports Med* 9:250, 1981.

50. Kujala UM, Kzist M, Heinonen MB: Osgood-Schlatter's disease in adolescent athletes: retrospective study of incidence and duration, *Am J Sports Med* 13(4):236, 1985.

51. Larsen E, Lauridsen F: Conservative treatment of patellar dislocations, *Clin Orthop* 171:131, 1982.

52. Larson RL: Subluxation-dislocation of the patella. In Kennedy JC (ed): *The injured adolescent knee,* Baltimore, 1979, Williams & Wilkins.

53. Levi JH, Coleman CR: Fracture of the tibial tubercle, *Am J Sports Med* 4:254, 1976.

54. Lieb FJ, Perry J: Quadriceps function: an anatomical and mechanical study using amputated limbs, *J Bone Joint Surg* 50A:1535, 1968.

55. Lieb FJ, Perry J: Quadriceps function: an electromyographic study under isometric conditions, *J Bone Joint Surg* 53A:749, 1971.

56. Libscomb A, Anderson A: Tears of the anterior cruciate ligament in adolescents, *J Bone Joint Surg* 68A:19, 1986.

57. Lipscomb P, Lipscomb P Sr, Bryan R: Osteochondritis dissecans of the knee and loose fragments, *J Bone Joint Surg* 60A:235, 1978.

58. Lombardo S, Harvey J: Fractures of the distal femoral epiphysis, *J Bone Joint Surg* 59A:742, 1977.

59. Manzione M et al: Meniscectomy in children: a long-term follow-up study, *Am J Sports Med* 11:111, 1983.

60. Maybar II: Avulsion fracture of the tibial tubercle apophysis with avulsion of patellar ligament, *J Pediatr Orthop* 2:303, 1982.

61. McCarroll Jr, Rettig AC, Shelbourne KD: Anterior cruciate ligament injuries in the young athlete with open physes, *Am J Sports Med* 16(1):44, 1988.

62. McCarty DJ: *Arthritis and allied conditions,* ed 9, Philadelphia, 1979, Lea & Febiger.

63. McConnell J: The management of chondromalacia patellae: a long-term solution, *Aust J Physiother* 32(4):215, 1986.

64. McDermott A, Langer F, Pritzker K: Fresh small fragment osteochondral allografts, *Clin Orthop* 197:96, 1985.

65. McGinty JB, McCarthy JC: Endoscopic lateral release: a preliminary report, *Clin Orthop* 158:120, 1981.

66. McLennan JG: The role of arthroscopic surgery in the treatment of fractures of the intercondylar eminence of the tibia, *J Bone Joint Surg* 64B:477, 1982.

67. Medlar RC, Lyne GD: Sinding-Larsen-Johansson disease, *J Bone Joint Surg* 60A:1113, 1978.

68. Medlar RC, Mandiberg JJ, Lyne ED: Meniscectomies in children: report of long-term results (mean 8.3 years) of 26 children, *Am J Sports Med* 8:87, 1980.

69. Meyers M, McKeever F: Fracture of the intercondylar eminence of the tibia, *J Bone Joint Surg* 41A:209, 1959.

70. Meyers M, McKeever F: Fractures of the intercondylar eminence of the tibia, *J Bone Joint Surg* 52A:1677, 1970.

71. Micheli LJ: Overuse injuries in children's sports: the growth factor, *Orthop Clin North Am* 14:337, 1983.

72. Micheli LJ et al: Patella alta and the adolescent growth spurt, *Clin Orthop* 213:159, 1986.

73. Minkoff J, Patterman E: The unheralded value of arthroscopy using local anesthesia for diagnostic specificity and intraoperative corroboration of therapeutic achievement, *Clin Sports Med* 6(3):471, 1987.

74. Morrissey RT et al: Arthroscopy of the knee in children, *Clin Orthop* 162:103, 1982.

75. Murakami Y: Intraarticular dislocation of the patella: a case report, *Clin Orthop* 171:137, 1982.

76. Ogden J: *Skeletal injury in the child,* Philadelphia, 1982, Lea & Febiger.

77. Ogden JA: The anatomy and function of the proximal tibiofibular joint, *Clin Orthop* 101:186, 1974.

78. Ogden JA, McCarthy SM, Jokl P: The painful bipartite patella, *J Pediatr Orthop* 12:263, 1982.

79. Ogden JA, Southwick WO: Osgood-Schlatter's disease and tibial tubercle development, *Clin Orthop* 116:180, 1976.

80. Ogden JA, Tross RB, Murphy MJ: Fractures of the tibial tubercle in adolescents, *J Bone Joint Surg* 62A:205, 1980.

81. Osgood RB: Lesions of the tibial tubercle occurring during adolescence, *Boston Med Surg J* 148:114, 1903.

82. Potts H, Noble J: Arthroscopic surgery in the very young, *J Bone Joint Surg* 71B:541, 1989.

83. Roberts JM: Avulsion fractures of the proximal tibial epiphysis. In Kennedy JC (ed): *The injured adolescent knee,* Baltimore, 1979, Williams & Wilkins.

84. Ross AC, Chesterman PJ: Isolated avulsion of the tibial attachment of the posterior cruciate ligament in childhood, *J Bone Joint Surg* 68B:747, 1986.

85. Sanders W, Wilkins K, Neidre A: Acute insufficiency of the posterior cruciate ligament in children, *J Bone Joint Surg* 62A:129, 1980.

86. Sandow MJ, Goodfellow JW: The natural history of anterior knee pain in adolescents, *J Bone Joint Surg* 67B:36, 1985.

87. Schlatter C: Verletzungen des schnabelfoermigen fortsatzes der oberen tibiaepiphyse, *Beitr Klin Chir* 38:874, 1903.

88. Shelton WR, Canale ST: Fractures of the tibia through the proximal tibial epiphyseal cartilage, *J Bone Joint Surg* 61A:167, 1979.

89. Sinding-Larsen MF: A hitherto unknown affection of the patella, *Acta Radiol* 1:171, 1921.

90. Smillie IS: *Injuries of the knee joint,* ed 5, New York, 1978, Churchill Livingstone.

91. Soren A, Fetto JF: Pathology, clinical findings, and treatment of Osgood-Schlatter's disease, *Orthopedics* 7:230, 1984.

92. Steiner M, Grana W: The young athlete's knee: recent advances, *Clin Sports Med* 7(3):527, 1988.

93. Thomas NP, Jackson AM, Aichroth PM: Congenital absence of the anterior cruciate ligament, *J Bone Joint Surg* 67B:572, 1985.

94. Torg JS, Pavlov H, Morris VB: Salter-Harris type III fracture of the medial femoral condyle occurring in the adolescent athlete, *J Bone Joint Surg* 63A:586, 1981.

95. Watson-Jones R: *Fractures and joint injuries,* ed 4, vol 2, Baltimore, 1955, Williams & Wilkins.

96. Weaver JK: Bipartite patella as a cause of disability in the athlete, *Am J Sports Med* 5:137, 1977.

97. Wiley JJ, Baxter MP: Tibial spine fractures in children, *Clin Orthop* 225:54, 1990.

98. Wolf J: Larsen-Johansson disease of the patella: seven new case reports; its relationship to other forms of osteochondritis: use of male sex hormones as a new form of treatment, *Br J Surg* 23:335, 1950.

99. Woolfrey BE, Chandler EF: Manifestations of Osgood-Schlatter's disease in late teenage and early adulthood, *J Bone Joint Surg* 42A:327, 1969.

100. Wroble RR et al: Meniscectomy in children and adolescent, *Clin Orthop* 279:180, 1992.

101. Wu C, Huang S, Liu T: Sleeve fracture of the patella in children *Am J Sports Med* 19(5):525, 1991.

102. Yamashita F et al: The transplantation of an autogenic osteochondral fragment for osteochondritis dissecans of the knee, *Clin Orthop* 201:43, 1985.

103. Zarienznyj B: Avulsion fracture of the tibial eminence: treatment by open reduction and pinning, *J Bone Joint Surg* 59A:1111, 1977.

104. Ziv I, Carrol N: Role of arthroscopy in children, *J Pediatr Orthop* 2:243, 1982.

ADDITIONAL READINGS

Aglietti P et al: Arthroscopic drilling in juvenile osteochondritis dissecans of the medial femoral condyle, *Arthroscopy* 10(3):286, 1994.

Apple DF Jr: Adolescent runners, *Clin Sports Med* 4:641, 1985.

Binazzi R et al: Surgical treatment of unresolved Osgood-Schlatter lesion, *Clin Orthop* 289:202, 1993.

Brody TA, Russell D: Interarticular horizontal dislocation of the patella: a case report, *J Bone Joint Surg* 47A:1393, 1965.

Cahill B: Treatment of juvenile osteochondritis dissecans and osteochondritis dissecans of the knee, *Clin Sports Med* 4:367, 1985.

Huberti HH, Hayes WC: Patellofemoral contact pressures: the influence of Q-angle and tendofemoral contact, *J Bone Joint Surg* 66A:715, 1984.

Hughston JC, Hergenroeder PT, Courtenay BG: Osteochondritis dissecans of the femoral condyles, *J Bone Joint Surg* 66A:1340, 1984.

Kennedy JC (ed): *The injured adolescent knee*, Baltimore, 1979, Williams & Wilkins.

Libscomb AB et al: Fracture of the tibial tuberosity with associated ligamentous and meniscal tears, *J Bone Joint Surg* 66A:790, 1984.

Lubowitz JH, Graver JD: Arthroscopic treatment of anterior cruciate ligament avulsion, *Clin Orthop* 294:242, 1993.

McManus F, Rang M, Heslin DJ: Acute dislocation of the patella in children: the natural history, *Clin Orthop* 139:88, 1979.

Medler RC, Jansson KA: Arthroscopic treatment of fractures of the tibial spine, *Arthroscopy* 10(3):292, 1994.

Molander ML, Wallin G, Wikstad I: Fracture of the intercondylar eminence of the tibia: a review of 35 patients, *J Bone Joint Surg* 63B:89, 1981.

Moretz JA et al: Long-term follow-up of knee injuries in high school football players, *Am J Sports Med* 12:298, 1984.

Mubarak SJ, Carroll NC: Juvenile osteochondritis dissecans of the knee: etiology, *Clin Orthop* 157:200, 1981.

Nicholas JA: Dynamic causes of patellar pain, *Orthop Rev* 11:33, 1973.

Nicholas JA, Veras G, Goldberg B: Sports medicine—pediatric perspective, *NY State J Med* 78:1978.

Nicholas JA et al: Children's sports injuries —arc they avoidable? *Orthop Trans* 3:88, 1979.

Outerbridge RE: Osteochondritis dissecans of the posterior femoral condyle, *Clin Orthop* 175:121, 1983.

Roberts JM, Lovell WW: Fractures of the intercondylar eminence of the tibia (proceedings of the American Academy of Orthopaedic Surgeons), *J Bone Joint Surg* 52A:827, 1970.

Singer KM, Henry J: Knee problems in children and adolescents, *Clin Sports Med* 4:385, 1985.

Stanitski CL: Anterior knee pain syndromes in the adolescent, *J Bone Joint Surg* 75A(9): 1407, 1993.

Zaman M, Leonard MA: Meniscectomy in children: results in 59 knees, *Injury* 12:425, 1981.

CHAPTER 57 Injuries to the Hip and Pelvis

Lawrence I. Karlin

Although athletic injuries to the hip and pelvis are uncommon, seemingly benign injuries to the hip and pelvis in children may lead to lifetime disability because of peculiarities of the local anatomy and the growth process. In addition, serious disease states that are unrelated to trauma may occur and be misinterpreted as a posttraumatic event.

To understand the cause and treatment of childhood athletic injuries, it is helpful to classify them as acute, macrotraumatic injuries or repetitive, microtraumatic or overuse injuries. The concept of overuse syndromes is relatively new to children's orthopaedics. Tendinitis, stress fractures, and apophysitis are all results of repetitive microtrauma and constitute a truly unique sports-related injury. If preventive medicine is to be applied, the factors that predispose the child to injury must be appreciated. This allows intelligent counseling as to choice of events, earlier diagnosis, and prevention of more serious injuries.

PREDISPOSING FACTORS

The risk factors unique to children are growth cartilage, differential growth rate between bone and muscle, and malalignment. Growth cartilage is located on the joint surface, the epiphyseal and apophyseal plates. An increase in susceptibility of the growing articular cartilage to shear forces has been proposed as a predisposing factor in osteochondritis dissecans.[94] The relative weakness of the physis makes it more susceptible to injury than the adjacent ligaments; a youngster is more likely to sustain an epiphyseal fracture than a sprain. The same predisposition of the apophysis also affects the hip and pelvic area.

Another important but less popularized factor in childhood injuries is the growth process itself.[92] The musculotendinous units and ligaments lengthen in response to longitudinal osseous growth. Soft-tissue lengthening lags behind skeletal growth, and during growth spurts an increase in musculotendinous tightness occurs, resulting in loss of flexibility and increase in susceptibility to overuse injuries. In a related way, imbalance between muscle groups, for instance, the quadriceps and hamstrings, also predisposes to injury.[17]

The most common malalignment conditions affecting the hip and pelvis are excessive lumbar lordosis and femoral anteversion. The increased lumbar lordosis may be a result of factors within the lumbar area, such as increased sacral inclination or spondylolisthesis, or it may be a compensation for structural abnormalities elsewhere, such as increased thoracic kyphosis or hip flexion contractures. The change in pelvic alignment can result in relative tightness of the hip flexors or the hamstring musculature and increases the risk of tendinitis or apophysitis.

Femoral Anteversion

Excessive femoral anteversion is a common finding in children. In the normal individual the femoral anteversion measures 30 to 40 degrees at birth and resolves gradually with growth to 8 degrees in the male and 14 degrees in the female at skeletal maturity. In the affected individual the torsion declines at a slower rate and presumably remains increased throughout life. The clinical manifestations include toeing-in and, at times, an awkward running style. Little anatomic change can be expected after approximately 8 years of age, although further clinical improvement may result from dynamic compensation.[134]

A number of reports relate increased femoral anteversion to structural pathologic conditions, most notably degenerative arthritis of the hip. The evidence is often anecdotal or inconclusive.[51,77,114,129,132] Significant functional problems are likewise rare. Running may be characterized by internal rotation of the lower extremities during the swing phase, which in severe cases may appear ungainly and be a source of embarrassment to the child. In a small study, Staheli, Lippert, and Denotter[135] demonstrated no relationship between femoral anteversion and impaired physical performance as measured by running, static balance, speed of limb movement, and explosive strength. Certainly, activities that require excessive hip rotation, such as ballet dancing, may be limited by the torsional problem. This can result in poor perfor-

mance or an overuse syndrome, since excessive external tibial torsion and foot pronation are substituted for hip turnout. Leg pain or night cramps may result. Buttock pain may also occur and is thought to be secondary to overuse of the external rotators during dynamic compensation.

Clearly, excessive femoral anteversion should be identified in the young athlete. The clinical examination should include a torsional profile (Fig. 57-1). This profile should take into account (1) foot progression angle, (2) internal and external rotation of the hip, (3) thigh-foot angle, and (4) forefoot adduction. The anteversion may be quantitated by clinical, radiographic, and computed tomographic methods.[35,74,118,122,147]

Treatment and Prevention

The management of the problem is controversial. Shoe modifications, splints, and braces all have their propo-

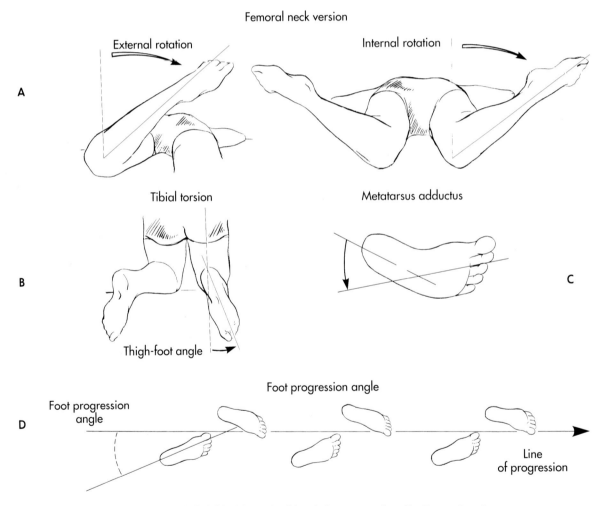

FIG. 57-1. Evaluation of all child athletes should include a torsional profile. Femoral neck version is measured clinically by internal and external rotation of hip. Child is prone with knee flexed to 90 degrees **(A).** Tibial torsion or version is quantitated by angle between longitudinal axis of foot and thigh. Child is prone with knee flexed to 90 degrees **(B).** Metatarsus adductus is evaluated by inward deviation of forefoot on longitudinal axis of hindfoot **(C).** Foot progression angle describes toeing-in or toeing-out as seen in gait. It is the angle formed by longitudinal axis of foot at stance with line of forward progression of body **(D).** Significant malrotation may cause stress-related symptoms. If diagnosis is made early, proper stretching program may be preventive.

nents, but no treatment has been shown to improve the natural history of the condition. Some form of exercise is often prescribed. There is some evidence that ballet dancers have increased external rotation of the hips, and ballet is often suggested as a therapeutic activity for those with excessive internal rotation.[94] Nonetheless, anatomic improvement in the bony structures has not been documented, and it is likely that the increased external rotation is caused by soft-tissue adaptation. The only true anatomic remedy is derotation osteotomy, and its rather high complication rate of 10% to 20% must be considered in respect to the operative benefits.[134]

Preventive measures involve proper counseling with respect to potential problems related to malalignment. Relative inflexibility is treated by careful stretching exercises. All growing athletes require daily stretching of the gastrocsoleus, quadriceps (including rectus femoris), hamstring muscles, and lumbodorsal fascia. Relative imbalance between opposing muscle groups must be corrected by a strengthening program.

Children with excessive femoral anteversion should strengthen the external rotators of the hip and the pronators and evertors of the foot and ankle to avoid the overuse problems of dynamic compensation.

RADIOGRAPHIC ANATOMY

Knowledge of the anatomic peculiarities of the child's pelvis and hip is mandatory for proper interpretation of radiographs. The multiple epiphyseal and apophyseal centers in the region are all areas of potential injury (Fig. 57-2). (They cannot be visualized radiographically before ossification.) Common anatomic variations are present and further confuse the picture, leading to misinterpretation and improper treatment.

The **pelvic apophyses** ossify during adolescence and fuse shortly thereafter. The iliac crests may show an irregularity beginning at age 2 or 3 years that persists to puberty. Segmental ossification may occur with interceding clefts misinterpreted as fracture fragments.[19] The apophysis begins to ossify from anterior to posterior, beginning at age 12 or 14 years. Complete ossification of the crest may take up to 3 years, although on the average is complete by 1 year. Fusion of the apophysis to the ilium is complete by age 19 years.[48,116]

Ossification of the **ischiopubic synchondrosis** is quite variable in timing and pattern. Radiographic enlargement usually accompanies closure and is present unilaterally in 57% and bilaterally in 40% of 7-year-old children (Fig. 57-3). Irregular mineralization and super-

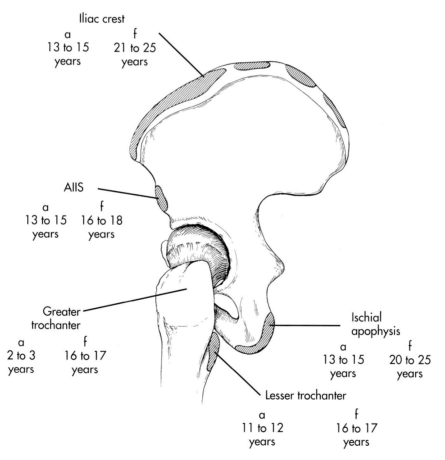

FIG. 57-2. Approximate age of appearance (*a*) and fusion (*f*) of iliac and proximal femoral apophyses. (From Caffey J: *Pediatric x-ray diagnosis*, ed 5, Chicago, 1967, Year Book Medical Publishers; and Tachdjian MO: *Pediatric orthopedics*, Philadelphia, 1972, WB Saunders)

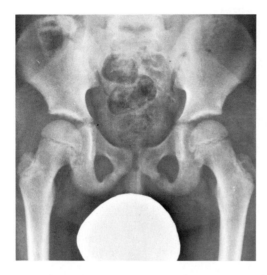

FIG. 57-3. Radiographic enlargement usually accompanies closure of ischiopubic synchondrosis, as shown in this 7-year-old boy. It may be unilateral in 57% of youngsters and should not be confused with fracture or tumor.

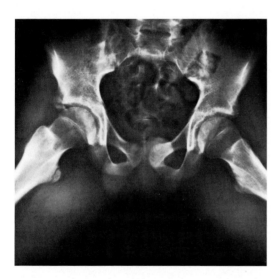

FIG. 57-4. Os acetabuli in 14-year-old boy. Radiograph was obtained after fall on right hip, and original diagnosis was an acetabular fracture. Tracing of left acetabular margin conformed perfectly to the right.

numerary ossification centers occur infrequently. In the preadolescent the outer edges of the lateral ischium and inferior pubic ramus show a variable irregularity in radiographic shape and density. During growth and before fusion with the apophysis, this area is a provisional zone of calcification.[19]

The **os acetabuli** is a bony center that appears radiographically in the cartilaginous rim of the posterior segment of the acetabulum. It is present in 20% of children and fuses with the ilium within several years. In some cases it persists as a separate ossicle, either unilaterally or bilaterally.[105] Confusion with an avulsion fracture or soft-tissue calcification is not uncommon (Fig. 57-4).

The surface of the acetabular cavity itself may also appear irregular during growth.[19]

The ossific nucleus of the **capital femoral epiphysis** is often stippled or granular.[105] Multiple centers may appear, and a cleft may be visible if the epiphysis has been formed from two separate ossification centers. The **trochanteric aphophysis** also frequently develops from multiple foci, which are usually irregularly mineralized.[19]

The diagnosis of apophyseolysis or osteochondritis without high clinical suspicion must be made with reservation in sites where irregular mineralizations appear to be a normal variation. These include the iliac crests, roof of the acetabulum, body of the pubic bones, ischiopubic synchondrosis, and lateral ilium.

Sites of irregular ossification

- Iliac crests
- Actabular roof
- Body of pubis
- Ischiopubic synchondrosis
- Lateral ilium

STRESS FRACTURES

Although the early studies derive from military experience,[45,58] stress fractures are now well recognized among athletes, and the diagnosis must always enter into the differential diagnosis of any stress-related symptom.[6,37,86,131,137] The injury is quite unusual in the area under consideration and especially rare in the individual with open epiphyses. Stress fractures may involve the femoral neck and ischiopubic junction.

Femoral Neck

Femoral neck stress fractures are almost unheard of in children. Wolfgang[155] reported a right femoral neck stress fracture in a 10-year-old girl but found only one previously reported case in a child in a review of 131 femoral neck stress fractures. In the older population the sports that are usually involved with the injury are long-distance running, jumping events, and hiking.[67,79,86] A surprisingly high incidence has been reported in ballet dancers.[125]

Femoral neck fractures have been classified into compression and distraction varieties. The distraction form is characterized by a small crack beginning in the superior surface of the femoral neck. The compression fracture is found in a younger age group and occurs in the inferior portion of the neck. Radiographically it appears as a haze. If weight bearing continues, callus increases and eventually a small, linear radiolucency can be seen.

The presentation is one of gradual onset of hip or anterior thigh pain associated with vigorous activity. Groin pain or pain referred to the knee may occur.[11,79] Initially, the pain is stress related and is relieved by rest, but later it may become constant. Chronicity of symptoms is common. Physical examination usually reveals tenderness

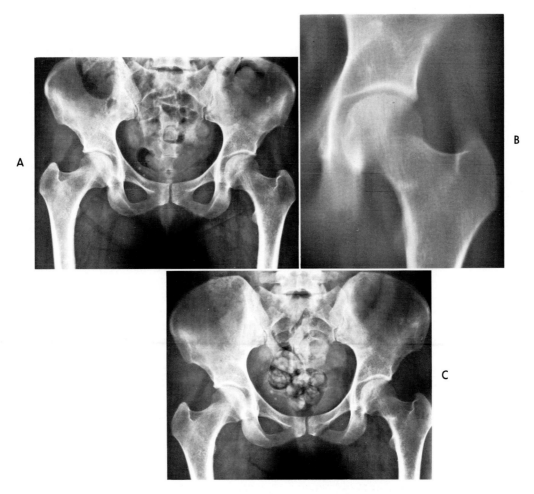

FIG. 57-5. Young adult woman who experienced right anterior hip pain when walking. Only after repeated questioning did she recall that pain began after hiking trip 3 months previously. Her initial film **(A),** taken 3 months after onset of pain showed osteopenia of left proximal femur with thinning of medial femoral neck cortex and reduced trabecular pattern. Bone scan was positive at base of neck, and a tomogram, **(B),** revealed stress fracture. After 6 weeks of bed rest and toe-touch ambulation, healing was obvious **(C).**

over the anterior hip and occasionally slight swelling or induration. There is pain at the extremes of motion especially flexion and internal rotation. Percussion or compression over the greater trochanter may be painful.[11] The gait is slightly antalgic. Displaced fractures usually occur while running and are seen as acute injuries.

Radiographs are frequently negative for up to 3 or more weeks after the injury, with a 71% false negative rate reported (Fig. 57-5).[123,151] The distraction and compression varieties produce a characteristic appearance. The differential diagnosis includes osteoid osteoma, osteomyelitis, or osteosarcoma. A pathologic fracture through a cystic or metastatic lesion is another possibility.

Bone scintigraphy seems a far better screening measure in patients with stress-related symptoms. Prather et al[109] analyzed 42 patients with possible stress-related injuries. Of the 16 with a negative scan, none developed positive radiographs at follow-up. The zero false negative rate has also been reported by Wilcox, Moniot, and Green.[150] The false positive rate is 24%.

To evaluate a lower extremity complaint, the bone scan should encompass the pelvis, both lower extremities, and the lumbar spine. **Examinations limited to the symptomatic area do not detect lesions producing referred pain.** In addition, the scan often demonstrates unsuspected remote lesions. Of the stress-related abnormal scans in the series of Rosen, Micheli, and Treves,[121] 46% were multifocal, with the associated radiographic abnormalities present in only 28%.

A femoral neck fracture that goes on to displacement has the usual complications of coxa vara, avascular necrosis, and late degenerative changes. To avoid these consequences, the earlier diagnosis afforded by bone scanning makes this the proper screening technique. Bargren and Tilson[4] have shown an impressive improvement in early diagnosis and prevention of displacement when physicians were sensitized to stress-related symptoms.

The treatment of femoral neck stress fractures is controversial. The distraction form is often treated symptomatically, but cases of displacement have occurred during bed rest, making internal fixation the preferred choice.[29-32] The compression variety is also frequently treated conservatively. Devas[30,31] claims that displacement does not occur even if weight bearing continues. Evidence to the contrary exists. Lombardo and Benson[79] reported a marathon runner with a compression-type stress fracture that displaced when weight-bearing activity continued. The 10-year-old child reported by Wolfgang[155] showed slight varus angulation. It seems that this variety of fracture could be approached conservatively in the older and more reliable patient. Rest should be instituted until the patient is asymptomatic, followed by protected touch-down ambulation. Enforced, monitored bed rest is required in the younger and unreliable patient. Careful and frequent clinical and radiographic evaluations are required. Any signs of progression are an indication for internal fixation.

Pelvis

Stress fractures may also occur in the pelvis. Devas[30] reported stress fractures at the ischiopubic junction in five children aged 5 to 8 years. The clinical presentation was an antalgic gait, painful hip abduction, and external rotation. There was associated tenderness. This entity seems similar to ischiopubic osteochondrosis juvenilis, as described by VanNeck.[19] In both conditions the radiographic changes said to be characteristic are found in many asymptomatic children and may be normal radiographic variants.

Regardless of the cause, symptomatic youngsters improve on a program of restricted activity. In Selakovich and Love's series[128] of older patients, four of five patients required only 4 to 5 weeks of crutch ambulation for complete resolution of symptoms. Activity should be curtailed to alleviate the acute symptoms. Isometric exercises are performed as tolerated, and less stressful activities, such as swimming, are instituted to maintain strength. Appropriate stretching of tight structures and strengthening when muscle imbalance exists may begin on the opposite side and proceed to the involved side when symptoms allow.

The risk of stress fractures is reduced by a proper training program that involves a gradual increase in physical demands. Stress-related symptoms must be thoroughly evaluated. Bone scanning of the entire pelvis, lower extremities, and lumbar spine should be used early as a screening test.

SOFT-TISSUE INJURIES

Soft-tissue injuries include contusions, strains, sprains, and tendinitis. These are, in general, far more common in adults and must be carefully differentiated in the youngster from the uniquely pediatric injuries of apophyseal avulsion and apophysitis.

Strains

Groin strains involve the muscles arising in the area of the symphysis pubis, the adductor longus, adductor brevis, and gracilis. Running activities, such as those en-

countered in track and football, are usually involved in the mechanism of injury. There is often a violent external rotation of the thigh while the leg is abducted and the foot planted.

A study of ice hockey players demonstrates the well-known association of muscle imbalance and injury.[90] Eight players with groin strain were reported. In all, a 25% power imbalance existed between the two legs, and the weaker leg was injured in each case. Although the usual mechanism of injury occurs during push-off, when the thigh is forcefully abducted and externally rotated, another interesting mechanism was suggested in this particular study. Of the eight injured athletes, seven played a wing position. In six of these, the stepover thigh was injured, implicating active adduction stress as the cause of the injury.

Actual adductor avulsions may also occur at the symphysis pubis. The radiographic findings based on an analysis of the injury in five athletes aged 17 to 23 years have been reported.[126] There was unilateral irregularity in the form of bone destruction and sclerosis involving the pubis and extending in some cases to the inferior pubic ramus. Separate bony fragments were not identified. The radiographic appearance is similar to that of an infection or neoplasm, but the proper diagnosis can usually be made once the history of a relationship to athletic injury is established.

Hamstring strains also occur with some frequency. They are often seen in the sprinter and hurdler. Predisposing factors include strength ratio imbalance between the flexors and extensors of the knee, as well as a strength differential between the two legs.[17] Several other etiologic considerations have been theorized. One is based on the variable attachment of the short head of the biceps femoris to the linea aspera. An extensive attachment is hypothesized as being a predisposition to injury. The dual innervation of the biceps femoris is also proposed as a possible factor in injury caused by simultaneous contractions of the quadriceps and the hamstrings.[18]

Iliopsoas strains are also common. There is usually forced extension of the flexed hip, such as occurs in a football tackle. This must also be differentiated from an avulsion fracture. Musculotendinous disruptions usually cause pain and tenderness in the groin, whereas injuries at the lesser trochanter itself cause pain at the proximal anteromedial thigh. Groin pain may also be caused by strains of the abdominal muscle attachments along Poupart's ligament. The differential diagnosis also in-

---

Differential diagnosis of groin pain

- Adduction strain and apophyseal injury
- Iliopsoas strain and apophyseal injury
- Abdominal muscle strain along Poupart's ligament
- Inguinal hernia
- Lymphadenitis
- Phlebitis
- Epididymitis

cludes inguinal hernia, lymphadenitis, phlebitis, and epididymitis.[26,138]

In general, these strains have typical findings on physical examination with pain on passive stretching and active contraction of the muscles involved. Tenderness is localized to the area. Soft-tissue swelling may occur when a significant musculotendinous injury has occurred.

The treatment is usually supportive and related to the severity of the injury. The initial treatment is rest and ice. This is followed by protected ambulation. Moderate and severe strains involve significant musculotendinous tears, and in this case, 2 or more weeks of protected ambulation is necessary. Later, rehabilitation is added in the form of gentle stretching and then strengthening. The athlete progresses along the rehabilitation schedule as comfort allows. Preventive methods involve correction of muscle imbalance and proper stretching programs.

Contusions

The **greater trochanter** is the most frequently contused area of the hip. Treatment of this in children, as well as an iliac crest contusion or hip pointer injury, is similar to the treatment in the adult. Ice is applied initially, and if necessary, rest is prescribed. Stretching and strengthening are initiated, and return to function is based on the individual's progress. In contact sports, properly padded equipment is used.

AVULSION FRACTURES OF THE PELVIC AND FEMORAL APOPHYSES

Avulsion fractures of the pelvis are most often caused by athletics.[53,72] They typically occur in the adolescent age group after the radiographic appearance but before the fusion of the apophyseal ossific nucleus—the apophyseal phase. Initially the collagen fibers flow smoothly from the tendon into the perichondrium and cartilage of the apophysis. Apophyseal ossification introduces a disruption and produces a stress riser in the unit adapted to tensile load.[102,104]

Sites of apophyseal injury

- Ischium
- Anterior superior iliac spine
- Anterior inferior iliac spine
- Iliac crest
- Lesser trochanter

The gradual evolution of the anatomy and the increasing demands made by the size and vigor of the athlete produce injuries of variable severity. At one end of the spectrum are acute macrotraumatic events such as sudden complete avulsion fractures. At the other extreme are microtraumatic injuries that represent microscopic distractions at the sites of tendon insertions. The pathologic condition is probably similar to that found in Osgood-Schlatter disease (Fig. 57-6).[103] When early symptoms are ignored, more serious injuries may occur. The classic example is the sprinter who complains of vague buttock pain over the course of several months and then sustains a complete ischial apophyseal avulsion fracture. This somewhat disabling injury can be avoided if the prodromal symptoms are recognized.

In general, excellent clinical outcomes following pelvic and femoral apophyseal injuries can be anticipated with appropriate individualized nonoperative treatment.[102,117,145] The thick periosteum and perichondrium usually prevent significant displacement. A successful program must protect the injured area to allow healing and avoid further displacement and encourage a gradual rehabilitation to allow return to activity without reinjury. Such a program has been outlined (Table 57-1).[91] It progresses through five phases with advancement monitored by six clinical assessments: pain, tenderness to palpation, range of motion, muscle strength, level of activity, and radiographic appearance. Functional impairment can occur in rare cases of pelvic avulsion injuries, and surgery may be a viable option in selected individuals.

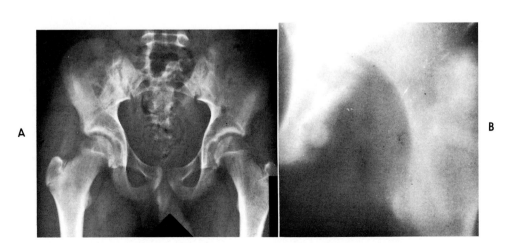

FIG. 57-6. A, A 15-year-old with persistent stress-related buttock pain 3 months after "pulling his hamstrings." Fragmentation and irregularity of ischium, shown best in tomogram, **(B),** bears striking resemblance to Osgood-Schlatter disease. I believe a similar mechanism is involved.

TABLE 57-1 Phases of treatment

Treatment Phase	Days after Injury	Subjective Pain	Tenderness	Range of Motion	Muscle Strength	Level of Activity	Radiographic Appearance
I	0 to 7	Moderate	Moderate to severe	Very limited	Poor	None, protected gait	Osseous separation
II	7 to 20	Minimal	Moderate	Improving with guided exercise	Fair	Protected gait, guided exercise	Osseous separation
III	14 to 30	Minimal with stress	Moderate	Improving with gentle stretch	Good	Guided exercise, resistance	Early callus formation
IV	30 to 60	None	Minimal	Normal	Good to normal	Limited athletic participation	Maturing callus
V	60 to return	None	None	Normal	Normal	Normal	Maturing callus

From Metzmaker JN, Pappas AV: *Am J Sports Med* 13:349, 1985.

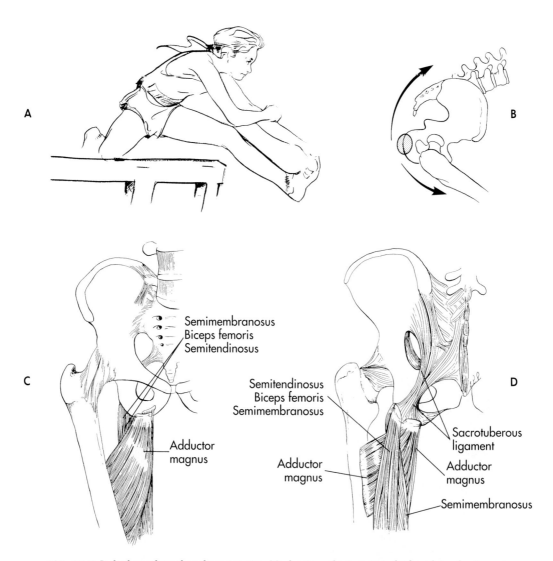

FIG. 57-7. Ischial apophyseal avulsion injuries. Mechanism of injury in ischial avulsion fractures is well demonstrated in hurdler (**A**). Counterforces are generated by pelvic and hip flexion (**B**). Muscle group involved in distracting force is hamstrings, although adductor magnus plays variable degree depending on amount of abduction of leg (**C** and **D**). Note how sacrotuberous ligament serves to provide some stability and how pressure over this structure may cause pain following avulsion injury.

Ischial Apophysis

The ischial apophysis ossifies between ages 14 and 16 years and fuses at 18 to 25 years.[19] It is divided into two portions for the attachment of the posterior portion of the adductor magnus and the hamstrings. The biceps femoris and semitendinosus arise via a common tendon from the posteromedial surface of the distal ischial tuberosity and the semimembranosus by a flat tendon from the posterolateral segment (Fig. 57-7). The apophysis may actually be larger than the tuberosity, extending toward the junction with the pubis and therefore including the anterior and the posterior portion of the adductor magnus.[57]

Avulsions are apt to be partial when the mechanism involves either the hamstrings or adductors preferentially, for example, hurdlers with hamstring injuries as compared with cheerleaders doing splits and injuring the adductors. The sacrotuberous and sacrospinous ligaments brace the ischium and help prevent wider detachment of the ischial apophysis.

A number of mechanisms are probably involved. One involves a powerful hamstring contraction with the pelvis fixed in flexion and the knee in extension. This occurs in anteroposterior splits and is responsible for some of the more severe displacements. Uncoordinated muscle action explains the events involved in ischial avulsions that occur in the athlete who steps in a hole or on uneven ground and attempts to right himself; a sudden, powerful contraction of the knee extensors precedes knee flexion relaxation. The ischial apophysis is then avulsed by the overstretched hamstrings. Similarly, the hamstrings may initiate knee flexion before extensor relaxation. Disproportionate development of the quadriceps and hamstrings has also been mentioned (Fig. 57-8).[52]

Milch[93] proposed a mechanism based on the lever principle. In the erect position the femoral head is considered the fulcrum and the pubic and ischial rami the force and weight arms. The pubic force arm is subject to a flexion force via the iliopsoas and pubofemoral muscles and an extension force by the anterior abdominal muscles. The ischial arm is extended by the forces of the hamstrings and gravity. The sacrotuberous and sacrospinous ligaments resist the force and, in the clinical setting, decrease the displacement of any fracture.

Predisposing abnormalities have been suggested, including endocrine dysfunction, predisposition to osteochondritis or epiphyseolysis, and rickets.[52] DePalma and Silberstein[28] presented two cases of avulsion of the ischial tuberosity in siblings, one of whom was thought to have evidence of an old slipped capital femoral epiphysis.[127]

Ischial avulsion injuries represent events along a continuum of pathologic processes. Recurrent microtrauma, subclinical fractures, and persistent stress-related vague symptoms are at one end; and complete avulsion is at the other. A number of cases with prodromal symptoms are illustrative.[119] Martin and Pipkin[83] described a 15-year-old boy who had vague right hip pain for 2 months before a sudden snap and severe right buttock pain were incurred while broad jumping. An ischial avulsion injury was later diagnosed. Renonapoli[115a] described a fencer with pain in the right buttock after each practice session during a 2-week period. An acute avulsion followed a forward lunge during a competitive match.[52]

Detachment in stages is demonstrated in a number of cases, with at least two distinct episodes of stress-related pain. DeLucchi[27a] reported on a 15-year-old boy who developed severe left buttock pain after completing 80 yards of a 100-yard dash. He finished the race at a lower speed. Two years later, in the same event there was recurrence of the symptoms, which at this time were so severe that he was unable to continue and fell to the ground.[52]

The injury occurs primarily during running, as demonstrated in a retrospective sampling of reported cases with known mechanisms (Table 57-2). The mechanism in football is usually open field running or cutting. In sprints the injury may occur at the starting blocks, the midportion, or during the final kick and lunge at the finish line. Broad jumpers and hurdlers are also often affected.

TABLE 57-2 Ischial apophyseal avulsion injuries*

Incurring Activity	Number of Cases
Running	13
Broad jump/hurdling	11
Football	10
Dance	5
Skating	4
Basketball	2
Baseball	1
Horseback riding	1
Soccer	1
Non-sports related	10
TOTAL	58

Data from Barnes ST, Hinds RB: *J Bone Joint Surg* 54A:645, 1972; Cohen HH: *J Bone Joint Surg* 19:1138, 1937; DePalma AF, Silberstein CE: *Clin Orthop* 38:120, 1965; Martin TA, Pipkin G: *Clin Orthop* 10:108, 1957; McMaster P: *J Bone Joint Surg* 27:493, 1945; Milch H: *Clin Orthop* 2:184, 1953; Schlonsky J, Olix ML: *J Bone Joint Surg* 54A:641, 1972; and Young LW: *Am J Dis Child* 134:885, 1980.
*Based on a review of a number of series that produced 58 cases of ischial apophyseal avulsion injuries of known cause.

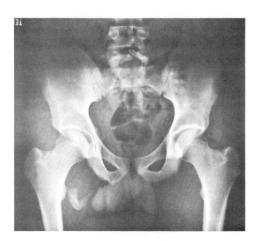

FIG. 57-8. Ischial fracture with this amount of displacement is quite likely to cause late symptoms. Internal fixation is suggested in serious athletes.

TABLE 57-3 Avulsion injuries of the apophysis: a classification and treatment program

Classification	Treatment
Apophyseolysis*	Protection
Avulsion fracture	
Minimal displacement	Protection
Wide displacement	Protection ± reduction, fixation in selected individuals
Old avulsion fracture—symptomatic	Excision

Modified from Martin TA, Pipkin G: *Clin Orthop* 10:108, 1957.
*"Apophyseolysis" and "apophysitis" are essentially synonymous.

The usual presentation is a young athlete between the ages of 13 and 17. The youngest in Hamada and Rida's review[52] of the literature was age 8, and the oldest was age 24 years. Delay in presentation and diagnosis is common. The symptom complex may be variable. It is best understood and rational treatment is more easily established when the injury is divided into stages. The classification of Martin and Pipkin[83] is (1) apophyseolysis, (2) avulsion fracture, and (3) nonunited avulsions (Table 57-3).

The youngster with an apophysitis is seen with mild to moderate pain. The gait is often antalgic. There is tenderness over the ischial tuberosity, and pain is exacerbated by passive stretching and active-resisted motion of the hamstrings or adductor magnus. The area of maximal damage may be further differentiated. The more medial attachment of the adductor is stressed more by passive abduction and active-resisted adduction, whereas the more lateral origin of the hamstrings is involved with active-resisted knee flexion during hip extension and passive straight leg raising. Pressure over the sacrum or sacrotuberous and sacrospinous ligaments may cause pain by traction on the fragment.[93]

The acute avulsion fracture is similar but more painful on physical examination. The gait, when walking is possible, is severely antalgic. Swelling over the ischium and ecchymosis may occur.

Nonunions are frequent, although not all are symptomatic.[5,104,154,157] Symptoms either persist following an injury or recur later. Episodic, vague hip and buttock pain is caused by activity. Inability to sit comfortably on the enlarged tuberosity is quite characteristic. Local tenderness is most often mild, and pain with range of motion is less marked.[93]

Diagnosis is confirmed radiographically. Only rarely does the injury occur before the appearance of the apophysis. In apophyseolysis, there may be irregularity or fragmentation (Fig. 57-6). The differential diagnosis includes osteomyelitis and Ewing's sarcoma. A crescentic fracture is noted under the body of the ischium in the acute avulsion injury. Determination of the amount of displacement is critical to the treatment plan (Fig. 57-8).

In late cases the radiographic appearance is a large, bony mass with exuberant callus inferior to and often in contact with the ischial tuberosity. In two thirds of the cases a well-delineated radiolucent line of nonunion is present.[5]

The radiographic appearance of exuberant bone may be confusing. Differential diagnosis includes myositis ossificans, calcified hematoma, osteochondroma, enchondroma, and chondrosarcoma.[105] In several reported cases surgical excision has been performed because of suspicion of malignant neoplasm.[5] The diagnosis of avulsion is favored by the history of previous trauma and the finding of a radiolucent nonunion line (Fig. 57-9).

Treatment is individualized to the severity of the injury and the demands of the individual. Cases of apophysitis and minimally displaced avulsions have excellent results when treated according to the suggested protocol. Local steroid injections should be avoided. Inflammation represents the normal healing mechanism and should not be adversely influenced.

The treatment of widely displaced avulsion fractures is controversial. Most authors suggest a nonoperative approach.* Recommendations in the literature are often based on inadequate analysis and follow-up. The functional results are rarely documented. In a severely dis-

*References 24, 52, 73, 88, 91, 93, 117, and 145.

Treatment of ischial apophyseal injury

Apophyseolysis	Rest
	Ice
	Protected ambulation
	Isometrics (as tolerated)
	Stretching ⎱ Added when isometrics
	Progresive resistance ⎰ are well tolerated
Avulsion fractures	
Minimum displacement	As above
	Return to sports after radiographic evidence of healing
Marked displacement	As above
	± Open reduction–internal fixation in selected individuals
	Return to sports following healing and rehabilitation
Nonunion	Surgical excision of the nonunited fragment and repair of the muscle attachments

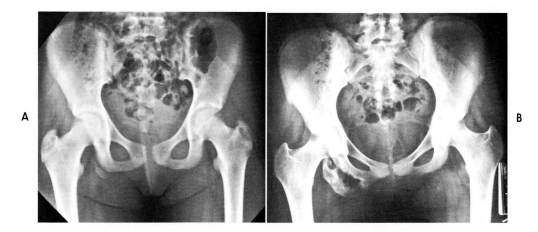

FIG. 57-9. A 15-year-old gymnast sustained ischial avulsion fracture while doing splits (**A**). After 3 years typical picture of enlarged bony mass with probable fibrous union is evident (**B**). This particular patient has no symptoms. Occasionally, avulsion involves cartilaginous tissue only, and radiograph is negative.

placed avulsion, radiographic evidence of osseous healing may require 1 or more years, and some evidence suggests that preinjury function is difficult to reestablish.[124]

Nonunion is a common sequela and is often symptomatic. Barnes and Hinds[5] reported a 68% nonunion rate in their series of 39 cases. Of 14 cases treated surgically, 10 were late excisions of the bony mass for pain. Prolonged rehabilitation, possible diminished athletic capability, and late symptoms of nonunion all favor aggressive treatment in the elite, highly competitive athlete.

Although closed reduction has been reported,[83] open reduction is the surest method of treatment. Several approaches have been described.[93,119] These involve a curved incision in the gluteal fold, a longitudinal incision along the hamstrings, or a peroneal incision. Fixation by screws provides the most stability.

Cases of symptomatic nonunion are best treated with surgical excision of the nonunited fragment and repair of the muscle attachments. Relief of symptoms is the usual course.[83]

Anterior Superior Iliac Spine Apophysis

The ossific nucleus for the anterior superior iliac spine (ASIS) apophysis appears radiographically between the ages of 13 and 15 years and fuses between ages 21 and 25.[19] Virtually all reviewed cases of avulsion fractures fall within this age group. Christopher[22] found 45 reported cases in his 1933 review of the literature. Carp[21] noted an age distribution of 15 to 23 years, excluding a single case of a 70-year-old man. Nearly all the injuries are related to sports.

The ASIS serves as the origin of the sartorius, tensor fasciae latae, and inguinal ligament (Fig. 57-10). Attached to the inguinal ligament are the external and internal obliqui and transversalis muscles. The mechanism of the acute macrotraumatic avulsion is via a severe contraction, stretch, or combination involving the opposing muscle groups. Sudden contracture of the sartorius or hyperextension of the trunk is usually involved. The pre-

dominant causative sport is sprinting, but noncontact football injuries are second. Most often the athlete is affected while in the middle of a running event.[95] Sprint starts are a less frequent cause, but they do allow a study of the probable mechanism.

In the usual history, a young sprinter feels a sudden, sharp pain in the right groin immediately on starting a race. There is an explosive stretching of the hip flexors along with a sudden extension of the trunk, resulting in strong forces acting in opposition to one another. The usual starting position with the right leg flexed may be one reason for the dominating right-sided frequency of the injury. Microtraumatic injuries are characterized clinically by aching pain that is initiated or exacerbated by exertion. Cross-country running is a typical sport associated with this mode of injury.[34]

On physical examination the athlete demonstrates an antalgic gait with a listing both forward and laterally to the affected side. The athlete depicted in Fig. 57-11 demonstrates the typical findings that are expected from the local anatomy. There is local tenderness over and inferior to the ASIS. Pain is exacerbated by passive hip extension and further increased by knee flexion. Active hip flexion and abduction against resistance, as well as attempting to sit up while in the supine position, exacerbate the pain. Radiographic evaluation may require oblique views to demonstrate the small avulsed segment (Fig. 57-12). Findings consistent with apophyseolysis, such as irregularity and fragmentation, may be encountered in those with microtraumatic injury. Displacement is usually not significant.

As a rule, treatment is conservative, with excellent results uniformly reported.[21,22,34] In Carp's series[21] the length of disability averaged 20 days.[34] In the series of Dulabal, Brunelte, and Haddad,[34] two internal fixations were performed. Their criteria for surgery involved displaced fragments in high-performance athletes.

Preventive measures involve thorough stretching and strengthening exercises of the hip flexors. Prodromal

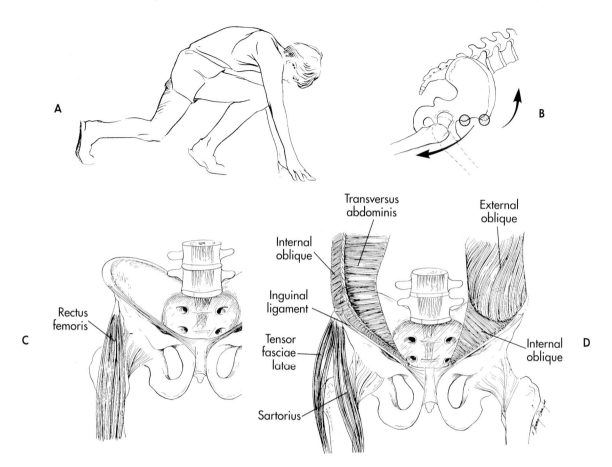

FIG. 57-10. Anterior superior and anterior inferior iliac apophyseal avulsion injuries. These injuries occur through a similar mechanism, which is well demonstrated by sprinters (**A**). **B,** Pelvic and hip extension provide opposing motion. **C,** Distracting muscle force is provided by rectus femoris in anterior superior iliac avulsion. Combination of forces is involved in superior spine injury. Superior distraction is provided by abdominal muscles via inguinal ligament. Distally directed force is generated by tensor fasciae latae and sartorius (**D**).

symptoms should be appreciated and proper conditioning prescribed.

Anterior Inferior Iliac Spine Apophysis

Fractures of the anterior inferior iliac spine (AIIS) are unusual and occur much less frequently than those of the ASIS.[25] Gallagher[41] thought that the injury was more common than is usually acknowledged. He described two cases in a small community that occurred within a 7-month period. The apophysis appears at age 13 to 15 years and fuses between 16 and 18 years.[19] It accepts the origin of the straight head of the rectus femoris, which is responsibile for the avulsion force (Fig. 57-10).[57]

The relative infrequency of AIIS injury with respect to the ASIS was explained by Weitzner.[149] He believed that the sartorius went into action earlier and generated more force than the rectus femoris and that the earlier age of fusion decreased the length of time during which the AIIS apophysis was susceptiblc to injury. Hc also believed that the attachment of one as opposed to three different muscles diminished the stress.

The mechanism of injury is similar to that of an ASIS injury. Again, this is a sprinter's injury with the apophysis avulsed suddenly by flexion stress. In the series of Dulabal, Brunelte, Haddad,[34] both of the AIIS injuries occurred in sprinters at the starting blocks. The sprinters in Gallagher's series[41] became symptomatic well into the races. Reports of prodromal symptoms of mild pain preceding acute injury demonstrate the overuse nature of these cases (Table 57-4).

The patients are seen with sudden pain in the groin area during a sporting event. There is an antalgic gait, tenderness, and pain with active hip flexion. Radiographs, including oblique views, show the injury. Displacement is usually minimal.

Treatment of apophysitis and minimally displaced fragments is conservative, and healing without functional impairment is the usual result. Irving[62] presented two cases of exostosis formation following the injury. In one case this resulted in a limp and limited rotation in abduction. Excision was performed.

Treatment of the widely displaced fracture is controversial. Conservative treatment is suggested by most, but

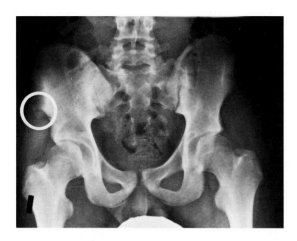

FIG. 57-11. This 16-year-old boy bruised his right hip on a door-knob. Pain prevented him from attending baseball practice for 1 week. He then returned on the day of a game and played without discomfort. While sliding into second base, he reinjured the hip. He had attempted to "take out" the second baseman, and in so doing, slid well to left of base. His hips and trunk were therefore fully extended, and his knee was flexed; these maneuvers put maximal tension on muscle groups inserting and originating on anterior superior iliac spine (ASIS). There was sudden pain and inability to ambulate. Physical examination was classic for ASIS avulsion. There was markedly antalgic gait. Active trunk flexion, hip flexion, and hip abduction were extremely painful, as were passive hip adduction and extension. There was point tenderness over ASIS. Radiographs confirmed diagnosis. He was treated with bed rest for several days, followed by protected weight bearing on crutches with toe-touch gait. After 3 weeks there was no longer any point tenderness. At that time, stretching exercises could be performed without pain and were initiated. One week later, resisted exercises were begun when these could be performed without any discomfort. At 6 weeks, fracture was healed radiographically and athlete was allowed to return gradually to competitive sports. In this case minor injury may have set stage for more severe avulsion fracture. Localized hemorrhage and muscle tightness resulted from initial injury. In addition, discomfort prevented exercise that week. He then returned to competitive sports and did not perform a thorough warm-up. Here, training errors and some slight local tightness combined to cause injury.

the number of cases in any series is small. The report of Irving[62] demonstrates that definite functional impairment may occur. Dulabal, Brunelte, and Haddad[34] treated one of their two AIIS avulsions with open reduction and internal fixation. They believed that the possibility of exuberant healing with resultant limited motion was an indication for the procedure. This may be true in the high-performance athlete.

Iliac Crest Apophysis

The iliac crest apophysis ossifies at 13 to 15 years of age and fuses to the ilium at 21 to 25 years. Ossification begins anterolaterally and progresses medially. Complete excursion takes an average of 1 year, while 2 to 3 years are required for fusion of the apophysis to the underlying ilium. The ossification may develop in fragments.[19,116] The muscles responsible for the avulsion force are the abdominal obliquus, tensor fasciae latae,

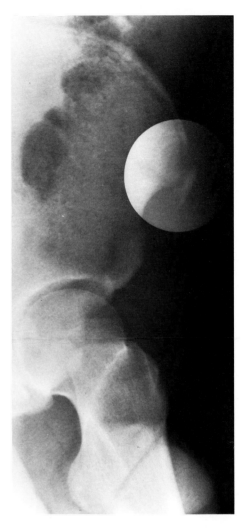

FIG. 57-12. Anterior superior iliac spine avulsion in 17-year-old sprinter.

TABLE 57-4 Avulsion injuries of the anterior inferior iliac spine apophysis*

Incurring Activity		Number of Cases
Track		12
Sprints	8	
Cross-country running	2	
Long jump	1	
Other	1	
Football		6
Baseball		2
Wrestling		1
Dance		1
Falls (nonsport)		2
TOTAL		24

Data from Corlette CE: *Med J Aust* 2:682, 1927; Dulabal TA, Brunelte ME, Haddad RJ: Avulsion fractures of the lower extremity in the adolescent athlete. Paper presented at American Academy of Orthopaedic Surgeons Annual Meeting, Anaheim, Calif, 1983; Gallagher JR: *Am J Surg* 102:86, 1935; Irving MH: *J Bone Joint Surg* 46B:720, 1964; and Weitzner I: *AJR* 33:39, 1935.
*Based on a review of representative reports that revealed 24 cases of known mechanism.

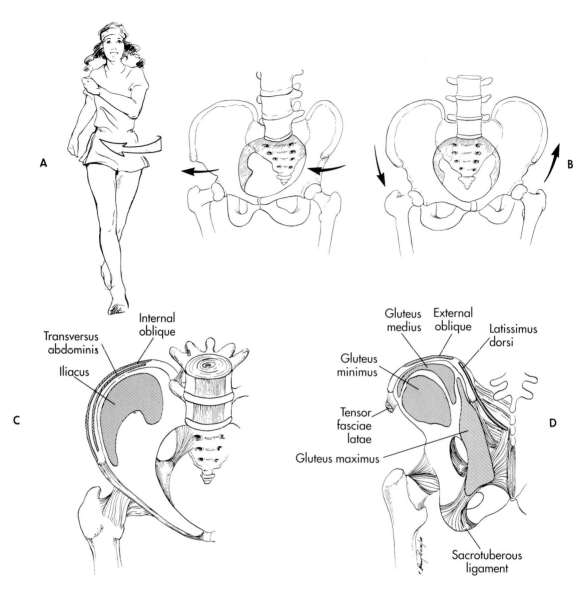

FIG. 57-13. Iliac crest apophyseal avulsion injuries. Commonly involved sport seems to be distance running (**A**). There is repetitive stress caused by rotational and translational motions of pelvis in concert with forces generated by trunk and hip muscles (**B** to **D**).

and gluteus medius, which attach on the anterior portion, and the latissimus dorsi and gluteus maximus, which are found posteriorly (Fig. 57-13).[57]

There are three forms of injury: acute contact, acute noncontact, and overuse.[34] The contact injury is essentially a hip pointer. This usually occurs in football when a direct blow over the crest results in a compression fracture.

The noncontact injuries are avulsions. In the acute variety, this usually occurs when a sudden, severe abdominal contraction is opposed by the tensor fasciae latae and gluteus medius in a set and planted leg. A common event is a sudden change in direction while running. Godshall and Hansen's case[44] is indicative. A 14-year-old baseball player rounded third base and suddenly reversed direction. He experienced acute pain in the anterior aspect of

the left iliac crest. A posterior crest injury may occur when the trunk acutely flexes forward, as in the lunge at the finish of a sprint (Fig. 57-14).

Most commonly, the iliac crest avulsion presents subacutely as an overuse syndrome in runners. The pelvis is subjected to multiplane motion during running, which results in repetitive stresses across the iliac crest by the opposing muscles (Fig. 57-13). Rotation occurs through the longitudinal axis of the body. There is a proportional relationship to the amount of rotation and arm swing. Bringing the arms across the trunk increases this rotation and the stress involved.[16] In the frontal plane the pelvis dips on the unsupported side, while flexion and extension occur in the lateral plane and are exaggerated by uphill and downhill running.

The repetitive trauma may result in an actual avulsion

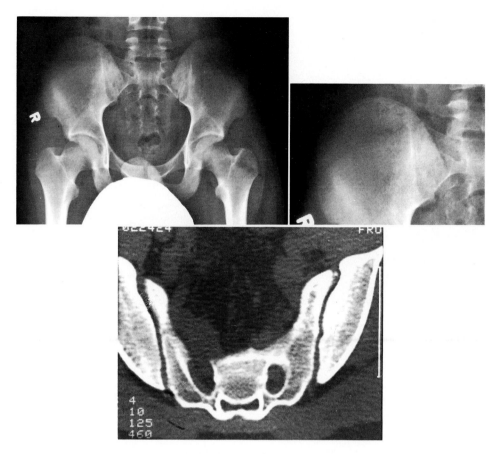

FIG. 57-14. This 17-year-old sprinter developed sudden severe low back pain as he lunged forward at finish line of 100-yard dash. He was seen several months later complaining of recurrent back pain when he tried to return to athletics. Examination demonstrated tenderness at posterior superior iliac spine and mild pain with sacroiliac joint stress. Plain films were suggestive of small avulsion at posterior iliac crest. While this could not be verified by computed tomography scan, vacuum phenomenon in sacroiliac joint is indicative of distraction injury. He was able to return to sports after an 8-week rest.

or a subclinical avulsion or apophyseolysis. Clancy and Foltz[23] found the subacute injury to be relatively common in track. Of 310 track-and-field injuries encountered over a 2½-year period, there were three avulsion fractures of the anterior iliac crest apophysis and 13 cases of apophysitis. The age range was 14 to 17 years. Typical of the group is a 17-year-old middle-distance runner with a history of pain of gradual onset in the region of the right anterior iliac crest. There was no history of acute trauma. The examination revealed localized tenderness and pain associated with resisted abduction of the hip. An avulsion fracture was noted on radiographs. The patients with apophysitis had similar histories and findings without apparent fractures on the radiographs.

In this same series five track athletes were diagnosed as having a posterior iliac apophysitis. The pain was localized to the posterior inferior spine and was duplicated by resistance to abduction with the hip flexed. Clancy and Foltz[23] hypothesized that this mechanism was either an inflammatory reaction of the injured iliac apophysis caused by the repetitive muscular contraction or a response to a subclinical stress fracture.

The radiographic findings may be minimal (Fig. 57-

15). In the case of contact injuries small lucent lines perpendicular to the apophysis are often diagnosed as compression fractures. Caution must be exercised because radiographic peculiarities are common to the area. Radiographic abnormalities of the iliac crest in adolescents have recently been described.[80] In 9 out of 13 patients seen with the diagnosis of hip pointer, radiographs showed discontinuity of the apophysis at the junction of the middle and outer third. The finding was bilateral in all cases, although only two had bilateral symptoms. This discontinuity disappeared at skeletal maturity in all patients.

The clinical presentation is variable, with gradual onset in the overuse group and sudden onset of pain in the acute cases. There is tenderness to palpation and pain to resisted abduction. In Clancy and Foltz's group[23] of overuse syndromes the time of onset to presentation varied from 2 to 8 weeks, with the average being 2 to 3 weeks.

Treatment is conservative, and no functional impairment has been reported. All reported cases returned to full function after 6 weeks of treatment.

Preventive measures are indicated. The running tech-

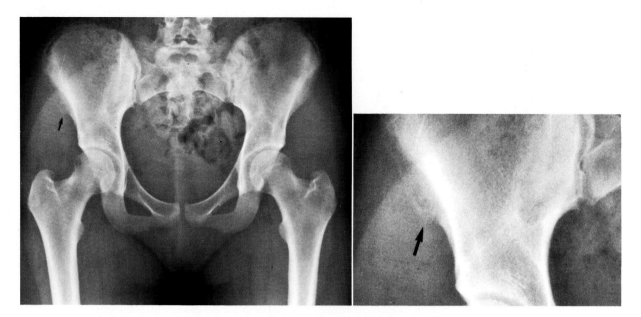

FIG. 57-15. This 15-year-old girl had persistent activity-related pain of insidious onset 1 month after start of soccer season. There was tenderness over anterior iliac crest. Radiographs demonstrate slight displacement of right crest with minimal fragmentation (*arrows*). She recovered and returned to soccer after 1 month of protected ambulation on crutches.

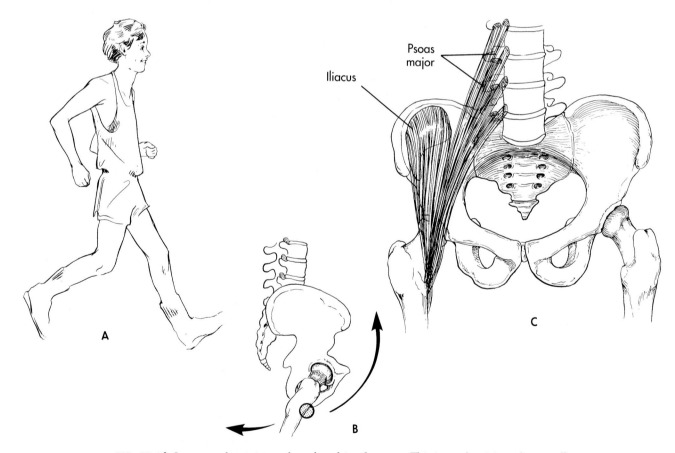

FIG. 57-16. Lesser trochanteric apophyseal avulsion fractures. This is another injury that usually occurs in runners (**A**). Counteracting skeletal motions are pelvic and hip extension (**B**). Iliopsoas serves as distracting force, often acting against planted lower extremity with extended hip (**C**).

nique should be evaluated, and motion that increases the stress should be avoided. The arm swing should not excessively cross the trunk, and the body should be fairly perpendicular to the running surface. In adolescents uphill and downhill running should be eliminated if possible. Proper padding is required in contact sports.

Lesser Trochanter Apophysis

Wilson, Michele, and Jacobson[152] found 78 cases of lesser trochanteric apophyseal avulsions in their review of the literature from 1854 through 1939. Of these cases 90% occurred in adolescents between the ages of ossification and fusion of the lesser trochanter. In Dimon's series,[33] 22 of the 26 cases of known mechanism occurred during sports.

The lesser trochanteric apophysis appears at age 11 to 12 years.[139] It accepts the tendinous insertion of the iliopsoas (Fig. 57-16). The fibers of the iliacus span it and the subjacent femur.[57] This muscular attachment may be instrumental in preventing wider separations following the avulsion injuries.

The avulsion occurs via the contraction of the iliopsoas muscle against resistance. The insult usually takes place during vigorous running. In Dimon's series,[33] football and track headed the etiologic list.

The classic presentation is a teenage athlete who experiences a sudden, sharp pain in the anterior hip area while running. The pain usually forces the athlete to stop running immediately and fall to the ground. Usually, the patient is able to arise with aid. But over the next few days, limping, pain, and stiffness increase. The pain may radiate into the groin, flank, or hip joint. This symptomatology may be variable.

The physical examination is characterized by a short-stance phase and an antalgic gait on the affected side. The leg is often held in external rotation. Tenderness to deep palpation is elicited over the anteromedial hip joint. The athlete is unable to straight leg raise fully when supine, and pain increases with hip flexion against resistance. Passive extension and internal rotation are painful.

Radiographs confirm the diagnosis (Fig. 57-17). A supine anteroposterior view of the pelvis for the hips allows a comparison view. Slight external rotation places the lesser trochanter in profile and affords the best view. The apophysis is displaced proximally and medially. A good lateral x-ray study is required as well to ensure that the injury does not extend into the neck or shaft.

Treatment suggestions vary. Mercer and Duthie[89] suggested bed rest in a sitting position. Key and Conwell[71] used a hip spica cast with the hip flexed to 90 degrees and externally rotated slightly. Others recommend open reduction and internal fixation with cortical or cancellous screw for displacement of greater than 2 cm.[117] There is no good evidence that anything other than symptomatic treatment is needed. In Dimon's series[33] the patients were treated symptomatically, used crutches for 7 to 14 days, and then progressed to unprotected ambulation. By 6 to 8 weeks most were back to activities as tolerated. The athlete is allowed light running and jogging at 6 to 8 weeks and full speed and contact sports by 12 weeks. There is no improvement gained by trac-

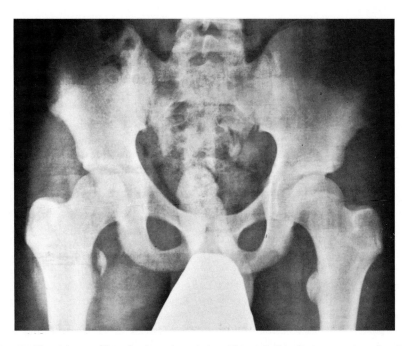

FIG. 57-17. This 14-year-old ice hockey player injured his right hip during practice when "one leg went one way and the other went the other way." Apparently the right hip hyperextended, causing lesser trochanteric avulsion fracture. There was sudden, sharp pain radiating down anterior medial thigh to knee. Following conservative treatment with protected ambulation for 6 weeks, he had complete return to his previous function.

tion, casting, or open reduction. Furthermore, there is no relationship of return to function or temporary disability based on the amount of displacement.

TRAUMATIC DISLOCATION OF THE HIP

Traumatic dislocation of the hip in the child bears little resemblance to the same injury in the adult with respect to incidence, mechanism, and treatment results. It is a relatively unusual injury in children. In Epstein's series[38] of 830 traumatic dislocations over a 48-year period, there were 75 pediatric dislocations in 74 patients, representing 9% of the total. The age ranged from 2 to 15 years, with 15 chosen as the pediatric age limit for the study. Approximately 75% occurred in boys. There were 11 dislocations in the 2- to 4-year-old age group, 13 in the 5- to 7-year olds, 18 in the 8- to 12-year-olds, and 33 in the 13- to 15-year-old group.

Dislocations are classified as anterior, posterior, and central, based on the relationship of the femoral head to the acetabulum. Further subdivisions based on exact location and presence of concomitant fractures have been proposed.[38,104] Posterior dislocations predominate. In Epstein's series[38] there were 8 anterior and 67 posterior injuries. Of these, 8 were fracture-dislocations.

The mechanism is variable and age dependent. The severity of the trauma varies proportionately with age because of changing anatomic considerations. In the young the acetabulum is largely pliable cartilage, and ligamentous laxity is greater. Little force may be required to cause a dislocation. With increasing age, greater portions of the acetabulum ossify and joint laxity diminishes, leading to a more stable condition. More violent trauma is required to cause a dislocation.[104]

A hip dislocation in the child under age 5 is usually caused by a fall with minimal trauma, such as tripping or slipping while walking (Fig. 57-18). Athletic injuries predominate in the 6- to 10-year-old group. Football was the most common sport in Pearson and Mann's review.[106] In these young children the diminished violence makes the injury more benign than its adult counterpart. In the older child, motor vehicle accidents are the most common cause.[112]

The clinical presentation is that of a child with severe pain and inability to bear weight after the traumatic event. The pattern of findings varies with the type of dislocation. In the **posterior dislocation** the hip is held in flexion, adduction, and internal rotation. Extension, abduction, and external rotation are restricted and painful, although external rotation may be possible if the iliofemoral ligament is torn.[26] The limb demonstrates shortening.

Anterior dislocations are much less frequent. The mechanism seems to be a forced abduction in external rotation. Frequently, there has been a fall from a height with the impact on the posterior aspect of the thigh, which is held in abduction and external rotation. A direct blow to the greater trochanters is another common mechanism. The leg is held in abduction, external rotation, and slight flexion. There may be some difficulty in palpating the greater trochanter. There is an apparent

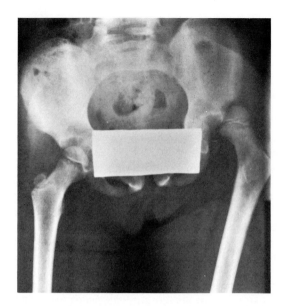

FIG. 57-18. Rare complication of excessive femoral anteversion. This 4½-year-old child was advised to pursue ice skating to correct her toeing-in. She subsequently fell while skating and complained of left knee pain. She was unable to walk. Radiographs of knee were performed at local hospital and were read as negative. Leg was placed in knee splint. She was then seen on referral for persistent and constant knee pain and inability to ambulate over the ensuring week. Left leg was adducted, internally rotated, and slightly flexed. Radiographs demonstrated posterior dislocation of hip. She underwent closed reduction under general anesthesia without difficulty, and leg was placed in a one-and-a-half hip spica cast for 1 month. This was followed by 1 week of split Russell traction and range of motion exercises. She continued on protected weight bearing for 3 additional weeks and made an uneventful recovery. Radiographs remain normal 7 years following her injury, and she continues to be asymptomatic.

lengthening, and the femoral head may be palpated in the obturator foramen. The motion is markedly restricted with almost no adduction or external rotation. The anterior capsule and the ligamentum teres are ruptured, but the iliofemoral ligament is usually spared. In the central dislocation, all motion is decreased, and the femoral head may be palpated on the rectal examination.[38,104,106]

A thorough evaluation for concomitant injury is mandatory. Special attention is given to the knee, patella, femur, and upper tibia, as well as the spine and abdomen. Hip dislocation is often difficult to detect when present with an ipsilateral femoral fracture. In one series hip dislocations associated with ipsilateral femoral shaft fractures were evaluated. The dislocations were appreciated at the initial examination in only 15 of 42 cases.[116]

A radiographic evaluation must be performed before any attempt at reduction. The type of dislocation and the presence of other injuries are determined. Anteroposterior, perineal lateral, and inlet and outlet views are performed. The gonadal shield should initially be omitted to avoid obscuring a pelvic ring fracture. Oblique views as well as laminagrams and computed tomography (CT) scanning are sometimes necessary. Radiographs of the femur, knee, proximal tibia, patella, and lumbar spine

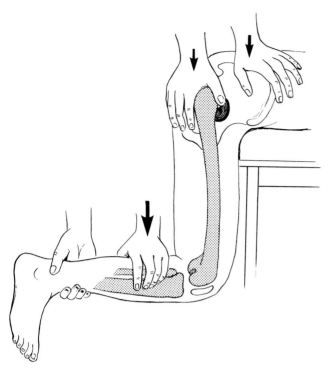

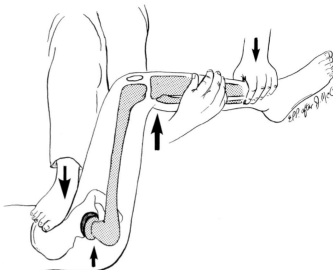

FIG. 57-20. Allis method. See text for details. (Modified from Tachdjian MO: *Pediatric orthopedics*, Philadelphia, 1972, WB Saunders.)

FIG. 57-19. Stimson method. See text for details. (Modified from Tachdjian MO: *Pediatric orthopedics*, Philadelphia, 1972, WB Saunders.)

should be included. Underlying the need for several views of the pelvis are a number of reported cases in which standard anteroposterior views demonstrated a concentrically reduced hip joint despite retroacetabular (posterior) dislocation.[104]

An acute traumatic hip dislocation must be treated as an emergency. General anesthesia to provide complete muscle relaxation is preferred. Reduction within the first 24 hours is associated with a decreased incidence of avascular necrosis.[43,107,112] Closed reduction is nearly always possible, and open reduction is reserved for the rare, neglected, or otherwise irreducible fracture.

Three classic maneuvers are used to reduce the posterior dislocation. Each uses flexion to relax the iliofemoral ligament, the chief obstacle to reduction, and approximate the femoral head to the level of the capsular tear.[139]

The **Stimson method** uses the assistance of gravity and is the most gentle method (Fig. 57-19). The patient is placed in the prone position with the lower extremities hanging freely over the edge of the table. The hip is flexed 90 degrees, and pressure is applied just distal to the knee while the pelvis is stabilized. Direct pressure on the femoral head and a rocking maneuver on the leg may assist.

In the **Allis method** the patient is in the supine position with the pelvis stabilized (Fig. 57-20). The involved hip and knee are flexed to 90 degrees with slight hip adduction and internal rotation. Direct vertical traction lifts the femoral head over the posterior acetabular rim,

through the capsular rent, and into the acetabulum. The hip and knee are then extended. If extension of the hip is difficult, soft-tissue interposition is probable and another attempt is made.

Bigelow described the **circumduction method** (Fig. 57-21). With the patient in the supine position the thigh is gently adducted and internally rotated. The hip is then flexed to 90 degrees and longitudinal traction applied in the direction of the deformity. While traction is maintained, the femoral head is levered into the acetabulum by a gentle rocking and rotating motion.

Failure to obtain a reduction may be caused by interposition of the torn capsule, a buttonhole lesion of the capsule, or iliopsoas or rectus femoris interposition. A greater trochanteric avulsion may accompany an anterior dislocation and requires an open reduction to restore the proper anatomy.[26,104]

After the reduction the hip should be taken through a gentle range of motion with the patient under anesthesia to ensure the stability and confirm the absence of any obstacle to motion. Radiographs should be taken with the patient still under anesthesia to ensure a complete and concentric reduction and to detect the presence of intraarticular or extraarticular fracture fragments, which may have been obscured on the original film or dislodged further by the manipulation. The width of the cartilage space is compared with the opposite side. Possible impediments to reduction, other than fracture fragments, are the capsule, inverted labrum, piriformis tendon, sciatic nerve, and cartilaginous fragments.[26,104] A computed tomography (CT) scan affords an excellent means of confirming a concentric reduction and may reveal intraarticular fragments not seen on the plain films (Fig. 57-22).

In the rare event that closed reduction is impossible or significant chondroosseous articular fragments are

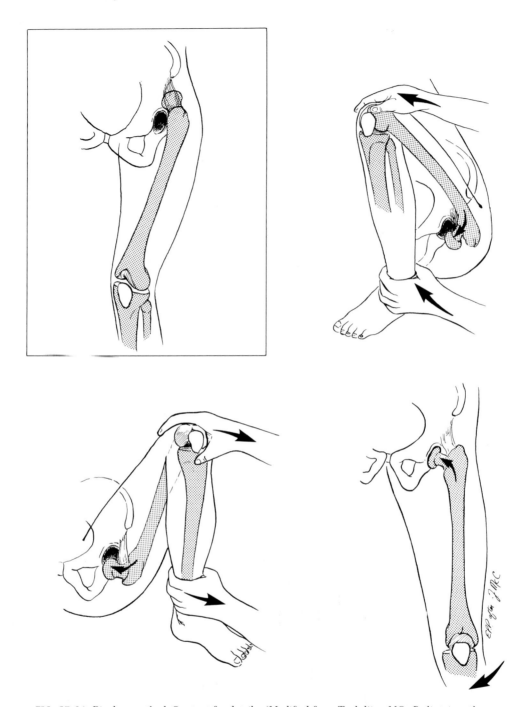

FIG. 57-21. Bigelow method. See text for details. (Modified from Tachdjian MO: *Pediatric orthopedics*, Philadelphia, 1972, WB Saunders.)

present, open reduction should be accomplished via a posterolateral approach. The fragments should be removed and the joint thoroughly irrigated. The capsule must be repaired. Fair results have been reported only in the open reductions.[26,38,104]

Treatment following reduction is aimed at allowing soft-tissue healing via immobilization. In the pediatric age group, split Russell's traction is usually applied with the hip gently flexed and abducted. This may be continued or followed by immobilization in a one-and-a-half hip

spica cast. After cast removal the hip is protected with a three-point crutch gait until full pain-free motion is obtained.[26]

There seems to be no good relationship between the clinical result and the length of non–weight bearing. Funk[40] proposed a relationship between the length of non–weight bearing and avascular necrosis. On the other hand, Glass and Powell[43] thought that weight bearing after 4 weeks was sufficient treatment. Pearson and Mann[106] allowed weight bearing 2 to 3 weeks after the

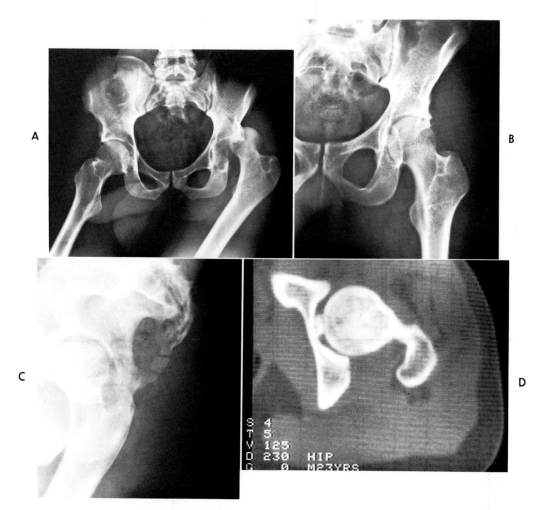

FIG. 57-22. This 20-year-old man sustained posterior fracture dislocation of left hip in motor vehicle accident (**A**). He underwent immediate closed reduction under general anesthesia and was placed in skeletal traction. His reduction appeared to be concentric and stable (**B** and **C**). Computed tomography scan demonstrated retained fracture fragment in medial joint, and open reduction with removal of fragment was performed (**D**). Uneventful recovery followed.

hip demonstrated freedom of pain with range of motion. Ogden and Southwick[104] proposed non–weight bearing for 1 month in children under age 6 years and for 3 to 4 months in the older child. They used synovial irritation as a guide to immobilization. Traction is enforced while acute signs of irritation and pain are present.

The results of treatment are better in children than adults. In the series in which results are followed to maturity, about one third of the hips show some abnormality. This may be somewhat misleading because the cases that develop problems are usually associated with factors that predictably cause poor results. In the Pennsylvania Orthopedic Society study[107] 16 of 51 hips were abnormal, but of these 16, 13 had an associated fracture or a delay in reduction of greater than 24 hours. In Epstein's series[38] all the results but one in the 2- to 12-year age range were good to excellent. The single fair result was in a 3½-year-old child who required an open reduction. The other fair and poor results were in older children

who generally had suffered trauma of greater severity and often sustained fracture-dislocations. Good results can be expected when a simple dislocation in the younger age group is treated by a closed reduction within 24 hours. Severe trauma, associated fractures, delayed reductions, and open reductions are poor prognostic signs.

A number of complications occur both early and late so that follow-up is required until skeletal maturity. The most common is avascular necrosis, which seems to occur in about 10% of the cases.[26,49,104,107] A definite age-related variation exists. In Glass and Powell's series[43] there was one case of avascular necrosis in 26 cases under age 10 years, and five in the 20 children aged 10 years or above. One theory is that the younger children have some protection against avascular necrosis because of the anatomic peculiarities of the vascular supply to the hip.[26] In addition, the trauma sustained to this younger age group seems less significant. A delay in reduction also bears a direct relationship to avascular necrosis. Rang[112] found avascular necrosis in only two cases where reduction was performed within 12 hours.

Other problems less frequently encountered are osteoarthritis, myositis ossificans, recurrent dislocations, sciatic nerve palsy, unrecognized epiphyseal separations, and coxa magna.[26,78,107]

SLIPPED CAPITAL FEMORAL EPIPHYSIS

In a slipped capital femoral epiphysis (SCFE) the femoral head displaces through the growth plate. The head remains within the acetabulum while the femoral neck rotates externally and migrates superiorly. This is not an injury specific to sports, but it may certainly occur during sports in a predisposed individual. Micheli and Smith[92] noticed an increase in frequency of new SCFE patients seen in their clinic each Fall at the start of football practice.

This injury almost always occurs in association with puberty, between the ages of 14 and 16 years in males and 11 and 13 years in females. The incidence has variously been reported between 0.71 to 3.41/100,000 and is higher in blacks.[10,68,69,78,81] It occurs bilaterally in 16% to 19% of cases, although the opposite side may be apparent at the initial diagnosis in 15% to 25% of cases.[22,68,153]

The predisposition of some children to this injury seems to be related to both mechanical and hormonal factors. There is a frequent association with both the Frolich adiposogenital body type and tall, thin individuals.[27,108,139,146] An absolute or relative increase in the ratio of growth hormone to sex hormone is probably involved. Harris[54] demonstrated experimentally an alteration in the thickness of the third layer of the epiphyseal plate secondary to growth and sex hormone variations. Growth hormone decreased, whereas sex hormone increased the sheer strength of the physis.

Hypothyroidism is the most commonly associated endocrinopathy. It is most unusual and should be suspected when the individual is younger than the usual case or demonstrates bone retardation or short stature.[15,82,111] There is a strong familial pattern with the incidence among family members higher than the general populations.[115] Some involvement of the immune system is suggested by the unique association of the synovitis found in SCFE with an immune complex.[99] Several mechanical factors may also be involved.[68,81,97,110] Increased stresses are caused by the enlarging adolescent size and the relative retroversion that seems present in these individuals.[42] Hypovascularity of the metaphysis at the time of the last growth spurt may also be involved in weakening the area.[141]

These children usually have both pain in the hip, groin, or knee and a limp. The pain may occur acutely, but more often it is of an insidious onset. Knee pain alone is a frequent complaint, and careful hip evaluation is mandatory when children in this age group complain of knee pain.[64]

It is helpful in terms of treatment to classify the injury based on the duration of the pathologic process. An

---

> **Classification of slipped capital femoral epiphysis**
>
> - Acute—< than 3 weeks duration
> - Chronic—> than 3 weeks[7] duration
> - Acute on chronic—acute further displacement of a chronic slip

---

acute slip is defined as 3 or less weeks old, chronic slips are greater than 3 weeks[7] duration, and an acute on chronic slip designates an acute displacement superimposed on a process present for greater than 3 weeks.

Radiographs are diagnostic. An anteroposterior view of the pelvis to show both hips and a lateral view are required. The frog lateral view is technically easier to perform but often shows asymmetry between the two sides because of the difficulty in positioning the painful leg. Additionally, there is some theoretic danger of further slip during the radiographic maneuver. A well-performed, true lateral view provides a more accurate and a safer assessment.

Minimal slips may be difficult to detect. A widened, irregular growth plate may be the only finding. The plate widens as removal of the hypertrophic cell layer is altered by a metaphyseal circulatory flow depressed by the minimal displacement.[141] **Trethowan's sign** is positive on the anteroposterior view.[78] The true lateral view is more sensitive. It detects small displacements because much of the translation is directed posteriorly. In this view the angle formed by the axis of the femoral neck and the physis should be approximately 90 degrees; a slip must be considered when the angle is less than 87 degrees.[45,46] A CT scan gives an accurate picture of the anatomy and should be considered when the plain radiographs are equivocal.

The goal of treatment is to stabilize the epiphysis, prevent further displacement, and avoid complications. In the absence of treatment-related complications most patients with SCFEs have an excellent result.[14,20] Slipping, once begun, continues. The only protection is plate closure. Treatment should be considered urgent. The established methods for maintaining position are hip spica cast immobilization, open epiphysiodesis, and pin fixation.[8,12,13,55,100]

Hip spica cast treatment avoids an open procedure but requires prolonged immobilization and has been associated with further slipping, chondrolysis, and pressure sores.[7] Open epiphysiodesis via an anteriorly placed bone graft avoids the dangers of pin penetration, but it is a

---

> **Treatment options in mild slipped capital femoral epiphysis**
>
> - Spica cast immobilization
> - Open epiphysiodesis
> - In situ percutaneous pin fixation

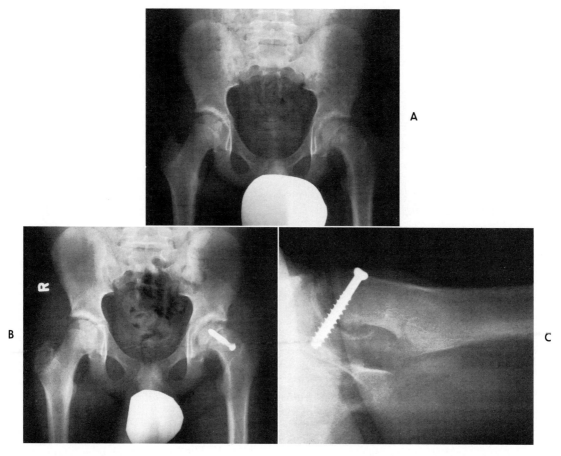

FIG. 57-23. This 13-year-old boy is 5' 10" tall and weighs 190 lbs. He has a 1-year history of left sided limp and episodic complaints of pain on left groin. Ideally diagnosis of slipped capital femoral epiphysis would have been made in acute stage so that fixation would have been performed when deformity was mild. Anteroposterior radiograph (**A**) demonstrates apparently widened physis. Displacement is predominantly posterior and its magnitude appreciated much better on true, or perineal, lateral view (**C**). Percutaneous screw fixation method allows entry into anterior femoral neck and permits a secure fixation (**B** and **C**).

much larger procedure and has a variable success rate.[1,143,148]

At present, the preferred method of treatment is in situ percutaneous fixation using a single partially threaded screw. This method has been thoroughly analyzed and perfected.[23,144] A single screw provides adequate stability, promotes premature closure, and is associated with significantly less pin-related complications than the multiple screw technique.[9]

The percutaneous method minimizes the surgical trauma and allows penetration of the anterior femoral neck, which permits the ideal placement of the screw perpendicular to the physis and into the midportion of the femoral head (Fig. 57-23).[99] To avoid osteonecrosis the screw should avoid the superior lateral aspect of the femoral head where the posterior superior retinacular vessels enter.[136]

Percutaneous pin placement is routinely performed on a fracture table using image intensification.[76,98] The fluoroscopic evaluation during hip motion ensures proper pin placement and detects pin penetration, which may

go unrecognized by routine anteroposterior and lateral radiographs.[120,158]

Reduction before fixation has been suggested in the past for unacceptable position; however, this is difficult to define. Reduction is associated with an increased risk of osteonecrosis. Numerous reports have documented improvement in range of motion to acceptable values through both soft-tissue and bony remodeling.[66,130,156] In addition, long-term studies reveal excellent function despite marked deformity. It appears that the risks of reduction outweigh the benefits. If reduction is to be performed, it should be for the acute displacement only and then either by gentle skeletal traction with internal rotation or by gentle manipulation under anesthesia at the time of surgery (Fig. 57-24).[39,50]

Extensive remodeling also seems to eliminate the need for corrective osteotomies at the time of initial treatment. Degenerative joint disease has been reported to occur in severe slips despite corrective osteotomies. It seems best, then, to delay these procedures for at least several years following surgery. At that time, these procedures are in-

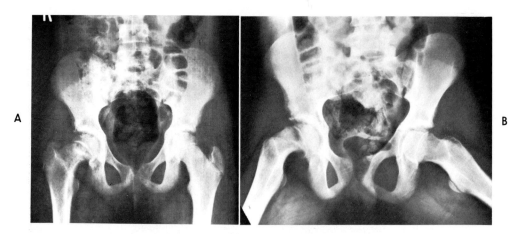

FIG. 57-24. This 12-year-old swimmer jumped into shallow water, landing on her heels, and experienced sudden severe pain in anterior right hip. Radiographs show obvious slipped capital femoral epiphysis (**A** and **B**), but this is most likely a long-standing deformity. There is femoral neck varus and buttressing, as well as wide lucent metaphyseal zone (**A**). Any attempt to improve this position is ill advised. In situ pinning is recommended.

dicated only in severe slips associated with functional impairment. Osteotomies performed through the femoral neck are closer to the true deformity but are associated with a significant risk of osteonecrosis. The intertrochanteric variety seems safer.[55,65,85,133]

The two main complications are avascular necrosis and chondrolysis. Avascular necrosis is reported in up to 15.6% of the cases.[50,153] Hall[50] noted this complication to have the greatest influence on end results. The hips at risk seem to be (1) acute slips of moderate severity that require reduction, (2) chronic slips subjected to manipulative reduction, and (3) severely displaced injuries treated with cervical osteotomy.[68,84]

Chondrolysis, or acute cartilage necrosis, is a rapidly progressive narrowing of the hip joint associated with limited motion.[36,63] It may have a much higher incidence in blacks.[70,140] The cause is unknown. A number of characteristics have been reported. There seems to be an association with unrecognized pin penetration.[142] It may occur at any time, although it usually does so within 1 year of the diagnosis of the slip. Most patients have moderate to severe slips, and many have had surgery with postoperative immobilization.[68]

The treatment is skeletal traction and physical therapy to improve the range of motion. Prolonged non–weight-bearing ambulation follows. A lengthy observation period with delay of surgical treatment is advisable because some cases have improved using the conservative regimen.[61,68,81]

FEMORAL NECK FRACTURES

Fractures of the femoral neck in children are extremely rare and usually are associated with severe trauma. Common causes are motor vehicle accidents and falls from heights. Other more serious associated injuries are present in 30% of cases. Occurrence during sports is most unusual.[78,87,96,112]

Rarely, the injury is trivial, and in such cases consideration should be given to a pathologic fracture. Possible causes are renal osteodystrophy, hypothyroidism, juvenile rheumatoid arthritis, septic arthritis, or neoplasm.[102]

Several factors distinguish the injury in children from adults. Periosteal and perichondral sleeves allow less displacement. Denser bones make internal fixation more difficult. The homogenous orientation of the cancellous trabeculae results in a smooth fracture line and allows less interlocking or impaction. Closed reductions are less stable. The vascular supply in the femoral head also plays a role in the high incidence of avascular necrosis.[26,102]

The usual presentation is a child in severe pain with an inability to raise the involved limb. There is shortening, external rotation, and mild abduction of the limb. Associated injuries, including pelvic fractures and concussion, must be sought and evaluated. Radiographs must include an anteroposterior and a true lateral view of the hip. The radiographic evaluation must include the lesser trochanter, the angulation of the fracture line, any varus or valgus alignment, and the position of the head in the acetabulum.

Femoral neck fractures have been classified by Delbet into transepiphyseal, transcervical, trochanteric or basal, and intertrochanteric fractures.[60]

Transepiphyseal fractures are the least common and carry the worst prognosis. In contrast to the SCFE, they occur through the previously normal growth plate, although this differentiation may be difficult. As noted already, Fahey and O'Brien[39] believed that only 17 cases of slipped epiphysis from the literature had trauma as the exclusive factor. Most of these occurred in an age group younger than that usually seen with SCFE. The trauma was severe, and associated injuries were common. Many of the injuries occurred in infancy.

Initial treatment usually involves skin traction with an internal rotation strap to prevent further displacement and relieve spasm. Skeletal traction may be preferable in

---

Classification of pediatric femoral neck fractures

- Transepiphyseal
- Transcervical
- Trochanteric (basal)
- Intertrochanteric

---

cases of more severe displacement. Aspiration of the intracapsular hematoma has been advocated to minimize compression of the intrasynovial blood supply.[68,112] Minimally displaced fractures may be treated with a one-and-a-half hip spica cast for 6 to 10 weeks, whereas displaced fractures usually require internal fixation.[60,73]

Treatment for **transcervical** or **trochanteric (basal) fractures** is more controversial. Undisplaced fractures are immobilized in a spica cast; the need for internal fixation to prevent loss of position is debated. Ratliff[113] reported coxa vara in only 2 of 40 undisplaced fractures, and Lam[75] thought that the deformity would remodel. Cast treatment alone is suggested by these authors. Loss of remodeling ability with age favors the suggestions of others to perform internal fixation in the older child. Some authors have attempted to select, via Pauwell's angle, those fractures at risk for displacement. Internal fixation is used when the angle is greater than 40 degrees.[102]

Intertrochanteric fractures have the best prognosis. Reduction via gentle manipulation or a short course of traction followed by spica immobilization is preferred. Internal fixation is used for nonreducible fractures or for

those in which other injuries prevent traction or cast treatment.[60,68,75]

Complications are unfortunately common. The most frequently seen are avascular necrosis, delayed union, nonunion, coxa vara, premature growth place closure, and shortening.

The incidence of avascular necrosis varies in major series from 17% to 46%.[50,68,75,102,113] No definite correlation to treatment has been made, although certain associations are suggested. In the Campbell clinic series avascular necrosis seemed to be related to age under 10 years, Type I or II fractures, and significant fracture displacement.[26] Ratliff[113] divided the pattern into three types based on the location of the vascular insult. The prognosis was based on this classification.

Coxa vara has been reported in up to 55% of the patients.[68,75,78,102,113] Probable causes are (1) failure to reduce the initial deformity fully, (2) loss of reduction while in spica immobilization, (3) gradual development caused by delay or nonunion, and (4) late deformity caused by growth plate retardation. Coxa vara associated with internal fixation seems to be less severe than with other forms of immobilization.[68] The mild forms seem to be compatible with a good result, whereas severe coxa vara was often progressive.

Nonunion is a less frequent complication. It is reported in transcervical fractures and in 85% of the cases in which Pauwell's angle was greater than 60 degrees.[102] Lloyd-Roberts and Ratliff[78] reported nonunion when treatment was subtrochanteric osteotomy.[113] Healing via secondary procedures is usually obtainable.

Limb shortening may be secondary to coxa vara or premature growth plate arrest. Lam[75] reported up to 1.3 to

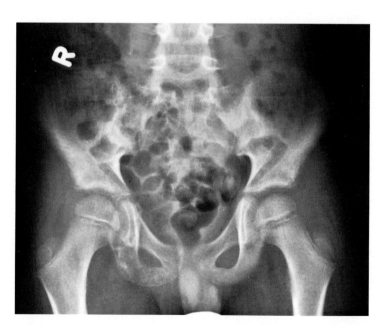

FIG. 57-25. This 8-year-old boy complained of right groin pain after he lunged after a ground ball at third base. He was able to walk off field but complained of constant pain exacerbated by any type of activity. He continued to complain of pain despite rest and limited activity but was reassured that this was only a strain. Six weeks after initial injury, radiographs were obtained. Permeative lesion in right inferior pubic ramus and ischium proved to be focus of acute leukemia.

3.2 cm of leg length discrepancy. Premature plate closure is often associated with coxa vara. Secondary problems are weak abductors and limited motion caused by greater trochanteric overgrowth.

OTHER PAINFUL CONDITIONS

A number of pathologic processes may occur in the region of the hip and pelvis. Frequently, the initial symptoms may be first noticed in association with athletics. These symptoms are often neglected or treated without thorough evaluation. Serious conditions are thereby allowed to progress to catastrophic results (Figs. 57-25 and 57-26).

Legg-Calvé-Perthes disease occurs in the 4- to 10-year age group. The initial presentation is a painless limp. Pain in the groin, anterior thigh, or knee follows. Radiographic findings are diagnostic but may be delayed. A bone scan shows either an increased or decreased uptake, depending on the stage of the disease.

Toxic, or **transient, synovitis** usually occurs in the child under 7 years of age. It too causes a limp with pain in the thigh or knee. There is a restricted hip motion. It is unilateral and self-limiting and shows a relatively prompt improvement with rest. Recurrences are quite unusual but have been reported.[59] This should be a diagnosis of exclusion.

Infectious processes include osteomyelitis and septic arthritis. Osteomyelitis of the pelvis or hip is seen with limited motion and an antalgic gait. Onset may be somewhat insidious, and radiographs are initially normal. An elevated white blood cell count and sedimentation rate is helpful in making this diagnosis. Occurrence following trauma may be related to bacterial seeding of a hematoma. Septic arthritis may involve either the hip or sacroiliac joint. Markedly limited hip motion is noted with a relatively short and rapid course. Fever, leukocytosis, and elevated sedimentation are present. The joint aspiration is diagnostic.

Benign and **malignant tumors** and **tumorlike lesions** may involve the area. Osteogenic sarcoma, osteoid osteoma, Ewing's sarcoma, bone cysts, fibrous dysplasia, and leukemia are among the possibilities. Although the need for earlier diagnosis of malignant growth is evident,

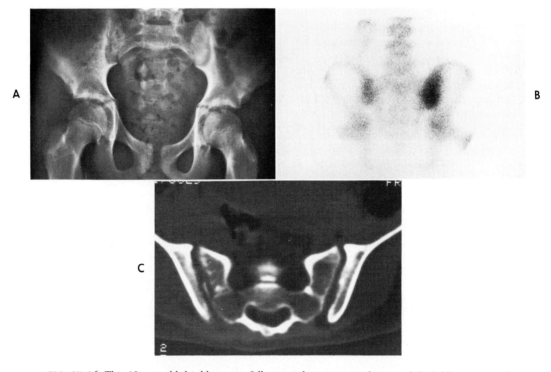

FIG. 57-26. This 12-year-old third basemen fell onto right greater trochanter while fielding a ground ball. He experienced immediate pain in hip and back, which prevented him from finishing the game. Diagnosis of strain was made by his local physician, and bed rest for several days and guarded ambulation thereafter were prescribed. The pain decreased over 5 days but then intensified on day six after 2-day bout with "the flu." At that time he demonstrated inability to bear weight and pain with hip motion. The most severe pain was in the area of the right sacroiliac joint and was duplicated by the Patrick maneuver and by compression of both greater trochanters. His blood examination revealed normal hematocrit and white count but markedly elevated sedimentation rate. Radiographs showed osteopenia in area of right sacrum (**A**). Bone scan was positive at right sacroiliac joint. (**B**), and computed tomography scan showed destruction and sequestration at right sacroiliac joint. **C,** Open drainage and debridement was performed for *Staphylococcus aureus* septic joint and adjacent osteomyelitis. He made an uneventful recovery and returned to full function in 3 months.

a benign process in the femoral neck may lead to a pathologic fracture and serious residual deformities.

Rheumatoid arthritis and **rheumatic fever** may be involved. There is usually no causal relationship with trauma.

REFERENCES

1. Aadalen RJ et al: Acute slipped capital femoral epiphysis, *J Bone Joint Surg* 56A:1473, 1974.
2. Aronson DD, Carlson WE: Slipped capital femoral epiphyses: a prospective study of fixation with a single screw, *J Bone Joint Surg* 74(A):810, 1992.
3. Aronson DD, Peterson DA, Miller DV: The case for internal fixation in situ, *Clin Orthop* 281:115, 1992.
4. Bargren JH, Tilson DH: Prevention of displaced fatigue fractures of the femur, *J Bone Joint Surg* 53A:1115, 1971.
5. Barnes ST, Hinds RB: Pseudotumor of the ischium, *J Bone Joint Surg* 54A:645, 1972.
6. Belkin S: Stress fractures in athletes, *Orthop Clin North Am* 11:735, 1980.
7. Betz RR et al: Treatment of slipped capital femoral epiphysis: spica-cast immobilization, *J Bone Joint Surg* 72:587, 1990.
8. Bianco AJ: Treatment of mild slipping of the capital femoral epiphysis, *J Bone Joint Surg* 47A:387, 1965.
9. Bianco JS, Taylor B, Johnston CE Jr: Comparison of single-pin versus multiple-pin fixation in treatment of slipped capital femoral epiphysis, *J Pediatr Orthop* 12:384, 1992.
10. Bishop JO et al: Slipped capital femoral epiphysis: a study of 50 cases in black children, *Clin Orthop* 135:93, 1978.
11. Blickenstaff LB, Morris JM: Fatigue fracture of the femoral neck, *J Bone Joint Surg* 48A:1031, 1966.
12. Boyd HB: Treatment of acute slipped upper femoral epiphysis. In *American Academy of Orthopaedic Surgeons instructional course lectures*, vol 21, St Louis, 1972, Mosby.
13. Boyd HB: Treatment of minimally slipped upper femoral epiphysis. In *American Academy of Orthopaedic Surgeons instructional course lectures*, vol 21, St Louis, 1972, Mosby.
14. Boyer DW, Mickelson MR, Ponseti IV: Slipped capital femoral epiphysis: long-term follow-up study of 121 partients, *J Bone Joint Surg* 63A:85, 1981.
15. Brenkel IJ et al: Hormone status in patients with slipped capital femoral epiphysis, *J Bone Joint Surg* 71(B):33, 1989.
16. Brody HB: Running injuries, *Ciba Clin Symp* 32:1980.
17. Burkett LN: Causative factors in hamstring strain, *Med Sci Sports Exerc* 2:39, 1970.
18. Burkett LN: Investigation into hamstring strains: the case of the hybrid muscle, *J Sports Med* 3:228, 1975.
19. Caffey J: *Pediatric x-ray diagnosis*, ed 5, Chicago, 1967, Year Book Medical Publishers.
20. Carney BT, Weinstein SL, Noble J: Long-term follow-up of slipped capital femoral epiphysis, *J Bone Joint Surg* 73:667, 1991.
21. Carp L: Fracture of the anterior superior spine of the ilium by muscular violence, *Ann Surg* 79:551, 1924.
22. Christopher F: Fracture of the anterior superior spine of the ileium, *JAMA* 100:113, 1933.
23. Clancy WG, Foltz AS: Iliac apophysitis and stress fracture in adolescent runners, *Am J Sports Med* 4:214, 1976.
24. Cohen HH: Avulsion fracture of the ischial tuberosity, *J Bone Joint Surg* 19:1138, 1937.
25. Corlette CE: Fracture of the anterior inferior spine of the ilium, *Med J Aust* 2:682, 1927.
26. Craig CL: Hip injuries in children and adolescents. *Orthop Clin North Am* 11:743, 1980.
27. Cruess RL: The pathology of acute neurosis of cartilage in slipping of the capital femoral epiphysis, *J Bone Joint Surg* 95A:1013, 1963.
27a. DeLucchi G: Distacco epifisario della tuberositá ischiatica, *Clin Ortop (Padova)* 6:245, 1954.
28. DePalma AF, Silberstein CE: Avulsion fracture of the ischial tuberosity in siblings, *Clin Orthop* 38:120, 1965.
29. Devas MB: Stress fractures in man and the greyhound, *J Bone Joint Surg* 43B:540, 1961.
30. Devas MB: Stress fractures in children, *J Bone Joint Surg* 45B:528, 1963.
31. Devas MB: Stress fracture of the femoral neck, *J Bone Joint Surg* 47:728, 1965.
32. Devas MB: *Stress fractures*, Edinburgh, 1975, Churchill Livingstone.
33. Dimon JH: Isolated fracture of the lesser trochanter of the femur, *Clin Orthop* 82:144, 1972.
34. Dulabal TA, Brunelte ME, Haddad RJ: Avulsion fractures of the lower extremity in the adolescent athlete. Paper presented at American Academy of Orthopaedic Surgeons Annual Meeting, Anaheim, Calif, Feb 1983.
35. Dunlop K et al: A new method for determination of torsion of the femur, *J Bone Joint Surg* 35A:289, 1953.
36. Eisenstein A, Rothschild S: Biochemical abnormalities in patients with slipped capital femoral epiphysis and chondrolysis, *J Bone Joint Surg* 58A:459, 1976.
37. Engh CA, Robinson RA, Milgram J: Stress fractures in children, *J Trauma* 10:532, 1970.
38. Epstein HC: *Traumatic dislocation of the hip*, Baltimore, 1980, William & Wilkins.
39. Fahey JJ, O'Brien ET: Acute slipped capital femoral epiphysis, *J Bone Joint Surg* 47A:1105, 1965.
39a. Fernbak SK, Wilkinson RH: Avulson injuries of the pelvis and proximal femur, *AJR* 137:581, 1981.
40. Funk FS Jr: Traumatic dislocation of the hip in children: factors influencing prognosis and treatment, *J Bone Joint Surg* 44A:1135, 1962.
41. Gallagher JR: Fracture of the anterior-inferior spine of the ilium. *Am Surg* 102:86, 1935.
42. Gelberman RH, Cohen MS, Shaw BA: The association of femoral retroversion with slipped capital femoral epiphysis, *J Bone Joint Surg* 68A:1000, 1986.
43. Glass A, Powell ADW: Traumatic dislocation of the hip in children: an analysis of 47 patients, *J Bone Joint Surg* 43B:29, 1961.
44. Godshall RM, Hansen CA: Incomplete avulsion of a portion of the iliac epiphysis *J Bone Joint Surg* 55A:1301, 1973.
45. Griffith MJ: Anatomical consideration in the treatment of slipping of the capital femoral epiphysis, master's thesis, Liverpool, 1972, University of Liverpool.
46. Griffith MJ: Slipping of the capital femoral epiphysis, *Ann R Coll Surg Engl* 58:34, 1976.
47. Griffs CG, Protzman RR: Stress fractures in men and women undergoing military training, *J Bone Joint Surg* 59A:825, 1977.
48. Gwinn J, Stanley P: *Diagnostic imaging in pediatric trauma*, Berlin, 1980, Springer-Verlag.
49. Haliburton RA, Brockenshire FA, Barber JA: Avascular neurosis of the femoral capital epiphysis after traumatic dislocation of the hip in children, *J Bone Joint Surg* 43B:43, 1961.
50. Hall JE: The results of treatment of slipped femoral epiphysis, *J Bone Joint Surg* 39B:659, 1957.
51. Halpern AA, Tanner J, Rinsky L: Does persistent fetal femoral anteversion contribute to osteoarthritis? *Clin Orthop* 145:213, 1979.
52. Hamada G, Rida A: Ischial apophysiolysis, *Clin Orthop* 31:117, 1964.
53. Hamsa WR: Epiphyseal injuries about the hip joint, *Clin Orthop* 10:119, 1957.
54. Harris WR: The endocrine basis for slipping of the upper femoral epiphysis, *J Bone Joint Surg* 32B:5, 1950.
55. Herndon CH: Treatment of minimally slipped upper femoral epiphysis. In *American Academy of Orthopaedic Surgeons instructional course lectures*, vol 21, St Louis, 1972, Mosby.
56. Herndon CH: Treatment of severely slipped upper femoral epiphysis by means of osteoplasty and epiphysiodesis. In *American Academy of Orthopaedic Surgeons instructional course lectures*, vol 21, St Louis, 1972, Mosby.
57. Hollinshead WH: *Anatomy for surgeons*, ed 2, vol 3, New York, 1969, Harper & Row.
58. Hopson CN, Perry DR: Stress fractures of the calcaneus in women marine recruits, *Clin Orthop* 128:159, 1977.
59. Illingworth CM: Recurrence of transient synovitis of the hip, *Arch Dis Child* 58:620, 1983.

60. Ingram AJ, Bachynski B: Fractures of the hip in children, *J Bone Joint Surg* 35A:867, 1953.
61. Ingram AJ et al: Chondrolysis complicating slipped capital femoral epiphysis, *Clin Orthop* 165:99, 1982.
62. Irving MH: Exostosis formation after traumatic avulsion of the anterior inferior iliac spine, *J Bone Joint Surg* 46B:720, 1964.
63. Jacobs B: Chondrolysis after epiphyseolysis. In *American Academy of Orthopaedic Surgeons instructional course lectures*, vol 21, St Louis, 1972, Mosby.
64. Jacobs B: Diagnosis and natural history of slipped femoral capital epiphysis. In *American Academy of Orthopaedic Surgeons instructional course lectures*, vol 21, St Louis, 1972, Mosby.
65. Jacobs B: Treatment of severely slipped upper femoral epiphysis by wedge osteotomy. In *American Academy of Orthopaedic Surgeons instructional course lectures*, vol 21, St Louis, 1972, Mosby.
66. Jones JR et al: Remodeling after pinning for slipped capital femoral epiphysis, *J Bone Joint Surg* 72(B):568, 1990.
67. Kaltas DS: Stress fracture of the femoral neck in young adults, *J Bone Joint Surg* 63B:33, 1981.
68. Katz JF, Siffert RS: *Management of hip disorders in children*, Philadelphia, 1983, JB Lippincott.
69. Kelsey J, Southwick WO: Etiology, mechanism, and incidence of slipped capital femoral epiphysis. In *American Academy of Orthopaedic Surgeons instructional course lectures*, vol 21, St Louis, 1972, Mosby.
70. Kennedy JP, Weiner DS: Results of slipped capital femoral epiphysis in the black population, *J Pediatr Orthop* 10:224, 1990.
71. Key JA, Conwell HE: *Management of fractures, dislocations, and sprains*, ed 7, St Louis, 1961, Mosby.
72. Reference deleted in proofs.
73. Labuz EF: Avulsion of the ischial tuberosity, *J Bone Joint Surg* 28:388, 1946.
74. LaGasse DJ, Staheli LT: The measurement of femoral anteversion: a comparison of the fluoroscopic and biplanar roentgenographic methods of measurement, *Clin Orthop* 86:13, 1972.
75. Lam SF: Fractures of the neck of the femur in children, *J Bone Joint Surg* 53A:1165, 1971.
76. Lindaman LM et al: A flouroscopic technique for determining the incision site for percutaneous fixation of slipped capital femoral epiphysis, *J Pediatr Ortho* 11:397, 1991.
77. Lloyd-Roberts GC: *Orthopaedics in infancy and childhood*, London, 1971, Appleton-Century-Crofts.
78. Lloyd-Roberts GC, Ratliff AHC: *Hip disorders in children*, London, 1981, Butterworth.
79. Lombardo SJ, Benson DW: Stress fractures of the femur in runners, *Am J Sports Med* 10:219, 1982.
80. Lombardo SJ, Retting AC, Kerlan RK: Radiographic abnormalities of the iliac apophysis in adolescent athletes, *J Bone Joint Surg* 64A:444, 1983.
81. Lovell WW, Winter RB: *Pediatric orthopaedics*, Philadelphia, 1978, JB Lippincott.
82. Mann DFC, Weddington J, Richton S: Hormonal studies in patients with slipped capital femoral epiphysis without evidence of endocrinopathy, *J Pediatr Orthop* 8:543, 1988.
83. Martin TA, Pipkin G: Treatment of avulsion of the ischial tuberosity, *Clin Orthop* 10:108, 1957.
84. Maurer RC, Larsen LJ: Acute necrosis of cartilage in slipped capital femoral epiphysis, *J Bone Joint Surg* 52A:39, 1970.
85. Maussen JP, Rozing PM, Obermann WR: Intertrochanteric corrective osteotomy in slipped capital femoral epiphysis: a long-term follow-up study of 26 patients, *Clin Orthop* 259:100, 1990.
86. McBryde AM: Stress fractures in athletes *J Sports Med* 3:212, 1976.
87. McDougall A: Fracture of the neck of the femur in childhood, *J Bone Joint Surg* 43B:16, 1961.
88. McMaster P: Epiphysitis of the ischial tuberosity, *J Bone Joint Surg* 27:493, 1945.
89. Mercer W, Duthie RB: *Orthopedic surgery*, ed 6, Baltimore, 1964, Williams & Wilkins.
90. Merrifield HH, Cowan RF: Groin strain injuries in ice hockey, *Am J Sports Med* 1:41, 1973.
91. Metzmaker JN, Pappas AM: Avulsion fractures of the pelvis, *Am J Sports Med* 13:349, 1985.
92. Micheli LJ, Smith AD: Sports injuries in children, *Curr Probl Pediatr* 12(9), 1982.
93. Milch H: Ischial apophysiolysis: a new syndrome, *Clin Orthop* 2:184, 1953.
94. Miller EB et al: A new consideration in athletic injuries, *Clin Orthop* 111:181, 1975.
95. Miller ML: Avulsion fractures of the anterior superior iliac spine in high school track athletic training, *Athl Train* 17:57, 1982.
96. Miller WE: Fractures of the hip in children from birth to adolescence, *Clin Orthop* 92:155, 1973.
97. Mirkopulos N, Weiner DS, Askew M: The evolving slope of the proximal growth plate relationship to slipped capital femoral epiphysis, *J Pediatr Othop* 8:268, 1988.
98. Morrissy RT: Slipped capital femoral epiphysis technique of percutaneous in situ fixation, *J Pediatr Orthop* 10:347, 1990.
99. Morrissy RT, Steele RW, Gerdes MH: Localized immune complexes and slipped upper femoral epiphysis, *J Bone Joint Surg* 65B:574, 1983.
100. Newman PH: The surgical treatment of slipping of the upper femoral epiphysis, *J Bone Joint Surg* 42B:280, 1960.
101. Nguyen D, Morrissy RT: Slipped capital femoral epiphysis: rationale for the technique of percutaneous in situ fixation, *J Pediatr Orthop* 10:341, 1990.
102. Ogden JA: *Skeletal injury in the child*, Philadelphia, 1982, Lea & Febiger.
103. Ogden JA, Hempton RF, Southwick WO: Development of the tibial tuberosity, *Anat Rec* 182:431, 1975.
104. Ogden JA, Southwick WO: Osgood-Schlatter's disease and tibial tuberosity development, *Clin Orthop* 116:180, 1976.
105. Ozonoff MB: *Pediatric orthopedic radiology*, Philadelphia, 1979, WB Saunders.
106. Pearson DE, Mann RJ: Traumatic hip dislocation in children, *Clin Orthop* 92:189, 1973.
107. Pennsylvania Orthopedic Society: Traumatic dislocation of the hip joint in children: a report by the Scientific Research Committee, *J Bone Joint Surg* 50A:79, 1968.
108. Ponseti IV, McClintock R: The pathology of slipping of the upper femoral epiphysis, *J Bone Joint Surg* 38A:71, 1956.
109. Prather JL et al: Scientigraphic findings in stress fractures, *J Bone Joint Surg* 59A:869, 1977.
110. Pritchett JW, Perdue KD: Mechanical factors in slipped capital femoral epiphysis, *J Pediatr Orthop* 8:385, 1988.
111. Puri R, Smith CS, Malhotra D: Slipped upper femoral epiphysis and primary juvenile hypothyroidism, *J Bone Joint Surg* 67B:14, 1985.
112. Rang M: *Children's fractures*, Philadelphia, 1974, JB, Lippincott.
113. Ratliff AHC: Fractures of the neck of the femur in children, *J Bone Joint Surg* 44B:528, 1962.
114. Reikeras O, Bjerkreim I, Kolbenstuedt A: Anteversion of the acetabulum and femoral neck in normals and in patients with osteoarthritis of the hip, *Acta Orthop Scand* 54:18, 1983.
115. Rennie AM: The inheritance of slipped capital femoral epiphysis, *J Bone Joint Surg* 64(B):180, 1982.
115a. Renonapoli E: Distacchi apofisari da trauma sportivo, *Clin Ortop (Padova)* 7:337, 1955.
116. Riser JL: The iliac apophysis: an invaluable sign in the management of scoliosis, *Clin Orthop* 11:111, 1958.
117. Rockwood CA, Green DP: *Fractures*, vol 2, Philadelphia, 1975, JB Lippincott.
118. Rogers SB: A method for determining the angle of torsion of the neck of the femur, *J Bone Joint Surg* 13:821, 1931.
119. Rogge EA, Romano RL: Avulsion of the ischial apophysis, *J Bone Joint Surg* 38A:442, 1956.
120. Rooks MD, Schmitt EW, Drvaric DM: Unrecognized pin penetration in slipped capital femoral epiphysis, *Clin Orthop* 234:82, 1988.
121. Rosen PR, Micheli LJ, Treves S: Early scintigraphic diagnosis of bone stress and fractures in athletic adolescents, *Pediatrics* 70:11, 1982.
122. Ryder CT, Crane L: Measuring femoral anteversion: the problem and a method, *J Bone Joint Surg* 35:321, 1953.

123. Saroca CJ: Stress fractures: a classification of the earliest radiographic signs. *Radiology* 100:519, 1971.
124. Schlonsky J, Olix ML: Functional disability following avulsion fracture of the ischial epiphysis, *J Bone Joint Surg* 54A:641, 1972.
125. Schneider JJ et al: Stress injuries and developmental changes of lower extremities in ballet dancers, *Radiology* 113:627, 1974.
126. Schneider R, Kaye JL, Glickman B: Adductor avulsion injuries near the symphysis pubis, *Radiology* 120:567, 1976.
127. Scott W: Nonunion of the ischial tuberosity associated with epiphysitis vertebrae, *J Bone Joint Surg* 28:862, 1946.
128. Selakovich W, Love L: Stress fractures of the pubic ramus, *J Bone Joint Surg* 36A:573, 1954.
129. Sharrard WJW: *Pediatric orthopaedics and fractures*, Oxford, England, 1971, Blackwell Scientific Publications.
130. Siegel DB et al: Slipped capital femoral epiphysis: a quantitative analysis of motion, gait, and femoral remodeling after in situ fixation, *J Bone Joint Surg* 73:659, 1991.
131. Skinner HB, Cook SD: Fatigue failure stress of the femoral neck, *Am J Sports Med* 10:45, 1982.
132. Somerville EW: Persistent fetal alignment of the hip, *J Bone Joint Surg* 39B:106, 1957.
133. Southwick WO: Treatment of severely slipped upper femoral epiphysis by trochanteric osteotomy. In *American Academy of Orthopaedic Surgeons instructional course lectures*, vol 21, St Louis, 1972, Mosby.
134. Staheli LT: Medial femoral torsion, *Orthop Clin North Am* 11:39, 1980.
135. Staheli LT, Lippert F, Denotter P: Femoral anteversion and physical performance in adolescent and adult life, *Clin Orthop* 120:214, 1977.
136. Stambough JL, Davidson RS, Ellis RD: Slipped capital femoral epiphysis: an analysis of 80 patients as to pin placement and number, *J Pediatr Orthop* 6:265, 1986.
137. Stanitski CL, McMaster JH, Scranton PE: On the nature of stress fractures, *Am J Sports Med* 6:391, 1978.
138. Symeonides PP: Isolated traumatic rupture of the adductor longus muscle of the thigh, *Clin Orthop* 88:64, 1972.
139. Tachdjian MO: *Pediatric orthopedics*, Philadelphia, 1972, WB Saunders.
140. Tilleman DA, Golding SR: Chondrolysis following slipped capital femoral epiphysis in Jamaica, *J Bone Joint Surg* 53A:1528, 1971.
141. Trueta J: *Studies of the development and decay of the human frame*, Philadelphia, 1968, WB Saunders.
142. Walters R, Simon SR: Joint destruction: a sequela of unrecognized pin penetration in patients with slipped capital femoral epiphysis. In The Hip Society: *The hip: proceedings of the eighth open scientific meeting of the Hip Society*, St Louis, 1980, Mosby.
143. Ward WT, Wood K: Open bone graft epiphysiodesis for slipped capital femoral epiphysis, *J Pediatr Orthop* 10:14, 1990.
144. Ward WT et al: Fixation with a single screw for capital femoral epiphysis, *J Bone Joint Surg* 74(A):799, 1992.
145. Watson-Jones R: *Fractures and joint injuries*, ed 5, Edinburgh, 1976, Churchill Livingstone.

146. Wattleworth AS et al: Pathology of slipped capital femoral epiphysis. In *American Academy of Orthopaedic Surgeons instructional course lectures*, vol 21, St Louis, 1972, Mosby.
147. Weiner DS et al: Computed tomography in the measurement of femoral anteversion, *Orthopedics* 1:299, 1978.
148. Weiner DS et al: A 30-year experience with bone graft epiphysiodesis in the treatment of slipped capital femoral epiphysis, *J Pediatr Orthop* 4:145, 1984.
149. Weitzner I: Fracture of the anterior superior spine of the ilium in one case and anterior inferior in another case, *AJR* 33:39, 1935.
150. Wilcox JR, Moniot AL, Green JP: Bone scanning in the evaluation of exercise-related stress injuries, *Radiology* 123:699, 1977.
151. Wilson ES Jr, Katz FN: Stress fracture: an analysis of 250 consecutive cases, *Radiology* 92:481, 1969.
152. Wilson MJ, Michele AA, Jacobson EW: Isolated fracture of the lesser trochanter, *J Bone Joint Surg* 21:776, 1939.
153. Wilson PD, Jacobs B, Schecter L: Slipped capital femoral epiphysis, *J Bone Joint Surg* 47A:1128, 1965.
154. Winkler H, Rapp IH: Ununited epiphysis of the ischium, *J Bone Joint Surg* 29:234, 1947.
155. Wolfgang GL: Stress fracture of the femoral neck in a patient with open capital femoral epiphysis, *J Bone Joint Surg* 59A:680, 1977.
156. Wong-Chung J, Strong ML: Physeal remodeling after internal fixation of slipped capital femoral epiphysis, *J Pediatr Orthop* 11:2, 1991.
157. Young LW: Radiologic case of the month, *Am J Dis Child* 134:885, 1980.
158. Zionts LE, Simonian PT, Harvey JP: Transient penetration of the hip joint during in situ cannulated-screw fixation of slipped capital femoral epiphysis, *J Bone Joint Surg* 73:1054, 1991.

ADDITIONAL READINGS

Collins HR: Epiphyseal injuries in athletes, *Clev Clin J Med* 42:285, 1975.
DeHaven K: Athletic injuries in adolescents, *Pediatr Ann* 7:704, 1978.
Fabry GI, MacEwen GD, Shands AR: Torsion of the femur: a follow-up study in normal and abnormal conditions, *J Bone Joint Surg* 55A:1726, 1973.
Goldberg B et al: Children's sports injuries—are they avoidable? *Phys Sports Med* 7:9, 1979.
Jackson DW: Injury prediction in the young athlete: preliminary report, *Am J Sports Med* 6:6, 1978.
Larson RL: Epiphyseal injuries in the adolescent athlete, *Orthop Clin North Am* 4:839, 1973.
Larson RL, McMahon RO: The epiphysis and the childhood athlete, *JAMA* 196:607, 1966.
Micheli LJ, Gerbino PG: Epidemiology of children's sports injuries, *Orthop Trans* 3:88, 1979.
Quinby WC Jr, Truman JT, Connelly JP: Athletic injuries in children, *Clin Pediatr (Phil)* 3:533, 1964.
Siffert RS, Ling RN: Athletic injuries in children, *Pediatr Clin North Am* 12:2027, 1965.

CHAPTER 58 Injuries of the Spine

Douglas W. Jackson
Wylie D. Lowery, Jr.
Jerome V. Ciullo

"Who knows the thoughts of a child?" (Nora Perry, "Who Knows?," American poet, 1832-1896.)

At times it may be confusing to assess spinal complaints in adults; this may be even more difficult in children and adolescents. Children infrequently complain of physical pain. Because of this, a child's complaint of backache must be associated with a significant attempt to determine its origin. The patient's medical history and physical examination often suggest the cause and determine if tests are needed to establish or confirm a diagnosis. A proper diagnosis is the key to subsequent therapy and treatment that determines when the young athlete may return to sports activity.

Nicholas, Grossman, and Hershman[43] directed our attention to the important concept of **linkage** of the upper and lower extremity motions with the vertebral column. Ciullo and Zarins[9] expanded on this concept, explaining upper extremity power amplification of the lower extremity athletic performance by crossed extensor reflexes built into the circuitry of the spine. Athletic performance may be seen as a combination of upper and lower extremity motions linked through the spine. Back pain and dysfunction can significantly diminish athletic performance. Conversely, sporting activity involving upper and lower extremity motion may result in back injury and pain, particularly when the vertebral column and supporting structures are inflexible or overloaded. The back may become the weak link in the chain.

Fortunately, spinal symptoms and injuries are relatively infrequent among young athletes compared with other musculoskeletal causes of pain. Most retrospective studies have shown that less than 10% of the reported sports-related musculoskeletal injuries involve the spine.[5] Although spinal injuries are infrequent, most of the fatalities and permanent spinal cord injuries occur in the 15- to 18-year-old age group. Spinal injuries occur in two peaks: one in children 5 years' old or younger, and one in those older than 10 years of age.[5,11] Zaricznyj et al[75] surveyed all sports-related injuries of school-age children in a single community during a 1-year period. Of those in the study group, 6% sustained injury during that year. Injury to the back composed only 4% of the entire series. The type of injury was sport specific. Apparently minor injuries, for example, strains and sprains, most commonly resulted from track and field events, whereas the highest incidence of serious injury occurred in horseback riding. Although the overall incidence of back pain is low in sports, it is higher in specific sports such as gymnastics, football, and racquet sports.[60] These sports combine repetitive, high-velocity twisting with bending and axial loading in extremes of motion, which greatly increase the risk of injury. Widespread athletic participation by all ages has resulted in more patients with sports-related back injuries.

Jackson, Rettig, Wiltse,[30] in a retrospective study of 100 top-level female gymnasts, reported that 50% of these athletes had sustained a self-limited episode of back pain at some time during their career. This is typical of most back pain occurring among athletes; such injuries are usually not severe. However, back problems have ended the careers of a few outstanding young athletes and have probably been associated with the initiation of longer term disabilities in others. In this same study, Jackson, Rettig, and Wiltse[30] revealed that 9% of preelite, 43% of elite, and 63% of Olympic-level gymnasts had spinal abnormalities on magnetic resonance imaging (MRI). Of all swimmers, 16% had spinal abnormalities on MRI. Increased intensity and length of training in the female gymnasts made them more prone to have MRI changes in their spines.

Specific practices within a sport may lead to an increased incidence of trauma. Duff[15] found injuries ranging from cardiac contusion to cervical spine injuries resulting from spearing or face blocking in youth football. Piggot[51] noticed a dramatic increase in major cervical spine injury in athletes in Great Britain while they were playing rugby. Dr. Piggot noted that a change had occurred in the "game's character," namely the technique of ball carrying and tackling. A recent change in coaching techniques in which the ball carrier was coached to run deliberately at the tackler was believed to have been the most important contributing factor for the increase in cervical spine injuries. Likewise, spinal injuries recorded in ice hockey players by Tator et al[67] were most commonly from a posterior check. This caused the player to be catapulted headfirst into the boards. These observations demonstrate how the physician dealing with the care of the young athlete must take an active role in identifying patterns of injury so that the preventive measures can be developed. These may include rule changes as well as changes in coaching techniques.

With the increased interest in fitness and the popularity of vigorous participation in sports, more athletes are being seen with acute and chronic back complaints. The evaluation of an injured back in the young athlete is no different from that for any other patient. It requires that a detailed history be taken and a thorough physical ex-

amination be performed. Knowledge of the biomechanics of the sport involved may be beneficial in the diagnosis of the underlying injury. Treatment programs should be tailored to the various stresses of different athletic activities. The passage of time and withdrawing the young athlete from vigorous activity assists in making a diagnosis. The physician must keep the entire differential diagnosis of all possible causes of back pain open, for example, tumors, which are rare in young athletes. These infrequent causes of symptoms are missed unless the physician has an index of suspicion, particularly in those back complaints that are atypical or persist longer than anticipated.

The differential diagnosis of back pain in young athletes includes sprains, strains, contusions, herniated disks, developmental or Scheuermann's kyphosis, apophysitis, degenerative processes, pathologic conditions of the pars interarticularis, facet syndrome, spinal stenosis, fractures or dislocations, neurologic sequelae, inflammation, disk calcification, diskitis, vertebral osteomyelitis, sacroiliac joint infection, rheumatoid diseases, spinal neoplasms, and somatoform pain disorder. Spinal disorders associated with skeletal dysplasias and metabolic diseases are not discussed in this chapter.

Differential diagnosis of back pain in young athletes

- Sprains
- Strains
- Contusions
- Herniated disks
- Developmental kyphosis
- Apophysitis
- Vertebral osteomyelitis
- Rheumatoid disease
- Somatic pain disorders
- Degenerative process
- Pars pathology
- Facet syndrome
- Spinal stenosis
- Inflammatory disease
- Disk calcification
- Diskitis
- Sacroiliac joint infection
- Spinal neoplasm

ANATOMY

Phylogenetically, primitive segmental somites of the mesoderm condense around the notochord, and each segment divides into a cranial and a caudal element. In vertebrates the cranial half fuses with the caudal half of the preceding segment, and the original segmental mesodermal orientation shifts by one half segment. The previous single segment muscles are now found to extend between vertebrae, and the blood vessels that once lay between somites are found to enter the middle of the vertebral bodies. The remains of the intersegmental notochord are condensed to form the nucleus pulposus of the intervertebral disk (Fig. 58-1). In the third month of fetal life, vertebral arches grow dorsally and meet in the

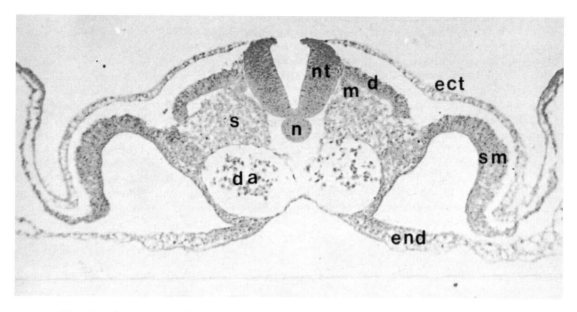

FIG. 58-1. Cross section of thoracic somite in chick embryo of 20 somite stage. Notochord (*n*) underlies neural tube (*tf*). Somite is divided into dermatome (*d*), myotome (*m*), and sclerotome (*s*). Lateral to this, somatic mesoderm (*sm*), endoderm (*end*), and ectoderm (*ect*) are displayed. Ventral to sclerotomes lie paired dorsal aortae (*da*). Transient myocele is apparent on right side between dermatome and myotome. (From Parke WW, Rothman RH, Simeon FA: Development of the spine. In Rothman RH, Simeone FA (eds): *The spine,* ed 3, Philadelphia, 1992, WB Saunders.)

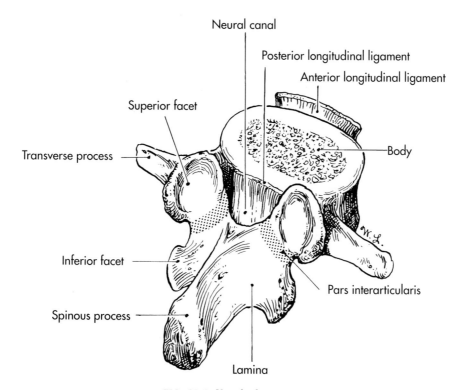

FIG. 58-2. Vertebral anatomy.

posterior midline (Fig. 58-2). Failure to fuse results in **spina bifida.**

Each half of a vertebra has a separate center of ossification. Failure of one of these ossification centers to develop results in a **hemivertebra.** Similarly, the individual sides of the arch ossify, fuse posteriorly, and then fuse anteriorly to the vertebral body. Failure of this latter fusion may result in **congenital spondylolysis.**

The apophyseal rings develop into the endplates of the vertebral body. The apophyseal rings are related to the intervening disk. Their growth, which occurs in the presence of the pressures and stresses associated with corresponding disks, lengthens the spine. Excess pressure may result in the herniation of disk material either through the apophyseal ring or into the vertebral body and produce a **Schmorl's nodule.**

The first two vertebral bodies, the atlas and the axis, develop differently. The odontoid process of C2 actually represents the body of the atlas, which is initially united to the axis by cartilage. This cartilage may remain intact between the two parts rather than progress as a normal epiphysis. If it persists, it represents a syndesmosis that leaves the odontoid process fragile in youth. The **os odontoidium** is an example of this. Although congenital segmentation variations of the cervical spine are common, they do not necessarily rule out participation in sports.

There are usually 7 cervical vertebrae, 12 thoracic vertebrae, 5 lumber vertebrae, 5 sacral segments, and 4 coccygeal segments (Fig. 58-3). Rarely there are 3 coccygeal segments instead of 4, 4 or 6 sacral vertebrae instead of 5, and in about 4% of spines, 6 lumbar vertebrae instead of 5. In 1% of spines the fifth vertebra is found completely fused to the sacrum. In 6.5% of spines the L5 or L6 vertebra is unilaterally fused to the sacrum; clinically, this variation is more likely to correlate with low back pain than any other anomaly previously mentioned. Congenital fusion does occur between vertebrae, most commonly between the second and third cervical bodies. Fusion may even occur between the atlas and occipital bone. In at least 5% of young athletes radiographs reveal evidence of anomalies of the lumbar spine; this does not necessarily preclude participation in sports.

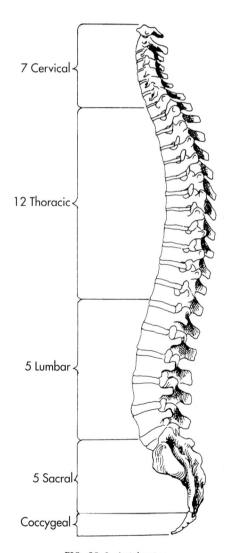

FIG. 58-3. Axial spine.

7 Cervical

12 Thoracic

5 Lumbar

5 Sacral

Coccygeal

Incidence of lumbosacral anomalies	
Anomaly	**Incidence %**
Lumbarization of S1	4
Sacralization (complete) of L5	1
Sacralization incomplete of L5 or L6	6.5

The intervertebral disks themselves contribute to spinal motion. The motion segment, which is composed of a disk and its surrounding vertebrae, has motion limited by the posterior synovial joints. Orientation of these facet articulations also defines rotation of the spine. Nevertheless, about 90% of cervical total rotation takes place at the atlantoaxial joint. Flexion and extension at the cervical spine takes place primarily between C5 and C6. In the thoracic region, motion is severely restricted by the anterior ribs and sternum, and the facet joints are oriented to best allow lateral bending and rotation. Sagittally placed facet joints in the lumbar region allow flexion and hyperextension but limit rotation to about 5 degrees (Table 58-1). Within the athletic population there is a wide variation of normal spinal motion. The extremes of motion varies between individuals and may be limited by age-related changes.

TABLE 58-1 Range of motion (in degrees) of the axial spine*

Segment	Flexion	Extension	Lateral Tilt	Rotation
Cervical	40	75	35	50
Thoracic	45	25	20	35
Lumbar	60	35	20	5
TOTAL	145	135	75	90

*Does not account for age-related difference.

The annulus fibrosus of the intervertebral disk and the anterior and posterior longitudinal ligaments unite adjoining vertebral bodies. Tension along the anterior longitudinal ligament resisting hyperextension results in traction osteophytes, which develop with age. The posterior longitudinal ligament is thicker at the midline than laterally and contributes to the clinical occurrence of posterolateral disk protrusion rather than midline protrusion. This posterior ligament is so thick that if a disk collapses, it may fold and actually impinge on the spinal cord. Denis[13] introduced the three-column theory in classification of acute thoracolumbar spine injuries. The anterior column includes the anterior longitudinal ligament, the anterior annulus fibrosus, and the anterior half of the vertebral body. The middle column, thought to be the key for stability, is formed by the posterior longitudinal ligament, posterior annulus fibrosus, and posterior half of the vertebral body. The posterior column comprises the pedicles, facet joints, laminae, spinous process, interspinous ligaments, and supraspinous ligaments. In the posterior column the facet joints bear approximately 20% of vertebral load, except at the lumbosacral joint, where the load is greater.

The strong, elastic, paired ligamenta flava span the distance between laminae. Forceful hyperextension, particularly in the cervical spine, causes them to buckle so that they can decrease the anteroposterior diameter of the vertebral canal by as much as 30%. Traction spurs or congenital stenosis of the spinal canal may contribute to making symptoms worse. The supraspinous ligaments attached to the spinous processes resist hyperflexion of the spine and extend down to the L4 vertebra and do not reach the sacrum.

Innervation and vascularity of the posterior structures of the spinal column retain the primitive organization that existed before the half-segment shift. The posterior rami of spinal nerves are thus seen to give off branches to the facet joint in their own interspace, as well as the interspace below in the lumbar region and above in the thoracic region. Like the joints the spinal ligaments are similarly innervated by two spinal nerves, and this leads to the confusion of mixed patterns of referred pain seen clinically.

A major function of the spinal column is to protect the delicate spinal cord. This cord is immersed in fluid within the relatively elastic dural sac. Because the spinal cord is fixed at either end, abrupt change of length, particularly with hyperflexion, may be associated with a stretch of substance of the cord. Vertebral impact may result in fracture fragments of vertebrae, endplates, and the disks, which may protrude into the spinal canal. Compression injuries may occur because the cross-sectional area of the spinal canal is limited.

Spinal cord damage can occur without evidence of skeletal injury. Particularly in young children and infants vertebral dislocation may reduce spontaneously without physical deformity or radiographic evidence. The only evidence of trauma may be residual spinal cord damage **(SCIWORA—spinal cord injury without radiologic abnormality).** Hyperextension of the cervical spine can lead to temporary dislocation and rupture of the anterior

longitudinal ligament and bulging of the ligamentum flavum. Bulging of the ligamentum flavum most commonly is found at C3-C4 and C5-C6 with cord damage most common at C5 to C7, since flexion and extension is most apparent in the C5-C6 area.

The ligaments within the young spine are strong, and vertebral fracture can occur before ligament rupture. The neural arch often fractures when the anterior longitudinal ligament ruptures by a hyperextension injury. The disks, joints, and ligaments are resistent to compression, distraction, extension, and flexion. They are more vulnerable to the rotation and horizontal shearing forces common in sports movements; hence the higher incidence of strains and sprains.

Many small intersegmental muscles are associated with the spine and include the interspinal and intertransverse muscles. Other muscles of the spine have multiple origins and multiple insertions. Because of such arrangements the back muscles are extremely complex, which explains why a spasm secondary to an acute muscle strain may be quite diffuse.

BIOMECHANICS

The substance of the intervertebral disk is known to imbibe water. This effect is limited by body weight and the effect of gravity. Cumulatively, the intervertebral disks account for 25% of the length of the vertebral column above the sacrum. With loss of fluid during the day and advancing age, there is progressive loss of height. It is interesting to note that astronauts who returned to Earth after approximately 80 days in space were found to be 1½ to 2 inches taller than at liftoff.

The nucleus pulposus has fluid characteristics. This forms an incompressible "marble" in youth when longitudinal pressure is more likely to result in endplate fracture or herniation into the adjacent vertebral body, a Schmorl's nodule, rather than the usual posterior or posterolateral clinical disk protrusion. As the annulus becomes increasingly inelastic with age, the adult disk protrusion pattern becomes more of a clinical problem.

Intradiskal pressure within the spine is about 30 lbs/sq inch unloaded with pressures of 200 to 300 lbs/sq inch when the back is used as a lever during lifting. The water-bearing property of the disk material seems to be a protective mechanism in that compression leads to loss of about 1 to 2 ml of water before adjacent vertebral endplate fracture. The nucleus pulposus itself is noncompressible; therefore with axial compression, vertebral endplates are found to bulge initially and then fracture. Roaf[54] noted that vertebral compression of the spine resulted in collapse of the vertebral endplate with rupture of the nucleus pulposus into the cancellous portion of the vertebra in such a way that the vertebral body disinte-

---

Intradiskal pressure

- 30 lbs/sq inch—unloading
- 200 to 300 lbs/sq inch—lifting

grates before disintegration of the disk itself. This leads to Schmorl's nodule development. With age, as the disk loses its turgor, the annulus tears before endplate effects occur.

Of torque resistance within the spine 35% is provided by the disk and the rest is provided by posterior joints and ligaments. Defects in the posterior structures thus increase the risk of disk failure. Facet joints protect the disk from excessive torsion and are able to carry compressive loads, thus stabilizing the effect on the motion segments in flexion and extension. The motion segment, defined as two adjacent vertebrae and the intervening soft tissues, is the essential functional unit of the spine.

Torque resistance within the spine

- Disk   35%
- Ligaments and posterior joints   65%

The anterior elements provide the major support of the spine and absorb impact. The posterior structures control patterns of motion. Together they protect the spinal cord, which lies posterior to the vertebral body and is surrounded by the neural arch. The disk is separated on both sides by hyaline cartilage endplates. These endplates influence nutrition of the disk, since the disk lacks vascular tissue and is fed by diffusion alone. Just as in articular cartilage, when the load of the disk increases, there is an outflow of fluid; and with decreased load, there is a fluid influx. With fluid influx comes proportional increase in stiffness of the disk.

The axial muscles work as shock absorbers. Increased muscle tone may have a profound effect on the ability to avoid athletic injuries. In contrast, training techniques may significantly influence patterns of injury. Schneider, Paps, and Alvarez[57] studied Acapulco high divers. The greatest bony change of posterior encroachment and spondylosis of the cervical spine was found in divers who had slightly longer necks and who struck the water with hands outstretched in such a way that they absorbed a good deal of shock directly on their heads. Those divers who clasped their hands over their heads at the time of impact with the water were not found to have severe spondylosis or cervical arthritis.

Cervical spine ligaments in children are extremely lax, with 4 mm of normal subluxation at C2-C3 and C3-C4. Longitudinal force can thus separate the vertebral bodies significantly, and it is possible to transect the spinal cord without fracture or dislocation.

The muscles of the trunk and abdomen provide considerable stability for the vertebral column. Since mobility is limited in the thoracic spine because of stable rib and facet orientation, flexion, lateral tilt, and extension maneuvers, when combined with rotation, lead to more mechanical breakdown than in the lumbar spine, where more functional motion occurs.

With normal posture and a balanced upright stance the weight of the upper trunk is supported by the spinal

---

Factors contributing to increased cervical mobility in young athletes

- Soft, cartilaginous endplates
- Horizontal attitude of facet joints
- Soft-tissue laxity

---

column, its ligaments, and the psoas muscle. With forward lean the effect of gravity imposes a turning moment that is counteracted by contraction of the extensors. The extensor muscles must provide sufficient moment to balance the increase in gravitational effect on the upper body until the posterior ligamentous complex is put into effect at about 60 degrees of forward flexion in the lumbar spine. Tension produced in the posterior structures at this point provides enough strength that no further extensor muscle activity is necessary, and in fact, these muscles are found silent in electromyelographic (EMG) study. The weight of the upper body exerts a compression force on all joints in the lumbar spine. In addition, a shear force is present at L5-S1. This may be an important developmental etiologic factor in spondylolisthesis.

The facet joints have two principal movements: they either slide or gap. When they slide on both sides simultaneously, the result is forward bending. When they slide on one side, the result is side bending. Rotation can occur by distracting on the side of one facet where the other facet becomes a fulcrum. This relationship between distraction and rotation explains why rotation is such an important element in the pathogenesis of facet injury, particularly subluxation and dislocation.

A number of authors have attempted to correlate specific anthropometric measurements to development of back pain in certain sports.[42,72] It is uncertain at this time whether these are self-selected attributes to certain sports or true cause and effect. The back, abdominal, and gluteal muscles combine to allow control of trunk motion and aid in support of the ligaments of the spine. The anterolateral prevertebral muscles in the lumbar region, including the psoas major and minor muscles, support the vertebral column. The quadratus lumborum also acts as a lateral flexor. The deep posterior vertebral muscles, which consist of the erector spinae, are subdivided into the transversal-spinal muscles and the sacral-spinal muscles. These muscles interact in extension, flexion, rotation, and lateral flexion.

Superficial back muscles cover the erector spine musculature, except over the lumbar region, where they insert into the thoracolumbar fascia. The superficial layer, the trapezius, the latissimus dorsi, and the lumbar segment of the gluteus maximus are involved in function of the extremities and are located far enough from the centers of motion to have important supportive roles in movement of the trunk and crossed extensor power amplification of extremity motion through the spine. In addition, the thoracic and abdominal musculature increases intracavitary pressure, which permits the thoracolumbar spine to withstand pressures that might otherwise result in injury.

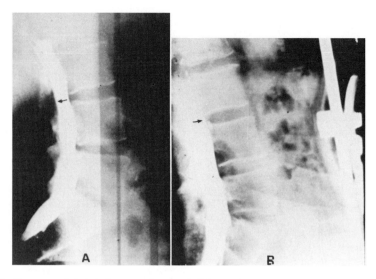

FIG. 58-4. Decrease of disk bulging with use of abdominal binder documented myelographically. **A,** Without binder, note disk bulge. **B,** With binder, bulge diminished. (Courtesy Harry Ingberg, Medical Director, Detroit Rehabilitation Institute, Detroit, Mich.)

Farfan[17] demonstrated that as muscles contract to extend the spine, the psoas and multifidus produce shearing forces in the intervertebral joints. The facet joints can resist 500 to 700 pounds of shear force. Greater shear than that can be encountered in normal lifting; therefore the facets and disks are protected by abdominal muscles, particularly the internal oblique muscles, which contract and actually produce negative shear in flexion. If the external oblique muscles and the contralateral internal oblique muscles contract together, they tend to rotate the spine. More important, symmetric contraction blocks rotation to reinforce the antirotational function of the facet joints and reduce shear force on the intervertebral joint. Thus the strong abdominal muscles work as a secondary support and reduce the load on the spine. This is why there is such an emphasis on abdominal strengthening during rehabilitation. Furthermore, these muscles must not be weakened in the recuperative period, or the cycle may worsen. The effect of binding or strengthening the abdominal muscles can be documented myelographically (Fig. 58-4).

CLINICAL HISTORY

Young athletes can often elicit the mechanism of their back injury and pinpoint the moment of onset. Such information may help delineate a diagnosis and emphasize the factors to be evaluated during subsequent physical examination. Other young athletes are reluctant to discuss the matter with a physician or may not remember the cause of injury; thus careful history-taking is mandatory. Specifically, the physician must try to elicit such factors as the circumstances leading to the onset of pain, the nature and severity of pain, how the patient ranks the degree of pain, changes in the character of pain since its initiation, and associated systemic complaints.

Establishing the time of onset of pain is important to

Important points in history-taking of young athletes with back pain
■ Mechanism of injury or onset of pain ■ Nature and severity of pain ■ Degree of pain ■ Changes in pain characteristics since onset ■ Systemic complaints

estimate the duration of pain. Frequently, a change in activity level, training technique, or athletic equipment is directly related to the onset of symptoms. This is particularly true at the beginning of the season.

The physician must establish how debilitating the pain is and how frequently it actually occurs. It is important to note whether it is related to activity, relieved by rest, or whether it radiates. Typical patterns leading to diagnosis of disk pain must be differentiated by atypical patterns that might indicate the presence of a tumor. Aggravation of pain with coughing or straining indicates an intraspinal cause. Response to medication must also be explored.

It is important to establish whether the pain has changed from the onset. Pain that initially follows activity and progresses to the point of interfering with activity may suggest an inflammatory condition. If other symptoms or problems were apparent before the onset of back pain, these should be recorded in the history. Changes of gait patterns or bowel and bladder habits, as well as peripheral muscle weakness, are factors that must be explored because their onset is usually gradual and may be ignored by the patient or parents.

Having the patient pinpoint areas of pain on a pain chart drawing may be helpful (Fig. 58-5). A child is often unable to easily rate pain so that the significance of

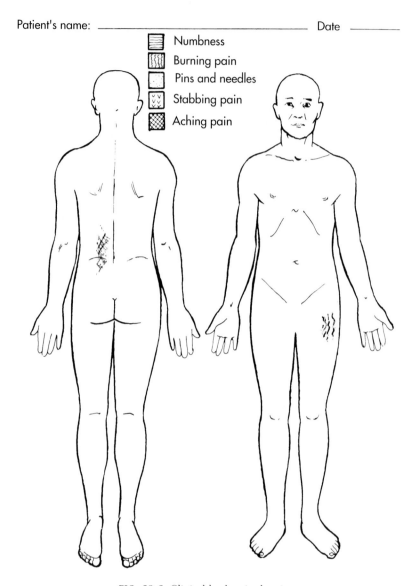

Patient's name: _____ Date _____

- ▤ Numbness
- ▨ Burning pain
- ▢ Pins and needles
- ⋁⋁ Stabbing pain
- ▩ Aching pain

FIG. 58-5. Clinical back pain drawing.

pain can be explored; thus it is helpful to relate back-ache to other experiences he or she may have had during childhood, such as a toothache, appendicitis, or a crushed finger. The coach can often be helpful in supplying information about the sports activity and the mechanism of injury.

CLINICAL EXAMINATION

Many physicians are involved in preparticipation sports assessments. Goldberg et al[22] found that the medical history and musculoskeletal examination are the highest yielding components of these assessments. The history may suggest specific areas for further investigation. The physical examination, particularly the back examination, must have the patient dressed properly, that is, with a hospital gown that opens in the back or in gym shorts.

The neck and back should be examined posteriorly to evaluate posture and structural deformity. Accentuated lumbar lordosis or thoracic kyphosis may be immediately obvious. A list in which the head is not centralized over the body may also be apparent. Cutaneous lesions associated with neurofibromatosis may be apparent, and a midline dimple, hair patch, or nidus might implicate intraspinous, congenital, or etiologic factors. A decrease of chest expansion and spinal motion in the young athlete with generalized spinal pain may indicate early spondylitis.

With forward bending, a rib or lumbar scoliotic hump may become apparent or thoracic kyphosis accentuated. Listing in forward bending might be related to scoliosis. The ability to bend forward and return to an upright position without ratcheting is important in normal function. If the one-legged hyperextension of the lumbar spine reproduces the pain the patient has experienced, particu-

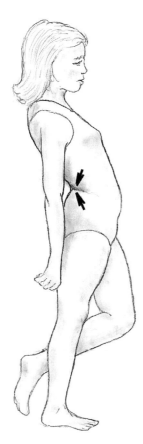

FIG. 58-6. One-leg hyperextension test: beltline pain implicates a pathologic condition of pars complex.

larly at the posterior belt line, a pathologic condition involving the pars interarticularis or posterior elements may be indicated (Fig. 58-6).

The physician should "lay hands on." Palpation determines if there is tenderness or the presence of muscle spasm; with the hands on the iliac crest, pelvic obliquity, possibly related to limb-length discrepancy, can be elicited. Palpation may help localize transverse process or spinous process fractures. Spinal percussion may be useful in the young athlete because it may suggest an inflammatory process such as abscess or diskitis. Nerve irritation may also be implicated by pain with palpation over the sciatic notch. Compression over the sacroiliac joint by direct pressure may help differentiate a pathologic condition; compression is best done with the patient in the supine position and flexing the hip 90 degrees with adduction of the leg across the midline. When a figure-4 or Patrick's test is performed, the patient may demonstrate contralateral sacroiliac joint pain.

Pathologic conditions of the hip may often aggravate or be misinterpreted as back symptoms. Because pathologic processes of the hip usually incur early loss of internal rotation, internal rotation of the hip should be tested. In addition, hip flexion and extension should be examined. A loss of hip flexion and extension has the potential to affect the lumbar spine. Neurologic examination is part of any spine examination. Hamstring spasm,

if present, must be distinguished from nerve root irritation. This can be distinguished by straight leg raising. The straight leg raising test is positive for referred pain when the radiation of pain is produced down the posterior aspect of the lower extremity (below the knee). When the radiation extends distally, it implicates nerve root irritation or an intraspinal pathologic condition. If results of the straight leg raising test are equivocal, it is not diagnostic. The direct femoral nerve stretch test may be evaluated with the patient in the prone position and with the knee in flexion and the hip in extension. The upper extremity is similarly evaluated with an excursion maneuver used to test for thoracic outlet pain; passive abduction, external rotation, and elevation of the arm producing radicular pain is pathognomonic of cervical nerve root irritation and is probably as reliable as the straight leg raising test in the lower extremity. Reflex evaluation and deep tendon reflex analysis must be done in upper and lower extremities, and visual examination combined with circumferential measurement and palpation can used to detect and document atrophy. Vibratory sensual changes or decreased sensation to pin prick can be used to delineate early neurologic change. The gait of the young athlete should be observed, noting stride length, limp, joint flexion, circumduction rate, and posture. Any abnormality necessitates further evaluation.

LABORATORY EVALUATION

Back pain in the child and young athlete should be approached with a high index of suspicion. The standard battery of tests for persistent, unexplained spinal pain should include a complete blood count, erythrocyte sedimentation rate test, and urinalysis. If a rheumatologic disorder is considered the rheumatoid factor, antinuclear antigen (ANA), and other serologic tests may be used. These specific tests are usually negative in the younger

---

Screening laboratory evaluation for unexplained back pain

- Complete blood count
- Erythrocyte sedimentation rate
- Urinalysis

---

athlete, even if an underlying collagen disease is present. Alkaline phosphatase isoenzyme levels measured by serum electrophoresis may demonstrate an elevated bone fraction in malignant disease.

RADIOLOGIC EVALUATION

In the past decade remarkable advances have occurred in diagnostic imaging with the introduction and refinement of computed tomography (CT), CT myelography, MRI, single photon emission computed tomography (SPECT), and ultrasound (US).

Radiographs

Plain x-ray studies are usually the first radiologic test requested in young athletes complaining of spine-related injuries or symptoms. Anteroposterior and lateral views should be supplemented with specific views. It is critical for patients with suspected cervical spine injuries to have radiographs that include the entire cervical spine including the C7-T1 junction. Pillar views are used in the cervical spine in evaluation of facet subluxation, and open-mouth views are often necessary to visualize the odontoid process. Lateral hyperflexion and hyperextension views aid in evaluation of ligamentous or segmental instability. Oblique films are important, particularly in the cervical and lumbar spine, to rule out foraminal entrapment, pars interarticularis injury, or facet joint disorders. If the clinical examination warrants, radiographs to evaluate scoliosis or kyphosis should be taken. With evaluation of the lumbar spine, a spot lateral view of the lumbosacral junction often yields increased definition in detail, and flexion-extension views may document instability. Films of the sacroiliac joint and pelvis can also be useful.

Linear Tomography

In some instances conventional tomography may be more helpful than CT. Tomograms can be used to investigate congenital fusions, anomalies, osteoid osteomas, and other tumorous conditions. In dens fractures tomograms generally show the fracture line clearly.

Computed Tomography

With the exception of certain trauma and complex congenital abnormalities, tomography has been replaced by CT. CT remains the superior method for detecting cortical bone injury or detecting calcification or ossification. CT is superior to routine radiography in assessing the degree of degenerative changes in the spine such as facet joint hypertrophy and spinal stenosis. CT supplements routine radiography in assessment of spinal fractures and dislocations. For example, a burst fracture of the vertebral body at the same level of a laminar fracture on CT usually signifies a dural laceration. CT is also valuable in assessing other pathologic processes such as osteoid osteomas, osteoblastomas, and aneurysmal bone cysts. For better soft-tissue definition or evaluation of intraspinal injury, contrast-enhanced CT may be used.

Magnetic Resonance Imaging

MRI has been found to be equally effective compared with contrast-enhanced CT in diagnosing intraspinal injury (e.g., neoplasia, disk herniation, and spinal dysrhaphism).[12,26,64] MRI is even more attractive in the pediatric and young athletic population because there is no exposure to ionizing radiation. It is noninvasive and is ideal for screening and serial examination of the lumbar spine when indicated. Although relatively expensive, MRI is the best technique for defining disk degeneration and neural element injury.[35] The MRI is helpful for defining a number of different anatomic patterns of cord injury. In addition, it is becoming the most widely used test for assessing disk herniation. Degenerative changes in the symptomatic immature spine have been docu-

mented. However, there have been no large studies documenting the incidence of MRI abnormalities in the asymptomatic immature spine. Gibson et al[21] found lumbar disk abnormalities in 4 of 20 asymptomatic adolescents. Powell, Wilson, and Szyeryt[52] found physiologic disk degeneration in 6% to 20% of asymptomatic subjects under the age of 20 using MRI studies.

MRI signal intensity is related to three parameters: the number of hydrogen protons in the tissue or proton density (M_0), the spin-lattice relaxation time (T1), and spin-spin relaxation time (T2). In the intervertebral disk, M_0 is related to the amount of disk hydration. T1 and T2 are related to the interaction between water molecules. In the normal disk the M_0 and T2 values are high in the nucleus pulposus and low in the annulus. When using T2-weighted images the nucleus pulposus (long T2) exhibits high intensity in contrast to annulus (short T2) with its low-intensity appearance. With disk degeneration the water content of the nucleus pulposus decreases with a resultant decrease in signal intensity on the MRI. This corresponds to decreased values of M_0, T1, and T2. Although disk degeneration can be an age-related phenomenon, such age-related changes should not be present in the adolescent. Therefore in this age group, changes in signal intensity generally reflect disk injury.

In addition to bone scans MRI is a sensitive test in the diagnosis of stress fractures. Atwell and Jackson[1] reported on subtle stress fractures of the sacrum in runners that are apparent on MRI scans.

MRI may be helpful in delineating infectious processes, giving abnormally high-signal intensity on T2-weighted images. Some authors have advocated its superiority to myelography and CT in evaluating such spinal infections such as myelitis, osteomyelitis, and disk space infections.[38,39] Nevertheless, both MRI and CT scans should be viewed as complementary technologies.

Scintigraphy

Bone scintigraphy is used to define bony reactions, such as spondylolysis, in the young athlete. It may help distinguish between established nonunions and healing defects in patients with back pain and spondylolysis. A gallium scan is helpful if infection is implicated. These tests often yield positive results before definitive changes can be seen on standard radiographs. However, a negative bone scan does not exclude infection.

Diskography

Diskography alone or combined with CT is still controversial, but it may be of value in assessing primary or recurrent disk herniations. At our institution diskography has been helpful in assessing atypical disk pain in young athletes. A degenerated nucleus shows irregularities and may be associated with abnormal mobility of the motion segment on flexion-extension analysis. Disk abnormalities in the young athlete may be associated with the development of Schmorl's nodules.

Ultrasound

US evaluation of the spinal canal is being used to study the spine in normal infants, spinal dysrhaphism, and patients with spinal cord tumors. Despite the development of high-resolution scanners, an intact osseous posterior spine acts as a barrier to US evaluation.[53]

MISCELLANEOUS EVALUATION
Electrodiagnostic Studies

EMGs and nerve conduction studies are not usually needed in the assessment of athletic injuries. EMGs are helpful with the differential diagnosis when multiple nerve roots may be involved and after recovery from nerve injuries.[35] The EMG is useful in the hands of someone skilled in its use. With such expertise, localization of the pathologic process may be possible in a high percentage of cases with neurologic involvement.

Needle Biopsy

Radiographic lesions with clinical correlation may necessitate a definitive diagnosis. The Craig needle biopsy may be useful in particular situations in evaluating questionable lesions in the spine. CT-guided needle biopsy is also helpful. Ackerman needle biopsy is similarly used under fluoroscopic control in evaluation of the cervical and lower thoracic spine. The midthoracic spine is not easy to evaluate fluoroscopically, and in such cases open biopsy through costotransversectomy is recommended.

Cystometrics

Early symptoms of urinary frequency, urgency, or enuresis may be signs of irritation of the sacral nerve roots. With signs of a neurogenic bladder, cystometrography should be considered. Small bladder capacity is noted early on; a large capacity with a high residual level indicates chronicity.

DISORDERS

We consider nine different etiologic categories in assessing the young athlete's back pain: idiopathic, congenital, soft tissue, anterior and middle column, posterior column, fracture or dislocation, inflammation, tumor, and somatoform pain disorders. In athletic patients, neck and back pain are usually related to the musculoskeletal system; however, visceral injury and patterns of referred pain should always be suspected.[27]

Idiopathic or Mechanical Disorders

In a number of young athletes, no particular mechanical etiologic factors can be found other than increased

clinical lordosis of the lower back, neck, or stooped shoulders (Fig. 58-7). Relief is occasionally obtained with a regimented exercise program. Sometimes with strict attention to clinical and radiographic findings, a more specific diagnosis can be elicited.

Micheli[39] stated that some lumbar pain could actually be considered "growing pain." He postulated that the adolescent athlete experiences a phase of transient overgrowth of the bony elements, as compared with the ligaments, tendons, and strong dorsal fascia, during the second growth spurt. The result is a combination of tight lumbosacral fascia and hamstrings and decompensation of the torso over the pelvis posteriorly and weak abdominal muscles anteriorly. The young athlete offsets structural imbalance by developing a mild roundback posture so that he or she may balance the torso forward over the pelvis. This compensatory kyphosis may lead to developmental wedging of the vertebral bodies. Treatment consists of flexibility exercises for hamstrings and lumbodorsal fascia and strengthening exercises for anterior abdominal musculature.

Congenital and Developmental Abnormalities

Many congenital abnormalities of the pediatric spine are inconsequential to any symptomatology. However, anomalies must still be included in the differential. As a

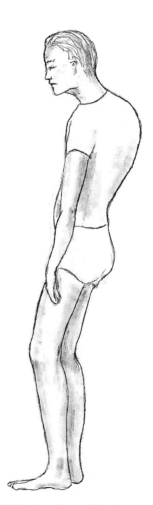

FIG. 58-7. Postural back pain.

Categoric grouping of back diagnoses

- Idiopathic conditions
- Congenital problems
- Soft-tissue injury and conditions
- Anterior and middle column dysfunction
- Posterior column disorders
- Fracture or dislocation
- Inflammation
- Tumor
- Somatoform pain disorders

rule the younger the child, the more obvious the anomalies must be to make the diagnosis.[18] Enuresis and extremity weakness may be subtle findings of dysrhaphism or diastematomyelia diagnosed in later childhood.

A detailed discussion of congenital and developmental abnormalities of the pediatric spine is beyond the scope of this chapter. However, in the cervical spine the differential should include cervical instability, congenital anomalies of the odontoid, and torticollis. Patients with certain bone dysplasias (e.g., achondroplasia and Morquio's syndrome) have a propensity for an occipito-cervical problem such as **basilar impression.** The C1-C2 articulation is the most mobile and hence the least stable joint of the spine. Of Down syndrome (trisomy 21) patients, 25% have **C1-C2 laxity** (Fig. 58-8). This is important in screening for participation in the Special Olympics. In Down syndrome patients a predens interval of less than 7 to 9 mm is usually managed by observation and avoidance of any contact sport or activity that may subject the neck to a load. The Committee on Sports Medicine of the American Academy of Pediatrics states

---

Special Olympics restrictions for athletes with trisomy 21

- Gymnastics
- Butterfly swim stroke
- Swimming dive start
- High jump
- Pentathlon
- Soccer
- Any warm-up exercise that places pressure on the head and neck

---

that Down syndrome patients who do not have evidence of atlantoaxial instability may participate in all athletic events.[70] The Special Olympics Committee more specifically recommends prohibiting Down syndrome individuals from "participating in any Special Olympics training or competition in gymnastics, butterfly stroke (in swimming), diving start (in swimming), high jump, pentathlon, soccer, and warm-up exercises that place pressure on the head and neck muscles."[59]

Rotatory subluxation of C1-C2 may follow an upper respiratory tract infection or be associated with rheumatoid arthritis or Down syndrome and present as torticollis. CT is helpful in making the diagnosis. Surgical stabilization is rarely necessary. The vast majority respond to rest, aspirin, and use of a soft collar. A halo may be needed if the subluxation continues more than 3 weeks.

Pseudosubluxation of C2 on C3 is common in children under 8 years of age (Fig. 58-9).[53] The child's spine has much more flexible soft tissue than the adult spine.

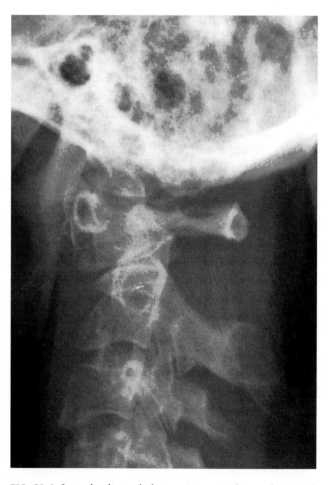

FIG. 58-8. Lateral radiograph demonstrates significant atlantoaxial instability in patient with Down syndrome. (From Clark CR: The cervical spine: pediatric and reconstructive aspects. In AAOS: *Orthopaedic knowledge update III*, Park Ridge, Ill, 1990, American Academy of Orthopaedic Surgeons.)

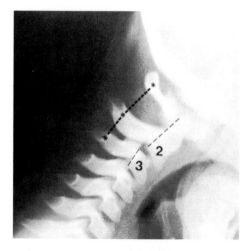

FIG. 58-9. Pseudosubluxation of C2 on C3. Hypermobility is common in children under age of 8 years. Specific measurements of movement of vertebral bodies (*thin dotted line*) are unreliable, whereas relationship with posterior elements (*thick dotted line*) is more consistent. In flexion, posterior arch of C2 normally aligns itself in a straight line with C1 and C3. (From Hensinger RN: Cervical spine: pediatric. In AAOS: *Orthopaedic knowledge update I*, Park Ridge, Ill, 1984, American Academy of Orthopaedic Surgeons.)

To differentiate physiologic processes from pathologic processes the posterior elements of C2 are normally aligned with C1 and C3.

Atlantooccipital fusion, although common, may cause problems if associated with C2-C3 fusion leading to C1-C2 instability. Surgical stabilization is usually needed in this case.

Os odontoideum is the most common congenital anomaly of the odontoid. The cause may be traumatic or congenital. If there is more than 10 mm of instability documented on lateral flexion-extension x-ray studies or evidence of neurologic progression, surgical stabilization should be considered; Otherwise, nonoperative treatment is sufficient.

Klippel-Feil syndrome is a congenital failure of segmentation of a portion or the entire cervical spine. The symptoms are usually associated with the unfused segment that is hypermobile. Although most Klippel-Feil syndrome patients respond to nonoperative treatment, a small percentage may require surgical stabilization (Fig. 58-10).

Vertebral disk calcification, although uncommon, may follow a history of trauma or upper respiratory infection. It may present with torticollis, decreased motion, and neck pain. The symptoms usually resolve spontaneously. Although it is rare, the disk may herniate anteriorly or posteriorly.

Soft-Tissue Injury

Acute or chronic **musculotendinous strains** and **capsular** or **ligamentous sprains** are the most common causes of backache in the young athlete. These in-

---

> **Factors contributing to back strains and sprains**
>
> - Improper body mechanics and form
> - Poor conditioning
> - Insufficient stretching
> - Overuse
> - Unbalanced trauma

---

juries may be precipitated by improper body mechanics and form, poor conditioning, insufficient stretching, overuse, or a traumatic event. An effort to strengthen and stretch the back must be made in all sports but is particularly valuable in high-risk sports in which twisting and rotation are an integral part of performance. Symptoms often include associated muscle spasm that usually is off the midline posteriorly and occasionally leads to a list or limitation in motion of a segment of the spine.

Minor strains of the cervical spine may involve the ligaments of the interspinal structures and facet joints. These injuries are not associated with instability of the spine, and they respond to simple therapeutic measures. The use of a felt collar for a limited period may be beneficial in the more symptomatic injuries. The collar should be used for as short a period as necessary, and it can be removed for active and passive exercise.

Patients who have more severe strains in the lumbar spine may require the initial treatment of bed rest, but in the young athlete minor strains can be treated symptomatically with a lumbar corset. The increased intraabdominal pressure afforded by such measures can de-

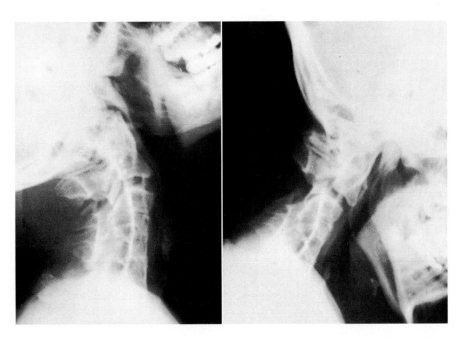

FIG. 58-10. Klippel-Feil syndrome. Clinically, patient maintains near-normal extension and flexion. Radiographically, majority of neck motion is occurring at C3-C4 disk space. With aging, this hypermobility can lead to frank instability or degenerative osteoarthritis. (From Hensinger RN: Cervical spine: pediatric. In AAOS: *Orthopaedic knowledge update I,* Park Ridge, Ill, 1984, American Academy of Orthopaedic Surgeons.)

Treatment of lumbar strains and sprains

Stage I
- Bed rest
- Lumbar corset
- Ice
- Analgesics

Stage II
- Lumbosacral stretching
- Paraspinal and abdominal strengthening
- Hip flexor stretching (if indicated)

Stage III
- Ultrasound
- Transcutaneous electric nerve stimulation
- Swimming
- Bicycling
- Continued stretching and strengthening exercises

Stage IV
- Graded return to sports
- Appropriate technique modification

---

crease force exerted on the spine. Ice in the initial stages of injury provides better relief than heat. This may be followed by US and transcutaneous electric nerve stimulation (TENS)[19] for the local areas of discomfort that persist after 24 to 48 hours. Analgesics and muscle relaxants are used as necessary, but sparingly. Rest constitutes the cornerstone of treatment and may be tailored to each individual and to each sport's requirements.[60] Jogging (repetitive pounding), racquet sports (twisting), and weightlifting (back stress) should be avoided. Swimming, bicycling, and a stair-climbing machine should be encouraged as pain allows.[35] Following the healing phase the phase of prevention of reinjury occurs. At the same time, gradual reentry into competition is permitted. This must include a careful analysis of the mechanisms of injury and appropriate change in technique where indicated. Assuming that this is achieved satisfactorily, exercises to increase endurance, strength, and flexibility are begun so that the athlete can resume previous levels of performance.[60]

A **contusion** is the result of an external force or blow. Contusions of the back are common in many athletic endeavors; infrequently, blunt trauma to soft tissue may lead to myositis ossificans, whereas if associated with fracture, may lead to pseudarthrosis or osseous bridging.[28] Contusions result in soft-tissue damage, leading to interstitial bleeding with tissue healing over time and the incorporation of scar. Initial activity should be limited to decrease hematoma formation. Most low back contusions resolve in 2 to 3 weeks with minimal treatment. It is important to use icing immediately after trauma to decrease swelling and hematoma formation. Ice is also effective for pain control and decreasing muscle excitability and spasm. This may be followed in 72 hours with heat.

With significant pain and spasm there may be flattening of the lumbar curve or an obvious list. Physical examination reveals unilateral or bilateral paraspinous spasm but a negative neurologic examination. Bed rest and medication are occasionally necessary to control pain. Physical therapists familiar with lumbar spine mobilization may offer early exercises on mobilization of the spine. Caution must be used in these techniques, but if used correctly the athlete may be able to return to activity earlier.

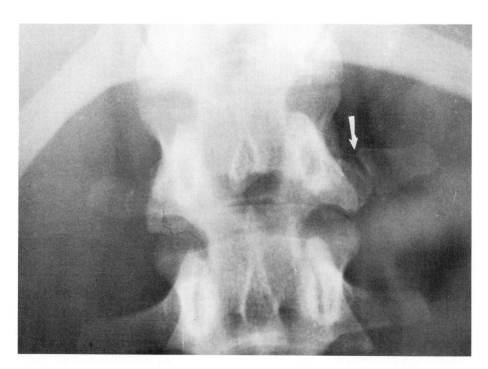

FIG. 58-11. Avulsion fracture, equivalent of severe sprain or strain, often heals with fibrous interposition.

Avulsion fractures of the transverse processes or spinous processes associated with insertions of tendons or ligaments do occur and are equivalent to the severe sprains in terms of disability. Clinical healing usually takes 4 to 6 weeks. Often, transverse process fractures heal merely by fibrous union (Fig. 58-11). Transverse process fractures often implicate a more severe injury; therefore the physician should have a high index of suspicion for associated injury, including a ruptured disk, other spinal trauma, or kidney or visceral injury. Bed rest is minimized, but it is used to control severe pain and spasm. The more significant sprains, strains, and contusions may require 6 to 8 weeks before full athletic activity can be resumed. Some may take longer. An abdominal binder can be used to increase the intraabdominal pressure and relieve pressure on the back while abdominal exercises are initiated. Stretching to maintain flexibility is mandatory but must be approached cautiously because flexion combined with some rotation is frequently the mechanism of the original injury. Thus rehabilitation must be tailored to the individual athlete.

Because soft-tissue injury heals with scar, stretching and regaining strength are necessary after injury to prevent reinjury. Following the initial phase of healing, such activities as swimming, cycling, and weight training may be substituted for the athlete's usual activity to maintain cardiovascular fitness and muscle tone until the athlete can return to the specific sport that caused the injury.

Anterior and Middle Column Dysfunction
Herniated Nucleus Pulposus

Of all symptomatic herniated disks diagnosed clinically, only 2% occur in young individuals. The diagnosis is often difficult to confirm initially because only one third of young patients complain of sciatica. Two thirds have atypical pain with symptoms related to the lower back. Use of the back pain drawing is helpful. When there is a dermatomal pattern to the pain in the extremity below the knee, the diagnosis of ruptured lumbar disk can be made with some confidence. Careful neurologic examination for subtle weakness in the extremity must be done. The fact that the initial symptoms of tumor mimic a lumbar disk injury should not be overlooked. A history of significant, associated trauma is present in approximately half of young athletes with pathologic conditions of the disk.

In the young athlete a ruptured disk not involving the endplate is usually associated with posterolateral herniation affecting adjacent neural elements. Symptoms and findings are acute and can respond rapidly to bed rest and supportive measures. Ehni and Schneider[16] described **posterior vertebral rim fractures** and associated disk protrusion in adolescence and thought that disk compliance and developing vertebral structure were the primary reasons for this unusual injury. Jackson[29] also demonstrated that a source of low back pain in the skeletally immature athlete was **disk herniation through the anterior ring apophysis** with subsequent narrowing of the disk space and altered disk mechanics at that level. This is most common at the thoracolumbar junction but may involve any of the lumbar vertebrae as well

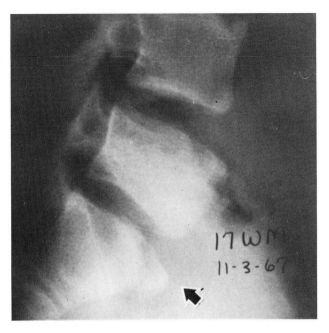

FIG. 58-12. Rupture of disk through endplate may result in disk narrowing.

(Fig. 58-12). It usually involves less than three vertebrae and may skip levels, in contrast with Scheuermann's kyphosis. It is most common in athletes who participate in vigorous training programs such as gymnastics and wrestling at an early age. Disk space narrowing is associated, and the altered disk mechanics seen on radiographs during bending can be significant. We find that the disk space narrowing often reverses itself if bracing is instituted and the aggravating activity is restricted.

On clinical examination, patients with a posterolateral disk protrusion herniation often demonstrate a positive contralateral straight leg raising test. This is indicative of nerve root compression. The patient is often found to have muscle spasm, decreased lumbar lordosis, limited forward flexion, and tight hamstrings. Just as in the adult, motor weakness of the foot dorsiflexors (L5) and quadriceps (L4) may be differentiated from a decreased or absent Achilles tendon reflex, which strongly suggests an S1 nerve root lesion.

Because two thirds of young athletes with disk disease have atypical symptoms, the workup varies. Griffin[25] stated that less than 15% of adolescents with leg pain caused by herniated disk recover satisfactorily with bed rest, exercise, and spinal orthoses. Our experience is to the contrary. We find muscle spasm and nerve root irritation quite pronounced in some young athletes. The onset of symptoms can be rapid, but resolution may be just as rapid in a majority of patients when bed rest is instituted. We have found decreased activity and supervised physical therapy, including abdominal strengthening, to be effective for many of the patients with atypical symptoms. If surgery is needed, interlaminal laminectomy without fusion is the procedure of choice.[14]

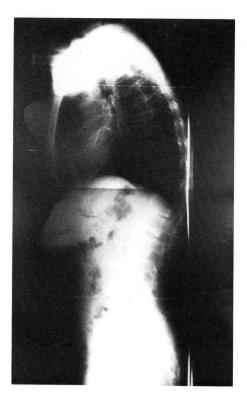

FIG. 58-13. Endplate irregularity with anterior wedging in Scheuermann's kyphosis.

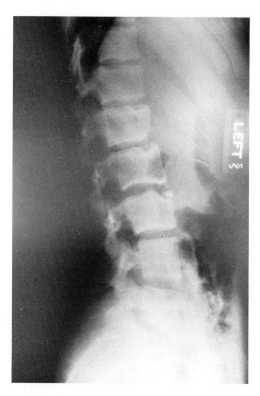

FIG. 58-14. Multiple level endplate irregularity of apophysitis. (Courtesy Anthony Melanoakos, MD, Monroe, Mich.)

Scheuermann's Kyphosis

According to Bradford et al[6] Scheuermann's kyphosis is an abnormal, fixed kyphosis associated with vertebral wedging that develops around the time of puberty. The patient complains of a dull, nonradiating fatigue-type pain at the apex of the kyphos. The pain is related to activity and is relieved by rest.

On physical examination, an obvious kyphos is demonstrated that is more prominent than in a simple roundback postural deformity. In forward bending the deformity is worsened. A protuberant abdomen is often obvious because of the increase in lumbar lordosis. The head and neck may appear to be thrust forward as a result of the thoracic kyphosis. Scoliosis can also be present.

Lateral view radiographs confirm the diagnosis (Fig. 58-13). Specifically, there is vertebral endplate irregularity present and herniation through the endplate with the formation of Schmorl's nodules. Classically, there is a wedging of at least 5 degrees anteriorly of at least three adjacent vertebrae, establishing a kyphos of greater than 35 degrees in the thorax and 60 degrees in the lumbar spine. A long anteroposterior radiograph is also useful to identify the 33% of patients with structural scoliosis. The radiographic findings differentiate this syndrome from simple roundback and postural pain.

The fact that this disease develops around the time of puberty may mean that this is a developmental problem. Possibly the vertebral endplate is at risk in this stage of growth because herniation through it by a resistant nucleus pulposus is common. However, the concurrent effect of trauma should not be overlooked.

We have seen butterfly-stroke swimmers whose symptoms and deformity are alleviated in a brace even when daily practice and swimming activity is allowed out of a brace (as long as the butterfly stroke itself is avoided). A similar treatment protocol can be established in any sport. Treatment consists of back flexibility and strengthening exercises and postural bracing. Sachs et al[55] found that kyphotic curves greater than 75 degrees were less responsive to bracing. Rarely, with rapid progression or in an older adolescent with severe pain, spinal fusion might be indicated.

Apophysitis

Symptoms ranging from vague pain to point tenderness along the back may be related to apophysitis. Pain is mechanical, made worse with activity, and relieved with rest. Radiographic evidence of changes of apophyseal irregularity at one or multiple vertebral levels without kyphotic deformity distinguish this from Scheuermann's kyphosis (Fig. 58-14). These radiographic changes may be related to excessive stress from vigorous activity during growth spurts when the endplates are particularly susceptible to injury. Treatment is by a combination of decreased activity, stretching, strengthening, and therapeutic modalities.

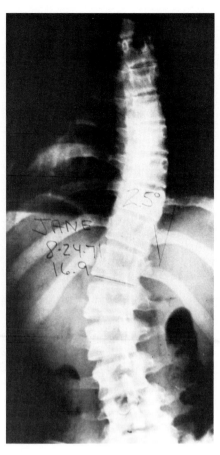

FIG. 58-15. Acute back pain may focus attention on preexisting but unrelated scoliosis.

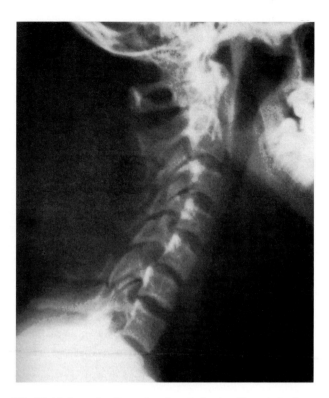

FIG. 58-16. Lateral radiographs of cervical spine. There is kyphotic deformity at C5-C6 with normal lordosis of most cervical spine above and below this level. An anterior displacement of 4 mm of C5 occurs on C6. Spinous process at C5-C6 is wider apart than at other levels. These findings were not recognized at initial visit to hospital. (From Paley D, Gillespie R: *Am J Sports Med* 14[2]:92, 1986.)

Scoliosis

Scoliosis is fairly common in youth, yet it is rarely symptomatic. If pain is evident, it is usually related to some other cause. Scoliosis itself may have only been noted because of back pain or some other cause. When symptomatic, scoliosis rarely causes more than mild fatigue pain, usually localized to the convex side of the apex of the upper curve or a vague pain in the lumbosacral area (Fig. 58-15).

> Idiopathic adolescent scoliosis is usually *not* a source of back pain!

Progression of adolescent idiopathic scoliosis is related to curve size, area of the spine involved, and physiologic age of the child. There are no specific contraindications for participation in sports in children with scoliosis.

Curvature of the spine may be (1) related to Scheuermann's disease, (2) a temporary phenomenon related to strain or sprain, (3) related to a pathologic process such as tumor or neurofibromatosis, or (4) related to an underlying painful process. If significant back pain is found in the presence of scoliosis, the workup should include more than the standard scoliosis radiographic series of long and bending films. It may include blood studies, radionuclide studies, CT, CT myelography, or EMG, if warranted.

Degenerative Processes

There have been a number of reports of degenerative changes in the spine of the immature athlete. Sward, Hellstrom, and Jacobsson[63] investigated 142 wrestlers, gymnasts, and soccer and tennis players (ages 14 to 25 years). Radiologic abnormalities representing chronic changes (reduced disk height, Schmorl's nodules, and vertebral body changes) were noted in 36% to 55% of the athletes and correlated with back pain found in 50% to 85% of the athletes. Paley and Gillespie[48] found that chronic repetitive, unrecognized flexion injuries may occur in high jumpers (high jumper's neck) (Figs. 58-16 and 58-17). Tertti et al[68] found MRI evidence of disk degeneration associated with Scheuermann's manifestations and spondylolysis in 3 of 35 young competitive gymnasts. Goldstein et al[23] found that 9% of preelite, 43% of elite, and 63% of Olympic level gymnasts and 15.8% of all swimmers had spinal abnormalities as seen on MRI. They found length and intensity of training and age to be associated with these abnormalities in gymnasts (Fig. 58-18).

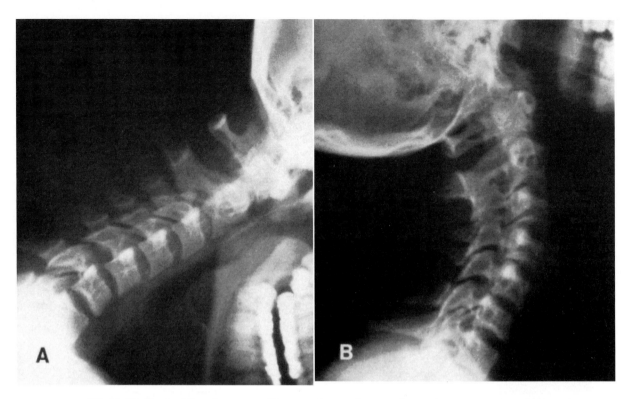

FIG. 58-17. Flexion (**A**) and extension (**B**) views of cervical spine. Abnormalities are accentuated by flexion. There is subluxation of both facets on C5 on C6 such that facets are almost perched in full flexion. With extension, C5 completely reduces on C6, reestablishing normal cervical alignment. (From Paley D, Gillespie R: *Am J Sports Med* 14[1]:92, 1986.)

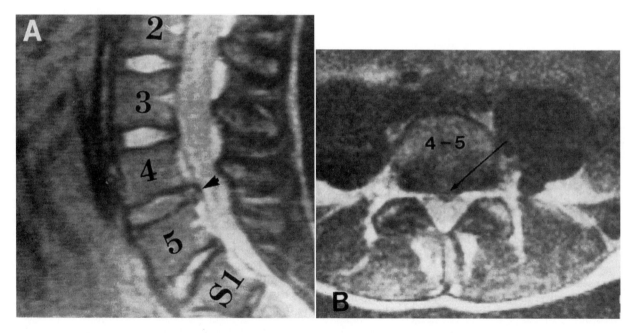

FIG. 58-18. A 19-year-old elite gymnast with symptomatic degenerative L4-L5 disk with central herniation. **A,** Sagittal lumbar magnetic resonance imaging (MRI) scan showing L4-L5 disk degeneration. **B,** Transverse MRI of L4-L5 disk showing central herniation. (From Goldstein JD et al: *Am J Sports Med* 19[5]:464, 1991.)

Collegiate women athletes with irregular menses during adolescence have been shown to have decreased bone density.[36] Whether this has any association with pathologic changes in the spine or development of spinal pain has not been shown.

Posterior Column Dysfunction
Pathologic Conditions of the Pars Interarticularis

A comprehensive classification of spondylolysis and spondylolisthesis was proposed by Wiltse, Newman, and MacNab.[72] The dysplastic (Type I) and isthmic (Type II) spondylolysis and spondylolisthesis are the most common in children and adolescents.

A stress fracture developing in the pars interarticularis may be the source of persistent, unexplained lumbar pain in the young athlete. These complaints should raise the possibility of an acute stress fracture developing in the pars interarticularis. We believe that this stress fracture can initiate the developmental sequence of spondylolysis.[32] Certain sports require repetitive jarring forces combined with hyperextension and rotation to cause an acute stress fracture to the lumbar spine. Pole vaulting, gymnastics, blocking and hitting in football, hurdling, pitching, diving, and even serving in tennis are particularly stressful to the lower back. Jackson et al[33] demonstrated an 11% incidence of pars defects in young female gymnasts, and similar high incidences were found in young male football players, wrestlers, and those involved in weight training.

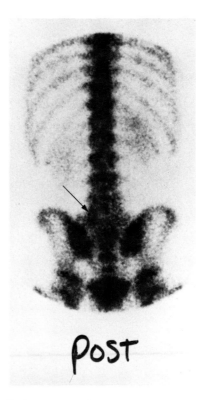

FIG. 58-19. Early pars stress fracture not seen on radiographs but demonstrated by bone scan.

Sports associated with pathologic conditions of the pars interarticularis
■ Pole vaulting
■ Gymnastics
■ Football (blocking and hitting)
■ Hurdling
■ Pitching
■ Diving
■ Tennis (serving)
■ Wrestling
■ Weight training

In the early onset of this entity the aching low back pain is usually unilateral and is aggravated by twisting and hyperextension motion. Neurologic deficit and nerve root tension signs are usually absent. In hyperextension, particularly on one leg, the young athlete can usually localize a 2- to 3-cm area of pain posteriorly and unilaterally at the belt line.

Standard radiography of the lumbar spine often yields negative results, but with persistent symptoms early confirmation can be demonstrated by technetium pyrophosphate bone scans (Fig. 58-19). A bone scan is unnecessary to make the diagnosis of stress fracture but is often helpful in delineating the problem, particularly if the patient and parents seem worried that an underlying tumor may be involved. A scan can be helpful in ruling out other bony lesions of the lumbar spine. Bellah et al[3] rec-

ommended SPECT to localize stress injuries to the pars interarticularis when planar bone imaging or radiography is negative.

In our experience, pain from the lesion of the pars interarticularis that is often demonstrated by scan lasts for about 3 to 8 months. Disability has been noted to last longer than this in some patients and even to recur at the same or another location. A stress reaction may progress to involve the pars interarticularis on the other side or even evolve into a radiographically demonstrable defect in young patients who elect to continue to perform in this sport despite the pain.

Spondylolysis. With the presence of pars interarticularis defects on initial radiographs and a negative bone scan, we think that the radiographic changes are probably old. These x-ray changes are of an established fibrous union. Fatigue fractures of the pars interarticularis differ from most stress fractures seen elsewhere in the athlete's body in that they generally do not show periosteal new bone formation and that there is a high incidence of fibrous union. This is probably related to the stability afforded by the opposite facet joint and anterior intervertebral joint (Fig. 58-20).

Flexion and extension views on radiography or cineradiography can often demonstrate abnormal segmental motion in evaluation of bilateral pars defects. Pars interarticularis defects are rare before a patient is age 5 or 6; however, they have been reported. The physician should look closely at the radiographic defect for signs of rounding or reabsorption to evaluate chronicity and to see if

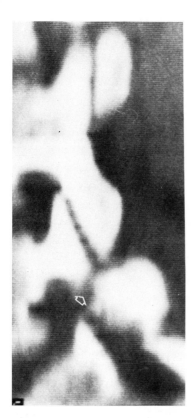

FIG. 58-20. Spondylolysis found on computed tomography scan. (Courtesy William Glenn, Jr, MD. Multi-Planar Diagnostic Imaging and Co, Torrance, Calif.)

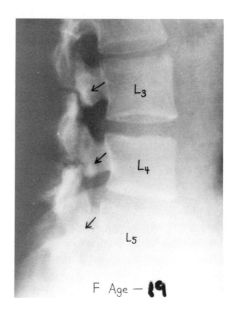

FIG. 58-21. Multiple level spondylolysis in young equestrian.

one side is more prominent than the other in bilateral defects. Defects can occur at more than one level and are best seen on oblique radiographic views (Fig. 58-21). Pars defects do not preclude a patient's participation in sports; however, flexibility and back and abdominal strengthening exercises should be encouraged to decrease the incidence of back pain. The average time for return to pain-free competition after developing an acute pars interarticularis stress fracture is approximately 7 months.[31]

Spondylolisthesis. Although the incidence of pars defects is higher in boys, the incidence of vertebral slippage appears to be higher in girls.[32] The role of decreased back and abdominal muscular strength may be implicated. A typical youngster with a high degree of slippage shows the spondylolisthesis build of a shortened torso, heart-shaped buttocks, and a rib cage that appears low; the iliac crests are high, buttocks flat, and sacrum vertical. Stance is altered by tight hamstrings, and with the vertical sacrum, the hips do not fully extend (Fig. 58-22). Sciatic scoliosis may be present. The patient may have tenderness to palpation in the low back. Adolescents with thoracolumbar Scheuermann's disease have a 32% to 50% incidence of spondylolysis.[73]

If pain is associated with athletic activity, normal activities of daily living on a baseline fitness level can be maintained until pain subsides. Short periods of bed rest may be necessary at the onset to relieve pain. Activity

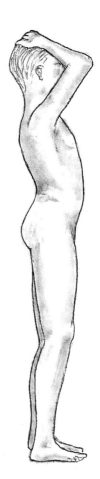

FIG. 58-22. Spondylolisthesis build.

should be determined and regulated by pain. Micheli, Hall, and Miller[41] advocated antilordotic bracing to relieve pain and restrict activity. Bell, Ehrlich, and Zaleske[2] treated 28 pediatric patients with Grades I and II spondylolisthesis with antilordotic braces for an average of 25 months. All of the patients were pain free at the end of treatment, and none demonstrated significant progression. We use measurement of anterior displacement as described by Wiltse and Winter[74] to assess the young athlete's ability to return to sports.

If the young athlete is initially seen with low back pain and spondylolisthesis of less than 30% forward slippage, he or she is restricted from further vigorous activity until both pain and muscle spasm have subsided completely. When the patient is symptom free, we allow him or her to return to all sports. If pain returns on return to sports then we suggest that the athlete stop that activity. If he or she is just an average player or interested in other sports, activity that carries less probability of back injury is suggested. We are not certain that boys with minor slips are any more susceptible to back injury than those without spondylolisthesis. Most athletes with spondylolysis or pars elongation with low-grade spondylolisthesis perform their sport without knowledge of the underlying structural abnormalities.

It has been our experience that severe progressive slippage is not the usual pattern in young athletes. As the number of young women participating in competitive athletics continues to increase, this observation may change to some degree. It is not well understood why this severe slippage occurs more often in girls or why a vertebral slippage progresses between the ages of 9 to 13. Once vertebral growth is complete, further slippage occurs, although minimally. However, we are familiar with a few patients who had slippage in their teens, then stabilized radiographically, and are now documented to have progressed during their late twenties. Low back symptoms, which continue in adult life, and disk degeneration are most likely to occur when spondylolisthesis is 25% or more.[31]

If the young athlete has back pain and spondylolisthesis of 50% or greater, we encourage a period of rest and avoidance of painful activity. We strongly suggest that the athlete choose sports that are less aggravating. It is noted, however, that successful participation in vigorous activities of patients having greater than 50% vertebral slippage is difficult because of the apparent loss of hip extension and sacral tilt associated with such slippage (Fig. 58-23). In young patients who have not completed growth, it is imperative that serial radiographs be taken to document progression of slip. A CT myelogram or MRI

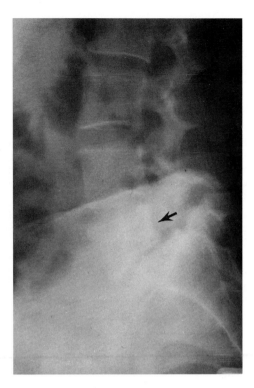

FIG. 58-23. Progressing spondylolisthesis in young gymnast before reduction and fusion.

should be considered in spondylolisthesis when patients have symptoms of nerve compression. If such documentation is obtained, or if there is persistence of pain in spite of adequate rest and conservative measures, a fusion with an attempt at reduction of the high-grade slippage is recommended. Although reduction is controversial in Grades IV and V spondylolisthesis, some authors have recommended in situ anterior interbody arthrodesis followed by posterior arthrodesis.[34] On occasion, following fusion some patients have been able to return to rigorous athletic competition successfully. The decision to allow full sports participation depends on the type and level of fusion or decompression and levels of potential segmental instability.[40]

Facet Syndrome

Although the facet joint had been considered as a source of pain in the early 1900s, it was not as well accepted until Pedersen, Blauck, and Gardner[50] demonstrated the pattern of nerve supply to these joints. Facet

Facet syndrome

- Low back pain
- Sclerodermal distribution (may radiate to knee)
- Intact neurologic examination
- Negative straight leg raising
- Pain with hyperextension
- Positive one-legged hyperextension test
- Morning stiffness
- Pain with pressure over the facets
- Pain relief with ambulation
- Positive injection test

joints are of the synovial type, and a pathologic facet condition may be a cause of atypical back and leg pain in the athlete.

In the facet syndrome the young athlete complains of low back pain, which may radiate distally as far as the knee without a classic radicular pattern. Straight leg raising yields negative results as does a neurologic examination, but there is pain with hyperextension so that the one-legged hyperextension test is usually positive. The patient may indicate that there is morning stiffness, pain with pressure over the facets, and relief of pain with ambulation.

Radiographs may show facet joint narrowing, irregularity, sclerosis, or cystic changes (Fig. 58-24). Although such findings are rare in youth, they are quite common in athletes in their early twenties. Computed axial tomography (CAT) scans may demonstrate cartilaginous changes and early arthritis before obvious change by standard radiographs.

Injection of the implicated facet joint can reproduce pain in the back and upper thigh. At the time of such a provocative test, if the facet above and below the affected level is also injected with lidocaine (as a result of cross innervation) symptoms may be relieved. We use 2 to 5 ml of lidocaine and 1 ml of methylprednisolone (DepoMedrol). This may yield relief for several reasons. Pinched synovial folds within the facet joints can be the cause of pain; injection pressure may push out such pinched tissue. Manipulation may have a similar effect. If instability is the cause of pain, the patient often complains of discomfort in various sitting positions. Morning stiffness, implicating arthritis, may develop over time. If there is no relief with facet injection or manipulation, facet rhizotomy as described by Mooney and Robeiton[42] can be considered.

Spinal Stenosis

The young athlete may suffer from congenital, developmental, or spondylolisthetic decrease in the size of the spinal canal. He or she complains of claudicatory or sciatic pain in the legs with hyperextension of the back. The athlete also has pain on standing, but sitting or lying supine relieves the pain. There may be cramping in the calves, paresthesia, or numbness related to walking. Walking uphill is easier than walking downhill; nevertheless, as symptoms worsen, gait may become unsteady. In contrast, there seems to be no difficulty in riding a bicycle. Hyperextension-type movements that are common in sports may become impossible because of the pain.

Young athletes with cervical stenosis may remain asymptomatic until a hyperextension injury, spondylolysis, or vertebral subluxation calls attention to the underlying abnormality. Pavlov et al[49] found that a spinal canal/vertebral body ratio of less than 0.82 indicates significant spinal stenosis. Any sport or activity that subjects the cervical spine to trauma is potentially dangerous to patients with spinal stenosis. Cheng et al[8] identified

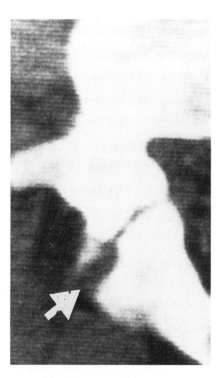

FIG. 58-24. Arthritic change associated with facet syndrome. (Courtesy William Glenn, Jr, MD, Multi-Planar Diagnostic Imaging and Co, Torrance, Calif.)

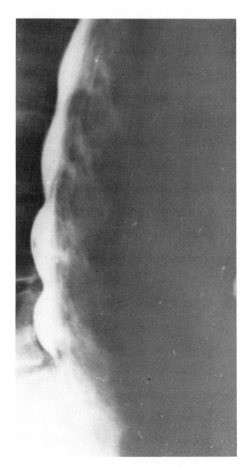

FIG. 58-25. Myelogram demonstrating spinal stenosis.

14 patients who suffered neurologic injury from body surfing. All had evidence of preexisting spinal stenosis. Grant and Puffer[24] described an 18-year-old linebacker with recurrent weakness and numbness in the C5-C6 distribution related to a hyperextension injury of the cervical spine. This progressed to temporary quadriparesis. Radiographs were interpreted as normal, but air myelogram disclosed no air passage from C4 to C6. Sagittal diameter at C5-C6 was 13 mm with greater than 14.5 mm being assumed normal. Under such circumstances the athlete should completely refrain from participating in the inciting activity.

Spondylolisthetic or congenital lumbar spinal stenoses are more commonly identified clinically. CT myelograms, CT, and MRI are the most valid testing procedures (Fig. 58-25). The CT myelogram can show central canal stenosis, whereas the CT scan may help define foraminal stenosis along nerve canals. Spinal fluid protein levels are often elevated.

It is assumed that pain develops when nerves are denied adequate nourishment as a result of pressure on the blood vessels that supply them. In standing with increased lumbar lordosis or in hyperextension, such vascular encroachment is worsened. Sitting and squatting increase the space within the lumbar canal, which explains why symptoms can be relieved by such maneuvers.

With developmental, spondylolisthetic, or congenital lumbar stenosis, symptoms may initially be handled conservatively. The patient is trained in proper methods of lifting and stooping and is given abdominal strengthening exercises in an attempt to limit abnormal stresses on the motion segment. An elastic back support may similarly decrease abnormal motion but should only be used for treatment of the acute injury in the young athlete. Manipulation of the spine after a cortisone injection or antiinflammatory medication may decrease inflammation of tissues irritated in this impingement process. Nevertheless, when symptoms become severe, we agree with Wiltse, Kirkaldy-Willis, and McIvor[72] that surgery should be considered.

Because congenital spinal stenosis tends to encompass several segments, surgical decompression must extend to all levels involved so that there is adequate space for the contents of the spinal canal. In the young child with a high-grade spondylolisthetic slip, fusion can be done without decompression because of adequate circulation and the potential of collateral circulation. In multilevel congenital stenosis, however, the canal may need to be decompressed before fusion. Decompression probably relieves leg pain and allows normal activities of daily living with some residual back pain, but athletic activity is permanently curtailed.

Fracture or Dislocation and Neurologic Sequelae

For children under the age of 16 years cervical injuries account for almost 70% of all serious injuries of the spine. Unsupervised diving and American football are the most common causes of injury in the pediatric spine.[11] Blitzer et al[4] reported that head and spine injuries composed 6.2% of the pediatric injuries in downhill skiing and were more prevalent in children than in adults. Thoracic and thoracolumbar injuries are rare before age 8 and usually result from hyperflexion with axial loading. Children younger than 8 years usually reconstitute their vertebral height after compression injuries.[11]

Seven major types of injury to the upper cervical spine have been described and include atlantooccipital dislocations, fractures of the lateral mass and occipital condyle, atlas (C1) ring fractures, atlantoaxial subluxation, atlantoaxial rotatory fixation, dens fractures, and traumatic spondylolisthesis of the axis, or C2 (Hangman's fractures). Traumatic injuries to the lower cervical spine are more commonly associated with some degree of neural compression because of the decreasing ratio of canal area to cervical cord. The major types of injury in the lower cervical spine include minor compression, avulsion, burst facet, and teardrop fractures.[46] A detailed discussion of each injury type listed above is presented in Chapter 50; however, the physician should understand that any of these injuries may occur in the young athlete's cervical spine.

Fractures and dislocation

Upper cervical spine
- Atlantooccipital dislocations
- Lateral mass and occipital condyle fractures
- C1 ring fractures
- Atlantoaxial subluxation
- Atlantoaxial rotatory fixation
- Dens fracture
- Traumatic spondylolisthesis of C2

Lower cervical spine
- Compression fractures
- Avulsion fractures
- Burst fractures
- Facet fractures
- Teardrop fractures

Holdsworth[27a] presented his classification scheme in which spinal injuries were categorized by four basic causative types of force: flexion, flexion and rotation, extension, or compression. These are the same forces that produce common athletic injuries. Spinal trauma may or may not be involved with neurologic compromise. Neurologic injury seems to be regulated by the associated stability of the spine. This stability most often is related to the integrity of the posterior elements. Nevertheless, it must be pointed out that the vertical arrangement of facet joints in the adult is developmental and, in fact, in the child may be found to be nearly horizontal. For this reason, dislocation can occur without fracture in a child with spontaneous reduction. All injuries resulting in severe neck or back pain must be treated for the potential of neurologic compromise when present.

Fracture or dislocation, common particularly in the cervical spine, can be found with associated head trauma. Therefore **in all head injuries with loss of consciousness the physician must suspect associ-**

Head injury with loss of consciousness
Treat for neck injury until proven otherwise

ated neurologic compromise. If neurologic compromise is suspected, the cervical spine should be protected against further injury by the use of sandbags, external splinting, and avoiding manipulation until radiography and definitive studies can be done.

Although the indications for surgery of the pediatric patient are not well established, they include nonreducible or grossly unstable injuries, significant subluxation without fracture, spinal cord compression with incomplete neurologic deficits, and unstable injuries after nonoperative management.[11]

Flexion Injury

The majority of spinal injuries, particularly of the cervical spine, occur in association with flexion movements. When the posterior articulations remain intact, the result may be a **vertebral body wedge compression fracture.** With significant trauma there may be an upward tilt of the spinous process, indicating bilateral laminar fracture as the posterior elements become involved. If both pedicles are fractured, the vertebral body may be pushed forward. When an unstable situation exists, a cervical fusion must be considered. Nuber and Schafer[44] reported on fractures of the spinous processes of the lower cervical area (**clay shovelers' injuries**) occurring in two high school football players. The mechanism is believed to be from an avulsion of the spinous process occurring from a hyperflexion injury. If cervical spine stability is present, treatment usually requires protection against forward flexion with a cervical orthosis for a period of 6 to 8 weeks. Following a flexion injury of the cervical spine, special attention should be directed to the facet fiber capsular mechanism, the posterior longitudinal ligament, and the posterior annulus fibrosus fibers. Without posterior element involvement, treatment is essentially conservative. Damage to the posterior elements may necessitate surgical decompression or fusion when there is evidence of instability. Instability may be on an acute or chronic basis and is demonstrated with hyperflexion and hyperextension radiographs in the lateral plane. Cineradiography is another technique that can help delineate associated instability. It is important to remember that the vertical facet arrangement in a child may allow dislocation and spontaneous reduction to occur; therefore neck and head injuries must be evaluated thoroughly.

Thoracic wedge fractures may remain untreated because of the strut support of the associated ribs; **lumbar compression fractures** may usually be treated in a lumbar corset (Fig. 58-26). If greater than 30% of the vertebral body is affected, posterior stability is reduced and stress occurs on the facet joints. In some of these cases there may be progressive neurologic injury. Surgical intervention may include a laminectomy, anterior interbody fusion, and decompression with a posterior fu-

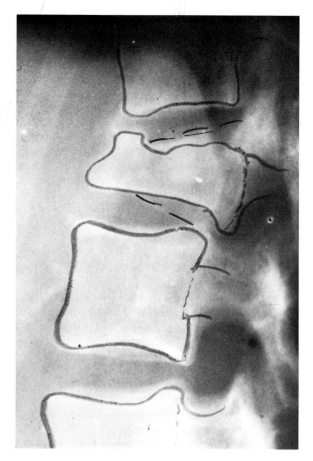

FIG. 58-26. Flexion injury: wedge fracture. Even with retropulsion here, myelogram was negative and posterior column intact.

sion if indicated. Osenbach and Menezes[47] found that most injuries to the spinal cord or vertebral column are successfully managed with nonoperative therapy. The prognosis is most closely correlated with the extent of the initial neurologic insult.

Flexion-Rotation Injury

Flexion and rotation injuries may result in **subluxation of the facet joints** or may cause the facet joints to slide, gap, or dislocate. Flexion-rotation injuries may lead to significant disruption of the posterior elements. Because the cervical spine is mobile, it is more common to find flexion-rotation injuries. The thoracic spine has the stabilization afforded by the ribs, which makes these injuries extremely rare. They do occur in the lumbar spine, but the amount of rotation necessary is great.

Unilateral pars or laminar fractures and **facet dislocations** require recognition and appropriate treatment. Unilateral facet dislocation in the young athlete in either the cervical or the lumbar spine can occur as described by Boger et al.[5] Significant trauma is necessary to develop such an injury with or without fracture. Reduction in traction or open reduction is followed by surgical fusion to afford stability (Fig. 58-27, B). Halovest immobilization is also commonly used for fractures with or without associated neurologic damage.

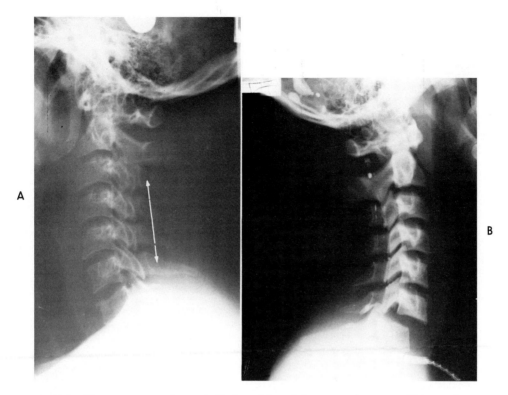

FIG. 58-27. Flexion-rotation injuries. **A,** Unilateral facet dislocation with associated laminar fracture suspected by malrotation of only a segment of posterior elements. **B,** Bilateral facet dislocation with neurologic (quadriplegic) compromise (spearing injury) in 16-year-old.

Rotatory dislocation of the atlantoaxial articulation is a common childhood injury. Because the syndesmosis of the dens to the C2 vertebra is visible radiographically, this is occasionally diagnosed as a fracture, but it must be recognized that odontoid fracture is more commonly an adult injury. The differential growth and ossification patterns that occur in the young athlete's cervical spine require special attention. Even with syndesmotic separation in children less than 7 years of age, there is decreased morbidity and decreased degenerative changes compared with the injury occurring in the older population.

Because of the amount of trauma associated with flexion-rotation injuries, particularly with spearing-type injury in football, diving, and trampoline injuries, quadriplegia does occur (Fig. 58-27, *A*). Early administration of high-dose corticosteroids is appropriate following spinal cord injury. The disabilities associated with tetraplegia are so devastating at the present time that prevention must be emphasized. The young athlete must be taught proper techniques to discourage such devastating injury. A football player should block with the shoulders and hands rather than block with the head or neck. The young diver must learn that locked hands should make contact with the water to dissipate the force transmitted along the spine.

Sprain injury of the facet capsular tissue or **strain injury** of the back may be associated with **transverse**

Transverse process fractures → Be alert to visceral trauma!

---

process fracture, spinous process fracture, or mere soft-tissue injury, which can be treated conservatively. A contiguous transverse process fracture must be watched for development of pseudarthrosis or myositis ossificans. If three or more transverse processes are fractured, significant underlying visceral trauma must be suspected.

Extension Injury

Distraction forces in the immature cervical spine usually involve the cartilaginous vertebral endplates because the intervertebral endplates and the intervertebral disks are stronger than the bone.

Generally, in an extension injury the posterior ligaments remain intact, but the bony elements (i.e., the laminae and pedicles) may fracture (Fig. 58-28). This is common in the cervical spine of young "midget" auto racers who sustain a whiplash-type injury. With hyperextension there may be decreased pain or temperature sensation by vascular compression or cord contusion. Schneider, Thompson, and Bebin[58] described the acute cord compression syndrome produced by hyperextension of the neck. There is a characteristic paralysis of the arms, more so than in the legs, and ascending improve-

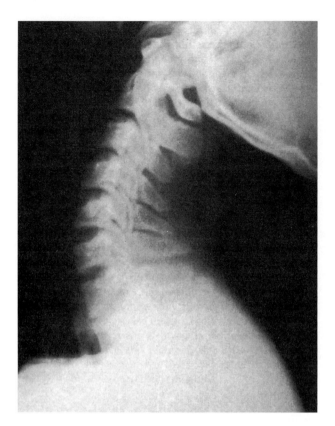

FIG. 58-28. Lateral radiograph displaying fracture of spinous process of C7. (From Nuber GW, Schafer MF: *Am J Sports Med* 15[2]:182, 1987.)

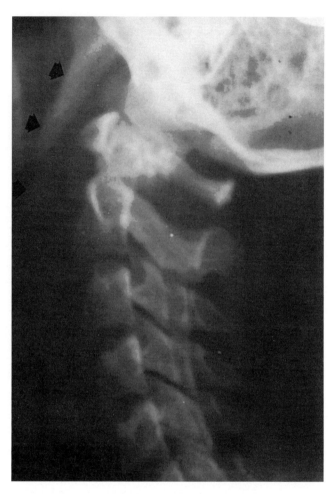

FIG. 58-29. Lateral radiograph demonstrates significant soft-tissue shadow resulting from fracture of anterior portion of ring of C1. Although there is little evidence on lateral radiograph of fractures, presence of this soft-tissue shadow (*arrows*) suggests that fracture of anterior portion of upper cervical spine is present. (From Levine AM, Lipson SJ: Cervical spine and cord trauma. In AAOS: *Orthopaedic knowledge update III*, Park Ridge, Ill, 1990, American Academy of Orthopaedic Surgeons.)

ment of bowel and bladder dysfunction followed by improvement of the lower extremities before improvement in the arms. It is important to recognize such injury because laminectomy may actually cause increased damage to the cord.

Compression Injury

Compression fractures are rare in the pediatric cervical spine. Before age 8 to 10 years the unossified vertebral bodies appear wedge shaped.

In longitudinal compression, such as in landing on the heels of a gymnastic dismount or a spearing injury in football, force may rupture the incompressible disk through a vertebral endplate. In such cases the ligaments generally remain intact so that the spine is stable. If a **vertebral body fractures in a bursting type pattern** in spite of stability, neurologic compromise may occur by posterior protrusion of vertebral fragment into the cord. C1 ring compression, or **Jefferson fracture,** can also occur, and if suspected because of the presence of spasm and high cervical pain, multiple radiographs are often necessary to disclose a fracture (Fig. 58-29).

Torg et al[69] analyzed 25 **axial loading injuries** to the middle cervical spine segment (C3-C4) and found that (1) the lesions do not usually involve the bony elements, (2) disk herniations are frequently associated with transient quadriplegia, (3) reduction at this level is difficult to maintain, and (4) unilateral facet dislocations are best

managed by closed reduction and bilateral by open reduction.

In addition to the chronic, repetitive, unrecognized flexion injuries of the cervical spine (high jumper's neck),[48] the "Fosbury flop" technique of landing on the back in high jumping has led to an increased incidence of wedge fractures and Schmorl's nodule formation (Fig. 58-30). In this group, as in all groups previously discussed, after osseous healing occurs, if there is no neurologic compromise and the posterior column remains stable, the young athlete should be able to return to sport activity. This is assuming that flexibility, strength, and agility have been regained before returning to sport. Attention should be directed to form because biomechanically unsound methods may result in repeat injury.

Growth Plate Fracture

Growth plate fractures involve the vertebral ring apophysis as seen most commonly in adolescents. The

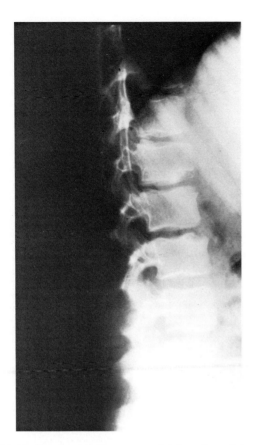

FIG. 58-30. Compression fractures and Schmorl's nodule formation in adolescent high jumper.

Growth plate injuries of the spine

- Simple separation (no bony fracture)
- Avulsion fracture
- Localized injury
- Fracture of entire vertebra

posterior-inferior aspect of the L4 vertebra is most commonly involved (Fig. 58-31).[11] Fujita et al[20] described a posterior dislocation of the sacral apophyseal ring in a 14-year-old soccer player. Takata et al[66] described four types of growth plate injuries to the spine. These include a simple separation with no evidence of associated large bony fracture, an avulsion fracture, a localized injury, and a fracture spanning the entire vertebra. These injuries have been seen in increasing frequency in young weight-lifters[7] and adolescent gymnasts (Fig. 58-32).[62]

Transient Neurapraxia

Contact sports such as American football are associated with injuries resulting in a neurapraxia of the cervical spinal cord. A neurapraxia of the cervical spine may vary from weakness to complete paralysis involving both upper and lower extremities. The episodes are usually transient and may be associated with spinal stenosis mentioned previously. Athletes with canal sagittal diameters of less than 14 mm at any level (C3 to C6) should be advised against participating in contact sports.[69] Surgery is not indicated. Such injuries occur with hyperex-

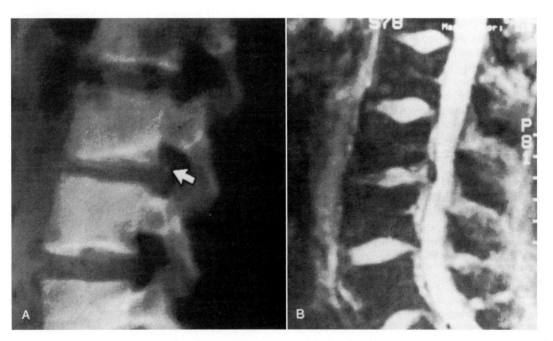

FIG. 58-31. A 13-year-old boy scaled a high fence and jumped down, sustaining pain to his back. He had radicular symptoms of L4-L5 distribution. Removal of large osteocartilaginous apophysis of inferior aspect of L3 gave immediate relief. **A,** True lateral radiograph of lumbar spine showing ossific density in spinal canal (*arrow*) posterior to inferior margin of L3. **B,** Magnetic resonance imaging scan illustrates rim fracture of posterior-inferior endplate of L3 vertebra with posterior displacement of fragment into spinal canal. Child underwent excision of vertebral endplate apophysis with complete relief. (From Crawford AH: *Orthop Clin North Am* 21[2]:325, 1990.)

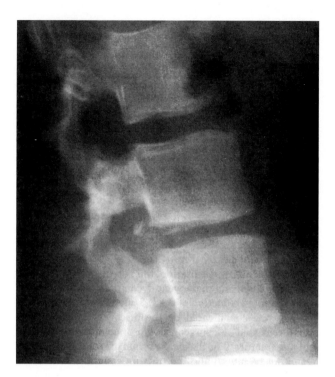

FIG. 58-32. Lateral radiograph of lumbosacral spine showing bony fragment at inferior border of L3. (From Browne TD, Yost RP, McCarron RF: *Am J Sports Med* 18[5]:533, 1990.)

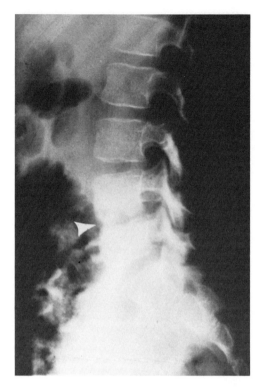

FIG. 58-33. Disk calcification 2 weeks after onset of back pain.

tension or neural foraminal encroachment and contusion of a nerve root by transient posterior overriding facets or transient posterior inward wrinkling of the ligamentum flavum. This is a common injury with head-butting or spearing types of tackling.

Transient neurapraxia can be differentiated from the flexion type of "pinched nerve syndrome" in which a traction or avulsion injury of the nerve root can occur or may be associated with cervical spondylosis with protruded disk fragment. When numbness and tingling down the upper extremity are associated with such an injury and are relieved spontaneously within a few minutes, the player can probably resume the sports activity. If this becomes a recurrent problem, the horseshoe-type collar or restricted motion equipment can be used with strengthening exercises if symptoms are infrequent. With frequent recurrence, however, the sports activity should be halted because fibrosis, nerve root avulsion, or nerve root injury can lead to permanent paralysis or weakness.

Inflammatory and Infectious Processes
Disk Calcification

The young athlete with midline tenderness, decreased vertebral column flexion, and corresponding muscle spasm may initially have no abnormal radiographic findings. Within 2 weeks, however, calcification of a disk in the area of tenderness may develop because of vascular or degenerative etiologic factors (Fig. 58-33). This is different from the generalized disk calcification seen in ochronosis, hyperparathyroidism, fluorosis, chondrocalcinosis, and hemochromatosis. Walker[71] found an in-

---

Differential diagnosis of disk calcification

- Idiopathic disk calcification
- Ochronosis
- Hyperparathyroidism
- Fluorosis
- Chondrocalcinosis
- Hemochromatosis

---

creased incidence in young males with an average age of 7 years and no evidence of an infectious cause. Findings included elevated temperature and increased sedimentation rate and white blood cell count. No specific therapy other than rest is required. Patients may return to sports after pain of the acute episode subsides.

Diskitis

Diskitis is an inflammatory or infectious lesion affecting the intervertebral disk. The infection is assumed to stem from the adjacent vertebral body, the source of the intervertebral disk's blood supply. Children affected are usually between the ages of 2 and 7 years. In a large series presented by Menelaus,[38] 14 patients were found to have their lumbar spine affected 74% of the time, the thoracic spine 24% of the time, and the cervical spine 2% of the time. The L4-L5 disk space was most commonly involved.

Symptoms of diskitis include back, abdominal, or gluteal pain. Parents may relate that the child has been irritable and restless or may have demonstrated a limp or

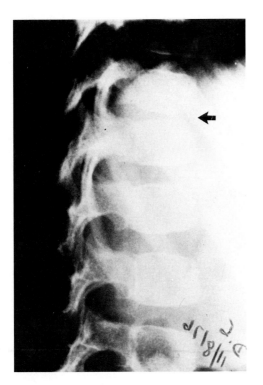

FIG. 58-34. Diskitis. (Courtesy Richard L LaMont, MD, Chairman, Department of Orthopaedic Surgery, Wayne State University, Detroit, Mich.)

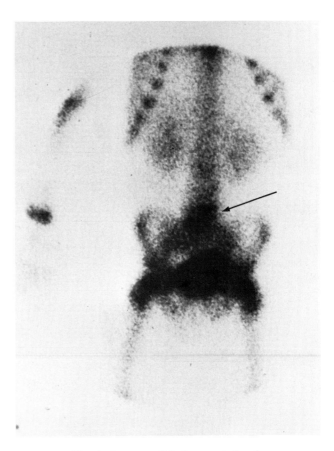

FIG. 58-35. Vertebral osteomyelitis documented on bone scan.

refusal to walk. A history of fever, malaise, or antecedent upper respiratory infection may be elicited. At times, systemic signs may not be pronounced.

On physical examination paravertebral muscle spasm is the principal finding. The patient may refuse to walk and may demonstrate decreased range of motion of the back with either increased or decreased lumbar lordosis and a diminished range of straight leg raising. Examination with the child in the prone position with the knees flexed 90 degrees may elicit pain and spasm with alternating hyperextension of the hips. No neurologic deficit is evident. With minor systemic complaints, laboratory and radiographic findings may aid in the diagnosis.

The erythrocyte sedimentation rate is elevated initially, but the white blood cell count is often normal. Blood cultures and a tuberculin test should be done, but they most likely prove negative. If cultures are positive the most common pathogen is staphylococcus. In the first 3 weeks of illness, radiographs are negative. At this point, according to Matthews, Wiltse, and Karbelnig,[37] disk space narrowing with mild irregularity and sclerosis of the vertebral endplates become evident (Fig. 58-34). Bone scans are positive, demonstrating increased uptake in the involved level. MRI may be helpful in differentiating between diskitis and vertebral osteomyelitis. More than one level is occasionally involved, and the differential diagnosis should include tuberculosis spondylitis, disk calcification, appendicitis, urinary tract infection, Scheuermann's kyphosis, spinal trauma, and pyogenic vertebral osteomyelitis.

The principal treatment is rest for 6 to 12 weeks. If symptoms persist past this time or if the patient does not respond to rest, antibiotics or needle biopsy should be considered.

Vertebral Osteomyelitis

Vertebral osteomyelitis is rarely a cause of back pain and is even less common in children than in adults. The clinical findings are similar to those described for diskitis. The source of infection is hematogenous, and a history of infection of another source is common. Symptoms may include a low-grade fever, malaise, vague abdominal complaints, and a gradual onset of back pain.

On clinical examination point tenderness is demonstrated at the level of the infected vertebrae and made worse with percussion. Associated muscle spasm is noted. Characteristically, back pain is nonmechanical and continuous. It is present with the patient at rest and accentuated by movement. Bed rest, antiinflammatory medication, and heat application do little to alleviate pain.

There may be an increased white blood cell count, sedimentation rate, or high serum globulin level. Blood culture results are generally positive during the acute phase and generally negative when back pain becomes subacute or chronic. If the blood culture yields negative results, a vertebral biopsy should be contemplated.

Radiographs are negative for the first 3 weeks at which time progressive collapse of the vertebral body may be

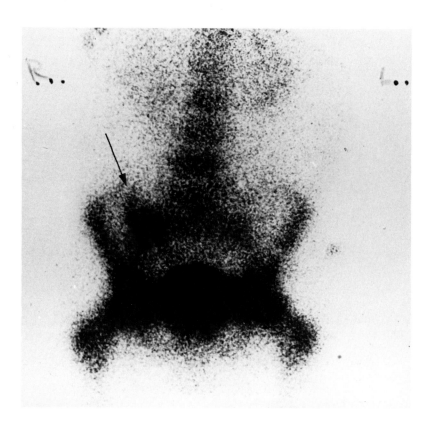

FIG. 58-36. Pyogenic sacroiliitis on bone scan; radiographic findings were negative. (Courtesy Richard L LaMont, MD, Chairman, Department of Orthopaedic Surgery, Wayne State University, Detroit, Mich.)

seen. Kyphosis may be a subsequent sequela. Laminograms show early bony destruction and the presence of soft-tissue abscesses. Radioisotope scanning shows increased uptake and helps identify septic processes during the acute and chronic phases (Fig. 58-35). MRI may be helpful by showing an abnormally high-signal intensity on T2-weighted images.

Treatment consists of antibiotic therapy, rest, and immobilization. The appropriate antibiotics depend on sensitivities of blood cultures or results of needle biopsy. The prognosis for patients with pyogenic vertebral osteomyelitis is good. Stauffer[61] stated that the disease process is followed by intense bony regeneration; in fact, new bone may be formed during the acute phase while concurrent destruction is occurring. Bone bridging and spontaneous fusion of adjacent vertebral bodies occur in about 80% of the cases. Some patients are identified in retrospect because they recover without treatment; other patients have been noted to have the infection recur after an interval of several years.

Sacroiliac Joint Infection

Pyogenic arthritis of the sacroiliac (SI) joint is uncommon, yet it must not be overlooked in the young athlete. The pain associated with acute infection may be localized in the lumbar, gluteal, or adductor areas. Pain demonstrates an inflammatory pattern, being relieved with exercise and worsened with rest. Perhaps the most de-

finitive clinical sign is unilateral pain in the affected sacroiliac joint. The pain can be reproduced, demonstrated by raising the ipsilateral leg and flexing the hip with adduction across the opposite leg. Infection or arthritis is also suggested as the basis of SI joint pain when it is reproduced by simultaneous forced abduction of the hips. Examination reveals tenderness specifically over the affected joint. Bone scans and coaxial tomography are extremely helpful in confirming the diagnosis (Fig. 58-36). Aspiration should be attempted if infection is thought to be a possibility, both for diagnosis and to decompress the joint. Other than drainage of a potential abscess, treatment includes recumbency and immobilization.

Rheumatoid Disease

Juvenile rheumatoid arthritis is uncommon, yet may be found as a cause of back pain in the young athlete.

A physical examination, radiography, bone scan, and nerve root tension signs may all be interpreted as normal in the young athlete with back pain. The possibility of seronegative spondyloarthropathy should not be overlooked in these individuals.

Arthritis resulting from seronegative spondyloarthropathy characteristically occurs in the axial skeleton. Occasionally, the large synovial joints of the hip and shoulder may also be involved. Compression over the sacroiliac joint may confirm on active sacroiliitis. Thoracolum-

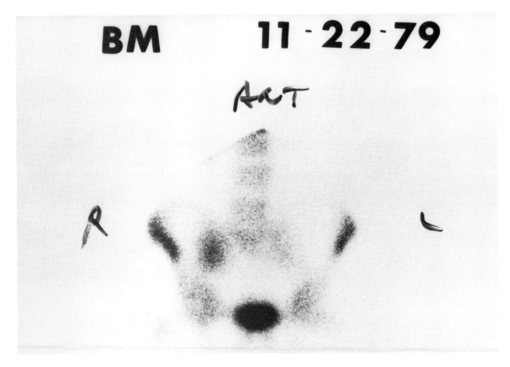

FIG. 58-37. Sacroiliitis on right, as seen on bone scan.

bar motion and chest expansion measured at maximal inspiration may be limited.

The generalized inflammatory process associated with seronegative spondyloarthropathy has a propensity for early fibrosis, calcification, and even ossification. Radiographic findings of periosteal new bone formation or erosion with reactive sclerosis at areas of tendon insertion can be found. The annulus fibrosus surrounding the intervertebral disk is commonly inflamed, leading to calcification, ossification, and even syndesmophyte formation.

Sacroiliitis is the most common clinical finding (Fig. 58-37). If this is radiographically documented bilaterally, this indicates ankylosing spondylitis. Only 30% of patients with Reiter's syndrome of even 5 years' duration demonstrate radiographic changes. The physician must closely scrutinize the lower two thirds of the SI joint for sclerosis, erosions, or bony fusion. Positive bone scan results indicating inflammation of the sacroiliac region may give evidence before radiographic findings are clear. If the ligamentous upper third of the joint is fused, diagnosis is certain. Radiographic changes in the peripheral joints differ from those changes of rheumatoid arthritis by their lack of symmetry and the presence of reactive sclerosis, periostitis, and small fluffy erosions.

Laboratory investigation to evaluate chronic inflammatory process and mild anemia should include tests for the following: complete blood count, white blood cell count, sedimentation rate, uric acid, serum proteins, rheumatoid factor, LE preparation, C-reactive protein, and HLA B-27 antigens. Nearly all white patients with ankylosing spondylitis or Reiter's syndrome have a positive HLA B-27 antigen; in colitic spondylitis or psoriatic arthritis

the incidence is lower but higher than the 6% to 8% incidence found in the general population. Macrophages found within the aspirate of swollen peripheral joints confirm the diagnosis of Reiter's syndrome.

Treatment of rheumatoid disease consists of antiinflammatory medication and appropriate activity selection. Patients with Reiter's syndrome, ankylosing spondylitis, psoriatic arthritis, and colitic sacroiliitis can participate in competitive sports when their pain and symptoms are medically controlled.

Spinal Neoplasm
Vertebral Tumor

Bone tumors of the spine in children are extremely rare. Nevertheless, the possibility of a tumor in a young athlete with back pain must not be overlooked. Clark and Stanish[10] presented a case of a 17-year-old sprinter who had acute onset of upper back pain. After exploring all diagnostic possibilities, a diagnosis of a highly malignant Hodgkin's lymphoma was made. As Tachdjian and Matson[65] stated, many of these lesions are benign or grow slowly; with early diagnosis, irreversible damage to the spinal cord may be prevented. In their large series of intraspinal tumors in children, surgical management frequently led to reversal of neurologic deficits. Long-term survival rates were encouraging.

The pain is usually well localized and frequently worsens at night. It is unlike mechanical back pain in that it is neither associated with activity nor relieved by rest.

On physical examination there may be tenderness with local palpation or percussion. Other neurologic signs, such as the straight leg raising, may be negative. Reactive scoliosis is a frequent radiographic finding. Lat-

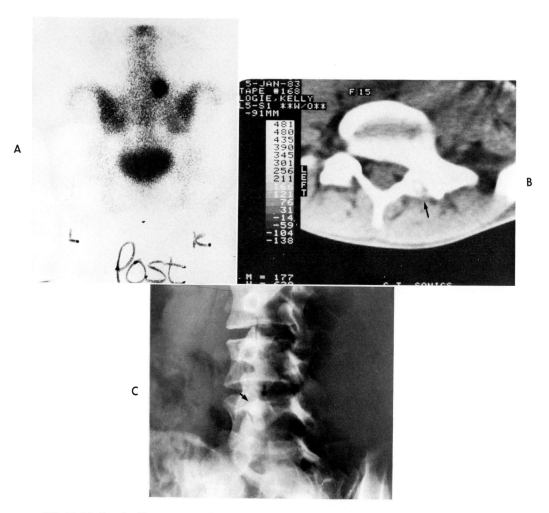

FIG. 58-38. Vertebral laminar osteoid osteoma. Documented on bone scan, **A,** substantiated on computed tomography scan, **B,** and seen in retrospect on plain radiograph, **C.** (Courtesy of Richard L LaMont, MD, Chairman, Department of Orthopaedic Surgery, Wayne State University, Detroit, Mich.)

eral deviation with forward flexion should raise the physician's suspicion.

The most common benign neoplasms in the spine include osteoid osteomas, osteochondromas, hemangiomas, eosinophilic granulomas, and giant cell tumors.

Osteoid osteoma and osteoblastoma most frequently occur in individuals in the second and third decades of life, but they have been found in young athletes. These tumors are common in the spinal elements. (Fig. 58-38). Complaints of back pain or painful scoliosis in the adolescent patient may be caused by tumors of the bony elements: aneurysmal bone cyst, osteoblastoma, or osteoid osteoma. Dramatic relief with aspirin may implicate an osteoid osteoma. When the lesion is not found or is found to be subtle on plain radiographs, tomography and bone scan are extremely useful.

Aneurysmal bone cyst may be found in the young athlete's spine with a characteristic "soap bubble" radiographic appearance. Treatment is resection or curettage.

Although uncommon, giant cell tumors have been re-ported, especially in the sacrum. Curettage and bone grafting are the treatment of choice.[56]

Vertebral hemangioma can be found in the vertebral body; trabeculae appear characteristically longitudinally on radiographs. Although surgery is rarely needed, the physician should consider preoperative embolization before surgical excision.

Osteosarcoma, non-Hodgkin's lymphomas and leukemia, and Ewing's sarcoma are the most common malignant lesions in the pediatric spine and may present with pain, neurologic deficit, and pathologic fractures.

Intramedullary Tumor

In children with persistent back pain the physician should also be suspicious of spinal cord tumors such as chordomas and solitary plasmacytomas. CT, CT myelography, bone scans, MRI, and arteriography may be helpful in better defining these lesions. After definitive diagnosis the management goals are maintenance of neural function and spinal stability. Tumors within the spinal

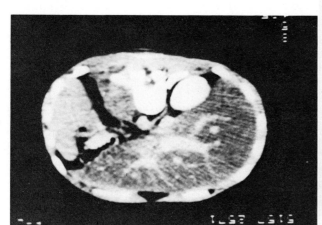
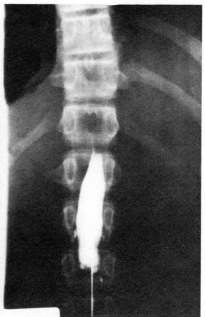

FIG. 58-39. A 14-year-old swimmer initially seen with atypical hip pain and antalgic gait. Back pain slowly developed and was found clinically to worsen with straight leg raising. Paravertebral round cell tumor (formerly called Ewing's extraskeletal tumor) was found within canal with computed tomography scan, **A,** and on myelogram, **B.**

canal frequently do not have as specific localizing signs. Persistent or intermittent pain in the back, trunk, neck, or extremities that is not readily explained by local trauma or other disease processes should lead the physician to rule out the rare intraspinal tumor. Pain is often poorly described and may be accentuated by physical activity, sneezing, coughing, straining, hyperflexion, hyperextension, or straight leg raising, thus mimicking a herniated disk. Motor weakness is a frequent clinical finding.

In their large series of intraspinal tumors, Tachdjian and Matson[65] found torticollis in 18%, scoliosis in 27%, and kyphosis in 15%. Incontinence, limp, or foot deformity such as claw toes, cavovarus, or cavus may indicate an intraspinal tumor. The straight leg raising sign is usually positive. Pathologic reflexes and sensory deficits may be present. Dermoid and epidermoid cysts may occur anywhere in the spinal canal and may actually connect to an external tract appearing as cysts on the back. Intraspinal neurofibromas may occur at multiple levels and may be the underlying cause of scoliosis. Astrocytoma of the cord is the most common tumor in childhood and usually occurs with pain and other neurologic findings.[18] MRI has revealed it to be cystic in nature. Paraspinal masses are more likely ganglioneuromas or neuroblastomas.

The physician must view radiographs for spinal deformity, reactive scoliosis, widening of the spinal canal, and thinning or erosion of pedicles with or without erosion of vertebral bodies, laminae, or ribs. A paravertebral mass with or without calcification may be demonstrated; if

suspected, CT scan or bone scan may aid in definition (Fig. 58-39). A CT myelogram is essential with concurrent examination of the cerebrospinal fluid. Lumbar puncture is contraindicated until a plain radiographic study of the entire spine has been done.

Analysis of cerebrospinal fluid almost always demonstrates increased protein and may even reveal tumor cells with cytologic examination. We must emphasize that history of repetitive trauma may sidetrack early diagnosis of spinal tumor; in such cases the physician must hold a high index of suspicion for tumor. Early recognition and treatment of tumor may decrease irreversible damage and increase life expectancy.

Somatoform Pain Disorder

Somatoform pain disorder (previously called psychogenic pain disorder) is characterized by pain in the absence of physical findings to account for the pain or its intensity. There is little to differentiate this disorder from other conversion symptoms in children. The pain usually appears suddenly and in about half of the cases is associated with physical trauma. It may occur at any age and is almost twice as frequent in females. There are no good studies documenting the prevalence of somatoform pain disorder. Biologic factors, psychodynamics, learning theory, emotions and communications, and family systems model are all theories describing its cause. This is primarily a diagnosis of exclusion, and if physical causes have been eliminated, a psychiatric referral may be appropriate.

PREVENTIVE MEDICINE

Prevention is an important aspect in the management of spinal injuries in the pediatric and adolescent athlete. Proper coaching techniques and form protect the spine. There is no protective equipment to protect the spine. Paying attention to the surrounding environment and avoiding dangerous techniques are important in any athletic program. Training of responsible personnel in the initial management of spinal injuries should be included in all athletic programs. Spine boards should be available at all activities that have the potential for spinal injury.

SUMMARY

Any young athlete who complains of acute or chronic back or neck pain with athletic activity should be listened to and be given a detailed examination. Pain in the spine in a child, especially a competitive individual involved in athletic endeavors, should be considered highly significant. A careful attempt to establish the correct diagnosis must be made. Many of the self-limited complaints may resolve without an exact diagnosis. Time and conservatism are on the side of the physician in coming to an accurate diagnosis. Relative or absolute rest usually provides a solution or diagnosis. Diagnostic testing should be individualized. In the young athlete after a few weeks the physician should avoid a "wait-and-see" attitude. On the athlete's return to activity the coach and trainer must be involved in analyzing form to help the athlete prevent reinjury by proper technique. It is technique and form that protect the spine the most. Return to competition must be gradual and steady so that the young athlete may be able to obtain and exceed previous performance levels without reinjury of the back. Serious spinal injuries are infrequent, but they do occur. Those responsible for the athlete should know basic transportation technique.

REFERENCES

1. Atwell EA, Jackson DW: Stress fractures of the sacrum in runners, *Am J Sports Med* 19(5):531, 1991.
2. Bell DF, Ehrlich MG, Zaleske DJ: Brace treatment for symptomatic spondylolisthesis, *Clin Orthop* 236:192, 1988.
3. Bellah R et al: Low back pain in adolescent athletes: detection of stress injury to the pars interarticularis with SPECT, *Radiology* 180:509, 1991.
4. Blitzer CM et al: Downhill skiing injuries in children, *Am J Sport Med* 12(2):142, 1984.
5. Boger D et al: Unilateral facet dislocation of the lumbosacral junction, *J Bone Joint Surg* 65A:1174, 1983.
6. Bradford D et al: Scheuermann's kyphosis and roundback deformity: results of Milwaukee brace treatment, *J Bone Joint Surg* 56A:740, 1974.
7. Browne T, Yost RP, McCarron RF: Lumbar ring apophyseal fracture in an adolescent weightlifter: a case report, *Am J Sport Med* 18(5):533, 1990.
8. Cheng CLY et al: University of Maryland, Baltimore: bodysurfing accidents resulting in cervical spinal injuries, *Spine* 17:257, 1992.
9. Ciullo J, Zarins B: Biomechanics of the musculoskeletal unit: relation to athletic performance and injury, *Clin Sports Med* 2(1):71, 1983.
10. Clark A, Stanish WD. An unusual cause of back pain in a young athlete: a case report, *Am J Sports Med* 13(1):51, 1984.
11. Crawford A: Operative treatment of spine fractures in children, *Orthop Clin North Am* 21(2):325, 1990.
12. Davis P, Hoffman J, Ball T: Spinal abnormalities in pediatric patients: MR imaging findings compared with clinical myelographic and surgical findings, *Radiology* 166:629, 1989.
13. Denis F: Spinal instability as defined by the three-column spine concept in acute spinal trauma, *Clin Orthop* 189:65, 1984.
14. Dillin WH et al: The child's spine. In Rothman RH, Simeone FA (eds): *The spine,* vol I, ed 3, New York, 1992, WB Saunders.
15. Duff J: Spearing: Clinical consequences in the adolescent, *Am J Sports Med* 2:175, 1974.
16. Ehni G, Schneider SJ: Posterior lumbar vertebral rim fractures and associated disc protrusion in adolescence, *J Neurosurg* 68:912, 1988.
17. Farfan E: Muscular mechanism of the lumbar spine and the position of power and efficiency, *Orthop Clin North Am* 6:135, 1975.
18. Fitz C: Diagnostic imaging in children with spinal disorders, *Pediatr Clin North Am* 32:1537, 1985.
19. Fox BJ, Melegach L: Transcutaneous electrical stimulation and acupuncture—comparison of treatment for low back pain, *Pain* 2:141, 1976.
20. Fujita K et al: Posterior dislocation of the sacral apophyseal ring: a case report, *Am J Sports Med* 14(3):243, 1986.
21. Gibson MJ et al: Magnetic resonance imaging of adolescent disc herniation, *J Bone Joint Surg* 69B:699, 1987.
22. Goldberg B et al: Preparticipation sports assessment, *Pediatrics* 66(5):736, 1980.
23. Goldstein J et al: Spine injuries in gymnasts and swimmers: an epidemiologic investigation, *Am J Sports Med* 19(5):463, 1991.
24. Grant T, Puffer J: Cervical stenosis: a developmental anomaly with quadriparesis during football, *Am J Sports Med* 4:219, 1976.
25. Griffin P: Protruded intervertebral lumbar disc in an adolescent, *Orthop Consult* 4:1, 1983.
26. Hall WA, Albright AL, Brunberg JA: Diagnosis of tethered cords by magnetic resonance imaging, *Surg Neurol* 30:60, 1988.
27. Henderson JM: Ruling out danger: differential diagnosis of thoracic pain: *Phys Sports Med* 20(9):124, 1992.
27a. Holdsworth FW: Fractures, dislocations, and fracture dislocations of the spine, *J Bone Joint Surg* 45B:6, 1963.
28. Jackson DW: Unilateral osseous bridging of the lumbar transverse processes following trauma, *J Bone Joint Surg* 67A:125, 1975.
29. Jackson DW: Low back pain in young athletes: evaluation of stress reaction and discogenic problems, *Am J Sports Med* 7(6):364, 1979.
30. Jackson DW, Rettig A, Wiltse L: Epidural cortisone injections in the young athletic adult, *Am J Sports Med* 8:239, 1980.
31. Jackson DW, Wiltse L: Treatment of spondylolisthesis and spondylolysis in children, *Clin Orthop* 117:92, 1976.
32. Jackson DW, Wiltse L, Cirincione R: Spondylolysis in the female gymnast, *Clin Orthop* 117:68, 1976.
33. Jackson DW et al: Stress reaction involving the pars interarticularis in young athletes, *Am J Sports Med* 9(5):304, 1981.
34. Jones AAM et al: Failed arthrodesis of the spine for severe spondylolisthesis: salvage by interbody arthrodesis, *J Bone Joint Surg* 70A:25, 1988.
35. Kurzweil PR, Jackson DW: When low back pain sidelines recreational athletes, *J Musculoskel Med* 9(1):24, 1992.
36. Lloyd T et al: Collegiate women athletes with irregular menses during adolescence have decreased bone density, *Obstet Gynecol* 72(4):639, 1988.
37. Matthews S, Wiltse L, Karbelnig M: A destructive lesion involving the intervertebral disk in children, *Clin Orthop* 9:162, 1957.
38. Menelaus M: Discitis—an inflammation affecting the intervertebral discs in children, *J Bone Joint Surg* 46B:16, 1964.
39. Micheli LJ: Low back pain in the adolescent: differential diagnosis, *Am J Sports Med* 7(6):362, 1979.
40. Micheli LJ: Sports following spinal surgery in the young athlete, *Clin Orthop* 198:152, 1985.
41. Micheli LJ, Hall J, Miller E: Use of modified Boston brace for back injuries in athletes, *Am J Sports Med* 8:351, 1980.

42. Mooney V, Robeiton J: The facet syndrome, *Clin Orthop* 116:149, 1976.
43. Nicholas J, Grossman RB, Hershman E: The importance of a simplified classification of motion in sports in relation to performance, *Orthop Clin North Am* 8:499, 1977.
44. Nuber GW, Schafer MF: Clay shovelers' injuries: a report of two injuries sustained from football, *Am J Sports Med* 15(2):182, 1987.
45. Orthopaedic knowledge update I, Park Ridge, Ill, 1984. American Academy of Orthopaedic Surgeons.
46. Orthopaedic knowledge update III, Park Ridge, Ill, 1990, American Academy of Orthopaedic Surgeons.
47. Osenbach RK, Menezes AH: Pediatric spinal cord and vertebral column injury, *Neurosurgery* 30(3):384, 1992.
48. Paley D, Gillespie R: Chronic, repetitive, unrecognized flexion injury of the cervical spine, *Am J Sports Med* 14(1):92, 1986.
49. Pavlov H et al: Cervical spine stenosis determination with vertebral body ratio method, *Radiology* 164:771, 1987.
50. Pedersen IL, Blauck L, Gardner E: Anatomy of lumbosacral posterior rami and meningeal branches of spinal nerves (sinuvertebral nerves) with experimental study of their functions, *J Bone Joint Surg* 38A:377, 1956.
51. Piggot J: The need to make rugby safer (letter), *Br Med J* 296:1260, 1988.
52. Powell MC, Wilson M, Szyeryt P: Prevalence of lumbar disc degeneration observed by magnetic resonance in symptomatic women, *Lancet* 2:1366, 1986.
53. Raghavendra BN, Epstein FJ: Sonography of the spine and spinal cord, *Radiol Clin North Am* 23(1):91, 1985.
54. Roaf R: A study of the mechanics of spinal injuries, *J Bone Joint Surg* 42B:810, 1960.
55. Sachs B et al: Scheuermann's kyphosis: follow-up of a Milwaukee brace treatment, *J Bone Joint Surg* 69A:50, 1987.
56. Savini R et al: Surgical treatment of giant-cell tumor of the spine, *J Bone Joint Surg* 65A:1283, 1983.
57. Schneider R, Paps M, Alvarez C: The effects of chronic recurrent spinal trauma in highdiving, *J Bone Joint Surg* 44A:648, 1962.
58. Schneider R, Thompson J, Bebin J: Syndrome of acute central cervical spinal cord injury, *J Neurol Neurosurg Psychiatry* 21:216, 1958.
59. Special Olympics Bulletin: *Participation by individuals with DS who suffer from atlantoaxial dislocation*, Washington, DC, 1983, Special Olympics.
60. Spencer CW, Jackson DW: Symposium on Olympic sports medicine: back injuries in the athlete, *Clin Sports Med* 2(1):191, 1983.
61. Stauffer R: Pyogenic vertebral osteomyelitis, *Orthop Clin North Am* 6:1015, 1975.
62. Sward L, Hellstrom M, Jacobsson B: Acute injury of the vertebral ring apophysis and IVD in adolescent gymnasts, *Spine* 15(2):144, 1990.
63. Sward L, Hellstrom M, Jacobsson B: Back pain and radiologic changes in the thoraco-lumbar spine of athletes, *Spine* 15(2):124, 1990.
64. Szalay E, Roach J, Smith H: Magnetic resonance imaging of the spinal cord, *J Pediatr Orthop* 7:291, 1987.
65. Tachdjian M, Matson D: Orthopaedic aspects of intraspinal tumors in infants and children, *J Bone Joint Surg* 47A:223, 1965.
66. Takata K et al: Fracture of the posterior margin of a lumbar vertebral body, *J Bone Joint Surg* 70:589, 1988.
67. Tator CH et al: Spinal injuries in ice hockey players, *Can J Surg* 34(1):63, 1991.
68. Tertti M et al: Disc degeneration in young gymnasts: an MRI study, *Am J Sports Med* 18(2):206, 1990.
69. Torg JS et al: Axial loading injuries to the middle cervical spine segment: an analysis and classification of twenty-five cases, *Am J Sports Med* 19(1):6, 1991.
70. Van Dyke DC, Gahagan CA: Down syndrome, C-spine abnormalities, and problems, *Clin Pediatr* 27(9):415, 1988.
71. Walker C: Calcification of intervertebral discs in children, *J Bone Joint Surg* 36B:601, 1954.
72. Wiltse LL, Kirkaldy-Willis W, McIvor G: The treatment of spinal stenosis, *Clin Orthop* 115:83, 1976.
73. Wiltse LL, Newman PH, MacNab I: Classification of spondylolysis and spondylolisthesis, *Clin Orthop* 117:23, 1976.
74. Wiltse LL, Winter R: Terminology and measurement of spondylolisthesis, *J Bone Joint Surg* 65A:768, 1983.
75. Zaricznyj B et al: Sports-related injuries in school-aged children, *Am J Sports Med* 8:318, 1980.

PART VI Neurovascular Injuries

CHAPTER 59 Neurovascular Problems

Kurt P. Spindler
Jim Pappas

This chapter represents a comprehensive review of chronic neurovascular conditions of the lower extremity, including chronic compartment syndromes, popliteal vessel entrapments, and entrapment neuropathies of the pelvis, hip, knee, leg, ankle, and foot. Acute compartment syndromes are only briefly addressed in the discussion of the differential diagnosis of leg pain. They are discussed in more detail in the respective anatomic chapter. Spinal nerve compressive neuropathies (herniated nucleus pulposus [HNP] or spinal stenosis [SS]) and vascular claudication (peripheral vascular disease [PVD]) are not discussed but should be considered in the differential diagnosis in acute (HNP) or chronic (SS or PVD) lower extremity pain.

Chronic neurovascular conditions of the lower extremity are uncommon causes of disabling pain in athletes, and diagnosis of these conditions is frequently delayed. The delay in diagnosis and effective treatment is frequently the result of omitting from the differential diagnosis these rare but important causes of persistent lower extremity pain. The information presented herein should aid the expert clinician in the diagnosis of pain of the lower extremity where the cause is not obvious.

CHRONIC COMPARTMENT SYNDROME

Pain in the leg while exercising is a common problem for athletes. Historically, a nonspecific diagnosis of shin splints was given to this condition. However, this pain with activity that is typically relieved with rest has many causes. The differential diagnosis includes chronic compartment syndrome (CCS), inflammatory reaction of the musculotendinous tissues, periostitis of the tibia, venous obstruction, stress fractures, obliterative arterial diseases, and pain from the central and peripheral nervous

---

Differential diagnosis of leg pain

- Chronic compartment syndrome
- Inflammation of muscle-tendon unit
- Periostitis of the tibia
- Venous obstruction
- Stress fracture
- Obliterative arterial disease
- Pain from central and peripheral nervous systems

---

systems.[99] Obviously, the appropriate treatment can be administered only if the correct diagnosis is made.

CCS was first described in an athlete by Mavor[65] in 1956, who labeled the condition *anterior tibial syndrome*. Other names given to this condition since that time include *anterior tibial pain, chronic anterior tibial compartment syndrome, anterior compartment syndrome, recurrent compartment syndrome,* and *exertional compartment syndrome*.[72,99] Mavor[65] described the plight of a professional athlete with bilateral exercise-induced leg pain. The symptoms spanned a period of 2 years and were found to increase when the intensity of exercise was increased. Ultimately, the patient gained relief after the completion of bilateral anterior compartment fasciotomies.

Clinical Findings

The subjective and objective findings as described by Mavor[65] are identical to more recent descriptions of CCS. Today the symptoms produced by CCS are well documented. They include pain with exertion, muscle fullness or tightness, cramping, weakness, and dysesthesias of the nerve crossing the involved compartment.[62] Short periods of rest during activity usually alleviate the symp-

---

Symptoms of chronic compartment syndrome

- Pain with activity
- Muscle fullness or tightness
- Cramping
- Weakness
- Dysesthesia of the nerve crossing the involved compartment

---

toms, and involvement is often bilateral.[62,63,82] Physical findings in the patient with CCS are sparse, particularly when the examination is performed at rest. One clinical finding that occurs with some consistency in CCS is the presence of a fascial hernia. The range of incidence of this finding is between 20% and 60%.[79] The examination should be performed immediately after exercise. Of patients in one study, 35% demonstrated sensitivity to pressure and compartment tenseness when evaluated immediately after strenuous exercise.[62]

Most of the information pertaining to CCS involves the anterior compartment of the leg.[7,28,62,101] The deep posterior compartment is also frequently involved, and symptoms are localized to the posteromedial aspect of the leg.[87] The superficial posterior and lateral compartments are less often involved.[48,73] Fig. 59-1 clearly demonstrates the normal anatomic compartments both schematically and by axial magnetic resonance imaging (MRI).

Pathophysiology
Acute Compartment Syndrome

Before the discussion regarding CCS is continued, CCS must be distinguished from acute compartment syndrome. Most often thought of in the setting of major trauma, acute compartment syndrome can occur in sports. The pathophysiology of acute compartment syndrome is well known.[11] Increased compartment pressures compromise the blood flow to the muscle and nerve tissue within the compartment. This ischemia produces symptoms and ultimately tissue necrosis if not treated. The symptoms begin as a dull ache and progress to severe pain. Distal pulses are generally maintained until late, and one of the earliest findings is significant pain with passive stretching of the involved muscle. Unlike

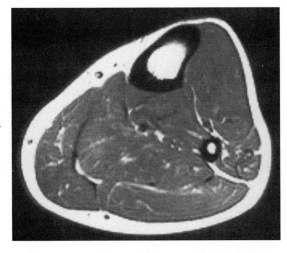

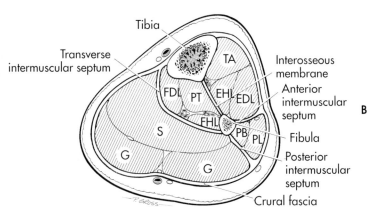

FIG. 59-1. Normal compartments of leg. **A,** T1-weighted magnetic resonance image clearly demonstrates normal four anatomic compartments in leg (anterior, lateral, superficial, and deep posterior). **B,** Schematic demonstrates individual muscles within each compartment and neurovascular structures. Anterior compartment (*TA,* tibialis anterior; *EDL,* extensor digitorum longus; *EHL,* extensor hallucis longus); lateral compartment (*PL,* peroneus longus; *PB,* peroneus brevis); superficial posterior compartment (*G,* gastrocnemis; *S,* soleus); deep posterior compartment (*FDL,* flexor digitorum longus; *PT,* posterior tibialis; *FHL,* flexor hallucis longus).

chronic compartment syndrome, cessation of activities, elevation, and ice do little to relieve symptoms. Immediate decompressive fasciotomies are required to prevent death of all muscles and nerves within the compartment.

Chronic Compartment Syndrome

Unlike the pathophysiology of acute compartment syndrome, that of CCS is speculative. The most common theory regarding the physiology of CCS is consistent with that of acute compartment syndrome. It is thought that with repeated contracture, an exercising muscle can increase its volume by 20%.[11] If this event occurs in a compartment surrounded by a noncompliant fascial envelope, compartment pressures are expected to increase. This increase in pressure then impedes blood flow and produces ischemic pain. This theory is supported by a study by Styf, Körner, and Suurkula[103] in which muscle blood flow was measured in patients with CCS. Their study showed that with prolonged activity, muscle relaxation pressures increased and muscle blood flow decreased. The tests were repeated following fasciotomies. The relaxation pressure and muscle blood flow were found to be normal after the fasciotomy. Increased lactate levels have been identified in the affected muscles, also supporting the theory of ischemia as being the cause of symptoms. Although this is the most widely accepted explanation for CCS, some controversy exists as a result of studies like that performed by Amendola et al.[2] Using a radioisotope to measure blood flow, the authors failed to show a difference in muscle perfusion between a group of patients with CCS and an asymptomatic control group.

Although there is one study reporting bilateral aberrant fascial bands as the cause of CCS in a single patient, the literature to date fails to identify any consistent anatomic or histologic fascial abnormalities as a contributing factor in CCS.[94]

Compartment Pressure Measurements

As stated previously, hard physical findings in patients with CCS are limited. In the past, many authors have stated that the diagnosis of CCS could be made by history and physical examination alone. Because of the lack of consistent physical findings and nonspecific manifestations, regular and accurate diagnosis of chronic compartment syndrome based solely on history and physical examination is impossible. In fact, Styf and Körner[101,102] reported that only 14% to 27% of athletes suspected of having CCS after having a clinical evaluation were found to have increased intracompartment pressures during and after exercise. As such, intracompartmental pressure monitoring is the most precise method for diagnosing CCS. Recently, MRI has been used to measure hydrogen proton density to confirm increased compartmental pressure that had previously been identified by slit catheter measurements.[2] Ultrasound has been used to aid in the placement of catheters for compartment pressure measurements and also to directly measure the change in compartment size with exercise.[31,111] Both MRI and ultrasound offer possible noninvasive methods of evaluation, but they have yet to replace the intracompartmental pressure monitoring.

Several techniques are available for intramuscular pressure measurement. These include the needle manometer, the constant infusion technique, the wick catheter method, the slit catheter monitoring system, and microtip pressure transducers with or without continuous infusion.[89] Although all these methods have been successful at measuring pressures while the limb is at rest, they are not all suitable for pressure measurement during exercise. Slit and wick catheters, for example, are more conducive to active measurements.

There is considerable controversy in the literature as to which phase of exercise produces the most diagnostic pressure readings. Some studies have suggested that resting pressures greater than 10 mm are indicative of CCS.[88] However, Styf, Körner, and Suurkula[103] thought that the wide range of resting pressures and the dependence of compartment pressure on foot position during rest made this parameter unreliable. Others have stated that dynamic pressure studies provide the most useful information. Puranen and Alavaikko[81] used the mean muscular pressure of 50 mm Hg as diagnostic when taking readings during exercise. The validity of the dynamic studies is in turn questioned. Fronek et al[28] reported that the depth of catheter placement and the intensity of muscular effort are variables that are difficult to control during dynamic testing. Also, with respect to *dynamic monitoring*, Bourne and Rorabeck[11] stated that in their study, careful statistical analysis failed to show a significant difference between CCS patients and the normal population. The authors placed diagnostic emphasis on increased intramuscular pressure that was generated by exercise and measured immediately following *cessation* of that exercise. They reported a significant difference between symptomatic patients and asymptomatic controls, 37 mm Hg vs. 18 mm Hg, respectively. Pedowitz et al[79] also emphasized postexercise pressures as important in diagnosis. They included a preexercise measurement with measurements at 1 minute and 5 minutes after cessation of exercise. They outlined the following pressure measurements for parameters in diagnosing CCS: (1) preexercise pressure greater than or equal to 15 mm Hg, (2) a 1-minute postexercise pressure greater than 30 mm Hg, or (3) a 5-minute postexercise pressure greater than or equal to 20 mm Hg. The normal resting pressure in asymptomatic controls is 4 ± 4 mm Hg.

Diagnosis of chronic compartment syndrome

Compartment pressure monitoring is imperative.

Compartment pressure in chronic compartment syndrome

Elevated pressure immediately after exercise and delay in return to baseline pressures are diagnostic.

The study by Styf and Körner[101] shows that all patients with CCS had pressures of more than 35 mm Hg after exercise, and these pressures remained elevated for more than 6 minutes. Thus Pedowitz et al[79] and Styf and Körner[101] not only pointed out the diagnostic finding of elevated compartment pressures immediately following exercise, but also introduced the concept that the delay in normalization of these pressures is diagnostic. In fact, although many authors argue about the significance of preexercise and dynamic pressure studies, most agree that a sustained elevated compartment pressure after the cessation of exercise is the most important parameter in diagnosing CCS.

Finally, in an effort to put the value of compartment pressure measurement in perspective, Styf, Körner, and Suurkula[103] stated that clinical observations serve only to select patients for pressure recordings, which in turn allow for diagnosis of CCS.

Treatment

Once the accurate diagnosis of CCS has been made, the next obvious step is the formation of a treatment plan. Various articles describe nonsurgical plans that include a trial of nonsteroidal antiinflammatory medications, local injection, cessation of sporting activities for a period of 4 to 6 weeks with subsequent graduated return to activities, shoe modifications, orthoses, and comprehensive stretching and icing programs.[28] With the exception of complete avoidance of the symptom-producing activity, the nonoperative treatment plans are for the most part unsuccessful.[28,82,88] The surgical option involves decompressive fasciotomies. The results of this procedure in the appropriate population are good. Of the limbs operated on in the study by Almdahl and Samdal,[1] 75% were reported to have excellent or good results after fasciotomy. Of those decompressed in the study by Rorabeck, Bourne, and Fowler,[88] 83% had significant improvement in exercise tolerance and pain relief, as did 92% of the patients in the study by Fronek et al.[28] Two important points in decompressive fasciotomies are, first, complete release of fascia overlying the compartment and, second, protection of the superficial peroneal nerve as it pierces the anterior intermuscular septum midway down the leg in the anterior compartment (where the majority of the decompression takes place).

Treatment of chronic compartment syndrome

- Nonoperative approaches, with the exception of complete elimination of activity, are seldom successful.
- Decompressive fasciotomies provide the best results.

Fronek et al[28] described a single-incision technique and used a fascitome to completely decompress the anterior and lateral compartments. Rorabeck, Bourne, and Fowler[88] described two separate longitudinal incisions separated by a 15-cm skin bridge. The two fasciotomies were then connected subcutaneously. Fascial hernias were included in the line of the fasciotomy to ensure complete decompression. As stated previously the deep posterior compartment is also often involved in CCS. Decompression of this compartment can also be performed through a single or double longitudinal incision just posterior to the medial border of the tibia. Care must be taken to avoid injury to the saphenous vein and nerve. Rorabeck and associates[89] also stated that the fascia about the tibialis posterior comprises a fifth compartment, which requires decompression in CCS involving the deep posterior compartment. Unlike fasciotomies for acute compartment syndrome the skin of patients with CCS can be closed immediately. Tight circumferential dressings are avoided, and patients are allowed to bear weight as tolerated. As soon as discomfort subsides, exercise is encouraged because it can expand and help maintain the new volume of the compartment after fasciotomy.

Surgical failures in those patients with documented elevated compartment syndrome can typically be explained in three ways. The first is failure to identify the appropriate compartments for decompression. An example of this is decompression of the anterior compartment without appreciating the involvement of the deep posterior compartment, particularly the tibialis posterior. Second, incomplete decompression of the compartment leads to persistent symptoms. Finally, Bell[7] reported on a group of five patients who had adequate decompressions but had persistent symptoms and elevated pressures. It was thought that because of rapid formation of scar tissue between the cut edges of the fasciotomy, the new size of the compartment was inadequate to accommodate the increased muscle volume during exercise. These patients were successfully treated with partial fasciectomy.

Failures of operative treatment

- Failure to identify appropriate compartment for decompression
- Incomplete decompression
- Rapid scar formation of fasciotomy edges preventing expansion of compartment

---

Complications

Reported complications after fasciotomies were few. Fronek et al[28] reported on one operative wound infection requiring debridement and split-thickness skin graft. A more tragic result was also described in the same paper. A 19-year-old woman had closure of her partial fasciotomy and developed an acute compartment syndrome. Myonecrosis ensued, and multiple reconstructive procedures were required. Styf and Körner[101] described pain from compression of the superficial peroneal nerve as a complication of decompression fasciotomy. They speculated that the swelling of the exercising muscle bellies could displace and entrap the superficial peroneal nerve as it comes through the fascia just lateral to the intermuscular septum.

Conclusion

The signs and symptoms of CCS are not specific enough to provide a diagnosis alone. Compartment pressure monitoring is mandatory to make the diagnosis. Although conservative treatment should be considered, it is seldom successful. Decompressive fasciotomy is the treatment of choice in CCS.

POPLITEAL ARTERY ENTRAPMENT SYNDROME

The first clinical case of popliteal artery entrapment syndrome was described by Hamming[38] in a 12-year-old boy with calf pain and foot paresthesias with exercise. Since then more than 300 cases have been reported in the world literature.[21] Although popliteal artery entrapment syndrome can present with a variety of symptoms, the most common one is a young individual with intermittent exercise associated claudication that responds to rest. The majority of cases are seen in individuals who have no history of atherosclerotic peripheral vascular disease and who are less than 40 years of age. Therefore for any young, fit individual who has exercise-induced calf or leg pain, popliteal artery entrapment syndrome should be included in the differential diagnosis. Surgical treatment is curative, and delay in diagnosis can not only compromise the long-term result of surgery, but also result in amputation.[110]

Stuart,[98] as a medical student, first described an abnormal course of the popliteal artery in 1879. The first clinical case was described by Hamming,[38] but the first case diagnosed before operation was reported by Servello[92] in 1962 by preoperative arteriography, which demonstrated an abnormal medial deviation of the popliteal artery secondary to the lateral insertion of the medial head of the gastrocnemius muscle. This is the classic type of popliteal artery entrapment syndrome reported in the literature to date, which includes a multitude of case reports,* two excellent review articles,[16,75] and three large retrospective reviews of treatment.[21,36,91]

The true incidence of popliteal artery entrapment syndrome is unknown but is believed to be higher than currently recognized. Bouhoutsos[10] found an incidence of 0.1% of symptomatic popliteal compression among all patients that had vascular compromise (33 of 2000 patients over 50 months). However, Gibson et al[32] found the anatomic abnormalities in popliteal artery entrapment syndrome to be 3.5% in 86 postmortem examinations.

Etiology

The exact cause of popliteal entrapment syndrome is unknown, but the findings of a case report in monozygotic twins[46] suggest that genetic factors may play a role. Besides the most common cause of popliteal artery entrapment syndrome, extrinsic causes of compression such as Baker's cyst,[77] fibular osteochondroma,[56] tibial osteochondroma,[49] and functional hypertrophy of the medial head of the gastrocnemius muscle with a normal

*References 6, 13, 15, 17, 25, 27, 37, 43, 50, 55, 57, 58, 60, 66, 76, 83, 85, 93, 96, 109, and 110.

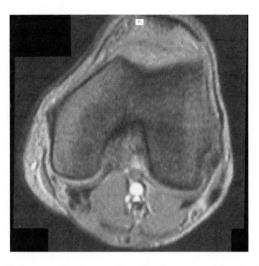

FIG. 59-2. Normal anatomy of popliteal artery and heads of gastrocnemius. Sequential flash two-dimensional magnetic resonance image clearly demonstrates normal relationship of popliteal artery (*bright white*) between medial and lateral heads of gastrocnemius on axial view.

arterial course have been reported.[85] The great majority of the causes described in the literature have been from an aberrant relationship of the popliteal artery to the medial head of the gastrocnemius muscle or a normal artery position with aberrant bands of the plantaris or gastrocnemius muscle.[75,91] The MRI in Fig. 59-2 demonstrates the normal course of the popliteal artery between the medial and lateral heads of the gastrocnemius muscle. Schurmann et al[91] have reviewed the many classification systems that can describe up to 10 subtypes of the relationship of the popliteal artery to the medial head of the gastrocnemius muscle as well as aberrant muscle slips. Because none of these classifications can accommodate all the anatomic findings, they have simplified the classifications into three types (Fig. 59-3). In Type I the popliteal artery, after leaving the adductor canal, lies medial to the medial head of the gastrocnemius muscle (normal relationship is lateral). The artery is compressed between the medial head of the gastrocnemius muscle and semimembranosus and the medial femoral condyle. In Type II the popliteal artery lies in its anatomically correct position; however, there are atypical insertions of muscle fibers, usually the medial head of the gastrocnemius muscle but sometimes slips of the popliteus or plantaris muscle. Type III is an intermediate type between Types I and II that comprises a combination of an abnormal location of the vessel as well as abnormal slips of fascia. It is the authors' opinions that this classification serves to highlight the major anatomic reasons for pop-

---

**Classification of popliteal artery
entrapment syndrome**

- Type I—atypical artery position
- Type II—abnormal muscle insertions or fibrous bands
- Type III—Elements of Types I and II

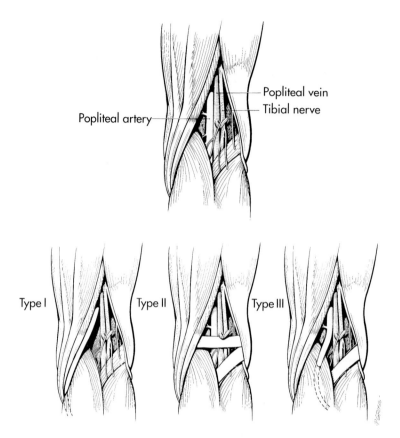

Popliteal vein
Tibial nerve
Popliteal artery

Type I   Type II   Type III

FIG. 59-3. Classification of popliteal artery entrapment syndromes. First diagram highlights normal course of artery *lateral* to medial head of gastrocnemius. Three types are defined: **Type I,** artery *medial* to medial head of gastrocnemius; **Type II,** tethering of normally positioned artery by anomalous insertions of gastrocnemius or fibrous bands; **Type III,** combination of Types I and II with abnormal artery position and anomalous insertions or bands.

liteal artery entrapment syndrome and correlates with the appropriate surgical principles that are discussed later.

Clinical Findings

The clinical features of the popliteal artery entrapment syndrome are dependent on the degree of damage to the popliteal artery and the activity level of the patient. Murray, Halliday, and Croft,[75] in their review of the literature, found a mean age of 28 years and a bimodal age distribution (peaks at 7 and 14 years) with two thirds of the patients under 35 years' old. There is a predominance of males (90%), and only 10% of the cases are women whose average age is 21. The exact percentage of bilateral involvement is unknown. It appears to be much greater than the documented incidence of approximately 30%. It appears that with new, sophisticated, noninva-

sive, diagnostic techniques (computed tomography [CT] and MRI scans) the presence of bilateral abnormality with or without symptoms on the contralateral limb may be as high as two thirds.[75] By far the majority (88%) of patients with popliteal artery entrapment syndrome have a slowly progressive unilateral calf claudication as a result of arterial insufficiency that is aggravated by exercise.[75] The claudication symptoms include a sensation of cramping, tightness, or fatigue, which requires them to stop exercise and resolves with a brief period of rest. Bachner and Friedman[4] stated that a reasonable index of arterial insufficiency is the distance a patient can walk with a normal stride before these claudication symptoms begin (see Chapter 28). If claudication occurs at a distance over 1800 feet (approximately six city blocks), this indicates mild disease, and significant occlusion is indicated when symptoms occur at less than 600 feet (two

---

Patient profile

- 67% < 35 years' old
- 90% Male
- 30% Bilateral

Popliteal artery entrapment syndrome

88% of patients have a slowly progressive unilateral calf claudication.

blocks). Occasionally a much smaller percentage of patients can have symptoms of acute or chronic limb ischemia. This is a result of embolization[27,40] or severe narrowing or occlusion of the popliteal artery. Rarely, patients may report symptoms of numbness, coolness, or paresthesias in the limb in a variety of postures that change with position of the knee. Rarely do patients have leg swelling after exercise or with deep venous thrombosis. These patients usually indicate popliteal vein and artery entrapment[10,20,24,39,84] (approximately 10%) or occasionally vein entrapment alone.[14,44] The history and symptom complex are critical to the diagnosis and indicate the need for further diagnostic work-up rather than the physical examination, which may be normal.

The physical examination findings depend on the degree of involvement. If there is severe occlusion of the artery, there may be diminished pulses that may or may not be diminished with active plantar flexion versus a passively dorsiflexed foot. At one time, pulse diminution with this maneuver was considered pathognomonic for popliteal artery entrapment syndrome,[30] but pulse diminution has also been shown to occur in normal individuals.[67] If abnormal physical examination findings are present, this represents a significant occlusion and degenerative changes of the vessel at the site of entrapment is present and has a worse prognosis. Therefore normal physical examination findings should not preclude further workup with the appropriate history.

Vascular Evaluation

To arrive at a diagnosis preoperatively and confirm suspicions based on history, angiography is established as a standard for diagnosis.[75] Recently, three noninvasive studies have been extremely helpful in screening for popliteal artery entrapment syndrome. di Marzo et al[20] think that duplex scanning studies performed both in the resting state and during active contraction of the calf muscles are positive if compression of the popliteal artery produces a decrease in flow. Thus duplex scanning can provide a quick, noninvasive screening tool to determine which patients need further dynamic angiography. Recently, CT[112] and MRI[19,29,68,69] have provided noninvasive methods for determining popliteal artery entrapment syndrome. It is the authors' opinions that given the superior soft-tissue contrast resolution of MRI, this becomes the noninvasive diagnostic procedure of choice compared with CT scanning. Furthermore, MRI can rule out other soft-tissue, intraarticular causes of leg pain or an extrinsic cause such as popliteal cyst besides identifying anomalous insertions and bands of the medial head of the gastrocnemius. Axial sections on either CT or MRI scans can show the position of the vessel in relationship

---

Diagnostic studies

- Duplex scanning
- Magnetic resonance imaging
- Computed tomography
- Angiography (gold standard)

---

to the medial head of the gastrocnemius (Fig. 59-2), easily confirming the anatomic variations consistent with popliteal artery entrapment syndrome.

At this time, however, the angiographic appearance of the popliteal artery remains the gold standard. In the review of the literature by Murray, Halliday, and Croft,[75] angiographic abnormalities were present in 98% of symptomatic cases. The most common abnormality was occlusion of the popliteal artery in 66% of the cases, followed by medial deviation of the artery in 29% of cases. Other less common findings included popliteal stenosis, 11%; poststenotic dilatation, 8%; and a lateral deviation of the artery in only two cases. Furthermore, it should be noted that of the 23 cases of bilateral popliteal artery entrapment syndrome reported in detail in the literature, 20 (87%) were found on preoperative monitoring to have identical anatomic lesions on both sides.[75] It is the authors' opinions that with the advent of newer, noninvasive diagnostic imaging in patients with popliteal artery entrapment syndrome on one side, the contralateral limb should be imaged with duplex scanning, CT, or MRI.

Pathophysiology

The pathophysiology of popliteal artery entrapment syndrome is a progressive damage to the artery at the site of compression, which if not corrected, leads to premature localized atherosclerosis with thrombus formation, occlusion, and potential embolization.[75] It is the progressive damage to the arterial vessel that necessitates early recognition and treatment.

Differential Diagnosis

The differential diagnosis of popliteal artery entrapment syndrome includes atherosclerotic vascular disease, Buerger's disease, trauma, popliteal aneurysms, adventitial cystic disease, extrinsic mass compression (e.g., popliteal cysts, osteochondromas, or posttraumatic deformity), and rarely, the entrapment is not in the popliteal fossa but at the adductor hiatus. If the patient has the clinical complex of intermittent claudication and the noninvasive studies are normal for the popliteal fossa, the physician should be careful to exclude compression of the superficial femoral artery at the adductor hiatus.[2,26,45,108] Occasionally, there is a tight fibrous band that constricts the vessel that is treated by surgical division.[2,26,45,108]

Treatment

It is almost universally accepted that the treatment for popliteal artery entrapment syndrome is surgical.[16,21,75,91,110] The principles of surgery are to release the entrapped vessel and restore it to its normal anatomic position with reestablishment of normal arterial flow. Reestablishing normal arterial flow depends on the degree of damage to the vessel. In the mildest forms or in the asymptomatic limb with popliteal artery entrapment syndrome, release of the entrapment may be all that is needed. With a greater degree of damage, a local procedure like endarterectomy may be sufficient, but if there is significant arterial damage or occlusion, a bypass with autologous vein graft has become the standard of treatment. At present the posterior approach is preferred. It is thought that a divided medial head of the gastrocnemius muscle should not be reattached to its muscle origin with little postoperative impairment.[75] There have been few long-term follow-up studies in the literature to determine the prognosis for this condition. There have been several case reports that demonstrate clinically patent vessels after surgical treatment; Schurmann et al[91] reported that surgical treatment consisting of either thromboendarterectomy or vein graft interposition in addition to decompression of the artery produced excellent results in 9 of 13 cases, but the length of the follow-up was not documented. Two of their patients have recurrent thrombosis, and in two others entrapment was not diagnosed until the patients were reoperated for aneurysms of the vein graft. It was the authors' conclusion that in selected cases freeing of the entrapped artery may be sufficient, but the majority probably required decompression and interposition of an autologous vein graft as the treatment of choice.[91] The largest long-term study on surgical treatment was by di Marzo et al,[21] who reported their surgical results in 31 cases in 23 patients. They found that a total of 10 different variants were seen, and abnormalities of the medial head of the gastrocnemius muscle were seen in 75%. Eighteen cases required only division of the aberrant musculotendinous tissue, 12 cases required vascular reconstruction, and the last additional case was explored without a specific procedure being warranted. There was a striking difference in the long-term patency rates; 94% of patients with simple

---

Treatment: surgery principles

- Restore normal anatomic course
- Release constricting muscle and bands
- Bypass graft for significant arterial damage

---

division of the musculotendinous tissue were patent at a mean follow-up of 46 months (2 to 120 months). This is in contrast to a 58% patency rate for the vascular reconstruction with a mean follow-up of 43.5 months (1 to 100 months). The authors concluded that early diagnosis is critical and that appropriate noninvasive screening should be performed even in patients with minimal symptoms because the early lesions can be treated by division of the musculotendinous structures alone with excellent long-term patency rates. They thought that a posterior approach was preferred and that vascular reconstruction was associated with a poor, long-term outcome.

Conclusion

Popliteal artery entrapment syndrome is a relatively rare entity that is often underdiagnosed or has an extensive delay in diagnosis. A history of intermittent claudication aggravated by exercise is paramount with physical examination findings that are subtle or entirely absent. It is recommended that any young patient with any

symptoms of intermittent claudication be noninvasively studied with either duplex ultrasonography, CT, or MRI, depending on the expertise at the attending physician's institution. If these noninvasive studies are suggestive, angiography should be obtained. Angiography should also be considered even if the diagnosis is not confirmed on the noninvasive studies but the history is appropriate to definitively exclude possible popliteal artery entrapment syndrome. Once the diagnosis is made, surgical treatment should be rendered, which consists of either simple division of aberrant fibrous bands and reestablishment of normal popliteal artery position vs. an autologous vein graft if there is significant arterial damage. The contralateral limb should also be noninvasively studied, and if a similar anatomic finding is noted, surgical release to prevent progressive arterial damage should be considered. If these lesions are diagnosed and treated early by division of the musculotendinous structures, the condition should be completely reversible and a normal result should be obtained for the remaining years of the individual's life.

ENTRAPMENT NEUROPATHIES

Entrapment neuropathies of the pelvis, hip, and lower extremity in athletes are relatively uncommon. Their symptoms and signs may be subtle or striking, depending on the specific nerve or the degree of involvement of that nerve. The majority of the literature involves a series of case reports on individual nerves. We take a regional approach that begins at the pelvis and hip, proceeds to entrapments around the knee, and finishes at the ankle and foot. We focus on chronic entrapments and injuries to the nerve that do not involve direct lacerations or are a result of dislocations of their respective joints. Injuries secondary to hip, knee, or ankle dislocations as well as penetrating trauma or fractures are the most common cause of nerve injuries in the lower extremity, and most physicians adequately recognize and treat these injuries. It is the chronic entrapments, however, with their paucity of physical findings and history, that may prove to be a difficult diagnosis and are the focus of this section.

Pelvis and Hip

The major motor nerves, including the sciatic, femoral, and obturator nerves, are rarely injured. The sensory nerves, including the lateral femoral cutaneous, posterior cutaneous, and pudendal nerves, are more commonly injured.

Sciatic Nerve

The sciatic nerve is rarely injured in sports. Stewart et al[97] reported a transient neuropathy in a cyclist after a prolonged bicycle ride. Venna, Bielawski, and Spatz[107] reported in a child a unilateral progressive sciatic nerve dysfunction that was caused by a fibrovascular band and that improved when it was surgically sectioned. Tsairis,[106] in a review of peripheral nerve injuries in athletes, believes that most lesions of the sciatic nerve are incomplete and present with a varying degree of deficits that usually recover. It is thought that the lateral (peroneal) trunk is more vulnerable than the medial (tibial) trunk because of the more variable location of the lateral trunk, and injuries to this branch can mimic a peroneal nerve injury at the knee.[104] Because the peroneal component of the sciatic nerve innervates the short head of the biceps femoris, electromyelogram (EMG) testing and involvement of the biceps femoris indicate a high lesion of the peroneal trunk and not an injury at the knee.

Piriformis syndrome. There has been great debate over the exact cause of the piriformis syndrome, which is believed to be compression of the sciatic nerve as it exits the external rotators of the hip. It is thought that direct trauma from the piriformis muscle accounts for the syndrome. The syndrome has recently been discussed by Pace and Nagle[78] and Solheim et al,[95] who recommended division of the piriformis muscle in refractory cases. However, the authors believe that the majority of buttocks pain with or without sciatic nerve type symptoms is the result of a herniated disk in the lumbar spine and not the piriformis syndrome. It is not until the diskogenic cause of the pain has been adequately tested for and ruled out that one should consider an attempt at sectioning the piriformis muscle. The use of a local anesthetic with or without corticosteroids to provide relief and diagnosis before surgery has been described but is not clearly defined. Also, the patients that may potentially benefit from surgery are not clearly defined. It is hoped that further research in this area will provide a more definitive answer.

Gluteal Nerve

Finally, in the buttocks region, Plihal et al[80] described two case reports of females with chronic gluteal pain without any paresthesias in which an EMG confirmed the diagnosis of entrapment of the superior gluteal nerve and its branches. They suggested that a local injection of corticosteroids is the treatment of choice initially, and if this does not cure the condition, consideration of surgical relief is warranted.

Posterior Cutaneous Nerve

An isolated lesion of the posterior cutaneous nerve has been reported in a cyclist from prolonged riding.[3] The presenting symptoms are paresthesias in the distribution of the nerve that covers the lower buttocks and posterior half of the thigh.

Pudendal Nerve

Compression of the pudendal nerve (pudendal neuritis) has also been reported from prolonged cycling with the symptoms including numbness and decreased sensitivity on half or all of the penis.[34] With proper adjustment of the seat as well as avoidance of protracted riding times these entrapments can be avoided.

Obturator Nerve

Tsairis[106] reported that injury to the obturator nerve is extremely uncommon in sports. The presenting symptoms could include weakness in adduction of the hip and paresthesias on the inner thigh.

Femoral Nerve

Brozin et al[12] and Miller and Benedict[70] have identified traumatic stretch injuries to the femoral nerve in dancers, gymnasts, judo practitioners, parachute jumpers, and athletes doing repeated somersaults. The causes and sites of injury have been theorized as compression of the nerve under the inguinal ligament during long periods of hyperextension or stretching of the nerve as it exits the lumbar plexus from sudden flexion and extension of the spine. The latter is thought to be the most common mechanism. Differentiation of the site of involvement can be determined clinically by evaluation of hip flexion strength (iliopsoas and L2-L3 nerve roots), which if abnormal, suggests a proximal lesion. EMG can evaluate the iliopsoas, hip adductors, and quadriceps muscles and can localize the lesion among a lumbar root, plexus, or femoral nerve. Isolated femoral neuropathies produce weakness of knee extension secondary to the innervation of the quadriceps muscles and a reduction in the knee jerk reflex (L4) and sensory loss over the anterior thigh and medial aspect of the leg. Analgesics for pain control and physical therapy to increase the strength of the quadriceps muscles and maintain hip joint mobility are recommended.[106] If a complete laceration or a bleeding disorder resulting in a hematoma of the iliopsoas muscle with compression neuropathy present, surgical exploration should be considered.[106]

Lateral Femoral Cutaneous Nerve

Perhaps the most common nerve injured around the pelvis and hip is the lateral femoral cutaneous nerve, which is a purely sensory nerve. This syndrome has been described as **meralgia paresthetica,**[23,59,106] which results in an altered sensation on the anterolateral aspect of the thigh. As previously stated, it is entirely sensory and there is no motor weakness in the quadriceps muscles. Clinical presentation includes either a burning sensation in the anterolateral aspect of the thigh or pain. The physical examination is significant for an altered sensation, which can either be an increased sensitivity to touch or a diminished response to light touch. This syndrome has been reported in weightlifters as a result of their tight corsets or belts[106] and in gymnasts from impacting their thighs on the parallel bars.[59] Tsairis[106] believes that the prognosis is dependent on the underlying cause. If a belt or corset has caused this condition, discontinuing the use of that constricting band allows the nerve to recover in most cases. If, however, the cause is unidentifiable, the prognosis is much more variable. As previously stated, this nerve is purely sensory and should not affect the function of that athlete in his or her respective sport. Rarely, a local anesthetic block may be beneficial and even curative, and even more rarely a surgical procedure to either free the trapped nerve or ablate it could be considered.[106] It is the authors' experience that once individuals with this lesion learn that it is purely sensory and has no affect on the muscle power in their leg, they can usually continue their sport with reassurance that they will not cause permanent functional deficit to their extremity. It is more difficult to identify the offending cause of the condition to correct the chronic compression.

Knee

The two nerves commonly entrapped in the knee region include the saphenous nerve, either as it exits the adductor canal[5,51,86] or near the pes anserine bursa,[40] and the peroneal nerve as it courses around the fibular neck and enters the peroneal longus muscle.

Saphenous Nerve

The main clinical finding is paresthesias in the distribution of the saphenous nerve on the medial aspect of the leg. Localization of the entrapment is by typical physical examination findings. Confirmation of entrapment is made by symptomatic relief with an injection of a local anesthetic. Treatment consists of an injection of a local anesthetic and a corticosteroid to stop the inflammation. Surgical release of the entrapment is rarely necessary.

Peroneal Nerve

Traction or stretch injuries to the peroneal nerve can occur with violent twisting activities of the ankle in sports or as a result of direct compression in its superficial location. After it winds around the fibular neck, the peroneal nerve divides into two components, a deep and a superficial branch. The deep branch provides motor function to the anterior compartment (Fig. 59-1), which consists of the anterior tibialis, extensor digitorum longus, and extensor hallucis longus. It then exits the superficial fascia and supplies sensation to the first dorsal webspace. The superficial branch of the peroneal nerve enters the lateral compartment (Fig. 59-1) and supplies the peroneal longus and brevis. It then exits to supply sensation to the top and the lateral side of the foot. Careful physical examination findings obtained after acute trauma usually provide a clear diagnosis. However, entrapments of the common peroneal nerve or its branches can be difficult to diagnose because they can lack abnormalities when the patient is at rest. Injuries to the peroneal nerve have been reported in runners[55,64,71,100] and in patients wearing tight ski boots or roller blades.[18] A common physical finding is a positive Tinel's sign at the site of the compression, and depending on the branch of the peroneal nerve involved, motor weakness or sensory change in that distribution can be present. However, the findings at rest may be entirely normal, and symptoms may appear only with exercise. Tsairis[106] thinks that most cases can be treated nonsurgically, and as long as recovery proceeds as expected, surgical intervention is not needed. However, Styf[100] and Leach, Punell, and Saito[55] have had excellent results in the majority of their patients with return to their previous level of activity without symptoms after undergoing a surgical decompression of the constricting fascia around the fibular neck. The physician should be wary of the overlap of a chronic anterior compartment syndrome with an entrapment of the deep peroneal nerve. Compartment pressure readings can help confirm or deny the diagnosis.

Unless the clinician is alert to potential entrapments of either the saphenous or the peroneal nerve, these rare causes of pain, which can be disabling, may be missed. The correct diagnosis is important because surgical release or removal of extrinsic compression can effectively return the athlete to his or her previous level of participation.

Ankle and Foot

Entrapment neuropathies of the foot and ankle are relatively common and often are undiagnosed or misdiagnosed, or diagnosis is extremely delayed. Entrapment neuropathies of the posterior tibial nerve and its three major branches (calcaneal, medial, and lateral plantar)[47,74] sural nerve,[42] interdigital nerves,[47,90,106] and dorsal sensory nerves[42] have been described in athletes.

It is commonly recognized that both foot and heel pain are common among athletes, especially runners. However, it is also not infrequent to find entrapment neuropathies in this same population, but the frequency of this condition is much lower than the more common overuse or tendinitis injuries to the foot and ankle. The key to the diagnosis of entrapment neuropathies is understanding the anatomy of the posterior tibial nerve and branches, the interdigital nerves, and the superficial cutaneous nerves (sural branches of the peroneal and saphenous nerves). Furthermore, the clinician must understand that the quality of the pain is different, and a sharper, more lancinating, radiating pain is typical of an entrapment vs. a more chronic aching for the more common overuse injuries. The examination and location of the pain, both a Tinel's sign and the distribution of the altered sensation or radiation, is specific for each type of entrapment. Finally, a diagnostic injection of lidocaine with or without an attempt at treatment with a corticosteroid can confirm the suspected entrapment.

Key features of entrapment neuropathies

- Differentiate motor vs. sensory nerve
- Positive Tinel's sign
- Either radiating sharp or dull pain
- Symptomatic during sports
- Often delayed diagnosis

Posterior Tibial Nerve

The posterior tibial nerve can be entrapped in the tarsal tunnel with any one of its branches, or the calcaneal medial and lateral plantar nerves can be independently entrapped. The tarsal tunnel consists of a closed space with an osseous floor covered by a roof consisting of the flexor retinaculum. The tunnel is located just behind the medial malleolus, and structures within the tunnel include the posterior tibial nerve and its branches; flexor digitorum longus; flexor hallucis longus; and tibial nerve, artery, and vein.[47] **Tarsal tunnel syndrome** is characterized by pain in the ankle or foot with or without paresthesias in the sole. This condition may result from injury to the ankle or foot in any sport and can occasionally become a chronic problem.[106] The initial treatment is conservative, consisting of antiinflammatory medication, correction of the biomechanical problems in the foot, and a trial of activity modification. For diagnosis and therapy, an injection of a lidocaine-corticosteroid is sometimes warranted. However, if this does not provide relief, surgical release of the retinaculum is indicated with good results.[74,106]

Calcaneal Nerves

Henrickson and Westlin[41] described chronic heel pain as entrapment of the calcaneal branch in runners and soccer players. All these individuals failed a conservative trial, and surgical decompression resulted in a resumption of athletic activity in slightly over 1 month.[42]

Plantar Nerves

Also, individual entrapments of the medial plantar nerve and the lateral plantar nerve can occur and follow the same general guidelines for treatment as for tarsal tunnel syndrome. Murphy and Baxter[74] reviewed their 10-year experience with 21 operations performed on competitive and recreational runners for recalcitrant foot and ankle neuralgia and described good results with surgical decompression of heel pain as a result of a compartment syndrome of the abductor hallucis muscles, compression of the deep peroneal nerve on the superior talus, and a tarsal tunnel as a result of compression of an os trigonum. The reader is referred to Murphy and Baxter[74] for a detailed discussion of these entrapments and their surgical technique and treatment.

Deep Peroneal Nerve

Jones and Singer[47] described entrapment of the deep peroneal nerve or anterior tarsal tunnel syndrome with four factors contributing to this condition. These factors include osteophytes in the medial and mid-tarus, fractures, tight shoes, and space-occupying lesions. It is believed that tight shoes may be the most common cause. Typical findings in patients complaining of pain on the dorsum of their foot include sensory changes in the first webspace and occasional atrophied extensor digitorum brevis.[47] It is recommended that radiographs be obtained to rule out a bony spur as a cause of the compression. An attempt should be made to identify a positive Tinel's sign on physical examination. Conservative therapy, which consists of removing the constricting stress and occasionally administering a corticosteroid injection should be tried initially.[53] If these conservative measures fail, surgical exploration with removal of the bony prominences and division of the compressing retinacular structures should be performed.

Superficial Peroneal Nerve

Jones and Singer[47] describe entrapment of the superficial peroneal nerve as it pierces the deep fascia just above the ankle to provide sensory innervation to the distal lateral part of the calf, dorsum of the foot, and toes. Anatomically, Kosinski[52] found that in a quarter of the cases it exits as two separate nerves. It is believed that ski boots, tight-fitting shoes, and sometimes trauma can entrap these cutaneous nerves with representative paresthesias and sensory changes on the foot. The treatment is usually conservative and consists of removal of the offending compression. The diagnosis can be confirmed by injection of a local anesthetic with or without corticosteroid. Rarely is fascia release or neurolysis performed.

Sural Nerve

The sural nerve can be entrapped in three locations. The first is an exit point in the fascia just above the ankle, the second is behind the lateral malleolus,[47] and the third is at the fifth metatarsal after a displaced fracture.[35] The symptoms and signs consist of a positive Tinel's sign, a variable degree of sensory changes in the distribution of the nerve, and sometimes an aching quality. The first line of treatment is to decide whether there is an intrinsic compression by some altered anatomy vs an extrinsic compression by a tight boot, shoe, or clothing. The treatment of extrinsic compression is to remove the offending structure. For the treatment of intrinsic compression, an injection of a local anesthetic and corticosteroid may be beneficial.

Dorsal Cutaneous Nerves of the Foot

Repetitive trauma to the dorsum of the foot can result in contusion neuropathies that involve the medial or intermedial dorsal cutaneous branches of the deep peroneal nerve.[42,113] These injuries may also involve the lateral dorsal cutaneous nerve, which is a continuation of the sural nerve as previously discussed. A positive Tinel's sign can sometimes be elicited with varying degrees of paresthesias and numbness in the distribution of these cutaneous nerves. Occasionally they may be caused by tight-fitting shoes, particularly the cutaneous nerve as it wraps around the fifth metatarsal. Treatment is based on relief of the offending trauma with proper shoewear or more protection within the shoe.

Interdigital Neuroma

The most common entrapment neuropathy in the foot is Morton's neuroma.[47] The pathophysiology is a degenerative process of the nerve characterized by fibrosis, neural edema, myelinization, and changes within the surrounding vessels that can lead to occlusion.[9,33,42,54,69,105] This condition was first described by Durlacher[22] in 1845. The exact cause of its appearance is still a matter of debate. One popular theory is pinching of the lateral plantar nerve between the fourth and fifth metatarsal heads.[8,18] Others have proposed a predisposition in flat feet or collapse of the metatarsal ligament. The most common location is in the third webspace between the third and fourth toes, which is believed to be caused by the connection of the branch from the lateral plantar nerve with a branch from the medial plantar nerve at a site between the metatarsal heads. Other theories have implicated a local vascular degeneration of the bursa within the webspace. Jones and Singer[47] believe that the athlete with a hypermobile foot with excessive pronation is the prime candidate for Morton's neuroma and that it is commonly seen in basketball players and runners. The clinical signs include pain in the plantar aspects of the foot, particularly during push-off that is relieved by rest. Pain may be dull and throbbing; however, more classically it may radiate into the adjacent toes; for example, with the most common neuroma in the third webspace, the third and fourth toes are affected. On physical examination there may or may not be some paresthesias within the webspace of the toes. There may also be a positive compression sign in which the metatarsal heads can be squeezed together with resulting pain and radiating symptoms within the toes. In our opinion, conservative treatment is only marginally effective. The patient can try a wider toe box and shoe, metatarsal pads, and oral antiinflammatory medications. If these do not resolve the symptoms, which is typical, an injection of a local anesthetic and corticosteroid may be helpful in treatment and to provide the diagnosis. If these methods fail, surgical excision has been shown to give excellent results, with most patients subjectively improved. The largest series, performed by Mann and Reynolds,[61] showed that over 80% of patients improved. They recommended that a dorsal incision be used to avoid disturbing the plantar aspect of the foot with potential painful scar. Surgery removes the neuroma and leaves a sensory deficit within those toes but should resolve the pain. Reasons for surgical failure include hematoma formation and a symptomatic stump neuroma, which may be difficult to handle at a second surgical procedure. One suggestion for avoiding surgical failure is to resect the neuroma proximal to the transverse metatarsal ligament by obtaining an adequate exposure. In summary, Morton's neuroma has a classic history and abnormal physical examination findings that usually do not respond to conservative therapy, but surgical excision yields excellent results and return of the athlete to prior level of function.

SUMMARY

Acute neurovascular injuries are much more prevalent than chronic neurovascular problems in athletes but are usually recognized early and treated appropriately. This is in sharp contrast with chronic neurovascular conditions like CCS, popliteal artery entrapment syndrome, and nerve entrapments in which the diagnoses are either entirely missed or frequently delayed. These chronic conditions now have a reasonable clinical data base upon which to make the diagnosis and offer some suggestions for the rationale for treatment. However, secondary to their infrequent nature, large series are not available on the majority of these conditions. The recognition of these sometimes severely disabling conditions is imperative when it may potentially save the athletic career, such as in the case of a CCS or popliteal artery entrapment syndrome, or simply alleviate an athlete's fears of a worse condition, as in the case of an entrapment of a sensory nerve. This chapter has provided a review and a detailed framework on the history, physical examination findings, radiographic studies, and recommended treatment plan for chronic neurovascular conditions of the lower extremity. It is hoped that with more awareness of these conditions, more clinical series will be forthcoming, particularly outcome studies so that as time goes on, early recognition, better treatment, and quicker return to athletic activities are achieved.

ACKNOWLEDGMENTS

We thank Holly Quick (editorial assistance), Debbie Chessor (photography), Paul Gross (illustrations), and Robert Couch and Pat Post for their assistance in preparation of this chapter.

REFERENCES

1. Almdahl SM, Samdal F: Fasciotomy for chronic compartment syndrome, *Acta Orthop Scand* 60(2):210, 1989.
2. Amendola A et al: The use of magnetic resonance imaging in exertional compartment syndromes, *Am J Sports Med* 18(1):29, 1990.
3. Arnoldussen WJ, Korten JJ: Pressure neuropathy of the posterior femoral cutaneous nerve, *Clin Neurol Neurosurg* 82:57, 1980.
4. Bachner EJ, Friedman M: Injuries to the leg. In Nicholas JA, Hershman EB (eds): *The lower extremity and spine in sports medicine,* vol 1, ed 2, St Louis, 1994, Mosby.
5. Balaji MR, DeWeesse JA: Adductor canal outlet syndrome, *JAMA* 245:167, 1981.
6. Barabas AP, Macfarlane R: Popliteal artery entrapment syndrome, *Br J Hosp Med* 304, 1985.
7. Bell S: Repeat compartment decompression with partial fasciectomy, *J Bone Joint Surg* 68B(5):815, 1986.
8. Betts LO: Morton's metatarsalgia: neuritis of the fourth digital nerve, *Med J Aust* 1:514, 1940.
9. Bliss BO: Morton's neuroma: regressive and productive intermetatarsal elastofibrosis, *Arch Pathol* 95:123, 1973.
10. Bouhoutsos J, Daskalakis E: Muscular abnormalities affecting the popliteal vessels, *Br J Surg* 68:501, 1981.
11. Bourne RB, Rorabeck CH: Compartment syndromes of the lower leg, *Clin Orthop* 240:97, 1989.
12. Brozin IH et al: Traumatic closed femoral nerve neuropathy, *J Trauma* 22:158, 1982.
13. Cassells SW, Fellows B, Axe MJ: Another young athlete with intermittent claudication, *Am J Sports Med* 11:180, 1983.
14. Connell J: Popliteal vein entrapment, *Br J Surg* 65:351, 1978.
15. Cowan I: Localized popliteal artery abnormalities in otherwise fit young adults, *Australas Radiol* 29:268, 1985.
16. Cummings RJ et al: The popliteal artery entrapment syndrome in children, *J Pediatr Orthop* 12:539, 1992.
17. Delaney TA, Gonzalez LL: Occlusion of the popliteal artery due to muscular entrapment, *Surgery* 69:97, 1971.
18. Dewitt LD, Greenberg HS: Roller disconeuropathy, *JAMA* 246(1):836, 1981.
19. Di Cesare E et al: Poplital artery entrapment: MR findings, *J Comput Assist Tomogr* 16(2):295, 1992.
20. di Marzo L et al: Diagnosis of popliteal artery entrapment syndrome: the role of duplex scanning, *J Vasc Surg* 13(3):434, 1991.
21. di Marzo L et al: Surgical treatment of popliteal artery entrapment syndrome: a ten-year experience, *Eur J Vasc Surg* 5:59, 1991.
22. Durlacher L: Treatise on corns, bunions, the diseases of the nails, and the general management of the feet, London, 1845, Simption, Marshall.
23. Ecker AD, Woltman HW: Meralgia paresthetica: a report of 150 cases, *JAMA* 110:1650, 1938.
24. Edmonson HT, Crowe JA: Popliteal artery and venous entrapment, *Am J Surg* 38:657, 1972.
25. Eurvilaichit C: Popliteal artery entrapment syndrome (angiographic finding in one case report), *J Med Assoc Thai* 71(5):274, 1988.
26. Ezaki T et al: Popliteal artery entrapment: an unusual case, *J Cardiovasc Surg (Torino)* 27:53, 1986.
27. Fong H, Downs AR: Popliteal artery entrapment syndrome with distal embolization: a report of two cases, *J Cardiovasc Surg* 30:85, 1989.
28. Fronek J et al: Management of chronic exertional anterior compartment syndrome of the lower extremity, *Clin Orthop* 220:217, 1987.
29. Fujiwara H, Sugano T, Fujii N: Popliteal artery entrapment syndrome: accurate morphological diagnosis utilizing MRI, *J Cardiovasc Surg* 33:160, 1992.

30. Gaylis H, Rosenburg B: Popliteal artery entrapment syndrome, *S Afr Med J* 46:1071, 1972.
31. Gershuni DH et al: Ultrasound evaluation of the anterior musculofascial compartment of the leg following exercise, *Clin Orthop* 167:185, 1982.
32. Gibson MH et al: Popliteal entrapment syndrome, *Ann Surg* 185:341, 1977.
33. Goldman F: Intermetatarsal neuroma: light microscopic observations, *J Am Podiatr Med Assoc* 69:317, 1979.
34. Goodson JD: Pudendal neuritis from biking, *N Engl J Med* 304:365, 1981.
35. Gould N, Trevino A: Sural nerve entrapment by avulsion fracture of the base of the fifth metatarsal bone, *Foot Ankle* 2:153, 1981.
36. Gyftokostas D et al: Poststenotic aneurysm in popliteal artery entrapment syndrome, *J Cardiovasc Surg* 32:350, 1991.
37. Haddad M et al: The embolus-type of popliteal entrapment syndrome, *Vasa* (Bern) 19:63, 1990.
38. Hamming JJ: Intermittent claudication at an early age due to an anomalous course of the popliteal artery, *Angiology* 10:369, 1959.
39. Hamming JJ: Obstruction of the popliteal artery at an early age, *J Cardiovasc Surg* 6:516, 1965.
40. Hemler DE et al: Saphenous nerve entrapment caused by pes anserine bursitis mimicking stress fracture of the tibia, *Arch Phys Med Rehabil* 72:336, 1991.
41. Henrickson AS, Westlin NE: Chronic calcaneal pain in athletes: entrapment of the calcaneal nerve? *Am J Sports Med* 12:152, 1984.
42. Hoadley AF: Six cases of metatarsalgia, *Chicago Med Rec* 5:32, 1893.
43. Insua JA, Young JR, Humphries AW: Popliteal artery entrapment syndrome, *Arch Surg* 101:771, 1970.
44. Iwai T et al: Popliteal vein entrapment caused by the third head of the gastrocnemius muscle, *Br J Surg* 74:1006, 1987.
45. Jaivin JS, Fox M: Thigh injuries. In Nicholas JA, Hershman EB (eds): *The lower extremity and spine in sports medicine,* vol 2, ed 2, St Louis, 1995, Mosby.
46. Jikuya T et al: Popliteal artery entrapment syndrome of the monozygotic twin: a case report and pathogenetic hypothesis, *Jpn J Surg* 19(5):607, 1989.
47. Jones DC, Singer KM: Soft-tissue conditions of the ankle and foot. In Nicholas JA, Hershman EB (eds): *The lower extremity and spine in sports medicine,* vol 1, ed 2, St Louis, 1995, Mosby.
48. Kirby NG: Exercise ischemia in the fascial compartment of the soleus, *J Bone Joint Surg* 52B:738, 1970.
49. Kirk SJ, McIlrath EM, Peyton R: Tibial osteochondroma and popliteal artery compression, *Br J Clin Pract* 42(4):170, 1988.
50. Kooster NJJ, Kitslaar P, Janevski BK: Popliteal artery entrapment syndrome, *Forschr Röntgenstr* 148(6):624, 1988.
51. Kopell H, Thompson WAL: Knee pain due to saphenous nerve entrapment, *N Engl J Med* 263(7):351, 1960.
52. Kosinski C: The course: mutual relations and distribution of the cutaneous nerves in the metazonal region of the leg and foot, *J Anat* 60:274, 1926.
53. Krause KH, Witt T, Ross A: The anterior tarsal tunnel syndrome, *J Neurol* 217:67, 1977.
54. Lassmann G: Morton's toe: clinical, light, and electron microscopic investigation in 133 cases, *Clin Orthop* 142:73, 1979.
55. Leach RE, Punell MB, Saito A: Peroneal nerve entrapment in runners, *Am J Sports Med* 17(2):287, 1989.
56. Longo JM et al: Popliteal vein thrombosis and popliteal artery compression complicating fibular osteochondroma: ultrasound diagnosis, *J Clin Ultrasound* 18:507, 1990.
57. Lowe JX, Whelan TJ: Popliteal artery entrapment syndrome, *Am J Surg* 109:620, 1965.
58. Lysens RJ et al: Intermittent claudication in young athletes: popliteal artery entrapment syndrome, *Am J Sports Med* 11:177, 1983.
59. MacGregor J, Moncur JA: Meralgia paresthetica—a sports lesion in girl gymnasts, *Br J Sports Med* 1:16, 1977.
60. Madigan RP, McCampbell BR: Thrombosis of the popliteal artery in a jogger, *J Bone Joint Surg* 64A:1490, 1981.
61. Mann RA, Reynolds J: Interdigital neuroma: a critical analysis, *Foot Ankle* 3:238, 1983.
62. Martens MA, Moeyersoons JP: Acute and recurrent effort-related compartment syndrome in sports, *Sports Med* 9(1):62, 1990.
63. Martens MA et al: Chronic leg pain in athletes due to a recurrent compartment syndrome, *Am J Sports Med* 12:148, 1984.
64. Massey EW, Pleet AB: Neuropathy in joggers, *Am J Sports Med* 6:209, 1978.
65. Mavor GE: The anterior tibial syndrome, *J Bone Joint Surg* 38B(2):513, 1956.
66. McDonald PT et al: Popliteal artery entrapment syndrome: clinical, noninvasive, and angiographic diagnosis, *Am J Surg* 139:318, 1980.
67. Reference deleted in proofs.
68. McGuinness G et al: Popliteal artery entrapment: findings at MR imaging, *J Vasc Intervent Radiol* 2(2):241, 1991.
69. Meachim G, Abberton MJ: Histological findings in Morton's neuroma: regressive and productive intermetatarsal elastofibrositis, *Arch Pathol* 95:123, 1973.
70. Miller EH, Benedict FE: Stretch of the femoral nerve in a dancer: a case report, *J Bone Joint Surg* 67A:315, 1985.
71. Moller BN, Kadin S: Entrapment of the common peroneal nerve, *Am J Sports Med* 15(1):90, 1987.
72. Mubarak SJ, Hargens SL: Exertional compartment syndromes. In Mack R (ed): *AAOS symposium on the foot and leg in running sports,* St Louis, 1982, Mosby.
73. Mubarak SJ et al: Acute exertional superficial posterior compartment syndrome, *Am J Sports Med* 6:287, 1978.
74. Murphy PC, Baxter DE: Nerve entrapment of the foot and ankle in runners, *Clin Sports Med* 4(4):753, 1985.
75. Murray A, Halliday M, Croft RJ: Poplital artery entrapment syndrome, *Br J Surg* 78:1414, 1991.
76. Ohta M et al: Popliteal artery entrapment syndrome: report of two cases, *J Cardiovasc Surg* 32:697, 1991.
77. Olcott C, Mehigan JT: Popliteal artery stenosis caused by a Baker's cyst, *J Vasc Surg* 4(4):403, 1986.
78. Pace JB, Nagle D: Piriformis syndrome, *West J Med* 124:435, 1976.
79. Pedowitz RA et al: Modified criteria for the objective diagnosis of chronic compartment syndrome of the leg, *Am J Sports Med* 18(1):35, 1990.
80. Plihal E et al: Mononeuropathie d'enclavement du nerf fessier supérieur, *Schweiz Rundschau Med (PRAXIS)* 78(12):326, 1989.
81. Puranen J, Alavaikko A: Intracompartmental pressure increase on exertion in patients with chronic compartment syndrome in the leg, *J Bone Joint Surg* 63A(8):1304, 1981.
82. Reneman RS: The anterior and lateral compartmental syndrome of the leg due to intensive use of the muscles, *Clin Orthop* 113:69, 1975.
83. Represa JAF et al: Popliteal artery entrapment syndrome, *J Cardiovasc Surg* 27:426, 1986.
84. Rich NM, Hughes CW: Popliteal artery and vein entrapment, *Am J Surg* 113:696, 1967.
85. Rignault DP, Pailler JL, Lunel F: The "functional" popliteal entrapment syndrome, *Int Angiol (Torino)* 4:341, 1985.
86. Romanoff M et al: Saphenous nerve entrapment at the adductor canal, *Am J Sports Med* 17(4):478, 1989.
87. Rorabeck CH: Exertional tibialis posterior compartment syndrome, *Clin Orthop* 208:61, 1986.
88. Rorabeck CH, Bourne RB, Fowler PJ: The surgical treatment of exertional compartment syndrome in athletes, *J Bone Joint Surg* 65A(9):1245, 1983.
89. Rorabeck CH et al: The role of tissue pressure measurement in diagnosing chronic anterior compartment syndrome, *Am J Sports Med* 16(2):143, 1988.
90. Sammarco GJ: Dance injuries. In Nicholas JA, Hershman EB: *The lower extremity and spine in sports medicine,* vol 2, ed 2, St Louis, 1995, Mosby.
91. Schurmann G et al: The popliteal artery entrapment syndrome: presentation, morphology, and surgical treatment of 13 cases, *Eur J Vasc Surg* 4:223, 1990.

92. Servello M: Clinical syndrome of anomalous position of the popliteal artery, *Circulation* 26:585, 1962.
93. Sieunarine K et al: Entrapment of popliteal artery and vein, *Aust N Z J Surg* 60:533, 1990.
94. Soffer SR et al: Chronic compartment syndrome caused by aberrant fascia in an aerobic walker, *Med Sci Sports Exerc* 23(3):304, 1991.
95. Solheim LF et al: The piriformis muscle syndrome: sciatic nerve entrapment treated with section of the piriformis muscle, *Acta Orthop Scand* 52:73, 1981.
96. Spitell JA Jr: Some uncommon types of occlusive peripheral arterial disease, *Curr Probl Cardiol* 8(8):1, 1983.
97. Stewart JD et al: Sciatic neuropathies, *BMJ* 287:1108, 1983.
98. Stuart TPA: Note on a variation in the course of the popliteal artery, *J Anat Physiol* 13:162, 1879.
99. Styf J: Diagnosis of exercise-induced pain in the anterior aspect of the lower leg, *Am J Sports Med* 16(2):165, 1988.
100. Styf J: Compression of the superficial peroneal nerve: results of treatment by decompression, *J Bone Joint Surg* 71B:131, 1989.
101. Styf J, Körner LM: Chronic anterior compartment syndrome of the leg, *J Bone Joint Surg* 68A(9):1338, 1986.
102. Styf J, Körner LM: Diagnosis of chronic anterior compartment syndrome in the lower leg, *Acta Orthop Scand* 58:139, 1987.
103. Styf J, Körner L, Suurkula M: Intramuscular pressure and muscle blood flow during exercise in chronic compartment syndrome, *J Bone Joint Surg* 69B(2):301, 1987.
104. Sutherland S: The relative susceptibility to injury of the medial and lateral popliteal divisions of the sciatic nerve, *BMJ* 41:2, 1953.
105. Tate RO, Rustin JT: Morton's neuroma: its ultrastructural anatomy and biomechanical etiology, *J Am Podiatr Med Assoc* 68:797, 1978.
106. Tsairis P: Peripheral nerve injuries in athletes. In Jordan BD, Tsairis P, Warren RF (ed): *Sports neurology*, Rockville, Md, 1989, Aspen Publishers.
107. Venna N, Bielawski M, Spatz EM: Sciatic nerve entrapment in a child: case report, *J Neurosurg* 75:652, 1991.
108. Verta MJ, Vitello J, Fuller J: Adductor canal compression syndrome, *Arch Surg* 119:345, 1984.
109. Wang-Jia-ju et al: Popliteal artery entrapment syndrome: a report of two cases, *J Cardiovasc Surg* 29:480, 1988.
110. White SM, Witten CM: Popliteal artery entrapment syndrome, *Arch Phys Med Rehabil* 71:601, 1990.
111. Wiley JP et al: Ultrasound catheter placement for deep posterior compartment pressure measurements in chronic compartment syndrome, *Am J Sports Med* 18(1):74, 1990.
112. Williams LR et al: Popliteal artery entrapment: diagnosis by computed tomography, *J Vasc Surg* 3(2):360, 1986.
113. Xethalis JL, Lorei MP: Soccer injuries. In Nicholas JA, Hershman EB (eds): *The lower extremity and spine in sports medicine,* vol 2, ed 2, St Louis, 1995, Mosby.

PART VII Sport-Specific Injuries

CHAPTER 60

Skiing Injuries

J. Richard Steadman
Robert R. Scheinberg

Each year, more Americans are traveling to ski resorts as the popularity of skiing continues to grow. As participation increases, so does the number of ski injuries. The incidence of total number of injuries, however, has decreased over the past 20 years.[32,33,36] Most skiers are between 20 and 35 years old and are healthy, relatively athletic, and participate skillfully in other sports when they are not skiing (Fig. 60-1). Physical activity and fitness are personally gratifying; therefore even after injury they

are unwilling to accept a sedentary lifestyle. Their loyalty to the sport makes a rapid and safe return to the slopes a matter of highest priority.

Because of the massive migration of skiers from warm weather areas to ski country, physicians in nonski areas must also be familiar with the management of skiing injuries, the physiologic demands of the sport, and the psychologic motivations of skiers. The injuries of both the competitive and dedicated recreational skier demand a dynamic regimen that treats the injury while maintaining cardiovascular and neuromuscular fitness during the healing period. Physicians also treat novice skiers for injuries. These injuries may be managed less aggressively, but in a manner that helps the patient to return to his or her chosen level of activity.

The skier's injury usually occurs away from home. Thus the treatment must be initiated out of the patient's local area, possibly creating several problems. The approach to a specific injury may be different in the ski area than in the location where the injury is followed up. With this in mind, treatment in the ski area should be correlated with follow-up care in the patient's home town. The physician in the ski area must determine what is an emergency and what is not a true surgical emergency. Indications for immediate surgical procedures are neurovascular complications, open wounds, or swelling to a dangerous degree. Rarely is a ligament repair a true emergency. Instead it becomes more an "emergency of convenience" that can be carried out either at the ski area or in the skier's home town.

This chapter provides a practical approach to the treatment of orthopaedic injuries that skiers sustain. Emergency procedures, surgical alternatives, rehabilitation programs, and other guidelines are described in the subsections, which are divided by anatomic site. The most commonly injured areas, the tibia and knee, are emphasized. These sections are preceded by an overview that provides some observations and information on the differences in ski terrain and equipment safety, physiologic requirements of the sport, and profiles of the ski patrol and the skier at risk. The references provide dimensions and information that cannot be incorporated into the scope of this chapter.

SKI TERRAIN AND EQUIPMENT

Skiers and ski area physicians are usually knowledgeable about the differences in ski terrain, snow conditions

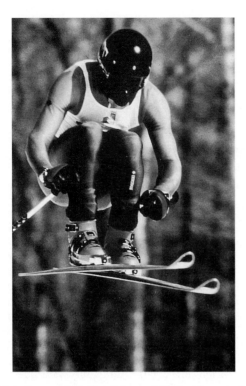

FIG. 60-1. Competitive skier airborne following jump in downhill race. (Photo by Tom Lippert.)

during the ski season, and equipment. Different ski techniques are required for hard-packed and soft snow; different techniques are also required for downhill and cross-country skiing. Skiers are alerted by the area management daily, sometimes hourly, of the ski conditions, and maps of slopes are available for beginning, intermediate, and advanced skiers. Skiers must choose the runs appropriate for their ability level. Skiers also have the responsibility of ensuring that their equipment is adequate and that the bindings are adjusted and in proper working order. Thus the skier assumes considerable responsibility for his or her own safety.

Factors affecting ski technique

- Hard-pack vs. soft snow
- Downhill vs. cross-country skiing
- Slope conditions
- Terrain variability
- Slope degree of difficulty
- Weather conditions

The physician treating skiers from the hard-packed slopes of Vermont and New Hampshire may see different injuries from the physician treating skiers on Western slopes that have softer snow conditions.[71] For example, Johnson et al[37] found that injuries to the thumb were almost exclusively caused by the pole strap; our experience in the West suggests that the injury to the ulnar

collateral ligament of the thumb is almost exclusively the result of jamming the outstretched thumb into soft snow.

In 1980 Johnson et al[37] reported that 80% of the lower extremity injuries were potentially equipment related. After 6 years the equipment-related injuries appeared to have decreased 37%. The improvement of binding function with regard to release and torques led Johnson and his associates to conclude that better binding function was directly related to the decrease in equipment-related injuries. They also observed that trail grooming, the safety consciousness of area management, and manufacturers' efforts to provide safety features in equipment may be factors related to the lower percentage of injuries.[37]

Ski equipment is being tested for safety and the improvement of safety features by such organizations as the American Society for Testing Materials (ASTM). This impartial group evaluates equipment and assesses research being conducted at universities or in the manufacturers' laboratories.

Several other factors account for the change in injury patterns. Skis themselves have changed and are generally shorter than they were years ago. Additionally, their composition and aerodynamic and biomechanical characteristics have been altered. Consequently, the "Arlberg" rotation style skiing of years past has been replaced by faster cutting and jumping techniques.

Changes in ski boot height and construction have also affected injury patterns (Fig. 60-2). The incidence of severe ankle injuries and "boot-top" tibia fractures has significantly decreased. This is, in part, a result of the higher, stiffer boots now in use. However, rotational injuries can still occur, causing injuries to the lateral malleolus and tibia. Knee injuries, particularly to the anterior cruciate ligament, have increased dramatically; these may also be related to boot height.[32-34,36,37]

PHYSIOLOGIC REQUIREMENTS

Skiing requires both aerobic and anaerobic conditioning. This has been documented in studies by Karlsson et al[38] and Eriksson, Nygaard, and Saltin.[21] The physiologic demands on the body during Alpine skiing require a skier to be in excellent physical condition before the skiing vacation. Activities that seem to correlate well with Alpine skiing include bicycling, uphill running, and ski-specific exercises for maintenance and improvement of proprioception and athletic agility. Sprinting is helpful, but is not specific as a training aid. Racquet sports appear to correlate fairly well with Alpine skiing. Downhill

---

Aerobic activities that correlate with alpine skiing

- Bicycling
- Uphill running
- Racquet sports
- Specific ski exercises
- Side-to-side agility exercises
- Downhill slalom running

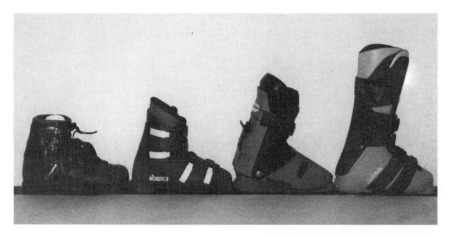

FIG. 60-2. Ski boot changes have affected injury patterns in skiing.

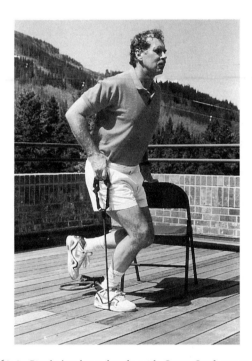

FIG. 60-3. Single-leg knee bends with Sport Cord using closed-chain kinetic exercise.

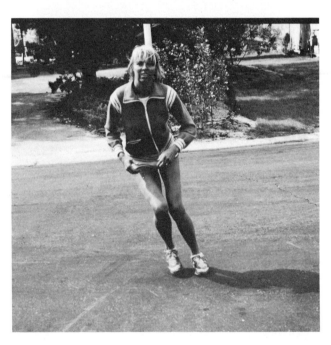

FIG. 60-4. Active preski exercise emphasizing absorption. Skier transfers from one foot to the other, emphasizing absorption and resulting in dynamic eccentric and concentric contractions.

slalom running is the most specific but tends to aggravate any preexisting knee problems.

A Sport Cord (surgical elastic tubing) program that uses closed-chain kinetic exercises, including double-leg knee bends, single-leg knee bends, and side-to-side agility drills, has been found to develop excellent muscle endurance and proprioception, concentrating on ski-specific muscles (Fig. 60-3).[41]

The U.S. Ski Team uses a year-round program that emphasizes maintenance of strength, power, endurance, and athletic agility. These skiers have demonstrated the importance of continuing exercise programs during the season and throughout the off season. Particular emphasis is placed on quadriceps muscle endurance because this muscle group maintains the body position in space. Because of the up-and-down nature of the sport, both concentric and eccentric contractions are emphasized (Fig. 60-4). Skiing places a high demand on the slow-twitch muscle fibers, particularly in the quadriceps muscle group. This is true not only in high-intensity skiing, but also in relaxed, recreational skiing. Consequently, quadriceps muscle endurance exercises are important in any skier's conditioning program.

Upper body and mid-body strength and power main-

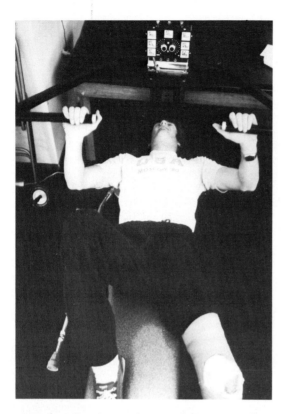

FIG. 60-5. Bench press for upper body conditioning.

tenance are also important in skiing. The athlete's ability to maintain an athletic position and to balance against gravitational forces requires upper body conditioning. This can be accomplished by concentrating on muscle endurance and strength exercises (Fig. 60-5).

Nutritional maintenance is also a factor in body conditioning for skiers. Eriksson, Nygaard, and Saltin[21] and others have shown that including complex carbohydrates in the diet during a ski vacation can help maintain the glycogen levels in muscle fibers.[10,42] Hence a restriction of carbohydrates during a ski vacation seems unwise.

SKI PATROL

The ski patrol is a group comprising 26,000 individuals working in the United States, Asia, and Europe. Members must pass annual refresher courses on rescue techniques, cardiopulmonary resuscitation (CPR), and first aid, which are administered by the local ski area

management. A majority of members of the ski patrol are volunteers. The volunteer status is usually determined by the local ski area management. As a prerequisite for being trained as a member of the ski patrol, the individual must have passed a winter emergency care course and hold a current CPR certificate.

The ski patrol carries emergency medical supplies and equipment for splinting. Procedures for transporting the injured skiers from the slopes are described in manuals and texts published by the National Ski Patrol System.

The physician at the local ski area should take the responsibility for working with the ski patrol in training them to differentiate between such injuries as hip dislocation and hip fracture. Splinting techniques and life- or limb-saving procedures should be taught as well. The physician's working relationship with members of the ski patrol may ultimately save skiers' lives. At the scene of an accident the ski patrol has the responsibility for immediate first aid, splinting, and transfer to a treatment facility. Unless requested by the ski patrol, advice from physician skiers on the mountain should be minimal.

SKIERS AT RISK

Persons who have not maintained body conditioning, who have not obtained and maintained proper equipment, who have not had adequate instruction, who attempt slopes beyond their ability, or who ignore the ski area's warnings of hazardous conditions are at risk of injury. These are all factors over which the skier has control.

Other persons at risk in the skiing population include skiers with degenerative conditions related to previous injuries; skiers with patellofemoral problems; skiers who have anatomic susceptibility, particularly internal femoral torsion and external tibial torsion that create patellar subluxation with resultant chondromalacia of the patella; or skiers with significant patella plica syndrome. Skiers with a previous meniscectomy, particularly the lateral, are at risk because executing a turn places great pressure on the lateral compartment (Fig. 60-6). Finally, skiers with ligamentous insufficiency within the knee run a considerable risk of injury.

For the less dedicated skier, a change to a less demanding and hazardous sport is preferable if he or she is in an at-risk category. For the dedicated skier, wearing prescribed knee braces to prevent excessive knee angulation and to protect insufficient ligaments is helpful. Supporting the unweighted arch with foot pads or orthot-

---

Skiers at risk

Factors under skier's control	Factors over which skier has no control
■ Poor physical condition	■ Degenerative joint disease
■ Improper equipment	■ Patellofemoral problems
■ Improperly maintained equipment	■ Anatomic susceptibility
■ Inadequate instruction	■ Previous meniscectomy (particularly lateral)
■ Poor choice of skiing terrain	■ Ligamentous insufficiency
■ Ignorance of hazardous conditions	

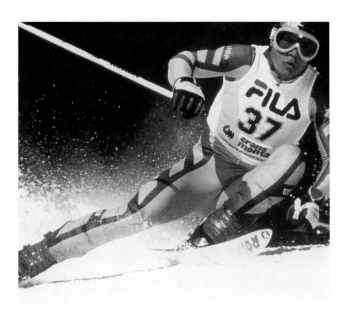

FIG. 60-6. Pressure is placed on lateral compartment while skiing. (Photo by Tom Lippert.)

ics can be protective in patients with patellofemoral problems. Wearing a neoprene sleeve with or without a patellar cup is helpful because it provides some stability and warmth. The at-risk skier's choice of well-groomed slopes instead of icy or heavily moguled ones increases the number of years he or she can enjoy skiing.

INCIDENCE AND EPIDEMIOLOGY

Ski injuries are generally reported as injuries per 1000 skier days. The overall incidence of ski injuries appears to be declining over the past several years from 7.4 injuries per 1000 skier days to 2.6 injuries per 1000 skier days.[32-34,36,37] Most of the decline is attributed to an approximately 60% decrease in lower extremity injuries.[34,37] In addition, the pattern of injury in the lower extremity has also changed. There has been marked decrease in ankle sprains and tibia fractures and an increase in severe ligamentous sprains to the knee.

Level of ability plays an important role in the incidence of injuries. Beginners are three to four times more likely to sustain an injury than experienced skiers.[8,18,19,34,37] Gender and age are also important factors. Women traditionally have a higher injury rate than men. Children have a slightly higher incidence of injury than adults, especially of spiral tibial fractures.[8,50,71] It remains unclear whether taking lessons can influence the incidence of ski injuries.[8]

In comparison to other sports, skiing is relatively safe. For example, per 1000 skier days skiing has an injury rate of 2.6, whereas high school football has an injury rate of 810, tennis has an injury rate of 30, and swimming has an injury rate of 10. The competitive skier, however, has a much higher incidence of injury than the recreational skier, and in fact, virtually all sustain an injury of some sort while skiing.

HIP INJURIES

The ski patrol must be able to differentiate between dislocations of the hip and fractures of the hip. A skier with a posterior hip dislocation has flexion and internal rotation; a skier with anterior dislocation has flexion and external rotation. The skier with a fracture of the hip has external rotation without flexion. The dislocated hip is a true medical emergency. A traction splint is contraindicated. The patient must be provided immediate transportation to a facility that can proceed with reduction of the dislocation. It is essential that this be done as soon as possible because it may prevent avascular necrosis.[20,47]

After immediate reduction with either intravenous sedation or general anesthesia the hip should be tested for stability. The patient then can be placed in Buck's traction for comfort until muscle spasm has subsided. A computed tomography (CT) scan of the hips can be performed to rule out loose bodies, femoral head, or acetabular lip fractures and to ensure a congruent reduction. Partial weight-bearing ambulation with crutches is allowed immediately. There is no general agreement as to when full weight bearing and sports can be resumed, but cardiovascular maintenance can continue with well-leg and upper body exercises. The patient should be monitored for avascular necrosis for 1 to 2 years after injury.

The skier with a fracture of the hip can be transported from the slope or splinted using either the uninjured extremity or a traction splint occasionally. The ski patrol should be aware that concomitant factors such as blood loss, effects of altitude, and wind chill are life threatening to the injured skier. After the diagnosis is confirmed, early open reduction is the treatment of choice. Criteria for selection of the fixation devices are the same as for other hip fractures. A compression hip screw is the generally accepted and widely used fixation device. Its use generally allows early motion and early ambulation. Closed nailing should be considered, particularly for the subtrochanteric area. Second generation interlocking nails have proved particularly helpful in this area.[17]

FEMUR FRACTURES

Femoral fractures are caused by rotatory forces or direct blows. Blood loss, soft-tissue injury, altitude, and wind chill factors make early evacuation from the site of injury as important with femoral fractures as with hip fractures. The skier should be transported from the hill with the extremity in a traction splint. At the hospital the physician should confirm the diagnosis and proceed with immediate stabilization of the fracture. Closed intramedullary nailing is the current method of choice for most femur fractures.[9] Interlocking nails have made treatment of spiral and comminuted fractures easier and have shortened the rehabilitation period. Early weight bearing and rapid progression to full weight bearing is encouraged with most fracture patterns. Alternative methods of treatment include plate fixation or traction. Plate fixation has the advantage of allowing early motion, but the disadvantage of requiring a prolonged non–weight-bearing period, extensive soft-tissue dissection, and a significant period of protection after removal of the plate and screws.

High altitude	
Higher incidence fat embolism	

The possibility of symptomatic **fat embolism** seems more likely at high altitudes as a result of the relatively low normal Po_2. The patient should be monitored closely for this during the first few days of hospitalization with regular checks for petechiae, sensorium changes, pulse rate, hemoglobin, hematocrit, and arterial Po_2. If symptoms develop, immediate oxygen therapy should be instituted. If severe symptoms develop, positive end-expiratory pressure (PEEP) should be initiated. Early fixation within the first 24-hour period has been shown to decrease the incidence of pulmonary embolus, reduce hospital costs, and reduce overall complications following femoral fractures.[7,31]

Rehabilitation should begin immediately following stabilization of the femoral fracture and should include hip and knee range of motion exercises, upper body exercises, and cardiovascular maintenance with well-leg cycling.

OTHER LOWER EXTREMITY FRACTURES, DISLOCATIONS, AND SPRAINS
Intercondylar Fractures

Intercondylar fractures are uncommon in skiing. Open reduction and internal fixation is required to exactly reapproximate the joint surfaces and allow for continued satisfactory range of motion. These fractures are generally fixed with a dynamic compression screw (DCS) or plate and screws.[52] Bone grafting may be necessary in severely comminuted fracture patterns. A cast brace or hinged brace can add some support during the healing process. The patient is usually not allowed to bear weight for approximately 3 months. If the fixation is rigid and the repair is stable, the patient can begin early range of motion exercises of the injured extremity. This precludes contracture, especially in the suprapatellar pouch, which is difficult to treat after immobilization of the knee. If the fixation is not rigid and the knee must be immobilized, motion should begin as soon as early union is apparent on radiographs. In either case, exercise of the opposite extremity and upper extremities combined with general body conditioning should begin immediately and be continued throughout the healing period. The patient should begin swimming as soon as possible and begin stationary bicycling at the first signs of union. Use of continuous passive motion is appropriate in the early non–weight-bearing period.

Patellar Injuries

Fractures and dislocations of the patella are relatively uncommon ski injuries. **Patellar dislocation** is a fairly minor injury in skiing, but because of its appearance beneath ski clothing, it must be differentiated from a complete knee dislocation. If the patella is dislocated (usu-

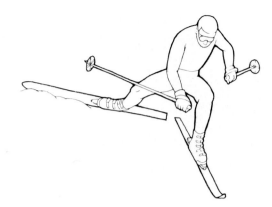

FIG. 60-7. Valgus external rotation injury resulting in patellar dislocation.

ally caused by a valgus and rotational force as a result of catching a ski edge in the snow) (Fig. 60-7), it may be reduced on the slope before the patient is transported to the clinic.

Fractures of the patella are treated surgically if there is displacement greater than 2 mm or if there is complete disruption of the extensor mechanism.[30,52] Treatment methods are the same for the skier's fractured patella as for treatment of the fractured patella of other athletes. Tension band wiring with Kirschner wires or screws is the treatment of choice.[74] This procedure permits the skier to begin early motion and flexion-extension of the knee. Through the surgical procedure the articular surface of the patella can be protected and reapproximated. This seems to give the best chance for return to skiing. Care must be taken to follow the rehabilitative range of motion exercises to avoid contracture, which interferes with skiing later.

Severely comminuted proximal or distal pole fractures should be treated by partial patellectomy and reattachment of either the quadriceps tendon or patellar tendon, respectively.[30] Rehabilitation, except for passive motion, is delayed for approximately 4 to 6 weeks to allow soft tissue–to–bone healing.

Occasionally, patellectomy is necessary. Skiing can continue after the patellectomy, but rarely at the same level as before surgery. This is preferable to the end-stage degenerative patella, which allows no activity requiring knee flexion and extension.

Dislocations of the patella are sometimes complicated by accompanying avulsion fractures and articular cartilage injuries. On the radiographic examination after reduction the physician should scan the films closely for the possibility of loose bodies in the joint. If these are identified, arthroscopy may be indicated; if not, closed treatment with a knee immobilizer, cylinder cast, or cast brace and later a patellar support brace is the treatment of choice. If dislocations become recurrent, a patellofemoral mechanism realignment may be necessary either by an open procedure or by arthroscopy with lateral release. Should locking symptoms develop, the knee must be examined for fragments of articular cartilage within the

---

**Criteria for return to skiing after
patellofemoral injury**

- Full range of motion
- Absence of quadriceps or hamstring contracture
- Documented muscle parity
- No effusion
- No tenderness

**Common types of tibial fractures encountered
in skiers**

- Tibial plateau fractures
- Distal tibial plafond fractures
- Avulsion fractures of the tibial spine
- Isolated tibial fractures
- Tibia-fibula fractures

---

joint that are not visible on ordinary x-ray films. If fragments are identified, the knee should be treated by an arthroscopic procedure. Magnetic resonance imaging (MRI) may help in diagnosing articular cartilage fragments within the joint that are not seen on ordinary x-ray films.

The skier with patellofemoral injury should not resume skiing until substantial function of the quadriceps mechanism is regained. Rehabilitation must include eccentric and concentric contractions of the quadriceps mechanism.

Tibial and Fibular Injuries

In the last few years the incidence of fractures of the tibia has been lower in skiers than previously reported.[34,37,71] Injuries to the tibia, however, are still seen frequently by ski area physicians. These include fractures of the tibial plateau, isolated tibial fractures, fractures of both the tibia and the fibula, and distal tibial plafond fractures. Avulsion fractures of the tibial spine are mentioned in the subsection Knee Joint Injuries and Their Mechanisms. A number of basic principles of treatment are common to all lower extremity injuries sustained by the skier. These include the principles of well-

leg exercise, upper extremity exercise, and general cardiopulmonary maintenance.

Tibial Plateau Fractures

Displaced tibial plateau fractures require accurate reduction and rigid internal fixation. The use of either a buttress plate and screws or buttress screws with or without bone grafting is indicated (Figs. 60-8 and 60-9).[52,63] The weight-bearing surface is evaluated radiographically and with tomograms or a CT scan, if necessary. A 10-degree caudad view or oblique views may also be of value to define the fracture anatomy and evaluate the joint surface. Ligamentous injuries are assessed by physical examination with or without anesthesia. Care should be taken not to compress the tibial plateau during the physical examination. The menisci may be evaluated either with an MRI or arthroscopically before fracture fixation.

Dye punch fractures and some lateral compression fractures can be treated with a combined arthroscopic and "mini open technique." The arthroscope is used to evaluate the articular cartilage step-off, whereas an anterior cortical window is used to elevate the depressed fragments. Bone graft can be inserted through the cortical window as well. With this technique the joint sur-

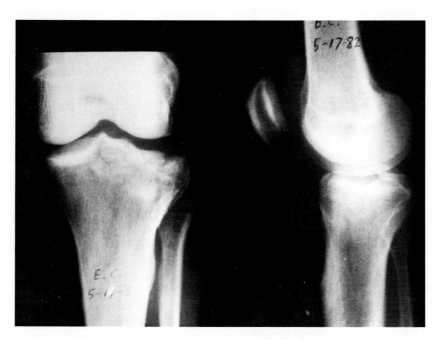

FIG. 60-8. Radiograph of comminuted tibial plateau fracture.

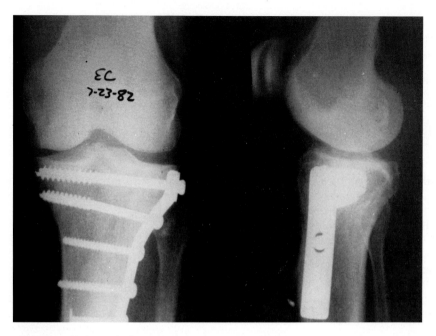

FIG. 60-9. Radiograph showing rigid fixation of tibial plateau fracture after bone graft.

face can be reduced anatomically with minimal soft-tissue interruption, and a buttress screw can be placed percutaneously, if needed.

If rigid fixation is obtained either with open reduction and internal fixation or by arthroscopic technique, a cast brace is used with early motion but without weight bearing for approximately 8 weeks. If rigid fixation cannot be obtained, distal tibial traction can be used with early motion. Use of continuous passive motion exercise seems particularly beneficial in comminuted intraarticular fractures because of its effect on articular cartilage.[60]

General body conditioning should be maintained with upper body, mid-body, upper extremity, and opposite leg exercise even during the period of non–weight bearing. If fixation is solid, riding on a stationary bicycle with no resistance is used to encourage joint articular cartilage nutrition, capsular compliance, and muscle tone. At approximately 8 weeks partial weight bearing is begun using crutches. This progresses to full weight bearing, which is governed by the radiographic appearance of the fracture site. Use of two crutches is encouraged during partial weight bearing to simulate more normal gait patterns. The minimum requirement for return to skiing is adequate remineralization as determined by radiographic evidence. The skier should resume the sport on smooth, groomed runs of soft snow. Skiing on hard-packed with ice and "chatter" should be avoided for approximately a year.

Isolated Tibial, "Explosion," and Combined Tibiofibular Fractures

Fractures of the skier's tibia usually is the result of a rotational force or occasionally a direct blow. On the slope the skier's leg should be brought into position for splinting (Fig. 60-10). Any dangers involved in this maneuver are counter-balanced by the likelihood of damage to soft tissues if the skier is transported with the limb unsplinted. Multiple splints are available. The old cardboard box splint is effective if properly applied. The air splint is another simple device used for protection of the extremity. After the limb is splinted at the site, the patient should be treated at a nearby facility. Swelling and compartment syndrome problems preclude transportation in one of the splints for long distances.

Emergency room treatment should include adequate radiographic evaluation and assessment of the fracture, soft-tissue swelling, and neurovascular status. The general condition of the patient should also be monitored. The physician must consider the distance the patient must travel in selecting treatment alternatives. We suggest that the patient be hospitalized locally for 1 to 3 days if travel distance is significant. During this time the patient is monitored closely for neurovascular or compartment complications, as well as for fat embolism.

Although the isolated tibial fracture may not be displaced significantly in the anterior, posterior, or lateral plane, generally, there is a rotational component. This should be checked carefully in the emergency room. The rotational deformity, if left uncorrected, can be a limiting factor in athletic and daily life. Reduction of an uncomplicated tibial fracture can be performed in the emergency room. Reduction may be delayed in cases where marked swelling in the extremity is present on arrival to the emergency room. These injuries are usually "explosion" fractures in which considerable energy is dissipated into the soft tissues of the leg at the time of the fracture (Fig. 60-11). These fractures can be splinted initially, placed in a bivalved cast, or placed in skeletal traction. Strict elevation is maintained until the neurovascular status is settled and reduction can be done.

If reduction is performed on admission, the patient is

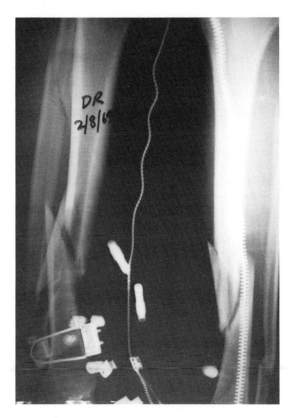

FIG. 60-10. Tibial fracture in position for splinting.

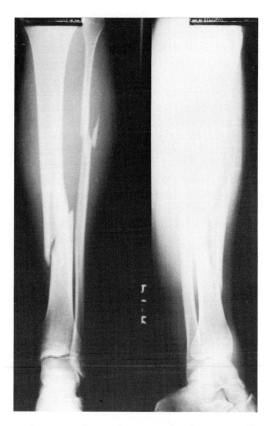

FIG. 60-11. "Explosion" fracture with soft-tissue swelling.

placed in a supine position on a gurney. The leg is hung over the side of the gurney with 90 degrees of flexion at the knee, and reduction is performed with light manual traction and rotation. This reduction can usually be done with intravenous analgesia or intravenous regional anesthetic. Occasionally, general anesthetic is required. A long leg cast is applied after verification of alignment, radiographically. The patient is hospitalized and observed for neurovascular status.

Acceptable alignment is generally considered to be less than or equal to 1 cm of shortening and an angular deformity of less than or equal to 5 degrees of varus-valgus angulation or anterior-posterior angulation. Rotational deformity is difficult to measure and evaluate; however, ± 5 degrees of rotational deformity is acceptable.[16,52,59,61]

If the neurovascular status is satisfactory, the patient can begin weight bearing immediately.[16,61] When the patient is not ambulating, the limb should be continuously elevated. If numbness or weakness develops in the

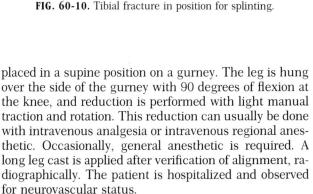

Acceptable tibial fracture position

- ≤ 1 cm shortening
- ≤ 5 degrees varus-valgus or anterior-posterior angulation
- ≤ 5 degrees rotational deformity

toes, the cast and cast padding should be opened. If there is any question of cast pressure, the cast and cast padding should immediately be relieved in the affected area.

If there is a question about closed **compartment syndrome,** a catheter should be placed in the limb compartments to monitor pressures, and the values should be followed closely.[45,51] If opening the cast or cast padding does not relieve the symptoms of a closed compartment syndrome or any other neurovascular complications that develop, immediate release of the compartment or other appropriate surgical intervention should be performed. If no signs of compartment syndrome or neurovascular complications develop, the patient is discharged from the hospital with a partial weight-bearing cast when the neurovascular status is stable and he or she is ambulatory. Diaphyseal fractures of the tibia and fibula are more likely to develop shortening and angular deformity. If shortening is suspected, leg length studies are frequently helpful in assessing leg length inequality. This is particularly important in patients who had preexisting leg length difference with the injured leg shorter before the injury. Without this information it is difficult to give the patient advice about the final outcome of the fracture treatment.

If angulation develops, wedging with the aid of an image intensifier can be done up until the stage of fibular healing, about 4 to 6 weeks after injury. If an anterior compression fracture is present, a closed reduction can be done, leaving the posterior angulation. The reduction can then be completed with an opening wedge placed anteriorly in the cast.

After 2 to 6 weeks the cast can be changed to a total contact cast. Once the contact cast has been worn for 2 weeks, which is approximately 5 weeks after the injury, the patient can usually begin full weight bearing. A cast brace can then be applied at this point and continued until clinical union is confirmed radiographically.[62]

Ambulatory treatment is almost universally successful in healing these fractures.[16,61,62] In ambulatory treatment the acceptance of a stable position usually creates an excellent environment for early union. The use of early weight-bearing techniques encourages the fracture to assume this stable position.

As in isolated tibial fractures the advantages and disadvantages of the early weight-bearing technique should be explained to the patient.

If any of these contradictory circumstances exist, open reduction or closed nailing must be considered. Fractures with metaphyseal involvement or articular cartilage

---

**Contraindications for ambulatory treatment
of tibial fractures**

- Patient's refusal
- Unwillingness to accept angular or rotational deformity
- Unacceptable alignment
- Closed compartment syndrome
- Extension of fracture into articular surface
- Multiple-injured patient
- Obesity

---

involvement or those with proximal comminution are particularly well suited for the AO-ASIF fixation plates and screws according to the techniques described by Müller et al[52] Diaphyseal fractures usually can be treated with a closed intramedullary nail using several alternatives in nails. Tibial interlocking nails have made the treatment of segmental and comminuted fractures much easier with the advantages of little, if any, soft-tissue stripping, ease of insertion, and a shortened rehabilitation period that allows early partial and full weight bearing (Figs. 60-12 and 60-13).[6,39]

External fixation with either a standard frame or an Ilizarov frame is rarely indicated in the treatment of ski injuries. These methods should be reversed for open fractures or severely comminuted metaphyseal fractures and for surgeons experienced with the application of these devices.

Rehabilitation varies slightly, depending on the method of fixation. The closed ambulatory group may begin active exercise for the injured extremity at the time of weight bearing. Stationary bicycling is increased and resistance is added as weight bearing progresses.

Patients with rigid fixation using A-O plates or screws can begin mobilization immediately, but they must delay weight bearing. Six weeks after the injury they can begin toe-touch exercises and progress to full weight bearing as bony union occurs. This is confirmed by radiographic and physical findings. Patients with intramedullary nailing may begin weight bearing as soon as they can tolerate it. Postoperative rehabilitation then coincides with the program for closed reduction cases. All patients, of course, should participate in upper body,

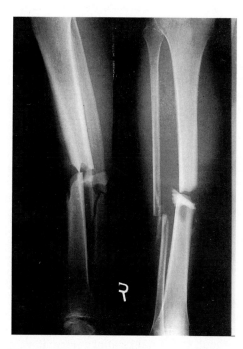

FIG. 60-12. Radiograph of comminuted tibiofibular fracture.

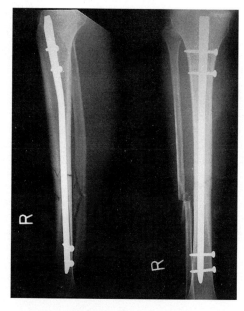

FIG. 60-13. Radiograph showing near-anatomic alignment of comminuted tibiofibular fractures after intramedullary nail fixation locked proximally and distally.

upper extremity, and uninjured extremity conditioning exercises throughout the period of recovery. Patients may return to skiing when the physician judges the density of the bone to be adequate and the fracture is healed as confirmed by radiographic and physical findings. It should be appreciated that a prolonged period of stress is required to obtain the elasticity that is helpful in avoiding a repeat fracture.

Distal Tibial Plafond Fractures

Intraarticular fractures of the distal tibial plafond are complicated in their treatment and rehabilitation. This is a "demand fracture" because it should be treated with open reduction and internal fixation if rigid fixation is possible. If not, traction and early motion should be considered.

The technique of fixation has been well described by Ruedi and Allgoweer.[58] First, the fibula is rigidly fixed internally; then the tibia is fixed rigidly through a separate incision. Spoon or T-plate fixation may be used in addition to interfragmental screw compression. Bone grafting is performed as needed. Kirschner wires are sometimes helpful in holding the fragments in reduced position. Prophylactic antibiotics are appropriate in these difficult fractures. Immediate postoperative treatment includes splinting in the neutral position and early passive and active motion (Fig. 60-14). The patient should be hospitalized until swelling is diminished and acceptable motion is obtained. The wound should be clean when the patient is discharged. Muscle tone across the joint can be maintained with light manual resistive exercises. After the patient regains 60% to 80% of motion in the ankle, the physician must decide if this extremity should be placed in a cast. A short-leg orthosis is suggested so that the patient may continue light resistive exercises. Stationary biking with slight resistance and swimming

---

Treatment of displaced tibial plafond fractures
■ Open reduction and internal fixation: first, rigid fixation of fibula, followed by rigid fixation of the tibia with bone graft, if necessary
■ Splint in neutral ankle position
■ Remove splint for early active and passive motion
■ Maintain muscle tone with light manual resistive exercises
■ When 60% to 80% of normal motion is regained, apply short-leg orthosis and continue resistance exercises
■ Stationary bicycle when motion and muscle tone are adequate
■ Weight bearing depending on radiographic evidence of healing

can be used as the ankle resumes its motion and protective muscle tone.

The patient should remain non–weight bearing for 8 weeks and then advance to partial and full weight bearing, depending on the radiographic evidence of healing. Using these principles, good results were obtained in 13 of 15 patients and fair results with the other two patients.[66,73]

Avulsion Fractures of the Tibial Spine

The important factor in treatment of avulsion fractures of the tibial spine is assessment of the anterior cruciate ligament (ACL). If no major stretching of the ligament has occurred, accurate relocation of the tibial spine, either by closed reduction or surgical intervention, should be performed. Closed reduction is usually successful by obtaining full extension of the knee. Aspiration of the hemarthrosis and intraarticular injection of lidocaine may make the patient more comfortable and facilitate the reduction. Surgical intervention, either open or arthro-

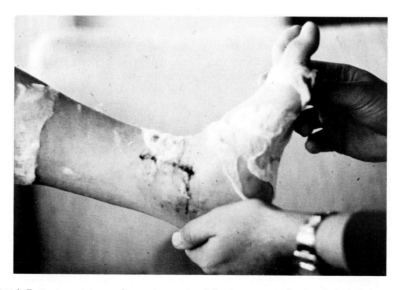

FIG. 60-14. Patient receiving early passive motion following surgery for distal tibial plafond fracture.

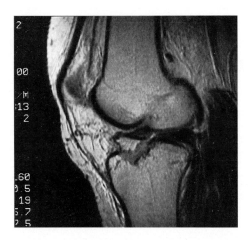

FIG. 60-15. Magnetic resonance imaging scan showing tibial spine fracture with attached anterior cruciate ligament.

scopic, is performed if the tibial spine cannot be adequately reduced while closed.

If the ACL fibers are found to be stretched, countersinking of the tibial attachment should be performed, either arthroscopically or open. Occasionally, a primary reconstruction is indicated. Arthroscopy may be required to adequately assess the fibers of the ACL, although MRI has been found to be accurate in defining these injuries as well (Fig. 60-15).[49]

If the ligament is damaged, the same precaution should be used as described in the cruciate injuries subsection to prevent deforming loads on this healing ligament. If no stretch is present in the cruciate ligament, this can be treated as a fracture and activities can begin as soon as healing of the fracture site has been accomplished.

Isolated Fibular Fractures

Isolated diaphyseal fractures of the fibula require only limited protection. These fractures were frequent when high ski boots were initially introduced because of their stiffness. Since the upper portion of the boot has been softened, these fractures have become infrequent. When they do occur, use of any extremely high boot that extends to just below the tibial plateau can avoid further stress at the fracture site and allow for earlier return to skiing.

Peroneal Tendon Dislocations

During the time when the low, soft boot was the one most commonly worn, dislocation of the peroneal tendons was a common skier injury. Since the adoption of the higher, stiffer boot, only severe forces cause peroneal tendon dislocations. Loose-fitting boots subject the skier to injuries of this type. This injury must be distinguished from injury to the lateral ligaments of the ankle. If the latter is suspected, stability of the peroneal tendons and their peroneal retinaculum behind the fibula must be defined first before beginning treatment for the ankle ligament.

If there is instability of the peroneal tendons and sur-

gical treatment is chosen, the groove, which is frequently shallow, should be deepened and the retinaculum repaired. Plain x-ray studies are occasionally helpful in identifying retinacular avulsion fractures (Fig. 60-16). If the lateral ligament is also injured, it can be repaired at the same time. Immobilization is continued for 1 week without bearing weight, followed by 5 weeks in a walking cast.

These injuries can be treated without surgery, but the simplicity of immediate repair combined with the relative difficulty of latent reconstruction make early surgical repair the preferred alternative.

Syndesmosis Sprain

Syndesmosis sprain is a relatively frequent injury caused by *external rotation* of the foot in skiing. The ankle twists to the outside, resulting in pressure on the syndesmosis. The key factor in diagnosis is tenderness in the syndesmosis area. If this is present, the return to skiing is delayed. This injury usually requires 6 weeks of protection to heal satisfactorily, but after 6 weeks the patient can generally return to the same level of skiing. If there is significant widening of the syndesmosis, surgery should be considered.

Ankle Fractures

Fractures of the ankle occur secondary to twisting or compression injuries. These may be less common than they were when skiers wore the soft boot, but they still occur. The majority are isolated to the lateral malleolus, but with the extension of rotational forces, bimalleolar and trimalleolar fractures can occur. Combination injuries with unimalleolar fractures coupled with ligament injuries must be suspected and ruled out when these unimalleolar fractures are present.

With no tenderness medially and a normal mortise, lateral malleolus fractures may be treated nonoperatively. More than 2 mm of lateral shifting and any shortening is not acceptable because either of these can lead to abnormalities of the ankle joint and accelerate degeneration.[43,52] Stable fibular fractures with less than a 2-mm shift can be treated with a short leg cast or orthotic device, and the patient should be not bear weight for 10 days. Weight bearing can then begin as tolerated, but the fracture should be reevaluated radiographically during the first 2 weeks to confirm that no shift at the fracture site or change in the mortise has occurred. If shortening or shift does occur, open reduction should be performed (Fig. 60-17).

Bimalleolar and trimalleolar fractures are demand fractures. Casting alone delays motion and can cause an unacceptable amount of stiffness or a poor anatomic result. Open reduction and internal fixation of both the medial and lateral malleoli, according to the A-O methods, is recommended.[52] A removable splint is used postoperatively. The limb should be mobilized, and the patient should remain in the hospital for approximately 3 days for this mobilization. Before any permanent immobilization the patient should regain 60% to 80% range of motion. Full weight bearing should not begin until about 2 weeks after immobilization. The timing of weight bearing de-

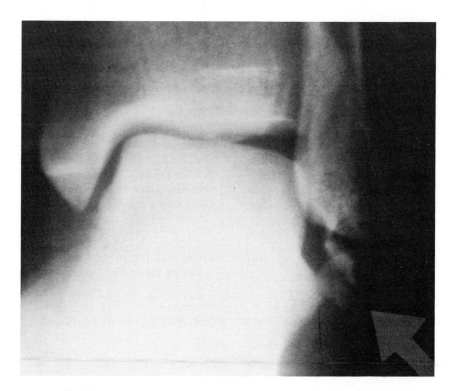

FIG. 60-16. Avulsion fracture of fibula created by dislocation of peroneal tendons.

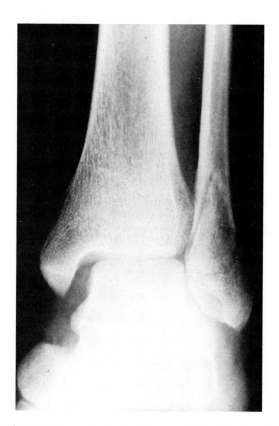

FIG. 60-17. Radiograph showing fracture of distal fibula with rupture of deltoid ligament.

pends on the security of the fixation. The posterior malleolus is stabilized with internal fixation if 25% or more of the joint surface is involved.[46]

The rehabilitation program is similar to the program for treatment of patients with tibial plafond fractures, although weight bearing can usually begin earlier for patients with ankle fractures.

Tarsal, Metatarsal, and Phalangeal Fractures

Fractures of the foot bones are so rare in skiers that treatment for these fractures are not be discussed in this chapter. (See Chapter 24 for discussion of foot fractures.)

Epiphyseal Fractures

The principles of treatment of epiphyseal fractures are the same in skiing as with any epiphyseal injury. Stress views or an MRI may aid in the diagnosis of subtle fractures. Fixation that does not cross the epiphysis is desirable. If a fixation device must cross the epiphysis, smooth pins are recommended. Delayed weight bearing is also helpful in these injuries. The use of spacers to allow continued growth has proven to be a great help in patients who have an epiphyseal arrest.

KNEE JOINT INJURIES AND THEIR MECHANISMS

This section emphasizes the injuries surrounding the knee joint that involve the ligamentous tissue, menisci, and plicae. The interrelationship of fractures discussed in the preceding section, particularly the intercondylar, patellar, and tibial plateau fractures, should not be minimized.

The more subtle physical findings that frequently went undiagnosed in the past are identified in this section.

Meniscal Injuries

All the properties of the meniscus are important to the skier, but particularly important are its stabilization effect, its energy-absorbing capacity, its ability to transmit load, and its ability to spare the intraarticular cartilage. Isolated meniscal injuries do occur in skiing. Either the medial or lateral meniscus may be torn. Accurate diagnosis, preferably confirmed with MRI and arthroscopy, is the key to determining the location of the injury, the extent of the tear, and the differentiation between meniscal injuries and other problems.[28] A preoperative MRI is particularly helpful when the point of tenderness is the posteromedial corner of the meniscus, the area most difficult to visualize arthroscopically. Other problems (e.g., medial plica, infrapatellar plica syndrome, and articular cartilage defects), simulate pathologic conditions of the meniscus.[25,55]

Arnoczky et al[4] have shown that the peripheral 15% to 30% of the meniscus has blood supply and can heal. The adverse long-term effects of meniscectomy and the favorable results of meniscal repairs have allowed more aggressive treatment of meniscal tears.[11,26,35,72] Historically, because of the available blood supply, the red-red and red-white tears were the only tears that were attempted to be repaired. However, Henning et al[26] reported various methods of repairing white-white complex and radial tears with some success. The torn edges of the meniscus are punctured and roughened using a needle or various rasps that provide vascular channels and a roughened surface that maintain a clot near the stabilized tear. This clot acts as a collagen bridge and increases the chances of healing.

When arthroscopy is considered for a skier who has sustained an injury to the meniscus, the physician should discuss with the patient the alternatives of meniscal repair vs. partial excision. Meniscal repair results in a longer delay in returning to activity. The long-term benefits, however, are significant as the meniscus regains its preinjury function. Partial meniscectomy has a shorter delay in return to activity, but it results in loss of the multiple protective effects of the intact meniscus.

Collateral Ligament Injuries
Medial Collateral Ligament Sprains, Grades I and II

Sprains of the medial collateral ligament (MCL) are common ski injuries and are more common in women than in men. The sprains usually result from the skis rotating with no binding release or the boots catching in snow after the binding releases. The force created that causes the MCL injury can also injure the ACL. With this in mind, patients who are treated for MCL sprains should be closely observed for the possibility of an ACL rupture. Once this is ruled out, treatment of the MCL injury can continue.

If the injury is limited to a Grade I sprain, no immobilization is needed. This precludes the expense of a hinged orthotic knee brace. The patient can be instructed in ambulating on crutches to allow weight bear-

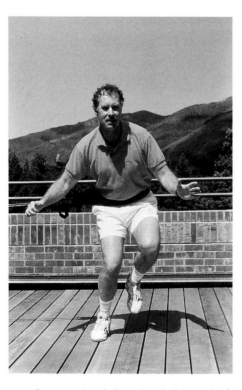

FIG. 60-18. Agility drills with aid of Sport Cord.

Treatment of Grade I medial collateral ligament injuries in skiers

Stage I
- Initial immobilization with a simple knee immobilizer or nothing
- Weight bearing as tolerated
- Stationary bicycling
- Early active extension-flexion exercises
- Closed-chain kinetic exercises

Stage II (pain free)
- Ambulation and full weight bearing without protection
- Walking and running in water
- Progressive resistance exercises
- Stretching exercises

Stage III
- Kicking in water
- Proprioceptive exercises

Stage IV
- Agility drills (ski specific)
- Running straight ahead

Stage V
- Cutting
- Return to sports after documented strength gains, flexibility, and proof of athletic ability including eccentric loading, power, balance, and proprioception

ing to tolerance. If a knee immobilizer or splint is used, the splint can be removed for knee extension-flexion exercises and stationary bicycling. As soon as these activities can be performed pain free, the athlete can progress to walking without crutches and walking and running in water. Kicking in water should be the next step, followed by agility and proprioceptive exercises. Before returning to athletics, training should be done in both concentric and eccentric contractions, and athletic ability should be proven with a series of agility drills (Fig. 60-18).[65]

Treatment of Grade II medial collateral ligament injuries in skiers

Stage I
- Early protection of knee with a hinged orthotic knee brace (30 to 90 degrees of allowed motion)
- Remove brace for stationary bicycle
- Weight bearing as tolerated with crutches
- Active extension-flexion exercises in brace
- Closed-chain kinetic exercises

Stages II to IV
- Treatment identical to that for Grade I injuries

If the injury is diagnosed as a Grade II sprain, early protection of the knee within the 30- to 90-degree range with a hinged orthotic knee brace is preferable. The treatment is the same as for the Grade I injury with the exception of protection with the brace. The brace can be removed for stationary bicycling and then reapplied. This exercise can begin immediately after the injury. As with Grade I injuries the patient should refrain from skiing until ligament integrity and athletic ability are restored and proven.

Medial Collateral Ligament Sprains, Grade III

The severity of these sprains forces the physician and patient to decide on a surgical or nonsurgical course of

---

Criteria for return to skiing after medial collateral ligament injury

Grade I
- Equal quadriceps function in both legs
- Full range of motion
- Maintenance of physiologic conditioning through bicycling, swimming, etc
- No evidence of instability on reevaluation after initial spasm has resolved

Grade II
- All requirements for Grade I
- Evidence of stability on physical examination (usually 6 to 8 weeks)
- Athletic bracing may be desirable

Grade III
- All requirements for Grades I and II
- 12 or more weeks if nonoperative treatment was elected; approximately 24 weeks if operative course is chosen

---

treatment. If the patient has no other injury, the physician in the ski area can allow the patient to return home for further treatment.

If a nonsurgical course of treatment is chosen, a hinged knee brace in the 30- to 90-degree range may be applied.[67] Exercise can begin immediately after the injury. Increasing amounts of extension and flexion exercises can be done, using closed-chain kinetic exercises. The progression is the same as for Grade I and II sprains. In this case the brace is worn for 6 to 8 weeks. For Grade III MCL sprains with rotational laxity, examination of the knee with an MRI or arthroscopy (primarily to determine the condition of the meniscus) is recommended. If there is an anteromedial rotational instability and a peripheral detachment of the meniscus (assuming a knee in which the remainder of the joint is intact, including the cruciate ligaments), a posteromedial incision of 2 to 3 inches is made to repair the meniscus, the posterior oblique ligament, and the MCL. The procedure is essentially extraarticular with the exception of suture through the meniscus. This procedure has been successful in treatment of higher level athletes in whom fear of meniscus loss is great. After the operative procedure the patient's knee is immobilized in a hinged knee brace for approximately 8 weeks, allowing 30 to 90 degrees range of motion. At the conclusion of the immobilization, bicycling is begun and rehabilitation progresses in the same sequence as described for Grades I and II sprains. If no anteromedial instability or meniscus tear is present, a hinged knee brace may be used and rehabilitation can begin in the same sequence.

Approach to Grade III medial collateral ligament injuries in skiers with normal anterior cruciate ligament

- Magnetic resonance imaging or arthroscopic evaluation of meniscus, if indicated
- If anteromedial rotational instability is absent, treat meniscus appropriately and treat patient's ligament injury with a hinged knee orthosis as described for Grade II sprains
- If anteromedial rotational instability is present, repair all structures as necessary (medial collateral ligament, posterior oblique ligament, and medial meniscus)

Posterior Cruciate Ligament and Posterolateral Corner Injuries

Although injuries to the posterior cruciate ligament (PCL) and posterolateral corner are rare in skiers, they do occur. Accurate diagnosis is imperative. Instability of the posterolateral ligament complex is frequently missed or unappreciated.[5]

Diagnosis of PCL instability is made by a combination of tests, including posterior drawer, posterior sag, and hamstring effect at 90 degrees (quadriceps active test). Instrumented testing using either the KT-1000 (Medmetric, San Diego) or CA-4000 (Orthopaedic Systems

Inc., Hayward, Calif.) can help quantitate the posterior instability. Diagnosis of posterolateral rotatory instability is made by the external rotation recurvatum test, the posterolateral drawer test, and the reverse pivot shift test.[29] MRI is useful in defining the extent of the injuries to the PCL and the posterolateral corner and ruling out meniscal or other related knee injury.[28]

If the injury to the PCL is determined to be slight, as evidenced by MRI and instrumented testing showing ≤ 5 mm posterior side-to-side difference, conservative treatment is generally recommended. A hinged knee brace is applied and set at 0 degrees of flexion and extension. Passive motion is encouraged from 0 to 60 degrees for the first 2 weeks, and then 0 to 90 degrees thereafter.

Knee bends are started immediately at 0 to 20 degrees of flexion in the brace. A rehabilitation program emphasizing quadriceps strengthening is begun at 4 weeks. When meniscal injury is present, arthroscopic evaluation of the PCL can be performed and direct probing of the ligament can help determine whether further treatment is necessary. Patients with more severe injuries or greater than 5 mm posterior side-to-side difference or who fail conservative treatment are offered surgical repair or the reconstruction of the PCL.

At surgery an attempt is made to approach the PCL through the intercondylar area and a posteromedial arthroscopic portal. The intercondylar notch is widened medially, and the femoral and tibial attachments of the PCL are visualized. If the ligament is torn from the tibia or femur, it is possible through this widened intercondylar notch to pass drills from either the anterior tibia or the anterior femur into the appropriate point on the joint. ACL drill guides can aid in accurate placement of these drill holes. The area of femoral or tibial attachment is roughened, and a trough is made with a curet. Sutures are then pulled into the joint through drill holes, and the ligament is tightened from the anterior area. Occasionally a posterior approach is necessary.

Reconstruction of the PCL is performed using either an allograft or the central third of the patellar tendon as a bone-tendon-bone autograft. Bone tunnels are made in the tibia and femur after accurate arthroscopic placement of the drill guides. The bone blocks are secured using interference screws.

In cases of posterolateral rotational instability, the posterolateral complex is repaired. If there is some question about the stability, advancement can be done in this area.[5] For chronic cases a biceps tenodesis may be indicated to correct posterolateral instability.

Rehabilitation is started immediately. A hinged knee brace set at 0 degrees of flexion and extension is used.

Passive motion beyond this point can begin 4 weeks after the repair. The remainder of the rehabilitation program mirrors a rehabilitation program for ACL injuries, with the exception of deemphasis on the hamstrings and more emphasis on strengthening the quadriceps.

Anterior Cruciate Ligament Injuries

The ACL is frequently injured in skiing. *Complete ACL tears represent 66% of all knee injuries compared with 16% 15 years ago.*[34] The diagnosis was often missed in the past, but with better understanding of the pathomechanics, history, and examination, the proper diagnosis is now frequently correctly made. Equipment changes may have contributed to the increase in cruciate injuries. The higher, more supportive ski boot, coupled with binding improvements to diminish tibial fractures, may explain the relative increase in ACL injuries.

There are three common mechanisms of injury for ACL tears in skiing. First, and possibly the most common, is an external rotation valgus moment to the knee, which commonly occurs when the skier catches a ski tip on a gate or in the snow (Fig. 60-19). As the skier continues downhill on the opposite weighted limb, the moment arm caused by the unweighted ski places a larger torque across the knee joint, frequently resulting in MCL, meniscal, and ACL tears.

Another common mechanism is hyperextension–in-

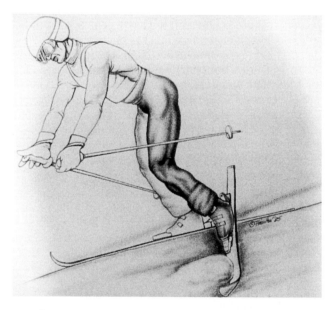

FIG. 60-19. External rotation and valgus stress of knee leading to ligament and possible meniscal damage.

Mechanisms of anterior cruciate ligament injury	
■ External rotation	Catching a ski tip on a gate or snow
■ Hyperextension–internal rotation	Crossing the ski tips or catching the outer edge of ski in the snow
■ Direct anterior translation	Landing from a jump or mogul

ternal rotation during a forward fall. This deceleration-type injury can occur when a skier crosses the ski tips or catches the outer edge of the ski in the snow, leading to sudden internal rotation and hyperextension of the knee. The internal rotation injury may also be associated with a "phantom fall" seen in beginner skiers. Their weight falls backward while their ski curves inward. As

the ski continues to internally rotate, the ACL subsequently ruptures (Fig. 60-20).

The third mechanism occurs from direct anterior translation of the tibia on the femur. This injury usually occurs in more advanced skiers during landing from a jump or a mogul. The skier falls backward as the back of the skis hit the snow, causing hyperflexion of the knee

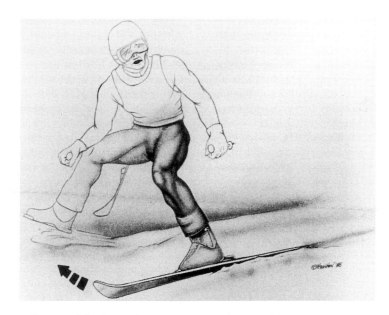

FIG. 60-20. "Phantom fall." Internal rotation stress on knee as ski carves a turn inward and skier falls backward, leading to rupture of anterior cruciate ligament.

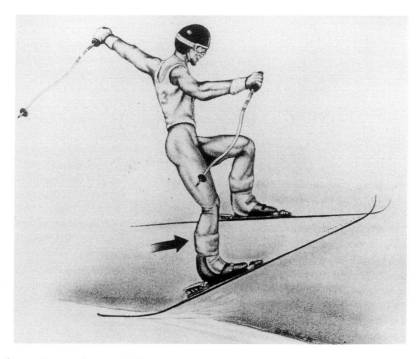

FIG. 60-21. Anterior forces of ski boot and quadriceps muscles in an attempt to recover from forced flexion leading to rupture of anterior cruciate ligament.

(Fig. 60-21). A combination of the anterior drawer produced by the anterior force of the boot top on the calf and the anterior pull of the quadriceps trying to recover from this hyperflexed position causes anterior subluxation of the tibia and subsequent rupture of the ACL.

The history and physical findings of ACL insufficiency have been described by Noyes, Bassett, and Grood[53] and DeHaven.[15] A "pop" in the joint and immediate effusion, coupled with a feeling of instability when first bearing weight on the extremity, are presumptive evidence of an ACL injury.

The Lachman test has proved more accurate than other tests in making this diagnosis.[40] Other tests, including the anterior drawer test, pivot shift maneuver, and rotational stress test, are also important in assessing the severity of the ACL injury. A large effusion can eliminate the physical findings and may require aspiration. Tight hamstrings may do the same thing and should be relaxed for the examination. Instrumented testing with either the KT-1000 or the CA-4000 can help quantitate the anterior translation of the tibia on the femur and more accurately define the side-to-side difference in anterior translation (Fig. 60-22).[13,14] A side-to-side difference in anterior translation of more than 3 mm is thought to be significant and usually indicates a tear in the ACL. Radiographic findings, such as a lateral capsular sign, indicate a possible anterolateral rotational injury with a resultant avulsion fracture of the distal attachment of the lateral capsular ligament.[75] Radiographs may also show avulsion fractures of the tibial spine avulsed by the ACL. They also rule out tibial plateau fractures and loose bodies.

MRI is extremely accurate in detecting ACL injuries.[28] MRI can determine whether the ligament is torn from its tibia or femoral attachments or if it is a midsubstance tear or has intrasubstance changes, representing a stretching of the ligament. MRI is also helpful in detecting other knee injuries frequently associated with ACL injuries such as meniscal tears, collateral ligament sprains, condylar defects, or bone bruising.

If MRI is not available or if the diagnosis is still in doubt, arthroscopy allows direct visualization of the ligament and allows probing to make a definitive diagnosis of the degree of cruciate ligament injury. The menisci can also be evaluated and repaired if tears are identified.

The extent of examination and the determination of whether the patient should be treated at the local ski medical facility depend on a number of factors, primarily the length of time the patient will be in the area. If the patient plans to travel home immediately, then treatment should be undertaken at home. If the patient elects to remain in the area, a complete examination and treatment can be initiated.

The timing of ACL reconstruction remains controversial. Several papers have shown an increased incidence of arthrofibrosis following reconstruction when surgery was performed during the acute period, 0 to 3 weeks following the injury.[24,48,64] However, if the patient shows negligible swelling and satisfactory range of motion, surgery need not be delayed. An active postinjury protocol can help diminish swelling and improve range of motion. A hinged knee brace allowing 10 to 90 degrees of range of motion, ice, elevation, passive range of motion exercises, and stationary bicycling can decrease the patient's pain, swelling, and stiffness, allowing earlier treatment of the injured ligament.

Although Higgins and Steadman[27] reported good success with repair of the injured ACL in elite skiers, most authors currently recommend reconstruction for complete tears. The advantage of quicker return to skiing

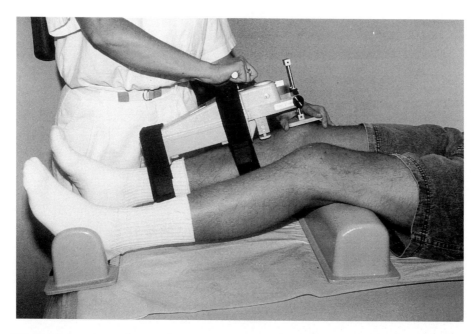

FIG. 60-22. Instrumented testing for anterior translation of the tibia using KT-1000. (Courtesy Medmetric, San Diego.)

with a repair or a ligamentodesis has been negated by recent advancements in ACL reconstruction and rehabilitation techniques. Immediate graft fixation, the superior pull-out strength of interference screws, and the superior strength of bone–patellar tendon–bone autograft have all allowed earlier range of motion and more aggressive rehabilitation, including early weight bearing and quadriceps strengthening.[56,58] These advancements have significantly shortened the time from injury to return to skiing. Therefore repairs are currently only recommended in rare cases.

ACL reconstruction is generally recommended to patients who demonstrate ACL insufficiency and plan to continue to ski or continue an active lifestyle that involves running, jumping, or cutting sports. Age should not dissuade a patient from reconstruction because recent reports have shown excellent results following ACL reconstruction in patients over the age of 40.[44] Before reconstruction, patients must be fully aware of the 6- to 12-month healing time required before their knee is fully recovered, and they should be willing to make an extreme commitment to their knee during this period. Alternatively, patients can be treated nonoperatively with rehabilitation. If they continue to have symptoms of instability, an ACL reconstruction can be performed at that time.

Patients with ACL insufficiency who do not plan on continuing to ski or who plan to have a lifestyle that is relatively sedentary should not be encouraged to undergo a reconstruction. Rather, they should be taught a rehabilitation program that emphasizes hamstring and quadriceps strengthening and encouraged to use a functional knee brace during vigorous activities or work.

Partial injuries to the ACL, as evidenced by instrumented measurements of no more than 3 mm of side-to-side difference, minimal or no pivot shift, MRI evaluation, or direct visualization and probing arthroscopically, are generally treated conservatively or by arthroscopically creating a fracture or a healing response at the anatomic site of avulsion. A hinged knee brace is applied, allowing 10 to 90 degrees of range of motion. Full weight bearing is encouraged, and standard ACL rehabilitation, described in the next section, is started immediately. Patients can begin light sporting activities with a functional knee brace 3 months following injury.

ACL reconstruction is recommended to patients with complete or partial ACL tears as evidenced by instrumented measurements showing at least 3 mm side-to-side difference, a gross pivot shift, MRI evaluation, or direct visualization and probing of the ligament showing significant fiber disruption. Reconstruction is performed using the central third of the patella tendon as a bone-tendon-bone autograft. Fixation is usually performed with interference screws.

Immediate postoperative protocol includes a hinged knee brace allowing 10 to 90 degrees of range of motion, cryotherapy, continuous passive motion, and antiinflammatory medication while the patient is in the hospital (Fig. 60-23). This protocol decreases postoperative swelling and pain and facilitates painless range of motion. Weight bearing is progressed from partial to full as the patient tolerates it. Passive range of motion from 0 to 120 degrees must be obtained and maintained before discharge from the hospital.

Rehabilitation plays a major role in the outcome of ligament reconstruction surgery. Early motion, weight bearing, and functional rehabilitation, which have been made possible by the improvements in the surgical technique of ACL reconstruction, are the cornerstone for a successful rehabilitation program.[56,68]

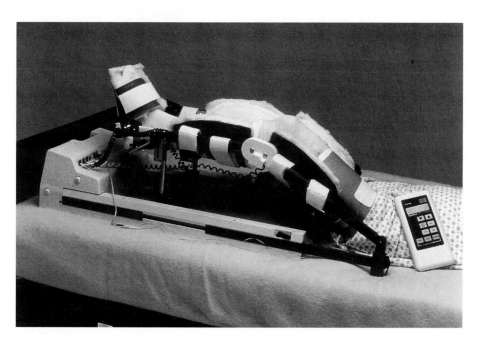

FIG. 60-23. Patient's lower extremity resting in continuous passive motion machine.

TABLE 60-1 Closed-chain vs. open-chain exercise

Category	Open Chain	Closed Chain
Axis of motion	Motion only distal to axis of joint	Motion is both proximal and distal to axis of joint
Muscle contraction	Emphasis is concentric	Concentric, eccentric, isometric
Movement	Usually isolated	Functional; muscles working in unison
Loads	Skeletal loads are artificial and are often abnormal	Normal physiologic loads are created through skeletal system
Stress and strain	Biomechanically inconsistent stress and strain within soft tissues and joints	Biomechanically consistent stress and strain within tissues and joints
Stabilization	Provided through artificial means	Provided through normal postural means
Planes of motion	Typically occurs in one of the cardinal planes of motion	Combination of motion occurs in all three planes, consistent with motion of joints and structures
Reaction	Provides action and less reaction to movement	Provides both action and reaction to certain movements
Balance and coordination	Typically requires no balance and little coordination during activity	Requires both balance and coordination during activity

Motion, which was once discouraged during the early rehabilitation period, has been found to be helpful for ligament healing, articular cartilage nutrition, and soft tissue and capsular contraction prevention.[1-3,54] Stress without deformation is desirable for collagen healing and stimulates formation of the collagen along the lines of stress.

These principles, coupled with **closed-chain kinetic physical therapy** have improved the outcome of ACL reconstruction. The concept of closed-chain kinetics described by Sterndler[70] in 1955 refers to a combination of several successively arranged joints in which the terminal joint meets with some considerable resistance, prohibiting or restraining it from movement. Weight-bearing activities are closed chain, whereas free knee extensions are open chain. Greg[23] described the advantages of closed- vs. open-chain kinetics (Table 60-1).

Rehabilitation encompassing closed-chain kinetics and early range of motion should be started immediately postoperatively. A hinged knee brace allowing 10 to 90 degrees of range of motion is recommended for the first 6 weeks. These brace settings essentially allow full extension but prevent hyperextension or hyperflexion, thus avoiding rupture or stretching of the graft. Full weight bearing and full passive range of motion are encouraged immediately. Double-leg, one-third knee bends and seated quadriceps and hamstring strengthening with a Sport Cord for resistance is started on the first day postoperatively. Well-leg bicycling is also started as soon as possible, and upper body, trunk, and aerobic conditioning are continued throughout the rehabilitation course (Fig. 60-24).

At 2 weeks after the injury, both-leg bicycling and deep-water running with a buoyancy vest are allowed. The deep-water running allows excellent aerobic exercise and range of motion while eliminating the adverse effects of impact encountered during weight-bearing exercise.

The patient is progressed to single one-third knee bends and forward and backward walking with elastic re-

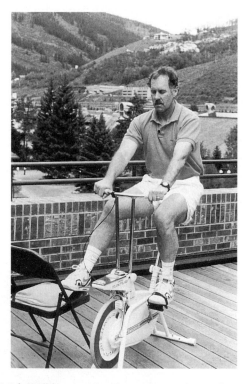

FIG. 60-24. Well-leg exercises for cardiovascular conditioning can be performed on stationary bicycle.

sistance from 6 to 12 weeks. Rowing, increased resistance bicycling, and use of a stair-stepper are also incorporated at this time. Side-to-side movement and light agility exercises with elastic resistance are begun at 12 weeks. Strength and endurance exercise with free or machine weights and low-level athletic skills are added at 20 to 24 weeks if range of motion and strength allow. Generally, skiers are ready to return to groomed skiing at 5 to 6 months and aggressive skiing at 6 to 8 months. A functional knee brace that limits hyperextension and may add proprioception is recommended for approximately 1 year.

The rehabilitation protocol should be modified as treatment of associated injury, such as meniscal tears or articular cartilage defects dictate. Repaired vertical meniscal tears generally allow full weight bearing and range of motion, but these patients may not be allowed to participate in water therapy until 6 to 8 weeks. Patients with repaired radial or complex meniscal tears are generally kept from bearing weight and are restricted on range of motion and water therapy.

Articular cartilage defects are frequently associated with ACL tears and dramatically alter the rehabilitation program. These defects are currently treated by attempting to stimulate ingrowth of fibrocartilage into the defects.[57] This is done by making multiple microfractures through the subchondral plate with a curved awl in the area of the defect. This allows blood to pool in the area, providing a clot and a medium for fibrocartilage to form. Continuous passive motion, which has been shown to have a beneficial effect on healing cartilage, is continued for 8 weeks and patients are kept non–weight bearing for this period as well. Water exercise and gentle bicycling are encouraged and begin between 0 and 2 weeks.

Knee Dislocation and Its Ramifications

Knee dislocation is a serious injury for anyone, particularly a skier (Fig. 60-25).[69] When a skier is injured on the slope, the limb should be splinted in its dislocated position, and the skier should be evacuated immediately to a facility where diagnostic studies can be done to determine the extent of the injury. During evacuation the ski patrol should be aware of limb-threatening factors such as neurovascular status.

At the local facility the patient's neurovascular status should be determined before examination of the injury. The evaluation of pulses and neurologic function is mandatory and can be limb saving. A Doppler apparatus is helpful in differentiating the normal pulse from a collateral pulse. The knee should then be reduced and once again neurovascular status evaluated. If pulses are absent or even diminished, immediate arteriogram is indicated. If the limb is pulseless and arteriography is not available or would delay arterial repair for longer than 6 hours after injury, immediate exploration should be considered. If neurovascular status is clinically adequate, the patient's knee is placed in a brace set at 30 degrees of flexion. Surgery is postponed until it is proved that no delayed vascular occlusion is present and swelling diminishes, usually in 3 to 7 days. The extremity is elevated, and neurovascular evaluation continues. If the knee has sufficient stability, a range of 15 to 30 degrees of motion can be continued while the patient is in the brace in anticipation of surgery. If not, quadriceps sets and electric stimulation can be used to maintain the muscle tone across the joint and to encourage mobilization of fluids.

Even if emergency surgical exploration is necessary to reestablish vascular function, ligament repair should be delayed for 3 to 7 days. An extensive procedure could put the arterial repair in jeopardy. However, if the knee has

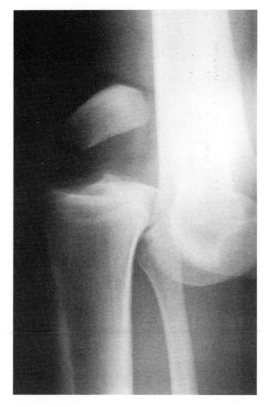

FIG. 60-25. Radiograph showing anterior dislocation of knee. Patient also had ruptured popliteal artery and required a vein graft.

severe ligamentous instability after arterial repair, this could also jeopardize the repair. In this case pins can be placed across the joint until a secondary repair is performed 3 to 14 days later. Usually, however, the stability is adequate without pins being applied. In performing repairs of knee dislocations, less obvious areas of injury must be considered. The most commonly missed areas are the posterolateral ligament complex, including the popliteus tendon and patellar dislocations. All torn ligaments and tendons should be repaired, if possible, and the meniscus should be retained if at all possible. Reconstruction of the ACL can be performed during this time frame, but PCL reconstruction should be delayed or deferred until the patient shows signs or symptoms of posterior instability.

To avoid stiffness of the joint, a hinged knee brace can be applied so that motion can be performed during the first 8 weeks after ligament repair. Continuous passive motion is used in the acute period. Later rehabilitation procedures are the same as those for patients with MCL and cruciate ligament injuries.

REHABILITATION

In skiing and other athletic activities, three factors have significant overall effect on the rehabilitation process: psychology, physiology, and restoration of the injured extremity (Table 60-2).

Psychologic factors are influenced by the patient's in-

TABLE 60-2 Important factors in the rehabilitation of skiers

Psychologic	Physiologic	Restorative
Innate drive for sports participation	Site of injury	Cooperation
Rapport with physician and rehabilitation staff	Innate healing capacity	Time commitment
Maturity	Morphologic factors (general looseness vs. tightness)	Appropriate secondary gains
Patient's cooperation	—	—

nate drive to participate in sports, rapport with the physician and rehabilitation staff, and maturity to accept healing time for an injured part while keeping uninjured parts in condition with alternative activities. Patients' cooperation and determination seem to reinforce physiologic factors in rehabilitation.

Physiologic factors are influenced by the site of injury, the patient's body healing mechanisms, psychologic motivation, and cooperation with the recuperative program prescribed by the physician.

Restoration of the injured part reflects the psychologic and physiologic factors. Skiers are notably cooperative and are willing to devote time to rehabilitation. All secondary gains seem to be related to their goal of return to skiing.

Cardiovascular conditioning in the phase after injury is a reinforcement for the physiologic recovery process. This gives the patient an outlet for pent-up energies and provides a psychologic reinforcement by promoting a sense of well-being. Activities that offer cardiovascular conditioning to the upper extremities, torso, and opposite lower extremity while the injured limb is healing are recommended. Guidelines are suggested in a number of places in the chapter.

The precise program must be prescribed by the physician for the individual skier. However, certain features of joint protection, range of motion, and muscle contraction are essential for the person returning to skiing, particularly the competitive skier. For example, in the early phases, rest, isometric contractions, passive exercise, and restriction of active extension to 10 degrees may be emphasized in ACL injuries. As the injury heals, particularly the knee, the joint motion may be controlled by an orthotic device. It is essential for the skier to regain control of joint motion by eccentric and concentric contractions. Also, redeveloping equal weight bearing on both extremities and avoiding hamstring spasm from limping is necessary before the patient can progress to jogging. Cutting is not begun until the patient can run pain free in the straight-ahead position. Curl, Markey, and Mitchell[12] have outlined some drills and events appropriate for the skier with a knee injury. Garrick[22] has diagrammed a simple approach to ankle injury rehabilitation.

Physical therapists help the patient through the early stages of treatment when the physician prescribes passive range of motion or specific active exercises. They must instruct the patient in crutch walking and oversee

---

Conditioning program

Aerobic and endurance
- Bicycling (stationary or street)
- Uphill running
- Downhill running (precluded if previous knee problems or symptoms occur)
- Side-to-side agility drills with Sport Cord (surgical elastic tubing)
- One-third knee bends

Games
- Racquet sports
- Soccer

Strength, power, and endurance
- Knee extension against resistance (avoid crepitation or patellofemoral pain)
- Knee flexion against resistance

Flexibility
- Static stretches designed for lower extremity, low back, and upper extremity

---

exercise on equipment such as the stationary bicycle, Sport Cord, or water therapy. Later, the competitive skier is followed up by the trainer and coach. Reevaluation of the injured extremity by the physician is scheduled at prescribed intervals or as indicated by symptoms.

SUMMARY

Even physicians who do not live near ski areas may be called on to treat lower extremity injuries sustained by skiers. Recreational and competitive skiers live in many parts of the country.

The best way for a skier to prevent injury to the lower extremities is good preparation for skiing, such as body conditioning year round, having custom-fitted equipment, respecting conditions on the slopes, and skiing within the limits of his or her abilities. The best protection against reinjury is preparation for returning to skiing by body conditioning of the uninjured parts during recovery of the injured part and following the physician's program for rehabilitation without trying to accelerate the use of the injured limb before adequate healing has been confirmed.

In this chapter some guidelines for physicians treating lower extremity ski injuries have been provided. Emphasis is clearly placed on the necessity of early, accurate diagnosis of the injury, basic principles of management and rehabilitation from the time of injury on the slope to the skier's return to skiing, and factors that differentiate skiers and their injuries from other persons with similar injuries but other interests.

REFERENCES

1. Akeson WH: An experimental study of joint stiffness, *J Bone Joint Surg* 43(A):1022, 1961.
2. Akeson WH, Amiel D, Woo SL: Immobility effects on synovial joints: the pathomechanics of joint contracture, *Biotechnology* 17:95, 1980.
3. Akeson WH et al: Collagen cross-linking alterations in joint contractures, *Connect Tissue Res* 5:15, 1977.
4. Arnoczky SP et al: The microvasculature of the meniscus and its response to injury: an experimental study in the dog, *Trans Orthop Res Soc* 6:177, 1981.
5. Baker CL, Norwood LA, Hughston JC: Acute posterolateral rotatory instability of the knee, *J Bone Joint Surg* 65A:614, 1983.
6. Bone LB, Johnson KD: Treatment of tibial fractures by reaming and intramedullary nailing, *J Bone Joint Surg* 68A:877, 1986.
7. Bone LB et al: Early versus delayed stabilization of femoral fractures: a prospective randomized study, *J Bone Joint Surg* 71A:336, 1989.
8. Bouter LM, Knupschild P: Causes and prevention of injury in downhill skiing, *Phys Sports Med* 17:81, 1989.
9. Bucholz RW, Brumbeck RJ: Fractures of the shaft of the femur. In Rockwood CA, Green DP, Bucholz RW (eds): *Fractures*, Philadelphia, 1991, JB Lipincott.
10. Costill DL et al: The role of dietary carbohydrates in muscle glycogen synthesis after strenuous running, *Am J Clin Nutr* 34:1831, 1981.
11. Coutts MD et al: Symposium: the diagnosis and treatment of articular cartilage injuries, *Contemp Orthop* 19(4):401, 1989.
12. Curl WW, Markey KL, Mitchell WA: Agility training following anterior cruciate ligament reconstruction, *Clin Orthop* 172:133, 1983.
13. Daniel DM et al: Instrumented measurement of anterior knee laxity in patients with acute anterior cruciate ligament disruption, *Am J Sports Med* 13:401, 1985.
14. Daniel DM et al: Instrumented measurement of anterior laxity of the knee, *J Bone Joint Surg* 67(A):720, 1985.
15. DeHaven KE: Diagnosis of acute knee injuries with hemarthrosis, *Am J Sports Med* 8:9, 1980.
16. Dehne E et al: Nonoperative treatment of the fractured tibia by immediate weight bearing, *J Trauma* 1:514, 1961.
17. DeLee J: Fractures and dislocations of the hip. In Rockwood CA, Green DP, Bucholz RW (eds): *Fractures*, Philadelphia, 1991, JB Lippincott.
18. Ekeland A, Holtmaen A, Lystad H: Skiing injuries in alpine recreational skiers. In Johnson RJ, Mote DC Jr, Binet MH (eds): *Skiing trauma and safety: seventh international symposium*, Philadelphia, 1987, AMSTM.
19. Elleson A: Skiing injuries, *Clin Symp* 29(1):2, 1977.
20. Epstein HC: Traumatic dislocations of the hip, *Clin Orthop* 92:116, 1973.
21. Eriksson E, Nygaard E, Saltin B: Physiological demands in downhill skiing, *Phys Sports Med* 5:29, 1977.
22. Garrick JG: "When can I . . .?" a practical approach to rehabilitation illustrated by treatment of an ankle injury, *Am J Sports Med* 9:67, 1981.
23. Greg GW: *Chain reaction: successful strategies for closed-chain testing and rehabilitation*, Albino, Mich, 1989, Wynn Marketing.
24. Hannon CD, Paul JJ, Fu FH: Loss of knee motion following arthroscopic anterior cruciate ligament reconstruction. Paper presented at the American Academy of Orthopaedic Surgeons, Anaheim, Calif, March 8, 1991.
25. Hardaker WT, Whipple TL, Bassett FH: Diagnosis and treatment of the plica syndrome of the knee, *J Bone Joint Surg* 62A:221, 1980.
26. Henning CE et al: Arthroscopic meniscal repair using exogenous fibrin clot, *Clin Orthop* 252:64, 1990.
27. Higgins RW, Steadman JR: Anterior cruciate ligament repairs in world class skiers, *Am J Sports Med* 15(5):439, 1987.
28. Jackson DW et al: Magnetic resonance imaging of the knee, *Am J Sports Med* 16(1):29, 1988.
29. Jakob RP, Hassler H, Staebli H-U: Observations on rotary instability of the lateral compartment of the knee, *Acta Orthop Scand (Suppl)* 52:191, 1981.
30. Johnson EE: Fractures of the patella. In Rockwood CA, Green DP, Bucholz RW (eds): *Fractures*, Philadelphia, 1991, JB Lippincott.
31. Johnson KD, Cadambi A, Siebert GB: Incidence of adult respiratory distress syndrome in patients with multiple musculoskeletal injuries: effects of early stabilization of fractures, *J Trauma* 25:375, 1985.
32. Johnson RJ: Prevention of cruciate ligament injuries. In Feagin JA (ed): *The crucial ligaments*, New York, 1988, Churchill Livingstone.
33. Johnson RJ, Ettlinger CF, Shealy JE: Skier injury trends. In Johnson RJ, Mote DC Jr, Binet MH (eds): *Skiing trauma and safety: seventh international symposium*, Philadelphia, 1989, AMSTM.
34. Johnson RJ, Pope M: Epidemiology and prevention of ski injuries, *Ann Chir Gynaecol* 80:110, 1991.
35. Johnson RJ et al: Factors affecting late results after meniscectomy, *J Bone Joint Surg* 56A:719, 1974.
36. Johnson RJ et al: Knee injury in skiing: a multifaceted approach, *Am J Sports Med* 7:321, 1979.
37. Johnson RJ et al: Trends in skiing injuries: analysis of a six-year study (1972-1978), *Am J Sports Med* 8:106, 1980.
38. Karlsson J et al: *The physiology of alpine skiing*, Park City, Utah, 1978, The United States Ski Coaches Association.
39. Klemom KW, Barner M: Interlocking nailing of complex fractures of the femur and tibia, *Clin Orthop* 212:89, 1986.
40. Larson RL: Physical examination in the diagnosis of rotatory instability, *Clin Orthop* 172:38, 1983.
41. Lessnick D: *Ski slope: how to get fit for skiing*, Las Vegas, Nev, 1992, Pioneer Books.
42. Lickteig JA, Foster C: Nutrition in winter sports. In Casey MJ, Foster C, Hixson EG (eds): *Winter sports medicine*, Philadelphia, 1990, FA Davis.
43. Lindsjo V: Operative treatment of ankle fractures, *Acta Orthop Scand (Suppl)* 52:1, 1981.
44. MacKinley D, Fulstone HA, Steadman JR: Anterior cruciate reconstruction in the middle aged patient. Paper presented at the fifty-fifth annual meeting of the Western Orthopaedic Association, Tucson, Ariz, October 20-24, 1991.
45. Matsen FA III: *Compartmental syndromes*, New York, 1980, Greene & Stratten.
46. McLaughlin HL, Ryder CT Jr: Open reduction and internal fixation for fractures of the tibia and the ankle, *Surg Clin North Am* 1523, 1949.
47. Miller CH, Guatilo R, Tambornino J: Traumatic hip dislocation: treatment and results, *Minn Med* 54:253, 1971.
48. Mohtadi NG, Webster-Bogaerts S, Fowler PJ: Limitation of motion following ACL reconstruction, *Am J Sports Med* 19(6):620, 1991.
49. Monto RR et al: MRI evaluation of tibial eminence fractures in adult skiers, (in press).
50. Mote CD: Snow falls: the mechanics of skiing injuries, *Mechanical Engineering* 9:94, 1984.
51. Mubarak SJ, Hargens AR, Owen CA, Garett LP, Akeson WH: The Wick catheter technique for measurement of intramuscular pressure, *J Bone Joint Surg* 58A:1016, 1976.
52. Müller ME et al: *Manual of internal fixation*, New York, 1981, Springer-Verlag.
53. Noyes FR, Bassett RW, Grood ES: Arthroscopy in acute traumatic hemarthrosis of the knee: incidence of anterior cruciate tears and other injuries, *J Bone Joint Surg* 62A:625, 1980.
54. Noyes FR, Mangine RE, Baber S: Early motion after open and arthroscopic anterior cruciate ligament reconstruction, *Am J Sports Med* 15(2):149, 1987.
55. Patel D: Arthroscopy of the plicae: synovial folds and their significance, *Am J Sports Med* 6:217, 1978.

56. Paulos L et al: Knee rehabilitation after anterior cruciate ligament reconstruction and repair, *Am J Sports Med* 9:140, 1981.

57. Rodrigo JJ et al: Improvement of full-thickness chondral defect healing in the human knee after debridement and microfracture by the use of continuous passive motion, *Am J Knee Surg* (in press).

58. Ruedi TP, Allgower M: The operative treatment of intraarticular fractures of the lower end of the tibia, *Clin Orthop* 138:105, 1979.

59. Russell TA, Taylor JC, LaVelle DG: Fractures of the tibia and fibula. In Rockwood CA, Green DP, Bucholz RW (eds): *Fractures*, Philadelphia, 1991, JB Lippincott.

60. Salter RB et al: The biologic effect of continuous passive motion on the healing of full-thickness defects in articular cartilage: an experimental investigation in the rabbit, *J Bone Joint Surg* 62A:1232, 1980.

61. Sarmiento A: A functional below-the-knee cast for tibial fractures, *J Bone Joint Surg* 49A:855, 1967.

62. Sarmiento A: Functional bracing of tibial fractures, *Clin Orthop* 105:202, 1974.

63. Shatzker J, McBroom R, Bruce D: The tibial plateau fractures: the Toronto experience 1968-1974, *Clin Orthop* 138:94, 1979.

64. Shelbourne KD, Wilickins JH, Mollasbesky A: Arthrofibrosis in acute ACL reconstruction: the effect of timing of reconstruction and rehabilitation, *Am J Sports Med* 19(4):332, 1991.

65. Steadman JR: Rehabilitation of first- and second-degree sprains of the medial collateral ligament, *Am J Sports Med* 7:300, 1979.

66. Steadman JR: Rehabilitation of tibial plafond fractures after stable internal fixation, *Am J Sports Med* 9:71, 1981.

67. Steadman JR: Rehabilitation of acute injuries of the anterior cruciate ligament, *Clin Orthop* 172:129, 1983.

68. Steadman JR, Forster RS, Silverskiold JP: Rehabilitation of the knee, *Clin Sports Med* 8(3):605, 1989.

69. Steadman JR, Montgomery JB: Dislocation of the knee in the competitive athlete, In Spiegel P (ed): *Topics in orthopaedic trauma*, Baltimore, 1984, University Park Press.

70. Sterndler A: *Kinesiology of the human body*, Springfield, Ill, 1955, Charles C Thomas.

71. Tapper EM: Ski injuries from 1939 to 1976: the Sun Valley experience, *Am J Sports Med* 6:114, 1978.

72. Warren RR: Arthroscopic meniscus repair, *Arthroscopy* 1(3):170, 1985.

73. Watson R, Steadman JR, Fry PJ: Ankle fractures, Paper presented at the American Orthopaedic Society for Sports Medicine, San Francisco, 1977.

74. Weber MJ et al: Efficacy of various forms of fixation of transverse fractures of the patella, *J Bone Joint Surg* 62A:215, 1980.

75. Woods GW, Stanley RF, Tullos HS: Lateral capsular sign: x-ray clue to a significant knee instability, *Am J Sports Med* 7:27, 1979.

CHAPTER 61 Dance Injuries

G. James Sammarco

Dancing is a continuous movement of the body as it travels through a predetermined space in accordance with definite rhythms in a conscious effort. The result is an elegant, regular movement that may be accompanied by music or voice. Dance begins as the uncontrolled movement of children expressing themselves. When that movement of exuberance is directed toward a definite pattern by training and control, dance is elevated to a fine art form. There are several types of dance, including **classical ballet,** which is based on tradition developed through centuries and has a specific technique that includes turnout of the hips,[54,72] rising (up on the toes), elevation, beats (crossing the feet in the air in rapid succession), turns, and toe dancing. **Modern dance** includes barefooted dancing, asymmetry, and personal choreographic or dance styles. **Folk dance,** including jazz dance, is based on folk rhythms and traditional dance steps from a particular geographic region or ethnic origin. **Variety dance,** as in Broadway shows, includes all of these elements.

Training for dance begins when a child is about 5 years old or younger. The child must be both physically

---

Developmental and physical requirements for dancing *sur les pointes*

- Balance
- Coordination
- Maturity
- Concentration
- Strength
- Mastery of basic steps

---

and mentally mature enough to follow direction and control his or her body.[44] For classical ballet, girls are not permitted to go on to pointe dancing *(sur les pointes)* before they have developed the proper balance, coordination, and mental maturity to be able to concentrate for continuous periods of up to 1 hour (McLain D: Personal communication, 1983). Also, they must have mastered the basic dance steps and have developed physical strength.[3] This seldom occurs before the age of 11 years and requires at least 3 years of training. The dancer's advancement is a combination of these prerequisites to prevent injury, and this depends on teacher interaction with the student.[36] *Advancing a dancer beyond his or her ability and training can lead to both acute and chronic injuries.*[48] Artistic directors are trained in the aesthetic and physical aspects of dance and choreography, and they have often been dancers themselves. They are able to choose dancers who have achieved a level of proficiency and who are ready to advance to more sophisticated and demanding steps.

Advancing a dancer beyond his or her ability can lead to both acute and chronic injuries

---

Body type is important for professional dancers. Each artistic director may choose dancers who represent his or her own aesthetic taste. Thus the "ideal" shape for a dancer has changed over the years. Today's ideal classical ballet dancer has a small head, long neck, and slightly shortened torso with long thin legs, the so-called "Balenchine" dancer shape. Dancers with a minimal amount of fat are preferred. The percentage of fat to body weight in female dancers tends to be below the tenth percentile.[7]

FLEXIBILITY AND WARM-UPS

In preparing for each dance class it is important to develop flexibility in the joints and to prevent injuries as well as concentrate on muscles and joints that have been previously injured and are in the state of rehabilitation.[9,11,35,37] Classical ballet begins with barre exercises, a precise set of exercises performed while holding onto a rail.[3] However, the dancer should also perform certain stretching exercises related to the trunk, upper back,

neck, hips, thighs, knees, legs, and feet[17] (Table 61-1). Flexibility in the dancer tends to increase with training.[32-34] This is not related to hypermobility but to continual stretching with motion at the limits of range of motion. It is important that children begin a program of flexibility and warm-up for the barre exercises early in their training because many young dancers perform modern and ethnic dances in class. These dances are less structured and may permit the student to dance highly technical steps before being properly warmed up. This also leads to unnecessary muscle and ligament injuries.

Theatrical dance is not an endurance sport. In organized dance, rehearsal and performance typically consist of short-burst aerobic-anaerobic activities; thus it is not an endurance sport. However, some forms of dance are very much aerobic or endurance activities. These include **marathon dancing,** a profoundly exhausting endurance activity that was most popular in the 1930s. Also, **all-night disco dancing** and more recently **aerobic dancing** as a form of exercise have become popular. This type of "fitness dance" has led to specific injuries and overuse syndromes.[15] Close observation and intense study indicate that during rehearsal, and indeed performance when the dancer dances intensively, cardiac output may approach maximum.[34] This is only for a short period of time, a minute or two, after which the dancer rests or dances at a level considerably less intense. This occurs in spite of the fact that dance class and rehearsals in many schools and companies may last 6 hours a day for 6 days a week.[43]

FLOORING

Dance surfaces are important for the prevention of injuries. Floors made of hardwood with springs beneath offer the best dance surface.[66,67] The damping mechanism and elasticity of this surface provide an optimal cushioning effect that helps prevent chronic overuse syndromes in the legs. Certain coverings, which are made of a softer plastic, stored in rolls, and carried with touring dance companies, can be laid across a stage or rehearsal area. These coverings provide a surface that is smooth and has a consistent friction characteristic and some resiliency. However, when placed on concrete, this flooring does not provide enough of a cushioning effect to prevent injuries. A dance company may also buy a floor with Permalastic properties beneath it, that is, one with some spring.

This chapter presents certain conditions common in dance and describes their mechanisms of injury and mode of treatment. Dance, like medicine, is a fine art and an exact science.

SPINE
Characteristics

The body of the dancer differs from that of other athletes, particularly with respect to the spine of a classical dancer.[32] These dancers are trained to hold the body erect, often in a somewhat stilted, stiffened manner. All positions of the classical tradition require that the dancers stand with the shoulders squared and spine erect to

TABLE 61-1 Dance flexibility program

Joint/Muscle Group	Objective	Position	Description*
Low back and hip	Flexibility	Stand	Stand with feet 2 feet apart and hands on hips. Make a circle with the upper torso, keeping the hips motionless. Repeat with the upper body, making a figure 8 with the hips.
Groin	Stretch	Sit	Sit on the floor with the soles of the feet in contact with each other. Pull the feet toward the buttocks while pressing the outside of the knees to the floor. Relax. Repeat. Then with the legs spread apart as far as possible reach with both hands to grasp the right foot while leaning out over the right leg. Hold. Relax. Repeat with the left leg.
Lateral hip	Flexibility	Sit	Sit on the floor, and bend the left knee beneath the hip. Put the right foot on the left side of the left knee. Turn the body to the right and pull the right knee to the chest with left arm. Hold. Relax. Repeat for the left hip.
Hamstring and thigh	Stretch	Stand	Standing with legs straight, try to touch the toes with the fingertips: then bend the knees and put palms on the floor. Slowly straighten legs. Hold. Relax. Repeat.
Hamstring	Flexibility	Stand	Cross the right foot over and in front of the left foot. Bend at the waist to touch the toes with the fingertips, keeping legs straight. Hold. Relax. Repeat, crossing the left foot in front of and over the right foot.
Quadriceps	Stretch	Sit	Sit on the floor with the right leg straight ahead and the toes pointed upward. Bend the left leg, and place the left foot behind hip. Lean backward and hold. Lean forward, trying to touch the toes. Relax. Repeat. Repeat with the right leg.
Quadriceps	Stretch	Stand	Bend the left knee, and grab the ankle with the left hand, pulling the left foot toward the buttocks. Hold. Relax. Repeat. Repeat with the right leg.
Calf	Flexibility	Stand	With the feet together and facing a wall, lean the body at a 45-degree angle. Keep the heels flat on the floor and hold the stretch. Relax. Repeat.
Soleus and Achilles tendon	Flexibility	Stand	With the feet together and facing a wall with the heels on the floor, lean into the wall, bending the knees. Stretching is felt lower down the leg and in the Achilles tendon area. Hold. Relax. Repeat.
Ankle	Flexibility	Stand	Rotations: Keep the leg straight and make circles with the foot moving first clockwise, then counterclockwise. Repeat. Flex and point: Keep the leg straight. Bring the foot toward the face. Hold. Next point the toes. Hold. Repeat.

*Stretching movements are slow and smooth and are performed without bouncing. Hold each stretch for 10 seconds, relax, and stretch further the next time.

decrease the normal dorsal kyphosis. Likewise, straightening the lumbar spine is preferred in classical dance.[36] In examining the dancer's spine, it is not surprising to find that dorsal kyphosis and lumbar lordosis are somewhat less than is expected. Radiographs of the spine often reflect this (Fig. 61-1). This is not considered an abnormality but rather a characteristic of dancers.

Dorsal Spine
Periostitis

Modern dance, ethnic, and jazz dance often require the dancer to lie on his or her back on the floor. If this is done on a hard floor, periostitis can occur over the dorsal aspect of the spinous processes. This is simply caused by direct pressure over the tip of the bone, not unlike a "stone bruise." Symptomatic treatment helps, such as wearing a heavy sweatshirt during rehearsal and using

---

Characteristic classical dance posture

- Diminished thoracic kyphosis
- Diminished lumbar lordosis

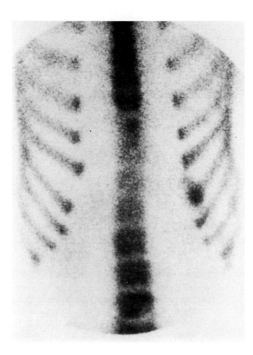

FIG. 61-1. Spine of ballet dancer in her fourth decade. Radiograph of spine is normal, but bone scan shows increased activity over lumbar spine. Dancers decrease lumbar lordosis by straightening of lumbar spine to have an aesthetic appearance on stage. (From Sammarco GJ: *Contemp Orthop* 8:15, 1984.)

Treatment of spinous process periostitis

- Heavy sweatshirt during rehearsal
- Mats
- Antiinflammatory medication
- Corticosteroid injection in selected cases

---

antiinflammatory medication. Injecting the dorsal spinous process with a corticosteroid solution may help but often produces skin atrophy because of the lack of adipose tissue in the subcutaneous tissue between the bone, ligaments, and skin. Mats are helpful if permitted by the instructor. The duration of symptoms varies and is related to the exercise, that is, the particular dance step that aggravates the condition, and to the vigor with which the dancer participates.

Scheuermann's Disease

The basic deformity in Scheuermann's disease is an increase in dorsal kyphosis along with symptoms of pain and stiffness in the dorsolumbar spine. Severe symptoms of pain and deformity preclude dance as a career, but dance, including aerobic dance, may be a therapeutic adjunct in the treatment of this condition to help maintain strength and flexibility of the paravertebral musculature. The symptoms usually dictate the level of participation.

Scoliosis

The development of scoliosis in a young dancer is not a reason to discontinue dance training.[1] Barre exercise and *adagio,* or center-floor, dance steps increase muscle strength and coordination and help maintain control and spinal alignment. Dancers with curvature greater than the upper limits of normal, 20 degrees, and even with significant rotation of the spine are often able to become professional dancers. The author has treated identical twin professional dancers with significant kyphoscoliosis but without symptoms and without significant deformity that prevents dance as a career. If the deformity is well hidden by the position of the curve in the dorsolumbar region, the dancer is able to compensate for the visual defect through technique and charisma. Of course, a significant deformity is noticed by an artistic director; thus the dancer may not make it through the process of auditioning, known as the "meat show," to be chosen for a company.

Lumbar Spine
Spondylolysis

Spondylolysis is characterized by a defect in the pars interarticularis that is often seen most clearly on oblique radiographs of the lumbar spine. Male dancers tend to begin dancing at a later age than females or may have participated in contact sports before choosing dance as a career or main avocation. Repeated acute trauma to the upper body with the spine in extension can lead to the development of such a defect. In *partnering,* that is, when a male dancer lifts a female dancer, certain specific strain is added to the male's lumbar spine. Such lifting often occurs at arm's length, and therefore additional strain from the leverage required to lift a 100-pound (45.35-kg)[8] female dancer with the arms extended 2 feet and using the lumbar spine as the fulcrum increases the stresses in the posterior elements of the vertebrae, causing symptoms. Repeated lifts by a tired dancer may aggravate symptoms of a stress fracture through the pars interarticularis. Treatment includes general instruction in a flexibility program and intensification of class studies in the technique of lifting and carrying the partner.

Spondylolysis is treated with nonsteroidal antiinflammatory drugs (NSAIDs) and improved dance technique. If symptoms include radiculopathy that is unrelieved by conservative measures, a laminectomy with appropriate nerve root decompression is indicated. In selected patients percutaneous diskectomy may be the treatment of choice. The dancer must be counseled on the risks of surgery and the length of time required to return to a full schedule of dance. This may be greater than 1 year. Such a condition may in fact be responsible for early termination of a dance career in spite of corrective surgery.

Spondylolisthesis

The diagnosis of spondylolisthesis includes general complaints of pain with or without radicular symptoms, local tenderness, and signs of a step-off at the level of involvement caused by vertebral slippage anteriorly. Tight hamstrings are often present with limited forward bending. Treatment depends on the significance of symptoms. Dance class and rehearsal time may be restricted until symptoms have subsided. NSAIDs, physical therapy, and a slow warm-up with appropriate stretching of the lumbar musculature are also indicated. If symptoms warrant, surgical intervention is indicated (see p. 1167). Although lumbar corsets and braces may be worn during classes and rehearsals, they are impractical during a performance and may give the dancer a false sense of security.

Herniated Disk

Continuous bending and twisting may lead to a herniation of the intervertebral disk. This may not necessarily be caused by poor technique (Callander J: Personal communication, 1983). A dancer is highly motivated and may ignore symptoms of pain until nerve root compression is significant enough to cause paralysis of affected muscle groups. This may be characterized by muscle weakness and calf atrophy. Appropriate diagnostic tests include computed tomography (CT), electromyography (EMG), and magnetic resonance imaging (MRI), which help to localize the lesion. When symptoms are acute and intractable, diskectomy is indicated. A small midline surgical incision or percutaneous diskectomy is preferred. During hemilaminectomy and disk excision it is not uncommon to find a free fragment of disk in the spinal canal. The incision and dissection should be so placed to minimize the disruption to the paravertebral musculature. In the immediate postoperative period a rehabilitation program is started that permits the patient to return to his or her premorbid level of activity as soon as possible.

Strain

Back strain is often caused by poor technique, dancing beyond the individual's ability, or lack of preparedness. Unsupervised horseplay may lead to unnecessary injuries.[29] Treatment is related to the symptoms and includes rest, use of NSAIDs, and reduction of rehearsal time while continuing a flexibility program. Strict adherence to the instructions of the dance teacher is extremely important to the aspiring young dancer.

Sacroiliac Joint

Lack of flexibility in the sacroiliac joint in the male and the female dancer characterizes the function of this joint.[5] In fact, except in women in the last trimester of pregnancy, the sacroiliac joint moves very little. Because dancers use the lumbar spine extensively, they tend to develop arthritis of this joint at a slightly earlier age than the general population. Treatment is directed toward relieving the symptoms and includes the use of NSAIDs as well as physical therapy modalities such as hot packs, ultrasound, and a muscle-stretching and power-building program designed to help support these broad pelvic joints during the daily rigors of dance class.

HIP
Training

Training for dance begins at an early age for girls. **Turnout** is a major part of classical ballet that is demonstrated by standing in first dance position with the hips externally rotated (Fig. 61-2). It is necessary to show the hip in external rotation during classical ballet so that position, intent, and movement may be implied without the dancer herself moving. Such positioning of the limb in profile with the dancer facing the audience has a long history that dates back before the beginning of classical ballet, which was 300 years ago (Fig. 61-3). In fact, Egyptian hieroglyphs dating back more than 3000 years show bas-relief figures in this manner. With training, the angle of anteversion may change until the dancer reaches age 11. After this time, even with training, a decrease in the anteversion angle at the hip will not occur. As a result, turnout is achieved by stretching the hip capsule over the head of the femur anteriorly.[21,55] A "good turnout" is the result of continued exercises, including stretching of the hip in external rotation through active muscle contraction. This contraction comes from the hip,

---

```
Causes of back strain in dancers

■ Poor technique
■ Dancing beyond capabilities
■ Lack of training
■ Poor conditioning
```

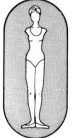 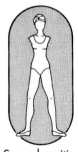 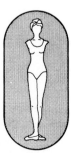 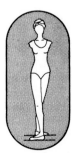 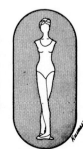

First position   Second position   Third position   Fourth position   Fifth position

FIG. 61-2. Five positions of lower extremities on which classical ballet dancing is based. (From Jahss M (ed): *Disorders of the foot,* Philadelphia, 1982, WB Saunders.)

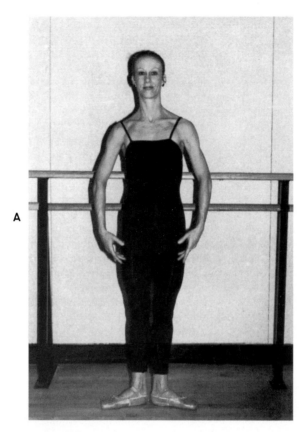

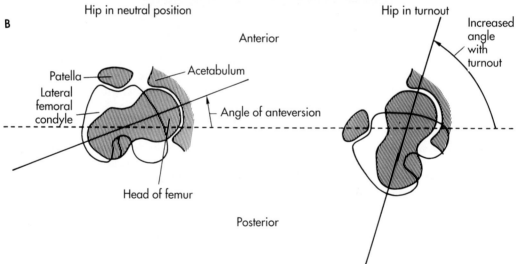

Hip in neutral position

Hip in turnout

Anterior

Increased
angle
with
turnout

Patella

Acetabulum

Lateral
femoral
condyle

Angle of anteversion

Head of femur

Posterior

FIG. 61-3. A, Dancer demonstrating turnout. Dancer faces forward, but hips are turned outward so that knee and foot appear in profile. **B,** Diagrammatic transverse cross-section through hip joint with knee superimposed demonstrates position of femoral head within acetabulum of dancer in turnout. This gives appearance of knee and leg in profile as dancer faces audience. (From Sammarco GJ: *Clin Sports Med* 2:489, 1983.)

and a dancer's attempts to increase it by manipulating the knees and feet cause problems in those joints.[57]

Soft-Tissue Conditions
Bursitis

Bursitis can occur in the region of the anterior hip, beneath the iliopsoas tendon, or over the greater trochan-

ter. Bursitis anterior to the hip is characterized by pain deep in the groin, whereas bursitis of the greater trochanter is characterized by pain in the region of the greater trochanter that is felt during turning, landing, and even walking. Palpation of the appropriate area reveals tenderness. Treatment includes the use of NSAIDs and hot packs and restricting dance steps that aggravate

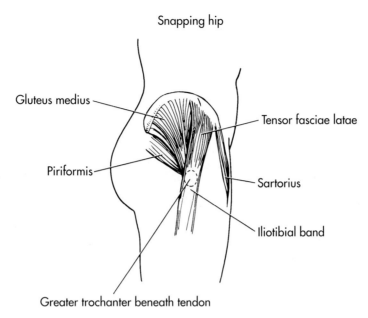

Snapping hip

Gluteus medius

Tensor fasciae latae

Piriformis

Sartorius

Iliotibial band

Greater trochanter beneath tendon

FIG. 61-4. Iliotibial band snaps over greater trochanter as dancer lands from a leap, giving a jerky unaesthetic appearance to the step. (From Sammarco CJ: *Clin Sports Med* 2:494, 1983.)

the condition. Symptoms usually subside within 10 days. A program of slow warm-up, including instruction in stretching the abductors and flexors of the hips, is an important adjunct to therapy. Occasionally, a local corticosteroid injection is indicated if other conservative measures fail.

Anterior Hip Click

The iliopsoas is the strongest flexor of the hip. During flexion, abduction, and external rotation the tendon may snap across the anterior hip capsule as the hip is brought from the abducted position back into first position. A click is felt and often heard.[57] This is common in the dancer and is usually asymptomatic. It can, however, be accompanied by symptoms of pain and be disabling enough to require cessation of dance until symptoms subside. This is seen mostly in young, female dancers who are highly motivated and occasionally in those who are advanced beyond their strength to withstand long periods of rehearsal and dance technique. The diagnosis is made through deep palpation of the iliopsoas muscle at the anterior hip. With the patient supine the hip is flexed with the knee bent, abducted, and externally rotated and then brought back to neutral position. The characteristic click is felt. Treatment includes reducing the rehearsal regimen, prescribing NSAIDs, and performing stretching exercises for the hip flexors. These must be done in a slow and gentle manner during the warm-up period.[9] In severely symptomatic cases the prognosis must be considered guarded.

Abductor Snap

Abductor snap occurs as the dancer lands from a leap. This is not a particular property of dance only. It is seen in various forms of high jumping from vertical to rota-

tion and in sports with a high frequency of jumping. It is characterized by the tight iliotibial band snapping from anterior to posterior over the greater trochanter (Fig. 61-4). On landing, the dancer suddenly finds the pelvis slipping into lordosis. As the dancer rises after having landed, the iliotibial band may snap forward again as it goes from posterior to anterior across the greater trochanter. This is unaesthetic because it is seen by the audience as a jerky movement. It may also be painful. Conservative measures over a period of several weeks are usually sufficient to correct this condition. These include strengthening the abductors and the gluteal muscles with prolonged periods of warm-up by having the dancer lie on the opposite side while the affected hip is elevated in abduction and then flexed and extended in its elevated position about 2 feet above the floor. If continued therapy, muscle strengthening, and stretching do not lessen the condition, incising the iliotibial band through a small posterolateral incision over the greater trochanter may be necessary.

Iliacus Tendinitis

Iliacus tendinitis occurs in the iliacus portion of the iliopsoas muscle of young dancers (Fig. 61-5). The muscle narrows as it passes into the floor of the femoral triangle. When the hip is brought into flexion, abduction, and external rotation, as during the dance step of *developpé* (Fig. 61-6), the tendon of the iliopsoas, the strongest flexor of the hip, must turn outward at an acute angle as it exits the pelvis.[57] Overzealous dancing, particularly in younger female dancers, causes acute tendinitis. Although often asymptomatic, it is characterized by pain in the groin and crepitus on palpation over the muscle. Treatment consists of decreasing the rehearsal regimen, use of NSAIDs, and following a program of phys-

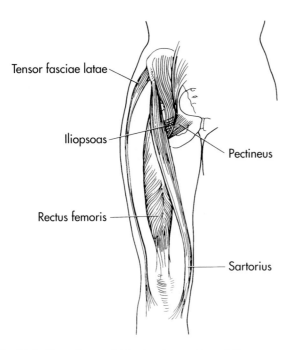

FIG. 61-5. Musculature of hip showing position of iliopsoas muscle. Crepitus (iliacus tendinitis) is palpable inferior and medial to anterior superior iliac spine. (From Sammarco GJ: *Clin Sports Med* 2:496, 1983.)

ical therapy to the hips, including instruction in slow stretching of the iliopsoas muscle. The condition is self-limited and does not prevent dancing.

Femoral Nerve Neurapraxia

Femoral nerve neurapraxia is an unusual condition found in dancers that may be produced by unusual posturing and stretching of the back and hips. Although it has been reported with *hinging* (i.e., backward bending while sitting on the floor with knees bent beneath the body), it also occurs in pure modern dancers.[45,64]

The onset is insidious, occurring over a period of days or weeks without trauma. It is characterized by a progressive weakness in hip flexion and knee extension. EMG localizes the weakness to muscles served by the femoral nerve. Crutches are required, and NSAIDs may be of help. Dance is discontinued until strength in the affected limb returns to above 90% of the well leg. This is a unilateral condition that is self-limited. However, several months may be required before the dancer is permitted to take class again.

Posterior Hip Strain (Piriformis Syndrome)

Posterior hip strain has been variously called *piriformis syndrome, posterior hip syndrome,* and *posterior hip capsulitis.* No clear-cut evidence of tendinitis has been found, and in the absence of radiculopathy from impingement or trauma to the sciatic nerve or its branches, it is most likely a bursitis overlying the posterior hip capsule. It may be present for months. NSAIDs and a gentle stretching program with gluteal exercises are recommended. Occasionally, an injection of steroid or local anesthetic (i.e., betamethasone [Celestone] with 1 mg of

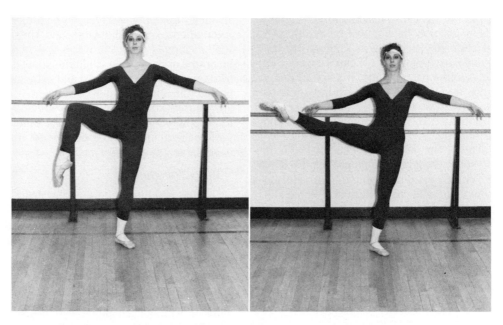

FIG. 61-6. Dancer demonstrating classical ballet dance step of *developpé.* Hip is abducted, flexed, and extremity rotated as knee is flexed and brought upward. Dance step is completed as extended leg is brought back into first position. Iliacus tendinitis is best diagnosed with dancer performing this step.

1% lidocaine [Xylocaine]) may be helpful. The condition is rarely severe enough to discontinue dance.

Muscle Strain

Generalized muscle strain occurs most commonly in the hip adductor and at the origin of the hamstring muscles at the ischial tuberosity.[59] These are self-limited conditions requiring a decrease in dance schedule, NSAIDs, and gentle stretching therapy until symptoms subside.

Bony Conditions
Stress Fracture

Great leaps and turns in the air, *grande tours jeté,* done repeatedly by dancers who are clearly dancing beyond their training or ability and who are tired can lead to the development of stress fractures. Such stress fractures occur characteristically in the neck of the femur.[17] Symptoms are insidious and may begin 2 to 3 weeks after changing technique or dancing a new role. There may be symptoms for several months before the dancer seeks medical attention. Standard radiographs of the hips may not reveal the fracture. Bone scan and tomograms of the hip are helpful in making the diagnosis (Fig. 61-7).[25] Treatment requires that the dancer stop dancing until the symptoms completely subside and the fracture heals. Such stress fractures are uncommon in dancers. I have not had to perform surgery on dancers for this injury. If surgery is required for complete fracture, the insertion of multiple pins in situ is recommended through a small incision. Return to full dance routine may require up to a year.

Arthritis

Arthritis of the hips is often found incidentally when the dancer has an x-ray examination for another problem. Many dancers attempt to increase their turnout by lying prone on the floor with the hips fully flexed and abducted and having another dancer press down with a foot on their pelvis. In young dancers this has been called

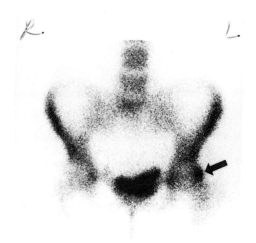

FIG. 61-7. Bone scan of dancer demonstrating stress fracture (*arrow*) of femoral neck that is not visible on radiographs.

the frog. Such forced passive stretching of the hip capsule may cause damage. The characteristic osteophyte formation at the periphery of the acetabulum and femoral neck tends to occur at an younger age in dancers than in the average population, that is, during the third decade of life. It is usually asymptomatic until the late fourth or early fifth decade. Because many male dancers begin dancing at the end of adolescence or in the beginning of their third decade of life and then rapidly advance as their talent and training permit, arthritis secondary to this sudden, intense use can develop within a few years and cause a painful decrease in joint motion. This may bring a tragic and premature end to the dancer's career. The well-trained, mature professional dancer often compensates for the slight decreased motion from arthritis through technique and charisma with the audience and by emphasizing other dance steps. Ultimately, however, the hip stiffness and pain take their toll. Treatment of the mild condition includes symptomatic use of an anti-inflammatory medication and development of the full range of motion of the hip joints during warm-up periods, before barre exercises and warm-down periods, and after dance class and rehearsal, in which the dancer again goes through gentle stretching motions of the soft tissue about the hips.

KNEE
Meniscus Tears

The sudden rapid actions that characterize contact sports are much less common in dance.[16,53] Acute bucket-handle tears are less likely to occur in dancers unless they have previously been exposed to such activities or suffer a fall.[49] The fifth position of classical ballet is normally achieved at the hip by externally rotating both hips then crossing the legs so that the left medial arch lies flush against the lateral aspect of the right foot. Dancers with poor turnout have difficulty achieving this position at the barre. They attempt to force the position by flexing the knees and hips, "screwing the knee" (Fig. 61-8).[24] This applies a high rotational shear force on the meniscus as the tibial plateau is forced against the femur, causing a meniscal tear. The onset is insidious and may present over a period of several months and even years. It is important that screwing of the knee be watched for during training in the basic dance steps and eliminated before the meniscus is injured. The dancer tends to mask symptoms of pain until muscle atrophy is noticed by the artistic director and locking and giving way alter the dancer's style.

Excision of the torn meniscal fragments is performed through the arthroscope. A rehabilitation program should be started immediately in the postoperative period, that is, within a few days, as soon as the dancer is able to tolerate barre exercises at the bedside. The sound leg is used as the leg of support to bear the body weight. The affected leg may be used as the working leg, that is, the leg off the floor with active motion. As soon as the stab wounds heal, a "water barre" is begun.[57] Here the dancer is submerged to the nipple line in water, using the side of the pool as a barre. The sound leg is used as the leg

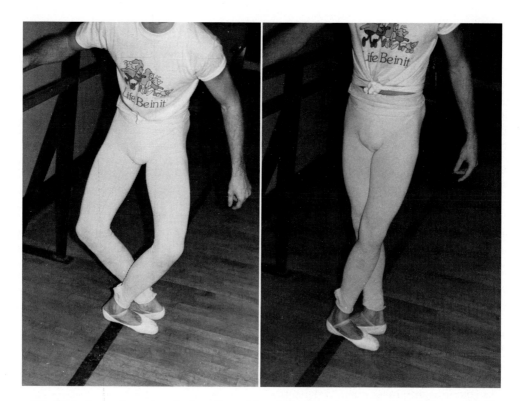

FIG. 61-8. Dancer "screwing the knees" to achieve fifth classical dance position. Because of stiff hips and poor turnout, dancer bends his knees to facilitate placing feet into fifth position. He then extends knees to hold that position. This commonly performed, dangerous maneuver is a fault that often leads to internal derangement of the knee.

of support and the injured leg as the working leg. Barre exercises are then performed. Return to a full schedule of dance and ultimately performance requires at least 90% of normal strength in the muscles that control knee motion.

Muscle Strains and Ruptures
Quadriceps Avulsion at Patella

Avulsion of the lateral portion of the quadriceps tendon from the superior lateral pole of the patella is common in weightlifters and football players but occurs less commonly in dancers performing *grande tours jeté* (Karlholm S: Personal communication, 1978). Treatment for minor injury includes immobilization in extension for a period of 10 days followed by gentle flexion under the supervision of a physical therapist. A program of quadriceps stretching and power building is then instituted 2 weeks after injury. Within 3 weeks the dancer may return to barre exercises and rehearsal as tolerated. If the tear is massive, operative repair is necessary with progressive mobilization beginning 2 weeks postoperatively in an adjustable hinge knee immobilizer (Bledsoe). In 6 weeks a full rehabilitation program is initiated. Return to dance may take at least 6 months.

Partial Patellar Tendon Avulsion

Partial avulsion of the patellar tendon fibers from the inferior pole of the patella causes symptoms of tenderness at the inferior pole of the patella with pain on leap-

ing. The onset usually begins over several hours or days but seldom as an acute, traumatic episode. A lateral radiograph of the knee may show a relative osteoporosis at the inferior pole of the patella with periosteal reaction or calcification in the proximal portion of the patellar tendon. Treatment includes decreased dance schedule, use of NSAIDs, and a training program of stretching exercises and power building. Symptoms may be doggedly persistent and last several months. If the tender area can be localized, surgical excision of this painful, tender, pea-sized mass of granulation tissue can be achieved. A local anesthetic is injected into the skin, followed by making a 2-cm incision. The tender area is again localized in the patellar tendon with a needle, through cooperation of the patient, by probing the tendon until the tender granuloma is found (Quirk R: Personal communication, 1984). This area is then anesthetized locally, the tendon is incised in the direction of its fibers, and the small mass is removed. The dead space is obliterated and the wound closed with a subcuticular absorbable suture. Rehabilitation is begun in the immediate postoperative period.

Lateral-Riding Patella

Attempting to increase turnout by improperly rotating the knee instead of the hips predisposes the dancer to symptoms related to a lateral-riding patella. Other causes may also be present, including hyperextended knees, patella alta, or laterally placed tibial tubercle. The symptoms, which include medial or lateral parapatellar pain and tenderness on palpation, alter the dancer's style and endurance. Treatment includes correcting ballet technique and building power of the quadriceps, particularly in the last 30 degrees of extension. The use of a knee support with a lateral pad to prevent subluxation is also of help. If symptoms are unrelieved by conservative measures, lateral retinacular release through the arthroscope is recommended. Patellar tendon reconstruction with medial and distal transfer of the distal insertion of the patellar tendon accompanied by lateral retinacular release is reserved for recurrent patella dislocation. Quirk[52] reported that 4.1% of his operative procedures were performed for this purpose.

Ligament Injuries

Acute vs. Subacute Ligament Pain

Medial or lateral ligament pain often occurs when the dancer changes technique, is given the responsibility of a principal role, or increases rehearsal schedule before an opening performance. Physical examination reveals the seriousness of such sprains. Treatment is usually symptomatic and includes whirlpool therapy, ultrasound, use of antiinflammatory medication, and a warm-up regimen of stretching that concentrates on the muscles and ligaments about the knee. An important adjunct to rehabilitation of any injury to the knee includes the use of the water barre,[57] because it eliminates gravity. The dancer does a complete set of barre exercises immersed in a pool, using the side of the pool as the barre. The injured leg is used as the working leg, and the barre exercises are performed with gravity eliminated. The water barre is discontinued when the dancer and the therapist are confident that sufficient strength and stability have returned to the injured knee or hip to permit the addition of gravity to the exercise regimen.

Gross Ligament Injuries

Severe ligamentous injuries to the knee occur infrequently in dance. However, when they do occur, the dancer usually gives a history of a previous significant injury. If the knee is unstable, the prognosis is poor. Injuries requiring major ligament repairs with or without primary ligament reconstruction require cast immobilization, including cast bracing and a vigorous rehabilitation program. Braces with hinges may be used during water barre and barre exercises on return to class, but a hinged brace must be discarded before center floor or adagio dance steps can be permitted. Because no such supports may be worn during a performance, the dancer cannot be permitted to rely on such braces for confidence.

LEG

Periostitis

Periostitis is caused by dancing on floors that are too hard, fatigue, vigorous dancing, or changing technique without lessening the intensity of the dance schedule. It most commonly occurs along the posteromedial border of the tibia at the distal third of the shaft (Fig. 61-9). It

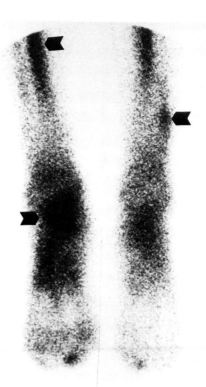

FIG. 61-9. Bone scan of dancer showing periostitis of tibia (*upper left arrow*), stress fracture of fibula (*right arrow*), and synovitis of ankle (*lower left arrow*). (From Sammarco GJ: *Clin Orthop* 187:176, 1984.)

may be extremely annoying and persistent. If the onset occurs over several weeks, the recommended treatment includes hot packs or a warm shower before rehearsal followed by a warm-up program designed to gently stretch the muscles of the leg and calf. Antiinflammatory medication is an important adjunct. If symptoms are severe, an ice pack applied to the affected area after rehearsal may lessen the pain and decrease local edema. Occasionally, a transcutaneous nerve stimulator unit is beneficial.

Compartment Syndrome

Anterior compartment syndrome is rare in dancers and indicates gross misconduct in the dancer, such as unsupervised horseplay or dancing for extended periods without warming up or resting.

Myositis and Acute Muscle Tears

Myositis in the calf can occur following any change in technique and often occurs after a laying-off period in which the dance company is dismissed for a period of at least a month and the dancer does not do warm-ups on a daily basis during this time. An abrupt change in dance technique may cause the muscles of the calf to become inflamed. Treatment includes whirlpool therapy, use of antiinflammatory medication, general stretching, and massage. Symptoms generally subside within 5 days. Dance class may be restricted at first, but as symptoms subside the dancer is permitted to take barre exercises and finally return to a preinjury level of participation.

Partial tears at the musculotendinous junction of the triceps surae are more common in the male dancer who performs leaps.[56] Treatment includes immobilization in a splint until the acute pain subsides, usually 7 days, followed by a program of gentle stretching, whirlpool therapy, and use of antiinflammatory agents. Technique must be perfected, including *balloon,* the graceful landing from a leap that immediately connects with another dance step and provides a graceful transition from one step to another.

Achilles Tendon Rupture

Complete rupture of the Achilles tendon usually occurs only after symptoms of tendinitis have been present for a few weeks.[71] It is the general consensus that to maintain length of the gastrocsoleus complex equal to that of the opposite leg, open repair is indicated (Callander J: Personal communication, 1983).[9,38,39,69,73] Postoperative cast immobilization should be continued for at least 4 weeks and be followed by an adjustable walker boot (Bledsoe), increasing the range of motion at 10-degree intervals twice a week for 2 more weeks. This should be followed by a slow-stretching and rehabilitation program of supervised therapy. There are several cases of dancers returning to a full active schedule as a principal dancer following such a severe injury. This requires up to 1 year. Prognosis may be guarded for achieving the level of preinjury performance.

Stress Fracture

Of all injuries below the knee, one of the most difficult to assess, diagnose, and treat is stress fracture. Stress fractures are often multiple and bilateral. Symptoms may mimic anterior compartment syndrome and periostitis for several months. Indeed, bone scan may be equivocal for several months before symptoms, signs, and diagnostic tests localize enough to present one or several stress fractures.[65,69] In women the occurrence has been linked to associated menstrual abnormalities.[28,70] Multiple stress fractures, that is, transverse partial fractures through the proximal, middle, and distal shaft of the tibia or fibula, may be present several months or even years before diagnosis is made (Quirk R: Personal communication, 1984) (Figs. 61-9 and 61-10).* The cause of stress fractures is a heavy work schedule, poor technique, and dancing on many different surfaces, some of which may be concrete and others of which are poor and made of uneven wood with no springs. The highly motivated, artistic personality of the dancer often overcomes the pain experienced during rehearsal and performances, only for the dancer to be plagued by symptoms when resting or when beginning to warm-up for the following day's schedule. Stress fractures of the fibula characteristically occur 10 cm above the lateral malleolus in the distal shaft of that bone. Bone scan often localizes the site.

Physical examination reveals acute tenderness over a

---

*References 6, 13, 46, 60, 63, 69, and 72.

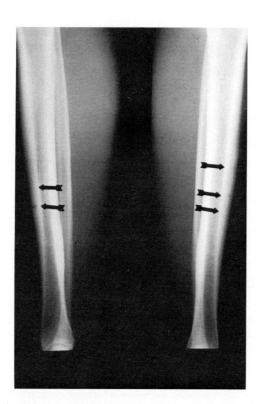

FIG. 61-10. Radiograph showing multiple stress fractures in midshafts of tibiae of a dancer. Symptoms were present 18 months before diagnosis.

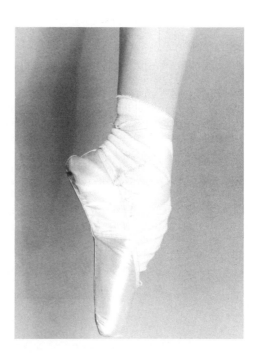

FIG. 61-11. Dancer with acute tendinitis of peroneus brevis. She is treated with elastic adhesive dressing and allowed to rehearse as symptoms permit.

discrete area on the anterior border of the tibia and at the fibula in the affected area. Treatment includes cessation of dance until symptoms subside and examination reveals tenderness has disappeared. A fibular fracture can be treated with an air splint and crutches with partial weight bearing on the affected limb. With tibial and fibular stress fractures, warm-ups are permitted. Symptoms may be such as to require fiberglass cast immobi-

lization. A water barre is permitted during this period so that the dancer does not lose flexibility and coordination in the rest of the body. Treatment may require restriction from dance for up to 6 months. If the dancer returns before appropriate healing or advances too quickly, symptoms will return. It is important that the dance surfaces be analyzed if a company has several such fractures (see Chapters 5 and 28).

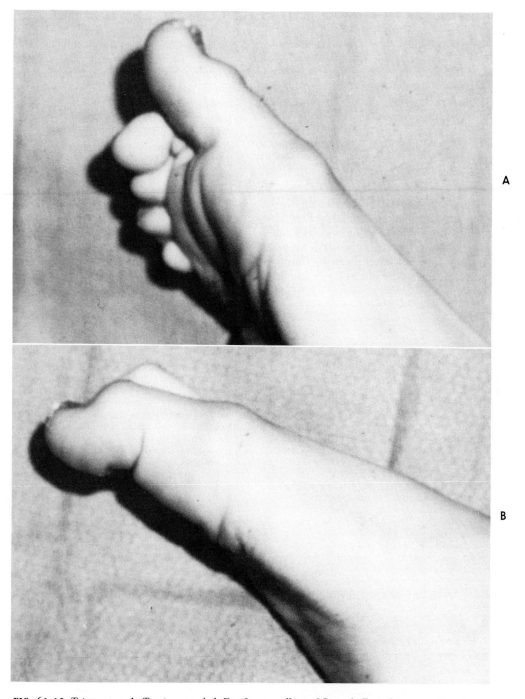

FIG. 61-12. Trigger toe. **A,** Toe is extended. Fusiform swelling of flexor hallucis longus tendon sits distal to pulley beneath sustentaculum tali. As hallux is flexed, flexor hallucis longus is pulled through retinaculum, causing toe to snap into flexion, **B,** where it remains until it is forced distally again by passive extension of the toe. (From Sammarco CJ: *J Bone Joint Surg* 61A:150, 1979.)

ANKLE
Tendinitis

Tendinitis is caused by returning to dance after long periods of laying off without performing a sufficient flexibility or warm-up regimen.[22,68,69] It can occur in any of the tendons about the ankle, but the most common is the Achilles tendon.[14,24,69] Flexor hallucis longus tendinitis, called "dancer's tendinitis,"[18] and tendinitis of the peroneus brevis and longus are also common (Fig. 61-11). Diagnosis is made by palpating over the specific painful anatomic area. The onset of symptoms is usually in the evening or the day after return to the schedule. Often this occurs when technique is changed or dance rehearsal regimen is increased. The treatment includes use of NSAIDs, whirlpool therapy or hot showers before dancing, a light compressive dressing with an elastic bandage, and whirlpool therapy and ultrasound after dancing. Although complete rupture of the peroneal brevis muscle has been reported in a dancer, it is accompanied by congenital absence of other lateral ankle supporting structures.[12]

Trigger Toe

Trigger toe is caused by a partial rupture of the flexor hallucis longus tendon with fusiform swelling of the tendon (Fig. 61-12).[61] It occurs most commonly in female classical ballet dancers and is characterized by pain when descending from the *demi-pointe* position to foot-flat, that is, standing on the ball of the foot and descending to the floor. The symptoms include triggering of the hallux as the fusiform swelling in the flexor hallucis longus tendon snaps to and from through its pulley at the posteromedial compartment of the ankle from beneath the sustentaculum tali (Fig. 61-13). Occasionally, the tendon may lock distal to the tendon canal thus preventing the dancer from using the strength in her hallux when standing *en pointe*. This can be dangerous because it prevents standing *sur les pointes* and predisposes the dancer to additional strains and other injuries of the foot. Diagnosis is made by palpating the tendon deep in the posteromedial compartment of the ankle at the ankle joint line anterior to the Achilles tendon and feeling the snap as the hallux and ankle are flexed and extended. Crepitus may also be palpable. Treatment includes use of NSAIDs and slow gentle stretching of the tendon before barre exercises. Surgical release of the ligamentous portion of the flexor hallucis longus canal at the posterior ankle and repair of the rent in the tendon effect a complete cure. Active range of motion is encouraged in 48 hours, and the dancer is permitted to return to pointe dancing after 8 weeks. At least 3 to 6 months are necessary for the dancer to return to the high level he or she had attained before the development of the syndrome.

Fractures and Dislocations

Performing a *fouette en dehors,* that is, turning on the leg of support, when the dancer is tired or unprepared can cause an ankle fracture of external rotation with or

---

Ankle exercises

Non–weight-bearing exercises

- Sit on floor with affected leg straight in front of you. Place a belt around the ball of foot and pull foot forward, slowly stretching the muscle and tendon in the calf. Pull with right hand to bring foot to right, then left hand to bring foot to left.
- Sit on floor with knees straight out in front of you. Dorsiflex ankle and curl toes at the same time. Then point foot and flex and extend ankle. Put feet flat against wall, pull toes toward you. Hold. Repeat with knees bent at 30 degrees.
- Sit in chair with knees flexed to 90 degrees and raise toes, pressing heels to floor. Progressively move feet back beneath chair until it is impossible to keep raising toes while heels are down. Then raise heels keeping all toes flat on floor and press forward.
- Sit with knees flexed to 90 degrees and feet flat on the floor. Raise right toes, then left toes; raise right heel, then left heel. Alternate until rhythmic pattern develops.
- While sitting, slide feet forward, keeping toes and heels in contact with floor. Keep heels in place while pulling foot upward, then downward with toes curled.
- Sit with feet flat on floor and pull medial sides of feet inward, keeping lateral aspects on floor. Hold, flatten feet, then reverse, keeping medial sides on floor including big toe. Do not move knees.

Weight-bearing exercises

- Stand between two chairs with one foot in front of the other, 12 inches apart. Rock forward onto front foot, leaving the back foot in contact with floor (toes on floor, heel lifted). Rock back so that front foot is on heel and toes are pulled back. Change position of feet and repeat.
- Stand with back to wall, feet directly under shoulders, and weight evenly distributed. Slowly bend your knees, without raising heels. Go down to point of maximal stretch and hold. Repeat. At bottom of the knee bend, roll onto balls of feet, then roll back and straighten up.
- Stand on step with feet parallel and heels hanging off the edge. Drop down so that the calves are maximally stretched. Slowly pull up onto the ball of foot, then slowly lower all the way down to maximum stretch again. Repeat with feet turned out, then turned in. Progress to using 5- to 10-pound ankle weights with exercise.
- Standing with weight on one leg, bend knee down, then straighten knee and pull up to a full arch. Slowly lower the heel, keeping the knee straight. Repeat.
- Standing, rock back on heels, claw toes, and walk on heels. Repeat. Use 1- to 3-pound weights wrapped around the forefoot.
- Stand on balls of feet. Weight should be on outer borders of feet with knees 4 inches apart. Role weight from the fifth metatarsal to the big toe in circular motion. Repeat with feet turned in, then with feet turned out.
- *Plié.* (a) Parallel—Standing, keeping knees parallel and directly over feet and shoulders over hips, squat progressively toward floor. Keep heels in contact with floor as long as possible on the way down, and put them down on floor on the way back up to straight-leg position; (b) Turned-out—Do the same as above with legs turned out from hips so that heels are together, toes fanning out, and knees directly over feet.

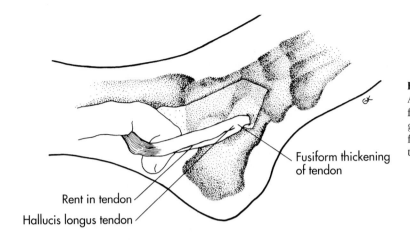

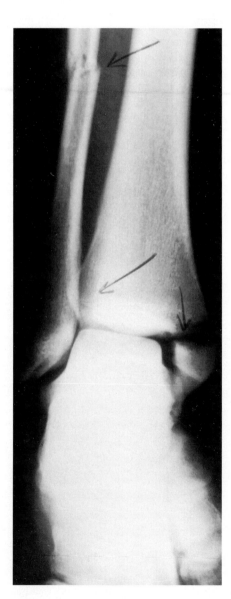

FIG. 61-13. Diagram showing injury of trigger toe. A 3-cm rent in flexor hallucis longus tendon and fusiform thickening of tendon distally alter smooth gliding at ankle, causing tendon to impinge at flexor pulley as it passes beneath sustentaculum tali.

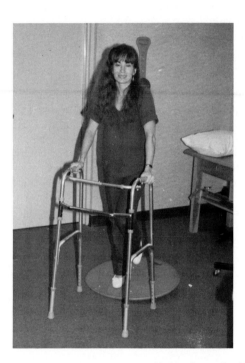

FIG. 61-15. Dancer demonstrating use of biomechanical ankle platform system (BAPS) board. This is an important part in rehabilitation of any injury to foot or ankle because it helps develop proprioception, coordination, and strength in muscles of calf and foot.

FIG. 61-14. Severe fractures of ankle (*arrows*) caused by external rotation during dance step of *fouetté*. Injured leg is used as leg of support. Fractures of medial malleolus and fibular shaft with disruption of syndesmosis are the result of injury to leg of support caused by *fouetté*.

without dislocation, disruption of the syndesmosis, or tear of the deltoid ligament (Fig. 61-14). For treatment of this injury, anatomic reduction must be achieved, preferably by closed manipulation and application of a cast for at least 6 weeks. Reduction may have to be performed by open means. This should be followed by the use of an adjustable walker cast, air splint (Aircast), or cast brace. Active range of motion is then encouraged so that ankle motion can return as quickly as possible. Even under the best of conditions, rehabilitation is prolonged and may require up to 2 years before the dancer is able to again proficiently perform *sur les pointes*.

Emboité is a rapid succession of steps in which one foot is brought from behind to in front of the opposite foot and then the other foot in turn is brought forward.

If the foot and ankle invert and rotate inward, fracture of the lateral malleolus or medial malleolus may occur. Such severe injuries occur after long periods of rehearsing and the dancer is tired. This happens particularly if the dancer has a tendency to sickle the foot, that is, curve the foot inward while dancing. This injury is also caused by trying to perform steps beyond the dancer's proficiency level. Treatment includes a closed anatomic reduction with cast immobilization for 4 weeks followed by an air cast or fracture brace and a rehabilitation program to increase flexibility, strength, and coordination. A biomechanical ankle platform system (BAPS) board (Fig. 61-15) used to exercise the foot and ankle is an important adjunct to therapy and should be used to help the dancer obtain proprioception and range of motion as well as strength. Return to dance is permitted after 6 weeks, but preinjury level of skill may take several months to attain. Dorsiflexion of the ankle is usually compromised following such an injury.[60]

Arthritis

Arthritis of the ankle may occur following injury but is seldom disabling. The dancer often changes style or technique slightly to accommodate the loss of motion. The technique of dance protects the ankle by the slow, steady control of motion and the development of strong muscles to protect the joint. However, osteophytes may form on the dorsal aspect of the talar neck.[31] If the osteophytes prevent dorsiflexion of the ankle joint, as during *plié,* and the graceful bending of the knees and ankles, the bending may be asymmetric. Surgical excision of such osteophytes from the neck of the talus and the anterior border of the tibia may be necessary. Arthroscopy is the preferred method to excise these impending osteophytes. Rehabilitation may take at least 2 to 3 months. The dancer should be warned of continued loss of ankle motion, particularly dorsiflexion, and of the long rehabilitation required before returning to dance.

Synovitis

Synovitis of the ankle may develop subsequent to a mild ligamentous injury and may persist for several months and even years (Fig. 61-9). It is characterized by swelling and tenderness at the joint. If it becomes chronic, the prognosis is guarded. Treatment includes use of NSAIDs, compressive ankle support, whirlpool therapy, and a prolonged warm-up before barre exercises that concentrates on developing flexibility.

Os Trigonum Syndrome

Although the os trigonum syndrome is present as an accessory bone in 8% of the population, it is seldom symptomatic except in dancers (Fig. 61-16). Pointing the foot requires that the ankle joint be plantar flexed to its limit. This compresses the os trigonum when it is present, and may in fact fracture it by crushing it between the posterior tibia and the calcaneus (Quirk R: Personal communication, 1984).[4,20,25,51] If symptoms are persistent, surgical excision through a small lateral incision anterior to the Achilles tendon effects a cure. The entire os trigonum must be excised and a stretching program begun as soon as the edema of surgery has begun to subside, 3 days postoperatively. Return to a full dance schedule may take 6 weeks, and it may take several

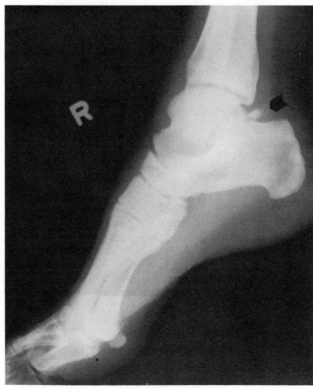

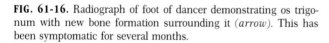

FIG. 61-16. Radiograph of foot of dancer demonstrating os trigonum with new bone formation surrounding it *(arrow).* This has been symptomatic for several months.

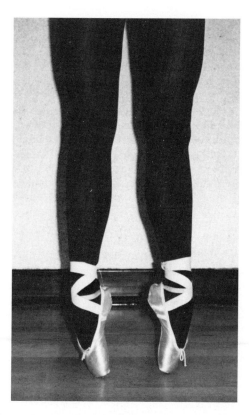

FIG. 61-17. Dancer standing *sur les pointes* in first position, demonstrating sickling in. (From Jahss M [ed]: *Disorders of the foot*, Philadelphia, 1982, WB Saunders.)

months to achieve a preinjury level of proficiency, particularly for pointe dancing because of restricted range of ankle motion.

Ligament Injury

Sickling is a technical fault of dancing in which the foot is turned inward with the heel in varus. This can lead to lateral ankle joint laxity (Fig. 61-17). Because the foot is in varus, the poor position and fatigue predispose the dancer to inversion injuries.[73] Grades I and II lateral ligament injuries are treated with a compressive dressing for a period of 2 weeks followed by an air splint and a rehabilitation program that includes the use of the BAPS board and power-building exercises (see p. 505).

Complete disruption of the ligaments of the ankle with gross instability requires surgical repair if the dancer's career is to continue.[19,74] In dance, however, complete acute tears of the ligaments with gross instability are uncommon and surgery is seldom indicated. If repair is indicated, the prognosis is guarded because of possible postoperative loss of motion (Fig. 61-18).

FOOT
Acute Myositis and Ligament Sprains

Acute myositis and ligament sprains may occur as the result of dancing a full schedule when a dancer is ill prepared to withstand the strain because of laziness or poor training during periods of laying off. Antiinflammatory medication, massage, and whirlpool therapy as well as

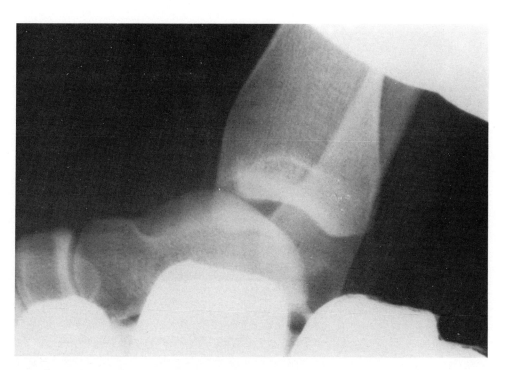

FIG. 61-18. Stress radiograph of dancer with chronic ligamentous instability of ankle. Note subluxation of talus anteriorly. Patient, a prima ballerina, refused surgery and continues to dance with minimal, if any, symptoms.

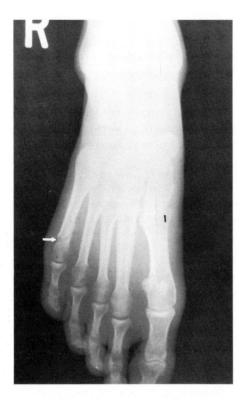

FIG. 61-19. Fracture of neck of fifth metatarsal *(arrow)*, most common fracture of foot in dancers. This may require 5 months to heal and may also require open reduction to achieve satisfactory alignment.

elevation and active range of motion bring prompt relief of the spasm and return the dancer to rehearsal within 48 hours. Sprains of the tarsal-metatarsal joints can be annoying, particularly those about the cuboid. Although **subluxation of the cuboid** has been reported, no documentation with CT or MRI has been found. This condition appears to be a result of peroneus longus tendon subluxation beneath the cuboid as observed by Marshall and Hamilton[42] and others (Baxter D: Personal communication, Houston, 1992). It is important that the dancer exercise on a daily basis even when not performing. Certain conditions can predispose the dancer to this problem, such as modern dance in which no shoes are worn.

Plantar fasciitis occurs as a result of increasing schedule and changing technique without properly preparing the foot. If symptoms become chronic and do not respond to general conservative measures of rest, therapy, and antiinflammatory medication, a leather orthosis with a high longitudinal arch may be inserted into a ballet shoe. It is not recommended for use in the pointe shoe because of its bulk.

Fractures

Acute fractures of the foot in dancers usually occur in the metatarsals, the most common site being the fifth metatarsal (Fig. 61-19).[27] Jones[27] has observed a dancer performing an entire ballet with such acute fracture without being aware of the injury. These fractures are usually the result of an inversion injury caused by physical fatigue; the dancer's timing is off, and the outside of

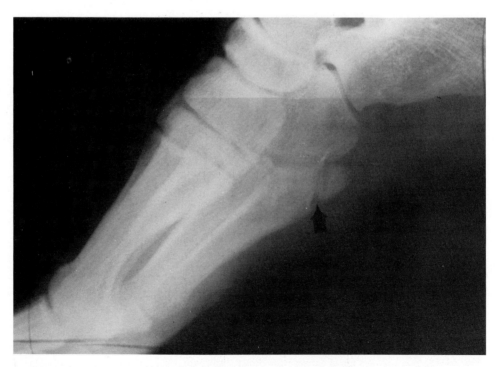

FIG. 61-20. Avulsion fracture of fifth metatarsal styloid through apophysis *(arrow)*. This fracture is uncommon in serious dance students and professionals because of their level of conditioning.

the foot is caught when landing from a leap or turn. The most common fracture site is at the junction of the neck and shaft. These fractures are usually spiral but may be transverse or comminuted. Treatment includes closed manipulation to effect an anatomic reduction. If there is displacement of the fracture and deformity can be predicted, open reduction with pin fixation is indicated to ensure a proper fit in the ballet or pointe shoe after healing. Postoperatively, the foot is held in a cast until bony union is present on radiographs. Healing of a nondisplaced fracture takes a minimum of 2 months until bony bridging is visible radiographically. The BAPS board is used following cast removal to develop proprioception and coordination, condition muscles, and increase range of motion. Exercises to increase intrinsic muscular strength in the foot are prescribed. It takes approximately 5 months to return to a full dance schedule following open or closed reduction.

Fractures through the base of the fifth metatarsal are somewhat less common, as are styloid, or Jones, fractures (Fig. 61-20). The styloid fracture initially described by Jones[27] in 1902 occurred when Jones sustained one while dancing the Viennese waltz. Professional dancers, on the other hand, seldom sustain this fracture because of the extensive conditioning of their feet.

Sesamoid Fracture

Transverse fractures of the sesamoids are common (Fig. 61-21). Acute fractures are usually transverse and occur as the dancer lands from a leap, or *jeté*. Treatment consists of using a ½-inch thick horseshoe-shaped felt pad shaped so that the open U area is large enough to provide relief around the fracture site. Danc-

ing is restricted until symptoms subside, which usually takes about 3 weeks. Gentle active and passive exercises of the toes and foot can be initiated by 2 weeks, as soon as the initial pain subsides. When symptoms subside, the dancer may return to class even though radiographs indicate that the fracture is not completely healed. A pad should be worn until symptoms of pain cease completely.

Chronic compression fractures of the sesamoids develop over a much longer period of time, up to 18 months, before diagnosis is made. They are the result of high stresses placed on the ball of the foot with the toe in a hyperextended position, such as during an ethnic dance step like the kowtow in which the dancer kneels with the body weight on the ball of the foot and the forehead touching the floor. Tangential radiographs of the sesamoid often show this fracture graphically, whereas it may be completely missed on the standard views of the foot (Fig. 61-22). Bone scans and tomograms are also useful. Treatment includes a ⅜-inch U-shaped felt pad with relief in the area of the sesamoid taped to the foot. The pad should be worn in street shoes also. Because the problem may be long-standing, dancing should be restricted following diagnosis until symptoms have been significantly reduced. NSAIDs are an adjunct to treatment.

Dislocation

Acute dislocation of a lesser toe is uncommon and usually occurs when the dancer strikes a piece of furniture while exiting from the well-lit stage into the poorly lit stage wing. Closed manipulation with splinting to adjacent toes for 3 weeks is the treatment of choice. Dancing is restricted until symptoms of pain subside, and lim-

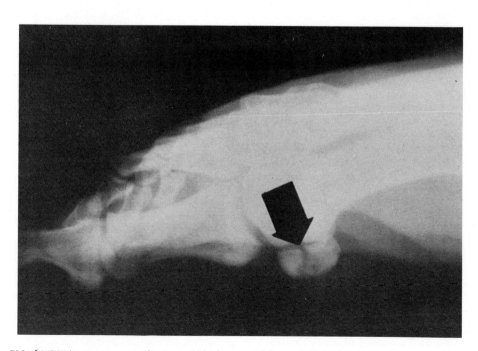

FIG. 61-21. Acute transverse fracture of tibial sesamoid (*arrow*). This often occurs on improper landing from a leap but heals within a few weeks to become asymptomatic.

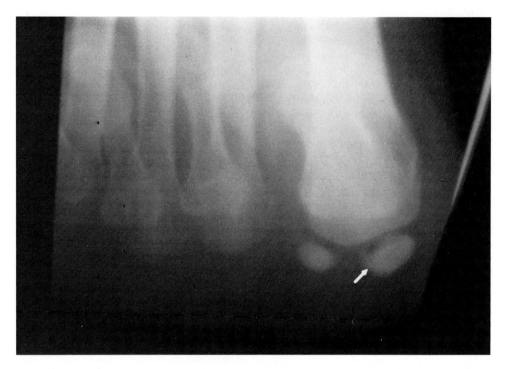

FIG. 61-22. Compression fracture of tibial sesamoid (*arrow*) as seen on tangential radiograph of foot. This fracture was symptomatic for 18 months before diagnosis.

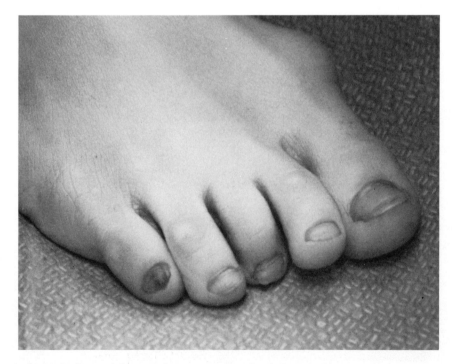

FIG. 61-23. Professional dancer in her teens with no family history of bunions demonstrating early bunion formation. This is common in dancers. It causes minimal symptoms and seldom requires surgical correction.

ited barre exercises are permitted thereafter. Whirlpool therapy, active range of motion of the toes, and use of antiinflammatory medication may be necessary for 3 months until the dancer is comfortable with use of the foot. The dancer may return to a full schedule before that time if symptoms have subsided.

Bunion

Hallux valgus and bunion develop at a younger age in dancers than in the general population (Fig. 61-23).[2,62,63] This may be because of the increased time they spend on the ball of the foot in dancing as well as the external constriction of a ballet pointe shoe.[23,47,50] However, the existence of these conditions in modern and folk dancers, who do not wear a constrictive shoe, suggests that dynamic muscle forces and a variety of dancer positions also contribute to their formation. Pain over the medial head of the first metatarsal usually subsides after a few hours of rest. Antiinflammatory medication and elevation control the symptoms. A foot and ankle flexibility program with the use of a proper-fitting shoe and appropriate padding with lamb's wool or felt helps lessen symptoms during dance class. Surgery is rarely necessary. A surgical procedure shortens and stiffens the toe, and convalescence is long, often a year. The dancer must be made aware of this possibility so as to participate in the decision with a knowledge of the career risks involved.

Hallux Rigidus

The increased time spent on the ball of the foot causes chronic stresses across the metatarsophalangeal joint and in the capsule and collateral ligaments of the hallux.[26] Infrequently, calcification in the ligaments and arthritis in the joints may cause hallux rigidus. Although

this may sometimes be mistaken for chronic stenosing tendinitis, radiographs indicate the true nature of the condition. The condition develops over a period of time, and the mature dancer accommodates his or her dance style to the decreasing hallux motion often without major symptoms as visible signs of altered dance technique. However, as symptoms of stiffness increase, the dancer is unable to dance in demi-pointe position or perform a *grand plié* without placing the foot in some varus. This is usually compensated for with style and technique so that it is not noticed by the audience. Pain may develop eventually, and technique may be compromised to accommodate for the stiffness. Treatment should be directed toward relieving the symptoms with physical therapy and the use of antiinflammatory medication before surgical cheilectomy is performed. I do not recommend Silastic arthroplasty. Although dancing may be resumed, the prognosis is guarded because of the pain and limited range of motion that may persist.

Subluxation of the Toe

Chronic subluxation of the metatarsophalangeal joint is characterized by pain beneath the ball of the foot in a lesser toe. As the dancer rises to the demi-pointe position on the ball of the foot, subluxation of the affected toe occurs slightly dorsally. This permits an increased load to be carried across the respective metatarsal head (Fig. 61-24). Symptoms increase over months and may even cause the dancer to stop dancing (Ronconi P: Personal communication, 1983).* Laxity in the dorsoplantar plane is demonstrated by manipulating the toe with the foot in the neutral non–weight-bearing position. If symptoms persist and pain is not relieved, excision of

---

*Physician to Ballet della Roma.

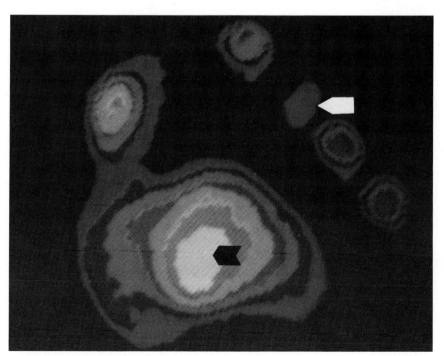

FIG. 61-24. Foot imprint demonstrating pressure beneath foot of dancer standing in demi-pointe position. Dancer has subluxation of third metatarsophalangeal joint. Lightest area shows most pressure and darker areas show least pressure. Impression made by subluxation of third toe shows no concentric rings beneath toe tuft (*upper arrow*) because it is exerting only minimal pressure on floor. However, high area of concentrated pressure is localized beneath third metatarsal head (*lower arrow*). (Courtesy D Ronconi, MD, Rome.)

20% of the proximal portion of the proximal phalanx is indicated. The capsule may then be drawn over the head of the metatarsal. This ensures that the plantar capsule remains beneath the metatarsal head. Rehabilitation requires at least 3 months. I prefer to use an axial Kirschner wire across the joint for 3 weeks to splint the toe in proper position during the healing phase, which prevents it from riding dorsally. Following removal of the pin, active range of motion is encouraged in the toes; however, a full rehearsal schedule is not recommended until edema and pain have completely resolved. Limited barre exercise, whirlpool therapy, and passive stretching are initiated 4 weeks postoperatively.

Interdigital Neuromas

Interdigital neuromas in dancers are treated initially using appropriate felt padding with relief in the area of tenderness. Corticosteroid injection into the pad of the foot in the region of the neuroma is *not* recommended because this may cause lysis in the supportive tissues of the fat pad beneath the metatarsal heads and cause development of a crystal granuloma consisting of sequestered corticosteroid vehicle. Excision is recommended in cases of persistent pain.

Avascular Necrosis

Avascular necrosis of the head of the metatarsal occurs insidiously and is aggravated in the dancer by long periods of time in the demi-pointe position (Pipkin G: Personal communication, 1975). Symptoms include pain and gradual onset of metatarsophalangeal stiffness (Fig. 61-25). Prognosis is guarded unless motion can be restored to the joint. Debridement of the metatarsophalan-

geal joint and, in particular, the osteophytes of the metatarsal head without disturbing the articular cartilage is recommended. However, if deformity is significant, the proximal 20% of the proximal phalanx is resected with debridement but not excision of the metatarsal head. The capsule is sutured over the metatarsal head to maintain soft tissue with the dancer in the demi-pointe position (Fig. 61-26). A Kirschner wire is used to secure the toe in alignment postoperatively. The wire is removed 3 weeks postoperatively, and active range of motion and barre exercises using the operated leg as the working leg are begun. Prosthetic replacement of the base of the phalanx in this condition results in stiffness and carries a poor prognosis.

Acute Flexion Injury of the Hallux: Tripping

Acute flexion injury of the hallux is caused by landing on the tip of the toe, which forces the hallux into sudden hyperflexion. This tears the mediodorsal capsule and ligaments. Acute tenderness directly over the metatarsophalangeal joint on flexion and indirectly in the same area when the hallux is flexed is diagnostic. There is no loss of stability at the joint. Treatment includes a compressive dressing followed by taping in 10 days when symptoms subside. Restricted activity is required for 3 weeks before the dancer is able to return to a full schedule.

Stress Fractures

Dancers who have poor technique and have not developed the ability to control their balance and coordination may develop a stress fracture of the foot. This may happen after rapid advancement of study or following ad-

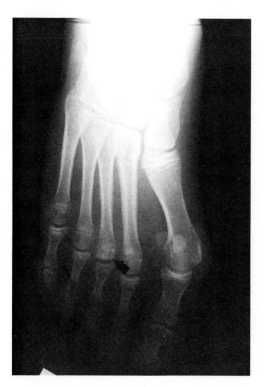

FIG. 61-25. Radiograph showing avascular necrosis of head of third metatarsal (*arrow*). Symptoms were present for 3 months before radiographic evidence was seen. Stiffness ensued.

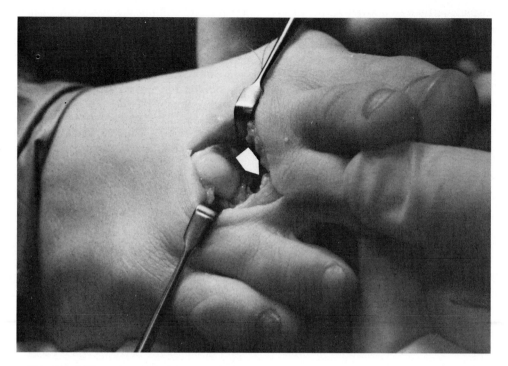

FIG. 61-26. Foot of patient with avascular necrosis of head of third metatarsal. Proximal 20% of proximal phalanx was excised *(arrow)*. Suture is present in plantar plate so that it can be secured to remaining synovial tissue.

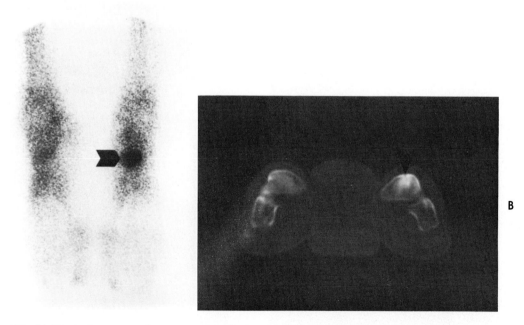

FIG. 61-27. A, Bone scan of patient previously diagnosed and treated as having tendinitis for 3 months. Tarsal navicular is "hot," indicating stress fracture *(arrow)*. **B,** Computed tomography scan of same patient showing transverse section through midfoot. Stress fracture *(arrow)* is seen extending from dorsal to plantar in tarsal navicular bone. (From Sammarco GJ: *Clin Orthop* 187:176, 1984.)

vancement from the corp de ballet to become a principal dancer. Unsupervised horseplay on a poorly conditioned foot or a hard floor can also lead to stress fracture. These fractures have been reported in every bone and through most of the articular surfaces of joints in dancers. Broadway show dancers get calcaneal fractures through the posterior part of the bone from dancing in "character shoes," which have a 2-inch (5-cm) heel. They also occur through the proximal portions of the second or third metatarsal and tarsal bones, such as the navicular and cuboid. The most rigid portion of the foot comprises the navicular, cuneiforms, and second and third metatarsals.[10,40,41,58] Most stress fractures occur in this area. Bone scans, CT scanning, and laminagrams are of prime importance in confirming the diagnosis (Fig. 61-27). Symptoms may be present for up to 1 year before diagnosis. On physical examination, tenderness may at first be diffuse and may localize to a specific, pinpoint area only in ensuing months. Treatment includes decreased weight bearing with elastic support and use of NSAIDs and crutches. Electric bone stimulation has been attempted with some success. Occasionally, open repair with bone grafting may be necessary. This requires at least 6 months for recovery. As the symptoms subside over a period of 6 to 8 weeks, the dancer may continue barre exercises in a swimming pool, that is, the water barre, and may be started in physical therapy using the BAPS board. The dancer should not return to a full schedule of dance until the fracture is healed and pain is gone.

SKIN
Fissuring

Shoes are not worn in modern dance, but in other types of dance the thin ballet slippers, pointe shoes, character shoes, or tap shoes may be used. The skin easily adapts to these coverings. Fissuring may be present at the skin flexion creases of the sole and toes. This occurs in modern dancers who dance barefoot. It is the result of increased friction at the foot-floor interface. To achieve better traction a dancer may put rosin on the feet, which increases the tension at the flexion creases. This condition is seldom disabling and is easily treated with gentle cleansing after class. Proper foot hygiene is stressed.

Corns and Calluses

Corns and calluses are a natural reaction of the body to increased pressure. Female classical ballet dancers often pad their toes. It is normal for classical ballet dancers to have calluses over the hallux and on the dorsal skin of the toes because the points of the toes bear weight when in a pointe shoe. Tender corns are treated with appropriate doughnut-shaped closed-cell foam padding, which the dancer shapes himself or herself. A single layer of micropore paper tape is recommended to fix the pad to the toes; this permits the skin to breathe (Fig. 61-28). Changing the pads repeatedly through rehearsal is also important. The dancer may choose to put lamb's wool in the point of the shoe to more evenly distribute the loads across the toes while dancing *sur les pointes*.

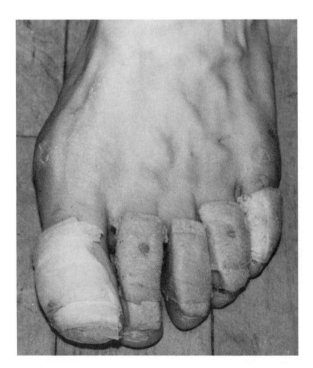

FIG. 61-28. "Normal" feet of classical ballet dancer showing use of pads and felt-shaped doughnuts to protect weight-bearing areas while dancing en pointe.

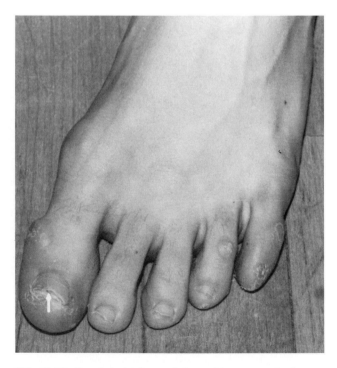

FIG. 61-29. Onycholysis of toenail (*arrow*) is common in dancers because they use the top of toe as weight-bearing surface.

Soft Corns

Soft corns between the toes are treated in a similar manner but with gentle cleansing, prophylactic antibiotic, and doughnut- or U-shaped felt pads. Care must be taken to prevent abscess formation in the web space because this can be disabling. If abscess occurs, incision and drainage are necessary. When surgical intervention is required, use of appropriate antibiotics is based on cultures taken at the time of surgery. Postoperatively, the dancer is encouraged to perform barre exercises even during the immediate postoperative period to maintain flexibility. Healing occurs within 2 weeks, and the patient should be able to resume full activity within 3 weeks.

TOENAILS

Subungual Hematoma: Black Toe

The dancer's toenails are subjected to increased stresses, and this may cause subungual hematoma. Although usually asymptomatic, if it is painful, it may be drained by drilling a small hole through the dorsal aspect of the hallux toenail to decompress the subungual blood. The hallux toenail should *not* be removed because it takes 1 year to regrow, and the bed remains tender during that period.

Onycholysis

Onycholysis commonly occurs in dancers because the tip of the nail has become weight bearing (Fig. 61-29). The nail bends forward and backward, causing delamination. This is usually painless and requires no treatment.

Paronychia

Paronychia should be treated with surgical incision and drainage and appropriate antibiotics. Cultures should be taken at the time of surgery and the patient given coverage with a gram-positive spectrum antibiotic until identification of the pathogen is made. At the time of surgery, irrigation of the wound with an antibiotic solution should be performed.

Ingrown Toenails

Ingrown toenails result from ill-fitting shoes or poor technique of pedicure, which permits the distal peripheral portion of the nail to remain intact while the central portion is removed. As the nail digs into the skin, inflammation occurs. Granulation tissue builds up and makes it difficult to dance. The lateral 20% of the nail may be removed surgically and the granulation tissue curetted. The bed is packed with Adaptic gauze to permit additional drainage. The dancer is restricted from dancing until the wound heals and is then counseled in the proper technique of nail trimming. The entire toenail should not be removed because it requires 1 year to regrow, and the bed remains tender during that period.

REFERENCES

1. Akella P et al: Scoliosis in ballet dancers, *Med Prob Perf Art* 6(3):84, 1991.
2. Ambre T: Degenerative changes in the first metatarsophalangeal joint of ballet dancers, *Acta Orthop Scand* 49;317, 1978.
3. Beaumont CW, Idzikowski S: *A manual of the theory and practice of classical theatrical dancing,* New York, 1970, Dover Publications.
4. Brodsky AE, Khalil MA: Talar compression syndrome, *Am J Sports Med* 14:472, 1986.
5. Brooke R: Sacroiliac joint, *J Anat* 58:299, 1924.
6. Burrows JJ: Fatigue infraction (incomplete fracture) of the middle of the tibia in ballet dancers, *J Bone Joint Surg* 38B:83, 1956.
7. Calabrese L, Kirkendall DG: Nutritional and medical consideration in dancers, *Clin Sports Med* 2:539, 1983.
8. Callander J: The dancer's spine. Paper presented at the fourth annual Dance Medicine Seminar, Cincinnati, 1982.
9. Cobb S, Sammarco GJ: Flexibility program for the dancer. Clinic for the Performing Arts. Paper presented at the Fifth Annual Dance Medicine Symposium, Cincinnati, 1983.
10. Collis WJM, Jayson MIV: Measurement of pedal pressures, *Am Rheum Dis* 31:317, 1972.
11. Como W: *Raoul Gelabert's anatomy for the dancer with exercises to improve technique and prevent injuries,* New York, 1964, Danad Publishing.
12. Cross MJ et al: Peroneus brevis rupture in the absence of the peroneus longus muscle and tendon in a classical ballet dancer, *Am J Sports Med* 16:677, 1988.
13. Devas MB: *Stress fractures,* Edinburgh, 1975, Churchill Livingstone.
14. Fernandez-Palazzi F, Rivas R, Mujica P: Achilles tendinitis in ballet dancers, *Clin Orthop* 257:257, 1990.
15. Garrick JA: Ballet injuries, *Med Prob Perf Art* 1(4):123, 1986.
16. Garrick J, Fillien D, Whiteside P: The epidemiology of aerobic dance injuries *Am J Sports Med* 14:67, 1986.
17. Grahame R, Jenkins JM: Joint hypermobility—asset or liability: a study of joint mobility in ballet dancers, *Ann Rheum Dis* 31:109, 1972.
18. Hamilton WG: Tendinitis about the ankle joint in classical ballet dancers, *Am J Sports Med* 5:84, 1977.
19. Hamilton WG: Sprained ankles in ballet dancers, *Foot Ankle* 3:99, 1982.
20. Hamilton WG: Stenosing tenosynovitis of the flexor hallucis longus tendon and posterior impingement upon the os trigonum in ballet dancers, *Foot Ankle* 3:74, 1982.
21. Hamilton WG et al: A profile of the musculoskeletal characteristics of elite professional ballet dancers, *Am J Sports Med* 20:267, 1992.
22. Hardaker WT et al: Ankle sprains in theatrical dancers, *Med Prob Perf Art* 3(4):146, 1988.
23. Hardy RH, Clapham JC: Observations on hallux valgus, *J Bone Joint Surg* 33B:376, 1951.
24. Howse AJG: Orthopaedists aid ballet, *Clin Orthop* 89:52, 1972.
25. Howse AJG: Posterior block of the ankle joint in dancers, *Foot Ankle* 3:8, 1982.
26. Howse AJG: Disorders of the great toe in dancers, *Clin Sports Med* 2:499, 1983.
27. Jones R: Fractures of the fifth metatarsal bone, *Liverpool Med Surg J* 42:103, 1902.
28. Kadel NJ: Stress fractures in ballet dancers, *Am J Sports Med* 20:445, 1992.
29. Kerr G, Krasnow D, Mainwaring L: The nature of dance injuries, *Med Prob Perf Art* 7(1):25, 1992.
30. Kirkendall DT, Calabrese L: Physiological aspects of dance, *Clin Sports Med* 2:525, 1983.
31. Kleiger B: Anterior tibiotalar impingement syndromes in dancers, *Foot Ankle* 3:69, 1982.
32. Klemp P, Chalton D: Articular mobility in ballet dancers, *Am J Sports Med* 17:72, 1989.
33. Klemp P, Learmonth ID: Hypermobility and injuries in a professional ballet company, *Br J Sports Med* 18:143, 1984.
34. Klemp P, Stevens JE, Isaacs S: A hypermobility study in ballet dancers, *J Rheumatol* 11:692, 1984.
35. Laws K: Physics and the potential for dance injury, *Med Prob Perf Art* 1(3):73, 1986.
36. Lawson J: *Classical ballet: its style and technique,* New York, 1960, MacMillan Publishing.
37. Lee SA: Patterns of choice, bias, and belief: report from a pilot study on dancers and health care, *Med Prob Perf Art* 7(2):52, 1992.

38. Lindholm A: A new method of operation in the subcutaneous rupture of the Achilles tendon, *Acta Chir Scand* 117:261, 1959.

39. Lynn T: Repair of the torn Achilles tendon, using the plantaris tendon as a reinforcing membrane, *J Bone Joint Surg* 48A:268, 1966.

40. Mann RA: Biomechanics of the foot. In American Academy of Orthopaedic Surgery: *Atlas of orthotics: biomechanical principles and applications*, St Louis, 1975, Mosby.

41. Manter JT: Distribution of compression forces in the joints of the human foot, *Anat Rec* 96:313, 1946.

42. Marshall P, Hamilton WG: Cuboid subluxation in ballet dancers, *Am J Sports Med* 20:169, 1992.

43. McNeal AP et al: Lower extremity alignment and injury in young preprofessional college and professional ballet dancers: dancer-reported injuries, *Med Prob Perf Art* 5(2):83, 1990.

44. Messerer A: *Classes in classical ballet*, New York, 1975, Doubleday.

45. Miller EH, Benedict FE: Stretch of the femoral nerve in a dancer, *J Bone Joint Surg* 67:315, 1985.

46. Miller EH et al: A new consideration in athletic injuries—the classical ballet dancer, *Clin Orthop* 3:181, 1975.

47. Nikolic V, Zimmerman B: Functional changes of tarsal bones of ballet dancers, *Rad Med Fak Zegrebu* 16:131, 1968.

48. Nixon JE: Injuries to the neck and upper extremities of dancers, *Clin Sports Med* 2:459, 1983.

49. O'Donoghue DH: *Treatment of injuries to athletes*, ed 4, Philadelphia, 1984, WB Saunders.

50. Pelipenko VL: Specific characteristics of the development of the foot skeleton in pupils of a choreographic school, *Arkh Anat Gistol Embriol* 64:46, 1974.

51. Quirk R: Talar compression syndrome in dancers, *Foot Ankle* 3:65, 1982.

52. Quirk R: The Australian experience, *Clin Sports Med* 2:507, 1983.

53. Quirk R: Knee injuries in classical dancers, *Med Prob Perf Art* 3(2):52, 1988.

54. Rambert M: *Quicksilver*, London, 1972, Macmillan Publishing.

55. Reid DC et al: Lower extremity flexibility patterns in classical ballet dancers and their correlation to lateral hip and knee injuries, *Am J Sports Med* 15:347, 1987.

56. Sammarco GJ: The foot and ankle in classical ballet and modern dance. . In Jahss MH (ed): *Disorders of the foot*, Philadelphia, 1982, WB Saunders.

57. Sammarco GJ: The dancer's hip, *Clin Sports Med* 2:485, 1983.

58. Sammarco GJ: Diagnosis and treatment in dancers. *Clin Orthop* 187:176, 1984.

59. Sammarco GJ: The hip in dancers, *Med Prob Perf Art* 2:5, 1987.

60. Sammarco GJ, Burstein AH, Frankel VH: Biomechanics of the ankle: a kinematic study, *Orthop Clin North Am* 4:75, 1973.

61. Sammarco GJ, Miller EH: Partial rupture of the flexor hallucis longus in classical ballet dancers, *J Bone Joint Surg* 61A:440, 1979.

62. Sammarco GJ, Miller EH: Forefoot conditions in dancers. Part 1. *Foot Ankle* 3:85, 1982.

63. Sammarco GJ, Miller EH: Forefoot conditions in dancers. Part 2. *Foot Ankle* 3:93, 1982.

64. Sammarco GJ, Stephens MM: Neuropraxia of the femoral nerve in a modern dancer, *Am J Sports Med* 19(4):413, 1991.

65. Schneider JH et al: Stress injuries and developmental change of lower extremities in ballet dancers, *Radiology* 113:627, 1974.

66. Seals J: A study of dance surfaces, *Clin Sports Med* 2:557, 1983.

67. Seals J: Dance floors, *Med Prob Perf Art* 1(3):81, 1986.

68. Sparger C: *Anatomy and ballet*, ed 5, London, 1970, Adam and Charles Black.

69. Stojanovie S, Marenie S, Ukropina D: Disease in ballet dancers, *Srp Arh Celok Lek* 91:903, 1963.

70. Strudwick WJ: Proximal fibular stress fracture in an aerobic dancer, *Am J Sports Med* 20:481, 1992.

71. Tomasen E: *Diseases and injuries of ballet dancers*, Copenhagen, 1982, Universitetsforlaget I Arhus.

72. Vaganova A: *Principles of classical ballet*, New York, 1969, Dover Publications.

73. Volkov MV: Principles of diagnosis, treatment, and prevention of occupational injuries in ballet dancers. *Vestn Khir* 114:87, 1975.

74. Volkov MV, Badnin IA: Surgical treatment of certain occupational injuries and diseases of bones and joints, *Khirurgiia (Mosk)* 5:137, 1975.

75. Wilcox JR et al: Bone scanning in the evaluation of exercise-related stress injuries, *Radiology* 123:699, 1977.

CHAPTER 62 Basketball Injuries

John G. Yost, Jr.
Daniel W. Schmoll

Basketball is a popular sport in America that is closing in on its centennial as an organized sport. Basketball was first played at Smith College in Northampton, Massachusetts, in 1894. It remained a women's sport only until 1920 at which time it was added to the men's sport curriculum. It has since developed worldwide popularity and has been included as an Olympic sport since 1936. Basketball ranks thirteenth in the United States in sports participation with an average of 25,323,000 participants according to a 1982 survey by the A.C. Nielsen Co. It is a sport that requires speed, strength, endurance, quick reflexes, coordination, balance, agility, and excellent peripheral vision.[2,44] The role of somatotype is greater in basketball than in any other sport. On a competitive level, in general, individuals are tall and tend toward a more ectomorphic or mesomorphic body type.[42,46]

EPIDEMIOLOGY

For many years an increasing amount of body contact has been allowed in basketball, first on the professional level and now in college and high schools. Consequently, the injuries incurred in basketball are a combination of contact injuries from collisions and falls similar to those in football and ice hockey and overuse injuries from running, jumping, and quick acceleration and deceleration similar to those seen in track and field events.

Basketball is a limited contact sport in which the predominant motion is running. It poses a significant burden on the musculoskeletal system, and musculoskeletal injuries are common. The incidence of injuries by the area involved at the adolescent and elite levels are shown in Table 62-1. On the high school level the ankle is the sight most often injured, followed by the knee, thigh, shoulder, and hand. Sprains, strains, and contusions are the most common types of injuries. Reports by Moritz and Grana,[26] Zelisko, Noble, and Porter,[50] and others[45] comparing male and female basketball injuries showed a much higher incidence in females. It is hypothesized by these authors that poor initial conditioning accounted for this difference because most of the injuries in the female players occurred early in the season (Table 62-2).[26] The injuries of Swedish elite basketball players surveyed by Colliander et al[7] also demonstrates a slightly higher incidence of injuries among women and correlates well with the types of injuries seen in professional American basketball. However, the frequency of injuries on the

TABLE 62-1 Percent of incidence of injury by anatomic location in the lower extremity and spine

	Back	Hip and Thigh	Knee	Ankle	Foot
Henry et al	11.5	10	14	18.2	6
Apple et al	14	—	18	14	6
Yde and Nielson	—	5	5	33	0
Zelisko et al					
Male	8.2	9.2	18	20.3	2.1
Female	13	14.8	19.3	17.9	6.7
Moritz and Grana					
Male	0	0	12	36	12
Female	5	18	11	30	8
Colliander et al					
Male	5	2	19	48	5
Female	1	3	17	56	8

Data from Henry JH, Lauear B, Neigut D: *Am J Sports Med* 10:16, 1982; Apple DF, O'Toole J, Annis C: *Phys Sports Med* 10(1):81, 1982; Yde J, Nielsen AB: *Br J Sport Med* 24(1):51, 1990; Zelisko JA, Noble HB, Porter M: *Am J Sports Med* 10:297, 1982; Moritz A, Grana WA: *Phys Sports Med* 6:91, 1978; and Colliander E et al: *Orthopedics* 9(2):225, 1986.

TABLE 62-2 Frequency of injuries throughout the season

	Number of Injuries	
	Boys	Girls
November	2	14
December	2	12
January	2	12
February	2	2
March	0	3

From Moritz A, Grana WA: *Phys Sports Med* 6:91, 1978.

TABLE 62-3 Relationship of type of injury and player position

	Guard		Forward		Center	
	Henry et al	Apple et al	Henry et al	Apple et al	Henry et al	Apple et al
Back	11%	12%	<10%	13%	<10%	24%
Knee	48%	22%	<10%	21%	17%	12%
Ankle	<10%	10%	<10%	14%	14%	16%
Foot	12%	<10%	<10%	<10%	<10%	12%

Data from Henry JH, Lauear B, Neigut D: *Am J Sports Med* 10:16, 1982; and Apple DF, O'Toole J, Annis C: *Phys Sports Med* 10(1):81, 1982.

whole is much lower among these elite amateurs when compared with American professionals.

Studies of professional athletes by Apple, O'Toole, and Annis[2] and Henry, Lauear, and Neigut[12] show that 67% to 69% of players sustain at least one injury in a season. The knee, back, and ankle were areas most commonly involved (Table 62-3).[2,12] Most injuries occur early in the season. Apple, O'Toole, and Annis[2] found that 46.7% of the injuries occurred during practice and the first 27 games of an 82-game season. Henry, Lauear, and Neigut[12] found that most injuries occurred in game situations. Injuries during practice were second most common (Table 62-4). In these studies and those by Colliander et al,[7] injuries to the knee resulted in the longest restriction from participation and required the greatest number of surgical procedures. Ligamentous and meniscal injuries were seen in addition to contusion and overuse problems.

Ankle sprains represent the most common traumatic injury at all levels of play.[2,7,12,47,50] By the time a competitive athlete gets to the professional level, he or she usually has a history of several ankle injuries to both ankles and often has evidence of early degenerative changes as well. Other common problems include back injuries of which strains and sprains are most common,

"jumper's knee," thigh contusions, groin strains, hamstring strains, and Achilles tendinitis. In general, stress fractures of the fifth metatarsal and the tarsonavicular and sprains of the tarsometatarsal ligaments are infrequent injuries, but they have a high incidence in basketball players.[7,14,40,41]

BACK INJURIES

Depending on the study, injuries to the lumbar spine reportedly represent the second or third largest group of injuries among basketball players followed by ankle and knee injuries.[7,12,50] Centers were most commonly involved in one series.[2] Basketball requires an exceptional amount of jumping and twisting, often with outstretched arms. This increases the stress forces (compression, flexion, and lateral rotation) on the lumbar disks and vertebrae.[36] Types of back injuries included lumbosacral sprains and contusion, stress fractures, and disk injuries.

Lumbosacral contusions are the result of direct trauma and are common to all contact sports. The treatment should consist of ice, compression, rest, and as symptoms resolve, gentle range of motion exercises. Early return to competition is usually allowed. Lumbosacral sprains, stress fractures to the pars interarticularis, and disk in-

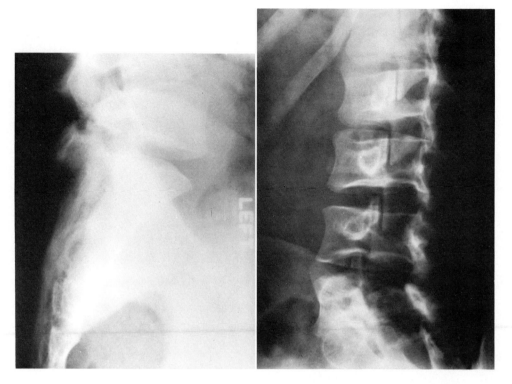

FIG. 62-1. Spondylolysis with Grade I spondylolisthesis in professional basketball player.

TABLE 62-4 Relationship of activities to injuries

Situation	Percentage of Injuries
Game	45.0
First quarter	8.0
Second quarter	15.0
Third quarter	11.0
Fourth quarter	11.0
Practice	23.0
Warm-up	6.0
Scrimmage	0.2
Other	25.8

From Henry JH, Lauear B, Neigut D: *Am J Sports Med* 10:16, 1982.

Contributing factors to back injuries in basketball

- Poor conditioning
- Improper body mechanics
- Overuse
- Poor preworkout stretching
- Incomplete rehabilitation of injuries of the lower extremity
- Unrecognized or untreated previous injury

---

jury are associated with high-velocity running, twisting, or bending and a high-moment force applied to the lumbar spine.[39] These injuries occur, for example, when a player comes down from a rebound slightly off balance and tries to maintain a central center of gravity or jumps off balance and decelerates with the back in flexion. These injuries occur in basketball players of all ages, and they cause the symptoms of back pain. Successful treatment of these problems lies in early recognition and treatment of the specific problem. Back injuries may be precipitated by poor conditioning, improper mechanics, overuse, or poor preworkout stretching. In addition, incompletely rehabilitated injuries of the lower extremities or unrecognized or untreated prior injuries can fatigue more quickly than the rest of the body during activity, putting greater strains on the lower back. Prevention of many injuries is possible by having the athlete work on stretching of the lumbosacral muscles and strengthening of the abdominal musculature and by rehabilitation of any deficiencies in the lower extremities.[39]

Examination of the injured player may show abnormal posture with a lumbar list, limitation of motion, flattening of the lumbar spine, and reproduction of symptoms with flexion, extension, and lateral bending. Injuries to the pars interarticularis (spondylolysis or spondylolisthesis) are usually associated with repetitive stresses over a period of time (Fig. 62-1). In our experience spondylolysis is rare in collegiate and professional players. Athletes with symptomatic spondylolysis are "weeded out" by their back problems before they reach high levels of competition. Lumbosacral sprains are treated initially with rest, ice, support, and as symptoms resolve, gentle range of motion exercises. Spondylolysis is seen in younger athletes, usually adolescents. On examination, the player has pain on hyperextension. Oblique radiographs often show the defect, which is most commonly in the pars interarticularis of L5. It can also occur at level L3 or L4. If

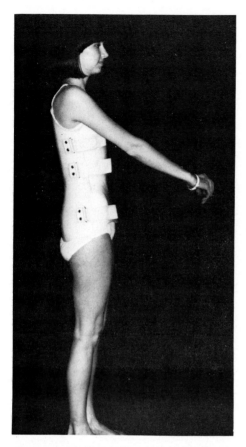

FIG. 62-2. Anterior-opening Boston brace for spondylolysis.

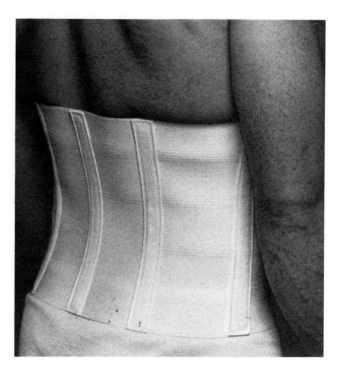

FIG. 62-3. Basketball player in lumbosacral corset.

radiographs are inconclusive, a bone scan has been found to be of great assistance in making the diagnosis. The treatment usually consists of rest until symptoms resolve and strengthening and stretching exercises for the spine and lower extremities. Bracing has been used successfully; it allows early resumption of activities.[25] An anterior-opening antilordotic polyethylene brace was used in 52 young athletes, 12 of whom had spondylolysis. Of these, 8 had excellent results and 4 had good results. The brace, which is a semirigid orthosis, lessens the loading on the spine by decreasing the lumbar lordosis and increasing intraabdominal pressure and, at the same time, limiting pelvic torsion of the trunk (Fig 62-2). A flexibility and muscle strengthening exercise program is used in conjunction with the brace. The brace is worn for an average of 3 to 6 months. In patients with a positive bone scan, it is recommended that the brace be worn until the bone scan is negative.[25]

If symptoms of a back injury include radiculopathy and increased pain with coughing or sneezing and examination reveals positive straight leg raising or bowstring signs, the athlete should be considered to have a disk injury until proven otherwise. With a severe disk injury, extrusion or protusion of the nucleus pulposus can injure the nerve root, resulting in a sensory or motor deficit. Hospitalization for absolute bed rest, antiinflammatory medication, analgesics, and muscle relaxants are necessary. As symptoms improve, gentle exercises for ab-

TABLE 62-5 Graded return to basketball following back injury (including postoperative patients)

Steps*	Activity
I	Running
II	Dribbling and cutting
III	Jumping and shooting
IV	Practice sessions (half-court initially, then full-court)
V	Limited playing time
VI	Full activity

*Note: Advancement between stages is dependent on pain-free activity in each stage. Length of time is variable in different players and types of injuries.

TABLE 62-6 Criteria for return to play following back injury

Symptoms	Examination Findings
No pain	Normal flexibility
No spasm	Normal strength
No neurologic complaints	No abnormal neurologic findings

dominal strengthening and back flexibility are started. Calf and hamstring stretching exercises should also be performed if they are not painful. Swimming is an excellent rehabilitation exercise and is recommended. The sidestroke, crawl, and backstroke are usually well tolerated.

If symptoms are unabated after 10 to 14 days, epidural

injections can be started. A standard dose of 5 ml of 1% lidocaine and 40 to 80 mg methylprednisolone (Depo-Medrol) is used. Epidural injections can be spaced out over several days or weeks; however, no more than three injections should be given. If symptoms of sciatica persist after 3 months or if the patient has a progressive weakness of the dorsiflexors, plantar flexors, hip abductors, or more rarely, quadriceps muscles, high-resolution computed tomography (CT) scanning, magnetic resonance imaging (MRI), or lumbar myelography should be performed to confirm the diagnosis. Surgical disk excision can then be performed. Postoperatively, the patient is allowed out of bed as tolerated and a corset is applied (Fig. 62-3). At 3 weeks the athlete can begin a gentle stretching and strengthening program for the back if symptoms have abated. This is followed by a supervised, graduated increase in activity as outlined in Table 62-5. The entire course of rehabilitation after back surgery is 4 to 6 months. The time before returning to basketball depends on rehabilitation of strength, power, endurance, and flexibility of the legs and spine following surgery. The criteria for allowing complete resumption of basketball are outline in Table 62-6.

HIP, GROIN, AND THIGH INJURIES

Injuries of the hip, groin, and thigh are less common than other injuries to the lower extremities in basketball players.[2,7,12,50] Contusions and muscle strains are the most common injures in this area.

Contusions

Contusions are common in basketball because of the large body area that is unprotected by special equipment. Mechanisms of injury include blunt trauma from an opponent's knee or elbow, particularly during aggressive rebounding with the elbows held away from the body. Contusions from blunt trauma can lead to formation of a large hematoma, which may progress to myositis ossificans (Fig. 62-4). To prevent this complication, all contusions should be treated with ice, compression, and rest. In the case of a large hematoma, protective weight bearing is added. Stretching exercises are started as soon as possible to prevent contracture in the involved muscle group. For example, quadriceps stretching and iliotibial band stretching exercises are used for an anterolateral thigh hematoma (see Chapter 45). Progressive resistance exercises for the involved muscle group are started as soon as symptoms allow. In addition, all components of the extremity must be rehabilitated. Progressive resistance exercises are included for hip adduction, hip abduction, quadriceps strengthening, hip flexion, knee extension, and dorsiflexion and plantar flexion of the ankle.

Muscle Strains

Quadriceps, hamstring, rectus femoris, and adductor muscle strains occur from excessive tension on a contracted muscle fiber that causes it to tear.[49] This develops into a fibrous scar tissue, which, as it matures, develops contractures. Contractures result in a net loss of excursion in the muscle unit with a decrease in func-

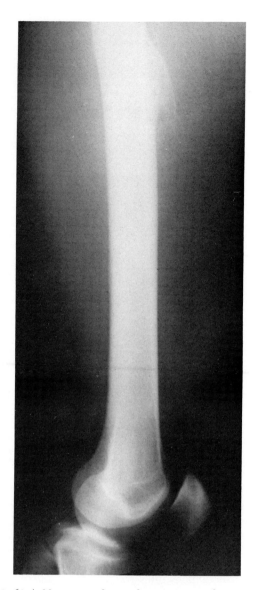

FIG. 62-4. Myositis ossificans of vastus intermedius muscle.

tion and an increase in the risk of reinjury. The most common area involved in the quadriceps muscle is the middle portion of the rectus femoris. The most common areas in the groin are the upper portions of the adductor longus and adductor magnus. The lower and middle portions of the biceps femoris are the most commonly involved portions of the hamstring. The mechanism of injury is a forced overload during an eccentric muscle contraction. This occurs when the muscle is contracting against a strong external force or when a sudden uncoordinated force is applied while the muscle is in a state of maximal contracture.[49] Weakness may also predispose to muscle strains because the protective mechanism of strength is lost. Muscle strains can be graded by the amount of tissue damage. Grade I is designated as the mildest, and Grade III is the most severe, characterized by complete tissue disruption. The severity of the strain dictates the amount of time out of activity. A Grade III muscle strain is usually a 4- to 6-week injury.

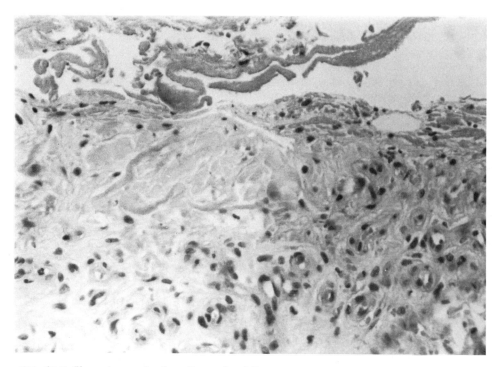

FIG. 62-5. Photomicrograph of patellar tendon following spontaneous rupture. Note degenerative fraying with moderate hypercellularity and vascular proliferation (hematoxylin and eosin stain).

The treatment includes rest, ice, compression, and elevation (RICE). When symptoms improve, stretching within the bounds of pain to maintain normal muscle excursion is begun. This is followed by a progressive resistance exercise program to attain normal strength in comparison to the opposite extremity. This is followed by organized and supervised resumption of activity.

Stress Fractures

If a player demonstrates symptoms of vague thigh pain that is originally presumed to be a quadriceps strain but symptoms do not improve with physical therapy and reduction of activities as described previously, a stress fracture of the femur should be considered. Symptoms characteristic of a stress fracture of the femur include vague thigh pain, diffuse tenderness, and no antecedent history of trauma. Early definitive diagnosis can be made by radionuclide scanning or, if symptoms have been present for a sufficient period of time, plain radiography. In a case study of a professional basketball player, conservative therapy enabled the athlete to return to play within the same season without symptoms or difficulties.[13]

LOWER EXTREMITY TENDINITIS AND TENDON RUPTURES

Tendinitis and tendon rupture are associated with the constant jumping and quick acceleration and deceleration that are inherent in basketball. Tendinitis around the knee is more common in basketball players than any other athlete. Numerous investigators have addressed this issue by trying to understand what places the bas-

ketball player at higher risk for such an injury. Studies such as those by Sommer[38] have attempted to show that intrinsic factors or abnormalities of the knee extensor mechanism may play a role. On the other hand, Ferretti[9] has shown that extrinsic factors including the type of playing surface and the duration of play are also important in the etiology of this condition. The most common areas involved in the lower extremity are the quadriceps, patellar, and Achilles tendons. Blazina et al[4] coined the term "jumper's knee" to describe the tendinitis of the patellar and quadriceps tendons that they found to occur most commonly in basketball players. Tendinitis is an inflammation of the tendinous portion of the musculotendinous unit and is caused by repetitive trauma. It should be considered a pathologic condition of the bone-tendon junction. Microscopic tears occur, followed by inflammation, degeneration, and replacement with scar tissue (Fig. 62-5). In a microscopic study of specimens obtained during surgery for jumper's knee, Ferretti et al[10] found that the main abnormalities were pseudocystic cavities at the borderline between mineralized fibrocartilage and bone, increased thickness of the fibrocartilage, myxomatous metaplasia of the fibrocartilage, mineralization and ossification far from the tidemark, and disappearance of the tidemark. Roels et al[31] described different findings in their patients with jumper's knee. They reported a mucoid degeneration, fibrinoid necrosis, mineralization in areas of regeneration, and fibroblast capsular proliferation in the patellar tendon. These patients, however, had received repeated local injections of corticosteroids. Ferretti et al[10] had similar findings in one patient in their series who had received local injections of steroids. In

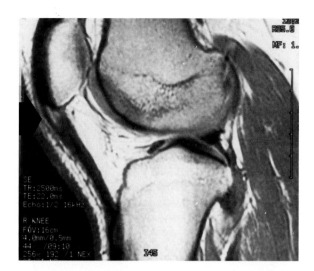

FIG. 62-6. Patellar tendinitis with abnormal magnetic resonance imaging signal (*arrow*).

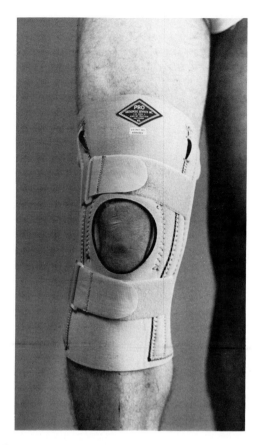

FIG. 62-7. A neoprene patella-restraining brace that is useful in a variety of patellofemoral disorders.

an experiment on rabbit patellar tendons Kennedy and Willes[17] clearly demonstrated that steroids injected directly into a normal tendon weakened it significantly for 2 weeks. They thought that this biomechanical disruption was directly related to collagen necrosis. This phenomenon was followed by the formation of a relatively acellular amorphous material. Bodne et al[5] have demonstrated the value of MRI in the evaluation of tendon disorders. They have used MRI to detect thickening and to illustrate areas of focal involvement as well as reveal chronic tears in the tendons of basketball players (Fig. 62-6).

Quadriceps Tendinitis

Quadriceps tendinitis is an overuse syndrome that is common in basketball players. It is caused by repetitive jumping. It is most often seen in older basketball players, particularly those older than 30 years of age. It can be bilateral and tends to be chronic in the older athlete. The tendon undergoes repetitive trauma with running, and quadriceps tendinitis is associated with a tight muscle-tendon unit, inadequate flexibility, and improper strengthening exercises. Dull aching pain and a burning sensation along the insertion of the tendon are common complaints, and tenderness to palpation of the tendon-bone junction is found on physical examination. In chronic cases and older patients, rupture can occur. Treatment of quadriceps tendinitis is conservative and consists of limitation of activities (while symptomatic), heat, and use of oral antiinflammatory medication. Quadriceps stretching exercises are begun immediately. Tight hamstrings are also common in these patients. As flexibility increases and pain resolves, quadriceps, hip abductor, and hip flexor strengthening exercises are started in a progressive resistance manner using weights with the knee in full extension. This prevents the repetitive loading of the injured area during rehabilitation that occurs with the knee flexion-extension exercises with weights. When the patient's strength in both lower extremities is

equal, activities are resumed on a supervised basis. A patella-restraining brace is helpful and should be worn when activity is resumed (Fig. 62-7).

Patellar Tendinitis

Patellar tendinitis is seen more is basketball players than in any other athlete. Blazina et al[4] found it to be one of the three most common injuries in college basketball players. The patellar tendon is strong, and it has been demonstrated that the forces necessary to rupture the tendon equal 17.5 times body weight.[4] In spite of this, spontaneous ruptures of this tendon have been reported, most commonly associated with chronic pain in the older athlete. Patellar tendinitis is seen in players of all ages. It usually has a slow onset with an aching, burning pain in the area of the inferior aspect of the patella. On examination, there is tenderness at the insertion of the tendon into the inferior pole of the patella. A patellar tendon may be normal in appearance or slightly enlarged, and in chronic cases it may be smaller on palpation than the unaffected side. In addition, tight, weak hip flexors are often found on examination of patients with patellar tendinitis.

Patella alta is commonly seen in patients with patellar tendinitis (Fig. 62-8). Osgood-Schlatter disease, which is thought to be a benign entity resulting from partial avulsion of the growing tibial tubercle with subsequent avascular necrosis, may also be found.[33] Sindig-Larsen-

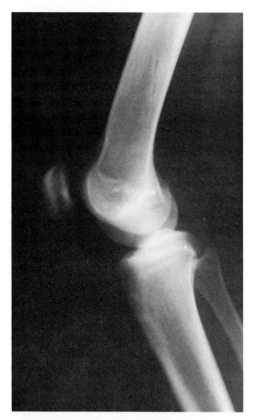

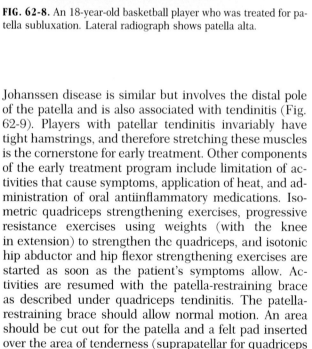

FIG. 62-8. An 18-year-old basketball player who was treated for patella subluxation. Lateral radiograph shows patella alta.

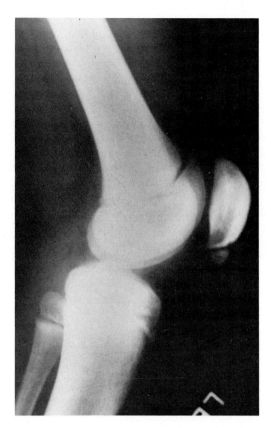

FIG. 62-9. A 13-year-old basketball player clinically diagnosed with "jumper's knee." Lateral radiograph shows Sindig-Larsen-Johanssen disease.

Johanssen disease is similar but involves the distal pole of the patella and is also associated with tendinitis (Fig. 62-9). Players with patellar tendinitis invariably have tight hamstrings, and therefore stretching these muscles is the cornerstone for early treatment. Other components of the early treatment program include limitation of activities that cause symptoms, application of heat, and administration of oral antiinflammatory medications. Isometric quadriceps strengthening exercises, progressive resistance exercises using weights (with the knee in extension) to strengthen the quadriceps, and isotonic hip abductor and hip flexor strengthening exercises are started as soon as the patient's symptoms allow. Activities are resumed with the patella-restraining brace as described under quadriceps tendinitis. The patella-restraining brace should allow normal motion. An area should be cut out for the patella and a felt pad inserted over the area of tenderness (suprapatellar for quadriceps tendinitis and infrapatellar for patellar tendinitis).

Achilles Tendinitis

Achilles tendinitis ranks only behind patellar tendinitis in frequency among overuse injuries in basketball players. The tendon undergoes repetitive trauma with running. This condition is associated with a tight muscle-tendon unit, inadequate flexibility of the hamstrings, and improper strength conditioning of the entire lower extremity. Pain and a burning sensation along the insertion of the tendon are common complaints. Tenderness is palpated in the same area. The tendon may become large in chronic cases, and partial or complete rupture can occur. The treatment of Achilles tendinitis is conservative and consists of rest, heat, and use of oral antiinflammatory medication with limitation of activities. A heel lift is inserted into the shoe. Heat treatments or hot-and-cold contrast treatments are used. A stretching exercise program for the hamstrings and Achilles tendon is started with a progressive resistance exercise program for the entire lower extremity. When strength is equal in both lower extremities, the patient returns to activity with a felt insert in the shoe. On the court, running is started with dribbling and no cutting. The athlete is then permitted to try jumping and shooting, and if this is tolerated well, cutting and progression to a full-court, game-type situation are instituted.

Injection of steroids in the tendons is not recommended. Ferretti et al[10] found mucoid degeneration and fibrinoid necrosis on histologic examination of tissue from a patient with patellar tendinitis who had undergone steroid injections. Kennedy and Willes[17] studied rabbit Achilles tendons 7 days after injection and found that strength was 35% lower than controls and remained lower until approximately 2 weeks later. These findings imply that injection into the tendons can cause weakening of the tendon structure and put the player at risk for complete disruption of the tendon.

Tendon Ruptures

A tendon rupture in a collegiate or professional basketball player is a catastrophic injury and should be treated aggressively once the diagnosis is made. A tendon rupture usually has a history of sudden sharp pain, as if the individual had been kicked, usually during an activity in which the player has just undergone a quick acceleration or deceleration. Some may consider this an end stage of jumper's knee. With **quadriceps tendon rupture** there is a palpable defect at the superior pole of the patella.[34] The player often has an extension lag; however, if the retinaculum is still intact, the athlete can perform a straight leg raise. Kelly et al[15] point out that these quadriceps tendon ruptures are usually partial, involving mainly the rectus femoris tendon. A rupture of the **inferior pole of the patella** has a similar history, and on examination there is a palpable defect at the inferior pole of the patella. An extension lag is usually present, and the player is unable to do a straight leg raise if the retinaculum is torn. The patient with a ruptured **Achilles tendon** has a positive Thompson test in addition to the palpable defect. Rosenberg and Whitaker[32] have even documented a case of bilateral infrapatellar tendon rupture in a basketball player with jumper's knee who had no underlying systemic disease. Cases reported by Frankl, Wasilewski, and Healy[11] and Maar, Kerneck, and Pierce[21] on the younger athlete illustrate that the avulsion fractures of the tibial tubercle may also be seen.

Operative repair is required for all tendon ruptures. In cases of chronic disease in which there is a great deal of degeneration and tissue damage to the patellar tendon, it may be necessary to augment the patellar tendon using the semitendinosus. If a large defect remains after resection of the degenerated Achilles tendon, the plantaris tendon or a turned-down flap of the Achilles tendon is used to reinforce the defect in the Achilles tendon.[19,23,24] This is followed by cast immobilization.

A repair of a quadriceps or patellar tendon rupture is augmented by stainless steel suture to relieve tension on the repair site, and immobilization is maintained in a cylinder cast for 6 weeks. At 6 weeks the suture is removed and the patient is started on active, assisted range of motion exercises. Strengthening exercises for the plantar flexors and dorsiflexors of the foot are started immediately. When the player has full extension and at least 90 degrees of flexion, progressive resistance exercises for the hamstrings and quadriceps are started. Protected ambulation and, in cases requiring augmentation, a knee orthosis is used until the patient has a full range of motion. When quadriceps and hamstring strength are equal in both lower extremities, the patient has a normal range of motion, and there is no tenderness in the area of the repair, running in a patella-restraining brace is started. This is followed by running, dribbling, and cutting. Jumping is added last. When this is well tolerated, the player is allowed back into practice. Game time should be limited with a gradual progression of playing minutes as tolerated. Any signs of increased pain and swelling in the area of the repair require immediate reduction in activities until the symptoms have resolved.

Following repair of the Achilles tendon the extremity is placed in a long leg cast for 3 weeks. At that time the sutures are removed and the patient is changed to a short leg non–weight-bearing cast for 3 additional weeks. When the cast is removed, range of motion exercises are started and protective weight bearing is continued until a normal range of motion is attained. Strengthening exercises are added as soon as the patient has a normal range of motion. When strength is normal in both lower extremities, the patient is allowed to run with a heel lift. If running is well tolerated, cutting and shooting are added. Finally, practice, scrimmage, and limited game time are allowed. Total recovery time from Achilles tendon rupture to a high level of basketball performance is a minimum of 1 year. Few athletes at a high level of competition are able to attain their preinjury status following a rupture of the patellar, quadriceps, or Achilles tendon.

KNEE INJURIES

The knee joint ranks only behind the ankle joint in frequency of injury in basketball players.[7,12,47,50] Knee injuries were responsible for most games missed in one series,[12] and accounted for more injuries than ankle injuries in another series.[2] Ligament injuries, meniscal injuries, plica syndrome, patellar subluxation and dislocation, patellofemoral pain syndrome, and osteochondral lesions are common in basketball players.

Ligament Injuries

Ligament injuries can occur from a direct blow that imparts abnormal varus, valgus, hyperextension, or rotational force to the knee. Ligament injuries can also occur without contact, as when the athlete lands on the leg off balance, which produces a high force on the knee. The most common mechanism in basketball is a deceleration, valgus, and external rotation injury. The second most common mechanism is a hyperextension injury. In addition, a direct anterior-to-posterior force can cause ligament damage, but this is rare in basketball. Ligament sprains are classified by degree. The first-degree injury is a tear of a minimal number of fibers with localized tenderness and no abnormal laxity. A second-degree sprain is an injury with more torn ligamentous fiber, more loss of function, and more effusion. No noticeable instability is seen. A third-degree sprain has more disruption of fibers and demonstrable laxity. This group is further classified as to the degree of laxity noted in one-plane stress testing.[28] In Grade I injuries (mild disruption) there is less than 5 mm of opening of the joint space. Grade II injuries (moderate disruption) have less than 10 mm of opening at the joint space. In Grade III injuries (severe disruption) there is more than 10 mm of opening at the joint space.

An acute ligament disruption involving the anterior cruciate ligament (ACL) or the posterior cruciate ligament (PCL) usually results in an immediate effusion unless there is complete capsular disruption. Aspiration of the knee joint yields blood that can also be seen in an osteochondral fracture or peripheral or capsular meniscal tear. On examination of the knee, a positive Lachman test, Losee test, and pivot shift are seen with a torn ACL.[6,16,20] A positive posterior drawer sign, drop back sign, asymmetric recurvatum, and posteromedial and posterolateral instability are seen with a torn PCL.[28]

In reality, no injury causes damage to one specific ligament; rather there is damage to ligament and capsule often associated with meniscal or osteochondral damage. However, treatment is directed to the most serious area of involvement. Depending on the extent of the injury to the ligamentous or associated structures, operative or nonoperative management is undertaken.[48]

Treatment

In basketball players isolated Grades I and II collateral ligament injuries are initially treated with a brief period of immobilization. This is followed by range of motion exercises, modality therapy, and immediate progressive resistance exercises to strengthen the quadriceps, hip abductors, and hip flexors. Protective weight bearing is continued for 2 weeks or until symptoms have totally resolved. Grade II injuries are protected by a brace during therapy and the initial period of returning to play (Table 62-7).

Isolated Grade III medial collateral ligament (MCL) injuries are immobilized for 6 weeks. This is followed by progressive resistance exercises, range of motion exercises, and protection in a brace. When Grade III collateral ligament injury is associated with an injury to the ACL or PCL, resulting in instability in a single or multiple planes, a ligamentous reconstruction and repair are performed after examination with the patient under anesthesia. Diagnostic arthroscopy is used as an adjunct to the examination in these ligament injuries unless a complete capsular tear is suspected in which case arthroscopy is deferred. With complete capsular disruption, extravasation of fluid into the soft tissues makes the ensuing reconstruction difficult. It should be mentioned that arthroscopy should not be performed without a thorough history and physical examination and a working diagnosis. Isometric quadriceps and hamstring strengthening exercises for the knee are started as soon as the patient can tolerate them. All patients are begun on protected early range of motion usually at 3 weeks. These athletes are kept non–weight bearing for the first 6 weeks and then advanced to protective weight bearing until the range of motion is 5 to 100 degrees. Isotonic strengthening exercises are done by the player at home on a daily basis. This is augmented by isokinetic work and supervised by a physical therapist at least 3 times a week. We prefer to use both high-speed, low-resistance and low-speed, high-resistance isokinetic exercises. In addition, we have the athletes use a stationary bicycle ergometer to help with range of motion and endurance. The seat should be placed as high as possible to minimize pain in the area. Isotonic exercises for the quadriceps are done with the knee in extension, but knee extension exercises are avoided if patellofemoral pain symptoms should arise. A brace is worn during rehabilitation and for all activity

TABLE 62-7 Treatment of Grade I and II isolated medial collateral ligament injuries in basketball players*

Modality	Stage				
	I	II	III	IV	V
Knee immobilizer	X	X			
Crutches (partial weight bearing)	X	X			
Ice	X				
Compression	X	X			
Elevation	X				
Contrasts		X			
*Active range of motion		X			
Isometric exercises		X			
Hydrotherapy		X	X		
Ultrasound		X	X		
Muscle stimulation		X			
Well leg and upper extremity exercise		X	X		
Isotonic and isokinetic work			X		X
Stretching			X	X	X
Aerobic activity			X	X	X
Balance and coordination drills				X	X
Running straight				X	X
Figure-8 running					X
Dribbling and cutting					X
Practice					X
Limited playing time					X
Full activity					X

*Note: Grade II injuries are protected with an orthosis throughout therapy.

TABLE 62-8 Criteria for return to play following knee ligament injury

Symptoms	Examination Findings

Pain free	Muscle parity
	  Quadriceps
	  Hamstrings
	  Hip flexors
	  Hip abductors
	  Ankle dorsiflexors
	  Ankle plantar flexors
	No effusion
	Full range of motion
	Satisfactory brace fit (if brace is indicated)

for the first year (Fig. 62-10). The criteria for return to play after ligament surgery in a basketball player are outlined in Table 62-8.

Meniscal Injuries

Meniscal lesions are common in basketball players and have been reported extensively in the literature.[2,3,4,16,18] They can occur is association with cruciate and collateral ligament injuries and with dislocation of the patella. They also occur as a primary lesion with minimal associated injury. The study by Baker et al[3] shows a predominance for injury to the medial meniscus of the right knee. The right knee was thought to be involved at a higher frequency than the left because the predomi-

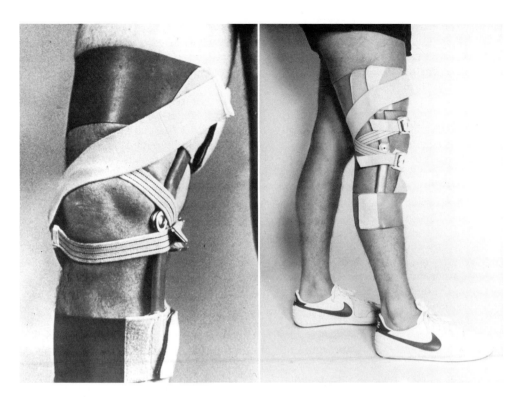

FIG. 62-10. Lenox-Hill derotational brace.

nance of players are right handed and prefer to jump, land, and cut predominately with the right leg. However, in a study by Krinsky et al[18] the lateral meniscus was reported to be injured at a higher frequency than the medial meniscus in professional basketball players followed up over 6 years. A possible explanation offered by the authors is that the lateral meniscus is more vulnerable to chronic damage from repetitive microtrauma, and the professional athlete, who is more likely to be injured in a game situation, plays a significantly greater number of games than the amateur.

There is no pathognomonic sign of a specific meniscal tear; thus the history and physical examination must be viewed as a complete picture when deciding on a diagnosis and treatment plan. On examination of the knee, palpable medial or lateral joint line tenderness is highly suggestive of a torn meniscus. When the patient is examined in the prone position, lack of complete extension or complete flexion may also be present. MRI is useful for evaluating these injuries. When a diagnosis of a torn meniscus is made, the patient is started on immediate quadriceps strengthening exercises. In addition, the player undergoes an examination under anesthesia and diagnostic arthroscopy to elucidate any other associated injuries. After arthroscopic confirmation of the lesion, partial meniscectomy is performed. In an acute peripheral separation a repair is performed. This is especially important in female basketball players or males with ligamentous laxity because the meniscus adds a certain amount of stability to the knee, and total meniscectomies usually result in some residual instability. Following arthroscopic partial meniscectomy the

players are kept on crutches for approximately 5 days. They are started immediately on isometric quadriceps strengthening exercises. At 72 hours the bulky Jones dressing is removed, adhesive strips are applied over the wounds, Ace bandages are wrapped around the knee, and the patient is begun on active range of motion exercises. At 5 days, if the wounds are healed, the sutures are removed and the patients are allowed to begin full weight bearing as tolerated. The remainder of rehabilitation to return to play is outlined in Stages IV and V in Table 62-7.

Patellar Subluxation and Dislocation

Patellar subluxation and dislocation occur in basketball players. A laterally directed force to the patella is the most common traumatic cause of patellar malalignment. As the patella is forced laterally, the medial retinaculum is stretched or torn. Patellar dislocation can usually be diagnosed by direct observation. However, if there is any question, radiographs should be obtained.

Reduction of the patella can usually be obtained with the help of a muscle relaxant and an analgesic. Following reduction the patient's knee is immobilized in extension, and quadriceps strengthening exercises are started immediately. The patient is kept non–weight bearing. At 4 weeks range of motion exercises are started as is partial weight bearing with the player in a patella-restraining brace (Fig. 62-7). The return to activity is outlined in Table 62-7. In cases of recurrent dislocation with a history of more than three dislocations of the patella, a reconstruction is recommended. This is rarely seen on the professional or collegiate level. In adolescent female basketball players a patellar malalignment syndrome may develop following an episode of subluxation or dislocation with persistent pain and instability that is refractory to conservative treatment. Lateral retinacular releases have been used in these individuals with good results.

Patellofemoral Pain Syndrome

With the constant acceleration, deceleration, and jumping that are required in basketball, the patellofemoral joint may become symptomatic as a result of high joint reaction forces. Patellofemoral pain syndrome and plica syndrome have been reported in basketball players.[50] These injuries are frequently seen particularly on the high school level but are common at all levels of competition. Pain is the primary complaint. Swelling, locking, and buckling are rare and should alert the examiner to look for other pathologic conditions. Tenderness is usually present under the medial patellar facet and occasionally on the lateral patellar facet and lateral femoral trochlea. The symptoms can usually be treated with progressive resistance exercises in extension, ice, oral antiinflammatory medication, and a patella-restraining brace.

Occasionally, a medial patellar plica or suprapatellar plica may become thickened and fibrotic and produce clicking, snapping, and pain to palpation. These problems usually respond to conservative treatment. If, however, this condition fails to improve with conservative treatment for more than 6 months, arthroscopy is indicated to confirm the diagnosis and excise the plica. This usually gives good results.

In cases of patellofemoral pain syndrome that are refractory to conservative treatment for more than 6 months, arthroscopy is performed to confirm the diagnosis and an arthroscopic lateral release is done if patellar tilt or a tight lateral retinaculum is present. Following surgery the patient is started on quadriceps strengthening exercises as soon as tolerated. Partial weight-bearing status is allowed when the player is able to do straight leg raising exercises. This is followed by range of motion exercises and strengthening of the entire lower extremity. Before resumption of activities, all players must have good flexibility in both lower extremities and symmetric strength in both quadriceps. A patella-restraining brace is worn during activity (Fig. 62-7).

SHIN AND CALF INJURIES
Contusions

The shin and calf are rarely injured in basketball players. Blunt contusions are the most frequently encountered injuries in this area, and early treatment with ice, compression, and oral antiinflammatory medication usually yields good results. Range of motion and progressive resistance exercises are started early, and the athletes are allowed to return to activities as tolerated.

Stress Fractures

A prolonged period of pain in the area of the shin or calf may indicate a stress fracture involving the tibia.

Stress fractures have been shown to involve both the posteromedial cortex of the tibia and the anterolateral cortex, although much less frequently. Rettig et al[30] point out two potentially significant complications of the anterolateral stress fracture. The first is delayed union that is thought to result from the poor blood supply of the anterior tibial cortex because of its subcutaneous location. The other is the increased risk of progressing to a complete fracture, which is known to occur with stress fractures on the tension side of the bone more so than those involving the compressive side. This study emphasizes an extended period of conservative treatment including rest and external electric stimulation before considering surgical intervention. Surgical treatments described include bone grafting of defects on the anterior tibial cortex and closed intramedullary nailing.

ANKLE INJURIES

Ankle injuries are common in basketball. In a review by Henry, Lauear, and Neigut[12] the ankle was the most injured joint and accounted for 105 of 576 (18.2%) of all injuries. However, only 18% of the missed games in their series were caused by ankle injuries.

Acute Sprains
Classification

Ankle sprains are classified as first-degree, second-degree, or third-degree sprains. In a first-degree sprain there is minor tearing of the ligament fibers. There is mild pain and point tenderness with little or no swelling and minimal hemorrhage. No abnormal motion is present. In second-degree sprains there is an incomplete tearing of the ligament fibers. Moderate pain and point tenderness are present. There is a moderate amount of swelling and hemorrhage, and abnormal motions are slight to moderate. Complete rupture of the ligament is defined as a third-degree sprain. Marked tenderness, swelling, and hemorrhage are present. Deformity, including dislocation, can be present. Abnormal motion is marked.

Functional Anatomy

The primary ligamentous restraints to the ankle are the deltoid ligament complex medially, the lateral collateral ligament complex laterally, and the syndesmosis. The deltoid ligament is divided into two primary portions, deep and superficial. The deep portion attaches to the talus and courses in a horizontal direction helping to resist lateral displacement. The superficial portion is a broad triangular band that has insertions on the calcaneus, navicular, and talus. The lateral collateral ligament complex consists of three ligaments. The anterior talofibular ligament arises from the anterior aspect of the lateral malleolus and inserts onto the neck of the talus. It is the prime stabilizer preventing anterior displacement of the talus.[22] The calcaneofibular ligament is the largest ligament in the complex and passes posteriorly and inferiorly from the lateral aspect of the distal fibula to insert on the lateral aspect of the calcaneus. This ligament resists inversion of the ankle and is tightest when the ankle is in dorsiflexion.[27] The posterior talofibular liga-ment extends from the posterior portion of the tip of the fibula and runs backward and slightly downward to at-tach to the lateral tubercle of the posterior process of the talus. This is the strongest of the three ligaments in the lateral collateral ligament complex and helps resist ante-rior and medial displacement of the foot.[22] The syn-desmosis ligaments hold the distal tibia and fibula to-gether. The syndesmosis ligaments consist of the ante-rior tibiofibular ligament, the posterior tibiofibular liga-ment, and the interosseous ligament, which is a thickening of the interosseous membrane between the tibia and fibula located approximately 2 cm above the an-kle joint. Syndesmosis disruption most commonly occurs with an external rotation type component to the injury.

Mechanisms of Injury

Injuries to the ankle occur primarily with inversion or eversion (which, in basketball, are commonly associated with a plantar-flexed foot) and an external rotation force (Fig. 62-11). The most common mechanism of an ankle sprain in a basketball player is plantar flexion with in-version of the foot. This occurs with a cutting or turning maneuver when the player is pushing off (e.g., cutting to the left and pushing off with the right foot).[22] Ever-sion injuries are less common in basketball players. The ankles can be everted and externally rotated when a player is coming down and lands on an irregular surface such as another player's foot. Other injuries to the foot

and ankle can occur with ligamentous injuries to the an-kles. These include a fracture of the os trigonum and an osteochondral fracture of the talus.

Evaluation

The player who injures his or her ankle usually gives a history of the foot being turned under, immediate pain, and often a sensation of a snap or a pop. On initial ex-amination, local tenderness is usually appreciated. Mo-tion may or may not be restricted. An early indication of the severity of the injury is the player's ability or inabil-ity to bear weight. In most Grade I and Grade II ligament sprains the player is able to bear weight. In a more se-vere injury where the patient is unable to bear weight, the initial decision involves differentiating a sprain from a possible fracture. The area around the ankle joint should be palpated to see if there is tenderness over the fibula, the medial malleolus, or the medial and lateral lig-amentous complexes. In addition, the area of the fifth metatarsal and the forefoot should be palpated to rule out an avulsion fracture of the fifth metatarsal or a possible midfoot sprain. Initial radiographs should differentiate between a fracture and a ligament injury. The clinician must determine whether this is a stable or unstable in-jury. We have found stress radiographs of the ankle to be of great assistance in this determination. A local an-esthetic (1% lidocaine) is injected into the area of ten-derness. Stress radiographs of the affected ankle and the opposite ankle are then obtained for comparison (Fig. 62-12). A lateral radiograph is also obtained for an anterior drawer test (Fig. 62-13). Evidence of opening of the mor-

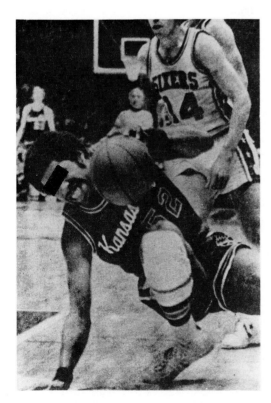

FIG. 62-11. National Basketball Association player sustaining an-kle injury. Mechanism of injury is equinus, eversion, and external rotation. (Courtesy World Wide Photos, Associated Press.)

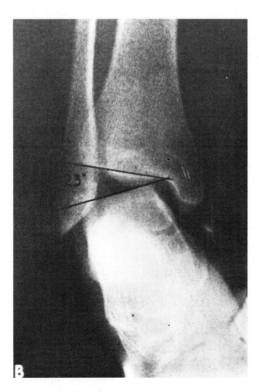

FIG. 62-12. Stress view of ankle showing lateral ligament instabil-ity.

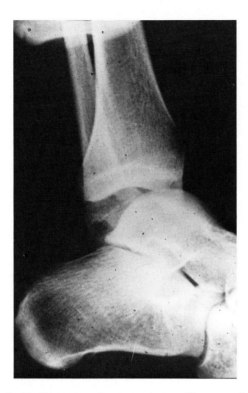

FIG. 62-13. Stress view showing anterior subluxation of talus.

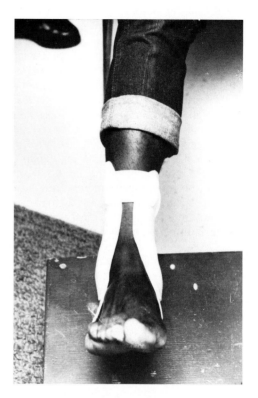

FIG. 62-14. Air splint used to stabilize ankle.

tise of greater than 7 degrees is thought to be significant, and 30 degrees of opening is compatible with disruption of the entire lateral collateral ligamentous complex. If there is a fracture of the fibula, a rupture of the deltoid ligament should be suspected and eversion stress radiographs should be obtained. If radiographs show widening of the mortise on the medial side, the syndesmosis may be disrupted. The more external rotation that is involved, the more proximal the injury can extend. Disruption can occur as far proximal as the neck of the fibula. Once the joint has been classified and stability determined, the course of treatment can be started.

Treatment

The treatment of Grade I and Grade II injuries is conservative.[43] Ice, compression, and elevation are started immediately. Grade II injuries are initially protected on crutches with an air splint (Fig. 62-14). Ice treatment, electrogalvanic stimulation, and range of motion exercises are started as soon as pain and swelling allow. Isometric exercises are started immediately and, as range of motion increases, isotonic and isokinetic progressive resistance exercises can be started to strengthen the dorsiflexors, plantar flexors, inverters, and everters. Weight bearing is allowed when the player has a full range of motion and no limp. When strength and endurance of the muscles of both lower extremities are equal, the player may begin running with support taping and a supervised increase in activity is started (Table 62-9). When the player resumes running after an inversion ankle injury, an orthotic with a lateral heel wedge is some-

TABLE 62-9 Final stages in rehabilitation following ankle injury

Stage*	Activity
I	Walking on toes
II	Running
III	Dribbling and cutting
IV	Jumping and shooting
V	Practice (half-court initially)
VI	Limited playing time
VII	Full activity

*These stages follow appropriate strength and range of motion gains.

times used. If an orthotic is used, it should be a full-length orthotic because a half-length orthotic slides up and down in the shoe with the constant acceleration and deceleration that are inherent in basketball.

Grade III ligament injuries are rare in basketball players and may require operative repair. Only one Grade III sprain in a basketball player has been described in the literature.[4] When operative intervention is necessary, the ankle joint should be opened, examined, and lavaged to remove any osteochondral fragments of the talus from the ankle joint space. The fibular fracture or tibiofibular ligament avulsion is fixed internally with the A-O technique; the ligaments are sutured, and the ankle is casted for 6 weeks. The rehabilitation protocol following immobilization is described in Chapter 26.

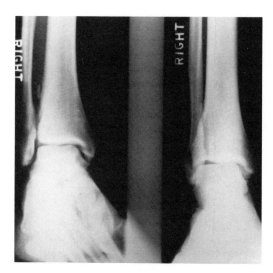

FIG. 62-15. Degenerative changes involving ankle joint following chronic ankle injury. Note calcification in deltoid ligament, calcaneofibular ligament, and syndesmosis.

Chronic Laxity

Most players on the professional level already have radiographic evidence of degenerative change in their ankles caused by previous ligamentous injuries (Fig. 62-15). For this reason we think that a rehabilitation program to strengthen the muscles around the ankle is important. The program is started during the preseason with professional players and consists of isotonic or isokinetic progressive resistance exercises if the players have access to a Cybex or Orthotron machine to strengthen the dorsiflexors, plantar flexors, invertors, and evertors. We place special emphasis on the strengthening of the evertors because they are capable of absorbing the stress and protecting the lateral ligamentous complex from injury. In our experience, taping prevents recurrent injuries and is used during the season. Furthermore, high-top shoes are worn on the professional

---

Muscle groups to be rehabilitated in ankle instability

- Ankle evertors (especially)
- Ankle invertors
- Ankle dorsiflexors
- Ankle plantar flexors

Supplementary devices for ankle sprains in basketball players

- Lateral heel and sole wedges
- Taping (see p. 252)
- High-top athletic shoes (with leather or canvas upper)
- Ankle brace

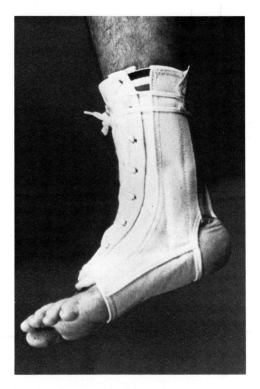

FIG. 62-16. Ankle brace used for chronic ligament instability.

level. A nylon upper, although light, is prone to stretch, and the player can literally roll out of the shoe. In cases of chronic ligament instability, an ankle brace is worn (Fig. 62-16). Training athletes to land with a wider stance may be beneficial in preventing ankle injuries by placing the foot more lateral to the falling center of gravity and therefore reducing the risk of inversion stress.[37]

Stress Fractures

Subacute and chronic ankle pain with clinical signs of tenderness over the medial malleolus and ankle effusion suggests the possibility of a stress fracture of the medial malleolus.[35] Radiographs are often normal, and nuclear scintigraphy is necessary to identify the lesion. Interval fixation with a compression screw is appropriate for those athletes with delayed healing despite appropriate immobilization.

FOOT INJURIES
Fractures

Foot injuries are common in basketball. In the study of Henry, Lauear, and Neigut,[12] 12% of all injuries to centers were foot injuries. Common foot injuries seen in basketball players include fractures of the base of the fifth metatarsal, stress fractures of the tarsal navicular, stress fractures of the metatarsals, strains of the tarsometatarsal joint, plantar fasciitis, and first metatarsophalangeal joint arthritis. These injuries are caused by overuse and repetitive jumping. In the reports of Torg et al[41] on stress fractures of the tarsal navicular, 8 of 21 cases presented were basketball players. In the report of Kav-

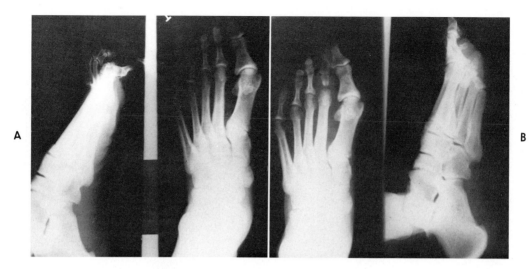

FIG. 62-17. A, Severe hammertoe deformity in professional basketball player resulting in dislocation of second metatarsophalangeal joint. **B,** This was treated with resection arthroplasty and had excellent result.

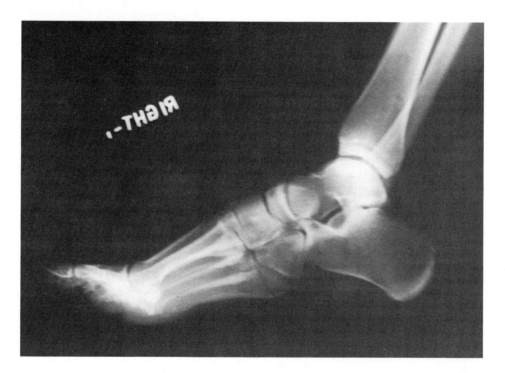

FIG. 62-18. Avulsion of base of fifth metatarsal.

anaugh, Brown, and Mann[14] on the Jones fracture, 10 of 21 cases were basketball players. In the report of DeLee, Evans, and Julian[8] on stress fractures of the fifth metatarsal, 6 of the 19 cases were basketball players.

Professional basketball players commonly have abnormalities of the forefoot, including hallux valgus, pes planus, hammertoes, and soft and hard corns. Corrections should not be attempted on these problems unless the deformity is functionally disabling (Fig. 62-17).

Fracture of the Base of the Fifth Metatarsal

Avulsion fractures of the base of the fifth metatarsal involve an avulsion of the peroneus brevis from its insertion (Fig. 62-18). This is caused by forced inversion and plantar flexion from a position of eversion and dorsiflexion. These injuries usually heal with a conservative treatment regimen consisting of compression, ice, weight bearing as tolerated, and range of motion exercises. This is followed by progressive resistance exercises as tolerated.

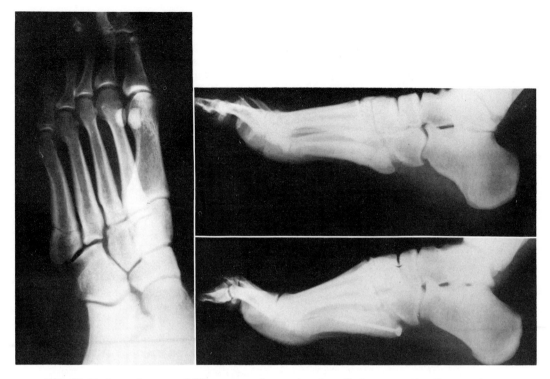

FIG. 62-19. Jones fracture of fifth metatarsal treated with malleolar screw. Excellent result was achieved with return to activity in 8 weeks.

Jones Fracture

A fracture of the fifth metatarsal distal to the articulation between the fourth and fifth metatarsals (Jones fracture) is a common basketball injury that has received a great deal of attention in the sports medicine literature.[8,14,41] The Jones fracture can be a tremendously disabling injury for an athlete. This fracture differs from an avulsion of the fifth metatarsal tuberosity in two respects. First, it is not caused by an inversion injury; rather, players who have sustained this injury described elevation of the heel, breaking at the metatarsophalangeal joints, and maximum load over the lateral aspect of the foot.[14] Second, this fracture is difficult to treat. The period required for immobilization is prolonged, and the incidence of delayed union and refracture is high. In the series of Kavanaugh, Brown, and Mann,[14] 9 of the 16 fractures treated conservatively had not healed after a period of 6 months. Rather than being the result of one specific insult, the Jones fracture appears to be a stress fracture with classic radiographic signs (Fig. 62-19). Kavanaugh, Brown, and Mann[14] reported that 41% of the patients had clinical pictures consistent with a stress fracture that was evident on the initial radiographs, which usually appeared as a small lateral cortical defect. Many patients reported a prodromal period of approximately 2 weeks of aching and discomfort in the area before they came for treatment. With the poor success of immobilization as treatment of these injuries and the prolonged immobilization required, several authors have recommended open reduction and internal fixation of this injury in the high-level, competitive athlete. DeLee, Evans, and Julian,[8] in a series of 10 athletes with stress fractures of the fifth metatarsal, obtained union in all patients in an average of 7.5 weeks with a return to their sports in an average of 8.5 weeks postoperatively. In the series of Kavanaugh and colleagues,[14] who reported on 13 athletes, all cases were clinically healed in 6 weeks and radiographically united 3 months after the operation. Complication rates from the surgery were low in both reports. We agree that open reduction and internal fixation is the treatment of choice in competitive athletes with this particular problem. We perform the open reduction and internal fixation using an A-O cancellous screw through a straight incision at the proximal end of the fifth metatarsal as described by Kavanaugh, Brown, and Mann.[14] Postoperatively, we maintain non–weight bearing to tolerance in a cast shoe for the next 2 to 4 weeks. Return to athletic competition is outlined for ankle injuries in Table 62-9 and usually requires 6 to 10 weeks.

Tarsal Navicular Stress Fractures

Stress fractures of the tarsal navicular occur rarely in recreational, amateur, and professional athletes but are reported more frequently in basketball players.[40] Players sustaining this injury are physically active and give a history of insidious onset of pain on the dorsum of the foot, in the medial aspect of the longitudinal arch, or both. The pain is a nonspecific soreness or cramping sensation that is aggravated by activity. The area directly over the tarsal navicular is often tender to palpation. There is usually little discoloration in the area and no swelling or limp. Dorsiflexion of the ankle, inversion and eversion of

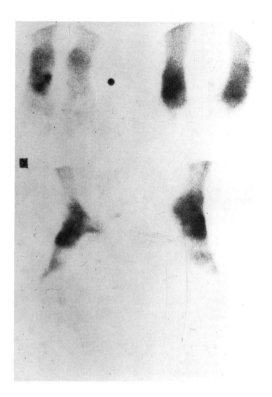

FIG. 62-20. Bone scan showing increased uptake in tarsal navicular, confirming diagnosis of stress fracture.

the subtalar joint, or both may be limited. Foot abnormalities, including a short first metatarsal and metatarsus adductus and limited dorsiflexion of the ankle and subtalar motion, have been reported in these patients. Standard anteroposterior radiographs of the foot may not show the lesion, but radionuclide bone scans usually show the stress fracture (Fig. 62-20).[29] To attain ideal images of the area, tomograms are obtained with the forefoot lifted off the table with a wedge so that the navicular is in anatomic anteroposterior alignment. On this view the central third of the navicular, where the stress fracture is located, can be seen.[40] Microangiographic studies of the tarsal navicular demonstrate avascularity of the middle third of the bone.[41] Once the diagnosis is made, treatment consists of immobilization in a cast and non–weight bearing for 6 to 8 weeks. If at 8 weeks the patient is clinically healed and radiographs show evidence of bony healing, the patient begins range of motion exercises and weight bearing as tolerated in an orthopaedic laced Oxford shoe with a scaphoid pad. When the player has a normal range of motion and normal strength in the lower extremity muscles, a supervised activity program as outlined for ankle injuries in Table 62-9 is begun. Surgery is appropriate for nonunions.

Metatarsal Stress Fracture

Stress fractures of the metatarsals in basketball players usually occur early in the training program because of the sudden increase in running and jumping. These injuries cause pain on activity and palpable tenderness. Radiographs do not usually show the fracture until reactive bone formation is seen as a sleeve of periosteal cal-

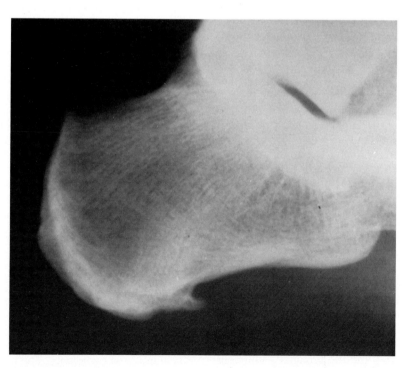

FIG. 62-21. Heel spur secondary to plantar fasciitis in professional basketball player treated conservatively with two missed games.

lus at 6 weeks. If there is a question as to the diagnosis, a bone scan can be performed. Treatment is rest, followed by an orthotic to unload the area, and increased activity as tolerated. Jumping is added just before return to play.

Sprains
Tarsometatarsal Ligament Sprain

A sprain of the tarsometatarsal ligament is a severely disabling injury. It results from landing on the foot off balance, which results in dorsiflexion, rotation, and eversion. In addition, diastasis with separation and displacement medially or laterally may occur. The player sustaining this injury is unable to bear weight on the affected foot and complains of pain in the area. There is usually pain to palpation in the tarsometatarsal region; adduction or abduction of the forefoot reproduces symptoms. Careful evaluation of anterior, posterior, lateral, and oblique radiographs is essential to evaluate displacement. If there is displacement, open anatomic reduction is required and Kirschner wires are inserted to close the diastasis. If this is not done, the injury results in a chronic, painful instability of the tarsometatarsal area that limits jumping and running. Nondisplaced injuries are treated with immobilization and non–weight bearing for 2 weeks followed by weight bearing as tolerated in an orthopaedic laced Oxford shoe with a full-length orthotic insert. The foot and ankle are taped for activity. As comfort allows, range of motion and progressive resistance strengthening exercises are started. The player is then allowed to resume activity in a supervised program for ankle injuries as outlined in Table 62-9.

Arch Sprains

Sprains of the arch are caused by improper jumping mechanics and result in injury to the plantar fascia, the intrinsic muscles of the foot, and the ligaments of the midfoot. The presenting complaint is pain with tenderness under the arch. This injury is more common in players with pes planus. Ice, oral antiinflammatory medication, taping (see p. 262), and orthotics with arch supports are prescribed. Activity is allowed as tolerated.

Heel Spurs and Plantar Fasciitis

The terms "heel spur" and "plantar fasciitis" are synonymous. The injury is a stressful response to overuse localized at the insertion of the plantar fascia on the calcaneus. It is associated with tight hamstrings and heel cords. The heel spur develops secondarily, and it is not the true cause of pain (Fig. 62-21). The pain is related to the inflammatory response caused by the repeated traction of the plantar fascia on its insertion.[1] The diagnosis is made by direct palpation over the plantar aspect of the heel. A lateral radiograph may show secondary spur formation on the calcaneus. The treatment is heat; use of oral antiinflammatory medication; flexibility exercises for the hamstrings, heel cords, and plantar fascia; and a soft heel support. In persistent cases a molded, rigid-heel arch support is helpful. Surgical release of the fascia has not been indicated in our experience.

Metatarsophalangeal Joint Problems
Hallux Rigidus

Hyperextension injury to the first metatarsophalangeal joint, or "turf toe," occurs in basketball players.[12] This can lead to degenerative changes and hallux rigidus. Pain with activity, especially running and jumping, is a major complaint. Also, there is pain with forced dorsiflexion of the first metatarsophalangeal joint. Redness and swelling may be apparent, and exostoses are palpable in chronic cases. Ice, use of oral antiinflammatory medication, and taping to prevent hyperextension constitute treatment. The player resumes activity as tolerated, and jumping is added just before return to play. A rigid arch support to protect the first metatarsophalangeal joint is prescribed and worn in the shoe. Cheilectomy can be performed for those athletes whose conservative therapy failed.

Sesamoiditis

Sesamoiditis is seen in basketball players and is common in planovalgus feet. It is also associated with degeneration of the first metatarsal head. Tibial bipartite sesamoiditis has also been reported in professional athletes as an accessory finding. Treatment for sesamoiditis is conservative and should consist of ice, use of antiinflammatory medication, and orthotic supports. Orthotics are placed proximal to and just under the sesamoids to provide relief. The players are allowed to resume activity as tolerated.

SUMMARY

The management of lower extremity injuries in basketball players is approached in three phases: prevention, diagnosis and treatment, and rehabilitation. Prevention is sine qua non in sports medicine, and the physician's role should begin in the preseason. The physician should work with the trainers, equipment managers, and players to ensure as safe a program as possible. We use an

TABLE 62-10 Off-season conditioning program

Type of Conditioning	Activity
Flexibility	Stretching program for lower extremities with emphasis on hip adductors, hamstrings, Achilles tendon, and planter fascia. Performed daily for 20-30 minutes
Endurance	Continuous exercise for cardiopulmonary fitness. Athlete's preference of running, cycling, swimming, or aerobic dance performed four times a week for 20-30 minutes
Strength	Power program with emphasis on hip abductors, hip flexors, quadriceps, hamstrings, gastrocnemius and soleus; combined with upper body program. Performed three times a week per muscle group
Skills	Free throws, shoot-around for 30 minutes five times a week at end of daily program. Supervised scrimmage or league games for two of five weekly sessions

off-season program that emphasizes three primary areas: strength, flexibility, and endurance (Table 62-10). The physician must continue his or her role after the season as well to monitor rehabilitation and recommend appropriate modifications as necessary. Basketball is a contact sport that is played on hard surfaces. It requires quick acceleration and deceleration, rapid changes in direction, and a great deal of jumping. Consequently, the physician who treats injuries in basketball players must be well versed in contact and overuse injuries in the musculoskeletal system.

ACKNOWLEDGMENTS

Special thanks to Donna L. James for assistance in completing this chapter.

REFERENCES

1. Andrews JR: Overuse syndromes in the lower extremities, *Clin Sports Med* 2:137, 1983.
2. Apple DF, O'Toole J, Annis C: Professional basketball injuries, *Phys Sports Med* 10(1):81, 1982.
3. Baker BE et al: Review of meniscal injury and associated sports, *Am J Sports Med* 13(1):1, 1985.
4. Blazina M et al: Jumper's knee, *Orthop Clin North Am* 4:665, 1973.
5. Bodne D et al: Magnetic resonance images of chronic patellar tendinitis, *Skeletal Radiol* 17:24, 1988.
6. Brown T: *Manual of orthopedic surgery*, Chicago, 1979, American Orthopedic Association.
7. Colliander E et al: Injuries in Swedish elite basketball, *Orthopedics* 9(2):225, 1986.
8. DeLee JC, Evans R, Julian J: Stress fracture of the fifth metatarsal, *Am J Sports Med* 11:349, 1983.
9. Ferretti A: Epidemiology of jumper's knee, *Sports Med* 3:289, 1986.
10. Ferretti A et al: Jumper's knee, *Am J Sports Med* 11(2):58, 1983.
11. Frankl V, Wasilewski SA, Healy WL: Avulsion fracture of the tibial tubercle with avulsion of the patellar ligament, *J Bone Joint Surg* 72A:1411, 1990.
12. Henry JH, Lauear B, Neigut D: The injury rate in professional basketball, *Am J Sports Med* 10:16, 1982.
13. Hershman EB, Lombardo J, Bergfeld JA: Femoral shaft stress fractures in athletes, *Clin Sports Med* 9(1):111, 1990.
14. Kavanaugh JH, Brown TD, Mann RV: The Jones fracture revisited, *J Bone Joint Surg* 60A:776, 1978.
15. Kelly DW et al: Patellar and quadriceps tendon ruptures—jumper's knee, *Am J Sports Med* 12(5):375, 1984.
16. Kennedy JC, Stewart R, Walker DM: Anterolateral rotatory instability of the knee joint: an early analysis of the Ellison procedure, *J Bone Joint Surg* 60A:1031, 1978.
17. Kennedy JC, Willes RB: The effects of local steroid injections on tendons: a biomechanical and microscopic correlative study, *Am J Sports Med* 4:11, 1976.
18. Krinsky MB et al: Incidence of lateral meniscus injury in professional basketball players, *Am J Sports Med* 20(1):17, 1992.
19. Lindholm A: A new method of operation in subcutaneous rupture of the Achilles tendon, *Acta Chir Scand* 117:261, 1959.
20. Losee ER et al: Anterior subluxation of the lateral tibial plateau: a diagnostic test and operative repair, *J Bone Joint Surg* 60A:1015, 1978.
21. Maar DC, Kerneck CB, Pierce RO: Simultaneous bilateral tibial tubercle avulsion fracture, *Orthopedics* 11(11):1599, 1988.
22. Mack RP: Ankle injuries in athletes, *Clin Sports Med* 1:71, 1982.
23. Marglis SW, Lewis MN: Bilateral spontaneous concurrent ruptures of the patella tendon without apparent systemic disease: a case report, *Clin Orthop* 136:186, 1978.
24. McLaughlin HL, Francis KC: Operative repair of injuries to the quadriceps extensor mechanism, *Am J Surg* 91:651, 1956.
25. Micheli LJ, Hall JE, Miller ME: Use of modified Boston brace for back injuries in athletes, *Am J Sports Med* 8:351, 1980.
26. Moritz A, Grana WA: High school basketball injuries, *Phys Sports Med* 6:91, 1978.
27. Nemeth VA, Throsher E: Ankle sprains in athletics, *Clin Sports Med* 2:217, 1983.
28. Nisonson B et al: The knee. In Scott WN, Nisonson B, Nicholas JA (eds): *Principles of sports medicine*, Baltimore, 1984, Williams & Wilkins.
29. Pavlov H, Torg JS, Freiberger RH: Tarsal navicular stress fractures: radiographic evaluation, *Radiology* 148:641, 1983.
30. Rettig AC et al: The natural history and treatment of delayed union stress fractures of the anterior cortex of the tibia, *Am J Sports Med* 16(3):250, 1988.
31. Roels J et al: Patellar tendinitis (jumper's knee), *Am J Sports Med* 6:632, 1978.
32. Rosenberg JM, Whitaker JH: Bilateral infrapatellar tendon rupture in a patient with jumper's knee, *Am J Sports Med* 19(1):92, 1991.
33. Salter RB: *Textbook of disorders and injuries of the musculoskeletal system*, Baltimore, 1970, Williams & Wilkins.
34. Scuderi C: Ruptures of the quadriceps tendon: study of twenty tendon ruptures, *Am J Surg* 95:626, 1958.
35. Shelbourne KD et al: Stress fractures of the medial malleolus, *Am J Sports Med* 16(1):60, 1988.
36. Shultz A et al: Loads on the lumbar spine, *J Bone Joint Surg* 64A:713, 1982.
37. Smith RW, Reischl SF: Treatment of ankle sprains in young athletes, *Am J Sports Med* 14(6):465, 1986.
38. Sommer HM: Patellar chondropathy and apicitis, and muscle imbalances of the lower extremities in competitive sports, *Sports Med* 5(6):386, 1988.
39. Spencer CW, Jackson DW: Back injuries in the athlete, *Clin Sports Med* 2:191, 1983.
40. Torg JS et al: Stress fractures of the tarsal navicular: a retrospective review of twenty-one cases, *J Bone Joint Surg* 66A:700, 1982.
41. Torg JS et al: Fractures of the base of the fifth metatarsal distal to the tuberosity, *J Bone Joint Surg* 66A:209, 1984.
42. Vaccaro P, Clarke DN, Wrenn JP: Physiological profiles of elite women basketball players, *J Sports Med Phys Fitness* 19:45, 1979.
43. Vegso JD, Harmon LE: Nonoperative management of athletic ankle injuries, *Clin Sports Med* 1:85, 1982.
44. Verma SK, Mohendrov SR, Kansal DK: The maximal anaerobic power of different categories of players, *J Sports Med* 19:55, 1979.
45. Whiteside PA: Men's and women's injuries in comparable sports, *Phys Sports Med* 8:130, 1980.
46. Withers RT, Roberts RGD, Davies GJ: The maximum aerobic power, anaerobic power, and body composition of south Australian male representatives in athletics: basketball, field hockey and soccer, *J Sports Med* 17:391, 1977.
47. Yde J, Nielsen AB: Sports injuries in adolescents' ball games: soccer, handball, and basketball, *Br J Sports Med* 24(1):51, 1990.
48. Yost JG et al: Intraarticular iliotibial band reconstructions for anterior cruciate insufficiency, *Am J Sports Med* 9:220, 1981.
49. Zarins B, Ciullo JV: Acute muscle and tendon injuries in athletics, *Clin Sports Med* 2:167, 1983.
50. Zelisko JA, Noble HB, Porter M: A comparison of men's and women's professional basketball injuries, *Am J Sports Med* 10:297, 1982.

CHAPTER 63 Football Injuries

Dean Fochios
James A. Nicholas

HISTORY OF FOOTBALL

In 1892, when William "Pudge" Hefflefinger was openly paid $500 by the Allegheny Athletic Association to play a game of football against the Pittsburgh Athletic Club, professional football was born. In 1922 the Na- tional Football League (NFL) was formed, replacing the American Professional Football Association, which had been formed in 1919. The popularity of football is repre- sented by the fact that over 133.4 million people in the United States alone viewed Super Bowl XXVII on televi- sion in 1993. Super Bowls comprise 9 of television's 10 most watched programs, with the final episode of *M*A*S*H* in 1983, which attracted 121.6 million view- ers, as the lone exception. It is estimated that 2.5 billion people watched the 1992 Olympic games, and over 1.6 billion people watched World Cup Soccer in 1990.

Athletes with a wide range of ability and at all ages and levels of competition, not just professional individu- als, play football each year. In 1982 the A.C. Nielson Company estimated that football ranked twenty-first in sports participation in the United States. Sixteen million individuals out of the U.S. population of 235 million play some type of football each year. This number is remark- ably high when considering that football is one of the most violent of all contact sports and has an injury rate that affects 80% of all men who have finished college and try out for the professional league.[53]

Professional football is now played in leagues in Eu- rope and the Far East. Attendance and interest in such games are rising. It is likely that international leagues spanning the globe will develop over the next decade. As a result, sports medicine societies made up of physicians throughout Europe and Japan are stimulated to study in- juries, treatments, and rehabilitation in football.

Football has many beneficial effects on its participants from physical development to development of social be- havior and team work. These attributes account for the popularity of the sport. It is an unfortunate and undis- putable fact that the risk of injury is an inherent part of the game. Thus football has served as an early labora- tory for the study of athletic injuries in many ways. In no other sport can severe injuries readily be seen at the moment they happen, studied on film, treated, and fol- lowed until the player returns to action. In addition, this process from injury to reentry into the game can be fol- lowed in a greater number of individuals in football than in other team or individual sports.

Over the last 30 years a unique relation has formed and grown between professional and college football and television. The degree of the electronic technology has exploded during this period making multiple cameras, camera angles, and variable film speed and direction common sights every weekend on televised games. This technology is also available to the football teams and is used to film and study games, practices, and individual players. Sports medicine as a field has also grown in popularity and exposure during this period. The technology mentioned above and computer-assisted graphics and analysis have provided the field of sports medicine a large scientific and clinical database. All sports and the risk-benefit ratios should be part of a physician's training and part of the training of the large number of young people seeking careers in sports medicine.

ETIOLOGY OF FOOTBALL INJURIES

The reasons for injury in football are that it is both a contact and a collision sport. The nature of the game itself calls for specific athletic abilities to be performed in many off-balance positions (Fig. 63-1). Players can become directly or indirectly involved in contact or collision with other players or the ground. The flow of the play, position of the individual, and peripheral awareness determine if the contact is anticipated or not. Each play involves 22 football players. Each player has an assignment that may involve deception, direct contact, and surprise.

This may pit individuals of varying size, speed, and maturity against each other and can lead to physical contacts producing forces of great magnitude.

The rate of injury reported in the literature has been variable and depends to a large extent on whether the injury is minor and requires a minimal time loss or major and requires hospitalization. Major injuries may result from a direct force that is greater than the supporting structures can stand before failure, or it may result from a subclinical cumulative trauma that has substantially weakened a structure before it was stressed. Proper astute diagnosis, evaluation, and rehabilitation of microtrauma is just as important, if not more important, than the rehabilitation of an acute macrotrauma.

A factor that must be considered in the assessments is the natural selection process. The natural selection eliminates many individuals from participation, starting at the prepubertal and pubertal levels, when the first major jump in injuries during play is manifested. At each school-age level, injury takes its toll. In examining the college draft players, it is readily apparent how many individuals have already been injured. These athletes bear scars that are the results of arthroscopy, ligament sur-

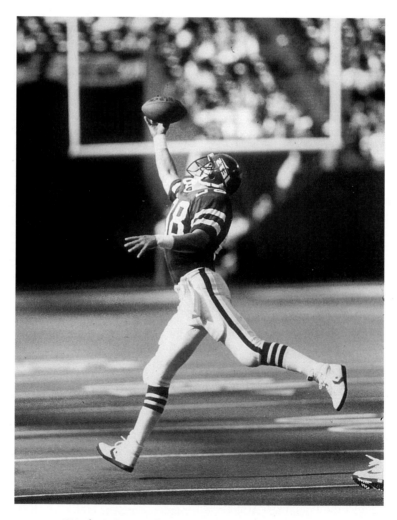

FIG. 63-1. Pass catching in vulnerable off-balance position.

gery, shoulder repair, or other surgery on various parts of the body. In addition, many exhibit asymmetric laxity, strength, and flexibility as a result of previous fractures, muscle strains, or ligament sprains. If they are carefully searched for, pathologic conditions can be found in 80% of all football players by the time they reach college.[53] In a review of college seniors selected in the professional football draft over 6 consecutive years, less than 20% have been injury free in their careers. In this instance an injury is being defined as a loss of playing time greater than 2 weeks. The remaining 80% of these young athletes have had different injuries in various combinations that have prevented them from participating in a contact situation. These players are at an increased risk of reinjury because the game on a professional level is played at a more intense level in which the size, speed, and deception of the players are greater.

ADDITIONAL SOURCES OF INJURY

Injuries in football may be caused by player-to-player contact, player-to-ground contact, overuse injury, or noncontact, high-force ligament tear or muscle strain (intrinsic overload). Football is a game played with great speed and high-speed acceleration that develops great forces. The offense attempts to fool the defense, and vice versa, in such a fashion that individuals are singled out to be blocked or put out of play. The use of questionable techniques occurs and leads to injuries despite these techniques being outlawed. These include "spearing," "battering" (with the helmeted head into the chest), "leg whipping," and "chop blocking." Simple, direct contact or overpowering with the arms, such as with chopping, holding, tripping, or even sticking fingers into the eyes, produces injuries to the unsuspecting or ill-prepared individual. These injury-producing techniques, despite the strict penalties, are seen at all levels of competition as a result of the emphasis on winning. At sophisticated levels of competition, these illegal techniques have already been learned by the players. Many can retaliate, and the veteran (those with 3 or 4 years of professional experience) seem to be able to anticipate such techniques. The younger athletes may be taught these techniques by coaches who are out to win at any cost.

EQUIPMENT

Improvements in helmet design have sharply reduced injury to the head, but unfortunately, helmets have become so solid that if another player is struck by one, the injury can be severe. These injuries can range from fractures and dislocations to severe contusions and sprains. In an effort to protect against such injuries, protective padding is worn around the shoulders, hips, and thighs. These pads also protect the body from contact with the ground and the padded parts and helmets of the opposing players. In most organized settings these pads are mandatory (Fig. 63-2). Even so, for players in positions emphasizing speed or agility (e.g., defensive backs, wide receivers, and quarterbacks), padding may be of an inappropriate dimension, and strength is sacrificed to permit the player maximum mobility. In some instances the cost of the equipment may be prohibitively high. This is seen most often at the public high school level. In these athletes dangerous cracks may be painted over on the helmets, and the protective padding may themselves be improperly fitted. This is usually done to save money but does not take into account what one head injury can cost. In these instances preventable injuries may occur, justifying codification of equipment, length of use, and condition.

Fixation of the foot in the turf by long cleats on grass and mud was the source of injury some years ago. Modification of cleat size and configuration coupled with changes in the playing surface, such as synthetic turf, have changed the pattern of injury. Multiple-studded cleats to prevent foot fixation are being used; however, the game has been "sped up" with the addition of artificial turf. Thus fractures are more common, although they can occur on any surface if sufficient force is applied (Fig. 63-3).

Although there is a perception that artificial turf causes more injuries than natural surfaces, there is no conclusive evidence to substantiate this thought. In a recent study on the NFL experience, injury and reinjury statistics were broken down comparing the different offensive and defensive positions. No clear-cut pattern or significance could be placed on the playing surface alone. This includes career-ending knee and spine injuries, as well as minor abrasions, contusions, and muscle

---

Illegal techniques that may contribute to injury

- Spearing — Using the head as a "battering ram" when making a tackle. The helmet is driven into the chest of the opponent.
  Potential area of injury: neck
- Chop blocking — Offensive man (e.g., tackle) is engaged in a block with a defensive man (e.g., end). A second offensive player (e.g., tight end) hits the defensive man below the waist. The second man is chop blocking.
  Potential areas of injury: knee and ankle
- Leg whipping — An offensive man is down on the ground (e.g., offensive tackle down on all fours after a block). As a defensive player runs by (e.g., blitzing linebacker), the man on the ground throws out his leg, attempting to trip or kick the rushing opponent.
  Potential area of injury: knee
- Butting — Using the helmeted head as a weapon by bringing it forcefully into an opponent's head while blocking
  Potential areas of injury: head and neck
- Clipping — Blocking from the back side below the waist
  Potential area of injury: knee

NFL UNIFORM AND EQUIPMENT RULES

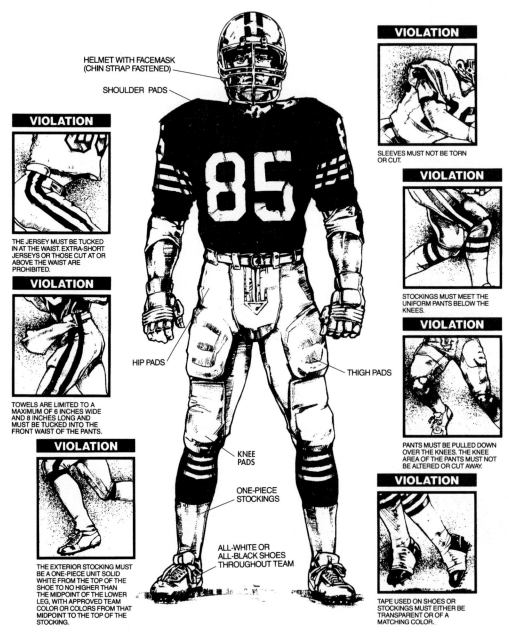

HELMET WITH FACEMASK
(CHIN STRAP FASTENED)

SHOULDER PADS

VIOLATION

SLEEVES MUST NOT BE TORN
OR CUT.

VIOLATION

THE JERSEY MUST BE TUCKED
IN AT THE WAIST. EXTRA-SHORT
JERSEYS OR THOSE CUT AT OR
ABOVE THE WAIST ARE
PROHIBITED.

VIOLATION

STOCKINGS MUST MEET THE
UNIFORM PANTS BELOW THE
KNEES.

VIOLATION

TOWELS ARE LIMITED TO A
MAXIMUM OF 6 INCHES WIDE
AND 8 INCHES LONG AND
MUST BE TUCKED INTO THE
FRONT WAIST OF THE PANTS.

VIOLATION

PANTS MUST BE PULLED DOWN
OVER THE KNEES. THE KNEE
AREA OF THE PANTS MUST NOT
BE ALTERED OR CUT AWAY.

VIOLATION

THE EXTERIOR STOCKING MUST
BE A ONE-PIECE UNIT SOLID
WHITE FROM THE TOP OF THE
SHOE TO NO HIGHER THAN
THE MIDPOINT OF THE LOWER
LEG, WITH APPROVED TEAM
COLOR OR COLORS FROM THAT
MIDPOINT TO THE TOP OF THE
STOCKING.

VIOLATION

TAPE USED ON SHOES OR
STOCKINGS MUST EITHER BE
TRANSPARENT OR OF A
MATCHING COLOR.

HIP PADS

THIGH PADS

KNEE
PADS

ONE-PIECE
STOCKINGS

ALL-WHITE OR
ALL-BLACK SHOES
THROUGHOUT TEAM

FIG. 63-2. Uniform codes are designed to protect players from injury, as well as prevent injury to opposing players. (Courtesy National Football League.)

NFL UNIFORM AND EQUIPMENT RULES

[The following are the uniform/equipment rules important to NFL players:]

GENERAL POLICY Throughout the game-day period while in view of the stadium and television audience, including during pregame warm-ups, all players must dress in a professional manner under the League's uniform standards. They must wear suitable padding and other equipment offering reasonable protection to themselves while reasonably avoiding risk of injury to other players. And they generally must present an appearance that is appropriate to representing their individual clubs and the National Football League. The term uniform, as used in this policy, applies to every piece of equipment worn by a player, including helmet, shoulder pads, thigh pads, knee pads, and any other item of protective gear, and to every visible item of apparel, including but not limited to pants, jerseys, wristbands, gloves, stockings, shoes, visible undergarments, and accessories such as head coverings worn under helmets and hand towels. All visible items worn on game day by players must be issued by the club or the League, or, if from outside sources, must have approval in advance by the League.

MANDATORY EQUIPMENT, APPAREL All players must wear the equipment and uniform apparel listed below, which must be of a suitably protective nature, must be designed and produced by a professional manufacturer, and must not be cut, reduced in size, or otherwise altered unless for medical reasons approved in advance by the Commissioner; provided, however, that during pregame warm-ups players may omit certain protective equipment at their option, except that helmets must be worn.

Helmets, Face Protectors Helmet with chin strap fastened and facemask attached. Facemasks must not be more than 5/8-inch in diameter and must be made of rounded material; transparent materials are prohibited. Plastic face shields, either clear or lightly tinted, for eye protection are optional, provided the League office is supplied in advance with appropriate medical documentation that the shield is needed. No visible identification of a manufacturer's name or logo on the exterior of the helmet or any attachment to a helmet is permitted unless provided for under a commercial arrangement between the League and manufacturer; in no event is identification of any helmet manufacturer permitted on the visible surface of a rear cervical pad.

Jerseys Jerseys that cover all pads and other protective equipment worn on the torso and upper arms, and that is appropriately tailored to remain tucked into the uniform pants throughout the game. Tearaway jerseys are prohibited. Mesh jerseys with large fishnet material (commonly referred to as bullet-hole or port-hole mesh) are also prohibited. Surnames of players in letters of 21/2 -inches high must be affixed to the exterior of jerseys across the upper back above the numerals; nicknames are prohibited; and in cases of duplicate surnames, the first initial of the given name must be used.

Numerals Numerals on the back and front of jerseys as specified under NFL rules for the player's specific position. Such numerals must be a minimum of eight inches high and four inches wide, and their color must be in sharp contrast with the color of the jersey.

Pants Pants that are worn over the entire knee area; pants shortened or rolled up to meet the stockings above the knee are prohibited. No part of the pants may be cut away unless an appropriate gusset or other device is used to replace the removed material.

Shoulder Pads Shoulder pads that are completely covered by the uniform jersey.

Hip Pads Hip pads that are covered by the outer uniform; provided, however, that punters and placekickers may omit such pads.

Thigh Pads Thigh pads; provided, however, that punters and placekickers may omit such pads.

Knee Pads Knee pads; provided, however, that punters and placekickers may omit such pads. Basketball-type knee pads are permitted but must be covered by the outer uniform.

Stockings Stockings that cover the entire area from the shoe to the bottom of the pants, and that meet the pants below the knee. Players are permitted to wear as many layers of stockings and tape on the lower leg as they prefer, provided the exterior is a one-piece stocking that includes solid white from the top of the shoe to no higher than the mid-point of the lower leg, and approved team color or colors (non-white) from that point to the top of the stocking. Uniform stockings may not be altered (e.g., over-stretched, or cut at the toe or stirrups) in order to bring the line between solid white and team colors higher than the mid-point of the lower leg. No other stockings and/or opaque tape may be worn over the one-piece, two-color uniform stocking. Barefoot punters and placekickers may omit the stocking of the kicking foot in preparation for and during kicking plays.

Shoes Shoes that are of a standard football design. Kicking shoes must not be modified, and any shoe that is worn by a player with an artificial limb on his kicking leg must have a kicking surface which conforms to that of a normal kicking shoe. Punters and placekickers may omit the shoe from the kicking foot in preparation for and during kicking plays. All players on the same team must wear the same color shoe (either all white or all black, with all-white or all-black laces, whichever are applicable). Punters and placekickers are permitted, only on plays in which they line up to kick, to deviate temporarily from this rule, e.g., by wearing one black and one white shoe, or two black shoes while the rest of the team wears white.

OTHER PROHIBITED EQUIPMENT, APPAREL In addition to the several prohibited items of equipment and apparel specified above, the following are also prohibited:

Projecting Objects Metal or other hard objects that project from a player's person or uniform, including from his shoes.

Uncovered Hard Objects, Substances Hard objects and substances, including but not limited to casts, guards, or braces for hand, wrist, forearm, elbow, hip, thigh, knee, shin, unless such items are appropriately covered on all edges and surfaces by a minimum of 3/8-inch foam rubber or similar soft material. Any such item worn to protect an injury must be reported by the applicable coaching staff to Umpire in advance of the game, and a description of the injury must be provided.

Detachable Toe Detachable kicking toe.

Torn Items Torn or improperly fitting equipment creating a risk of injury to other players, e.g., the hard surface of shoulder pads exposed by a damaged jersey.

Improper Cleats Shoe cleats made of aluminum or other material that may chip, fracture, or develop a cutting edge. Conical cleats with concave sides or points which measure less than 3/8-inch in diameter at the tips, or cleats with oblong ends which measure less than 1/4-by 3/4-inch at the end tips are also prohibited. Nylon cleats with flat steel tips are permitted.

Improper Tape Opaque, contrasting-color tape that covers any part of the helmet, jersey, pants, stockings, or shoes; transparent tape or tape of the same color as the background material is permissible for use on these items of apparel. Players may use opaque white tape on hands and arms, provided it conforms to "Uncovered Hard Objects, Substances" above and "Improper Glove Color on Linemen" below. Opaque tape on shoes is permitted, provided it is the same color as the shoe, and provided it does not carry up into the stocking area.

Improper Glove Color on Linemen Gloves, wrappings, elbow pads, and other items worn on the arms below or over the jersey sleeves by interior offensive linemen (excluding tight ends) which are of a color different from that which is mandatorily reported to the League office by the club before July 1 each year. Such reported color must be white or other official color of the applicable team

Adhesive, Slippery Substances Adhesive or slippery substances on the body, equipment, or uniform of any player; provided, however, that players may wear gloves which have a tackified surface if such tacky substance does not adhere to the football or otherwise cause handling problems for players.

OPTIONAL EQUIPMENT Among the types of optional equipment that are permitted to be worn by players are the following:

Rib Protectors Rib protectors ("flak jackets") under the jersey.

Wrist Bands Wrist bands, provided they are white or in official team colors.

Towels Towels, provided they are plain white with no logos, names, symbols, or illustrations. Such towels also must be attached to or tucked into the front waist of the pants and must be no larger than six inches by eight inches (slightly larger size may be folded to these limits for wearing in game). A player may wear no more than one towel. Players are prohibited from discarding on the playing field any loose towels or other materials used for wiping hands and the football. Streamers or ribbons, regardless of length, hanging from any part of the uniform, including the helmet, are prohibited.

Head Coverings Head coverings worn under the helmet, e.g., sweat bands and bandannas, are permissible and may be visible in the bench area, provided that they are of solid color (white or official team color) and issued by the club, and further provided that no portion hangs from or is otherwise visible outside the helmet during play. Baseball-type caps may be worn in the bench area, provided they are in official team colors and issued by the club.

LOGOS AND COMMERCIAL IDENTIFICATION Throughout the period on game-day that a player is visible to the stadium and television audience (including in pregame warm-ups, in the bench area, and during postgame interviews in the locker room or on the field), players are prohibited from wearing, displaying, or orally promoting equipment, apparel, or other items that carry commercial names or logos of companies, unless such commercial identification has been approved in advance by the League office. The size of any approved logo or other commercial identification involved in an agreement between a manufacturer and the League will be modest and unobtrusive, and there is no assurance that it will be visible to the television audience. Subject to any future approval arrangements with manufacturer and subject to any decision by the Commissioner to temporarily suspend enforcement of this provision governing shoes, visible logos and names of shoes are prohibited, including on the sole of the shoe that may be seen from time to time during the game. When shoe logos and names are covered with appropriate use of tape, the logos or name of the shoe manufacturer must not be re-applied to the exterior of the tape unless advance approval is granted by the League office.

PERSONAL MESSAGES Throughout the period on game day that a player is visible to the stadium and television audience (including in pregame warm-ups, in the bench area, and during post-game interviews in the locker room or on the field), players are prohibited from wearing, displaying, or otherwise conveying personal messages either in writing or illustration, unless such message has been approved in advance by the League office. Items such as armbands and jersey patches worn to celebrate anniversaries of events, to promote charities, to recognize causes and campaigns, or to honor or commemorate personages are also prohibited unless approved in advance by the League office. Further, such armbands and jersey patches must be modest in size, tasteful, non-commercial, and non-controversial; must not be worn for more than one football season; and if approved for use by a specific team, must not be worn by players on other teams in the League.

GENERAL APPEARANCE Consistent with the League's equipment and uniform rules, players must otherwise present a professional and appropriate appearance while before the public on game day. Among the types of activity that are prohibited are use of tobacco products (smokeless included) while in the bench area and use of facial makeup.

FIG. 63-2, cont'd. For legend see opposite page.

strains.[55] Other studies have considered the playing field conditions regardless of the surface as an initiating factor to injuries.[6,56] Shoe and surface frictional resistance and torque generated between two opposing surfaces have also been examined as a source of injury without any clear-cut pattern established.[5,41,71] From the data available there is no one primary factor responsible for injuries; instead it is probably multivariant in nature.

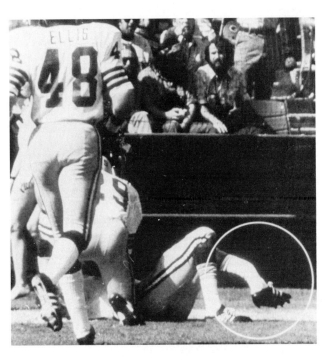

FIG. 63-3. Fracture of tibia and fibula from high-velocity collision.

CLASSIFICATION OF INJURIES

Injuries caused by football cannot be listed as different from those injuries that can be found in any textbook dealing with multiple trauma and fractures. However, many football injuries permit us to learn the specific mechanism of injury, how the injury could have been prevented, and how to tailor a treatment and rehabilitation program with specific goals and options. In describing these injuries it is usual to have some type of working classification. Injuries can easily be divided into those of lesser severity and those of greater severity.

Injuries of lesser severity are those that cause an individual to miss 2 consecutive weeks of practice and game participation. However, the individual can return successfully to play thereafter, and there should be no evidence of any permanent or residual sequelae that might require further intensive or invasive care. **Injuries of greater severity** range from lethal injuries, to injuries that require emergency care, to long-term injuries with permanent residual disability, which may or may not be amendable to aggressive intervention.

Injuries, whether minor or major, occur quite frequently in football. These are best discussed from the overall view of the musculoskeletal system as a series of links. This **linkage system** absorbs, dampens, accelerates, or transmits forces as they occur either self-generated or from collisions with the ground or other players (Fig. 63-4). Severe injuries can occur at any point in the linkage system as these forces are encountered. The contact requirements of the game differ such as in tackling, blocking, kicking, running, and for the quarterback, passing (Fig. 63-5). These different positions demand various athletic attributes that determine the overall success of the player and the potential situation for an injury to occur.

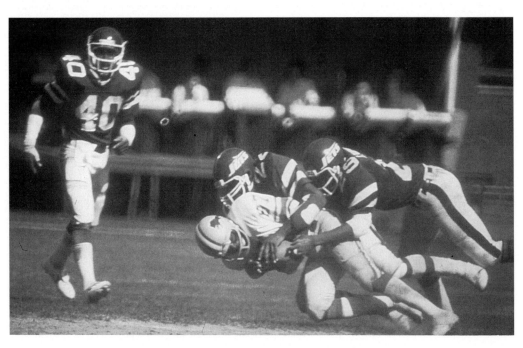

FIG. 63-4. Tackle being made on dirt portion of baseball infield.

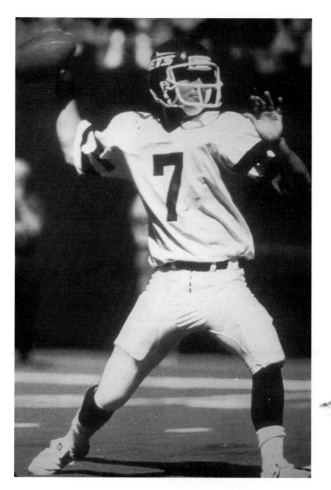

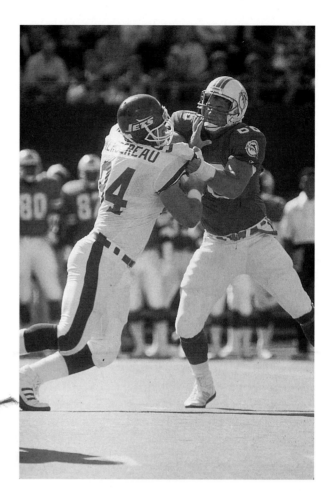

FIG. 63-5. Passing exposes lower extremities, abdomen, and thorax to unprotected hits.

FIG. 63-6. Blocking defensive lineman.

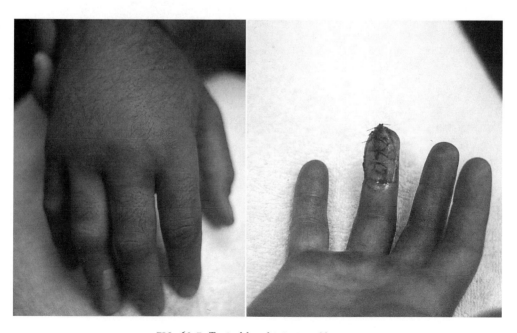

FIG. 63-7. Typical hand injuries of linemen.

Offensive and defensive linemen are the largest, heaviest players on the team. Their average sizes and weights range from a height of 6 feet 2 inches to 6 feet 8 inches and a weight of 240 to 320 pounds. Offensive linemen are larger and have more body fat than most other players. They tend to be serious weightlifters and are less flamboyant than their defensive counterparts (Fig. 63-6). Defensive linemen are aggressive and muscular, have particularly strong upper bodies, and have more explosive speed than offensive linemen.

Injuries to linemen include numerous hand injuries because their battles go unnoticed in the "trenches." These hand injuries may be serious, but they tend to be overlooked and taped up because they do not tend to impede the abilities necessary for them to continue playing their position (Fig. 63-7). Linemen also suffer knee and ankle injuries when other players are pushed and rolled into them unsuspectingly from the side and back while their focus of attention is centered toward their assignments for that play. These result in first- and second-degree collateral ligament sprains of the knee and cruciate ligament injuries. Many players wear knee braces as a protection against these injuries. The efficacy of bracing remains controversial as a protection against these knee injuries (see Chapter 44).

Linebackers are smaller with a height of 5 feet 11 inches to 6 feet 3 inches and an average weight of 215 to 245 pounds. They tend to have less body fat than linemen and are quicker in their movements. Lateral and backward agility are necessary qualities at this position. They also need good balance, great upper body strength, and an ability to read the play and react quickly (Fig. 63-8). They must be able to backpedal, move diagonally, and cut toward or away from the action during the play. In this age of specialization, football players are being substituted on the basis of field position, what down it is, and the yardage needed. This "new age" strategy is all done in an attempt to gain an advantage, however small, over the opposing team on every possible play.

Safeties and cornerbacks, who form the defensive secondary, are relatively small and have great speed. Their height averages from 5 feet 6 inches to 5 feet 11 inches, and their average weight is approximately 175 to 200 pounds. Their athletic abilities include those of linebackers, but they must be performed at a higher rate of speed because they cover the most playing area guarding against the wide receivers. Wide receivers and defensive backs tend to be the quickest players on the team. In addition to guarding the wide receivers, they also have a secondary responsibility to stop any players that have

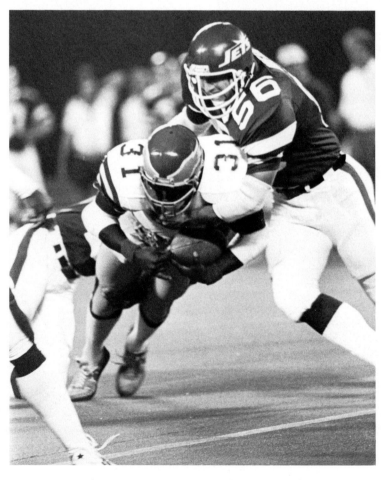

FIG. 63-8. Linebacker making tackle on running back.

broken through the front line of the defense (Fig. 63-9). The greatest mismatch is seen in these cases as these small defensive secondary players attempt to tackle larger oncoming running backs and blockers. Because they have less mass and are subject to high-accelerating

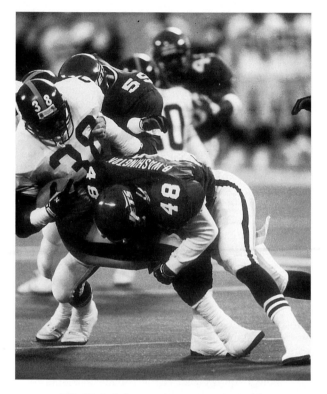

FIG. 63-9. Safety coming up to make tackle.

forces, they must use appropriate tackling techniques to avoid injuries.

The **quarterback** is the team leader and has to be reasonably articulate, have a strong sense of leadership, and must be able to throw, run, and jump. He must have some mobility and quick reactions to protect himself from being tackled or hit in a "blind-side" fashion. He has to learn to throw off either foot in pursuit and must handle the ball well. The quarterbacks, although their careers may last a long time, are frequently injured. Because of their talent and experience (qualities that are often hard to replace) most of them undergo surgery to perpetuate their careers if they are seriously injured. A good quarterback's career can last on the average 7 to 11 years. "Reading" the many combinations of defensive coverage and calling the correct offensive play options in 3.5 seconds obviously tests their reaction time. If they cannot do this, they are ineffective and tackled for a loss of yardage.

The **running backs** are divided into fullbacks and halfbacks. These athletes have short career expectancies, averaging between 4 and 7 years. This is a result of the constant pounding that they must take on every play in hitting the line, catching, passing, and blocking. They are usually smaller than the defensive lineman and linebackers that they are hitting. They have a low percentage of body fat and are usually muscular, compact, and quick. Running backs tend to work with their shoulders and head to deceive the defensive players. Their pelvis must remain balanced because their feet continually move in an effort not to be tackled. (Fig. 63-10). Most of their power comes from driving off their legs in various degrees of rotation at the spine, hip, ankle, and knee, and they learn to cut at right angles with both legs. Their ca-

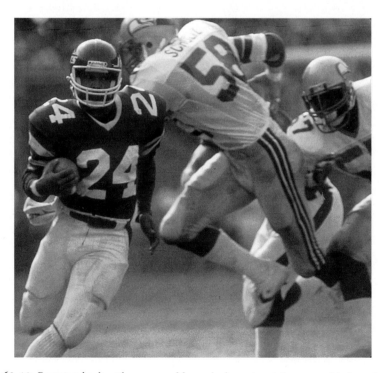

FIG. 63-10. Running back with upper and lower body parts rotating around balanced pelvis.

reers are often terminated by a knee or ankle injury that causes them to lose their speed and power, which are necessary as part of their position. Many have rotator cuff injuries and shoulder separations. They also suffer upper extremity sprains. Contused thighs and calves and adductor and hamstring strains are often frustrating to treat for the trainer and the physician.

The **receivers,** who catch passes, range in size from small, light individuals 5 feet 7 inches to 5 feet 8 inches tall and weighing 150 pounds up to large individuals from 6 feet 4 inches to 6 feet 8 inches and weighing up to 220 pounds. Receivers are apt to be injured when they are running patterns over the middle to catch passes, where collision is inevitable. High-speed, off-balance collisions occur as the tackle is being made, leading to injury (Fig. 63-11). Because these athletes depend so much on speed, hamstring, quadriceps, and groin injuries are particularly disabling to them. They are often hit in the flanks by a helmet, grabbed across the neck, and tackled while in full pursuit by the defensive players. Assessment of their injuries are gauged by how much of their speed is lost after each injury and throughout their career.

Over a 4-year period, 167 football players were studied and divided into four major groups: (1) linemen; (2) linebackers and tight ends; (3) running backs, quarterbacks, and kickers; and (4) wide receivers and defensive

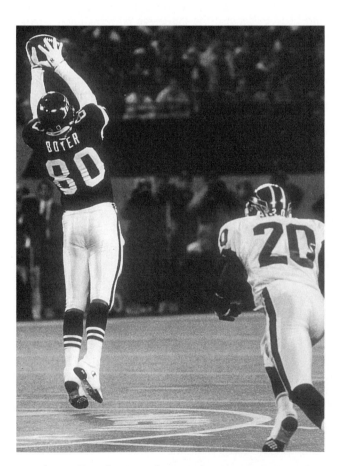

FIG. 63-11. Extending to make reception, receiver is exposed to injuries.

backs. These groups were then subdivided into rookies, veterans (nonstarters), and veterans (starters). Body characteristics and performance were then evaluated and analyzed. Group 1 players were taller, heavier, and had a higher percentage of body fat, whereas Group 4 players were smaller, lighter, and had the least amount of body fat. Cardiovascular parameters demonstrated the opposite trend; Group 4 players were the most fit. Although these trends were independent of the different subgroups, veteran starters were older and more cardiovascularly fit. The conclusion of the authors was that although measurable parameters were important, an unmeasurable quality was inherent that produced a successful player. This quality was not easily identifiable in a beginning player.[27,70]

PREPARTICIPATION ASSESSMENT

With the advent of physical fitness and awareness, preparticipation assessment has become commonplace in athletes on all levels of play from high school to professionals. The days are gone when just showing up to the first team meeting or making the last cut was all that was necessary to practice and participate in games. A review of college and high school sports consistently demonstrates that the highest proportion of injuries occur among male football players, and knee injuries are the most common.[22,46] Today medical, orthopaedic, and even psychologic data are gathered on players. Clandestine examinations of potential draft choices have given way to a cooperative, organized, combined evaluation of all collegiate players available for the professional draft. This medical information is then made available to all NFL coaches and management before the draft. Hiding physical impairments was once common, but it is now not desirable from either the management's or the player's viewpoint.

This profile, like all good medical records, provides a complete history of injuries, treatments, recovery time, and subsequent performance. This openness and detailed evaluation of the players from the time of injury to returning to action has provided the modern field of sports medicine with invaluable information on the cause and treatment of injuries. Throughout the course of a season, measurements of strength and flexibility can be recorded that help detect weakness and sites of possible injury. Following an injury, baseline data can be used to guide and evaluate progress in rehabilitation. Repeat physical examination, player performance, and updated testing measurements allow a timely return to action. It is not uncommon for the physician, trainer, physical therapist, and injured player to be drawn into a discussion of the risks and requirements needed for the best performance after an injury.

In addition, a new source of sports medicine data is now being generated on the late sequelae of various types of injuries. The natural history of these injuries can now be more carefully followed and the final outcomes assessed. This insight may then influence and play a role in changing certain attitudes toward the treatment of different injuries encountered.[52]

MOTIONS AND DEMANDS OF FOOTBALL

Football requires a maximum scale of motion, whether it is to walk, run, jump, kick, throw, or use stance. In studies done on the motions and demands of sports, football is at the top of the list.[54] Although football was not found to be as aerobic as speed or distance running, the diversity of motions and the exposure time, which is presumably only 6 to 8 actual minutes of contact per game (estimating 20 seconds per play), required maximum muscle strength, endurance, balance, agility, speed, coordination, alertness, rhythm, timing, reaction time, motivation, flexibility, steadiness, accuracy, discipline, and creativity. In addition, the type, amount, duration, and intensity of practice were the most important components of injury, as was defective and inadequate equipment.

Football entails a coaching process that demands continuous supervision, demonstration, practice, teaching, training, and standardizations of behavior as a team, which requires discipline. Because of this, football is one of the most demanding team sports, and it makes severe demands on movement and physical ability. For example, in running, there are many types of instantaneous adjustments to make. These include sprinting, jogging, right-angle pivots, outside-inside cuts, reverse or crossover steps, diagonal circles backwards, lateral zigzag steps, stop and go, run to jump, and jump to run. As a result of this, many types of injuries are seen in the lower extremities that are not seen in most other sports with the same frequency, with perhaps the exception of ice hockey and alpine skiing. This is because, in addition to these movements, the problems of contact and collision are generally contributors to injury.

Instantaneous adjustments during running

- Right-angle pivots
- Outside-inside cuts
- Reverse or crossover steps
- Circling
- Lateral zigzag steps
- Stop and go
- Run to jump
- Jump to run
- Speed adjustment

NONORTHOPAEDIC TRAUMA

Trauma other than to the musculoskeletal system is associated with football, and the team physician must be aware of this potential in every player. These injuries can be devastating, and the sports medicine practioner must constantly watch closely for their occurrence. Pneumothorax or hemopneumothorax is not an uncommon event and is often initially missed. Although rare, potential for major vascular injuries in the chest does exist on the football field. The physician must be alert to the widening of the mediastinum associated with fractures of the first and second rib or clavicle on chest radiographs. Abdominal injuries are always a source of concern. They may result in association with injuries to the trunk, spine, and pelvis and occur as a result of direct contusion from blocking or tackling while catching a knee in these areas. In particular, injuries to the spleen, kidneys, and liver occur often. Occasionally, altered states of consciousness from head injury may make a diagnosis of intraabdominal injury difficult. Also, intraabdominal injury may not show up initially in the locker room; symptoms can appear after the player has gone home. This is especially dangerous in amateur football in which there is no physical review process performed after the game.

Physicians dealing with football players must always maintain a high degree of suspicion for all these major injuries. Physicians responsible for the care of football players must also be aware of many complications that can be associated with musculoskeletal injuries. All kinds of injuries, including hip fractures and dislocations, knee dislocations, and ankle fractures and dislocations, occur during football and may be seen with vascular or neurologic compromise and compartment syndrome. These are commonly associated with serious soft-tissue injury and are always a source of difficulty in diagnosis. It is for this reason that during football games and practices, physicians who are aware of the management of trauma must be available.

The principles of trauma management should be known and appropriately applied; that is, how to establish an airway, how to provide oxygenation, how to understand volume deficit, and how to estimate the extent of blood loss with injury. The capability to evacuate an injured player from the football field should be prearranged, with the ambulance standing by and an emergency room on call. Whether a player is seen on the field, in an emergency room, or in a physician's office, players should be monitored for head, chest, abdominal, and other neurologic and vascular injuries. The four *R*'s that are important for the team physician are *r*ecognize, *r*eport, *r*epair, and *r*ehabilitate. In addition, compartment syndrome, infections from poorly healed abrasions, and embolism should be kept in mind, even in young athletes.

The four *R*'s

- Recognize
- Report
- Repair
- Rehabilitate

ORTHOPAEDIC INJURIES
Spine and Head Injuries

Up to 1.5 million men participate in organized football at all levels of play. Epidemiologic studies have demonstrated that injuries occur at higher rates in older athletes and on teams with the least amount of supervision and coaching. Approximately one half of all injuries occur in football during practice sessions. Lower extremity injuries account for 50% of all injuries, with the knee

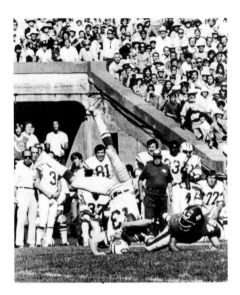

FIG. 63-12. The neck is vulnerable to injury as a result of contact in off-balance positions.

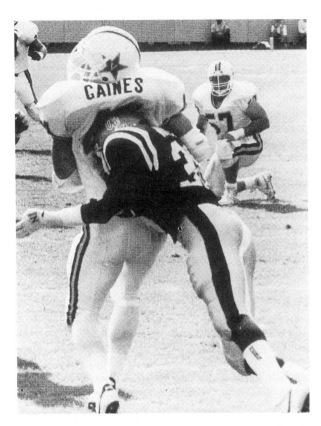

FIG. 63-13. Intercollegiate defensive back making head tackle, which resulted in axial loading injury to his cervical spine and quadriplegia. (From Torg JS, Vegso JJ, O'Neill MJ: *Am J Sports Med* 18:56, 1990.)

being involved in 36% of these cases. Upper extremity injuries accounted for another 30% of the injuries, with the remainder involving the head, neck, lumbar spine, and trunk. Soft-tissue sprains and strains involved 40% of all injuries, contusions 25%, dislocations 15%, fractures 10%, and concussions 5%.[67] In another review of 4551 sports injuries seen at the University of Rochester Sports Medicine Service over a 7-year period, football injuries were the most common. The number of football injuries observed were greater than 12 times the number of injuries seen in the next most common sport.[20]

Cervical Spine

Any athletic endeavor, especially sports played at high speeds with potential for collision and contact, can occasionally result in a catastrophic injury or fatality when the injury involves the head and neck. Perhaps the most visible injury in football, although by far not the most common, is the player who sustains trauma to the cervical spine. The lasting impression of a player with a cervical spine injury and resultant quadriplegia is not easily forgotten by the public and by all football players (Fig. 63-12). Because of the intense national media focus on each of these injuries, regardless of the level of play, the event and sequalae are etched emotionally in the minds of all.

From 1945 to 1984 84.6% of all football-related fatalities resulted from injuries to the head or cervical spine.[51] During the decade from 1965 to 1974 more of these injuries were reported than during any other period. Data collected since 1931 on football fatalities by the American Football Coaches Association and by the National Collegiate Athletic Association (NCAA) also demonstrate that head and neck fatalities steadily rose from 1960 and reached their peak incidence of 3.4 per 100,000 in 1968. Defensive players are at greater risk than offensive players for developing traumatic quadriplegia because most injuries occur during tackling.[14]

The National Football Head and Neck Registry was es-

tablished in 1975 to document the incidence of head and neck injuries in organized football. In the period from 1971 to 1975 there were 259 cervical spine injuries resulting in 99 cases of permanent quadriplegia.[75] Information from this organization and other studies provided the impetus for the 1976 NCAA rule change that prohibits initial contact with the head and face when blocking and tackling (Fig. 63-13). The first Professional Physicians Football Conference was held in 1968 and concluded that reduction in fatal head and neck injuries could be influenced greatly by four factors: (1) the rule changes prohibiting the use of the head in blocking and tackling, (2) coaches teaching proper fundamentals of blocking and tackling, (3) different football helmet standards, and (4) improved conditioning programs and close supervision by team physicians and trainers of every head and neck injury (Fig. 63-14). The decade from 1975 through 1984 was associated with the smallest number and percentage of head and cervical spine fatalities because these guidelines were implemented into all levels of organized football.[51] Unfortunately, these rule changes, regulations, and other factors have not completely eliminated neck injuries.

Mechanism of injury. In football, the neck is used to let the players see what is going on. As a result, it is vulnerable in many positions. It can be injured in rotation, flexion, and extension. The musculature of the neck provides support and protection for the cervical spine. In

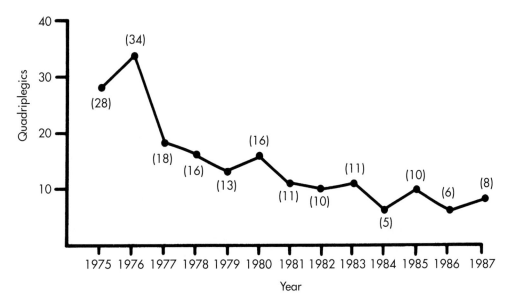

FIG. 63-14. Yearly incidence of permanent cervical quadriplegia for all levels of participation (1975 to 1987) decreased dramatically in 1977 following initiation of rule changes prohibiting use of head-first tackling and blocking techniques. (From Torg JS, Vegso JJ, O'Neill MJ: *Am J Sports Med* 18:56, 1990.)

particular, the short intrinsic muscles lie between the head and cervical spine (the longus capitus and the rectus capitus). These are small muscles with poor strength. The capital extensors, however, which include the rectus capitis major and minor, the obliquus capitis inferior and superior, and the suboccipital group, have little potential to develop much mechanical advantage; thus they are fortified by the long head extensors, including the longissimus, the splenius, and the semispinalis capitis. The importance of these muscles is their extensor power; when there is forward flexion, these muscles are capable of restricting motion with phasic contraction. As such, all football players should be taught to strengthen the neck musculature.

The mechanisms of injury to the cervical spine should be kept in mind by all individuals who take care of football players. These include (1) flexion with anterior compression and posterior distraction; (2) lateral flexion and rotation, which stretch the convex side and impinge on the rotating concave side; (3) extension with distraction anteriorly and compression posteriorly; and (4) direct axial compression.[83] Flexion and rotation injuries are commonly found in players such as the defensive linemen, receivers, and defensive backs, who are going downfield and following the flight of the ball. Suddenly, they may hit someone or be hit with their head in an off-center position and their muscles relaxed. This also can occur while tackling when there is no control of the neck as the player's head hits an individual or the ground.

Evaluation and early treatment. On-the-field examination of a player with a suspected neck injury is mandatory. Neurologic examination, including motor and sensory testing, can be carried out with the player in his initial position on the ground. Prevention of further injury to the cervical spine is paramount in the examination, stabilization, and transportation of the player from the field to the medical facility on call for the game (see

Chapter 48). Proper equipment is an absolute necessity with the supporting cast of physicians, trainers, and properly trained personnel working as a team to provide an organized delivery of primary care (Fig. 63-15). Cardiopulmonary resuscitation (CPR) with establishment and management of an airway in an unconscious player who is wearing a helmet is a situation not usually encountered but one that must be considered. The primary hospital on call should be notified ahead of time with a neurosurgeon and orthopaedic surgeon available to meet the athlete on arrival. At that time, adequate radiographic evaluation must be obtained during which time continued cervical spine precautions must be strictly adhered to. Visualization of C1 and C2 to C7 is imperative. At no point should a suboptimal radiograph be accepted (Fig. 63-16). If necessary and available, computed tomography (CT), myelography and magnetic resonance imaging (MRI) of the cervical spine to further delineate the amount of damage to the spinal cord may be obtained.

Previously, the mechanism of injury frequently implicated in cervical spine trauma has been forced hyperextension. More recently, with the evaluation of data gathered by the National Head and Neck Industry Registry and from biomechanical studies, the mechanism of injury to the cervical spine is now thought to be primarily one of **axial loading** (Fig. 63-17). When the neck is in a normal upright, anatomic position, the cervical spine demonstrates a natural, gentle cervical lordosis. When the neck is flexed forward 30 degrees, the cervical spine curve is flattened out and converted into a segmented column (Fig. 63-18).[76] In helmeted cadaver studies, stresses and strains were measured as forces were directed through various portions of the head. Forces directed through the crown of the head or the top of the helmet produced cervical spine fracture patterns that are commonly seen in football injuries and motor vehicle ac-

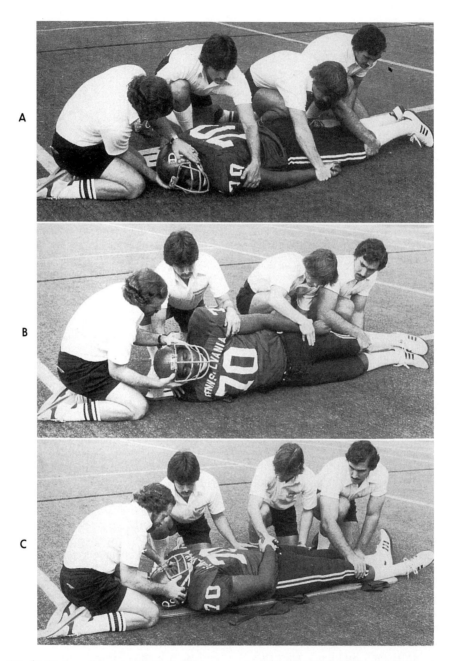

FIG. 63-15. Logroll to spineboard. **A,** This maneuver requires four individuals: one leader to immobilize head and neck and to command medical support team and three individuals positioned at shoulders, hips, and lower legs. **B,** Leader uses cross-arm technique to immobilize head. This technique allows leader's arms to "unwind" as three assistants roll athlete onto spineboard. **C,** Three assistants maintain body alignment during roll. (From Torg JS [ed]: *Athletic injuries to the head, neck, and face,* Philadelphia, 1982, Lea & Febiger.)

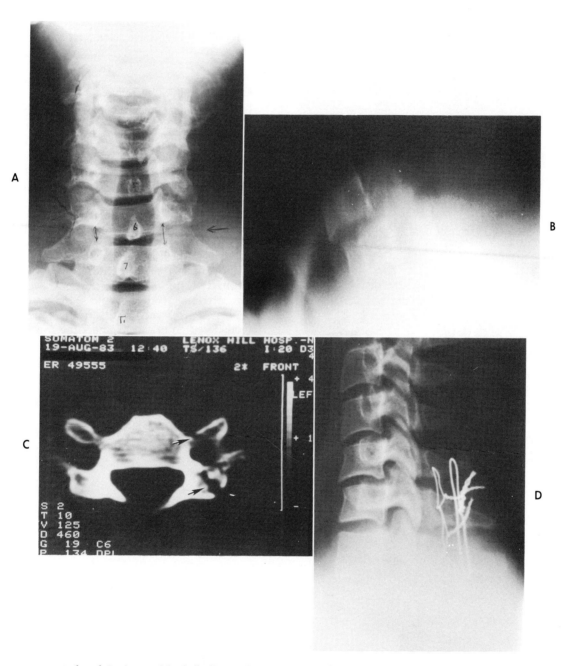

FIG. 63-16. Professional football offensive lineman sustained jumped facet and facet fracture during game. **A,** Anteroposterior view of injury. **B,** Lateral tomogram. **C,** Computed tomography scan demonstrating extent of fracture. **D,** Postoperative lateral view.

cidents involving head-on collisions (Fig. 63-19). These include isolated fractures, three-part, two-plane fractures (bursting fractures), dislocations (unilateral and bilateral jumped facets), fracture-dislocations, and soft-tissue injuries that involve ligaments and vertebral disks.*

The above injury patterns and the safety guidelines for treatment of these injuries were most recently demonstrated by an injury to the New York Jets defensive line-

---

*References 33, 44, 63, 64, 78, and 83.

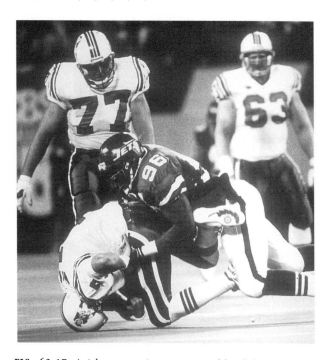

FIG. 63-17. Axial compression to crown of head during routine play.

man, Dennis Byrd. An unexpected head-on collision with the chest of a teammate produced a C4-C5 fracture-dislocation pattern with subsequent incomplete paraplegia. The response of the physicians and trainers and expedient delivery of emergency care produced an environment in which the initial injury pattern was not aggravated or worsened by his treatment. This team approach to on-field care, emergency and subsequent surgical stabilization, and aggressive rehabilitation have helped him make great improvements over his original neurologic status.[30]

Transient Neurologic Deficits

Partial transient neurologic deficits in the upper extremities are a result of **brachial plexus or nerve root traction injuries** sustained during tackling or in collision with the ground where the head and shoulder are stretched in opposite directions. This is characterized by sudden numbness and tingling and accompanied not infrequently with weakness in the upper extremity. These injuries are known as "burners" and "stingers." These injuries can range from a minor tingling in the upper extremity (with or without muscular weakness) to severe burning dysesthesias that may be associated with cervical cord contusion or bony injuries.[40]

Transient quadriplegia that involves upper and lower extremity motor weakness and paresthesias has been highly associated with an anatomic abnormality demonstrated on cervical spine x-ray studies. In a 1986 review by Torg et al[77] of 32 athletes with this condition, all involved some form of radiographic abnormality. Half of the athletes demonstrated cervical stenosis, whereas the other half was equally distributed with findings of degenerative disk disease, ligament laxity, and congenital anomalies.[31,77]

Cervical spine and neurologic injuries with or without

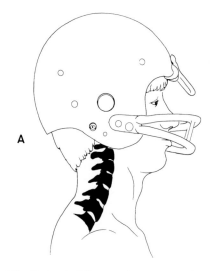
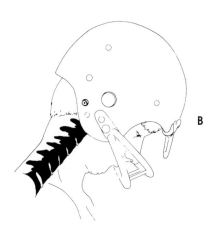

FIG. 63-18. A, When neck is in normal, upright, anatomic position, cervical spine is slightly extended because of natural cervical lordosis. **B,** When neck is flexed slightly to approximately 30 degrees, cervical spine is straightened and converted into segmented column. (From Torg JS, Vegso JJ, O'Neill MJ: *Am J Sports Med* 18:56, 1990.)

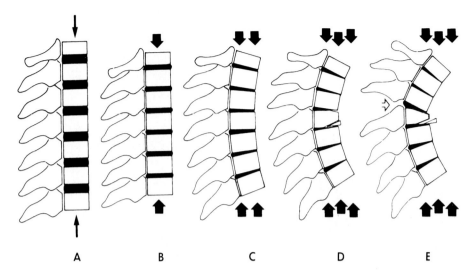

FIG. 63-19. Axial loading of cervical spine first results in compressive deformation of intervertebral disks (**A** and **B**) followed by maximum compressive deformation, and then angular deformation, and buckling occur. Spine fails in flexion mode (**C**) with resulting fracture, subluxation, or dislocation. **D** and **E,** Compressive deformation to failure with resultant fracture, dislocation, or subluxation occurs in as little as 8.4 msec. (From Torg JS, Vegso JJ, O'Neill MJ: *Am J Sports Med* 18:56, 1990.)

neurologic deficits present a complex issue in advising the athlete for return to contact sports. Torg and others[77] have provided general guidelines of the types of injury patterns seen and recommendations for management. Athletes with injuries of the cervical spine or spinal cord that are serious enough to cause a neurologic injury should not be allowed to compete in contact sports. Injuries involving transient neurologic deficits without bony injuries or with minor fractures without neurologic deficits may be allowed further participation in contact sports if asymptomatic, dynamic studies do not demonstrate any evidence of instability, and the above patterns of injury are not repeated. A gray area involves injured players who are now asymptomatic but who demonstrate radiologic abnormalities (e.g., cervical stenosis). These cases must be evaluated individually.[8]

Concussions

A new awareness of head injuries now includes concussions as a potential source of long-term disability. The pathophysiology of concussion is less well understood than that of severe cervical spine injuries and thus has received less attention. Concussion accounted for 75% of the total number of injuries involving the head area during the study of 49 college teams during a 7-year period. Concussion was characterized as a loss of consciousness or loss of awareness. Players with a previous history of loss of consciousness had four times the risk of a repeat episode than a player without a prior history. The highest risk of concussion was associated with offensive and defensive players involved in a block on a rushing play. Running backs demonstrated the highest risk of concussion regardless of activity.[13] Previously, guidelines for player evaluation after a concussion involved letting the player return to action if awareness to his surroundings was regained and if no severe headache

was present. Three thousand high school varsity athletes from Minnesota responded to a questionnaire regarding injury incidence patterns during their career. A general injury rate of 78 per 100 athletes was found with 19 of these injuries reported as being a concussion. Of those sustaining a concussion, as defined above, 69% were returned to play during the same game.

Awareness of long-term damage after concussion has always been difficult to assess because cellular microtrauma is not always detectable by MRI or CT scans.[72] Electroencephalographic evaluation of players with multiple concussions is just now being used. However, EEG patterns can be normal in the face of cellular microtrauma. It appears that the most sensitive testing for such low-level brain damage is neuropsychologic testing sessions. These sessions can pick up patterns suggestive of neural degeneration long before anatomic damage can be observed with scans. New guidelines for on-field evaluation of concussions, and more important, long-term evaluation of players with a history of concussions are forthcoming within the next decade.[38]

Lumbar Spine

The lumbar spine is a short segment of the vertebral column that connects the upper body and trunk with the pelvis and lower body. This small area is exposed to all the stresses generated within the linkage system through the upper and lower extremities. The forces through this area can be amplified by the player's weight, speed, off-balance movements, and collision or contact with the ground or other players. With this in mind, one can see why this area is at risk for injury in the athlete and also in the general population.[3] In a survey of 4800 intercollegiate athletes at the University of Wisconsin over a 10-year period, lumbar injuries were found to be most prevalent in football players and gymnasts. An injury rate of

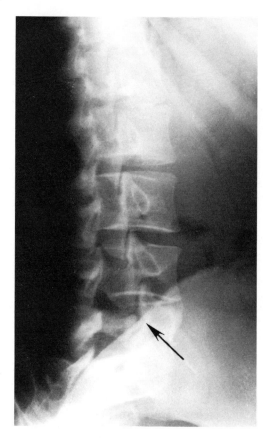

FIG. 63-20. Pars interarticularis defect in offensive lineman.

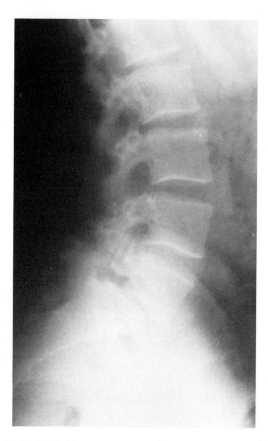

FIG. 63-21. Grade II asymptomatic and nonprogressive spondylolisthesis in professional football player.

7 per 100 participants was found. The majority of these injuries were muscular strains in the lumbar spine region.[37]

Pars interarticularis lesions. Of importance to the sport medicine provider is the incidence of **spondylolysis** and **spondylolisthesis.** Spondylolysis is a defect in the neural arch of the pars interarticularis (Fig. 63-20). Spondylolisthesis is a bilateral defect in this area that is accompanied by forward displacement of the vertebral body. Spondylolisthesis is a common structural defect that affects approximately 6% of the general population.[68] It is thought that repetitive athletic activities, especially where lumbar extension is involved, may contribute to the formation of spondylolysis. A prospective study evaluating 1445 freshman college players through their college years over a 5-year period was performed at a Division I school. A higher percentage of the pars defect was found than exists in the general population: 15.2% vs. 6%. Only 2.4% of these players were found to be symptomatic.[45] The presence of spondylolisthesis in an asymptomatic individual does not preclude their participation in organized football (Fig. 63-21). Semon and Sprengler[68] supported this view in their review of 506 college football players at the University of Washington from 1970 to 1977. From this group of players they compared one group of players with back pain and spondylolysis (N = 8) with a second group with back pain and an intact pars interarticularis (N = 12). They found that the players with spondylolysis did not have a significantly greater loss of time from games and practices than those with back pains but without spondylolysis.[68]

Some patients with spondylolysis or spondylolisthesis have significant protracted episodes of pain and stiffness with or without radiculopathy. Treatment of these patients may include spinal fusion to stabilize the slipped vertebrae. The decision of when to allow athletes with asymptomatic backs and spondylolysis or spondylolisthesis to participate in football is difficult. Certainly, if a neurologic deficit is present, participation in football is not permitted. As well, the presence of radicular signs, such as a positive straight leg raising test or a positive bowstring test, should limit participation in football until a final cure or arrest of symptoms can be achieved. Preventive measures that involve increasing the strength of abdominal muscles and maximizing the flexibility of the lower back may prevent some but not all of these injuries.

Disk injury. Disk injuries are not uncommon in football players. Generally they are seen as acute injuries with associated back pain and radiculopathy. Neurologic deficits may be present. Conservative treatment is appropriate initially for these problems. However, if neurologic deficits are present, consideration for diskectomy should be made.[19] If an individual is to undergo disk surgery, it is imperative to operate with minimal soft-tissue dissection and a small laminotomy. This provides minimal disruption of the bony and soft-tissue supports in the lum-

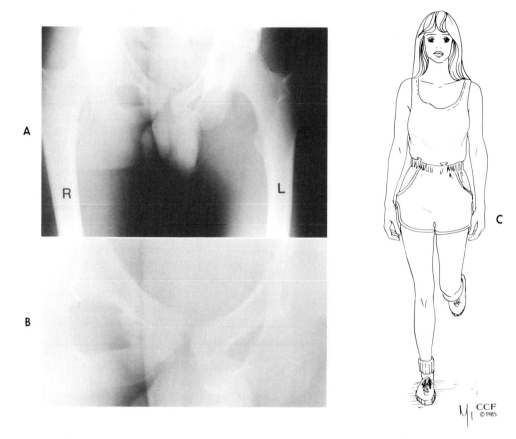

FIG. 63-22. Pubic symphysis diastasis sustained in high school football player when athlete slipped and performed a "split" on wet grass. **A,** Standing anteroposterior radiograph of pelvis (flamingo view). Support is on right leg only; left knee is flexed. **B,** Close-up view of pubic symphysis in **A. C,** Technique of flamingo view. If disruption of symphysis is present, pelvis drops on unsupported side. Only knee is flexed; hips remain in neutral. (**A** and **B** courtesy John Lombardo, MD.)

bar spine. A number of athletes are participating in professional football following lumbar laminotomy and diskectomy without any problems. A patient can resume play when he is asymptomatic and neurologically intact. The problem of disk herniation in adolescents is more complex, and results of treatment and surgery in this group are uniformly poor.

Pelvic Injuries

Injuries around the pelvic region may involve acute bony fractures of the pelvic ring, avulsion fractures, fracture-dislocations of the hip, stress fractures of the femoral neck, and numerous soft-tissue injuries. Except for the obvious traumatic bony fractures, soft-tissue injuries around the pelvis may produce only general symptoms of diffuse groin pain. The differential diagnosis of groin pain is long and varied. Included are infections, inguinal injury, abdominal processes with referred pain, nerve entrapment syndromes, and trauma to the anatomic complexes around the hip joint.[59]

Pubic symphysis injuries can occur in football. Although any athlete may be affected, soccer-style kickers are most commonly injured. Disruption of the symphysis can be seen as asymmetry or elevation of one side of the symphysis.[32] Acutely, this injury is painful with localized tenderness in the region of the symphysis (Fig.

63-22). Other signs include a lateral list on standing or one-leg hopping and pain with hip flexion and abduction against resistance. A local hematoma with scrotal extension may be present.

A rare but serious injury to the pelvic region is a **hip dislocation.** This may be anterior or posterior, and the position of the leg will indicate clinically the direction of the dislocation. Following radiographic evaluation, reduction is accomplished in the hospital with the patient under anesthesia (Fig. 63-23). Occasionally, subluxation of the hip can occur in practice or in a game situation and spontaneously reduce. A definitive diagnosis of the resulting groin pain may be initially elusive.[17] The sequelae of a traumatic dislocation of the hip can be serious and may not declare itself for many months or years after the initial injury.

Coccygeal pain in football players is not rare. Severe coccygeal joint pain from sprain of the coccygeal ligaments and the pubosacral ligaments is common and often unappreciated. For example, this injury can occur to a quarterback who is pushed backward and lands directly on the coccyx. In such individuals the usual measures that take weight off the coccyx when sitting are used. Whirlpool treatments and contrast therapy may be beneficial while healing occurs. Players are permitted to participate in football as tolerated with these injuries because there is no structural instability. It is important to check for anal sensation and spinal cord reflexes to be sure that an injury to the sacral plexus has not been missed. If pain persists, it is important to rule out chordomas, since these occur in the sacrum and athletes are not immune to tumors.

The **hip pointer,** a contusion to the pelvis, occurs from direct blows to the iliac crest and associated musculature with subsequent development of a hematoma. A large majority are caused by contact (Fig. 63-24). Protective padding has had some benefit in protecting hip pointers. Inappropriately placed padding when struck may actually further increase the soft-tissue damage. Football players who have suffered a hip pointer should

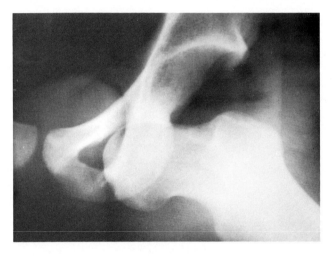

FIG. 63-23. Anterior hip dislocation that occurred during tackling in 18-year-old high school running back. Closed reduction was successful with patient under general anesthesia.

be fitted with appropriate, shock-absorbing, well-fitting pads to protect the region from further injuries on return to participation.

Another injury in the pelvic region that is often forgotten and disabling is the **strain** or **avulsion of the iliopsoas.** This occurs particularly in players who are charging or when trying to quickly get "off the ball" at the time of the snap. It usually results from excessive forceful contraction of the iliopsoas with the thigh fixed or forced hip extension with the foot and leg fixed. Preparticipation profiling may have demonstrated the existing tightness in the anterior thigh, hip flexors (Thomas test), quadriceps (Ely test), or iliotibial tract (Ober test). This injury is usually seen as acute onset of hip or groin pain. If the injury is left untreated, it could lead to flexion contracture, persistent disability, and excessive weakness of the entire limb. On examination, there is tenderness in the region of the lesser trochanter. Hip flexion against resistance is painful. Individuals with this injury generally hold their hips in a flexed, externally rotated position for comfort. Radiographs may show an avulsion of the lesser trochanter (Fig. 63-25). However, if an avulsion is not initially seen, follow-up films may show ossification in the region, corresponding to the tenderness felt in palpation of the iliopsoas. In addition to an avulsion fracture of the lesser trochanter or a strain of the iliopsoas tendon is the **painful snapping** that may occur as the tendons run over the pelvis. This can produce a deep anterior groin pain and an audible snapping sound. If symptoms persists, an iliopsoas lengthening can be performed to alleviate these symptoms.[35]

A troubling problem is a massive **rupture of the origin of the hamstrings or adductors.** This rupture occurs in individuals who have tightness of the adductors and hamstrings (Fig. 63-26). Muscle tightness can be

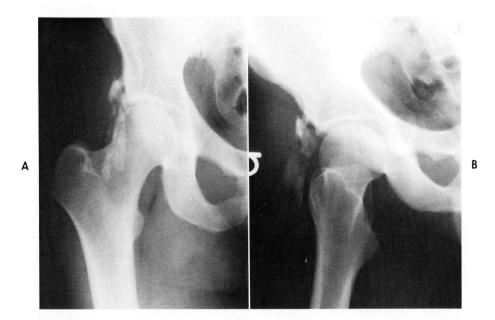

FIG. 63-24. Myositis ossificans of posterolateral hip muscles following hip pointer. **A,** Anteroposterior view. **B,** Lateral view.

determined in preseason screening examinations that include evaluation of the lotus position, sit and reach flexibility, and static stretch testing of adduction. Healing of major adductor strains can take up to 1 year. Occasionally athletes have residual hemorrhages, aching, and swelling.[18,29] Acutely, treatment includes rest, ice, pressure, contrast therapy, and gentle stretching. As symptoms abate, residual weakness in the hip musculature

must be resolved by participation in a progressive resistant exercise program of the surrounding muscle groups. The iliotibial band must be stretched because a positive Ober test can develop from scarring on the opposite side of the leg with the adductor tear. Stretching, of course, continues throughout the strength portion of rehabilitation. The importance of obtaining radiographs early after injury cannot be overemphasized. Later, ectopic bone formation about the pelvis may be difficult to differentiate from a bone-forming sarcoma. Bone scans and CT scans may be useful in this regard if there are any questions.

Thigh Injuries
Contusions

Standard padding does not protect the thigh adequately because the knee and hip must be free to bend. Both areas are therefore exposed above and below the thigh pads. These areas are then vulnerable to contusion. Diagnosis is easily made by obtaining a history of a direct blow, observing the patient's limited quadriceps excursion, locating the region of injury by careful palpation, and noting the onset of localized swelling and ecchymosis. Thigh contusions are difficult to treat and should never be taken lightly. Muscle does not heal by new muscle but by scar tissue and bone formation. Delay in treatment or neglect of the condition can lead to many problems affecting the other muscle groups and the extremity in general. In particular, hip flexion, adduction-abduction, and quadriceps contracture can occur in association with weakness of the entire thigh and leg. Weakness is found in manual muscle testing of hip flexion and hip abduction. The hamstring and calf muscles maintain a large, high ratio power as compared with the antigravity muscles of the hip flexor and abductor group. Adequate diagnosis and specifically directed rehabilitation are therefore essential for return to full performance after thigh contusions.

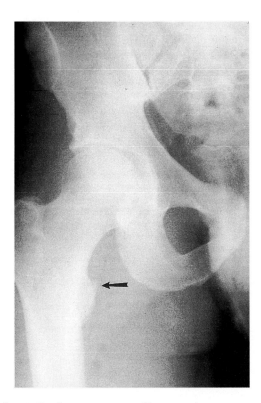

FIG. 63-25. Ossification in region of lesser trochanter, common sequela of hip flexor strain.

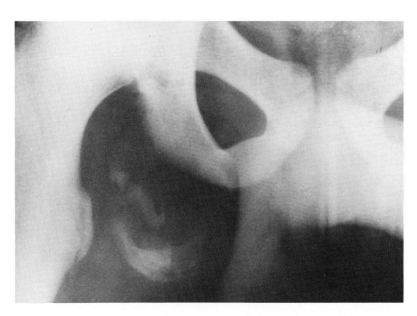

FIG. 63-26. Ischial spine avulsion that occurred during sprinting in adolescent football player.

The initial treatment of thigh contusions is rest, ice, compression, and elevation (RICE). For severe contusions crutches and flexion splinting may be required. Aspiration of the hematoma is not to be performed. Ice is continued intermittently for 24 to 48 hours.

Often an effusion develops in the ipsilateral knee. This sympathetic effusion need not be specifically treated other than with compression. However, specific knee injury that occurred at the same time as the thigh injury must be ruled out.

In an updated 3-year study of West Point cadets, 117 quadriceps contusions were classified and treated. Classification was based on knee range of motion 12 to 24 hours after injury. Treatment consisted of the previously described general regimen plus immobilizing the injured leg in flexion with emphasis on early flexion exercises rather than extension exercises. Mild cases (knee range of motion greater than 90 degrees) responded the quickest with minimal disability in less than 2 weeks. The moderate and severe contusions took 3 weeks for im-

provement to be seen.[66] These treatments must be tempered with overzealous attempts to stretch the injured quadriceps because this may lead to further hemorrhage and inflammation and may slow down the healing process.

The entire rehabilitation period may take 8 to 12 weeks before full motion is obtained. When the pain is absent and motion is almost full, isokinetic knee exercises and hip exercises are added. Finally, running straight ahead, figure-8 running, carrioca crossover running, and sprinting are resumed in a graduated fashion. The player may return to action when muscle strength and flexibility have returned and the athlete can perform agility drills without a problem (Table 63-1). A word of caution: endurance may still be a problem in the damaged leg during jumps of 20 inches, zigzags, and moveups. On return to action, an appropriate pad must be fabricated and well fitted to protect the injured area. Severe contusions can take up to 16 weeks to be completely resolved, and patience is required. As well, when the quadriceps tendon has been contused, the injury can take longer to heal

TABLE 63-1 Program for quadriceps contusions in football players

	Immediately After Injury (24 to 48 hr)	Early Rehabilitation	Intermediate Rehabilitation (90 Degrees' Flexion)	Advanced Rehabilitation (Pain Absent/Motion Almost Full)	Prereturn Sport-Specific Training	Maintenance
Rest	X					
Ice	X					
Compression	X					
Elevation	X					
Ice massage		X				
Quadriceps stretching		X	X	X	X	X
Hamstring stretching		X	X	X	X	X
Iliotibial band stretching		X	X	X	X	X
Quadriceps setting		X	X	X		
Seated hip flexion progressive resistance exercises			X	X		
Straight leg raising			X	X		
Straight leg hip abduction			X			
Straight leg hip adduction			X	X		
Hamstring progressive resistance exercises			X	X		
Leg Press			X			
Minisquats			X			
Isokinetic knee extension				X	X	X
Isokinetic knee flexion				X	X	X
Isokinetic hip flexion				X	X	X
Isokinetic hip abduction				X	X	X
Isokinetic hip adduction				X	X	X
Straight ahead running					X	
Figure-8 running					X	
Carrioca					X	
Striding (see p. 289)					X	
Sprinting					X	
Return to football						X
Protective pads (see p. 303)						X

and there is nothing that can be done to expedite it.

Myositis ossificans. General guidelines in the treatment of symptomatic myositis ossificans are as follows: (1) the athlete must refrain from any movement that causes pain, (2) no massage or manipulation treatment should be permitted once pain is present at the stage when myositis ossificans is present, (3) isometric exercises are performed at once, (4) the healing process often takes up to 6 months, (5) serial radiographs or bone scans are necessary to be sure there is no tumor, (6) the history of trauma is extremely important, and (7) if trauma is minimal, do not exclude the possibility of a tumor if there is a mass. If the physician resorts to a biopsy to make the diagnosis of myositis ossificans, it is important to inform

the pathologist whether the specimen is from the central or peripheral portion of the soft-tissue lesion and to provide an accurate history (Fig. 63-27).

Excision of myositis ossificans may be required if the mass is large and does not permit return of motion. Surgery on myositis ossificans should not be done before 1 year after the injury to allow full maturation. A premature operation produces a recurrence. In the same West Point study of 117 quadriceps contusions, 9% of the cadets developed myositis ossificans and five risk factors were identified. Risk of formation included: knee motion less than 120 degrees, injury occurring during football, previous quadriceps injury, delay in treatment greater than 3 days, and ipsilateral effusion.[66]

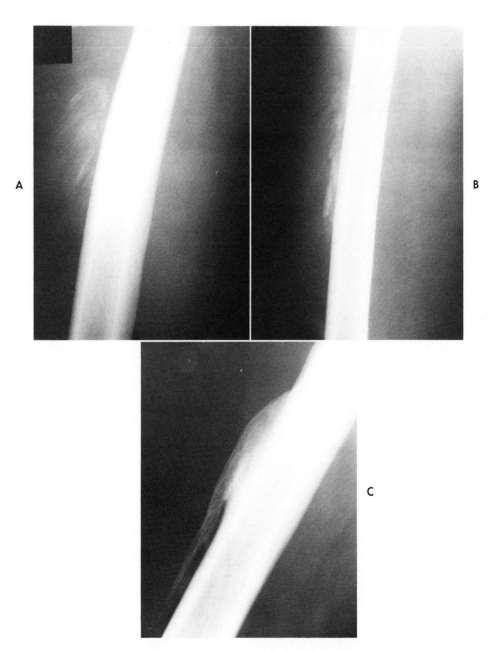

FIG. 63-27. A, Early, **B,** middle, and **C,** late, or mature, stages in formation of myositis ossificans.

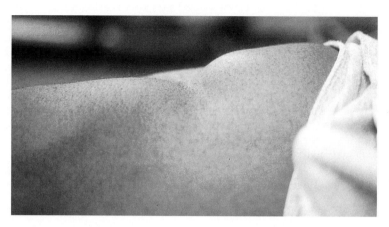

FIG. 63-28. Torn quadriceps with retracted muscle belly.

Quadriceps Strains

Muscle strain of the quadriceps are common in football. Mechanisms of the injury include forceful quadriceps contraction against the fixed leg, such as when a kicker gets a cleat caught in the ground, or forced knee flexion with the quadriceps contracting, which may occur during tackling. Often a player feels a pulling sensation in the anterior thigh at the time of injury.

Palpation may disclose a variety of findings. In mild strains no defect is present. Initial localization is made by noting the site of tenderness. With time, hematoma and swelling are observable. Minor tears, which are characterized by small defects, if any, can be localized by careful palpitation of the thigh with the knee flexed and the hip extended. This can easily be accomplished with the patient prone or laying the affected leg over the side of the table and flexing the knee. With severe strains a defect is usually palpable in the initial 12 hours. With time, hemorrhage and edema may obscure the defect, leaving only a large, swollen, ecchymotic, tender area.

Quadriceps strain should be treated conservatively with the initial treatment consisting of RICE. This is followed by ice massage and stretching until full motion returns. Quadriceps setting exercises can be done as tolerated. When pain and swelling are adequately diminished, strengthening exercises can be performed. Initially, hip flexion, hip adduction, hip abduction, and straight leg raising are used. With time, isokinetic and progressive resistance exercises are incorporated. Throughout the course of treatment an adequate stretching program must be performed for all the affected muscles and the surrounding muscle groups.

Grade III tears of muscle bellies are rarely operated on. Tears of the rectus are usually well tolerated from a functional point of view, although a bulbous mass may be present in the proximal portion of the muscle, representing the retracted proximal muscle belly (Fig. 63-28). In such tears the palpable defect is large and initially may be associated with an inability to extend the knee. Surgical repair of quadriceps muscle tears has not been found to dramatically change the final functional outcome.

If a partial or complete tear occurs close to the joint in the quadriceps tendon or the musculotendinous junction (up to 6 cm above the patella) and there is an extension lag, there is no question that this should be surgically repaired.

Hamstring Injuries

Hamstring injuries, from simple Grade I strains to avulsions, are responsible for a significant number of injuries on any given football team. It is thought that many of the recurrent injuries to the myotendinous units are a result of inadequate rehabilitation following the initial injury.[2,29] The hamstring/quadriceps ratio has also been implicated as a cause of injury with large imbalances, placing the athlete at risk.[73] Another theory is that two joint muscles in any area of the body are at risk for injury. This results from the demands made by two joints at different angles. For example, when the knee is hyperextended with the pelvis fixed, there is maximum stretch on the hamstrings as the hip is flexed. It is at this point, as in a punter with the body leaning forward, that hyperflexion of the hip occurs, and it is easy for a tear to occur in the hamstrings (Fig. 63-29). In football, in which kicking is such an important part of the game, a tight structured punter who is trying to get a high kick is liable to develop a hamstring strain. As a two-joint muscle the hamstrings are predominantly composed of Type II fibers. Garrett, Mumma, and Luvcaveche[25] have studied the histochemical morphology of hamstring strains, demonstrating that injury is repaired by scar formation without muscle repair.

The diagnosis of an acute hamstring strain is generally easy to make. The usual findings consist of localized tenderness, pain, and perhaps a palpable defect. As with quadriceps strains the initial defect may be obscured by swelling and hemorrhage, and it is therefore important to examine the player early after the injury. Occasionally, in patients with chronic hamstring tendinitis and hamstring pain, it may be difficult to differentiate between a tight hamstring problem that is causing pain in the buttock and sciatic problems. An area of localized tenderness on a portion of the hamstring associated with tightness of the hamstring muscles assists with this differentiation. A common location of hamstring injury is on the lateral side of the posterior thigh, adjacent to the lateral intermuscular septum. It is occasionally difficult to differentiate between an injury to the distal biceps and

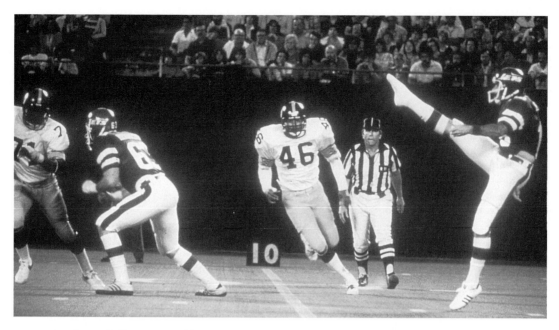

FIG. 63-29. Full extension of knee and hyperflexion of hip place hamstring muscles at risk for injuries.

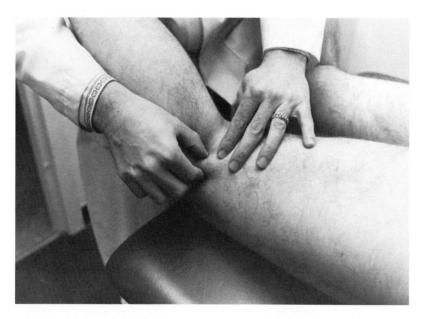

FIG. 63-30. Prone examination of distal hamstring folds. Athlete gently flexes knee against examiner's back to tense musculotendinous unit and allow examination for defects.

an inflammatory process centered around the iliotibial tract. To examine the area of the biceps, the knee must be flexed and the hip abducted to relax the iliotibial tract and palpate the biceps (Fig. 63-30). The examination of the hamstrings is most easily performed with the patient prone and the knees flexed to 90 degrees. The examiner then applies resistance, and the player gently flexes the knee. Palpation is performed up and down the entire hamstring group and includes palpation of the medial and lateral hamstring folds. In this fashion, small defects

in the hamstrings can be palpated. Another site for tear is the proximal semitendinosus, about 6 cm distal to the pelvis. It shows up in healing as a lump the size of a golf ball.

Treatment of hamstring strains acutely is identical to that of other strains. RICE is initially used. A posterior splint with the knee in extension and protected weight bearing with crutches may be necessary in severe strains. Following improvement in the initial pain and swelling, gentle hamstring stretching and ice massage

TABLE 63-2 Most commonly used rehabilitative progressive exercises for the thigh

Contracture	Weakness	Graded to Endurance
Quadriceps	Abductors	While weight training and
Iliotibial band	Adductors	stretching
Rotators of hips	Hip flexion	

are performed. Hamstring stretching, like stretching of other parts, should be done in a variety of positions. The leg is placed in neutral and internal and external rotation to allow the stretch to vary throughout the hamstring muscles. Additionally, the trunk is brought forward toward the knee in a medial-neutral position (centered over the patella) and a lateral position to vary the stretch. With these variations the player can easily feel which portion of the hamstring is tightest and which is the most functional stretch.

When the player begins running, a number of techniques can be used to speed along the return to sports. A brace or tape covering that provides limitation of terminal extension to perhaps 5 degrees short of full extension can be used to prevent full or hyperextension and help prevent unanticipated stretching of the injured hamstring. Also, a heel lift can be used to lengthen the limbs, making the player maintain the knee in a slightly flexed position. Occasionally, a pad over the hamstring strain can be incorporated into a wrap to provide a type of splint over the injured muscle. If the tears are in the superficial portion of the muscle belly, ultrasound, iontophoresis, and phonophoresis can be used in the rehabilitation process as well.

Midsubstance tears of the hamstring muscles respond well to conservative treatment. Surgical repair of the muscle belly itself is controversial as to its effectiveness. Adequate flexibility must be restored with return of power and excursion of all components of the leg before allowing the athlete to return to football (Table 63-2). If the tendinous portion of the hamstrings has ruptured in the distal thigh, it should be repaired. This is rarely required. Repairs should be performed within the first 2 weeks after injury and before retraction of the proximal muscle mass. Finally, once motion, excursion, and strength have been restored in all directions, workouts limited to 20 minutes and ¾ speed are emphasized for a week to avoid fatigue and prevent recurrence from overload situations.

Knee Injuries

As stated earlier in the chapter, out of all sports, football produces the most number of injuries seen. The knee joint is most often involved in approximately 25% to 45% of the cases.[60] Injuries may involve the four major ligaments of the knee, the medial or lateral meniscus, osteochondral fractures, muscle strains, tendinous overuse injuries, and dislocation of the patella or knee joints. The high incidence of knee injuries, coupled with the severe nature of many of these injuries, explains the tremendous exposure and awareness by the media and public.

Over the last 30 years the general public has seen a change in the initial evaluation, assessment, and outcome of knee injuries. Previously, a great percentage of serious knee injuries were career ending. An athlete undergoing surgery, rehabilitation, and a return to team play was an exception. A more common image was one of a player wrapping his knees up and limping onto and off of the field. Today the treatment of knee injuries has evolved with accurate, quick diagnosis and treatment being the rule. No longer are knee surgeries a rare and complex procedure limited to the elite athlete. The general public and the average weekend athlete with a meniscal tear are treated in a similar fashion as an all-star running back. This includes an expectation of return to action as soon as possible. These technical advances have placed more tools at the disposal of the sports physician, but they have also produced a greater burden because the players, coaches, and management expect preinjury levels of performance. In addition to the advancement of surgical techniques during this period, the clinical assessment, diagnostic scanning, and a better biomechanical appreciation of the structures involved have produced a plethora of knowledge and understanding making the knee joint the most studied.

Before the 1960s diagnosis was made basically on clinical grounds. Early operation was the treatment of choice for both the locked and unstable knee. O'Donoghue, Palmer, and Smillie correlated clinical examination and surgical pathology by advocacy of early surgery for torn ligaments and cartilage. In the middle 1960s, with refinements in arthrography, diagnostic accuracy was improved such that a physician could operate on the knee without having to explore it in layers by incision. In the early 1970s the advent of diagnostic arthroscopy, and later, operative arthroscopy, contributed immensely to further definitive diagnosis and treatment of knee injury. Through these periods the approach to knee injury continued to change, and further changes are still the norm. Many new treatments have been built on the old techniques. Outside of the operating room, refinements in bracing and rehabilitation and the implementation of early motion have also added a new dimension to the care of athletes.

Knee Motions and Demands

The knee is an important component of the linkage system, with forces passing from the ground through the knee to the trunk and upper extremity and reverse. In addition to its role of transmitting such forces, the knee must provide adequate motion for performance, as noted previously. This motion takes place in three planes: flexion-extension, varus-valgus, and internal-external rotation, the so-called X-Y-Z axis. In addition, a gliding motion occurs between the two surfaces of the knee joint.

X-Y-Z axis of knee motion

- Flexion-extension plane
- Varus-valgus plane
- Internal-external rotation plane

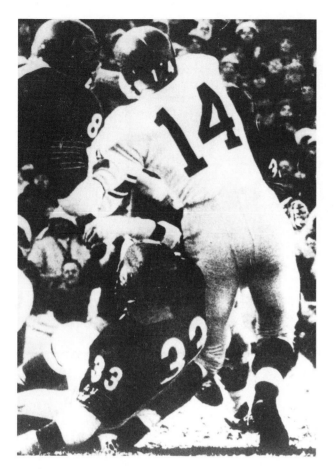

FIG. 63-31. Classification of knee injuries. This is considered acute valgus–external rotation in flexion.

These motions occur throughout the range of motion of the knee and are a result of bony topography, soft-tissue restraints, and active muscle forces. Any injured structure affecting these components can drastically change the normal pattern and create abnormal forces throughout the knee. These abnormal forces may seem relatively innocuous because they lead to no early symptoms, but they may lead to further problems. In other cases symptoms such as pain, buckling, and locking can occur quickly. A third pattern may be an asymptomatic knee that insidiously develops degenerative changes secondary to the altered biomechanics. There is as yet no clear-cut reason why these different patterns of response to injury occur, although it is apparent that a number of other factors play important roles.

Another point of interest more accurately being examined now is the long-term function and disability of the specific knee injury patterns. Examination includes the players with knee injuries who were treated either surgically or conservatively. In addition to evaluating the different types of treatment, the effects of the normal aging process must also be determined. Although there is no difference in the development of osteoarthritis between athletes and age-matched controls, there is a subset of injured athletes who demonstrate significant increases in knee joint degenerative changes.[49] Long-term follow-up studies on the newer techniques employed in

anterior ligament reconstruction are still pending. Long-term follow-ups of meniscal repair are also pending. Final outcome studies of isolated posterior cruciate ligament (PCL) injuries, cadaver allografts, new synthetic grafts, new rehabilitation protocols, and many others are all pending the test of time.

Athletic History

Compared with a detailed medical history the athletic history is usually more straightforward, with details being accurately relayed concerning the time of the injury, mechanisms and circumstances surrounding the injury, description of the sensation involved during the injury, immediate care provided (if any), ability to continue playing, subsequent swelling and pain patterns, medical care sought, treatment provided, and evaluation of the knee joint function since the injury. These facts can easily be elicited with careful, direct questioning. On-the-field examination often provides the best information concerning a knee injury because the mechanism of injury is observed and the examination is performed before the onset of reflex spasm, guarding, and effusion sets in (Fig. 63-31). This is much different from the examination done in the office 2 days or 2 weeks after the injury. A detailed history and careful knee examination, even late, provide information for the physician to piece together a clear picture of the injury. Each knee injury can then be classified into acute vs. chronic injuries. The mechanisms and forces involved in producing the injury and, most important, the examination provide anatomic information that allows an intelligent differential diagnosis to be formulated based on the facts gathered.[28,57]

Physical Examination

A basic, methodic evaluation of each knee injury provides the caretaker with an organized approach and thought process. The entire leg and knee should be exposed and observed. Is it grossly malaligned? Is there swelling involved? The entire knee should be palpated and any tenderness noted and documented. Observation of gait patterns and the ability to perform simple tasks such as taking on and off shoes and clothes may expose underlying pathologic conditions.

On the medial side, tenderness may be found in the posteromedial corner, in the anteromedial region, at the site of the femoral attachment of the medial collateral ligament (MCL), along the midsubstance of the MCL at the medial joint line, or along the tibial insertion of the MCL. The lateral collateral ligament (LCL) should always be palpated in extension and flexion, as well as with the leg crossed over the opposite leg, or the figure-4 position. A varus stress applied elicits any deficits in the integrity of this structure. Specific areas of tenderness on the lateral side, both above the knee and at the fibular head, are important to note, as well as the lateral joint line. The interval between the fibular head and proximal tibia should be palpated to determine if a diastasis of the proximal tibiofibular joint has occurred. Valgus and varus stress testing should be performed at 0 and 30 degrees. The opposite leg should always be examined to get a better sense of what the normal baseline is for each patient.

Examination of the knee should include a comprehen-

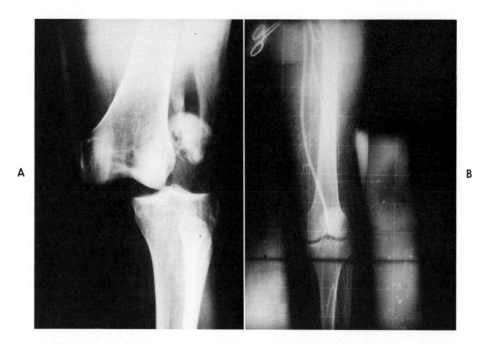

FIG. 63-32. A, Knee dislocation during football high-velocity collision injury **B,** Arteriogram demonstrated disruption of popliteal artery. Repair returned perfusion distal to knee. Posterior cruciate ligament was also repaired.

sive examination of the integrity of both cruciate ligaments. For the anterior cruciate ligament (ACL), the anterior drawer test and Lachman-Ritchie test should be performed. The physician may not always get a positive anterior drawer sign in the early phases of tears of the ACL, even though it may be completely torn. Indeed, the only finding that might be positive may be the Lachman-Ritchie test. The pivot shift sign or one of its many variations (jerk, Slocum, and Losee tests) should be sought as well to help in the determination of ACL injury. In our experience the presence of PCL injuries must never be overlooked. They are more common injuries in football than suspected. Examination of the posterior drawer test at 90 degrees and the drop-back test are performed to determine the integrity of the PCL. As well, the passive hyperextension test (external rotation recurvatum) is carried out.

Rotatory instability should also be tested in addition to the cruciate examination because it may be suggestive of a more extensive injury pattern. Drawer tests should be performed with the foot and leg in internal and external rotation. This test determines injury to the posteromedial corner, which is evidenced by forward rotatory motion of the tibia. Anterolateral rotational laxity is seen when the fibula comes slightly more forward and the tibial tubercle moves forward and medially. Rarely, posteromedial laxity can occur in which valgus and posteromedial rotation of the tibia occur from damage to the posterior capsule and posteromedial complex. This type of laxity often includes damage to the PCL. Posterolateral external rotational laxity in which the fibula drops backward in the popliteal space should be determined. The tibial tubercle moves laterally, the lateral tibial plateau rotates back, and the posterior drawer and sag signs are

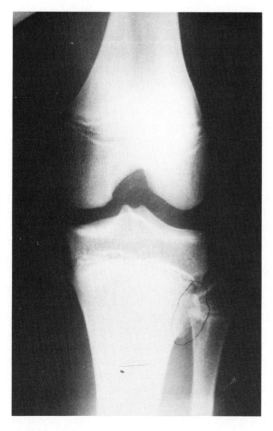

FIG. 63-33. Proximal tibiofibular diastasis with tibial avulsion.

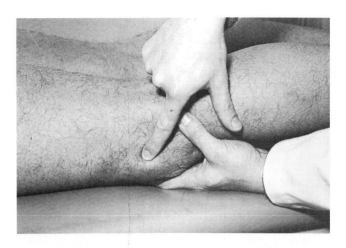

FIG. 63-34. Palpation of patella and its retinaculae can be accomplished easily with athlete prone, knee extended, and patella laterally or medially displaced.

minimal. This may suggest injury to the LCL and arcuate complex.

One of the more important parts of the examination is to rule out injury to the neurovascular structures of the limb. An acute knee injury can cause signs of peroneal nerve injury or vascular injury. This may have occurred during a subluxation or dislocation of the knee (Fig. 63-32) or tibiofibular diastasis (Fig. 63-33). The extreme nature of the injury may not be apparent to the initial examiner. For this reason, the physician must always check the distal pulses and motor and sensory functions for integrity.[39,69,79]

When the joint lines are palpated, it should be done carefully from the posteromedial and posterolateral corners forward. Flexion and extension movements of the knee are performed, noting snaps or clicks along the joint line. A meniscal snap must be differentiated from other knee noises, and the physician must always check the iliotibial band, patella, and the peripatellar soft tissues to determine the origin of the snap.

The popliteal space and posterior aspect of the knee should always be examined because popliteal swelling can rapidly occur in major injuries to the knee and is often unnoticed. To adequately examine this area, the individual is examined in the prone position. The knee can be allowed to hyperextend off the edge of the table to compare it with the opposite side and determine if there is laxity of the posterior capsule, recurvatum, excessive extension, or flexion contracture. While the patient is in the prone position, examination of the patella and patellar retinaculum can also be easily accomplished (Fig. 63-34). This can be a valuable way to displace the patella medially and laterally and feel the integrity of the patellar surface, the patellofemoral ligaments, and the patellotibial ligaments.

The entire extensor mechanism should also be thoroughly examined. For this the athlete must be asked to actively extend the knee to determine the integrity of the extensor mechanism. Rarely, an athlete with a history of jumper's knee can have a complete rupture of the infrapatellar tendon with traumatic patella alta, immediate

hemarthrosis, and a defect in the infrapatellar area. Inability to actively extend the knee will of course be present because, in general, the extensor retinacula are torn as well with this injury.

In addition, it must always be remembered that nontraumatic injury may exist in the knee of a football player. This is particularly true in high school and college athletes. Although trauma is often blamed as the inciting cause, a systemic disease may actually be present. For example, recurrent effusions may be an indication of pigmented villonodular synovitis. Thickened fat pad lesions (Hoffa's disease) can present as hemorrhagic synovitis and recurrent effusions. The patellar tendon is wide and crepitant, and the fat pad bulges. Rheumatoid arthritis, gout, and chondrocalcinosis must also be ruled out. Patterns of referred pain must always be remembered. Distal and proximal joints and bones should always be checked for injury. For example, a young adolescent football player may be suffering from a slipped capital femoral epiphysis with only knee pain as a symptom. Focusing only on the knee obviously misleads the examiner. In a patient with a chronic problem, additional portions of a total examination are included to supplement those techniques previously described.

The physician should always check the so-called screw-home mechanism in patients with chronic knee problems. As the patient extends the knee, the femur rotates medially and the tibia rotates laterally, increasing the Q angle as the tibial tubercle rotates laterally. This effect may be lost in patients with meniscal derangement or in patients who cannot fully extend the knee because of other pathologic conditions. The muscle power of the entire limb must be determined to assess the general state of well-being. Functional testing, toe-walking, heel-walking, squatting, and duck-walking are performed to determine any muscular deficits or joint contractures. With previous preparticipation evaluation data on hand, a high percentage of the specific diagnoses of the current status of an injury can be made.

Radiographic Evaluation

Radiographs should always be taken and should include a complete series. This consists of a standing anteroposterior and lateral view, tunnel view, and axial patella view. Oblique views may be necessary to visualize a patella fracture, femoral condylar fragments, and the proximal tibiofibular joint. Initial radiographs in the locker room may be inadequate to rule out all but a major bony problem. The physician must be careful to look for epiphyseal injury in the growing adolescent. Stress views may be necessary. The anterior tibial apophysis must be checked for a possible avulsion of the apophysis. The physician must not forget lesions that involve articular cartilage, which may or may not be visible on plain films. These can include osteochondral fractures if there has been a recent patellar dislocation.

A recent trend in the evaluation of the knee has been MRI. An MRI evaluates the molecular integrity of anatomic structures and constructs a picture based on these signals. A homogeneous structure such as a meniscus generates a certain signal and picture. By definition, an injury or degeneration of a homogeneous structure produces a mixed signal suggestive of an injury. The MRI scan is so sensitive that it can sometimes pick up changes in structures (suggestive of an injury) where in reality there may be none. MRI should not take the place of a careful physical examination.

Patellofemoral Problems

Examination of the football player with probable patellofemoral problems begins with careful observation of the muscle bulk of the vastus medialis and adductors. This is best done by having the athlete kneel on the ground and sit back on the buttocks. Atrophy of the thigh, especially of the adductor-quadriceps muscle masses, can easily be seen and felt with this maneuver. Any deficits can be observed more easily than with a tape measure. Evaluation of muscle mass is augmented by quantitative manual muscle testing. This quickly allows the determination of weakness in the hip flexors, abductors, adductors, extensors, and knee flexors. This is useful in providing a percentage of muscle deficit when related to the opposite leg. As rehabilitation progresses, strength gains can easily be documented by various methods such as Cybex isokinetic testing. Muscle testing can also be performed with a Nicholas manual muscle tester (MMT).[53] This may be helpful in programs with a limited budget. The presence of **patellar instability** can often be documented by examination and comparison of both knees. The examiner should move the patella medially, distally, proximally, and laterally and examine for patellar size and tightness as well as laxity of the medial and lateral patellofemoral ligaments. Tenderness of the medial and lateral patellar facets is also noted. Tightness of the iliotibial tract with a condensation of fibers directed toward the patella can be palpated. Proximal and vertical laxity is best found on testing with the knee bent at 90 degrees. A high-riding patella can be pushed down from above unless the quadriceps muscle is tight or there is bony incongruity. Instability can also be noted by having the patient flex and extend the knee. Abnormal patellar tracking can be observed in the terminal portions of extension. Whenever the physician examines for patella instability, the entire limb must be observed from the hip to the toes to determine the presence of increased external rotation, anteversion of the femur, or abnormal rotation of the tibia. The Q angle is measured with the patient supine and the quadriceps muscle relaxed. The patellofemoral compression test should be performed last because it is a provocative test and may be painful. The presence of grating, grinding, snapping, and pain should all be noted. The apprehension test, performed at 30 degrees by displacing the patella laterally, should always be performed.

Patellofemoral pain syndrome is particularly common in football players who lift weights frequently and excessively and in those who jump a great deal. This is often reflective of increased friction and decreased patellofemoral mobility, leading to a patellofemoral compression syndrome (Fig. 63-35). These individuals are best treated by a conservative therapy program that includes

quadriceps stretching. Deep-knee bending, deep-squat weightlifting, and excessive open-chain, full-arc knee extension strengthening should not be included in training programs to prevent these problems.

Rehabilitation is the primary therapy in patellofemoral pain syndromes associated with patellar instability. Knee range of motion exercises should only involve terminal extension short-arc ranges of 20 to 30 degrees only if they can be performed painlessly. Initial exercises us-

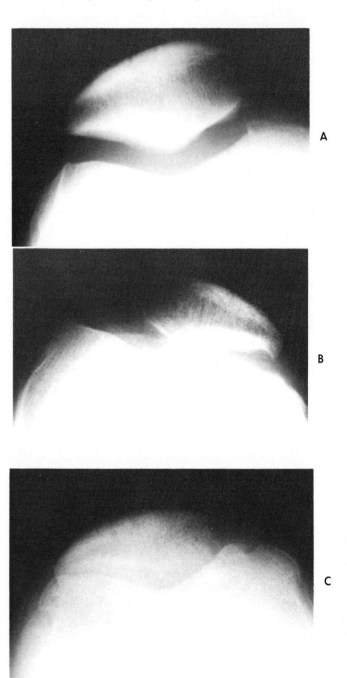

FIG. 63-35. Patellofemoral degenerative changes in football players. **A,** Medial facet and trochlea "kissing" osteophytes. **B,** Lateral facet overhanging osteophytes. **C,** Extensive patellofemoral disease affecting both medial and lateral facets.

ing progressive amounts of free weights include (1) hip abduction with the knee straight, (2) hip adduction with the knee straight, and (3) sitting hip flexion 6 to 8 inches high with the knee flexed at 90 degrees. The exercise program should not produce pain. As symptoms improve, straight leg raising can be included. These exercises are combined with stretching of the quadriceps, iliotibial tract, and hamstring muscles. Later, increasing use of Cybex and Nautilus equipment can be incorporated if the patient is asymptomatic. Cycling with low resistance and long duration can be added. A patella-restraining brace is beneficial for many of these players and allows controlled return to sports.

If malalignment is present and the patella is symptomatic, operative intervention can be considered if the patient has not improved on the rehabilitative program. Football players require a large amount of weight training to achieve rehabilitation of their muscles, and premature surgery must be avoided. The first surgical procedure to be considered should be arthroscopic lateral retinacular release. This provides symptomatic improvements in approximately 60% to 75% of the patients. In the group of patients who do not improve following lateral retinacular release, a more formal patellar realignment should be considered. This generally includes imbrication of the medial retinaculum, a lateral retinacular release, and occasionally, distal realignment.

Occasionally, in football players the physician can see the **fat pad syndrome,** also known as Hoffa's disease. Arthroscopically, this is probed and seen as thickening and fibrosis of the fat pad. On examination, there is tenderness medial and lateral to the patellar tendon. Occasionally, it is associated with thickening of the peritendinous area. Conservative treatment of this syndrome is often successful and consists of use of antiinflammatory

medication and a patella-restraining brace and restricted terminal flexion for about 3 months.

Patellar tendinitis, or jumper's knee, is common in athletes of football and other sports requiring jumping. It is most often seen at the lower pole of the patella. Occasionally, irregular calcification may be present on radiographs. This may be a difficult problem to treat in athletes. Initial treatment consists of the use of oral antiinflammatory medication and a patella-restraining brace and quadriceps stretching. The brace functions to limit proximal movement of the patella, thereby decreasing tension in the patellar tendon. Patient education in this condition is important, and the athlete should be instructed to avoid the movements that cause pain. Occasionally surgery is required for resistant cases of patellar tendinitis (Fig. 63-36). Resection of a focal area of degeneration can be performed through a local vertical split of the proximal patellar tendon. Patients can return to play in 3 months. In severe cases rupture of the patellar tendon can occur, and immediate surgical treatment is indicated. A primary repair of the tendon is performed, and the retinaculum, which is generally torn as well, is likewise primarily repaired. Often patients require 6 to 9 months for complete healing and rehabilitation.

Meniscal Injuries

Appreciation of meniscal function has grown as the number of arthroscopic surgeries in athletes and the general public has risen. A review of arthroscopic meniscectomies from 1973 to 1982 was tabulated by the University of Syracuse sports medicine service. The service found that meniscal injuries involved the medial side in 81% of the cases and the lateral side in 19%.[9,58] Symptomatic meniscal tears with effusion, locking, and catching are extremely common in football players. Arthro-

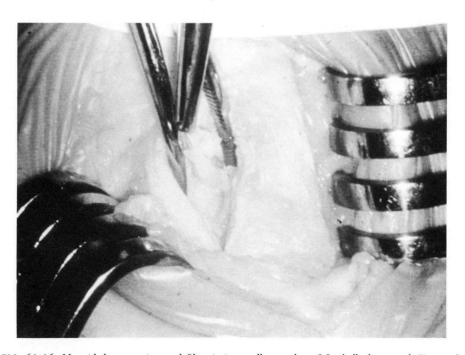

FIG. 63-36. Myxoid degeneration and fibrosis in patellar tendon of football player with "jumper's knee".

scopic surgery should be performed early in patients with symptomatic tears because of the necessity of getting the professional and elite player back to a high level of efficiency. It is unnecessary to perform early surgery in athletes with minimal symptoms. Meniscal lesions are often found in coaches because these injuries remain from earlier years of play and are associated with degenerative joint disease. This can lead to limited motion, pain, and recurrent swelling at an early age after retirement. Limitation of terminal motion in either extension or flexion is particularly worrisome in patients with symptomatic meniscal tears. The lack of full motion creates limited mobility and a potential for further injury. Following arthroscopy, a rehabilitation program is indicated to regain full strength in the lower extremity with special attention to quadriceps function. A restraining brace or knee sleeve may be useful in the early postoperative period to limit the effusion. At the time of arthroscopy the smallest amounts of meniscus should be excised to maintain the load-bearing and distributing capabilities of meniscus. Unfortunately, many players have other problems besides meniscal damage, including articular degeneration, chondromalacia patellae, loose bodies, and even absence of the ACL. At the time of arthroscopic surgery for a meniscal tear, the above mentioned pathologic conditions may be discovered. In spite of these other problems, their performance can be surprisingly good.

MRI has provided the sports physician with detailed information concerning the health status of the meniscus. There is an excellent correlation for high-grade meniscal injuries as seen with MRI when compared with arthroscopic findings. In addition, MRI has been able to establish and assess bone abnormalities not accessible to arthroscopic evaluation.[48,80] With MRI, longitudinal studies to evaluate the meniscus structure can now be performed. Meniscal structure of asymptomatic knees, as viewed by MRI, was evaluated over the course of one football season. In the study a significant progression of signal intensity was seen. These preliminary results suggested that observable degeneration can occur within the course of a season without an occult injury occurring.[61] In another study baseline evaluations of asymptomatic age-matched volunteers were compared with asymptomatic basketball and collegiate football players. Of asymptomatic athletes who had no previous surgical procedures on their meniscus, 25% demonstrated significant baseline MRI changes. These signal abnormalities could adversely affect scan interpretation in the face of an acute injury.[12]

Knee Ligament Injuries

The treatment of ligament injuries to the knee in football players requires careful and thoughtful analysis of a wide variety of factors. The first and foremost rule is to avoid a "tunnel vision" approach to ligament injuries. The dogma of one symptom, one diagnosis, and one treatment is to be condemned. The physician must evaluate each player individually. The player's position, size, strength, age, and level of competition must be considered in the decision process. This is in addition to the usual important facts that include a careful search of the patient's injury history, the anatomic diagnosis, and the athlete's ultimate goals. In chronic injury situations, what makes the knee unstable, how it becomes unstable, when it is unstable (off season or during the season), what exercises and bracing have been used, and what the player's plans for the future are all important considerations. A history sheet is important in this regard, and each player should fill one out annually and maintain it as part of the permanent record.

Much of the current literature regarding treatment of ligament injury is conflicting, and this controversy makes treatment decisions difficult. This is particularly true in the analysis of the effect of ACL injury and possible treatment modes. When it comes to knee stability, we must not delude ourselves by such statements as, "There is one key stabilizer." There is a tendency for ligament repair or reconstruction to be simple in concept, when actually the knee is a three-dimensional system that behaves differently in every position, as flexion, rotation, and varus-valgus motion occur, creating a unique series of biomechanical forces at every instant of motion and angle.

Collateral ligament injuries. Medial collateral ligament injuries are common in football players and may occur as isolated ligamentous injuries or in association with meniscal or cruciate damage. The most frequent mechanism of injury is a contact-induced valgus stress to the knee with the foot fixed (Fig. 63-37). Grade I injuries demonstrate tenderness anywhere along the MCL with no demonstrable increased laxity at 0 degrees and 30 degrees. They are treated symptomatically. The player is initially placed in a knee immobilizer for comfort and allowed to bear weight as tolerated. After 48 hours of immobilization the athlete is begun on range of motion and strength exercises. When a full range of motion has been achieved and muscle parity is evident, the player may return to participation. A derotation-type knee brace or a similar device does not have to be worn unless the player wishes.

Grades II and III injuries are indicative of a more serious injury to the MCL. In the more severe grades (Grade III), concomitant cruciate ligament damage must be ruled out. This can be done on clinical grounds or with examination under anesthesia or arthroscopy. Once a cruciate ligament injury has been ruled out, all MCL injuries of Grades II and III are treated conservatively. The player is fitted with a derotation type brace for approximately 1 week after injury and begun on range of motion exercises and strength rehabilitation as tolerated. In both Grades II and III injuries players may return to participation when swelling is absent, tenderness is gone, a full range of motion is present, and close to normal muscle strength has been achieved. It is important to remember in all three grades of injury that rehabilitation includes the entire limb. The hip flexors, hip abductors, and hip adductors must be included in the rehabilitation program. Players are allowed to return in a relatively short time (average 6 to 10 weeks) with adequate stability and mobility achieved through conservative treatment. For return to sports in the more severe injuries a

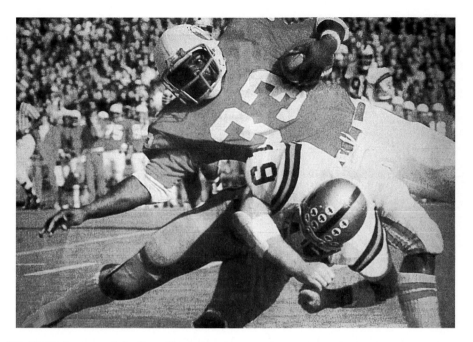

FIG. 63-37. Severe medial collateral ligament injury with foot fixed to ground and valgus stress placed on knee.

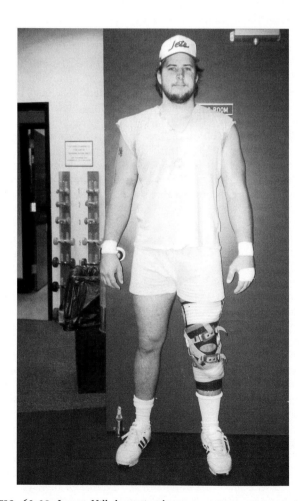

FIG. 63-38. Lenox Hill derotation brace worn to prevent anterior subluxation of tibia.

derotation brace, such as the Lenox Hill brace, is worn for protection during activity for approximately 12 weeks or more. Many players wear the brace every year for possible prevention against further injury. The efficacy of the brace in preventing an injury if the forces encountered are great has yet to be proven (Fig. 63-38).

Lateral collateral ligament injuries do not respond as well to conservative therapy for the higher grade strains. The attachment sites on the femoral epicondyle and fibular head are more distinct than the broad attachment sites of the MCL. The lateral ligament structure is more defined and has a cordlike feel compared with the broad sheet of thick collagenous tissue common on the medial side. A high-grade tear of the LCL usually denotes a serious injury and is often associated with a tear of the ACL, PCL, or posterolateral structures of the popliteus and the arcuate complex. If this is the case, surgical repair or reconstruction should be performed at the same time as repair of the collateral ligament. Postoperative rehabilitation is modified, depending on which structures were injured.

Anterior cruciate ligament injuries. In the case of a football player with a torn ACL it is important to recognize that several injury patterns can occur. The presence or absence of injury to the medial and lateral stabilizers and meniscus has important bearing on the treatment choices. In the 1960s and 1970s some authorities, including Hughston, Kennedy, and Slocum, thought that adequate function could be obtained from accurate extraarticular repairs of the posteromedial capsule and meniscal complex. This may be especially true in individuals who have adequate muscle strength, particularly in muscles such as the hamstrings that protect the tibia from anterior displacement. Among football players the offensive linemen often fall into this category, particu-

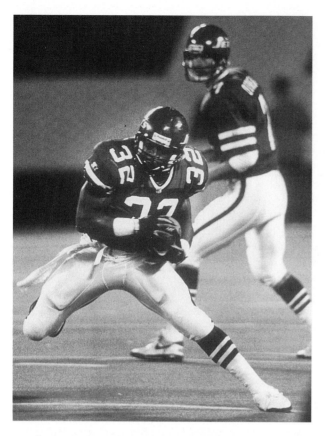

FIG. 63-39. Anterior cruciate ligament–deficient knees are unable to withstand this type of rotation maneuver.

larly tackles and centers. They cover a limited area, and their necessity for lateral movement is less than their teammates. Thus the demands on the knee without an ACL are less than that of a running back or receiver.

The indication for primary operative intervention is a grossly unstable knee. The amount of instability can be magnified by the position of the player. Wide receivers, defensive backs, and linebackers all require the ability to plant their feet and cut, and they do not tolerate a complete tear of the ACL injury associated with clinically apparent instability (Fig. 63-39). Often, multiple anatomic structures demonstrate injury on immediate clinical testing, and the presence of a multiple ligament injury is an indication for operative treatment.

In the limited number of cases in which bony avulsion is present, primary repair of the avulsion is carried out. This most often occurs in the younger adolescent football player. The results of surgical treatment of these avulsions are generally excellent.

Midsubstance tears represent, by far, the majority of ACL injuries. The results of midsubstance repairs alone have been poor. Although controversy exists about this, repair is therefore performed with augmentation if repair is considered at all. Results of primary repair with augmentation by a distally based, tubed graft of iliotibial tract brought over the top have been satisfactory for some. By far the most common procedure in ACL-deficient knees is the central third of the patellar tendon graft with bony plugs (see Chapters 38 and 39).

At the time of surgery an examination under anesthesia should be performed to confirm the diagnosis and to evaluate the collateral ligaments and the integrity of the PCL. ACL injuries with concurrent MCL sprains are reconstructed only after the MCL has healed and rehabilitation is completed with a full range of motion achieved. LCL injuries, if torn distally or proximally from their bony insertions, should be surgically reattached at the time of ACL reconstruction.

Posterior cruciate ligament injuries. Treatment of PCL injuries in football players has produced a twofold experience. Those players who *have* had surgical treatment have had a dismal return to function after surgery. The ability to restore high performance in any football player in a running position who has undergone an acute repair of an isolated PCL injury, even when it appears to be a simple avulsion of the femoral condyle, is difficult. However, conservative treatment of PCL injuries has yielded surprisingly satisfactory results (Fig. 63-40). Individuals with a positive posterior drawer sign or sag sign have done well in professional football with asymptomatic, long-term follow-up. The only exception is when there is some posterior tibial or femoral condyle injury. Therefore as long as the medial and lateral compartments are strong and the ACL is stable, individuals can function well without a PCL in football for many years at an all-pro level in some cases. However, if the patient is symptomatic, an isolated PCL reconstruction may have to be performed.

Additionally, it is important to recognize that with the size of the players today, injuries can occur around the knee from noncontact or minimal contact episodes. This is because great forces are generated through the linkage system.

Rehabilitation. Thigh muscle function has been shown to be adversely affected after cruciate or collateral ligament injuries.[23,42,43] Recent studies have demonstrated muscle strength deficits at high-speed, isokinetic movements.[36] They recommend rehabilitation using exercises in this range. Also, closed-chain vs. open-chain rehabilitation techniques are also being examined to determine which is the best method for rehabilitation. Fatigability and endurance levels should be evaluated preoperatively and followed closely postoperatively. After reconstructive surgery and progressive rehabilitation the player is returned to action. Although their reconstruction may be healed and mechanically sound, their return to practice may be slow. Their proprioceptive abilities and muscle strength must also be returned to a competitive level, and this may take several months. Advanced aggressive rehabilitation of surgically repaired or reconstructed knee ligaments is commonplace today in the general public. This rehabilitation is a direct outgrowth of the constantly modified, progressive programs that were first applied to athletes.

Summary. The lessons we have learned regarding instability are clear. We are on a roller coaster regarding the best method of ligament injury treatment. Between 1948 and 1963 early repair of all ligaments held sway. Most of the attention was placed on what O'Donoghue had described as the "triad," and medial instability was commonly found with the pivot shift lacking emphasis

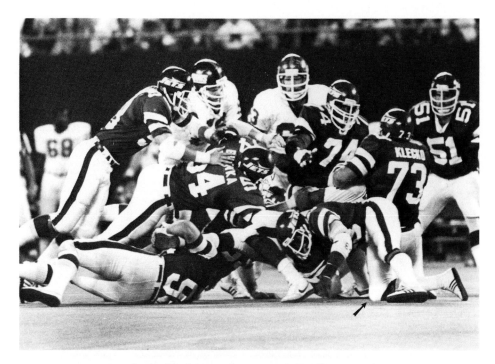

FIG. 63-40. Mechanism of posterior cruciate ligament injury.

or recognition. Between 1963 and the early 1970s extraarticular repair of the rotating corners without repair of the ACL was a dominant theme, and classification for accurate diagnosis of the X-Y-Z axis was emphasized. In the 1960s it was thought that the meniscus should be removed, and this contributed to the arthritic process in many cases. In the early 1970s the emphasis began to shift again to the ACL and especially to anterolateral instability. Since then, a host of operations have been designed or redesigned to repair, augment, or replace the ACL. Also, the menisci, as they relate to the protection of the joint, and the interaction between the menisci and the capsular structures have been better appreciated. With the emphasis on the ACL, rotation has to some extent been deemphasized. Rotatory instability exists and must not be ignored. The complete operation should include focus on both the intraarticular and extraarticular restraints and the triaxial functions of the knee.

Treatment should always be on the basis of diagnosis. The knees of football players can be worsened iatrogenically by poor diagnosis, poor indications for surgery, poor surgical technique, willingness to rely on inadequate examination, and failure to modify expectations for both the player and the physician. The earlier the player is seen after injury, the greater the chances for successful treatment. Treatment must include protection and successful rehabilitation. Close follow-up to detect progressive joint deterioration and appropriate intervention, which may include modification of activities, is imperative. At this time many advances and emphases have been placed on improving the classification of instability, physical examination, arthroscopy, and diagnostic scanning. However, some great athletes have played with significant ligamentous injury in both knees that were treated nonoperatively and have played for many years with minimal arthritis. Others have had numerous operations that have terminated their careers despite flawless surgical technique. For this reason the problem of the unstable knee has not yet been solved.

Leg Injuries

There are a number of conditions below the knee that occur in football players. The lower leg, ankle, and foot are relatively small compared with the body as a whole. These structures are involved at the start of the linkage system as it pertains to the biomechanics of running, cutting, and jumping. The ground reactive forces generated through these areas are amplified by the great weight and speed of the players. Some unique aspects concerning these areas in football players are discussed here.

Stress Fractures

Fatigue fractures of the skeletal system in athletes constitute approximately 3.3% to 4.6% of all overuse injuries. Delayed diagnosis is usually caused by a combination of continued hard physical activity while symptoms persist and a low degree of suspicion. In a study of competitive basketball players by Shelbourne et al,[69] an average of 4.4 months passed until an accurate diagnosis was made.[34,62] This time frame of injury and diagnosis is probably similar for football players who compete at the smaller collegiate and high school levels. Stress fractures in nonathletes also produce a similar delay in diagnosis if suspicion is low.[7] Diagnosis of stress fractures with professional football players is usually made sooner because there is closer contact between the player, trainer, and physician.

There are several current theories as to the risk factors producing tibial (including foot and hip) stress frac-

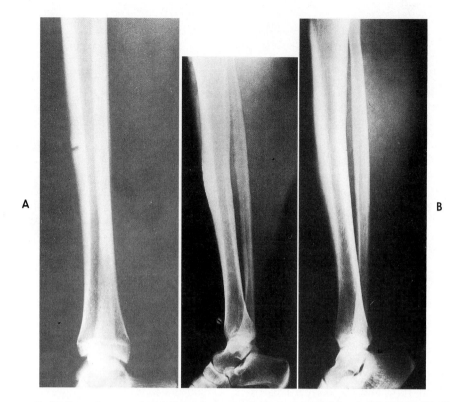

FIG. 63-41. Stress fracture tibia. **A,** Lateral x-ray study demonstrating "dreaded black line." **B,** Union after conservative treatment.

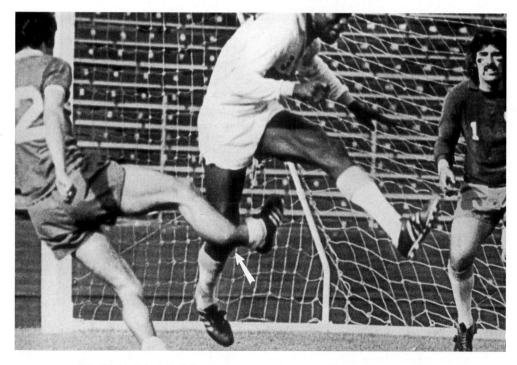

FIG. 63-42. Tibial shaft fractures occur in soccer and rugby as well as football.

tures. These theories include repetitive overuse patterns producing weakness and degeneration until a stress fracture becomes clinically evident. Additional theories involve changes in the normal forces transmitted through the linkage system. These include increased flexibility of sports shoes, the differing components of playing surfaces, and the different moments of inertia around the tibia.[4,47,81]

Classical symptoms of stress fractures involve pain along the anterolateral cortex of the midshaft of the tibia while running or jumping. A careful detailed history of pain with activity in a localized area can assist in making the diagnosis. Plain films and bone scans may also be used to confirm the diagnosis and to rule out other possible disorders.

Treatment involves rest, ice, and the use of antiinflammatory medication with a gradual return to sports activity as the symptoms subside. Delayed or nonunion stress fractures produce a difficult management problem. At this time x-ray findings may demonstrate the "dreaded black line" of an anterior tibial nonunion stress fracture (Fig. 63-41). Conservative treatment with or without electric stimulation is continued for a period of 3 to 6 months. At this time surgical intervention may be necessary. This may include bone grafting, drilling, and debridement of the nonunion site with or without placement of an unlocked intermedullary rod.[10]

Tibial shaft fractures are commonly seen in other contact sports in addition to football (Fig. 63-42). A prospective study examined 90 cases of tibial shaft fractures in rugby players, and the outcome of closed conservative treatment vs. intermedullary rodding was compared. Of the surgical group, 98% demonstrated fracture union at 14 to 18 weeks. Of these players, 62% had returned to work and were able to play their sport the next season. In the conservatively treated group, 53% demonstrated a solid union during the same time period, and only 22% had returned to work and were playing sports by 6 months. Internal fixation for competitive athletes provided a quicker, less complicated avenue for returning to work and sporting activities. Moreover, reduction can be anatomically achieved with surgery.[1]

Soft-Tissue Conditions

Contusions of the gastrocnemius and soleus are common and are treated in a fashion similar to other muscle contusions, that is, with rest, ice, compression, use of antiinflammatory medication, stretching, and strengthening.

Inflammatory conditions in the heel cord area, such as Achilles tendinitis, are a bothersome problem for many football players. Hard turf, excessive running, poorly fitted shoes, excessive taping, tight calf muscles, tight hamstrings, inadequate stretching programs, osteophytes at the insertion of the Achilles tendon, Haglund's deformity, and inadequate periods of rest are all causes of this particular problem. The inflammation is frequently bilateral and is a stubborn problem. Occasionally, nodules can be felt in the distal portion of the tendon. Rest is the treatment of choice and is coupled with heel elevation using either cowboy boots or 2- to 3-inch

heel lifts. Elevation should continue for 1 or 2 months with gradual stretching and strengthening of the legs. Occasionally, surgery is required, at which time the Achilles tendon is split in the direction of its fibers and an area of cystic degeneration may be noted. If a nodule is present, it generally takes 4 to 6 months for complete healing to occur. Complete ruptures of the Achilles tendon, which often follow repeated episodes of tendinitis, require operation. Good function and return to football in a year following this major injury can be expected.

Ankle Injuries
Sprains

The ankle joint includes the articulation and movement of the distal end of the tibia, fibula, and talus. These three bones form the ankle mortise, which is approximately 2 to 3 inches wide. The ankle is not an inherently stable joint when compared with a ball-and-socket joint. It derives its stability by the ligamentous structures surrounding these articulations. It is these structures that are placed at risk of injury during the high forces generated during running, cutting, twisting, and jumping movements that are common in football. They are also placed under stress during tackling or collisions, when the foot may be trapped on the ground while the body is twisting above.

Ankle injuries most commonly sustained in football can be classified into two general types: lateral ankle sprains involving the calcaneofibular ligaments and syndesmotic sprains (high ankle sprain) involving the anterior tibiofibular ligament. Lateral ankle sprains are more common and relatively less serious than high ankle sprains. Playing time lost, practices missed, and treatments received were all greater with syndesmotic ankle sprains in a review of a professional football team over a 6-year period.[11] Heterotopic bone ossification of the syndesmosis is a common sequela of high ankle sprains (Fig. 63-43).[74]

Diagnosis and differentiation of lateral and syndesmotic ankle sprains can easily be made during physical examination. Lateral ankle sprains are tender to palpation around the tip of the fibula and lateral calcaneus. Pain is reproduced with inversion of the foot. High ankle sprains are tender over the anterior aspect of the distal fibula at the level of the ankle joint. This ligament routinely pulls off of the fibula rather than the tibia. Pain is reproduced with plantar flexion-inversion or in dorsiflexion-rotation as the mortise is wedged open and the injured ligament stressed. Treatment for a severe high ankle sprain may include initial immobilization for the first 3 to 5 days to rest the ankle and control swelling. Then an aggressive range of motion protocol is instituted with contrast baths and ultrasound. The player should be non–weight bearing followed by progressive weight bearing. Straight ahead walking and jogging are allowed before cutting drills. This injury can linger and recur if the player is permitted to return to action before being pain free. Also, running backs and receivers can take a longer time to recover than linemen because their position demands a greater stress across the ankle joint.

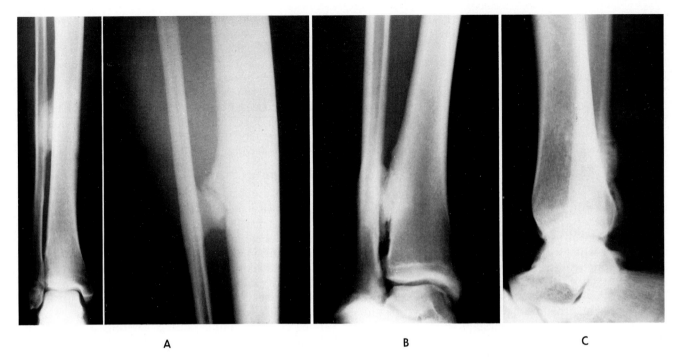

FIG. 63-43. Interosseous ossification. **A,** Middle third. **B,** Junction of middle and distal thirds. **C,** Distal third. Occasionally, excursion of tibialis anterior or common long toe extensor can be impeded beneath retinaculum.

Tendon Injuries

Tendon injuries about the ankle are often a result of overloading and repetitive microtrauma stemming from training errors, poor techniques, and the use of inappropriate surfaces and equipment. This can produce inflammation of the tendon sheath and tendon. Rest, ice, use of antiinflammatory medication, and correction of the offending factors mentioned above allow this type of injury to heal properly. Repeated episodes of injury and inflammation can place the structures at risk for rupture.

Tendon injuries can also include peroneal tendon subluxation and dislocation, which are not uncommonly seen in football players as the torque generated around the lateral side of the ankle during cutting places the peroneal retinaculum at risk for tearing. Symptoms most often include clicking and visible snapping of the peroneal tendons out of their groove, both behind the lateral malleolus and just distal to it. Often it is associated with spurs of the distal fibula or, in cases of chronic instability, anterior osteophyte formation of the talus. Repeated subluxation or dislocation has necessitated surgery for many patients with replacement of the tendons in their groove. In cases of chronic instability, a formal lateral ankle reconstruction is needed. This is followed by cast immobilization for approximately 8 weeks and a subsequent rehabilitation program that emphasizes strengthening of the lateral compartment muscles. The overall treatment in this fashion commonly takes 4 to 6 months for a player to return to sports participation.[16,21,24]

Repeated soft-tissue injuries around the ankle also place the bony structures at risk for damage. Osteochondral lesions of the talus are common occurrences of these

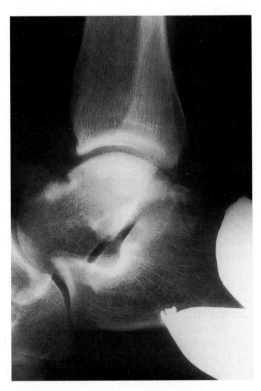

FIG. 63-44. Anterior osteophyte on talus suggestive of chronic ankle instability.

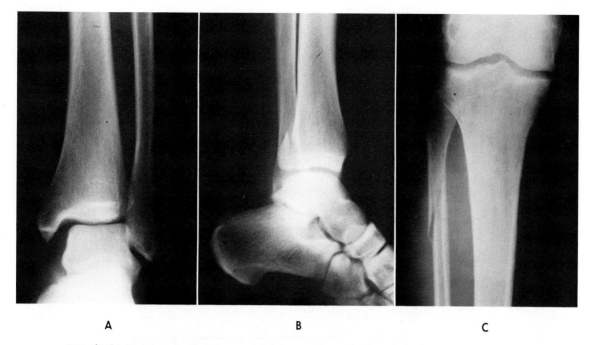

A   B   C

FIG. 63-45. Maisonneuve fracture sustained during pile-on. **A,** Note shift of mortise on anteroposterior view. **B,** Lateral view. **C,** Anteroposterior view of proximal fracture.

traumatic ankle injuries and instability. Ankle arthroscopy may then be necessary for removal of loose bodies, or chondroplasty may be performed, although its benefits remain questionable.

Osseous Problems

Talotibial impingement about the ankle caused by driving off the foot or chronic ankle instability is a common finding in individuals who have been playing football for 10 to 15 years, especially running backs and linemen. These spurs are sharp triangular osteophytes that extend forward (Fig. 63-44). In addition, they often communicate with the anterior tibiofibular ligament when there has been a previous diastasis. They are often sclerotic lesions that interfere with the nutrition of the articular cartilage of the tibia. If the spurs are symptomatic, they should be operated on. Resection of the anterior spurs allows increased dorsiflexion.

Fractures about the ankle are not uncommon in football. Unstable fractures should be treated with open reduction and rigid internal fixation (Fig. 63-45). Early motion is advised to hasten the recovery period.

Foot Injuries

Fractures of the midfoot can occur from direct compression as one player steps on another's foot (Fig. 63-46). As healing occurs in these nondisplaced fractures, custom footwear can be created to facilitate return to football.

Forefoot diastasis is a commonly overlooked injury (Fig. 63-47). Standing anteroposterior x-ray studies of the foot are necessary to make the diagnosis if the clinical index of suspicion is high. These athletes are seen with foot pain with weight bearing. Tenderness is located at Lisfranc's joint. Passive motion of the distal metatarsals

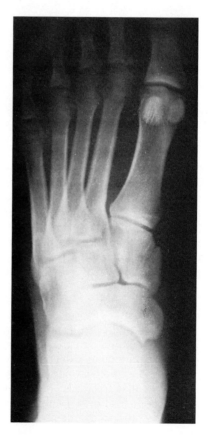

FIG. 63-46. Fracture of medial cuneiform bone in wide receiver. Player resumed participation 4 weeks after injury using customized protective shoes.

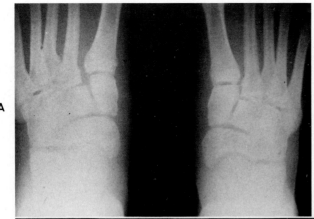

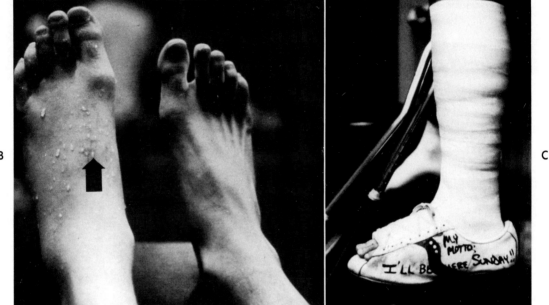

FIG. 63-47. **A,** Diastasis of first and second metatarsals in offensive center. Film was obtained in standing position. **B,** Location of tenderness *(arrow).* **C,** Treatment was by cast immobilization. Note enthusiastic player comment on cast boot.

helps localize the injury. Undisplaced or minimally displaced injuries are treated with cast immobilization. In these cases recovery generally takes 4 months. If significant displacement is present, closed or open reduction and percutaneous pinning is required.

Sore heels, metatarsalgia, and bruises about the foot are caused by cleats, improper footwear, and heel cord contractures. Orthotics may be required in some instances for relief of symptoms.

Stress fractures of the fifth metatarsal base can be troublesome (Fig. 63-48). These fractures occur in a zone called "no-man's land," just distal to the fifth metatarsal styloid. These fractures can proceed to a nonunion fracture and may require open reduction, internal fixation–bone grafting if symptoms persist longer than 2 months. Tarsal navicular fractures, when present, are not as bothersome but heal over a long period of time. Some, however, may proceed to a nonunion fracture and therefore must be treated appropriately (Fig. 63-49).

Toe Injuries

Injury to the **metatarsophalangeal joint of the great toe** is commonly known as turf toe. Synthetic

surfaces and flexible, lighter athletic shoes have been implicated as a source of this injury. Other factors were associated with formation of turf toe; these included the player's age, the number of years in playing organized football, and the active range of ankle dorsiflexion.[65]

Forced hyperextension of the toe results in damage to the plantar capsule and dorsal impingement. With recurrent injury, dorsal osteophyte formation occurs and limitations of motion result. Conservative treatment includes ice, taping, and use of antiinflammatory medications with gradual return to activity as symptoms allow.[15] Chronic injuries necessitate orthotics or the use of a steel shank in the sole of the shoe to limit motion at the joint.

Sesamoiditis or **stress fractures of the sesamoid** should be treated with rest, antiinflammatory medication, if appropriate, and an adequately high, proximally based, doughnut-shaped pad to decrease the forces across the sesamometatarsal joint (Fig. 63-50). Excision or injection is not indicated until all nonoperative forms of treatment have been thoroughly exhausted.

Nail bed injuries may result from a single overwhelming traumatic event or chronic repeated minor in-

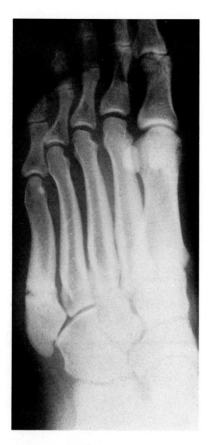

FIG. 63-48. Fracture of fifth metatarsal with obvious nonunion in linebacker. This injury was treated by conservative measures. We prefer fracture compression using internal fixation if delay in union is evident.

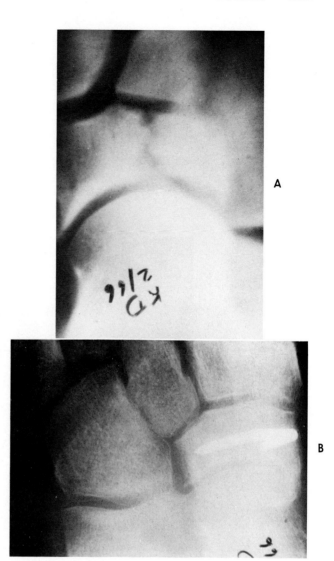

FIG. 63-49. A, Unusual nonunion of tarsal navicular. **B,** Treatment by bone grafting and fixation with staple. Player resumed college football career with no problem. (Courtesy Martin Blazina, MD, Los Angeles, Calif.)

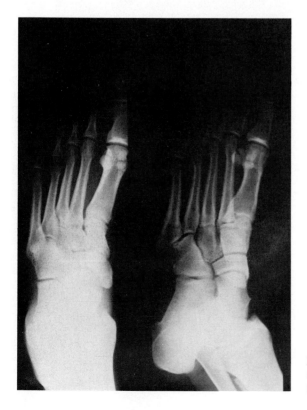

FIG. 63-50. Bipartite medial and lateral sesamoids. Treatment of sesamoiditis including padding, shoe modification, use of antiinflammatory medication, and rest.

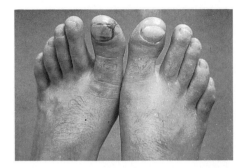

FIG. 63-51. Nail bed injuries. Acute bleeding *(left)*; subacute *(right)*.

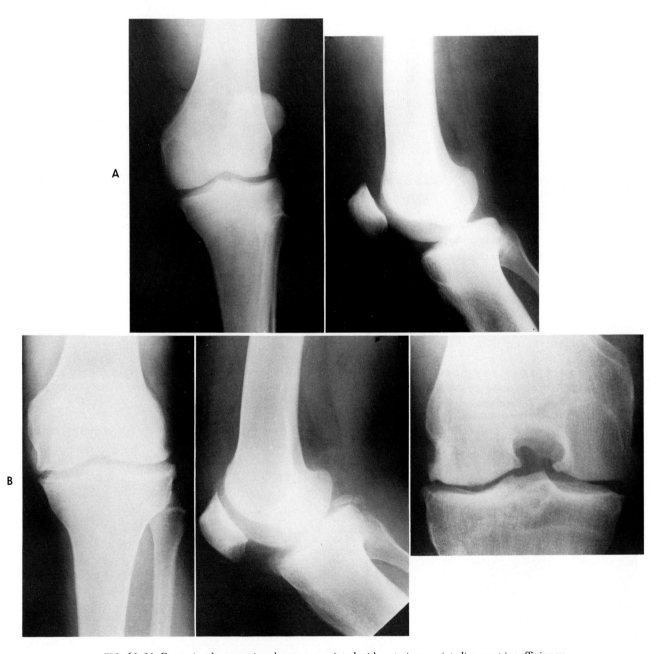

FIG. 63-52. Extensive degenerative changes associated with anterior cruciate ligament insufficiency and meniscectomy. **A,** Radiographs taken at time of preparticipation evaluation, following college graduation. **B,** Extensive joint destruction following 8 years of professional football. This patient in the intervening years had meniscectomies and extraarticular reconstructions.

juries. Nail bed injuries can occur on artificial turf when sudden cessation of movement occurs and the foot slides forward within the shoe (Fig. 63-51). The nail bed can hemorrhage, and the tuft of the distal phalanx can fracture. With chronic injury, spur formation at the interphalangeal joint of the great toe can occur. In many cases the nail may have to be removed. Prevention includes appropriate fitting of footwear.[50]

LATE SEQUALAE OF FOOTBALL INJURIES

The late sequelae of chronic injury to the neck, back, knee, and other joints, including those injuries leading to instability, tracking problems, fractures, and meniscal problems, are compressive and shearing lesions of the articular cartilage. A study of football players over a 25-year period revealed that 75% of them had developed arthritis in varying degrees as determined by x-ray studies and clinical findings in the spine, knee, hip, ankle, and great toe.[53] Many of these individuals, who no longer play football, are now attempting to stay in shape. With time, some may develop bowing of the legs with medial joint compartment injury in the knee where instability or meniscal injury had been present (Fig. 63-52). Repeated ankle injuries can produce ectopic bone and spur formation with arthritic changes. Hallux rigidus is common. Early arthritis of the hips and spine is characteristic of these large men who have been pounding and have been pounded on while playing sports for many years. Many of these individuals are candidates for joint replacement later in their lives. By the time they are 40 years old, they may require debridements and resections to allow the functional activities of daily living. Some knees that have undergone repair are so badly damaged that early arthroplasty may be indicated, but this brings with it its own set of problems.

The essence of athletic injuries in football is that they are high-speed, unexpected, high-impact injuries and that a number of injuries are to be expected in each individual. Unless an injury is so serious that it does not allow a return to football, these athletes do not give up easily and continue to play until it is too late. Continuous monitoring of injuries in each individual is important because an accumulation of minor problems can add up to chronic long-term disabilities. Monitoring should be done by someone well versed in sports medicine and football injuries, especially in injuries to the skeletally immature player. Injuries in this age group, with continued play, can place a young player at risk for a life-long problem. The competitive nature of these individuals, peer pressure, and parental pressure drive these athletes to play and continue playing beyond sensible endpoints. The sports physician can help maximize their performance and concurrently help minimize long-term sequelae.

REFERENCES

1. Abdel-Salam A, Eyres KS, Cleary J: Internal fixation of closed tibial fractures for the management of sports injuries, *Br J Sports Med* 25(4):213, 1991.
2. Agre JC: Hamstring injuries: proposed aetiological factors, prevention, and treatment, *Sports Med* 2(1):21, 1985.
3. Alexander MJ: Biomechanical aspects of lumbar spine injuries in athletes: a review, *Can J Sport Sci* 10(1):1, 1985.
4. Anderson EG: Fatigue fractures of the foot, *Injury* 21(5):275, 1990.
5. Andreasson G et al: Torque developed at simulated sliding between sport shoes and an artificial turf, *Am J Sports Med* 14(3):225, 1986.
6. Andresen BL, Hoffman MD, Barton LW: High school football injuries: field conditions and other factors, *Wis Med J* 88(10):28, 1989.
7. Aspegren D, Cox JM, Benak DR: Detection of stress fractures in athletes and nonathletes, *J Manipulative Pysiol Ther* 12(4):298, 1989.
8. Bailes JE et al: Management of athletic injuries of the cervical spine and spinal cord, *Neurosurgery* 29(4):491, 1991.
9. Baker BE et al: Review of meniscal injury and associated sports, *Am J Sports Med* 13(1):4, 1985.
10. Beals RK, Cook RD: Stress fractures of the anterior tibial diaphysis, *Orthopedics* 14(8):869, 1991.
11. Boytim MJ, Fischer DA, Neumann L: Syndesmotic ankle sprains, *Am J Sports Med* 19(3):294, 1991.
12. Brunner MC et al: MRI of the athletic knee: findings in asymptomatic professional basketball and collegiate football players, *Invest Radiol* 24(1):72, 1989.
13. Buckley WE: Concussions in college football: a multivariate analysis, *Am J Sports Med* 16(1):51, 1988.
14. Cantu RC, Mueller FO: Catastrophic spine injuries in football (1977-1989), *J Spinal Disord* 3(3):227, 1990.
15. Clanton TO, Butler JE, Eggert A: Injuries to the metatarsophalangeal joints in athletes, *Foot Ankle* 7(3):162, 1986.
16. Cohen I, Lane S, Koning W: Peroneal tendon dislocations: a review of the literature, *J Foot Surg* 22(1):15, 1983.
17. Cooper DE, Warren RE, Barns R: Traumatic subluocation of the hip resulting in aseptic necrosis and chondrolysis in a professional football player, *Am J Sports Med* 19(3):322, 1991.
18. Cossi CG et al: Apophysealolysis and osteochondrosis of the ischial tuberosity: criteria of differential diagnosis, *Ital J Orthop Traumatol* 12(4):515, 1986.
19. Day AL, Friedman WA, Indelicato PA: Observations on the treatment of lumbar disk disease in college football players, *Am J Sports Med* 15(1):72, 1987.
20. DeHaven KE, Lintner DM: Athletic injuries: comparison by age, sport, and gender, *Am J Sports Med* 14(3):218, 1986.
21. Duddy RK et al: Tendon sheath injuries of the foot and ankle, *J Foot Surg* 30(2):179, 1991.
22. DuRant RH et al: Findings from the preparticipation athletic examination and athletic injuries, *Am J Dis Child* 146(1):85, 1992.
23. Elmqvist LG et al: Knee extensor muscle function before and after reconstruction of anterior cruciate ligament tear, *Scand J Soc Med* 21(3):131, 1989.
24. Frey CC, Shereff MJ: Tendon injuries about the ankle in athletes, *Clin Sports Med* 7(1):103, 1988.
25. Garrett WE, Mumma M, Luvcaveche CL: Ultrastructural differences in human skeletal muscle fiber types, *Orthop Clin North Am* 14:413, 1983.
26. Gerberich SG et al: Concussion incidences and severity in secondary school varsity football players, *Am J Public Health* 73(12):1370, 1983.
27. Gleim GW: The profiling of professional football players, *Clin Sports Med* 3(1):185, 1984.
28. Hastings DE: Knee ligament instability—a rational anatomical classification, *Clin Orthop* 208:104, 1986.
29. Heiser TM et al: Prophylaxis and management of hamstring muscle injuries in intercollegiate football players, *Am J Sports Med* 12(5):368, 1984.
30. Hershman E: News brief, *Phys Sports Med* 21(3):19, 1993.
31. Herzog RJ et al: Normal cervical spine morphometry and cervical spinal stenosis in asymptomatic professional football players: plain film radiography, multiplanar computed tomography, and magnetic resonance imaging, *Spine* 16(6):178, 1991.
32. Heuck F: Roentgen morphology of sport injuries to the pelvic apophyses, *Radiologe* 23(9):404, 1983.
33. Hodgson VR, Thoma LM: Mechanism of cervical spine injury

during impact of the protected head. Twenty-fourth Stock Car Crash conference, 1980.

34. Hulkko A, Orava S: Diagnosis and treatment of delayed and nonunion stress fractures in athletes, *Ann Chir Gynaecol* 80(2):177, 1991.

35. Jacobson T, Allen WC: Surgical correction of the snapping iliopsoas tendon, *Am J Sports Med* 18(5):470, 1990.

36. Kannus P, Jarvinen M: Thigh muscle function after partial tear of the medial ligament compartment of the knee, *Med Sci Sports Exerc* 23(1):4, 1991.

37. Keene JS et al: Back injuries in college athletes, *J Spinal Disord* 2(3):190, 1989.

38. Kelly JP et al: Concussions in sports: guidelines for the prevention of catastrophic outcome, *JAMA* 266(20):2867, 1991.

39. Kremchek TE, Welling RE, Kremchek EJ: Traumatic dislocation of the knee, *Orthop Rev* 18(10):1051, 1987.

40. Lee CJ, Kim KS, Rogers LF: Sagittal fracture of the cervical vertebral body, *AJR* 139:55, 1982.

41. Levy IM, Skovron ML, Agel J: Living with artificial grass: a knowledge update. Part 1. Basic science, *Am J Sports Med* 18(4):406, 1990.

42. Lorentzon R et al: Thigh musculature in relation to chronic anterior cruciate ligament tear: muscle size, morphology, and mechanical output before reconstruction, *Am J Sports Med* 17(3):423, 1989.

43. Lutz GE et al: Rehabilitative techniques for athletes after reconstruction of the anterior cruciate ligament, *Mayo Clin Proc* 65(10):1322, 1990.

44. Maiman DJ, Sances A, Myklebust JB: Compression injuries of the cervical spine: a biomechanical analysis, *Neurosurgery* 13:254, 1983.

45. McCarroll JR, Miller JM, Ritter MA: Lumbar spondylolysis and spondylolisthesis in college football players: a prospective study, *Am J Sports Med* 14(5):404, 1986.

46. Meeuwise WH, Fowler PJ: Frequency and predictability of sports injuries in intercollegiate athletes, *Can J Sport Sci* 13(1):35, 1988.

47. Milgrom C et al: The area moment of inertia of the tibia: a risk factor for stress fractures, *J Biomech* 22(11):1243, 1989.

48. Mink JH, Deutsch AL: Occult cartilage and bone injuries of the knee: detection, classification, and assessment with MR imaging, *Radiology* 170:823, 1989.

49. Moretz JA et al: Long-term follow-up of knee injuries in high school football players, *Am J Sports Med* 12(4):298, 1984.

50. Mortimer PS, Dawber RP: Trauma to the nail unit including occupational sports injuries, *Dermatol Clin* 3(3):415, 1985.

51. Mueller FO, Blyth CS: Fatalities from head and cervical spine injuries occurring in tackle football: 40 years' experience, *Clin Sports Med* 6(1):185, 1987.

52. Nicholas JA: The value of sports profiling, *Clin Sports Med* 3:127, 1984.

53. Nicholas JA: Unpublished data, 1985.

54. Nicholas JA, Grossman RB, Hershman EB: The importance of a simplified classification of motion in sports in relation to performance, *Orthop Clin North Am* 8:499, 1977.

55. Nicholas JA, Rosenthal PP, Gleim GW: A historical perspective of injuries in professional football: twenty-six years of game-related events, *JAMA* 260(7):939, 1988.

56. Nigg BM, Segesser B: The influence of playing surfaces on the load on the locomotor system and on football and tennis injuries, *Sports Med* 5(6):375, 1988.

57. Noyes FR, Grood ES: Classification of ligament injuries: why an anterolateral laxity or anteromedial laxity is not a diagnostic entity, *Instr Course Lect* 36:185, 1987.

58. Paar O, Fürbringer W, Bernett P: Injuries of the posterior end of the medial meniscus and the posterior oblique ligament: classification and therapy, *Chirurg* 55(1):49, 1984.

59. Polglase AL, Frydman GM, Farmer KC: Inguinal surgery for debilitating chronic groin pain in athletes, *Med J Aust* 155(10):674, 1991.

60. Pritchett JW: A statistical study of knee injuries due to football in high-school athletes, *J Bone Joint Surg* 64A(2):240, 1982.

61. Reinig JW, McDevitt ER, Ove PN: Progression of meniscal degenerative changes in college football players: evaluation with MR imaging, *Radiology* 181(1):255, 1991.

62. Rettig AC et al: The natural history and treatment of delayed union stress fractures of the anterior cortex of the tibia, *Am J Sports Med* 16(3):250, 1988.

63. Roaf R: A study of the mechanics of spinal injuries, *J Bone Joint Surg* 42B:810, 1960.

64. Roaf R: International classification of spinal injuries, *Paraplegia* 10:72, 1972.

65. Rodeo SA et al: Turf-toe: an analysis of metatarsophalangeal joint sprains in professional football players, *Am J Sports Med* 18(3):280, 1990.

66. Ryan JB et al: Quadriceps contusions: West Point update, *Am J Sports Med* 19(3):299, 1991.

67. Saal JA: Common American football injuries, *Sports Med* 12(2):132, 1991.

68. Semon RL, Sprengler D: Significance of lumbar spondylolysis in college football players, *Spine* 6:172, 1981.

69. Shelbourne KD et al: Low-velocity knee dislocation, *Orthop Rev* 20(11):995, 1991.

70. Shields CL Jr, Whitney FE, Zomar VD: Exercise performance of professional football players, *Am J Sports Med* 1(6):455, 1984.

71. Skovron ML, Levy IM, Agel Y: Living with artificial grass: a knowledge update. Part 2. Epidemiology, *Am J Sports Med* 18(5):510, 1990.

72. Sortland O, Tysvaer AT: Brain damage in former association football players: an evaluation by cerebral computed tomography, *Neuroradiology* 31(1):44, 1989.

73. Stafford MG, Grana WA: Hamstring/quadriceps ratios in college football players: a high-velocity evaluation, *Am J Sports Med* 12(3):204, 1984.

74. Taylor DC, Englehardt DL, Bassett FH: Syndesmosis sprains of the ankle: the influence of heterotopic ossification, *Am J Sports Med* 20(2):146, 1992.

75. Torg J, Truex R, Quedenfeld CC: The National Football Head and Neck Injury Registry: report and conclusions, *JAMA* 241:1477, 1979.

76. Torg JS, Vegso JJ, O'Neill MJ: The epidemiological, pathologic, biomechanical, and cinematographic analysis of football-induced cervical spine trauma, *Am J Sports Med* 18:56, 1990.

77. Torg J et al: The National Football Head and Neck Injury Registry: 14-year report on cervical quadriplegia, 1971-1984, *JAMA* 254:3439, 1985.

78. Torg JS et al: The axial load teardrop fracture: a biomechanical, clinical, and roentgenographic analysis, *Am J Sports Med* 19(4):355, 1991.

79. Treiman GS et al: Examination of the patient with knee dislocation: the case for selective arteriography, *Arch Surg* 127(9):1056, 1992.

80. Tyrrell RL et al: Fast three-dimensional MR imaging of the knee: comparison with arthroscopy, *Radiology* 166(3):865, 1988.

81. Walz D, Craig BM, McGinnis KD: Bone imaging showing shin splints and stress fractures, *Clin Nucl Med* 12(10):822, 1987.

82. Weir MR, Smith DS: Stress reaction of the pars interarticularis leading to spondylolysis: a cause of adolescent low back pain, *J Adolesc Health Care* 10(6):573, 1989.

83. White AA, Punjabi MM: *Clinical biomechanics of the spine*, Philadelphia, 1978, JB Lippincott.

CHAPTER 64

Running Injuries

David M. Brody

Recent surveys indicate that interest in running has been maintained at a high level. Thirty million Americans are running at various levels of intensity. The orthopaedic surgeon and sports medicine expert are faced with patients who want immediate relief of symptoms so that they can return rapidly to their previous mileage levels. The information available to the injured runner in the lay press may not be applicable to the injury; thus the physician may be faced with treating an injury that has been rendered more intractable as a result of the patient's own continued "running through" the injury or injudicious home remedies. This chapter discusses the causes, biomechanical basis, prevention, and treatment of these injuries and some thoughts on the rehabilitation of the injured runner through "alternative training."

Although running-induced injuries may affect as many as 45% of all runners, these are usually not of a serious nature. In addition, no evidence suggests that running leads to degenerative arthritis of the hip, knee, or ankle joints.

Physicians who treat runners should be familiar with the "runner's language" but not necessarily be runners themselves. They should be aware that running is an important aspect of the patient's life* and be empathetic

---

*Editors' note: *Runner's mentality* varies from temporary enthusiasm to a methodical, compulsive, addictive behavior in an individual whose "life support system" is running, without which he or she cannot happily exist.

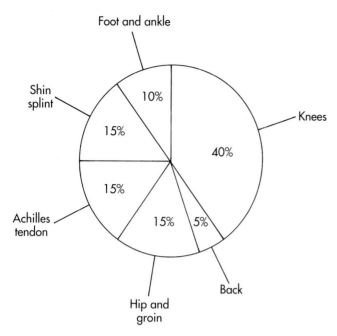

FIG. 64-1. Injuries to runners.

with the patient's desire to resume running as quickly as possible after an injury. Because a runner may resist undergoing blood studies; standard radiography, bone, or computed tomography (CT) scans; and therapeutic injections, the physician must carefully explain the need for such methods before proceeding.

Since early 1977 I have had the opportunity to treat over 8000 runners. An overview of the injuries seen (Fig. 64-1) indicates that the knee is by far the most commonly injured body part. The environment producing the injury (Fig. 64-2, *A*) may involve just one factor but is usually a combination of factors. The physician must understand at the outset, however, that preexisting conditions, either acquired, congenital, or biomechanical may dictate the final outcome of treatment. It is best that the runner be made aware of these conditions before getting heavily involved or "hooked" on running so as to be directed to other sports activities. For example, runners with arthritic knees do better to participate in some non–weight-bearing aerobic activity rather than develop pain as they increase their running mileage.

CLASSIFICATION OF RUNNERS (Fig. 64-2, *B*)

Injuries most commonly occur when runners begin a running program or when they progress too rapidly from one level of running to another. The level I jogger, or recreational runner, runs 3 to 20 miles a week at a pace of 9 to 12 minutes per mile. The level II, or sports, runner runs 20 to 40 miles a week and may participate in local fun runs or races of 5 to 10 km. The level III, or long-distance, runner runs 40 to 70 miles per week at a pace of 7 to 8 minutes per mile and is usually a competitor (10,000 m to the marathon). Finally, the level IV, or elite, runner is usually highly competitive and runs any-

where from 70 to more than 160 miles a week at a 5- to 7-minute per mile pace. In our series of running injuries the distribution of injuries as related to level of running is as follows (percentage of all injuries): level I, 25%; level II, 30%; level III, 35%; and level IV, 5%. If we consider the number of runners in this country today, approximately 70% of them sustain an injury sufficiently severe or painful to prevent running for a week to 10 days.

Seventy percent of runners sustain an injury sufficiently severe or painful to prevent running for 1 week to 10 days.

Shin splints, patellofemoral pain syndrome ("chondromalacia"), muscle soreness, hamstring strain, and low back pain are more likely to occur than stress fractures in the level I runner because of poor training techniques and improper shoes. Biomechanically induced injuries such as patellofemoral arthralgia and posterior tibial tendinitis are commonplace at level I but almost unheard of at level III or level IV. The overuse syndromes to soft tissue and bone occur when the runner progresses from one level of training to another, increasing mileage or speed. The runner simply overuses his or her body, not allowing it to adapt to a higher level of stress. Plantar fasciitis and Achilles tendinitis are often seen in the level I runner, who, along with the long-distance runner, is also susceptible to stress fractures. The long-distance runner sustains more serious muscle injuries in the thigh, calf, and back, sustains more sciatica and adductor tendon pulls, and is particularly susceptible to heat and cold injuries during competition. Stress fractures, acute muscular strain in the back, sciatica, and fatigue from overtraining may occur in the elite marathon runner.

Biomechanical malalignment, or imbalance, in the structures of the foot and lower extremity is frequently responsible for injuries in the recreational and sports runner. However, structural abnormalities are not gen-

---

Relationship of level of intensity to injury

Intensity level	Common injuries
■ Level I	Shin splints
	Patellofemoral pain syndrome
	Muscle soreness
	Hamstring strain
	Low back pain
	Posterior tibial tendinitis
	Plantar fasciitis
	Achilles tendinitis
■ Level III	Heat and cold injury during competition
	Adductor strains
	Sciatica
■ Level IV	Stress fracture
	Acute muscle strain
	Sciatica
	Fatigue from overtraining

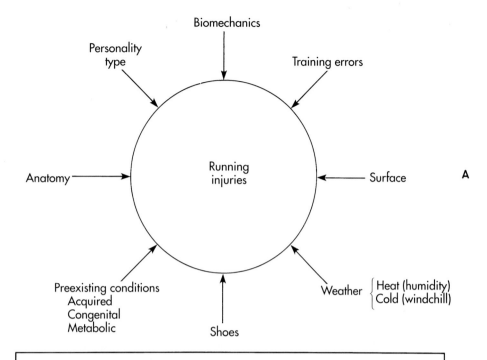

FIG. 64-2. A, Runner's environment. **B,** Classification of runners: Level I, Level II, Level III, Level IV, and Level V—triathlon (100 to 300 miles per week of swimming, bicycling, and running).

erally seen in the long-distance runner and marathoner, who would not have achieved their level of performance if there were any biomechanical problems.

MECHANISMS OF INJURY
Training Errors

Training errors are the most frequent cause of running injuries. Excessive mileage and intensive workouts with interval training and rapid increase in mileage over-

---

Common training errors

- Excessive mileage
- Rapid increase in mileage
- Intensive interval training
- Inadequate warm-up
- Faulty stretching
- Improper running surface

whelm the body's ability to adapt to new levels of stress. Inadequate warm-up and faulty stretching can also lead to overstress injuries.

For example, the recreational runner who decides to train for a marathon (26.2 miles, or 42 km) usually spends 2 months at 20 to 25 miles per week as a mileage base. They then do *peak* training at 45 miles per week for the 8 weeks before the date of the marathon and *taper* to 25% of their weekly mileage over the last 10 days to 2 weeks before the day of the marathon. The *peak* training period includes long runs of 18 to 20 miles (hopefully not closer than 4 weeks before the marathon day). Experienced marathoners also include "speed" sessions or interval training during the peak period. Too rapid a build up of mileage or the number of running sessions per week is a major cause of overuse injuries in this group of runners.

The running surface is important. The sine qua non of a good surface is that it be level from side to side. Ideally, a soft surface such as a dirt path is ideal, but most people wind up running wherever they can and wherever is most convenient to their home or office. The canter to the roadway can itself often produce problems in and about the lateral hip, knee, medial tibial area, and plantar fascia. Running on concrete sidewalks and up and down curbs exaggerates the impact loading in the lower extremities. Most grassy surfaces are irregular, and certainly sand is unstable. A sloping or banked surface such as a beach or a road shoulder forces the foot on the

higher part of the slope to pronate excessively and increases the time spent in pronation. In an individual who already tends to pronate, that surface may be the difference between a successful and a disastrous running career. Uphill running strains the Achilles tendon and muscles of the lower back, and downhill running significantly increases impact loading on heel strike. Recreational runners who begin their careers wearing inappropriate shoes, such as sneakers or tennis shoes with their poor cushioning and lack of stability, certainly have difficulty because of the repetitive shocks of running. Running shoes must be in good repair. Level III and IV runners may forget to repair an excessively worn-out outer heel on their running shoe, causing imbalance in heel strike and thereby causing lateral knee pain.

Biomechanical Factors

Running gait is a repetitive, cyclic movement that involves the entire body and produces a sequence of support and airborne (nonsupport) phases. The support phase includes heel strike, midstance, and toe-off. The airborne phase includes follow-through, forward-swing, and foot descent (Fig. 64-3). The runner's feet collide with the ground 5000 times per mile over 50 to 70 times per minute for each foot at a force of two to three times the body weight, depending on the terrain and the runner's weight. The impact at the foot-surface interface is absorbed by the running shoe or transmitted directly to the leg and back. Minor anatomic and biomechanical ab-

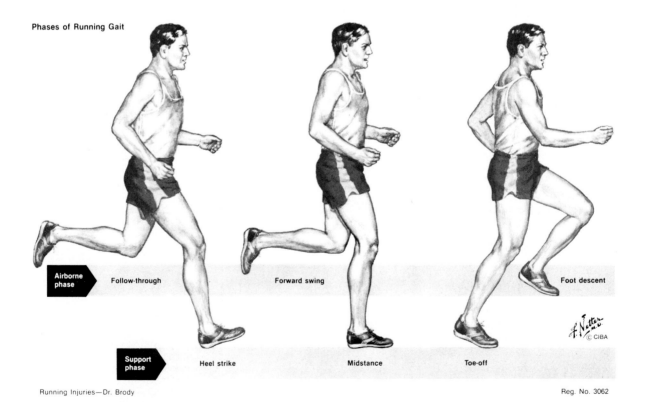

FIG. 64-3. Running gait. (© Copyright 1980, CIBA Pharmaceutical Company, Division of CIBA-GEIGY Corporation. Reprinted with permission from *Clinical Symposia,* illustrated by Frank H. Netter, M.D. All rights reserved.)

normalities that are of no functional significance in walking can produce injury while running.

Heel Strike

The long-distance runner usually lands slightly heel-toe or flat-footed. In the accomplished marathoner, the ball of the foot and the heel are touching the ground almost instantaneously. Most joggers and sports runners land on the lateral heel. Attempts by the novice to run on the toes may lead to such injuries as chronic anterior compartment syndrome or stress fracture. Heel-toe gait at this level of training offers more shock absorption than a flat-footed gait.

Pronation and Supination

Pronation and supination are complex motions that involve not only the subtalar joint, but also all of the structures of the lower extremity. Pronation unlocks the foot for surface adaptation and shock absorption during running, and supination locks the foot, allowing stabilization at heel strike and propulsion at toe-off. Approaching heel strike, the foot is slightly supinated and the tibia is externally rotated. After heel strike the foot pronates for 55% to 60% of the support phase. The subtalar joint then supinates for toe-off and stays in this position through the airborne phase. During pronation the tibia rotates internally on the talus in proportion to the amount of pronation.

The quadriceps angle (Q angle), which is the angle formed by the line of pull of the quadriceps muscle and the patellar tendon as they intersect at the center of the patella, changes with pronation and supination. At heel strike, the tibia is externally rotated and the patellar tendon is angulated laterally. When the foot pronates, the Q angle is reduced, indicating the amount of internal tibial rotation.

Any interference with sequential timing and extent of pronation and supination places abnormal stress on the lower extremity. If pronation is excessive or prolonged, the ankle sags medially and the obligatory internal tibial rotation increases, straining the structures of the knee and foot. Excessive pronation also prevents the foot from returning to the more stable, supinated position for toe-off. Hyperpronation is a compensatory mechanism for tibia vara, tight Achilles tendon, gastrocnemius, and soleus muscles, and hindfoot and forefoot varus.

Knee Extension and Flexion

The runner's knee usually flexes 20 to 40 degrees in midstance, depending on the stride length and terrain. Runners who take short steps may flex the knee only 15 to 20 degrees; most of the propelling force is generated by dorsiflexion and plantar flexion of the ankle and the lever action of the foot. The knee reaches maximum extension just after toe-off, accelerating the body into the airborne phase.

Foot Rotation

Some runners rotate the foot and lower extremity inward or outward (toeing in or out), which increases the amount of pronation and internal tibial rotation. The amount of foot rotation in midstance is primarily determined by (1) the amount of external and internal rotation of the hips, and (2) the amount of torsion in the hips and femoral neck anteversion (femur and tibia). A runner whose foot rotates may try to run with the foot pointing forward, but, with fatigue, may revert to the usual foot placement. Because the runner cannot consciously compensate for these motions, he or she may need an orthotic device to passively stabilize the foot and prevent abnormal motions.

Pelvic Motions

The pelvis rotates on the longitudinal axis of the body in proportion to the amount of arm swing (Fig. 64-4, *A*). Swinging the arms across the body rather than parallel to the line of progression rotates the pelvis and trunk excessively, which may cause pain at the attachment of the thoracolumbar muscles to the iliac crest. The pelvis also tilts upward and downward in the frontal plane (Fig. 64-4, *B*). In midstance the unsupported side of the pelvis tilts downward. This applies a shearing force to the sacroiliac joints and to both sides of the pubic symphysis, sometimes producing an osteitis pubis with overtraining. Excessive forward flexion of the lumbar spine in uphill running ("leaning into the hill") tips the pelvis anteriorly, which limits forward flexion and puts greater stress on the muscles of the lower back (Fig. 64-4, *C*). In downhill running the lumbar spine is hyperextended and the pelvis is tipped posteriorly. This may cause low back pain, especially in a runner with lordosis.

Carriage

Ideally the runner should maintain an upright posture with the trunk perpendicular to the running surface. The upper body, neck, and arms should be relaxed, the elbows flexed 90 to 100 degrees, and the hands held loosely (Fig. 64-5). Flexing the elbows to 145 to 150 degrees and clenching the fists can cause pain in the shoulders and trapezius and pectoralis muscles of the upper body. The sprinter has learned to use the arms in a pumping action, whereas the long-distance or level IV runner has learned to relax the upper body and use the arms very little, except in propelling up hills or in an all-out effort during the run. Upper body relaxation is a learned behavior and should be part of every runner's training session. If a runner runs "uptight" he or she is essentially producing isometric contractions for the upper arm musculature, trapezius, and pectorals. This causes fatigue much more quickly than if the runner learns in training to relax the upper body by maintaining a relaxed hand and "dropping" the elbows.

EVALUATION OF THE INJURED RUNNER

The orthopaedic surgeon must understand that, as in all athletes who take their sport seriously, the runner views running as an important part of his or her life. Therefore the physician should allow enough time in the office or the clinic for the runner to present his or her complaints, explain training methods, and give a history of previous injuries and treatments. All this information

Pelvic Motions in Running

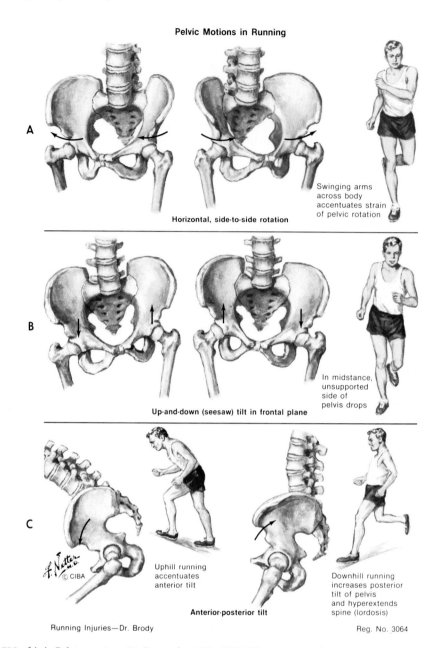

FIG. 64-4. Pelvic motion. (© Copyright 1980, CIBA Pharmaceutical Company, Division of CIBA-GEIGY Corporation. Reprinted with permission from *Clinical Symposia*, illustrated by Frank H. Netter, M.D. All rights reserved.)

can be included on a runners' clinic form with the history. Physicians are suspect in the eyes of many runners, and a hurried evaluation in a busy office setting by a brusque examiner confirms the runner's suspicion. A runners' clinic with a schedule of seeing only runners in an organized time frame is ideal. We find it helpful to have available videotaping television equipment, a treadmill, and orthotic fabricating equipment. Nevertheless, for the interested physician without specific equipment, a separate session devoted to seeing runners on a scheduled basis makes this a less harried experience than seeing these patients during regular office hours.

History

It is important to obtain a thorough medical history and carefully question the patient about any preexisting cardiac problems or musculoskeletal conditions in the lumbar spine, pelvic area, or lower extremity. Many conditions become symptomatic only when the patient begins running or increases mileage beyond a few miles a day. The patient may well have forgotten an injury acquired in college or high school sports that has caused no problems whatsoever in his or her sedentary lifestyle. Now that the patient is running, pain in these areas or injury may occur. Congenital conditions that may produce pain

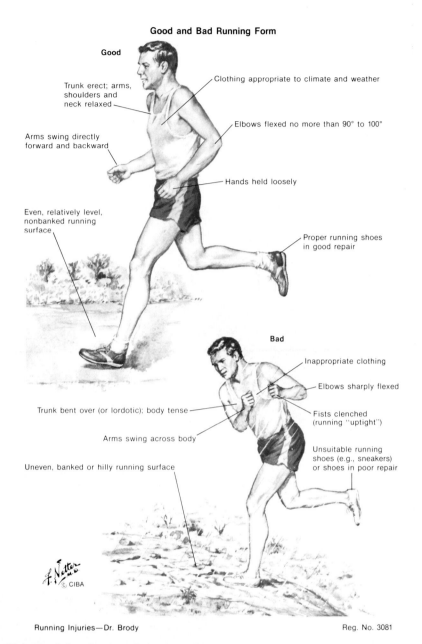

Good and Bad Running Form

Good

Trunk erect; arms, shoulders and neck relaxed

Clothing appropriate to climate and weather

Elbows flexed no more than 90° to 100°

Arms swing directly forward and backward

Hands held loosely

Even, relatively level, nonbanked running surface

Proper running shoes in good repair

Bad

Inappropriate clothing

Elbows sharply flexed

Trunk bent over (or lordotic); body tense

Fists clenched (running "uptight")

Arms swing across body

Unsuitable running shoes (e.g., sneakers) or shoes in poor repair

Uneven, banked or hilly running surface

Running Injuries—Dr. Brody

Reg. No. 3081

FIG. 64-5. Gait (relaxed or "uptight"). (© Copyright 1980, CIBA Pharmaceutical Company, Division of CIBA-GEIGY Corporation. Reprinted with permission from *Clinical Symposia,* illustrated by Frank H. Netter, M.D. All rights reserved.)

on running include spondylolysis and spondylolisthesis. Acquired conditions causing pain may be infectious, traumatic, developmental, or metabolic. The physician should determine not only when the symptoms appeared, but also what increases or decreases their severity.

The visit therefore essentially begins with the examiner reading the patient's questionnaire and focusing on the current problem. When and at what mileage level do the symptoms occur? Was the onset sudden or gradual? What type of surface was it, level or canted? What kind of shoes was the runner wearing? Was there any change in the runner's route, pace, or total weekly mileage? The runner usually offers this information to the examiner, who must listen but guide the discussion and allow the runner adequate time to present the history. Finally, were there any symptoms in the painful area before the individual's running career? It is common for runners with buttock pain or classic sciatica to have a history of low back pain that is unassociated with their running careers. Preexisting knee problems may also cause pain that appears at level I running.

Physical Examination
Static Examination

The runner is examined standing, lying down (both supine and prone), and kneeling on the examining table. During this examination the runner is wearing running clothes. The runner also should bring the last several pairs of running shoes to this examination.

In examining the foot and ankle, the physician should note any calluses, blisters, or deformities of the forefoot such as hallux valgus, metatarsus adductus, and dorsal bunion, and of the hindfoot such as subtalar varus or valgus. Callus and blister formation may indicate not only an ill-fitting shoe, but also a biomechanical imbalance.

Three foot types are commonly responsible for running injuries: cavus, hyperpronated, and Morton's. The cavus foot (Fig. 64-6) is highly arched and rigid, with limited subtalar motion and pronation. This foot does not adequately absorb shock or adapt to the running surface. Physicians frequently see Achilles tendinitis or plantar fasciitis associated with this type of foot. The hyperpronated foot (Fig. 64-7), however, is flexible and is thus associated with excessive subtalar motion. It suggests a

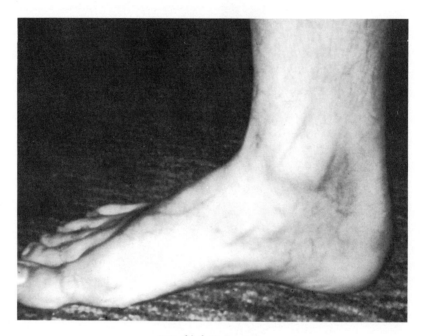

FIG. 64-6. Cavus foot.

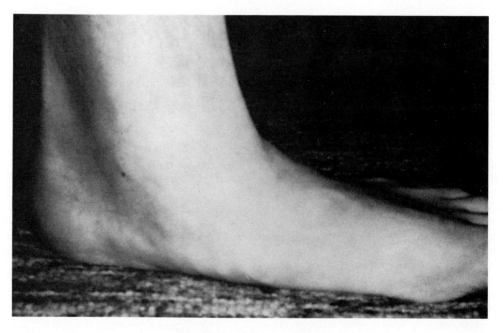

FIG. 64-7. Hyperpronated foot.

high degree of correlation between patellofemoral pain syndrome and medial tibial pain. The so-called Morton's foot, which is characterized by an excessively mobile first ray and an elongated second metatarsal, is frequently associated with hyperpronation in many high-stress injuries. In a study by Drez, there was no difference in the incidence of stress fracture between this particular foot type and the neutral foot.

Standing Examination

The physician should observe the patient with the patient's feet 5 inches apart and the knees together. The overall contour of the spine reveals the presence of any abnormal curvature or pelvic tilt. The general alignment of the lower extremities on weight bearing exhibits the presence of knee varus or valgus and "malicious malalignment syndrome" (broad pelvis, femoral anteversion, knee valgus, external tibial torsion, and pronation). The foot can be identified as cavus, neutral, or pronated.

Supine Examination

Evaluation for discrepancy in leg length is performed with the examiner measuring from the umbilicus to the inferior margin of the medial malleolus (apparent leg length) and from the anterior superior iliac spine to the same point (true leg length). The physician tests range

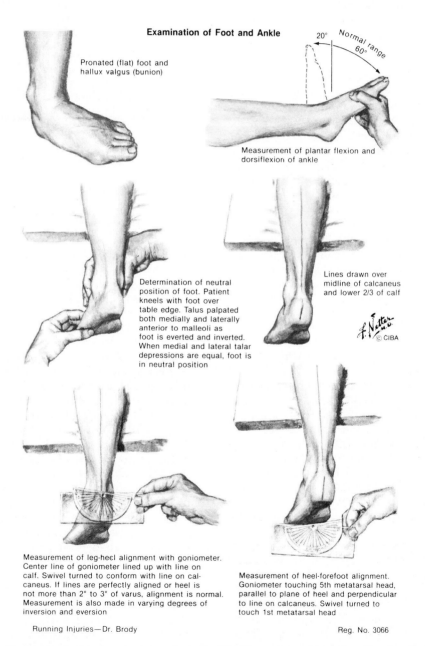

Examination of Foot and Ankle

Pronated (flat) foot and hallux valgus (bunion)

20° Normal range 60°

Measurement of plantar flexion and dorsiflexion of ankle

Determination of neutral position of foot. Patient kneels with foot over table edge. Talus palpated both medially and laterally anterior to malleoli as foot is everted and inverted. When medial and lateral talar depressions are equal, foot is in neutral position

Lines drawn over midline of calcaneus and lower 2/3 of calf

Measurement of leg-heel alignment with goniometer. Center line of goniometer lined up with line on calf. Swivel turned to conform with line on calcaneus. If lines are perfectly aligned or heel is not more than 2° to 3° of varus, alignment is normal. Measurement is also made in varying degrees of inversion and eversion

Measurement of heel-forefoot alignment. Goniometer touching 5th metatarsal head, parallel to plane of heel and perpendicular to line on calcaneus. Swivel turned to touch 1st metatarsal head

Running Injuries—Dr. Brody

Reg. No. 3066

FIG. 64-8. Swivel goniometer. (© Copyright 1980, CIBA Pharmaceutical Company, Division of CIBA-GEIGY Corporation. Reprinted with permission from *Clinical Symposia,* illustrated by Frank H. Netter, M.D. All rights reserved.)

of motion of the hips (flexion, extension, internal and external rotation, abduction, and adduction), knees (flexion, extension, and any pathologic instability), and ankles (dorsiflexion and plantar flexion). This measurement of the intrinsic ankle motion and the degree of calf muscle flexibility is done with the knee in full extension. Adequate calf muscle flexibility is indicated by 20 degrees of dorsiflexion.

Prone Examination

With the knees flexed to 90 degrees, tibial leg lengths can be assessed. At this point the midline of the calcaneus and the midline of the calf are marked with a water-soluble, broad-nib art marker, as is the most prominent portion of the tarsal navicular bone. These reference points are used in determining the range of motion of subtalar joint inversion and eversion, the neutral position of the subtalar joint, and forefoot varus or valgus.

Kneeling Examination

The runner is instructed to kneel on the examining table so that his or her body is upright with the ankle extending over the end of the examining table. The examiner is able to measure heel eversion and inversion with the use of a swivel goniometer (Fig. 64-8). The normal ratio of inversion/eversion is 2:1 to 3:1. A total subtalar motion of 30 degrees is normal, but many asymptomatic runners exhibit a range of motion of only 10 to 20 degrees.

The examiner measures leg-heel alignment by drawing one line over the midline of the lower two thirds of the calf and another line over the midline of the calcaneus at the insertion of the Achilles tendon. If these lines are aligned or parallel or the heel does not have more than 2 or 3 degrees of varus, leg-heel alignment is normal. Heel-forefoot alignment is normal if a line drawn over the midline of the calcaneus is perpendicular to the plane of the metatarsal heads. A defect in either of these alignments may cause abnormal motions in running, particularly hyperpronation.

The relationship between the plane of the hindfoot and that of the forefoot is measured by resting the goniometer on the head of the fifth metatarsal (plantar aspect) and rotating the swivel to touch the first metatarsal head. This measurement is best done with the subtalar joint held in a neutral relaxed position, using the neutral position of congruency of the subtalar joint. Normal forefoot varus is approximately 3 degrees.

To determine the neutral position of the subtalar joint by the technique of congruency, place the thumb and index finger on either side of the ankle (tibiotalar joint). In examining the left ankle the examiner's index finger is just in front of the anterior aspect of the fibula and the thumb just anterior and inferior to the medial malleolus. By inverting and everting the hindfoot and ankle, the examiner senses that the depressions felt by the index finger and thumb are equal (Fig. 64-9). This is the neutral position of the subtalar joint and the position of optimal function of the foot. This position is used in making prescription orthotic devices and in determining navicular drop.

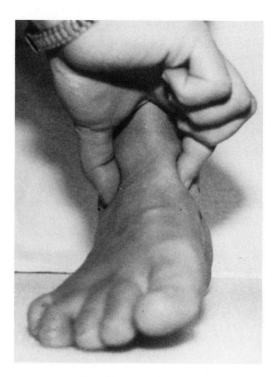

FIG. 64-9. Position of congruency.

The determination of **navicular drop** as described by Schuster has been helpful in evaluating the significance and amount of pronation in a runner's foot. I am frequently asked how much pronation is abnormal. Certainly, in the biomechanics of running, the amount and time spent in pronation in midstance may produce painful symptoms in the ankle, medial tibia, knee, hip, and low back. With the patient standing barefoot on a firm surface with the midline of the heel, lower half of the calf, and the navicular bone marked, the standing foot is placed so that the subtalar joint is in the neutral position (as palpated by the examiner's thumb and index finger, as previously explained) (Fig. 64-10). With a card placed on the inner side of the hindfoot, the level of the navicular is marked on the card. Then the foot is allowed to relax with weight bearing, and the resulting lower position of the navicular is also marked on the card. The distance between the original height of the navicular (with the subtalar joint in neutral) and its final weight-bearing position is the navicular drop (Fig. 64-11). This office procedure is a practical method of determining the amount of pronation in a runner's foot. Normal amounts of navicular drop are ⅜ inch, or approximately 10 mm. Drops greater than ⅝ inch, or about 15 mm, have been found in my clinic to correlate well with injury in the hyperpronated individual. Another technique is to have the runner hop on one foot so as to land on the plantar surface rather than just the forefoot. From the heel and navicular markings, the degree of navicular drop can be appreciated. The finding that this measurement is abnormal may be helpful in deciding whether an orthotic device is indicated for the symptomatic runner.

The runner's shoes should be examined if possible

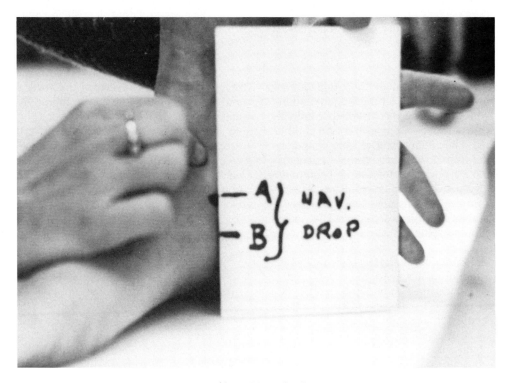

FIG. 64-10. Navicular drop.

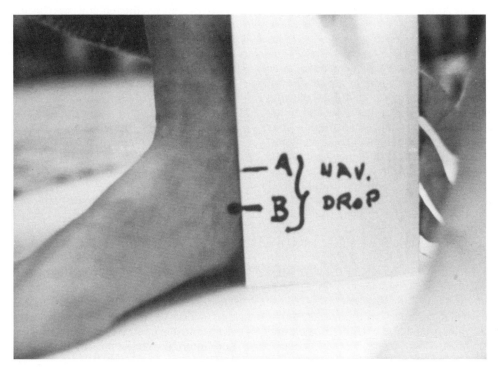

FIG. 64-11. Navicular drop.

Wear in the forefoot area indicates that he or she runs on the toes, and wear on the outer heel and sole indicates a supinated foot. Wear on the lateral heel is common, and if severe may be the cause of lateral knee pain (iliotibial band syndrome) or lateral hip pain.

Radiographic Examination

Plain radiographs are essential in the evaluation of many running injuries. The need for these examinations must be explained to the runner because many individuals are as suspicious of radiography as they are of other medical procedures. The anteroposterior, lateral, tangential ("sunrise"), and tunnel views are needed in diagnosing knee problems, especially preexisting conditions, malalignments, and patella tracking problems. Anteroposterior and lateral radiographs of the weight-bearing foot are most helpful for foot injuries. Standard five views for the low back (lumbar spine) are also helpful. Arthrography is rarely used for a runner except when he or she sustains a rotational injury. It is certainly indicated when a preexisting problem of meniscal origin is suspected.

The use of bone scans is most helpful in the early evaluation of stress fractures. CT scans and MRI scans have been helpful in eliciting changes and finding disk herniations in runners who are complaining of sciatica. These latter two tests should not be overdone not only because of their expense, but also because of the irradiation involved in CT scans. Bone scans are most helpful in and about the pelvis, where irradiation to the gonads is 100 times less than direct plain radiography and much more sensitive in diagnosing pelvic stress fractures. The MRI has been proven to be most helpful in the spine, hips, knees, and ankles in runners but should be used judiciously.

Dynamic Examination

For the past 15 years I have used videotape analysis and a treadmill to evaluate the running gait of the injured runner. This has been most helpful in allowing runners to visualize their own running gaits and to appreciate the biomechanics and mechanism that may have played a role in the development of their problems. However, this may be impractical in the average office.

The treadmill system has evolved over the years to use an elevated treadmill 4 feet long with a running belt 21 inches wide and a rear platform 33 inches wide. The treadmill is elevated on wheels for movement and is 11 inches off the ground. This is important for the video technique—if the running surface were floor level, the camera operator would have to lie on the floor to film the runner. The treadmill has speeds of 0 to 10 miles an hour and can automatically be elevated from a level position to 20 degrees of incline.

There are many video recorders on the market today. Our system uses ½-inch tape and a 19-inch black and white television. Most video recorders have regular speed, slow motion, and stop action (freeze frame), and tapes can be reused if necessary. No processing of film is necessary.

The runner, depending on the level of ability, is "run" at between 2½ and 5 miles per hour on a level surface.

The individual may be videotaped on a track or road surface, which is even more indicative of his or her normal gait. Videotaping with a hand-held camera is done from the front, recording movements of the foot and ankle and then, progressively, the tibia, knee, and pelvis. Next the camera (which has a 12-foot cord) is moved to the side to observe foot and knee movements and finally to the rear, beginning at the level of the lower spine and pelvis and gradually moving down to the thigh, knee, leg, and foot. The markings on the lower calf, heel, and navicular show well on the videotape and give an excellent picture of movement of the foot and ankle. Factors not obvious in the static examination may become plain on videotape playback, especially in slow motion and stop action. After a brief discussion of running in general, the examiner and runner review the tape together.

KNEE INJURIES
Patellofemoral Pain Syndrome

By far the most commonly seen knee problem in our runners' clinics is patellofemoral pain syndrome (patellofemoral arthralgia or anterior knee pain syndrome), a tracking abnormality of the patella frequently referred to as "runner's knee." This term has been used erroneously with the condition of chondromalacia.

The finding of true chondromalacia is best made as a pathologic diagnosis in which there are varying degrees of degenerative changes on the articular surface of the patella. During knee flexion and extension the patella tracks or glides in the groove between the femoral condyles. When the knee is fully extended, the patella is above the level of the femoral condyle and in contact with the fat pad of the suprapatellar pouch. As the knee flexes, there is greater contact between the articular surface of the patella and the groove of the femoral condyles. Tension in the patellar tendon increases as the knee flexes, increasing the compressive forces within the patellofemoral joint. The patella is maintained within the femoral groove by the height of the medial and lateral femoral condyles and by the muscular balance between the transverse and oblique fibers of the vastus medialis and the vastus lateralis muscles and the ligamentous part of the medial and lateral patellar retinacula and iliotibial tract.

Certain anatomic and biomechanical factors affect the normal tracking of the patella. Tightness of the vastus lateralis, iliotibial tract, and lateral retinaculum, coupled with weakness of the vastus medialis, moves the patella laterally when the knee flexes, causing pain of the quadriceps on contraction. Malicious malalignment syndrome is also associated with lateral displacement of the patella. The increased Q angle produces the bowstring effect on the quadriceps, pulling the patella laterally as the quadriceps muscle contracts at heel strike and as the tibia rotates internally on the pronated foot in midstance. Patella alta predisposes the patella to lateral stress and instability.

The typical runner with patellofemoral pain syndrome is a level I recreational runner who increases his or her mileage rapidly. The runner initially describes the pain as aching or soreness in the peripatellar area or under the kneecap, especially in the medial facet. The pain is aggravated by stair climbing or hill running. Symptoms may indeed abate during running, only to recur at the end of the run or later the same day. The first episode of pain may result from running after prolonged sitting, such as a long car or plane trip, or from a direct blow to the patella. "Running through" this injury invariably worsens the symptoms, which force the runner to seek medical attention. Stiffness after sitting or "giving out" of the knee may also bring the runner to the physician.

The patient may exhibit the malicious malalignment syndrome of poorly developed vastus medialis, squinting patellae, joint crepitus, or mild effusion. If the examiner attempts to move the patella laterally, the patient contracts the quadriceps (i.e., the positive anxiety or apprehension sign).* Extending the knee from 30 degrees of flexion to full extension against resistance reproduces the pain, as does compression of the patella against the femoral condyle.

Standard radiographs may yield normal results, but the tangential views may reveal an increased femoral sulcus angle, an inadequately developed lateral femoral condyle, and a "jockey cap" appearance of the patella.

Arthroscopy has developed into a most helpful tool in the treatment of many athletic injuries. However, runners do not usually sustain rotational injuries, and the incidence of Grades II or III chondromalacia is rare in the runner. The runner is usually complaining of patellofemoral arthralgia, and there is no visible articular damage to the surface of the patella. Any runner with preexisting patellofemoral pathologic change or chondromalacia is certainly a candidate for arthroscopy. At the time of arthroscopy the athlete who is found to have a cartilaginous injury of Types I, II, or III from a preexisting injury may see his or her running career end. There is often a lack of improvement following patellar or femoral condyle shaving in arthroscopy, so the athlete is unable to withstand impact loading in running.

Arthroscopy is usually not indicated except in cases that have failed to respond to conservative measures. The finding of a medial shelf and its treatment arthroscopically may produce a cure. However, pain around the patella can have many other sources; thus most individuals with even prolonged symptoms of patellofemoral arthralgia associated with a running career may have a negative arthroscopic examination.

In differential diagnosis the physician must consider rheumatoid arthritis, sepsis, osteochondritis dissecans, pigmented villonodular synovitis, and synovitis of the knee. Hip or pelvis abnormalities may produce referred pain by femoral nerve distribution in the distal anterior thigh, which may be misinterpreted by the patient or physician as "knee pain." Nothing can be more shocking than to examine a patient who has a primary bone tumor of the ilium, hip, or femur and for whom an orthotic device for "runner's knee" has been prescribed.

Treatment

The painful inflammation must be eliminated before running is resumed (Fig. 64-12). For the runner seen soon after the first appearance of symptoms, the treatment includes rest, nonsteroidal antiinflammatory drugs (NSAIDs), and application of ice to the knee (ice massage*) (Fig. 64-13) until the skin turns red (10 to 15 minutes). After 24 to 36 hours, ice treatment is discontinued and moist heat is applied to the knee for 15 to 20 minutes several times a day for as long as needed.

---

*Editors' note: With the patient prone and the knee extended, the medial and lateral patellar surfaces can be palpated without causing the patient apprehension.

*Ice massage: A Styrofoam cup filled with water can be frozen. The top of the cup is then torn off, and the ice is applied in a rotational manner.

	Day 1	2	3	4	5	6	7	TOTAL
Week								
1	2	0	2	0	2	0	3	9 miles
2	0	3	0	3	0	4	0	10 miles
3	4	3	0	4	4	0	5	20 miles
4	4	0	5	5	0	6	5	25 miles
5	0	6	6	0	7	6	6	31 miles
6	0	7	7	8	7	0	9	38 miles

Return to previous level of running in 6 weeks

FIG. 64-12. Return to running after injury.

Flexibility training for runners

A flexibility program should be part of all running programs at all levels. The most appropriate exercises are as follows:

- Back stretch—Lie on your back with both knees bent. Pull one or both knees up to your chest and hold for 5 seconds. Repeat.
- Partial sit-up—Lie on your back with both knees bent. Curl your head and shoulders upward, reaching for your knees with both hands. Stop when the tips of your shoulder blades leave the floor. Hold this position for 5 seconds.
- Hamstring stretch—Sit on the floor with your feet straight in front of you. Reach for your toes until you feel a stretch in the backs of your thighs. Hold this position for 5 seconds.
- Adductor stretch—Sit on the floor with your knees straight and legs spread apart as far as possible. Bend forward until you feel a stretch in the inside of your thighs. Hold this position for 5 seconds.
- Quadriceps stretch—Stand facing a stationary object for support. Bend one knee back as far as possible, then reach back with your hand and grasp the foot. Pull the heel toward the buttocks until you feel a stretch in the front of the thigh. Hold this position for 5 seconds. *Do not arch your back.*

- Heel cord stretch—Stand facing a stationary object with your feet apart and your toes turned in slightly. Place your hands on the object and lean forward until you feel a stretch in the calf of your leg. Hold for 5 seconds. *Do not bend your knees or allow your heels to come off the floor.*
- Soleus stretch—Assume same position as for heel cord stretch. Place one foot forward and bend the knee. Lean forward, keeping the heel of the front foot on the ground. You should feel a stretch in the lower part of the calf of your forward leg. Hold for 5 seconds.
- Dorsiflexor strengthening—Sit in a chair with both legs out straight. Place the heel of one foot on top of the toes of the other foot. Pull the toes toward you, applying resistance with the heel of the other foot. Hold for 5 seconds, then repeat with the other leg.
- Quadriceps strengthening—Sit in a chair with both legs out straight. Place one leg over the other leg. Keeping the knee of the bottom leg straight, lift both legs 4 to 6 inches off the ground, applying resistance with the top leg. Hold for 5 seconds, then repeat with the other leg.

The supplemental use of weight training can be most helpful when done judiciously.

Rest from running is essential. Although the runner may say that he or she can alleviate the pain by running with the feet turned in (which decreases the Q angle), this can only be done until the runner becomes fatigued. The patient should also curtail activities that place the patella under compressive loading such as kneeling, excessive stair-climbing, and prolonged sitting. When the pain is gone, the patient begins a progressive resistance exercise program with the knees in extension to strengthen the quadriceps—especially the vastus medialis. The runner who does not do well with this type of program may benefit from high-voltage, galvanic, electric stimulation in physiotherapy.

The runner may begin a graduated program of running (Fig. 64-12) when he or she can run without pain. Immediately after a run, ice should be applied to the knee, followed several hours later by moist heat (Fig. 64-14). Weight training should be continued to avoid recur-

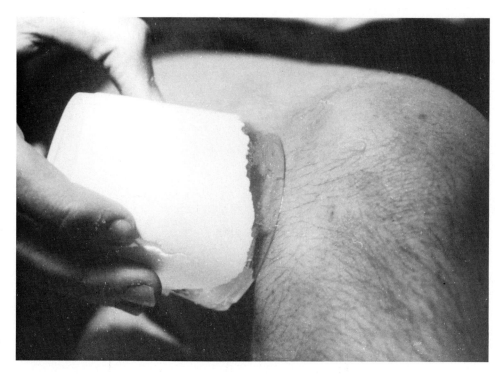

FIG. 64-13. Ice massage.

rence. Correction of a tracking problem frequently involves the use of a temporary orthotic device to block excessive pronation and internal rotation. This orthotic device can be made in the office and may wear out quickly, but it is an excellent clinical test (Fig. 64-15). This may necessitate the fabrication of a prescription orthotic device (Fig. 64-26). Results with orthotic devices in the

treatment of patellofemoral pain syndrome have been most gratifying.

Knee wraps, horseshoe braces, infrapatellar straps, and derotation braces have been used to relieve symptoms with varying degrees of success. Intraarticular injection of steroids may alleviate symptoms but is rarely used; it is preferrable to correct the biomechanical problem with exercises and orthotic devices. Surgery is rarely performed except in recalcitrant cases in which symptoms persist with normal daily activities. Arthroscopy may reveal a medial shelf, and in some difficult cases, a proximal realignment with an arthroscopic lateral release may be helpful. In the adolescent with chondromalacia with or without subluxation, correction of the biomechanical problems to allow running should be done only if the child can run painlessly. It may be wise to direct the child to another sport.

Iliotibial Band Friction Syndrome

The iliotibial band or tract is a thickened portion of tensor fasciae latae that passes down the lateral aspect of the thigh and inserts into Gerdy's tubercle on the lateral tibial condyle. As the knee flexes and extends during running, the iliotibial tract repeatedly rubs over the lateral femoral condyle, which may cause an inflammatory reaction. This is most commonly seen in the varus knee. The resulting lateral knee pain is above the joint line but is not as localized as the pain in popliteus tendinitis, which is a less common source of lateral knee pain. The iliotibial band friction syndrome usually occurs with rapid increase in mileage in a runner with tibia vara associated with either hyperpronated or cavus feet. The symptoms can occur if a runner fails to repair a worn

---

Running routine

Daytime

1. Moist heat (swimming)

2. Stretching

3. Running as prescribed

4. Ice massage (10 minutes)

Nighttime

1. Moist heat

2. Stretching

3. Weight lifting

4. Back exercises

FIG. 64-14. Running routine.

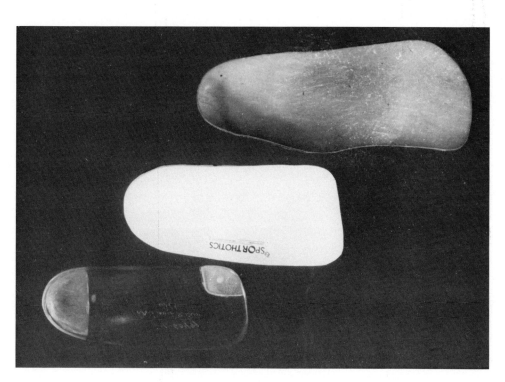

FIG. 64-15. Orthotic devices.

Factors associated with iliotibial band friction syndrome

- Rapid increase in weekly mileage
- Tibia vara
- Hyperpronation
- Cavus foot
- Worn outer heel of running shoe
- Iliotibial band contracture (positive result to Ober's test)

---

outer heel of the running shoe thus increasing varus loading on the lateral aspect of the knee.

Treatment

Therapy for the iliotibial band friction syndrome includes application of ice to the knee and ice massage for up to 5 minutes or until the area is numb. These measures are continued until symptoms subside. The use of NSAIDs may also be helpful. The modalities of ultrasound with 10% Hytone Creme (6 sessions) or the use of "friction massage" over the band has produced variable results in runners. This is followed by exercises to stretch the iliotibial tract (Fig. 64-16). These measures are continued until symptoms subside. In our experience the injection of steroids is helpful in this situation where the injection is given both superficial and deep to the iliotibial tract at the site of the femoral epicondyle. Surgery was performed in 11 recalcitrant cases in which symptoms persisted for over 1½ years. At the time of surgery an effervescent bursa was found deep in the tender area between the iliotibial tract and the femoral epicon-

dyle. This was excised, and a T-type tenotomy was performed on the iliotibial tract. Relief of the symptoms was complete in all 11 runners. It must be emphasized that surgery for this condition is rare, and most individuals are cured by correcting the worn lateral heel of the running shoe and using conservative measures. The use of orthotic devices for lateral knee pain of this type has not been found to be helpful.

Popliteus Tendinitis

Popliteus tendinitis is directly related to both hyperpronation and downhill running and is frequently seen in runners who run along the beach or other banked surfaces, which increase the pronation of the foot on the higher part of the slope. Internal tibial rotation applies traction to the attachment of the popliteus tendon to the lateral femoral epicondyle. Treatment of popliteus tendinitis is the same as the treatment for iliotibial band friction syndrome.

Patellar Tendinitis

Patellar tendinitis, either involving the midbody of the patellar tendon or the proximal attachment of the patellar tendon to the patella itself, is not a common injury in runners. The usual conservative treatment as outlined for popliteus tendinitis is most helpful. Medial pain in a runner's knee usually results from a preexisting medial meniscal injury or from a stress fracture involving the medial flare of the tibia. The latter may have to be diagnosed on the bone scan. Pes anserinus bursitis and strain of the medial collateral ligament (MCL) are uncommon but are seen in older runners and in women with marked genu valgum and increased to-and-fro femoral motion with the gynecoid pelvis.

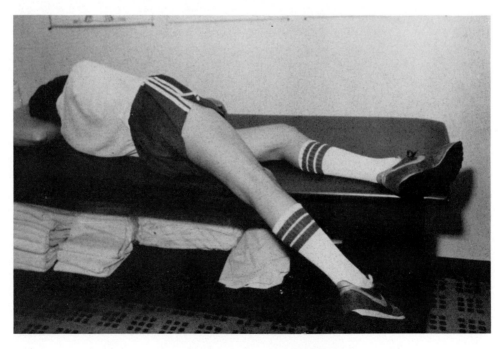

FIG. 64-16. Stretching iliotibial band.

LEG AND FOOT INJURIES*

Formerly the term "shin splints" referred to any pain from the level of the patellar tendon to the ankle that caused discomfort in the runner. Since the late 1960s and early 1970s, it has referred to pain on the medial aspect of the distal two thirds of the shaft of the tibia. Three separate diagnostic problems may produce pain in the medial distal two thirds of the tibia. The runner refers to these as "shin splints." However, they may be (1) posterior tibial tendinitis, (2) periostitis, or (3) a stress fracture of the tibia. Posterior tibial tendinitis is usually an

overuse syndrome in level I or II runners that usually develops early in their careers when conditioning is poor as a result of running on hard surfaces with poor shoes. It can also be caused by wearing improper running shoes or running on a banked track or shoulder of the road. Excessive femoral anteversion, external tibial torsion, hyperpronation, or increased eversion of the heel contributes to this injury.

A runner with a malalignment problem and who runs in poorly supporting shoes on a hard or banked surface repeatedly applies traction to the posterior tibial tendon at its attachment to the tibia and interosseous membrane (Fig. 64-17). This repeated stress produces **tendinitis.** When untreated, especially if the runner attempts to

*Also see Chapter 28.

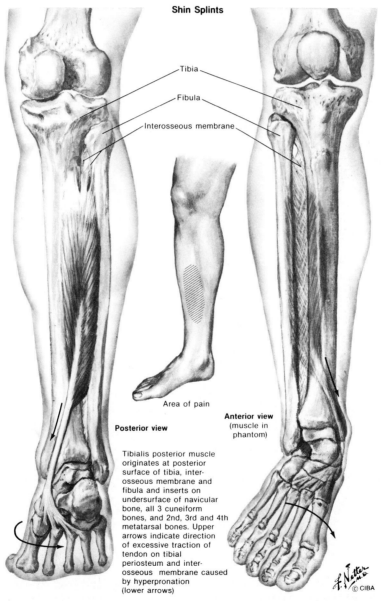

FIG. 64-17. Posterior tibial tendinitis. (© Copyright 1980, CIBA Pharmaceutical Company, Division of CIBA-GEIGY Corporation. Reprinted with permission from *Clinical Symposia,* illustrated by Frank H. Netter, M.D. All rights reserved.)

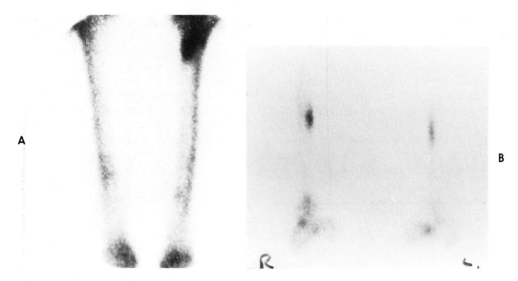

FIG. 64-18. A, Streaking seen in periostitis of tibia on bone scan (technetium-99). **B,** Localized uptake in stress fracture of tibia.

"run through it," there is a chronic traction effect on the periosteum, which produces periostitis. This latter diagnosis is usually made on bone scan with the "streaking" phenomenon evident (Fig. 64-18, *A*). If symptoms go on for a number of years, plain radiography shows irregularities in new bone formation at the attachment of both posterior tibial tendons and the interosseous membrane. The bone scan pattern, as mentioned previously, reveals increased longitudinal patterns of "streaking" as opposed to the localized accumulation of radioactive material, as is noted in a stress fracture. The latter is not an uncommon finding in the level II and even the level IV runner, who injudiciously increases his or her mileage rapidly in preparation for a race. Pain in posterior tibial tendinitis increases gradually with soreness after the run, but as training continues, the pain is present both during and after the run. In severe cases, walking and stair-climbing can become painful. There is usually tenderness along the distal third and occasionally the distal two thirds of the medial aspect of the tibia. Treatment involves rest, ice massage, and wrapping or taping of the leg for comfort in daily activities. Running must stop completely. When symptoms subside, the patient is aided a great deal by a simple commercial orthotic device to block hyperpronation and excessive rotation. If the runner adapts to increased training using this temporary device, he or she may not need a permanent device.

Periostitis, however, as mentioned previously, is usually caused by a prolonged attempt to "run through" posterior tibial tendinitis. In my experience it usually takes a great deal longer to heal. This usually occurs in the level III runner who is running 40 to 70 miles a week and is in an intensive training program in preparation for a race. The use of such conservative measures as alternating ice and heat, ice massage, cessation of all running, and the wearing of an orthotic device has been

helpful. The bone scan usually shows the previously mentioned streaking, and the treatment certainly includes use of NSAIDs. Local injections have not been advocated or thought to be advisable. I have carried out surgery on four athletes who had chronic periostitis for over 4 years. These individuals had classic histories of doing well at lower levels of mileage, but their symptoms recurred in direct relationship to their increased mileage. Open periosteal stripping of the attachment of the posterior tibial tendon and the periosteum to the tibia successfully eliminated symptoms in these four cases. There have been no recurrences of symptoms in these individuals, one of whom had a bilateral condition.

A **stress fracture** of the tibia (Fig. 64-18, *B*) is the third leading cause of medial distal tibial pain. The initial bone scan finding is usually negative. The sine qua non treatment of the stress fracture is rest. Essentially, the individual who has a stress fracture must be given some alternative means of training to maintain not only cardiovascular fitness, but also psychologic drive. The use of Nautilus equipment on the upper and lower body, swimming, running in water, cycling, and rowing are all appropriate while awaiting healing of the stress fracture.

Chronic Anterior (Tibial) Compartment Syndrome

Chronic anterior (tibial) compartment syndrome usually occurs when a runner changes from a flat-foot to a toe running style, begins interval training on a track or hill, or runs in a shoe with a sole that is too flexible. All of these overload the anterior compartment musculature, producing pain in this area along the extensor tendons of the ankle and foot. Anterior compartment syndrome caused by segmental artery spasm or by ischemia of the muscle or nerves from increased tension in the fascia compartments is rare in runners. Catheter studies (Fig. 64-19) have been helpful in making this diagnosis. Ath-

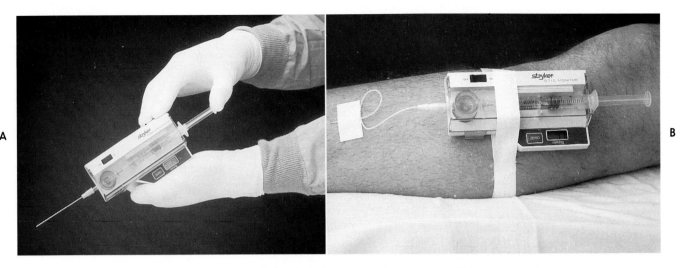

A

B

FIG. 64-19. A, Compartment catheter. **B,** Catheter inserted into anterior tibial compartment.

letes run on treadmills with catheters inserted in their anterior compartments to measure compartment pressures during the act of running.

Symptoms usually occur at a given distance and can be predicted by the runner, who notes increasing amounts of pain beyond a given distance, which forces him or her to stop running. Stopping the run causes the pain to gradually diminish.

Treatment

Successful treatment includes proper training techniques: wearing good shoes, running on a level surface, no excessive hill or speed work, stretching exercises, and strengthening exercises for the anterior compartment musculature.

Fasciotomy has been most helpful in the level III or level IV runner, allowing for expansion of the muscles in the anterior compartment. In the 11 operations I have performed, the results have been satisfactory, with all of the individuals returning to their previous levels of running. It should be mentioned that more than one compartment may have to be released at a given sitting because obviously similar problems may occur in the posterior compartment both superficially and deep.

In considering a differential diagnosis in a runner with anterior compartment syndrome, the physician should certainly consider a fibula stress fracture, thrombophlebitis, osteomyelitis, cellulitis, tumors, and intermittent claudication.

Lateral (Peroneal) Compartment Syndrome of the Ankle

Hyperpronation in the runner with or without a history of lateral ankle compartment sprains may cause lateral ankle pain as the individual increases mileage. The runner may report that his or her ankle "gives out." The treatment is an orthotic device to maintain the foot in a neutral position. A lateral heel wedge or a reinforced shoe upper stabilizes the foot and ankle. A

well-fitting rigid heel counter also helps maintain the heel in a neutral position and prevents eversion. The use of an ankle orthotic (AO) and a foot orthotic (FO) has been helpful in level I runners. In individuals who are only interested in low levels of running coupled with other sports, these orthotics have been found to be most satisfying. To strengthen the muscles of the lateral compartment, the runner should perform isometric exercises in which he or she pushes the foot against an immovable object while seated with the knee flexed and the ankle at a right angle, both in inversion and eversion. The use of a weight program to strengthen both the anterior and posterior compartments has been found helpful, as has grasping a towel with the toes of the bare foot resting on the floor. Careful evaluation with appropriate stress radiographs may have to be made for gross lateral ankle instability and to elicit a possible anterior drawer sign in the ankle. In my experience runners undergoing reconstruction of the lateral compartment for instability have not returned to any significantly high levels of running with or without an ankle-foot orthosis (AFO).

Achilles Tendinitis (Fig. 64-20)

Acute Achilles tendinitis is a painful inflammatory reaction of the pseudosheath about the Achilles tendon. The tendon does not have a true synovial sheath but is surrounded by a paratenon. Acute cases of tendinitis involve the paratenon and not the tendon itself. In severe or chronic Achilles tendinitis a nodule composed of mucoid degeneration with longitudinal fissures forms in the body of the tendon. The two most common training errors that lead to the development of Achilles tendinitis are running on hills and wearing shoes with rigid soles. Hill training, in which the runner lands with up to four times the body's weight on the heel running downhill and toeing off with an inflexible-soled shoe going uphill, can place abnormal stress on the Achilles tendon.

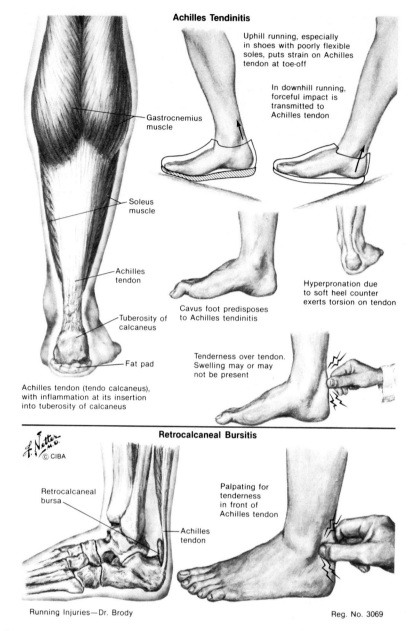

FIG. 64-20. Achilles tendinitis. (© Copyright 1980, CIBA Pharmaceutical Company, Division of CIBA-GEIGY Corporation. Reprinted with permission from *Clinical Symposia*, illustrated by Frank H. Netter, M.D. All rights reserved.)

Biomechanical problems such as tibia vara, functional talipes equinus, tight hamstrings and calf muscles, and a cavus foot are also associated with Achilles tendinitis. Heel or forefoot varus deformities cause the foot to land in an excessively supinated position and hyperpronate in midstance to compensate, which puts torque on the tendon. These repetitive stresses on the Achilles tendon at heel strike and toe-off and running on hills and uneven terrain inflict small cumulative tears in the paratenon that produce the inflammatory responses seen clinically. Initially, the patient complains of a burning type of pain during the run that becomes less severe as the run continues and worsens after the run. Early morning pain when the athlete gets out of bed and takes a few steps gradually subsides during the day. On examination, there is tenderness, usually 4 to 5 cm proximal to the insertion of the Achilles tendon into the calcaneus, but it may be diffuse along the tendon. In severe cases crepitus, swelling, and a tendon nodule develop. Measurement of subtalar motion shows absence of eversion in many of the biomechanical situations. The runner may have one or more of the biomechanical problems previously discussed: cavus foot, tight calf muscles, functional talipes equinus, pronated foot secondary to forefoot or hindfoot varus, or tibia vara.

```
┌─────────────────────────────────────────┐
│     Factors associated with Achilles tendinitis     │
│                                           │
│        ▪ Running on heels                 │
│        ▪ Shoe with rigid soles            │
│        ▪ Hill training                    │
│        ▪ Tibia vara                       │
│        ▪ Functional talipes equinus       │
│        ▪ Tight hamstrings                 │
│        ▪ Tight heel cords                 │
│        ▪ Cavus foot                       │
│        ▪ Forefoot varus or cavus          │
└─────────────────────────────────────────┘
```

Treatment

In acute cases, symptoms are treated with ice massage and antiinflammatory medication for the first several days. NSAIDs have been most helpful, but in our experience injections of steroids into and around the Achilles tendon are *contraindicated* because of the risk of tendon rupture. Cessation of all running is paramount. When symptoms start to subside, a gentle stretching program involving bent knee and straight leg exercises is most helpful and the patient begins a standard program of gradually increasing amounts of running with a new shoe, which must have a flexible sole, a well-molded Achilles pad, a heel wedge at least 15 mm high, and a rigid heel counter. A heel lift up to 2 inches inserted into everyday walking shoes also helps relax the Achilles tendon. In cases with excessive pronation, a prescription orthotic device is helpful in correcting the underlying malalignment. The cavus foot, however, is a more difficult problem. A heel wedge such as the Schuster type (Fig. 64-21) placed in the midsole of the heel of the shoe to essentially shorten the Achilles tendon has been most helpful. This helps not only to shorten the tendon but also to aid in absorbing impact at heel strike. High- and low-voltage galvanic stimulation have in certain instances been most helpful.

The level III or level IV runner who attempts to "run through" an acute Achilles tendinitis may convert this mild injury to a severe one with nodule formation, microtears, and mucoid degeneration of the tendon itself.

```
┌─────────────────────────────────────────┐
│       Treatment of Achilles tendinitis    │
│                                           │
│  Stage I (inflammatory)                   │
│    ▪ Rest                                 │
│    ▪ Ice massage                          │
│    ▪ Antiinflammatory medication          │
│    ▪ Heel lift in shoes                   │
│                                           │
│  Stage II (return to running sports)      │
│    ▪ Stretching                           │
│    ▪ Shoe modification                    │
│    ▪ Flexible sole                        │
│    ▪ Well-molded Achilles pad             │
│    ▪ Heel wedge                           │
│    ▪ Rigid heel counter                   │
│    ▪ Orthotic device, if appropriate      │
└─────────────────────────────────────────┘
```

This is a significant problem, especially when seen months or years later. The runner must stop running and go on an alternative program. Such chronic injuries may require surgical intervention with tenolysis and excision in areas of nodule formation. The degenerative material is excised and the remainder of the tendon sutured. In extreme cases the plantaris tendon is used to reinforce the repair. In our experience only 40% of runners who undergo this type of surgery go back to high-level performances.

Retrocalcaneal Bursitis

The runner's shoe may irritate a prominence on the calcaneus, causing a retrocalcaneal bursitis (Achilles bursitis), an inflammation of the bursa between the Achilles tendon and the calcaneus. Palpating with the thumb and index finger elicits tenderness anterior to the attachment of the tendon (Fig. 64-22). Radiographs may reveal a prominence in the calcaneus that in rare cases may have to be removed. The conservative measures used in treating Achilles tendinitis are also used in treating retrocalcaneal bursitis. Careful local injection of steroids into the region of the bursa may be helpful, but care must be taken to avoid injection into the Achilles tendon.

Plantar Fasciitis

Plantar fasciitis (heel spur syndrome) (Fig. 64-23) is the most common cause of heel pain in runners. It is an overuse syndrome involving an inflammatory reaction at the insertion of the plantar fascia into the calcaneus. The patient experiences pain with the first few steps taken in the morning. As in other overuse injuries, the pain develops in the beginning of a workout but diminishes during the run, only to recur at the finish or later that evening. On examination, palpation elicits point tenderness at the attachment of the plantar fascia to the heel, and radiographs may reveal a calcaneal spur. In my series the incidence of cavus foot is higher than that of hyperpronated foot, but there is increased eversion of the heel and a forefoot varus biomechanical problem.

Several conditions should be considered in differential diagnosis. In plantar arch strain the pain is located directly under the longitudinal arch. Certainly, rest and conservative measures effect a cure. If the treatment for plantar fasciitis is unsuccessful, the physician should suspect entrapment of the medial calcaneal branch of the tibial nerve. Pain is usually on the more medial side of the sole of the heel. Tarsal tunnel syndrome with entrapment of the tibial nerve causes pain on the medial aspect of the ankle and heel. Certainly the athlete who seeks help for plantar fasciitis has already tried heel pads, plastic heel cups, rest, and ice measures that certainly cure a great many heel injuries. If none of these measures is successful, the injection of steroids may relieve the pain but correction of the underlying imbalance is necessary for a cure. A ¼-inch felt heel pad, horseshoe-shaped pad, or Schuster heel wedge may help the runner with a cavus foot. A flexible laminated orthotic device ("leather laminate") has been successful in the pro-

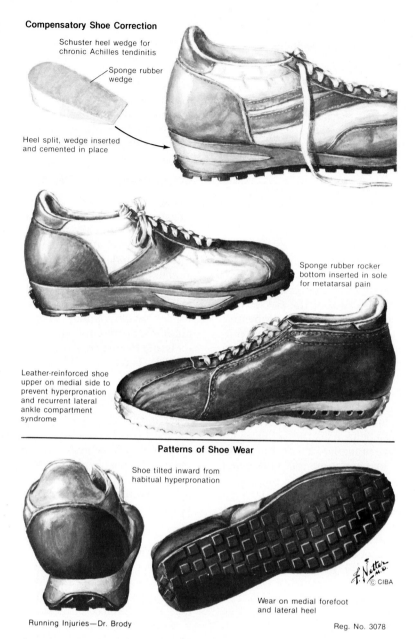

Compensatory Shoe Correction

Schuster heel wedge for
chronic Achilles tendinitis

Sponge rubber
wedge

Heel split, wedge inserted
and cemented in place

Sponge rubber rocker
bottom inserted in sole
for metatarsal pain

Leather-reinforced shoe
upper on medial side to
prevent hyperpronation
and recurrent lateral
ankle compartment
syndrome

Patterns of Shoe Wear

Shoe tilted inward from
habitual hyperpronation

Wear on medial forefoot
and lateral heel

Running Injuries—Dr. Brody

Reg. No. 3078

FIG. 64-21. Shoe corrections. (© Copyright 1980, CIBA Pharmaceutical Company, Division of CIBA-GEIGY Corporation. Reprinted with permission from *Clinical Symposia*, illustrated by Frank H. Netter, M.D. All rights reserved.)

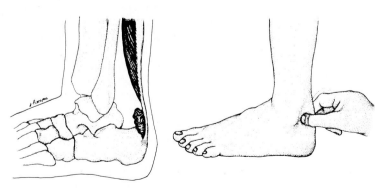

FIG. 64-22. Retrocalcaneal bursitis.

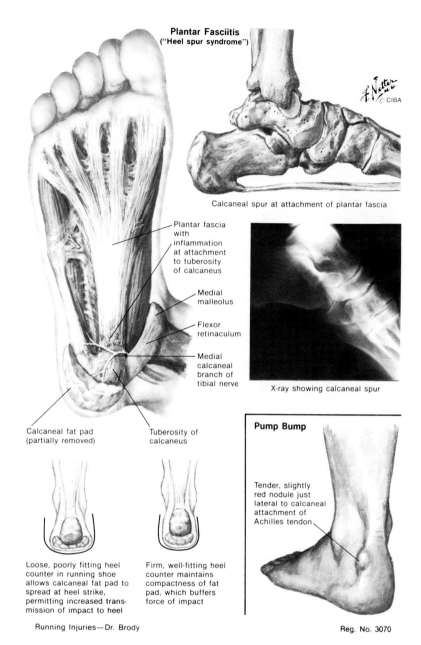

Plantar Fasciitis
("Heel spur syndrome")

Calcaneal spur at attachment of plantar fascia

Plantar fascia
with
inflammation
at attachment
to tuberosity
of calcaneus

Medial
malleolus

Flexor
retinaculum

Medial
calcaneal
branch of
tibial nerve

X-ray showing calcaneal spur

Calcaneal fat pad
(partially removed)

Tuberosity of
calcaneus

Loose, poorly fitting heel
counter in running shoe
allows calcaneal fat pad to
spread at heel strike,
permitting increased transmission of impact to heel

Firm, well-fitting heel
counter maintains
compactness of fat
pad, which buffers
force of impact

Running Injuries—Dr. Brody

Pump Bump

Tender, slightly
red nodule just
lateral to calcaneal
attachment of
Achilles tendon

Reg. No. 3070

FIG. 64-23. Plantar fasciitis.

nated foot. Bent leg stretches of the plantar fascia in the hyperpronated foot are most helpful. In rare cases surgical release of the attachment of the plantar fascia to the calcaneus, removal of the spur, and exploration of the medial calcaneal branch of the tibial nerve are indicated. The most serious problem here is the cavus foot in which it is essential that running be discontinued, the above-mentioned conservative measures tried, and a stable heel counter in the shoe prescribed.

Pump Bump

A pump bump is a painful bursa over a bony prominence lateral to the attachment of the Achilles tendon.

Inflammation develops here from poorly supported and poorly padded heel counters in the shoe, irritating a pre-existing enlargement of the calcaneus. The treatment is the usual conservative measures of NSAIDs plus the use of ice and gentle exercises, followed 2 to 3 hours later by warm soaks for 10 to 15 minutes. A runner with a severe injury may have to wear a backless shoe to help decrease the inflammation. The use of an orthotic device (Fig. 64-24) with a built-in heel counter cemented to the standard foot orthotic has been most helpful, with a cut-out heel cup allowing the area of the pump bump to be free of all pressure.

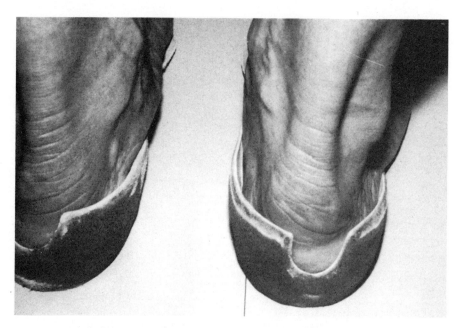

FIG. 64-24. Pump bump orthotic device. (© Copyright 1980, CIBA Pharmaceutical Company, Division of CIBA-GEIGY Corporation. Reprinted with permission from *Clinical Symposia*, illustrated by Frank H. Netter, M.D. All rights reserved.)

HIP, BUTTOCK, AND BACK PAIN

Back pain in runners makes up only about 5% of the running injuries that are seen. This is most frequently a result of preexisting degenerative disease in the lumbosacral spine in the middle-aged or older runner who increases mileage injudiciously and does abnormal amounts of hill training. Runners often complain of "hip" pain, but in many cases they are actually referring to symptoms or to an injury in the buttocks or pelvic area or referred pain from the lumbar spine. In determining the source of pain the examiner must differentiate between lateral hip injury (greater trochanteric bursitis or abductor muscle strain), true buttock pain (ischial bursitis, proximal hamstring injury), and lumbosacral spine disease producing buttock pain. Intrapelvic disorders, such as ovarian cyst and hernia, or any intraarticular problem, such as synovitis of the hip and femoral neck stress fracture, should also be considered when pain is felt in this area.

Differential diagnosis of hip and buttock pain

- Degenerative joint disease
- Referred back pain
- Trochanteric bursitis
- Abductor strain
- Ischial bursitis
- Hamstring strain
- Stress fracture
- Intrapelvic disorders

Lateral Hip Pain

There are several factors involved in lateral hip pain in runners, which may involve a strain of the distal attachment of the abductors, particularly the gluteus medius to the greater trochanter or the proximal attachment of the abductors to the iliac crest. These symptoms are usually seen in a runner with a broad pelvis and increased Q angle. A leg length discrepancy causing an abnormal pelvic tilt can also produce pain at the proximal portion of the gluteus medius. A gait problem in which the feet cross over the midline during running or running on and off sidewalks and curbs or on a banked surface may also produce pain in either the proximal or distal portion of the gluteus medius, pain and tenderness directly over the greater trochanter, or symptoms of greater trochanteric bursitis. Abductor muscle strain produces similar symptoms in the buttocks between the greater trochanter and the brim of the pelvis. Rest, ice applied immediately after running, and heat applied intermittently for 36 hours help to relieve the symptoms. Local steroid injection may also be used in chronic situations. A leg length discrepancy should be corrected with a lift inserted in the running shoe. It is not uncommon for a runner to develop gluteus medius strain on the side opposite the short leg because of abnormal pelvic tilt. Therefore a shoe lift for the nonpainful leg is a great help. As little as a ¼-inch leg length discrepancy should be corrected.

Iliac Apophysitis

Before fusion of the iliac apophyses in the adolescent runner, there may be pain at the attachments of the external oblique muscles and abdominal oblique muscles to the iliac apophysis. This is usually seen in the adolescent runner beginning a cross-country season who is running on irregularly canted surfaces. The treatment is cessation of all running until symptoms subside.

Ischial Bursitis

Ischial bursitis usually develops in an adolescent runner doing speed work. This condition can be associated with a fracture of the ischial apophysis caused by a violent contraction of the hamstring muscle. Tenderness directly over the ischium is caused by an inflammatory response at the attachment of the proximal hamstring muscles. The pain is aggravated by prolonged sitting, uphill running, and even carrying a wallet in the back pocket. Treatment is rest and application of ice followed by heat. Although rare in cases of ischial bursitis, a local injection of steroids may be considered in the adult.

Hamstring Muscle Injury

Symptoms of strain or partial tear of the proximal hamstrings, localized pain, or tenderness on bending or prolonged sitting appear suddenly if a hamstring muscle injury is caused by speed work or hill training. More commonly, symptoms develop slowly and are caused by inadequate stretching of these muscles before and after running. The treatment for acute hamstring injury in the proximal midthigh or distal thigh should initially be rest and application of ice, medication, and non–weight bearing. After that the patient can begin whirlpool bath therapy. When the symptoms abate, the runner can start gentle, active exercise. In a chronic hamstring strain, running, cycling, rowing, and prolonged driving should be stopped. Deep heat therapy, ultrasound, and electric acupuncture administered under the supervision of trained personnel can be used with supervised gentle hamstring stretching exercises.

Diskogenic Buttock and Back Pain

Radiculopathy with nerve root compression in the lumbar spine may produce and be the only cause of buttock pain with or without concomitant back pain. In a series of 11 level III and level IV runners complaining of buttock pain, all were found to have true disk ruptures diagnosed either by myelograms or CT scans. In only three of these athletes did back pain play a major role. Many of these runners had preexisting low back pain before their running careers began. (Running itself does not rupture disks.) Radiographs may reveal congenital anomalies such as spondylolysis and spondylolisthesis, degenerative disk disease with spinal stenosis, and nerve root entrapment syndromes. Stress fractures of the posterior elements of a lumbar vertebra have also been noted in this series. Certainly, treatment should involve rest, physical therapy, antiinflammatory medications, and further investigation as warranted using electromyography (EMG), myelography, and CT scanning. Many runners return to running after successful surgery. In returning from such an injury, running in water is most useful and swimming sidestroke and backstroke has been helpful. Freestyle swimming frequently aggravates the condition, as do cycling and rowing. Stress fractures of the pars in-

terarticularis have been seen in a number of young distance runners. This is usually associated with unilateral symptoms without radiculitis.

Piriformis Syndrome

The piriformis muscle may compress the sciatic nerve at the pelvis, causing localized tenderness in the buttock area between the ischium and the greater trochanter. However, this is a far less common cause of buttock pain than sciatic nerve involvement as with a herniated disk in the lumbar spine.*

Stress Fractures

Stress fractures are the most common overuse injury in running. These occur from the bone's inability to stand the repetitive force demanded of it by the poorly conditioned athlete's attempting to increase his or her mileage too quickly. These fractures may commonly occur from running too much or too fast with improper shoes and on a hard surface. The second most frequent victim is the level III runner getting ready for a marathon, who increases mileage from 40 to 70 miles a week over a 1- to 2-week period. Stress fractures have been seen in the lumbar vertebral bodies, pars interarticularis, sacroiliac joint, symphysis pubis (unilateral or bilateral osteitis pubis), iliac crest, neck of the femur, shaft of the proximal femur, medial proximal and medial distal tibia, distal fibula, lateral malleolus, and metatarsals. Most common sites are the metatarsal shafts, distal fibula, proximal tibia (medially), and symphysis pubis. Stress fracture may be suspected because of its ongoing pain even during walking, from a history of a recent increase in mileage, and from tenderness directly on a bone where the bone is palpable. Compartment syndromes and posterior tibial tendinitis or periostitis must be ruled out. Stress fracture may not appear on plain radiographs for 3 to 4 weeks after the onset of symptoms. Bone scans have been most helpful in the early diagnosis of stress fractures. A bone scan may remain positive for 14 to 24 months after injury and at times may not help determine whether a stress fracture has healed. The treatment of all stress fractures is *complete rest* from running. It should be remembered that stress fractures heal in varying amounts of time. Metatarsal stress fractures, if uncomplicated, heal anywhere from 4 to 10 weeks, distal fibula and tibial stress fractures in 6 to 10 weeks, fracture of the shaft of the femur in 3 months, and pelvic stress fractures in 1 to 1½ years.

The level I runner is particularly prone to fibular stress fractures because of the combination of possible hyperpronation or, most commonly, just excessive training. Injury is marked by the gradual onset of aching in the lateral ankle, absence of swelling, and point tenderness di-

---

*Editors' note: Before diskogenic disease was proved to be a major cause of sciatica by Barr and Mixter in 1931, piriformis tenotomy was a popular operation. Injection of the piriformis with a local anesthetic was the diagnostic test. If transient relief occurred with later recurrence of symptoms as the local anesthetic effect abated, the surgery was indicated. Occasionally this was found to be helpful, although only on an anecdotal basis.

rectly over, or three fingerbreadths proximal to, the tip of the lateral malleolus.

Stress fracture of the proximal medial tibia is commonly seen in runners with tibia vara. The fracture may involve just one cortex and may not be seen on radiographs for 4 to 6 weeks after the onset of symptoms. Pes anserinus bursitis is extremely rare, and physicians must consider a stress fracture of the medial flare of the tibia when individuals complain that the "inner side" of the knee hurts. On examination, the pain is *distal* to the joint line. An exact location is therefore essential in determining where the point of maximal tenderness is in these situations to rule out a medial compartment knee problem. In these stress fractures the treatment of choice is "benign neglect" and cessation of running. Athletes with significant pain may need the area immobilized for a period of time in a resin cast, which allows the runner with a stress fracture below the knee to run in water, cycle, or swim. An alternative training program of upper body training with Nautilus equipment or a similar upper body weight program, swimming, cycling, and rowing are certainly all advocated to maintain cardiovascular fitness while the stress fracture heals.

Pelvic Disorders

Osteitis pubis is a stress phenomenon involving the symphysis pubis, usually seen either unilaterally or bilaterally in runners at level II or level IV who increase their mileage or add interval training or speed work to their training routine. When one foot is in midstance, the opposite side of the pelvis drops, producing a rhythmic shearing force on the symphysis pubis. Small avulsion fractures occur at the attachment of the adductor tendons to the pubic bones and to the medial portion of the descending ramus. Abduction of the hip and abduction against resistance from the examiner's hand can produce pain. Radiographs reveal either unilateral or bilateral sclerosis of the pubic symphysis. Bone scans are obviously most helpful early after the onset of pain. When pelvic disorders are seen early, the treatment is complete cessation of all running and adductor stretching (which may in turn in the routine workout of the runner be helpful in preventing this problem). I have documented the same radiographic changes of osteitis pubis in runners over 40 years of age who have run from 15 to 20 years as in runners with pubic or groin pain caused by a sudden increase in training effort. Pain with osteitis pubis is usually located directly on the pubis with tenderness on palpation of this area.

In the differential diagnosis the physician must consider tumor, osteitis secondary to chronic prostatitis in men, traumatic delivery in women, adductor tendinitis (groin pull, which is characterized by tenderness on palpation of the tendons at their insertion), and fracture of the femoral neck (which is revealed on radiographs or bone scans). As mentioned previously, rest is the sine qua non of treatment. Heat therapy, including whirlpool or bath, is indicated. Steroid injections are not recommended. An alternate exercise program while this condition heals has been helpful. Upper body weight work and freestyle swimming (Australian crawl) using a flota-

tion device (pull-buoy) are the best substitute exercises. Swimming, using the frog or scissor kick, and bicycling may reproduce the symptoms. I have had no experience with surgery for osteitis pubis.

The prolonged pain resulting from pelvic stress fractures may be most disconcerting to level III or level IV runners. In my series of 43 cases of osteitis pubis, most were in these levels of running and eight were ultramarathoners. It is not uncommon for these individuals to take anywhere from 1 to 1½ years to recover from this injury and get back to their previous levels of running.

Abdominal Fascial Injuries

"Groin pain" above the level of the inguinal ligament may be caused by chronic fascial strain, which is difficult to alleviate because these strains are usually seen in high-intensity, level III and level IV runners. When such injuries are seen early, the conservative routine is cessation of running, antiinflammatory medication, and applications of ice and heat, or the standard physical therapy modalities such as ultrasound and electric stimulation have been helpful, but unfortunately many of these injuries are seen 1 to 2 years after the onset and are most difficult to treat. When injuries are in the distribution of the ilioinguinal and iliohypogastric nerves, steroid injection of these nerves has been helpful. Such injuries about the pelvis have been the most difficult of all running injuries to treat successfully.

Bone tumors in and about the pelvis, proximal femur, and distal femur certainly must be considered in diagnosing unusual pains in this area.

Iliac crest stress fractures and apophysitis of the anterior iliac crest similar to the "pointer" of adolescent football players occurs in adolescent runners who swing their arms across their bodies. Pain and localized tenderness develop over the anterior iliac crest at the insertion of the tensor fasciae latae, the gluteus muscle, and the external abdominal oblique muscles. Radiographs may yield normal results early in the displacement of the iliac apophysis. Posterior iliac crest apophysitis is less common than anterior injury and can be diagnosed during examination from the pain produced by abduction of the flexed hip while the patient is lying down. Injuries to the apophysis are treated with 4 to 6 weeks of no running, and the runner must carefully follow return-to-running instructions when running is resumed. Careful attention to proper upper body form is essential to prevent rotation of the torso on the pelvis. Because these are not uncommon to adolescent runners, the amount of hill running must be curtailed. Because these injuries are very common at the beginning of the cross-country season, a gradual build-up program over the summer and the ability to run distance is essential for the student athlete. The idea of beginning cross-country training with 3 miles on the first day of school is ludicrous.

PROBLEMS ASSOCIATED WITH RUNNING
Heat Injuries

Heat injuries can be among the most devastating of all injuries to runners because of their serious nature.

Heat cramps, heat exhaustion, and heat stroke must be identified and treated rapidly. The runner's body maintains a constant temperature by balancing the heat generated to produce energy with heat loss by radiation, convection, and the evaporation of sweat. When the level of exercise, air temperature, and relative humidity increases, evaporation of sweat becomes the principal means of dissipating heat. The runner can overheat by becoming dehydrated or when not enough perspiration is evaporated.

Heat Cramps

Heavy, prolonged sweating and inadequate replacement of water and salt in hot weather may cause muscle twitching, cramps, and spasms of the legs, arms, and back. Immediate treatment is to remove the athlete from the source of heat by placing him or her in a cool, shaded place to rest and by replacing water and electrolytes.

Heat Exhaustion

As body temperature rises, the signs and symptoms of heat exhaustion are evident with headache, light-headedness, confusion, restlessness, nausea, vomiting, and muscle cramps. The runner's skin is cold and clammy, and the pulse is weak and rapid. The runner usually finds it necessary to stop running. The feet should be elevated and the runner's body placed in a cool place with ice or cold towels around the neck, head, abdomen, and groin area. Intravenous solution of normal or half-normal saline solution with 5% dextrose may be used for initial fluid replacement. The runner may have to be transported to an emergency room if there are no adequate facilities at the race site. However, most marathons today have excellent medical coverage including emergency facilities with a medical staff and intravenous fluids available at the site.

Signs of heat stroke

- Temperature greater than 105° F
- Chills
- Irrational behavior
- Involuntary limb movement
- Seizures
- Cyanosis
- Vomiting

Heat Stroke

Acute loss of the normal regulatory mechanism leads to progressive hyperthermy and heat stroke. This is an acute medical emergency and can be fatal. Heat stroke usually occurs in long-distance races such as marathons or ultramarathons in which runners who have heat exhaustion push themselves too hard. Sweating stops, and the skin becomes hot and dry. Body temperature is usually over 105° F, and the runner exhibits chills, irrational behavior, involuntary limb movement and seizures, cyanosis, and vomiting; death may ensue unless treatment is sought at once. The patient must be

---

Signs of heat exhaustion

- Headache
- Light-headedness
- Confusion
- Restlessness
- Nausea
- Vomiting
- Muscle cramps

---

transported to the hospital immediately. While awaiting the ambulance, the medical officials should move the runner to a shaded area, remove the athlete's clothing, and fan the skin and keep it moist. Ice can be placed on the head and neck. Normal or half-normal saline solution with dextrose should be administered intravenously as quickly as possible and should be continued en route to the hospital.

Prevention*

Acclimatization to hot weather should be gradual. Depending on individual differences, this may take from 10 days to 6 or 8 weeks. During hot weather, training should be done early in the morning or late in the evening when the temperature is cooler. It is most appropriate to wear light-colored clothing, especially white. Runners must be sure that the waistbands of their shorts and the elastic part of their socks are not too tight. A white hat with a brim or beak may be helpful, or a terry cloth hat doused with water maintains the moisture during a long run. A runner should drink 6 to 8 ounces of water every 15 minutes before the training run and every 20 minutes or 2.5 miles during the run. Water is as good as any other replacement fluid. Liberal salting of food during hot weather is helpful, but salt tablets are not recommended. Before a race in hot weather, race officials should advise the runners to slow their pace far below normal and learn to recognize the signs of heat injury. The entire attending medical team should be instructed in detecting heat injuries in runners and be authorized to remove any runner who shows such signs during the race, *whether the runner agrees or not.*

In the planning of long-distance races such as marathons the medical staff and race officials must work closely together setting up communications between check points and treatment areas. They must enlist the aid of other health professionals, including nurses, podiatrists, and trainers, to set up triage areas so that the most serious problems, such as cardiopulmonary and heat or cold injuries, can be treated in one area and the orthopaedic and podiatric problems can be treated in another. Rapid access by ambulance support to nearby emergency rooms with prearranged commitments from

---

*Editors' note: Many runners older than 35 years take medication for various ailments. In particular, diuretics and beta-blockers for hypertension may lead to electrolyte imbalance, particularly potassium depletion. Appropriate monitoring of electrolytes and replacement therapy is always indicated in these individuals.

the hospital staff must be ensured. The *White Paper* produced by the American College of Sports Medicine is an essential document for the preparation of any race, and the understanding of it is essential to any race conducted in the warm-weather months.

Cold Injuries

Hypothermia may develop in the long-distance runner when cold, wind chill, and moisture are combined. If the runner's body temperature drops below 90° F, irrational behavior, uncoordination, and confusion result. The problem of hypothermia may become evident in triath-

lons because the water temperature varies significantly in different areas of the country. Wet suits have evolved and are used frequently in cold-water swims. The hypothermic runner, for example, responds well to rapid warming but may be hypovolemic, and rapid hospitalization and fluid replacement are essential. Lactated Ringer's solution is given rapidly with an initial dose of 300 ml with an additional 700 ml given over 1 hour. Heated, humidified oxygen is also recommended as part of the hospital treatment. Frostbite of varying dependent parts must be treated with appropriate warming.

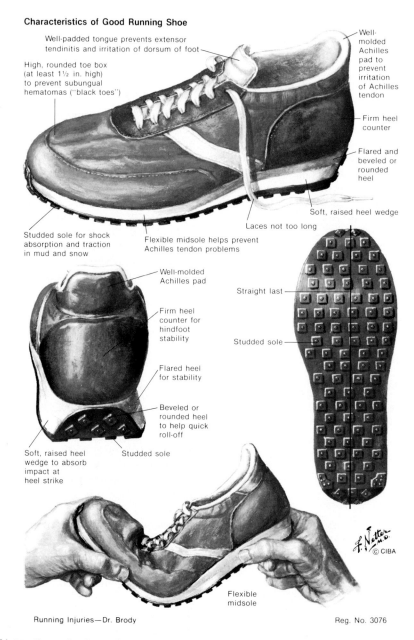

Running Injuries—Dr. Brody   Reg. No. 3076

FIG. 64-25. Shoes. (© Copyright 1980, CIBA Pharmaceutical Company, Division of CIBA-GEIGY Corporation. Reprinted with permission from *Clinical Symposia,* illustrated by Frank H. Netter, M.D. All rights reserved.)

Prevention

The runner training in cold weather already understands the concept of layering of clothing, as developed in cross-country skiing. In the coldest weather, thermal underwear (long johns or the more modern polypropylene underwear), a cotton turtleneck sweater, a nylon all-weather running suit of Gore-Tex, and gloves and a hat to cover the neck and ears are essential. If the weather warms, some of the clothes can be removed. Running shoes with studded or herringbone soles help secure traction in the snow. However, *the only contraindication to running is an icy surface.* Fluid intake during a run, even in cold weather, is important because fluid loss does occur.

RUNNING SHOES

Technologic new materials and newer design concepts have provided a wide range of training and racing shoes for the 1990s. Such names as dual- or triple-density compression moulded ethylene vinyl acetate (EVA), polyurethane, Tomolite (EVA and sponge rubber), Plastazote (orthotic device fabrication material), carbon rubber, blown rubber, solid rubber heel pegs, variable lacing system, last (board, slip, and combination), Sorbothane (viscoelastic material), and graphite are the new technology in materials. These materials have produced safer running shoes with improved shock absorbancy, rearfoot control, lighter weight, and more durability than those of the 1980s. There are more than 360 different models available (Fig. 64-25).

Terminology

Last: A wooden, metal, or plastic form over which the shoe is shaped. The shape of the last can be either curved or straight. The curved last is for the varus foot or the runner who supinates, as with a cavus foot. The straight last is for the neutral or flexible pronated foot. The shoe's upper is lasted in one of the following three ways (Table 64-1).
1. Conventional or board lasting: The upper is pulled over the last and cemented on the underside to a thin, flexible undersole board. The sole-midsole combination is then cemented to the board to provide maximum stability.
2. Slip lasting: The upper is stitched closed on the underside to provide maximum flexibility.

TABLE 64-1 Examples of running shoes based on "last"

Conventional (Board-Lasted)	Slip-Lasted	Combination Last
Nike Air Tailwind	New Balance 998	Saucony Grid Courageous
Avia 3020	Asics Gel-121	New Balance 530
Brooks Prodigy	Etonic Stableair VO-2	Adidar Torsion Revenge
New Balance 660	Saucony Jazz 4000	Avia 2075

3. Combination lasting: Rearfoot board and forefoot slip cast provides rearfoot stability and forefoot flexibility.
Uppers: Usually a combination of mesh nylon (for breathability) and leather (for stability and support), "Oxford nylon," Duramesh, or denier nylon. Lycra, neoprene, and Spandex provide the new stretch fit to the uppers.
Insoles: Arch support removable in most newer models for insertion of an orthotic device. "Sock-liners" (EVA polyethylene blend) mold to individual pressure pattern; Spenco (neoprene sponge).
Midsoles: Located between the upper and the outsole (outer sole), providing protection from impact forces.
Wedge: An additional ⅜- to ¾-inch cushion that extends under the heel, tapering into the midfoot. This provides increased shock absorption and helps elevate the heel to protect the Achilles tendon. Materials include EVA "gel," synthetic foam, cellogram, nusalite, carbon rubber, sponge rubber (expanded rubber compound); Tomolite (EVA and sponge rubber), Phylon (very light with more cushioning than EVA), and Sorbothane (viscoelastic polymer used in sole and heel padding).
Heel counter: Rigid material molded to the shape of the heel that is responsible for controlling rearfoot motion. Made of polyvinyl chloride (PVC).
External heel counter support: Polyurethane collar.
Stability saddle: Cording between upper and midsole; medial arch strap.
Outsole (outer sole): Contributes to cushioning and shoe stability; provides traction. Materials include solid rubber, Indy rubber, carbon rubber, and superflex carbon rubber, with the tongue of polyurethane foam.
The trend of running shoes in the early 1990s has been to provide a comfortable, lightweight shoe with the maximum in rearfoot stability and impact cushioning, combined with support in midstance and flexibility at toe-off. Although many observers think that the more flexible, pronated foot needs a more stable shoe and the more rigid foot a more flexible shoe, *comfort* is a primary consideration.

Shoe Modification

The rigid cavus foot and injuries associated with it are not usually amenable to orthotic correction; therefore, the running shoe itself must be modified (Fig. 64-21). For ongoing plantar fasciitis or Achilles tendinitis, a heel wedge (1 inch) placed between the inner sole and midsole of the shoe is helpful. This provides more cushioning for this rigid type of foot and helps relax the plantar fascia and Achilles tendon at heel strike. For individuals with ongoing metatarsal pain, a ¼-inch rocker bottom placed just proximal to the metatarsal heads within the midsole is most helpful. This allows the runner's foot to roll over the metatarsals without flexion of the metatarsophalangeal joints, permitting the inflammatory response to subside. Lateral compartment syndrome of the ankle may require modification of the upper part of the shoe in addition to an orthotic insert. The heel counter is made more rigid and is extended more proximal in the shoe to the base of the metatarsals. Many of the newer shoe designs incorporate these ideas in their makeup.

ORTHOTIC DEVICES (see also p. 519)

Orthotic devices compensate for biomechanical imbalances that cause injury. In the hyperpronated foot the device maintains a more neutral position. In the rigid cavus foot it provides better shock absorption. Such devices run the gamut from a simple rubber or piano-felt "cookie" to prescribed laminated devices made from a neutral cast of the foot. Over-the-counter devices sold by shoe size have been most helpful in level I runners with mild biomechanical imbalances.

Fabrication of Orthotic Devices (Fig. 64-26)

An orthotic device can be fabricated simply in the office. Equipment includes a toaster oven, sheets of ¼-inch Plastazote (white or black), stockinette, and surgical gloves. Rectangular pieces of Plastazote are cut from larger sheets of this material. Stockinette is placed over the foot and ankle while the Plastazote is heated in a toaster oven at 250 to 300° F (Fig. 64-26, *A*). When the Plastazote begins to curl (Fig. 64-26, *B*), it is applied to the plantar surface of the foot in the neutral position. While still in this softened state, it is molded well to the arch, heel, and web spaces (Fig. 64-26, *C*). During this process the foot rests on a pillow (Fig. 64-26, *D*) with the patient in the sitting position. As the material cools, it becomes firm. It is then trimmed (Fig. 45-26, *E*) and placed in the patient's running shoes. Some examiners prefer to wrap the softened material to the foot using roller gauze while maintaining the knee in full extension, the ankle at 90 degrees, and the foot in neutral position. In this position, pressing up on the plantar surface of the fourth metatarsal head keeps the neutral position of the foot.

An excellent office orthotic device can be fabricated

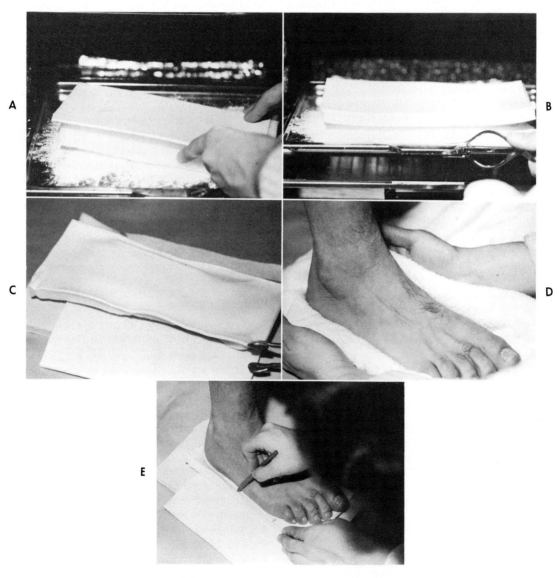

FIG. 64-26. Office orthotic device.

using an Aliplast 10 (⅛ inch thick) blank on top of the full Plastazote No. 2 (¼ inch) blank. Place this in a toaster oven set at 250 to 300° F. When this assembly is "marshmallow-like," it is ready to be molded to the patient's foot. Place a stockinette or towel over the foot as protection, check to be sure that the Aliplast surface is not too hot, and with the patient seated, the knee and ankle at 90 degrees, and the foot in neutral position on a firm pillow or foam casting pad, slowly press runner's foot into the hot assembly, which fuses upon heating. Mold well about the heel, longitudinal arch, metatarsal pad, and web spaces. The outline of the foot should be traced on the Aliplast before the molding and trimmed with scissors or a knife. Usually in runners the orthotic device is trimmed proximal to the metatarsal heads and scythed with a small drum sander.

If posting (balancing) is needed, post locks of ⅛-inch Aliplast or ¼-inch Plastazote No. 2 can be cemented to the bottom of the orthotic device with rubber cement (Barge contact cement). To ensure adhesion of the post to the device, abrade both surfaces before applying adhesive. With careful trimming, this device may be used immediately. The commercial insole material that comes with the running shoe (and is now removable in most newer models) should be removed before insertion of the newly fabricated orthotic device.

Prescription Orthotic Devices

Prescription orthotic devices (Fig. 64-27) are of three major types: flexible, semirigid (polyethylene), and rigid (polypropylene). The rigid orthotics are used only for high-mileage runners who need more control. These are fabricated in an orthotic laboratory from a plaster cast of the foot. The technique that we use for making these casts is as follows: the midlines of the calcaneus and navicular bones are marked with an indelible marker (Fig. 64-27, B). Plantar callosities are also marked. The patient sits on the examining table with the knee and ankle at 90 degrees of flexion and the foot resting on a firm pillow, which in turn rests on a foot stool (Fig. 64-27, C). Five thicknesses of 8-inch plaster of Paris are measured to the full foot. The plaster is dipped in water and placed squarely under the foot, which is held in neutral position. The rectangular plaster is then molded around the heel posteriorly and molded well in the arch and web spaces (Fig. 64-27, D to F). The plaster should be wide enough (hence the choice of 8-inch and not 6-inch plaster) so that the navicular marker is covered. The plaster mold is removed when dry (Fig. 64-27, G), and the imprints of the calcaneus, navicular bone, and plantar callosities should be highlighted with the indelible marker on the cast. The patient's name should be written on the outer side of the cast. It is then carefully packed and shipped to the laboratory.

In my clinics approximately 40% of the runners receive some type of orthotic device. For the problem of hyperpronation, I use the flexible runner's mold (leather, rubber, and cork). For plantar fasciitis, "laminated" (layered) runner's molds are most helpful in both hyperpronated and cavus feet. Semirigid and rigid orthotics are also used.

ALTERNATIVE TRAINING FOR THE INJURED RUNNER

While injured, the runner must be offered an alternative training program. This not only offers maintenance of the runner's cardiovascular level of fitness, but also provides some measure of positive mental feedback. One advantage triathletes have is their ability to change over to cycling or swimming, depending on the nature of the injury.

Swimming, cycling (stationary or road), rowing, and weight-training programs may be used. Running in water is a technique whereby the injured runner, wearing a water skiing vest or Styrofoam flotation belt, treads water in the deep end of a pool or diving well. In addition to moving the legs (the treading movement), the runner moves his or her arms without holding onto the sides of the pool and does not touch the bottom. This technique can be done in one of two ways: (1) long, slow distance or (2) intervals. In the former, running in water is carried out at a constant rate for 30 to 45 minutes. In the latter, the athlete moves the arms and legs as rapidly as possible in a "dog paddle" for a given period of time. Intervals of 60 to 80 seconds repeated 10 to 12 times between identical periods of rest maintain high levels of cardiovascular output.

Running in water coupled with freestyle swimming and cycling is excellent for the runner with a stress fracture, provided there is no irritation to the injured area. The individual with a stress fracture involving a metatarsal may cycle as alternative training, but rigid-soled cycling shoes are essential. The patient with patellofemoral arthralgia does well not to cycle but should concentrate on freestyle swimming using a "pull-buoy" between the thighs and not kicking at all. This, coupled with upper-body Nautilus, free, or Universal weights and progressive resistance exercises in extension, is helpful. Any type of cycling, rowing, deep squats, or swimming doing the "frog kick" exacerbates patellofemoral symptoms. Circuit training (moving rapidly from one weight station to the next) can provide cardiovascular conditioning.

RETURN TO RUNNING AFTER INJURY

Runners must be totally asymptomatic before running is resumed. Runners are asked, on a scale of 0 to 10, to rate their symptoms, with 10 being the worst and 0 being normal. When at 0, athletes are given a program that brings them back to their preinjury running level in 4 to 6 weeks. For the first 2 weeks they run every other day. On alternate days other types of training (e.g., swimming, running in water, cycling, weight training) are performed. For example, a level III runner (40 to 70 miles per week) begins at the 2-mile level (Table 64-2).

Training Routine

Associated with each training run there is a routine that should be followed. Moist heat is applied to the previously injured area for 5 minutes before the run. In addition, a warm-up program of calisthenics, low back exercises, and walking is followed by a period of 3 to 5 minutes of stretching. The muscles of the low back and ex-

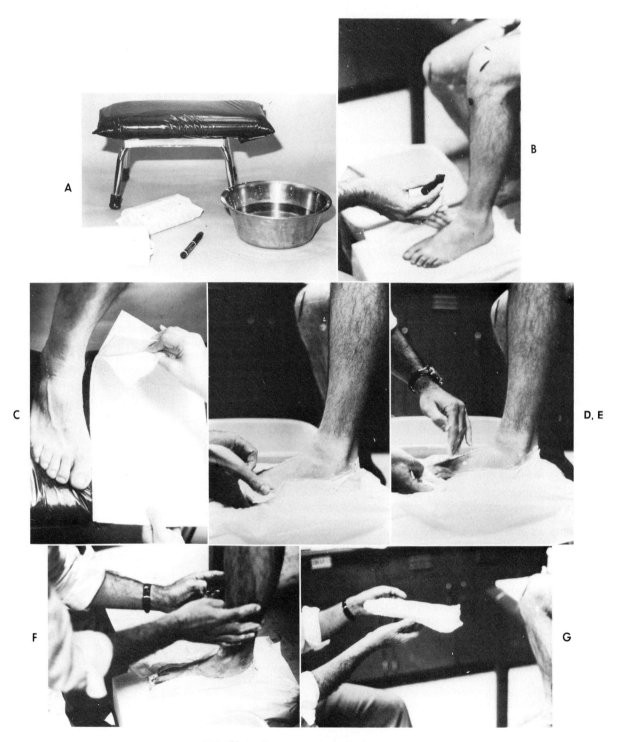

FIG. 64-27. Prescription orthotic device.

TABLE 64-2 Sample program for return to running

Week	Days of the Week							Total Miles Per Week
	1	2	3	4	5	6	7	
1	2	0	2	0	2	0	3	9
2	0	3	0	3	0	4	0	10
				If the patient is asymptomatic, this is increased to:				
3	4	3	0	4	4	0	5	20
4	4	0	5	5	0	6	5	25
5	0	6	6	0	7	6	6	31
6	0	7	7	8	7	0	9	38

tremities should be "warmed up" before the stretching takes place. This is followed by the prescribed run, then ice massage for 10 to 15 minutes over the previously injured area, even though there may be no pain. The ice causes a localized vasoconstriction initially, followed in 10 to 20 minutes by a reflex vasodilation if the massage is continued (see p. 208). Commercially available ice packs are more practical in the low back area but should not be applied to the bare skin without their coverings.

At a time unassociated with the run, moist heat is used for 10 to 20 minutes, followed by stretching or other prescribed exercises. For example, a runner advised to follow a low back exercise program (e.g., partial bent-knee sit-ups, pelvic tilts, or knees to chest) performs these at this time. A runner advised to do progressive resistance exercises in extension for patellofemoral arthralgia does these at night following the heat and stretching procedures.

ADDITIONAL READINGS

Achilles tendon problem increase, Round Table Symposium, *Phys Sports Med* 3:43, 1982.

Adelaar RS: The practical biomechanics of running, *Am J Sports Med* 14(6):497, 1986.

Apple D: Knee pain in runners, *South Med J* 72:1377, 1979.

Bordelon RL: Management of disorders of the forefoot and toenails in runners, *Clin Sports Med* 4:737, 1985.

Brody DM: Techniques in the evaluation and treatment of the injured runner, *Orthop Clin North Am* 13:541, 1982.

Brody DM: Running injuries, *Ciba Clin Symp* 39:3, 1987.

Brubaker EC, James SL: Injuries to runners, *Am J Sports Med* 2:189, 1974.

Campbell JW, Inmann VT: Treatment of plantar fasciitis and calcaneal spurs with UC-BL shoe insert, *Clin Orthop* 57, 1974.

Cavanagh PR: The shoe ground interface in running. In *AAOS symposium on the foot and leg in running sports*, St Louis, 1982, Mosby.

Clement DB: Stress fracture in athletes, *J Sports Med* 2:81, 1974.

Cox JS: Patellofemoral problems in runners, *Clin Sports Med* 4:699, 1985.

D'Ambrosia RD, Drez D: *Prevention and treatment of running injuries*, Thorofore, NJ, 1982, Slack.

D'Ambrosia RD et al: Interstructural pressure measurements in the anterior and posterior compartments in athletes with shin splints, *Am J Sports Med* 50:126, 1977.

Garfin S, Mubarak SJ, Owen CA: Exertional anterolateral compartment syndrome, *J Bone Joint Surg* 59A:404, 1977.

Gutten G: Herniated lumbar disk associated with running: a review of ten cases, *Am J Sports Med* 9:155, 1981.

Jacobs SJ, Berson BL: Injuries to runners: a study of entrants to a 10,000-meter race, *Am J Sports Med* 14:2, 1986.

James LL, Bates BJ, Osternig LR: Injuries to runners, *Am J Sports Med* 6:40, 1978.

Kaplan EB: The iliotibial tract, *J Bone Joint Surg* 40A:817, 1958.

Kennedy JC, Roth JH: Major tibial compartmental syndromes following minor athletic trauma, *Am J Sports Med* 7:201, 1979.

Konradsen L, BergHansen EM, Sondergaard L: Long-distance running and osteoarthritis, *Am J Sports Med* 18(4):379, 1990.

Leach R, Jones R, Silvia T: Rupture of the plantar fascia in athletes, *J Bone Joint Surg* 63A:537, 1981.

Lutter LD: The knee and running, *Clin Sports Med* 4:685, 1985.

Lysholm J, Wiklander J: Injuries in runners, *Am J Sports Med* 15(2):168, 1987.

Mann RA, Baxter DE, Lutter LD: Running symposium, *Foot Ankle* 1:190, 1981.

Mann RA, Moran GT, Dougherty SE: Comparative electromyography of the lower extremity in jogging, running, and sprinting, *Am J Sports Med* 14(6):501, 1986.

Marti B et al: On the epidemiology of running injuries: the 1984 Bern grand-prix study, *Am J Sports Med* 16(3):285, 1988.

McBryde AJ: Stress fractures in runners, *Clin Sports Med* 4:737, 1985.

Montgomery WH, Pink M, Perry J: Electromyographic analysis of hip and knee musculature during running, *Am J Sports Med* 22(2):272, 1994.

Mubarek SJ et al: Acute compartment syndromes: diagnosis and treatment with the aid of the wick catheter, *J Bone Joint Surg* 60A:1010, 1982.

Mubarek SJ et al: The medial tibial stress syndrome, *Am J Sports Med* 10:201, 1982.

Noble CA: The treatment of iliotibial band friction syndrome, *Br J Sports Med* 13:51, 1979.

Pavlov H et al: Stress fractures of the pubis ramus: a report of twelve cases, *J Bone Joint Surg* 64A:1010, 1982.

Renee JW: The iliotibial band friction syndrome, *J Bone Joint Surg* 57A:1110, 1975.

Schuster RO: Children's foot survey, *J Podiat Soc NY* 17:13, 1956.

Snook G: Achilles tendon tenosynovitis in long-distance runners, *Med Sci Sports Exerc* 4:155, 1962.

Sohn RS, Micheli LJ: The effect of running on the pathogenesis of osteoarthritis of the hips and knees, *Clin Orthop* 198:106, 1985.

Standish WD, Curwin S, Rubinovich M: Tendinitis: the analysis and treatment for running, *Clin Sports Med* 4:593, 1985.

Stanitski CL et al: On the nature of stress fractures, *Am J Sports Med* 6:391, 1978.

CHAPTER 65 Soccer Injuries

John L. Xethalis
Matthew P. Lorei

Hallux rigidus
Hallux valgus
Subungual hematoma
Abrasions

EPIDEMIOLOGY

The popularity of soccer is rapidly growing in this country, especially among youth. In 1994 the World Cup was played in the United States, generating further interest in soccer. Worldwide, soccer is by far the most popular sport, with an estimated 40 million participants.[71] In European countries, injuries sustained from this game account for about 40% of all sports-related trauma.[28] Because of its popularity, the epidemiology of soccer injury has been studied extensively.

The ultimate goal of sports medicine is the prevention of injury. Preventive medicine is best approached by the analysis of the epidemiology of disease or injury. Epidemiologic analysis involves the study of the classic agent-host-environment interaction. In the case of sports injury the agent is the immediate causative factor (usually an opposing player), the host is the athlete sustaining the injury, and the environment is the situation or conditions that may predispose or inhibit the injury (e.g., playing conditions, footwear, and protective padding).

In sports injury all three factors are variable, and appropriate control of the variables leads to injury reduction. For instance, the agent may be modified by installing rules to forbid dangerous play, the host may be modified by being properly conditioned, and the environment may be modified by wearing proper shoes or better protective padding.

Recently, there has been an explosion of reports on the epidemiology of soccer injury in the orthopaedic literature. The bulk of the work has originated from Sweden and Denmark. The thrust of these studies has been to examine the incidence and spectrum of injury and, to a lesser extent, the preventive measures and effects of injury.

One of the earliest attempts at epidemiologic study of injuries in soccer was presented in 1978 by McMaster and Walter,[42] who analyzed injuries sustained by an American professional soccer team in the course of one season. The authors drew several conclusions: (1) the injury rate of soccer was much lower than tackle football, (2) distribution of injury was spread evenly among players regardless of position, and (3) the most common injuries were foot and ankle sprains, with muscle strains running a close second.

The study by Sullivan and Gross[73] of 18 youth soccer clubs (ages 5 to 18) revealed several observations. Injuries in females were roughly twice the male rate, a finding that proved consistent with several subsequent studies. The under 10-year age group was only rarely injured. Less than one injury per 100 participants necessitated a loss from practice or competition. The incidence and severity of injury increased with the age of the participants. They also found the injury rate among secondary school

players to be roughly equivalent to that of basketball (7.7 injuries per 100 participants) and significantly lower and less severe than the injury profile for football. This study also served notice to the increase in the popularity of the game in the United States, since the number of players rose from 1800 in 1976 to 7800 in 1979.

A series of reports by Ekstrand et al[13,15,16] were some of the most significant published on the study of soccer injury. The authors studied the effects of training pattern on the occurrence of injury in 180 division 4, Swedish soccer players on 12 different teams. The authors defined several important concepts that have been widely used in the subsequent literature. They defined an injury as "any mishap occurring during scheduled games or practices that cause a player to miss a subsequent game or practice session." Injuries were classified into three grades of severity: minor (absence from training or games for less than 1 week), moderate (absence from training or games for 1 week to 1 month), and major (absence from training or games for more than 1 month). They also defined the concept of injury rate as injuries per 1000 hours of playing time (whether practice or game). They drew an important distinction between injuries occurring during practice and those occurring during games. The latter had a higher rate and severity of injury.

Ekstrand et al[13,15,16] observed the following. A higher incidence of injuries occurred at training camp. There was a highly positive correlation between team success and amount of training. A reduction in overall injury rate with increased training chiefly occurred by a decrease in traumatic injuries with overuse problems remaining constant. The authors also found that ligamentous sprains in the lower extremity are the most common injuries followed by muscle strains of the various thigh compartments. Last, they demonstrated less flexibility in soccer players than their reference peers.[13,15,16]

With the data gained from these preliminary studies Ekstrand et al[14] attempted a randomized study of an injury control program in the same population. By controlling several variables, such as optimum training and equipment, prophylactic ankle taping, exclusion of players with unstable knees, and supervision by medical staff, the authors were able to reduce the rate of injury by a remarkable 75% in the six test teams when compared with the controls.

In an attempt to further understand injury trends in the now defunct North American Soccer League (NASL), the Nicholas Institute of Sports Medicine and Athletic Trauma at Lenox Hill Hospital analyzed the injuries documented by the NASL in the 1979 season. Notable discoveries included the following. Of all injuries, only 12% involved the upper extremity; the remainder were all lower extremity injuries. Thigh strains accounted for 45% of all injuries. Major injuries accounted for only 4.3% of injuries. The number of fractures was significant at 15 injuries (Tables 65-1 to 65-4).[31]

Recently, two population-based studies of the incidence and severity of soccer injuries have been reported. In a study of injuries requiring evaluation at a hospital, Sadat-Ali and Sankaran-Kutty[64] found that 64% of all

TABLE 65-1 Types of injuries in soccer

	Number	Percentage (%)	
Strains	135	40.5	
Sprains	102	30.6	90.6%
Contusions	65	19.5	
Fractures	15	4.5	
Meniscal injury	12	3.6	9.3%
Dislocations	3	0.9	
Lacerations	1	0.3	
TOTAL	333	99.9	

TABLE 65-2 Percentage of injuries in time-loss categories

Time-Loss Category	Number of Injuries	Percentage (%)	
0 to 7 days	320	76.4	
8 to 14 days	62	14.5	
15 to 21 days	20	4.8	23.6%
Over 21 days (major)	18	4.3	
TOTAL	420	100.0	

TABLE 65-3 Injuries by body part

Body Part	Number		Percentage (%)	
Lower Extremity				
Thigh	156		45.2	
Ankle	66	80.5%	19.1	
Knee	56		16.2	90%
Lower leg	18		5.2	
Foot	15		4.3	
Upper Extremity and Torso				
Rib	13		3.7	
Torso	6		1.7	
Wrist	6		1.7	9.7%
Phalanx	6		1.7	
Elbow	3		0.9	
TOTAL	345		99.7	

sports injuries were soccer injuries. They noted a high incidence of fractures and dislocations (34%) as well as severe injuries requiring hospitalization (21%). Soccer injuries accounted for 6% of all emergency department attendances. The authors' findings are somewhat at odds with the rest of the literature, perhaps attesting to the ferocity of the game as it is played in the Middle East.

Hoy et al[28] performed a similar study in Denmark that revealed that soccer injuries accounted for 39% of all sports-related injuries seen in the emergency room with a hospitalization rate of 9% for all soccer injuries. This is more in line with the rest of the Western literature.[46]

From the results of numerous recent studies several facts become clear. The incidence of injury is exceedingly low in children under 12 (1 to 3 injuries per 1000 hours of competition),[47,66,73] increases steadily with age up to 18 years old when the rate equals that of divisional play (about 15 injuries per 1000 hours), and levels off from there.[26,34,46] The severity of injury also increases with age. Among elite players major injuries account for approximately 35% of all injuries, with a career-threatening injury occurring in 1 of 10 players during the course of a season.[19] The incidence of injury during practice is about one third that of competition.[18,19,46] The rate of injury in indoor soccer is significantly greater than that in outdoor soccer.[26,38] Chronic injuries consistently account for about 35% of all injuries and occur mostly in training camp or at the end of a season.[18,19,46] About one fourth of injuries are the result of rule violations.[19,28,46] Women are twice as likely to injure themselves as men, but the severity of injury is substantially less.[18,34,73] Overall, despite the increased participation in sports in the last decade there has been no associated increase in the pattern or incidence of soccer injuries.[75]

In terms of prophylaxis against injury, better conditioning, equipment, and policing of the rules have been shown to reduce the incidence of injury. Prophylactic ankle taping appears to have no benefit. Shin guards, although decreasing the frequency of shin contusions, are not protective against significant injury.[14,28]

TABLE 65-4 Injury types by position—lower extremity

Area/Type	Position				Total
	Defender	Midfielder	Forward	Goalkeeper	
Thigh/contusion	8	6	6	1	21
Thigh/strain	44	44	44	3	135
TOTAL	52	50	50	4	156
Knee/contusion	5	1	2	1	9
Knee/sprain	12	10	9	2	33
Knee/meniscal injury	5	5	2	—	12
TOTAL	22	16	13	3	54
Ankle/contusion	2	3	1	—	6
Ankle/sprain	18	20	16	2	56
Ankle/fracture	1	—	3	—	4
TOTAL	21	23	20	2	66
Foot/contusion	3	1	1	1	6
Foot/sprain	2	—	7	—	9
TOTAL	5	1	8	1	15
Leg/contusion	4	4	7	3	18

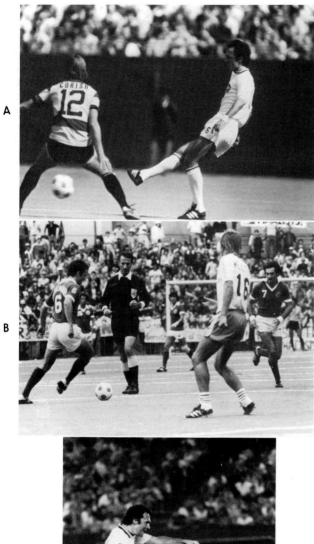

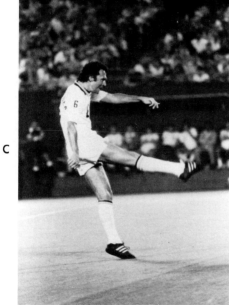

FIG. 65-1. Types of kicks. **A,** Inside kick. **B,** Outside kick. **C,** Straight-ahead kick.

ASPECTS OF THE KICK

The kick is the principal motion of the game. In an excellent biomechanical review of the kicking motion, Gainor et al[22] demonstrated that kicking activity involves the generation of extremely high values of kinetic energy

---

Soccer kicks

- Inside (power) kick
- Outside (control/lateral) kick
- Straight-ahead (place/dorsal) kick

---

in the lower extremity. They state that the primary risk of injury occurs immediately before foot strike on the ball and immediately following. The narrow analysis of the soccer kicking motion reveals that there are essentially three types of kicks involved in soccer: (1) the inside kick, or power kick; (2) the outside (lateral) kick, or control kick; and (3) the straight-ahead kick, or place or dorsal kick (Fig. 65-1). Other kicks seen in soccer include the bicycle kick and the side volley kick. The inside kick is primarily for power. The athlete uses the hip adductors; knee extensors; and anterior tibial, posterior tibial, and extensor hallucis longus muscles to drive the ball down the field. The outside kick is more controlled and relies on the fine motor muscles of the foot for passing the ball in shorter kicks. These kicks generally require less strength but more finesse and the use of the hip external rotators; vastus lateralis; peronei longus, brevis, and tertius; and extensor digitorum communis. The straight-ahead place kick involves forceful use of the knee extensors, hip flexors, and ankle dorsiflexors. By their definitions each kicking style entails a different biomechanical concept and results in different modes of possible injury to the lower extremity. As has been demonstrated in the literature by Gainor et al,[22] extremely high values of kinetic energy in the lower extremity are generated in both the inside and the straight-ahead place kick. Obviously, the energy is only partially transferred to the ball, and the rest must be dissipated by the leg during the follow-through. Energy dissipation is usually a smooth, well-coordinated process that uses the hip extensors, hamstrings, plantar flexors, and gravity to absorb the energy. During this critical zone of the kick, from immediately before striking the ball to the end of follow-through, the player is extremely vulnerable to extraneous loading. Injury occurs when the normal load dissipation is interrupted, whether by the ground, another player, or poor ball contact, resulting in extremely high-stress concentrations along the linkage system and ultimately failure or injury. Knowledge of the mechanics of the normal kicking motions helps to define the possible points of injury. Injury may be encountered anywhere from the pelvis to the foot. Failure at any point of articulation, either acutely or chronically, may produce injury.

Inside Kick

The inside kick, known to football enthusiasts as the soccer-style kick, is a moment of such explosive force that long bone fractures have occurred after errant kicks (Figs. 65-2 and 65-3). In one study a significant varus torque on the proximal tibia that ranged from 800 to 2000 inch-pounds was calculated before ball contact. Immediately after contact an equally large valgus torque on the tibia of about 1700 inch-pounds was measured as well.[22]

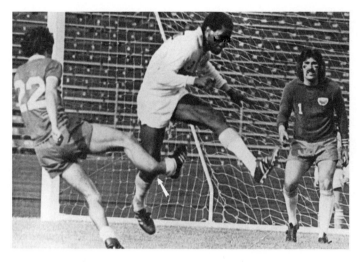

FIG. 65-2. Obvious fracture of tibia as result of high-velocity inside soccer kick.

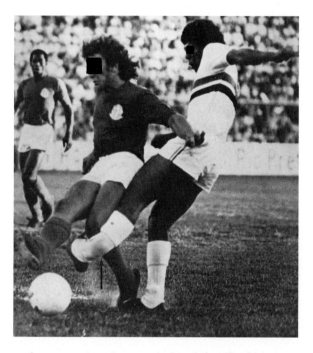

FIG. 65-3. Missed inside soccer kick ended in this fracture as result of contact.

Muscles used during the inside (power) kick

- Hip adductors group
- Quadriceps
- Tibialis anterior
- Tibialis posterior
- Extensor hallucis longus

Muscles used during the outside (control) kick

- Hip external rotators
- Vastus lateralis
- Peronei longus, brevis, and tertius
- Extensor digitorum communis

Muscles used during the straight-ahead (place) kick

- Hip flexors
- Knee extensors
- Ankle dorsiflexors

Indeed one wonders why injuries of more severe magnitude are not noted more routinely. Adductor and quadriceps strains are commonly seen as are avulsions of the anterior superior iliac spine, medial collateral ligament sprains, and midfoot injuries (Figs. 65-4 and 65-5).

Outside Kick

Although shots on goal are usually effected by the straight-ahead place kick or the forceful inside kick, the outside kick is used mostly in a finesse contest and for passing the ball short distances. As such, large torques are not usually generated and the likelihood of injury is significantly less. However, extremely agile players may certainly employ the outside kick to take shots. With the unique biomechanics of the outside kick, a constellation of injury may be encountered depending on the point of failure in the linkage system of the lower extremity. Common injuries attributed to this kick include hip abductor sprain, iliotibial tract tendinitis, lateral collateral ligament (LCL) injury, and peroneal sprains (Fig. 65-6).

Straight-Ahead Kick

The straight-ahead kick, also called the American kick, lacks the control of the inside kick and is therefore used much less frequently. However, because of the tremendous ball velocities that can be obtained, it is commonly

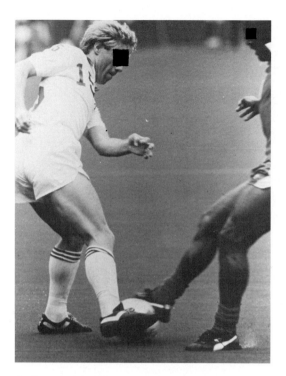

FIG. 65-4. Powerful inside kick simultaneously executed by opposing players. Injury occurs in any structure in linkage system of lower extremity from pelvis to interphalangeal joints of foot.

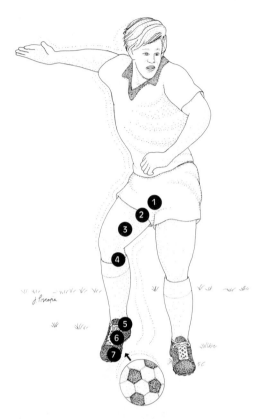

FIG. 65-5. Inside kick. Injury may occur at any point of linkage system that is stressed during this maneuver. *1,* Avulsion of anterior superior iliac spine; *2,* osteitis pubis (traumatic); *3,* adductor strain; *4,* medial knee ligament sprain; *5,* deltoid sprain; *6,* midtarsal joint injuries; *7,* forefoot injury.

used for clearing shots, on the volley, for long passing shots, and for short-range shots on goal (Fig. 65-7). Again, because of the tremendous torques created, injuries are commonly associated with this kick. Common injuries include anterior superior iliac spine avulsion, quadriceps strain, patellar tendinitis or rupture, and forefoot injuries.

PELVIS AND HIP INJURIES

Pelvis injuries in soccer are common and worrisome because they are often refractory to treatment (Fig. 65-8). The pelvis is predisposed to injury for two reasons: it is the site of attachment for all of the powerful muscles of the thigh, and as such, it is subject to strains and avulsions of their insertion sites (Fig. 65-9). Also, the pelvis contains many bony prominences that are susceptible to direct blows and contusion from a fall or player-player contact.

Hip Pointer

The hip pointer is a frequent injury in soccer athletes.[50] The cause of this common syndrome may be contusion of the periosteum or bone of the iliac crest or avulsion or strain of the muscles attached to the iliac crest (Figs. 65-9 and 65-10). The majority of hip pointers are produced when the soccer player falls on the ground and

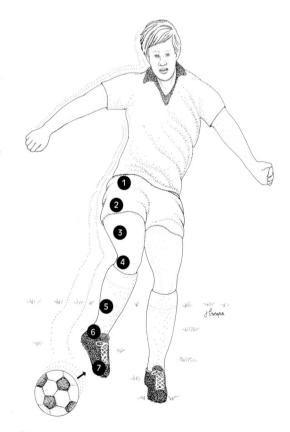

FIG. 65-6. Outside kick. Injury may occur at any point along linkage system. *1,* Hip abductor strain; *2,* iliotibial tract tendinitis; *3,* vastus lateralis strain; *4,* lateral knee injury; *5,* peroneal muscle strains; *6,* lateral ankle complex sprains; *7,* forefoot injury.

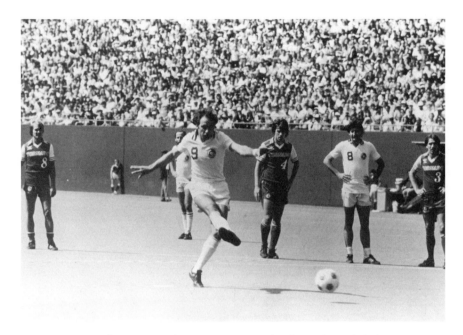

FIG. 65-7. Soccer player executing penalty shot with inside kick.

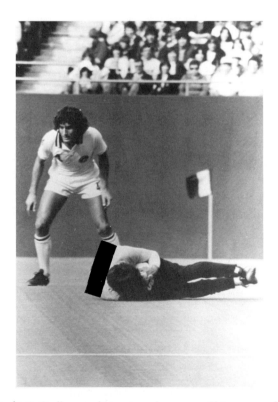

FIG. 65-8. Goalkeeper diving to make a save. This may produce injuries to pelvis and hip areas.

the prominent iliac crest is injured. Goalies are especially susceptible to this condition (Fig 65-8). Unlike football, soccer players usually do not wear protective padding for the iliac crest; protective padding may indeed reduce the incidence of this injury.

The injured player always complains of pain. The pain is never severe, however, and the player usually does not need to leave the field. Pain becomes more noticeable after a period of inactivity (e.g., during intermission or at the end of a game). On physical examinations, there is often a skin abrasion or ecchymosis as well as point tenderness over the iliac crest. By the next day a hematoma may be palpated. A radiograph should be taken to rule out iliac crest fracture or avulsion. The hematoma, if large, may be aspirated. An oral nonsteroidal antiinflammatory drug (NSAID) should be taken for several days. Ice packs should be intermittently applied to the area and compressed with an elastic bandage or pad. The player should wear a protective pad as long as tenderness persists. The player's tolerance should be a guide to return to sport.

Iliac Crest Apophysitis

Iliac crest apophysitis is the adolescent equivalent of a hip pointer. It represents a nondisplaced Salter I fracture of the iliac wing apophysis. Development of this condition is predicated by an open iliac crest growth plate. Closure of this apophysis usually occurs by age 14 in girls and age 16 in boys, although it may be delayed up to 4 years.[61] The injury is caused by direct trauma to the avulsion of the iliac crest. When this injury is secondary to a direct blow, it is often called traumatic iliac apophysitis. Usually, however, it is secondary to a traction force. The player complains of pain and tenderness over the iliac crest while running. There is usually no history of trauma.

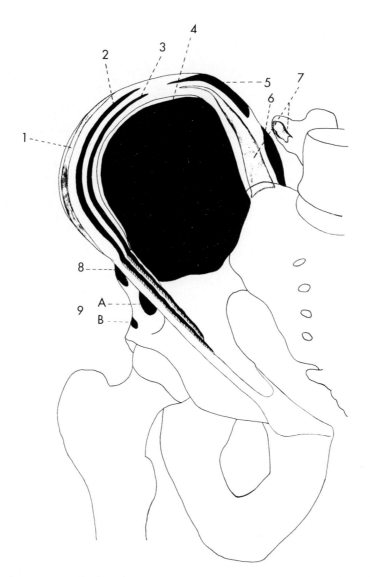

FIG. 65-9. Anterior view of pelvis. Artist's conception of origin and insertion of muscles and ligaments to pelvis. *1*, Insertion of external oblique abdominal muscle; *2*, origin of internal oblique abdominal muscle; *3*, origin of transversalis abdominal muscle; *4*, origin of iliacus muscle; *5*, origin of quadratus lumborum muscle; *6*, origin of erector spinae muscle; *7*, iliolumbar ligament; *8*, sartorius muscle; *9*, rectus femoris muscle with straight (*A*) and reflected (*B*) heads.

Mechanism of Injury

The mechanism of injury is thought to occur from repetitive muscular contractions, causing inflammatory apophysitis, or secondary subclinical stress fractures.[8,9] According to the symptoms present, it can be classified into two groups: (1) anterior, from repetitive contraction of the tensor fasciae latae, gluteus medius, or abdominal obliques (Fig. 65-9) or (2) posterior, from repetitive contraction of the gluteus maximus, quadratus lumborum, or erector spinae (Fig. 65-10).

Diagnosis

Tenderness on palpation of the iliac crest, especially with resisted abduction, suggests the diagnosis. Radio-graphs are usually normal but may reveal fragmentation or avulsion of the iliac apophysis. Diagnosis may be confirmed by radionuclide scan, but this is usually unnecessary.[62]

Treatment

Apophysitis is usually resolved with 2 to 4 weeks of rest. Following improvement of symptoms the athlete is begun on a stretching and strengthening program that is appropriate for the involved muscle groups.

Pelvic Avulsion Fractures

The following avulsion injuries can occur in the area of the pelvis in an adolescent player (Figs. 65-9 to 65-11):

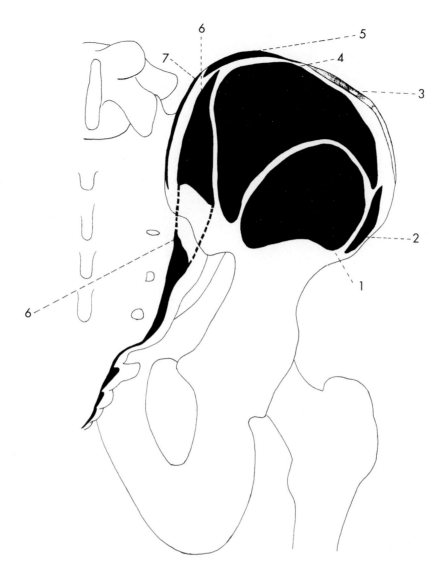

FIG. 65-10. Posterior view of pelvis. Artist's conception of insertion and origin of muscles. *1*, Origin of gluteus minimus muscle; *2*, tensor fasciae latae muscle; *3*, insertion of external oblique abdominal muscle; *4*, gluteus medius muscle; *5*, latissimus dorsi muscle; *6*, gluteus maximus muscle; *7*, erector spinae muscle.

I. Iliac crest fracture
   A. Fracture of the anterior iliac apophysis from the direct action of
      1. Internal obliquus
      2. External obliquus
      3. Transversalis
      4. Tensor fasciae latae
      5. Gluteus medius
   B. Fracture of the posterior iliac apophysis from action of
      1. Latissimus dorsi
      2. Gluteus maximus
      3. Quadratus lumborum
      4. Erector spinae
II. Anterior superior iliac spine fracture from action of
   A. Sartorius

   B. Tensor fasciae latae
III. Anterior inferior iliac spine fracture from direct action of the direct head of the rectus femoris (Fig. 65-11)
IV. Ischial tuberosity fracture from the action of the hamstrings
 V. Avulsion fracture of the pubis at site of origin of the pectineus, adductor longus, or gracilis muscle from strong contraction of the adductors or violent passive abduction of the extremity
VI. Lesser trochanter fracture from direct pull of the insertion of the iliopsoas

Treatment

The principles of treatment are similar regardless of location of the avulsion fracture. Bedrest with immobili-

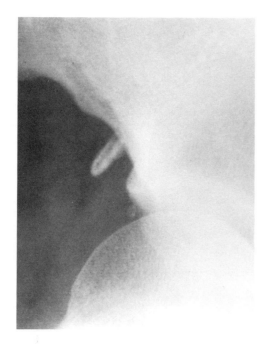

FIG. 65-11. Avulsion fracture of anterior inferior iliac spine.

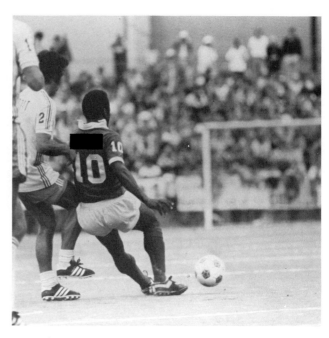

FIG. 65-12. Soccer player falling on his ischium during game.

zation of the extremity in a relaxed position to avoid tension on the avulsed fragment generally provides adequate relief from pain. The athlete may ambulate with crutches when he or she is able. The athlete can return to sports as tolerated, generally in 4 to 6 weeks. If a painful nonunion occurs, surgical reattachment of a large bony fragment or resection of a minor fragment with suturing of the attached tendon to its origin site may be required.

Greater Trochanter Bursitis

Greater trochanter bursitis is a common entity in the orthopaedic population and is frequently seen in soccer players. This bursa lies just deep to the tensor fasciae latae of the thigh and allows for smooth gliding motion of the tensor fasciae latae over the greater trochanter.[6] Injury to this structure in soccer players is thought to be the result of two inciting factors. First, with repetitive inside kicks there is increased friction over the tensor fasciae latae resulting in irritation of the bursa. This is compounded by recurrent blows and falls sustained to the bony prominence of the greater trochanter, contusing the bursa. The end result is chronic inflammation of the greater trochanteric bursa. It does not seem to be caused by gait abnormalities. Soccer players wear no padding over this area and so may be predisposed for this reason. In our experience this injury seems to increase when playing on artificial surfaces. Although this injury is not usually serious enough to preclude play, it may prohibit a player from performing up to capacity.

Diagnosis

The patient complains of pain and tenderness over the lateral aspect of the hip, especially with running or inside kicking. Pain and tenderness can be elicited over the greater trochanter, especially with passive adduction or resisted abduction of the involved extremity. The Ober test may be positive. Aspiration of the bursa yields serous, blood-tinged, or occasionally frank bloody fluid.

Treatment

The bursa may be aspirated if there is some degree of fluctuance present. An appropriate dosage of lidocaine and dexamethasone can be injected into the bursa. Ice and compressive dressing round out the treatment picture. Stretching the iliotibial tract can be useful for athletes with tightness in this structure.

Ischial Tuberosity Bursitis

Ischial tuberosity bursitis is another common entity in the soccer player. The mechanism of injury is thought to be a series of direct blows to the ischium from several falls (Fig. 65-12). Alternatively, it is also seen following drills that emphasize speed work. The symptom complex includes pain and tenderness directly over the ischial tuberosity that is exacerbated by sitting or jumping. Examination reveals both point tenderness over the ischial tuberosity and tight hamstrings.

Differential Diagnosis

Differential diagnosis of ischial tuberosity bursitis includes avulsion fracture of the tuberosity by the pull of the hamstrings in an adolescent player or a compression fracture of the tuberosity in an older individual. Therefore radiographs should be obtained to exclude these.

Treatment

Rest and use of NSAIDs and ice are the cornerstones of successful treatment in soccer players. If pain and tenderness persist, an injection of local anesthetic with cor-

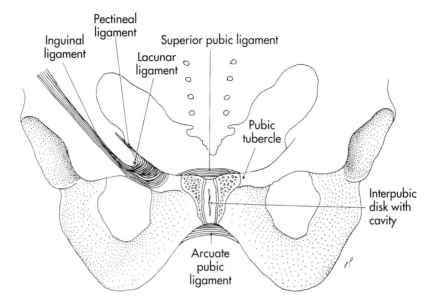

FIG. 65-13. Cross section of symphysis pubis.

tisone is advisable. We have never observed any spur formation or calcification as has been reported by others. Return to play is governed by the patient's tolerance.

Piriformis Syndrome

A tight piriformis muscle may compress the sciatic nerve. Anatomically, the sciatic nerve runs just deep to the piriformis muscle in the buttocks in approximately 85% of the population. In the remaining 15%, part or all of the sciatic nerve courses through or around the piriformis muscle.[27] Overuse or hypertrophy of the muscle may lead to impingement of the nerve. Symptoms include radicular pain or even tingling, numbness, or weakness of the lower extremity. Back pain is absent. Examination reveals point tenderness over the buttocks just medial to the greater trochanter. Extension and internal rotation of the hip exacerbate the pain. Differential diagnosis includes trochanteric bursitis, sacroiliac joint pain, and sciatica caused by lumbar disk herniation.

Treatment

Treatment consists of rest, ice, and stretching of the piriformis muscle (toe touching with the legs crossed). NSAIDs are often beneficial. In severe, persistent cases with radiculopathy, surgical release may be necessary.

Osteitis Pubis

Traumatic osteitis pubis is a syndrome of which its cause is unclear. It results in chronic pubic pain brought on by repetitive stress to the pubis. The vast majority of cases occur in soccer players, although other running athletes may occasionally be affected. This syndrome is variously referred to as osteochondritis of the symphysis pubis, gracilis syndrome, osteochondrosis of the pubis, pubalgia, osteitis necroticans pubis, rectus adductor syndrome, traumatic inguinal leg syndrome, anterior pelvic

joint syndrome, osteoarthropathy of the symphysis pubis, and Pierson syndrome.

Injury to the symphysis pubis area is a common and severe injury in soccer players. This type of injury is enigmatic in that neither its diagnosis nor treatment is well defined or understood. Injuries to the symphysis pubis are alarming because of their chronicity and resistance to treatment. They are often a career-ending injury for the elite player. Little is written about this syndrome in the English literature, although the entity is well described in the European literature. This syndrome was originally described by Beer[30] in 1924 after urologic surgery and since then has been reported with pregnancy and recently in association with trauma in athletes. In the 1950s Nescovic[30] described the first successful operative treatment.

Predisposition

Three primary predisposing conditions may be observed in players who are prone to this type of injury. The first characteristic is that of strong musculature and tight ligaments. The second characteristic is that the players are usually young, and it is likely that this is because the symphysis pubis reaches its adult maturity in the third decade[7] before there is some degree of motion obtainable at the symphysis. Almost all affected players are between the ages of 20 and 30 years[30]; it is exceed-

---

Factors that may contribute to traumatic osteitis pubis

- Well-developed, "tight" muscles and ligaments
- Young athletes most commonly affected
- Limitation of hip motion by degenerative joint disease

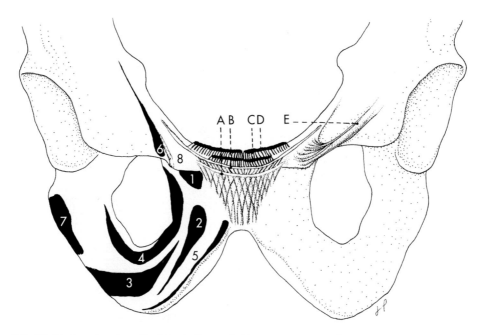

FIG. 65-14. Anterior view of pelvis. *A,* External oblique aponeurosis fibers crisscrossing in front of pubic symphysis before their insertion. *B,* Conjoint tendon or inguinal falx representing union of aponeurosis of internal oblique and transverse abdominal muscles. *C,* Pyramidalis muscle. *D,* Rectus abdominus muscle. *E,* Inguinal ligament. *1,* Adductor longus muscle; *2,* adductor brevis muscle; *3,* adductor magnus muscle; *4,* obturator externus muscle; *5,* gracilis muscle; *6,* pectineus muscle; *7,* quadratus femoris muscle; *8,* inguinal ligament insertion.

ingly rare in players over 30. The third predisposing characteristic is limitation of hip joint motion caused by degenerative hip disease in adolescents.[51,55,80] The players most frequently affected are strikers in the first division.[30] Other contributory factors include hard training, frequent competition, and poorly maintained grounds.

Anatomy

The symphysis pubis is a slightly movable joint that is constrained by three structures: the superior pubic ligament, the arcuate pubic ligament, and the interpubic disk (Fig. 65-13). The interpubic disk often contains a cavity, which usually appears after the tenth year of life, and has no synovial membrane lining. The pubis is the site of attachment of several major muscle groups, and it is thought that the imbalance among these muscle groups can lead to shearing forces across the symphysis leading to pain and degenerative changes of that structure.[39] The muscles of the anterior abdominal wall insert on the superior aspect of the pubis, and the adductors and short external rotators of the hip originate on the inferior surface of the pubis (Fig. 65-14).

Etiology

Although the presence of osteitis pubis complicating surgical procedures of the retropubic region is well documented in gynecology and urology, the cause of traumatic osteitis pubis is not so clearly understood. References in the literature date back to 1929, when Pierson[54]

reported a case in a 25-year-old man following repeated lifting of heavy boxes. Other references to the cause include documentation by Spinelli,[69] who described this entity among fencers. Occasional references in the literature followed, including that of Adams and Chandler,[1] who described changes in the symphysis pubis following isolated trauma and indicting either osteochondritis or infection as causative. Schwartzweller[68] referred to the lesion as the "gracilis syndrome" or "osteitis necroticans pubis," which he thought was secondary to degenerative changes in the gracilis at its origin on the pubic ramus.

Multiple theories have been proposed as to the cause of traumatic osteitis pubis among soccer players, and indeed traumatic osteitis pubis may be a conglomeration of several syndromes. The theories proposed as causes include (1) muscle strain with degenerative changes at the bony origin of the gracilis muscle, (2) tendinitis involving the gracilis muscle or other adductors at the inferior margin of the symphysis, (3) avascular necrosis of part of the pubis (osteochondritis dissecans), (4) unrecognized or subclinical subluxation of the symphysis with traumatic arthritis, (5) fatigue fracture of the pubis at the symphysis, (6) low-grade infection, and (7) avulsion fracture involving the gracilis tendon at its origin on the pubis.[79] Most authors agree that associated weakness of the abdominal wall musculature or fascia[30] usually leads to imbalance and shear stress across the pubis. Some propose the cause is merely a fascial defect in the abdominal wall, similar to a hernia.

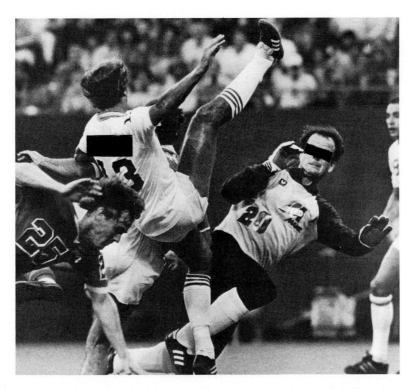

FIG. 65-15. Kicking leg is flexed, abducted, and externally rotated to reach ball. On impact, momentum of ball produces stress on origin of adductors.

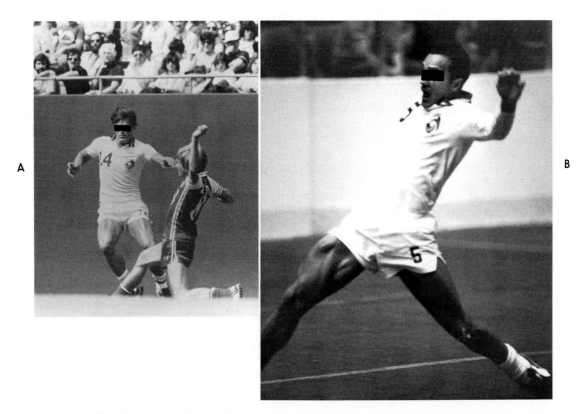

FIG. 65-16. Forceful abduction, flexion, and external rotation may produce strain of adductors.

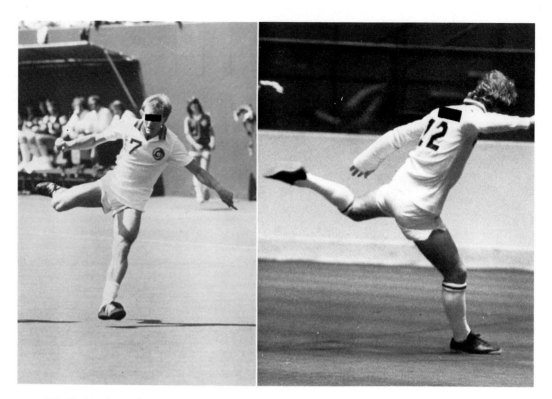

FIG. 65-17. Original position of thigh during hard inside kick (front and back views). Hip is extended, abducted, and internally rotated. Compare this with Fig. 65-7, in which at completion of follow-through, hip is externally rotated, flexed, and abducted.

Mechanism of Injury

With respect to the mechanics of soccer, three mechanisms actually produce this pubalgia of athletes. The first mechanism is a direct contusion to the area by an opponent's knee or by the ball. A second mechanism is an abnormal external rotation and abduction movement about the hip that overstretches the adductor muscle. This may happen when a player has one foot planted on the ground and brings the kicking leg forward in an abducted, flexed, and externally rotated position to reach the ball (Figs. 65-15 and 65-16). It may also occur during marking or checking of the opponent, if one foot of the player is forcefully abducted by the opponent during the dribbling phase when the other foot is planted on the ground. The third mechanism is repetitive trauma. This is the most common mechanism (about two thirds of all cases)[30] and it predominantly occurs in preseason, when the player lacks flexibility. It is thought to occur secondary to repetitive kicking on a poorly conditioned leg. Shooting practice, in particular, has been blamed. The player develops pain in the groin area that gradually increases. During shooting practice the player has to overextend and externally rotate the hip joint to kick the ball harder (Fig. 65-17), intensifying the rotational element of the adductors involved during the inside kick. Contributing factors may include a short warm-up and stretching period, cold weather, and a wet ball. It has been noted that a leather ball can be 20% heavier during wet weather. Synthetic balls are not significantly changed in weight by wet weather.

Clinical Appearance

Clinical appearance may vary according to the mechanism of injury. With the mechanism of contusion or adductor overstretching, the player usually develops severe pain in the groin area at the time of the injury. The player is usually unable to stand, and sometimes the pain is severe enough that the player is taken to the hospital for evaluation. With the mechanism of repetitive trauma, the player usually experiences a dull ache or mild, deep-seated pain in the groin region during kicking practice that gradually becomes more painful during the night. By the next morning the athlete is unable to kick the ball.

In the first few days during the acute phase the patient complains of severe pain in the lower abdominal musculature, the symphysis pubis, and the adductor tendon area. Pain is intensified on abduction and external rotation of the thigh or on resisted adduction. There is severe tenderness over the symphysis pubis, the adductor tendons, and the lower abdominal musculature. As the acute phase subsides and the player becomes more active, the athlete starts to experience some pain in the sacroiliac area on the injured side. The pain subsides within 2 or 3 weeks, but there is still tenderness on palpation of the groin area and symphysis pubis and resisted adduction elicits pain in the area (Fig. 65-18). As pain diminishes, the player becomes more active and is able to run but experiences pain in the pubic area on attempts to make a cut or kick the ball with the injured leg. As the athlete enters the chronic phase, he experiences pain

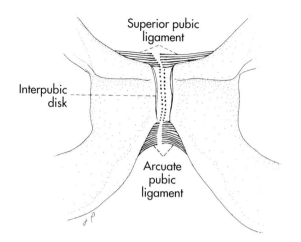

FIG. 65-18. Cross section of symphysis pubis with injuries to superior pubic ligament, interpubic disk, and arcuate pubic ligament during subluxation.

on cutting and pain becomes more severe in the groin area on attempts to kick the ball.

If the condition remains untreated and the player wants to continue playing despite the pain, the athlete may conceal the injury by kicking the ball directly in front of the body and by avoiding inside kicks. This mode of kicking uses mainly hip flexors and abductors and eliminates the use of the adductor musculature, thus lessening the shearing force across the symphysis. When, in the course of the game, these players kick the ball with the inside of the foot or cut while pivoting on the injured leg, they experience severe pain in the groin area. The clinician and the coaching staff should be watchful for the player with abnormal modes of kicking, especially in the professional who is extremely well trained in the fundamentals of the kick. Of course, if this situation is not alleviated and the player continues to use this "cheating" method of kicking, chronic injury occurs and ultimately is detrimental to the player's performance throughout the season.

Physical examination

On physical examination, there is usually tenderness over the adductor tendons and the symphysis pubis area. A combination of tenderness of the abdominal musculature and the adductor muscles is the most pathognomonic sign of an injury to the symphysis pubis. Imbert and Dupre-la-Tour[30] described three tests to confirm the diagnosis of osteitis pubis: (1) "relaxation" or loss of the normal integrity of the fascia of the anterior abdominal wall at its insertion on the pubis, (2) pain on resisted elevation of the leg in the supine position, and (3) tenderness and "relaxation" of the inguinal canal. Of these patients, 80% have tenderness in the adductor muscles. The patient should also be examined for evidence of decreased range of motion of the hip in comparison to the unaffected side because the incidence of hip arthropathy is high.[80]

Radiographic examination

Radiographs should include stress anteroposterior, inlet, and outlet views of the pelvis and stress anteroposterior views of the symphysis pubis. The stress views can be obtained by having the player stand first on one leg and taking a film centered on the symphysis and then changing legs and taking the same view (flamingo views). The two stress anteroposterior views are compared, and an instability is suggested if there is shifting of the relationships of the pubic bones between views.[69] Instability can also be assumed if there is anteroposterior or vertical discrepancy of the pubis on the inlet or outlet views. As pointed out by Schneider, Kaye, and Ghelman,[67] the x-ray changes that can be observed are changes of the pubic rami at the insertion of the adductor musculature in the form of osteolytic, erosion changes or avulsion fractures. It takes approximately 1 month following the initial injury for radiographic changes to manifest. The changes of the symphysis pubis joint can be manifested as instability in the stress views or slight widening with subarticular sclerosis and presence of traction osteophytes at the insertion of the superior pubic ligament. In severely unstable joints the osteophytes progress in an attempt to stabilize the joint (Fig. 65-19). Changes of the sacroiliac joint can be seen with narrowing or sclerosis of either or both sides of the joint. Changes of the hip joint may be seen.

Rispoli[60] described four stages of x-ray findings in the course of this injury. In Stage 1, or the florid stage, osteolytic changes occur in the os pubis at the insertion of the gracilis and adductor longus or brevis unilaterally or bilaterally, and erosions in the symphysis pubis and ischium take place. In Stage 2, or the transition stage, the symphysis is more affected, showing deeper erosions and asymmetry. In Stage 3, or the healing stage, the symphysis is more deformed, and arthrosis and avulsions are well developed. In Stage 4, the stage of secondary myositis ossificans, there may be evidence of myositis ossificans in the adductor longus and brevis, gracilis, obturator, and insertion of the internal and external obliques. Some calcifications of the healed osteonecrotic area of the os pubis may also be seen.

Other helpful diagnostic procedures include a technetium 99–pyrophosphate bone scan, which demonstrates increased bone metabolic activity in the area of the symphysis, although this is by no means pathognomonic.

Radiographic changes in osteitis pubis (after Rispoli)	
Stage 1 (florid stage)	Osteolysis of os pubis at the origin of the gracilis, adductor longus, or adductor brevis
Stage 2 (transitional stage)	Asymmetry and widespread erosions of symphysis pubis
Stage 3 (healing stage)	Arthrosis of symphysis pubis developing with deformity
Stage 4 (secondary myositis)	Myositis of adjacent muscles and calcifications of tissues around symphysis

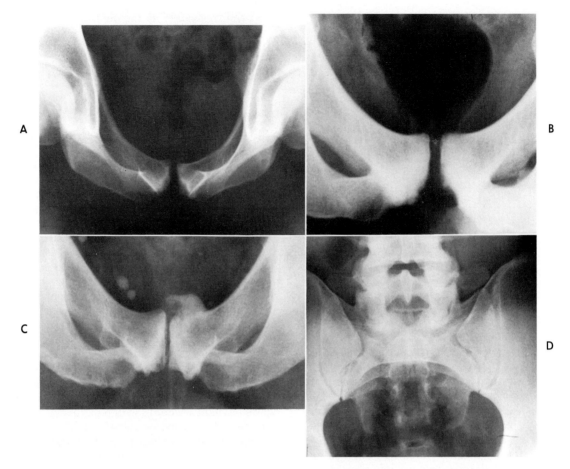

FIG. 65-19. Traumatic osteitis pubis of pelvis. **A,** Subluxation, slight widening, and subarticular sclerosis are observed 6 months after injury. **B,** Osteolytic changes of pubic rami at origin of gracilis muscles ½ year after injury (see Fig. 65-14). **C** and **D,** Radiographs of symphysis of professional soccer player and coach 15 years after injury. **C,** Note advanced osteophytes at origin of superior pubic ligament. In an attempt to stabilize the joint, advanced subarticular sclerosis of symphysis pubis is observed. **D,** Note narrowing and sclerosis of right sacroiliac joint.

Computed tomography (CT) is helpful, especially in the early stages of traumatic osteitis pubis, in demonstrating hematomas, soft-tissue swelling, and small avulsions not discernible on plain radiographs. We have not had much experience with magnetic resonance imaging (MRI) in the evaluation of these injuries, although it is likely to become a routine investigation in evaluating the patient with chronic groin pain in the near future because this syndrome is primarily a soft-tissue condition.

Treatment

Conservative. Conservative treatment is recommended in all cases for at least 6 months before any consideration of surgery. Treatment modalities have ranged from benign neglect to steroid injections, as outlined by Rispoli,[60] who noted spontaneous relief of symptoms after local infiltration with steroids. After the injury, ice packs or ice massage with cold cups should be applied to the groin area. Bed rest for 2 to 3 weeks is recommended for severe cases. Use of NSAIDs and analgesics is recommended as well. Local infiltration of the tender area with 5 to 10 ml of 1% lidocaine with methylprednisolone has been reported. The use of injectable glucocorticoids is controversial and may aggravate the condition or initiate a local necrosis. After the pain subsides, range of motion exercises are instituted with emphasis on gentle abduction of the hip joint and strengthening of the abdominal musculature.[60] Manual resistance is introduced when the range of motion is full and can be performed without pain. Players can start jogging gradually after 3 to 4 weeks, but running and cutting are not allowed until the eighth week, following proper stretching and strengthening of the adductor muscles and proper conditioning of the rectus abdominus and oblique muscles. Kicking the ball is introduced gradually.

Surgical. If conservative treatment, including ultrasound modalities, muscle rehabilitation, and reeducation fails and the player is still experiencing severe pain and discomfort in the groin area on kicking the ball or on trying to cut while running, surgical treatment may be considered. The literature is ambiguous with respect to surgical treatment. Surgical treatment has been noted in the

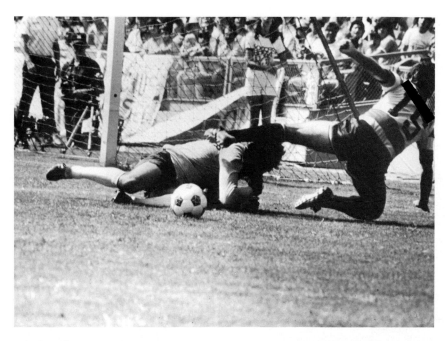

FIG. 65-20. Soccer combines features of running, kicking, and collision injuries.

literature dating back to Nescovic,[25,30] a Yugoslavian surgeon and former soccer player. Nescovic[25,30] believed that weakness of the anterior abdominal wall was to blame, and his operation involved reefing of the abdominal muscles to the pubis and Poupart's ligament.[30] In Europe most operations for chronic osteitis pubis are based on Nescovic's technique. In theory, his repair strengthens the fascia of the anterior abdominal wall, reinforces the floor of the inguinal canal, broadens the insertion area of the rectus, and aims at equilibriating the unbalanced muscular equilibrium acting on the pubis secondary to the strong adductors.[12,25] Dijan et al[12] (45 patients), Hermans[25] (69 patients), and Imbert and Dupre-la-Tour[30] (243 patients) have all reported good results with modifications of the Nescovic technique. Others have addressed their surgical approach based on the belief that the primary pathologic condition lies in the adductors. In the United States Schneider, Kaye, and Ghelman reported excellent results of one case treated by sectioning the gracilis tendon and removing a bony ossicle. Adams and Chandler[1] reported excellent results with arthrodesis of the symphysis. There has been no critical review of the surgical treatment of these injuries, and in our experience each case is individualized and surgery guided by the clinical symptoms and radiographic findings. If the symptoms are mainly in the adductor area and radiographs reveal avulsion fragments or erosion of the pubic rami, exploration of the groin musculature with a 1-cm tenotomy of the involved tendon and curettage of its insertion usually suffice. If the player has primarily suprapubic complaints, the inguinal canal and anterior abdominal wall may be explored and reinforced. For example, one player with radiographic findings of osteitis pubis and a 2-year history of chronic groin pain precluding play was found on CT scan to have a cyst in the midsubstance of the adductor longus tendon. On surgical exploration the cyst proved to be a chronic hematoma, which was resected without difficulty. The player's symptoms resolved completely 1 month postoperatively and was able to resume professional play. A second case involved a player with radiographic changes consistent with osteitis pubis and primarily inguinal complaints lasting for over a year. A defect in the rectus abdominus insertion was noted at operation, and a Nescovic-type repair was performed. Again, complete resolution of symptoms was obtained, and the patient was kicking a ball 3 months postoperatively. Regardless of the method of surgery, activities are routinely restricted for 8 weeks following operative treatment. After rehabilitation of the lower extremities the player is allowed to gradually participate in soccer.

ACUTE THIGH MUSCLE INJURIES

Strains and contusions of the thigh musculature have been shown to be exceedingly common in soccer and may account for up to 50% of all injuries in this sport. Injuries to the thigh in sport are common and may be incurred in one of several ways. In running and jumping sports (e.g., track, skating, and gymnastics) strains are relatively frequent. Contusion injuries are more common in the so-called collision sports (e.g., rugby, hockey, and football). Kicking provides yet a third element whereby strains and contusions may occur. Soccer combines the elements of running, collision, and kicking as well as poor protection to result in an unusually high rate of thigh injuries when compared with other sports (Fig. 65-20).

Simply put, a strain represents failure of the musculotendinous unit in tension, resulting in a tear commonly

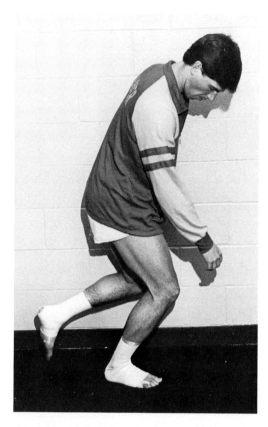

FIG. 65-21. Player squatting on injured extremity, eliciting pain at certain point of arc of motion.

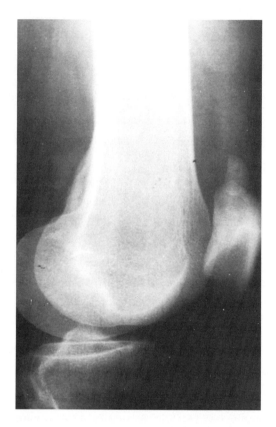

FIG. 65-22. Radiograph demonstrating complete rupture of insertion of quadriceps tendon and avulsion fragments of superior pole of patella.

of the musculotendinous junction and less commonly through the midsubstance of the muscle or tendon. A contusion is a compression injury of the muscle resulting from blunt trauma. The muscle belly is the usual site of this injury. Tendons are relatively resistant to contusion.[57]

Both contusions and strains are painful and tender. Tenderness and pain are proportional to the severity of injury. In Grade I injuries pain is minor and not constant, and symptoms can be elicited by having the player squat on the affected extremity (Fig. 65-21). At a certain point the injured part of the muscle comes into action, producing pain. Higher grade injuries are more self-evident.

Quadriceps Mechanism Injuries

Proximal quadriceps injuries usually represent either a strain caused by forceful contraction of the quadriceps muscle or an overstretch injury. Pain is referred to the region of the anterior hip or the anterior iliac spine. On physical examination, tenderness is elicited by hip flexion or knee extension against resistance. Swelling and occasionally ecchymosis may be seen. Radiographs help exclude avulsion fracture. Early return to activity should be encouraged as symptoms subside. Basic principles of orthopaedic rehabilitation are followed with gradual strengthening and stretching. Jogging progressing to running is done as tolerated. As with any rehabil-

itation process, pain should be the guide to progression. Surgical reattachment of avulsed proximal musculature is rarely indicated.[50]

Midthigh injuries are usually contusions; strains are rare. Injuries commonly occur secondary to a direct blow from a ball or an opposing player's knee or foot. Diagnosis is straightforward, with findings that include midquadriceps tenderness in the injured muscle and pain with active and passive knee motion. Edema is proportionate to the magnitude of the trauma. The goal of treatment is to minimize swelling and bleeding into the injured tissue.[41] Rest, elevation, and ice packs are employed for 24 to 48 hours. A compression bandage and flexed knee immobilizer are used (see p. 1014). Crutches are used, and isometric exercises of the quadriceps muscles are allowed as tolerated. After the player has full extension and gains at least 90 degrees of flexion, progressive resistive exercises are instituted. Disability from mild contusion averages 1 week, a moderate contusion 8 weeks, and a severe contusion 10 or more weeks.[33,41] The incidence of myositis ossificans is extremely high in these injuries and may complicate rehabilitation.[32]

Distal quadriceps injuries are usually strains and are caused by forceful contraction of the quadriceps muscle mechanism usually against resistance (e.g., when trying to kick the ball and instead striking the ground with the foot at midswing). The lesion causes pain with active or passive knee motion, and local tenderness occurs in the region. The lesion may be classified as follows: Grade I, minimal strain or stretch of the musculotendinous unit; Grade II, moderate strain or partial tear of the musculotendinous unit; and Grade III, suprapatellar avulsion with loss of continuity with the patella. Knee effusion may be seen with Grade II or Grade III lesions. Grade III injuries are readily apparent with a palpable defect in the quadriceps mechanism and inability of the patient to actively extend the knee. Radiographs may show a fragment of bone and a traumatic patella baja (Fig. 65-22). Grades I and II are treated in the usual manner with rest, ice, compression, and appropriate rehabilitation. In the Grade III injury, surgical repair is mandatory.

Adductor Injuries

Because of the amount of lateral movement in soccer as well as the mechanics of the inside kick, the adductor muscles are subject to frequent tensile loads. The adductor strain, or "pulled groin," is one of the most commonly seen injuries in soccer. Injury is often the result of a "reach" causing overstretch of the adductors or a forceful inside kick. Osteitis pubis is often confused with this lesion, and clearly there is some overlap. The patient complains of medial thigh and groin pain following the inciting maneuver, especially on attempted kicking. Examination reveals tenderness along the proximal adductor longus tendon and is exacerbated by passive abduction or resisted adduction of the leg. Treatment consists of the usual conservative measures of rest, ice, compression, and use of NSAIDs. The injury, per se, does not exclude the player from play, but it significantly hampers his abilities. Because of the propensity of this injury to go on to a chronic problem, abstaining from play for at least 1 week following the injury is customarily recommended. When acute pain resolves, stretching and strengthening exercises may be instituted. Taping of the thigh appears to have some benefit in the acute situation but is of little prophylactic value. Adequate adductor stretching appears to be the best prophylaxis against this injury, since adductor strains are associated with poor flexibility of these muscles.[15]

Hamstring Injuries

Strains or contusions of the hamstrings are common injuries in soccer players. Contusions mainly occur on the lateral hamstrings and usually in the distal one third because that area is more vulnerable to contact injuries (especially kicks or "kneeling" injuries). Strains of the hamstrings are more common on the short head of the biceps. The high frequency of hamstring strains in kicking may result from the fact that the hamstrings are responsible for slowing down the ballistic motion of the tibia and preventing hyperextension of the knee after a kick.

During a kick, 15% of the leg's kinetic energy is transferred to the ball to accelerate it. The remaining 85% of the force is absorbed mainly by the hamstring in an attempt to flex the knee and slow the ballistic motion of the leg. The most common causes of strained hamstrings are a violent kick, stretching to reach a ball, or a quick start. Associated causes of hamstring strains are poor flexibility, fatigue, inadequate warm-up, and imbalance of quadriceps and hamstring strength. Ideally, the hamstrings should be 60% to 70% as strong as the quadriceps group.[11]

Diagnosis

There is tenderness and swelling of the lateral hamstrings in a contusion. A strain usually reveals point tenderness over the proximal biceps femoris tendons and ischial tuberosity. Pressure and ice are applied after the injury to reduce bleeding and spasm. Oral enzyme treatment is popular in Europe but has no proven efficacy. After acute pain resolves, flexibility exercises should begin and the athlete should strengthen the hamstrings and quadriceps muscles. Taping and wrapping the injured area has some benefit for strains. Mild strains heal within 1 week, but severe strains may take more than a month. Hamstring contusions, like a quadriceps contusion, have a high incidence of subsequent myositis ossificans.

A surprising finding that we have noticed is the lack of flexibility in most European soccer players. Many of the successful international players have severe limitation in the hamstrings and low back. When questioned, their universal response is that they never spent time stretching. We have found that foreign players, when first coming to the United States, usually suffer some groin or hamstring strains. It might be said that the increased incidence of these strains is caused by unnatural playing surfaces or fatigue factors. In Europe soccer is played on natural grass and rarely more than once a week. The professional leagues in the United States play anywhere from one to three games a week. Therefore we consider an extensive stretching program a must for any foreign player. As part of pregame preparation the athlete must stretch the lower extremities, including the hamstrings, the quadriceps muscles, and the Achilles tendon.

Myositis Ossificans Traumatica

Heterotopic bone formation may follow hematoma formation in an injured muscle as a result of direct trauma or contusion; it is not seen with a strain injury. The most common location of myositis ossificans in the lower extremity is the quadriceps muscle.[29,32] In soccer the lateral hamstring is commonly involved as well. This follows logically as these two muscle groups are the most frequently contused. A severe thigh contusion should alert the clinician to the possible development of myositis. Diagnosis can be made clinically. After the swelling and acute pain stabilize, a focal site of acute inflammation sets in. On examination, there is a tender, firm, hot mass within the involved muscle, and range of motion of the adjacent joints is restricted. After the acute phase the mass is still palpable but painless. After 3 to 6 months the mass stabilizes. Aggressive rehabilitation should be avoided in favor of rest and immobilization until the acute inflammation resolves to avoid exacerbating the myositis. Play may be resumed only when the pain is

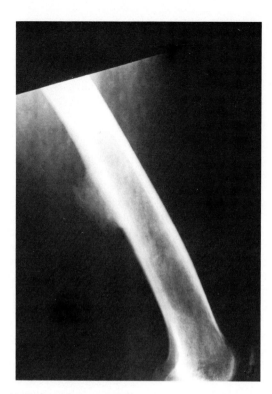

FIG. 65-23. Myositis ossificans located in lateral hamstrings in form of periosteal or broad-based type.

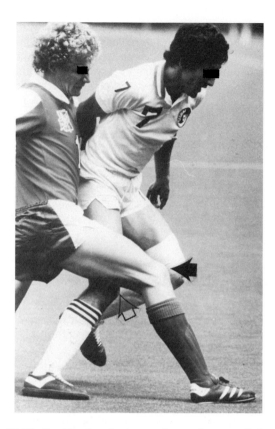

FIG. 65-24. Combination of valgus and varus forces applied to opponent's knee during marking. *Solid arrow,* varus; *open arrow,* valgus.

completely resolved and full range of motion has been restored—often up to 6 months. Radiographic examination within 2 to 3 weeks after the injury reveals a flocculation, which usually evolves into a corticated, well-defined, ossified mass (Fig. 65-23).[32] Soccer players usually do not complain of pain associated with matured myositis ossificans. Should the lesion become chronically symptomatic, surgical excision may be considered but only after 1 year has elapsed from the time of injury and a bone scan has demonstrated a lack of activity in the area. Excision before this may result in recurrence.

ACUTE KNEE INJURIES

Acute knee injuries are some of the most severe injuries sustained in soccer. Regrettably, they are also one of the more frequent injuries, especially at the professional level. It is estimated that one in five players at the elite level sustain a major knee injury in the course of one season.[19] The high incidence of these injuries is thought in part to result from the high-kinetic energies obtained in the leg during the kick and the various torques experienced across the knee that are somewhat unique to soccer.[22] Whereas in other sports most knee injuries are the result of a valgus load, soccer injuries are commonly caused by varus and hyperextension loads (Fig. 65-24). Because soccer is a sport requiring cutting or pivoting maneuvers, the players' knees are also subject to the usual noncontact injuries seen in other pivoting sports.

Medial Collateral Ligament Injuries

The mechanism of injury of the medial collateral ligament (MCL) is a severe valgus force across the knee joint. The ligament is commonly injured when the inside kick is interrupted by striking another player or a blocked ball or inadvertently hitting the ground with the foot (Fig. 65-31). This injury can also occur when a player is tackled on the lateral side of the support leg, similar to the clipping injury of American football. The injured player complains of pain that occurs just before making contact with the ball on an inside kick, and the injury is a result of the valgus torque created in the knee. This helps to differentiate this injury from medial meniscal tears in which the pain appears right after striking the ball. A medial meniscal tear is the result of varus torque compressing the meniscus. Diagnosis and management is as outlined in Chapter 38. Surgery has no role in the treatment of MCL injuries. Return to soccer is allowed when the player has full range of motion; is able to run, kick, and change directions without pain; and has no pain or instability to stress testing.[17,72] It should be noted that hinged knee braces are forbidden in most organized soccer games.

Lateral Collateral Ligament Injuries

In contrast with other sports, injuries of the LCL are common in soccer. The inside of the knee in soccer is

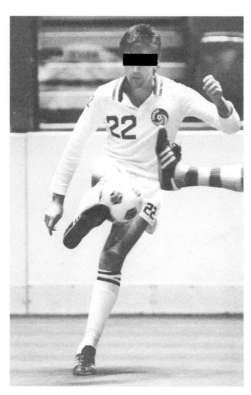

FIG. 65-25. Opponent's foot blocks adduction-flexion motion of thigh while ballistic motion of tibia continues, producing varus forces in lateral, posterolateral corner of right knee.

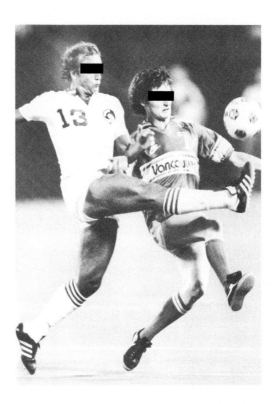

FIG. 65-26. Varus force produced on knee of kicking leg caused by immobilization of thigh by opponent's pelvis.

relatively unprotected, and varus forces are common as a result of contact and kicking mechanisms (Figs. 65-25 and 65-26). Injuries to the lateral structures are as common as injuries to the medial ligaments but are usually milder.

On physical examination the player has severe pain in the posterolateral corner of the knee. The athlete is unable to play, or in severe cases, to ambulate on the involved leg. There is tenderness over the LCL and insertion of the biceps tendon and posterolateral corner of the knee. Swelling may be observed within several hours.

Again, the specifics of management are discussed elsewhere (see Chapter 38). Suffice it to say that the injury is treated with rehabilitation aimed at restoring strength and full range of motion of the knee usually with protection in a hinged brace. Surgery has no role. Return to play is allowed when full range of motion is restored and the patient has no pain or instability to varus stress.

Anterior Cruciate Ligament Injury

Tears of the anterior cruciate ligament (ACL) are common in soccer and may result from several different mechanisms of injury. Hyperextension injury of the knee may produce ACL rupture, either as an isolated injury or in concert with a posterior cruciate ligament (PCL) rupture (Fig. 65-27).[49] Hyperextension may result as an opponent blocks the player's femur during the act of kicking. The femur is held fixed while the momen-

tum of the leg hyperextends the knee. Injury may also occur secondary to a valgus force or "clipping injury" as part of an unhappy triad (Fig. 65-28). Clipping injuries happen frequently during tackling. Last, an isolated ACL injury can be observed when the player tries to cut or twist, producing a valgus external rotation injury of the knee. This frequently occurs when dribbling the ball (Fig. 65-29).

Diagnosis and management are discussed in Chapters 38 and 39. It has been our common policy to offer reconstruction to all serious soccer players because the prospects for returning to their previous level of play are poor with conservative management. Our current technique is endoscopic ACL reconstruction with the central third of the patellar ligament. Postoperative management is discussed in Chapter 43. The knee is protected with a derotation brace, and the athlete is not allowed to kick the ball for 5 to 6 months. Full recovery and return to the starting lineup requires 12 months of rehabilitation.

Posterior Cruciate Ligament Injuries

As mentioned previously, the PCL may be damaged in conjunction with a ruptured ACL from a hyperextension injury (Fig. 65-27). Rupture of the PCL may also occur secondary to a posteriorly directed force on a bent knee (Fig. 65-30), resulting either from a fall or from a direct kick to the anterior surface of the tibia. PCL tears are uncommon.

Diagnosis and management are discussed in Chapters 38 and 39. Recently, we have become more aggressive

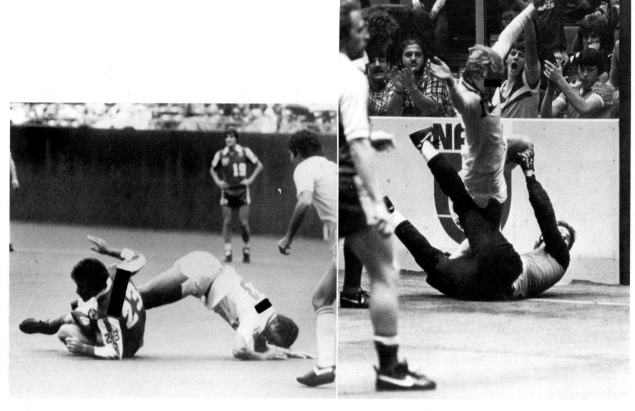

FIG. 65-27. Opponent blocks planted feet and tibia, forcing knee into hyperextension (two examples).

with PCL injuries, since the results of reconstruction have been encouraging when compared with conservative treatment or prior surgical procedures. Our current method is arthroscopic reconstruction with the central third of the patellar tendon. Rehabilitation is discussed in Chapter 43.

Meniscal Injuries

Meniscal injuries are common in soccer. According to Ricklin, Ruttiman, and Del Buono,[59] soccer accounts for the highest incidence of meniscal injuries among all sports (35%), followed by track and field (33%) and skiing (22%). Medial meniscal injuries occur with greater than twice the frequency of lateral tears.

Mechanism of Injury

Sudden rotation of the femur relative to the tibia causes indirect injury to the meniscus. The mechanism can be produced in a collision between players when a player's foot is fixed in the turf while trying to make a cut or when a player's foot is prevented from turning by another player or by the ball. The symptoms of a torn meniscus (pain, popping, and locking) presumably come from entrapment of the torn unstable portion of the meniscus between the tibial and femoral condyles. During kicking, a player with a torn medial meniscus experiences pain in the medial joint line right after contact with

Medial knee pain	
Medial collateral ligament injury (mild)	Pain just *before* ball contact during kick (acceleration phase and valgus force)
Medial meniscus injury	Pain just *after* ball contact during kick (deceleration phase and varus force)

the ball because of varus torque in the knee joint, which results in an increase in the pressure between the femoral and tibial condyles (Fig. 65-31). This is different from the pain experienced by a player with an MCL sprain that appears right before contact with the ball. Management is discussed in Chapter 37.

Patellar Dislocation

In soccer, lateral dislocation of the patella may occur secondary to a direct blow to the medial aspect of the patella often from a ball or an opponent's foot. Although rare in adults, this injury is frequent in youth leagues, especially among female players. The vast majority of dislocations spontaneously reduce (if the player is able to extend the knee) long before they are seen by the physician or trainer. If the patella remains dislocated, exam-

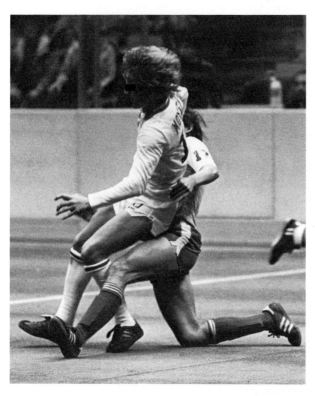

FIG. 65-28. Player's knee is hit from behind by opponent, which produces an anteriorly directed force.

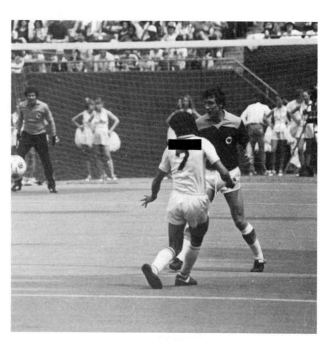

FIG. 65-29. Plant and cut noncontact injury to knee.

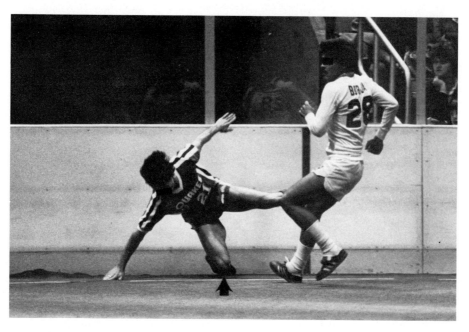

FIG. 65-30. Player falling on his flexed knee *(arrow)*, producing posteriorly directed force.

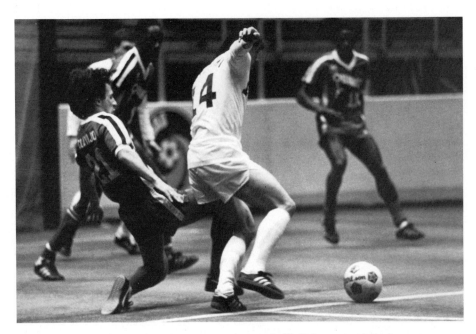

FIG. 65-31. Player hitting ground instead of ball during inside kick.

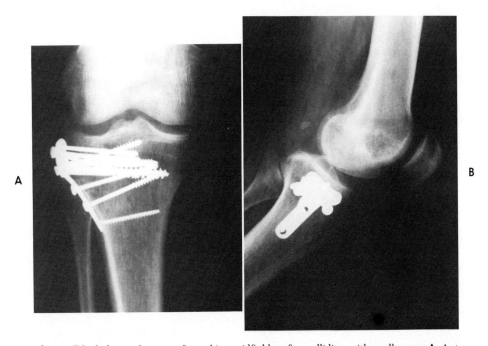

FIG. 65-32. Tibial plateau fracture of attacking midfielder after colliding with goalkeeper. **A,** Anteroposterior, and **B,** lateral postoperative radiographs following open reduction and internal fixation with A-O plate and screws.

ination reveals obvious lateral displacement of the patella. To reduce the dislocation, the hip is flexed to relax the quadriceps and the knee is then gently extended, which effects immediate reduction.

Examination of the injured player with a spontaneously reduced dislocation reveals a large effusion and greatest tenderness over the medial retinaculum, particularly in the region of the adductor tubercle. The patient has a positive apprehension sign. Range of motion is lim-

ited in flexion. Pain throughout range of motion or a locked knee suggests an osteochondral fracture.

Initial management includes aspiration and immobilization in extension to reduce the symptoms. Radiographs are taken to rule out osteochondral fracture. A cylinder cast is applied for a total of 5 weeks. Once the patient is out of the cast, aggressive quadriceps muscle rehabilitation is undertaken. Return to soccer is allowed when quadriceps muscle strength is 95% of the unaffected

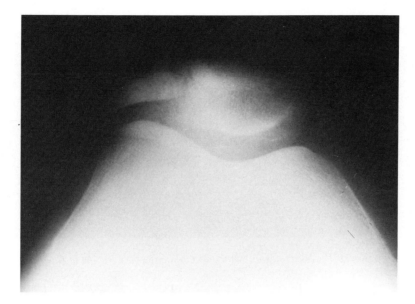

FIG. 65-33. Fractures through synchondrosis of bipartite patella after making contact with opponent's knee during game.

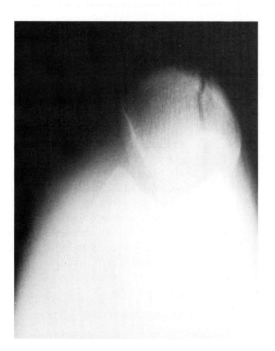

FIG. 65-34. Longitudinal fracture of patella in soccer player caused by direct fall to ground.

side. Recurrent symptoms necessitate surgical intervention.

Knee Joint Fractures

Fractures are relatively common in any type of contact sport; soccer is no exception. It is beyond the scope of this chapter to discuss the management of all the various fractures of the lower extremity. Suffice it to say that we have seen all types of fractures incurred as a result of this sport, including femoral and tibial shaft fractures, femoral condyle fractures, tibial plateau fractures (Fig. 65-32), and foot and ankle fractures. Below are entailed some of the fractures that are more unique to soccer. Standard principles of fracture management apply in all but a few circumstances.

Patellar Fractures

Fractures of the patella can be caused by direct force causing a primary longitudinal fracture line or indirect force causing a transverse fracture usually through osteoporotic bone. Longitudinal fractures are more common among soccer players than the general population (Figs. 65-33 and 65-34),[4] probably reflecting the high incidence of direct blows to the anterior surface of the knee during a game. Nondisplaced fractures with an intact extensor mechanism should be treated with a cylinder cast for 5 weeks. Displaced fractures require open reduction and internal fixation.

Intercondylar Eminence Fractures

Intercondylar eminence fractures represent an avulsion fracture of the ACL and are usually seen in adolescents. Injury often occurs secondary to hyperextension. Diagnosis is made radiographically (Fig. 65-35). Minimally displaced fractures may be reduced by placing the knee in extension and treating it in a cylinder cast. Displaced fragments require internal fixation. Open reduction is the standard of care, but recently we have been reducing these arthroscopically using a cannulated screw with good success. Alternative methods of fixation that do not violate the growth plate are necessary in the young athlete with an open tibial physis.

Tibial Tubercle Fractures

Fractures of the tibial tubercle represent an avulsion fracture from pull of the patellar ligament and can occur

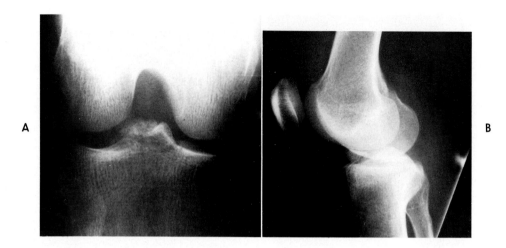

FIG. 65-35. Types II-III avulsion fracture of intercondylar eminence of tibia in **A,** anteroposterior, and **B,** lateral views.

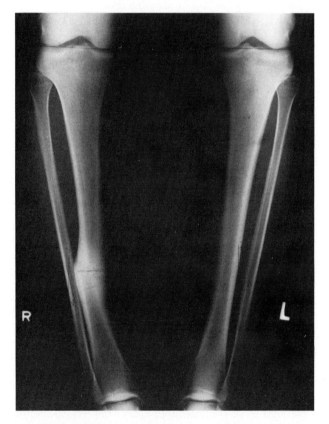

FIG. 65-36. Malunion of fractured tibia initially treated by closed reduction and plaster immobilization. This midfielder had recurrent hindfoot pain with prolonged play and was unable to resume upper division competition.

when the kick is interrupted by catching the turf or striking an opponent. This injury is common in 12- to 16-year-old athletes before proximal tibial growth plate closure. The injured athlete has extreme pain on attempts to actively extend the knee. Nondisplaced fractures are treated in a long cylinder cast and displaced fractures

with open reduction with internal fixation. Return to play is governed by presence of a healed fracture and normalized quadriceps muscle strength.

Tibial Shaft Fractures

Unfortunately, tibial shaft fractures are not uncommon in soccer. Injury is usually secondary to a direct force as the result of a kick or blow to the anterior surface of the tibia (Figs. 65-2 and 65-3). Diagnosis is usually obvious. Open injuries are rare. Immediate management of these injuries on the field consists of immobilization, ice, and mild compressive wrapping to reduce swelling. The incidence of compartment syndrome is small because these are relatively low-energy injuries; nonetheless, neurovascular integrity of the limb must be monitored. We have become more aggressive in treating these fractures with locked intramedullary rodding, since shortening or angulation is not tolerated in a soccer player (Fig. 65-36). Intramedullary rodding also allows for earlier rehabilitation and return to sport.

OVERUSE SYNDROMES
Iliotibial Band Friction Syndrome

Iliotibial band (ITB) friction syndrome is caused by excessive friction between the lateral femoral epicondyle and the ITB. The ITB lies anterior to the lateral epicondyle during knee extension but moves posterior to it during knee flexion. Formation of a bursa over the prominent lateral epicondyle of the femur can be caused by repetitive motion of the ITB over the epicondyle. Predisposing factors include a tight ITB, repetitive knee flexion and extension from running for prolonged periods, and direct trauma to the lateral aspect of the thigh or knee. The occurrence of this syndrome is not infrequent among soccer players, especially goalies. Goalies are forced to make many diving saves, and suffer from repeated contusions of this area (Fig. 65-37).

Symptoms include pain and a snapping sensation over the lateral aspect of the knee brought on by prolonged

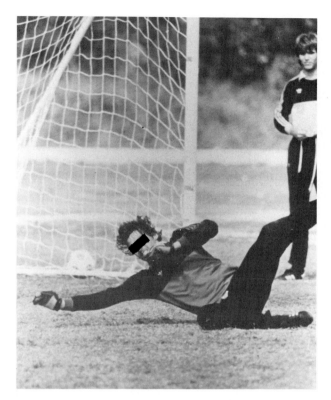

FIG. 65-37. Iliotibial band friction syndrome can be observed because goalkeepers are forced to make many diving saves.

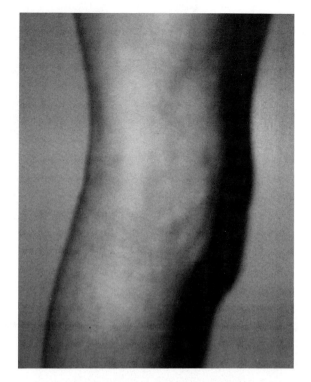

FIG. 65-38. Enlarged tibial tubercle in typical Osgood-Schlatter disease.

running. Examination may reveal a positive Ober test indicative of a tight ITB, tenderness over the lateral femoral epicondyle, and a popping sensation over the lateral aspect of the knee on flexion and extension. Symptoms may be elicited by having the athlete support all of his or her weight with the knee flexed at 30 degrees[58] or by having the athlete run on a treadmill until the pain recurs. If NSAIDs, stretching, rest, and local steroid injection produce no long-lasting relief, surgical release of the posterior fibers of the ITB may be considered.[48]

Jumper's Knee

Jumper's knee, or patellar tendinitis, is characterized by pain and tenderness on the superior pole or inferior pole of the patella or along the patellar tendon.[3] It is extremely common in the adolescent soccer player, perhaps secondary to repetitive running and kicking causing irritation of the extensor mechanism. On physical examination, there is pain on resisted extension of the knee and tenderness on the superior or inferior poles of the patella.[40] Radiography may reveal calcification in the tendon or changes in the poles of the patella.

Treatment consists of rest and abstention from sporting activity for a variable period. Quadriceps muscle strengthening exercises are instituted. Steroid injections are contraindicated.[77] Usually the symptoms are self-limited but are often recurrent. Return to soccer is allowed when the athlete can run without pain. If symptoms persist for greater than 1 year, surgical removal of the degenerated portion of tendon is indicated.[63] Al-

though rare, patellar tendon rupture has been reported in soccer players.[64,74]

Osgood-Schlatter Disease

Osgood-Schlatter disease is a common overuse injury in the young soccer player.[52] During the kick the powerful quadriceps complex, which inserts into the tibial tubercle, may partially avulse the tibial epiphysis, causing a chronic epiphysitis. The young soccer player complains of pain over the tibial tubercle and the patella tendon during and after the game. The kicking leg alone is usually affected, or, if bilateral, the kicking leg is usually worse. Kneeling is often painful. Examination reveals tenderness over the tibial tubercle with some crepitus and tenderness over the distal part of the patellar tendon. There may also be swelling and enlargement of the tubercle (Fig. 65-38). The quadriceps muscle mechanism is weak and tight in comparison with the other extremity. Radiographs may reveal soft-tissue swelling, enlargement, or fragmentation of the tubercle.[44] Treatment consists of temporary cessation of sports. When the acute pain resolves, stretching and strengthening exercises for the quadriceps muscles are instituted. Surgical excision of palpable loose bodies should be considered in persistent cases.[50]

Prepatellar Bursitis

Prepatellar bursitis can be observed in soccer players, mainly goalkeepers, because of the frequency with which they kneel or land directly on their knees (Fig. 65-

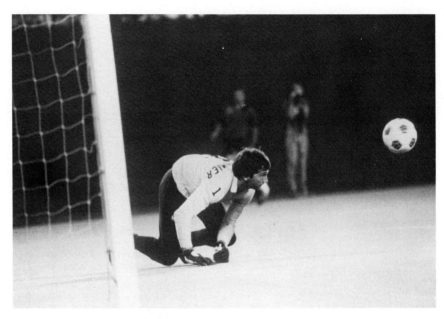

FIG. 65-39. Goalkeeper landing on his knees during a save.

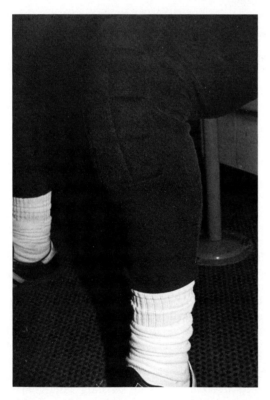

FIG. 65-40. Protective padding used to prevent prepatellar bursitis in goalkeeper.

39). On examination, there is swelling, erythema, and tenderness superficial to the patellar tendon, and the overlying skin becomes tense. For acute prepatellar bursitis, ice, immobilization, and NSAIDs are recommended. The bursa may be aspirated and injected with a steroid if symptoms persist. The key to preventing recurrence is proper knee padding (Fig. 65-40).

Pes Anserinus Bursitis

Pes anserinus bursitis has been observed in soccer players. It is an inflammation of the bursa that separates the pes anserine tendons (gracilis, sartorius, and semitendinosus tendons) from the anteromedial surface of the tibia. The cause is unclear but is probably secondary to direct trauma or overuse. Players complain of pain in the area on kicking the ball, running, or cutting. Signs include warmth, tenderness, erythema, and swelling over the anteromedial surface of the proximal tibia. This is usually managed with local treatments and an injection of a corticosteroid.

LEG INJURIES
Compartment Syndrome

There are two types of compartment syndrome of the leg: acute and chronic (exertional). Exertional compartment syndrome is discussed in Chapter 28. Compartment syndrome occurs in soccer players and should be differentiated from both tenosynovitis of the foot dorsiflexors and shin splints. If clinically indicated, a test of the compartment pressures during exercise should be performed.

Acute compartment syndrome of the leg in the absence of fracture is a true rarity, although it does occur. When it occurs, it is secondary to a direct blow usually to the anterior aspect of the leg from either an opponent's foot or a ball. The anterior compartment is most frequently affected. Tense swelling, pain out of proportion to findings, and pain with passive stretch are the classic findings of an early compartment syndrome. This entity can be easily recognized on the field if the possibility is kept in the differential. Measuring compartment pressures is not usually practical. In patients with suspected compartment syndrome the leg should be mildly elevated and iced. Treatment is on an emergency basis, and the

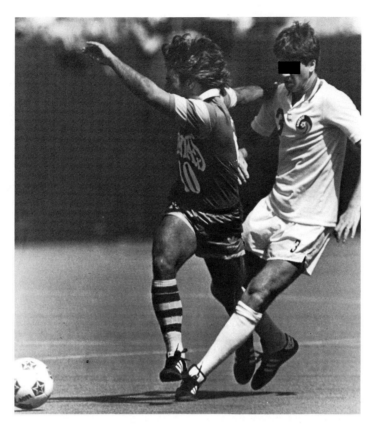

FIG. 65-41. Severe hyperpronation of foot from collision during running.

patient should be rapidly taken to a hospital for full evaluation and fasciotomy as indicated.

Peroneal Nerve Contusion

Direct contusion of the peroneal nerve as it crosses directly behind the neck of the fibula is the most common nerve injury seen in soccer. An errant kick in that area may compress the nerve against the underlying bone, causing at least temporary injury. Right after the kick the player experiences local pain from the contusion and pain (likened to an electric shock) radiating down the anterior leg into the dorsum of the foot. Numbness and paresthesias in the cutaneous distribution of the nerve may also be present. Locally, there may be skin abrasions or ecchymosis with tenderness of the underlying peroneal nerve. Local pressure may exacerbate the tingling. Usually this neurapraxia lasts only a few seconds or minutes, but if the injury is severe, the hypesthesia and weakness of the peroneals and dorsiflexors persist. These may inhibit the player from controlling the ball during the game. The player may even develop a drop foot. Most of the time the contusion of the nerve is minor, and usually the player recovers within 1 or 2 days after the injury. Treatment is supportive. Resumption of play is allowed when symptoms abate and there is no demonstrable weakness of the peroneals or dorsiflexors. Protective padding over the peroneal head area should be instituted to protect the nerve for a few weeks. An orthosis for a drop foot is rarely necessary.

Shin Splints

The term "shin splint" refers to a muscle, tendon, or periosteal inflammatory reaction that causes pain along either the anterior or the posterior surface of the tibia and is associated with running sports. Anterior shin splints result from repetitive trauma to the origins of the anterior tibialis, the extensor hallucis longus, and the extensor digitorum longus from excessive running on poorly conditioned legs. It is seen almost exclusively in preseason training. Soccer players seem to be particularly predisposed to this injury because of large active dorsiflexion and passive plantar flexion forces across the ankle that occur when kicking the ball, which cause stretching and tearing of the origins of the anterior compartment musculature on the anterior surface of the tibia.[52] This combined with the long distances that are run during the course of training results in a high incidence of injury. The athlete complains of pain on running, especially when slowing down. Pain and tenderness along the anterolateral border of the proximal tibia are noted. The pain is exacerbated by passive plantar flexion or resisted active dorsiflexion of the ankle. Treatment consists of ice, rest, and strengthening of the anterior compartment musculature.

Posterior shin splints are less well defined but appear to occur secondary to repetitive trauma to the origins of the muscles of the deep posterior compartment (the posterior tibialis, the flexor hallucis longus, and the flexor digitorum longus). This syndrome is much less common in soccer players, and when it occurs, it is usually secondary to hypermobile, pronated feet or a severe hyperpronation injury (Fig. 65-41). The player complains of posterior shin pain after running long distances and has tenderness over the posteromedial aspect of the tibia. Treatment consists of rest, ice, and an arch support, if appropriate.

ANKLE INJURIES
Tendinitis and Bursitis

Tendinitis around the ankle joint is common in soccer players. Its cause is a combination of overuse injuries and external mechanical irritation. A soccer player may run more than 7 miles per game with frequent jumping, acceleration, and stopping. The tendons around the ankle joint are used hundreds of times during the game to either transfer or absorb the tremendous amount of energy generated during the act of kicking. External mechanical irritation is the result of the repetitive direct trauma to which these structures are subject to during the game (Fig. 65-42).

Clancy's classification of tendon injuries

1. Tenosynovitis and tenovaginitis
   Inflammation of only the paratenon, either lined by synovium or not[25]
2. Tendinitis
   Injury or symptomatic degeneration of the tendon with a resultant inflammatory reaction of the surrounding paratenon
   a. Acute—symptoms present less than 2 weeks
   b. Subacute—symptoms present longer than 2 weeks but less than 6 weeks
   c. Chronic—symptoms present 6 weeks or longer
      (1) interstitial microscopic failure
      (2) central necrosis
      (3) partial rupture
      (4) acute complete rupture
3. Tendinosis
   Asymptomatic tendon degeneration caused by either aging or accumulated microtrauma or both
   a. Interstitial
   b. Partial rupture
   c. Acute rupture

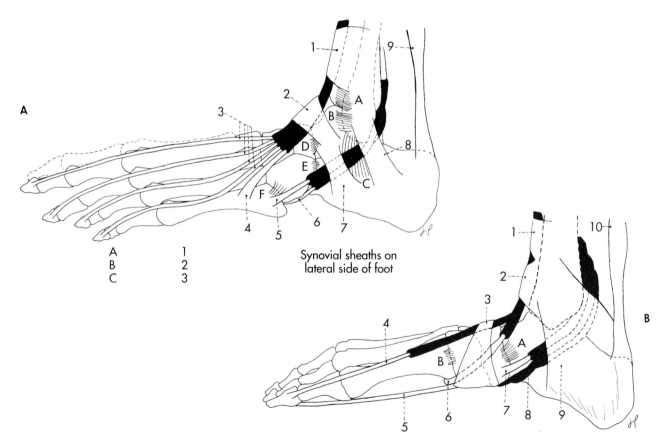

FIG. 65-42. A, Lateral view of tendons and synovial sheaths of foot and ankle. *1,* Superior extensor retinaculum; *2,* inferior extensor retinaculum; *3,* extensor digitorum longus; *4,* peroneus tertius; *5,* peroneus brevis; *6,* peroneus longus; *7,* inferior peroneal retinacula; *8,* superior peroneal retinaculum; *9,* Achilles tendon; *A,* lateral malleolus; *B,* talus; *C,* os calcis; *D,* navicular; *E,* cuboid; *F,* fifth metatarsal. **B,** Medial view of tendons and synovial sheaths of foot and ankle. *1,* Superior extensor retinaculum; *2,* superomedial band of inferior extensor retinaculum; *3,* inferomedial band of inferior extensor retinaculum; *4,* extensor hallucis longus; *5,* flexor hallucis longus; *6,* tibialis anterior; *7,* tibialis posterior; *8,* flexor digitorum longus; *9,* flexor retinaculum (laciniate ligament, medial annular ligament); *A,* talus; *B,* first metatarsal.

Achilles Tendinitis

Achilles tendinitis is one of the most common overuse injuries seen in soccer. It is frequently seen in leagues of athletes older than 25 years. Predisposing factors include cavus or varus feet, running on hard surfaces, and a tight gastrocsoleus muscle group. Patients complain of pain in the posterior aspect of the ankle, especially with prolonged running. Examination reveals point tenderness over the Achilles tendon, usually within 5 cm of its insertion on the calcaneal tuberosity. There is often marked restriction of passive dorsiflexion of the ankle. Treatment consists of decreasing play or practice time, gentle gastrocsoleus stretching, and the use of a ½ -inch heel lift during play. Ice should be used at the completion of play or practice. Steroid injections are strictly forbidden. Careful attention to this syndrome is warranted because of the risk of spontaneous rupture if left unchecked.

Achilles Tendon Rupture

The Achilles tendon usually ruptures at the zone of poor circulation, which is located 2 to 6 cm proximal to its insertion on the calcaneal tuberosity. Most of the time the athlete has a history of Achilles tendinitis. Typically the player feels like someone kicked him in the back of the leg or ankle and is associated with an audible snap and the development of severe pain. Signs include pain and swelling over the Achilles tendon with a palpable defect and a positive Thompson sign.[76] All acute ruptures in soccer players are routinely repaired because we believe the athletes have much better power and speed than they would if their injury were treated with an equi-

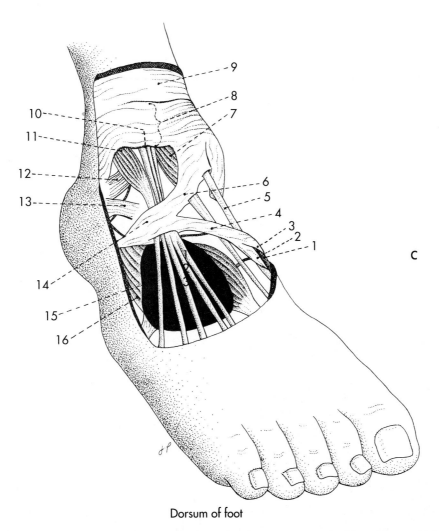

Dorsum of foot

FIG. 65-42, cont'd. C, Tendons and synovial sheaths of anterior aspect of ankle and foot. *1,* Abductor hallucis muscle; *2 and 3,* deep and superficial layers of oblique inferomedial band of inferior extensor retinaculum; *4,* oblique inferomedial band of the inferior extensor retinaculum; *5,* tibialis anterior tendon; *6,* oblique superomedial band of the inferior extensor retinaculum; *7,* extensor hallucis longus; *8,* superior extensor retinaculum; *9,* superficial aponeurosis of leg; *10,* extensor digitorum longus; *11,* peroneus tertius tendon; *12,* anterior inferior tibiofibular ligament; *13,* anterior talofibular ligament; *14,* stem of inferior extensor retinaculum; *15,* bursa or space located on dorsum of foot behind extensor digitorum longus tendon; *16,* extensor digitorum brevis muscle.

nus cast. A Bunnell-type repair is made with heavy, non-absorbable suture.[56] Lately, we have gotten away from using a pull-out wire with no compromise in results. We routinely treat players in a short leg cast for 8 weeks postoperatively and then with a heel lift for the subsequent 2 to 3 months. Kicking and light running are permitted at 6 months. Return to competition is not permitted until the following season. We have had no recurrences with this regimen.

If the rupture is only partial, that is, there is a negative Thompson sign, surgery should be avoided. These patients do well when treated with ice and immobilization. When the acute pain and swelling subside, a heel lift and gradual stretching exercises are prescribed. Return to sport is permitted when the patient is pain free and has full passive dorsiflexion of the foot. We routinely have these patients play with a heel lift for the remainder of the season.

Subcutaneous and Retrocalcaneal Bursitis

A bursa lies between the subcutaneous tissue and the Achilles tendon, and a retrocalcaneal bursa lies between the Achilles tendon and the calcaneus. Acute inflammation of these bursae are common in soccer players because the area is exposed to kicking injuries during the game. Also, soccer players tend to wear tight-fitting shoes, often two sizes smaller than their normal size, which significantly increases the friction in these bursae. A prominent posterior tubercle of the os calcis may be an additional cause of the bursitis. Examination reveals tenderness over the posterior aspect of the ankle, but unlike Achilles tendinitis, there is also marked swelling and erythema. Conservative treatment includes ice, rest, shoewear modification, and occasionally a steroid injection.[36] In persistent cases, exploration of the Achilles tendon is performed with excision of the enlarged posterior tubercle.

Posterior Tibialis Tendinitis

Posterior tibialis tendinitis is seen much more frequently in soccer players than in other athletes. This is probably because the posterior tibialis tendon of a soccer player is subject to more frequent microtrauma from repeated hyperpronation during the game (Fig. 65-41). Also, this tendon is relatively superficial and may be subject to direct contusion by an opponent's kick (Fig. 65-43) or by blocking a ball (Fig. 65-4). The player with this problem has constant pain in the medial aspect of the foot. Pain is mainly in the area of the navicular with radiation to the posterior aspect of the medial malleolus and along the posteromedial border of the tibia (Fig. 65-42, B). Running, jumping, attempting to hit the ball hard with an inside kick, or trying to block a ball increases the pain. The player limps during the play and is unable to accelerate or cut during running. Palpation of the tendon elicits tenderness along its course from behind the medial malleolus to its insertion on the navicular. Resisting supination or passively pronating the foot accentuates the pain. Treatment consists of ice, use of NSAIDs, calf stretches, and a medial heel wedge. This syndrome usually does not preclude play.

Anterior Tibialis Tendinitis

Many structures along the anterior aspect of the ankle, including the anterior tibialis, extensor hallucis longus, extensor digitorum longus, peroneus tertius, and extensor retinaculum, may become inflamed in a soccer player (Fig. 65-42, C). These structures are subject to direct trauma from the ball or an opponent's foot and microtrauma from repetitive kicking. Swelling, tenderness, and erythema are present. The complaints are increased by passively plantar flexing the ankle and toes or by resisting dorsiflexion of the ankle or toes. Treatment is conservative, and the results are prompt. Ice applied right after the game, use of NSAIDs for 5 to 7 days, and rest suffice. Taping with protective padding (Lace pad) is recommended.

Peroneal Tendinitis

Soccer players are subject to peroneal tendinitis as a result of contusion of those tendons from a direct kick or strain from outside kicking. Pain and tenderness along the course of the peroneal sheath is observed (Fig. 65-42, A). Symptoms are accentuated by resisting eversion or passive inversion of the foot. The main differential is a lateral ligament sprain. These two injuries are often concurrent. Treatment is conservative with ice, use of NSAIDs, and a progressive power program for the peroneal musculature. Ankle taping may be of some benefit.

Ankle Sprains

Although ankle sprains are covered thoroughly elsewhere, because they are exceedingly frequent in soccer, several points bear emphasis with regard to soccer. Ankle sprains are the most common injuries in most soccer leagues and in some series account for up to 36% of all

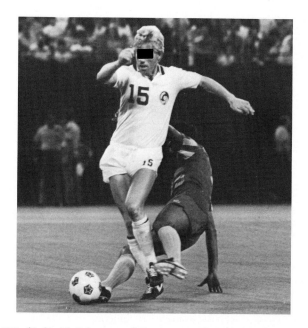

FIG. 65-43. Medial aspect of tibia is exposed to contact with opponent's feet during marking.

injury.[18,28,46,64] Ekstrand et al[15] noted that nearly one out of every two Danish senior players had a history of at least one lateral ankle sprain. Proper treatment of these injuries is vital because these sprains are prone to recurrence with subsequent development of chronic ankle instability. Of all ankle sprains, 56% are recurrent injuries[15] and one out of three elite women soccer players has a positive anterior drawer sign of the ankle.[37] Some authors argue that the high incidence of instability and persistent symptoms suggests that the standard treatment is inadequate for soccer players.[15] Injury commonly occurs secondary to inverting or "turning" the ankle while running or cutting or from a severe plantar flexion injury (Figs. 65-44 and 65-45) from falling on a plantar-flexed ankle or kicking a blocked ball (Fig. 65-4).

Radiographs are routinely obtained for all second- and third-degree sprains. We believe that stress radiographs are not helpful in the acute period but are important in the patient with suspected chronic or recurrent instability. The initial management of all acute ankle sprains consists of elevation, compression, and ice. Protected weight bearing is begun immediately with the use of crutches. As soon as pain subsides, active and gentle passive range of motion exercises are instituted. Progressive weight bearing is encouraged. Peroneal-, dorsiflexor-, and plantar-flexor strengthening exercises are begun when full motion has been obtained and pain has resolved. The most important part of rehabilitation is proprioceptive training exercises with a tilt board or the like.[20,21,79] Running is permitted when strength and motion are normalized.[70] All recent sprains are protected with a stirrup-type support or firm taping. We have had good experiences with treating acute, third-degree sprains conservatively alone and do not advocate operative treatment. For chronic instability the Chrisman-Snook reconstruction yields the best results in elite players.

Ankle sprains may be prevented with proper stretching, proprioceptive training, proper footwear, and well-maintained playing fields. Prophylactic ankle taping is one of the most widely used preventive measures in soccer; however, its use is a matter of great debate. In a study of injuries in soccer players over 1 year, Engstrom et al[19] found that taping an uninjured ankle had no benefit in preventing sprains. Ekstrand et al,[14] however, found taping to be instrumental in the prophylaxis of an-

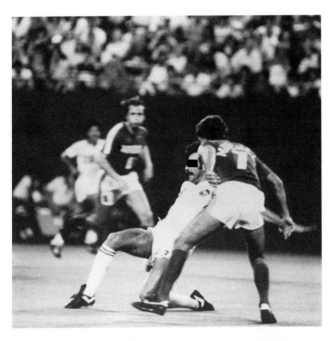

FIG. 65-44. Player falling on his plantar flexed-ankle joint.

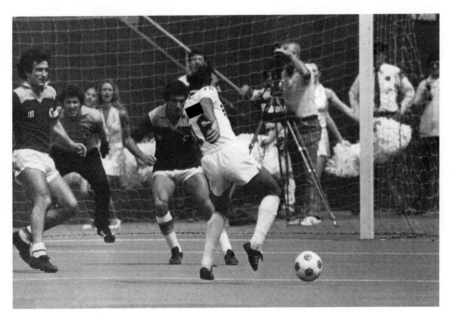

FIG. 65-45. Ball (injury-producing force) makes contact with foot while ankle capsule and ligaments are in severe tension.

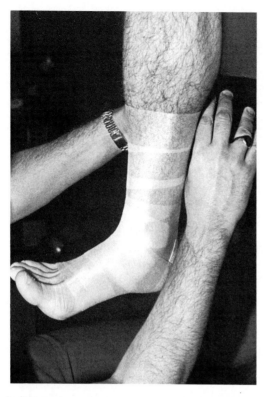

FIG. 65-46. Ankle is covered with pretape underwrap that covers all exposed skin and hair.

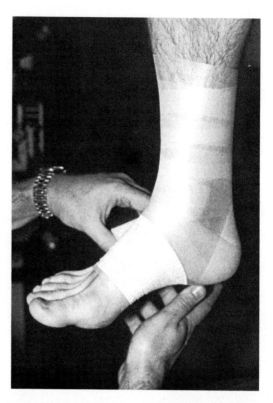

FIG. 65-47. Conform (Bike) applied just at level of metatarsal arch.

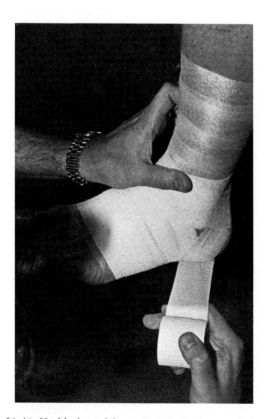

FIG. 65-48. Heel locks and figure-8s with Conform applied in one continuous motion.

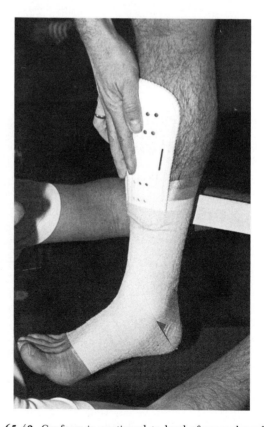

FIG. 65-49. Conform is continued to level of musculotendinous junction. Shin guard is incorporated.

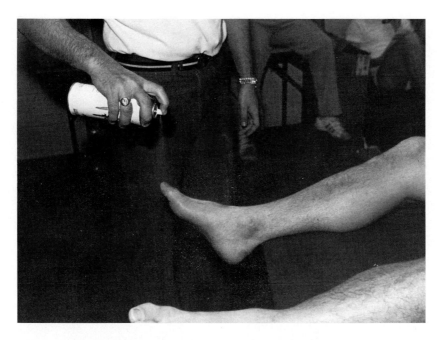

FIG. 65-50. Spraying of foot and leg with skin toughener.

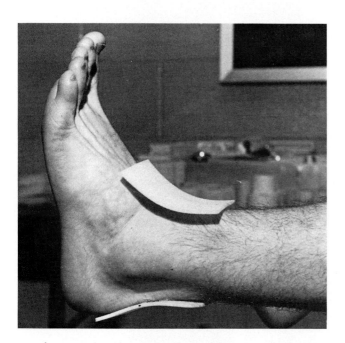

FIG. 65-51. Heel and lace pads with skin lubricant are applied over prominence of Achilles and extensor tendons of ankle joint.

kle sprains. The player is generally allowed to make his or her own decision, and about 80% of professional players elect to have some form of taping when there is no history of injury.

Ankle Taping

For prophylactic taping, the ankle is first covered with a pretape underwrap that should cover all exposed skin

and hair (Fig. 65-46). Conform (Bike) is applied just at the level of the metatarsal arch and circled up the ankle (Fig. 65-47), at which time heel locks and figures of eight are applied in one continuous motion (Fig. 65-48). The conform is then continued up the lower leg to the level of the musculotendinous junction (Fig. 65-49). A small piece of white tape prevents the Conform from unwrapping.

In the presence of injury the nature and severity dictate the type of therapeutic taping to apply. The most common is the traditional ankle strapping using white cloth tape. Heel and lace pads are applied with a skin lubricant followed by an underwrap (Figs. 65-50 and 65-51). Two anchor strips are applied at the lower leg, and two or three stirrups are placed first on the noninjured side pulling toward the injured side (Fig. 65-52). They are anchored individually. Figures of eight and heel locks are applied, preferably well behind the head of the fifth metatarsal. In some instances a combination using Elastikon as stirrups with tape anchors is preferred by some soccer players because of the degree of restriction white tape alone can create. In taping a soccer player's ankle it is important to stop the tape short of the midfoot because controlling the ball requires unimpeded mobility of the foot.

Talotibial Impingement Syndrome

The development of painful osteophytes on the anterior or posterior surfaces (Fig. 65-53) of the talocrural joint in the absence of degenerative joint disease has been given a variety of names. Among these include talotibial exostoses, athlete's ankle, footballer's ankle, and ankle or talotibial impingement syndrome.[24,35,43,45,53] The latter is now the most commonly used term. This disease is more common in soccer than

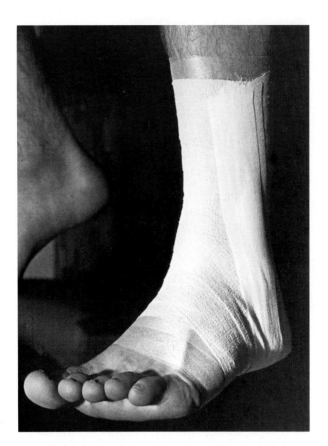

FIG. 65-52. Stirrups pulling toward injured side.

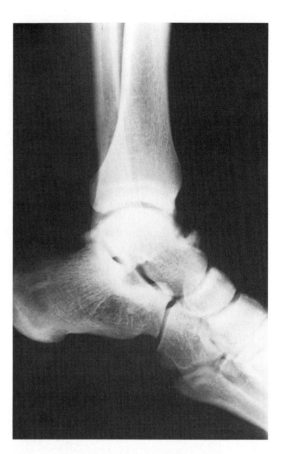

FIG. 65-53. Talotibial impingement. Note extensive osteophytes of talus anteriorly and posteriorly and osteophytes on anterior edge of tibia.

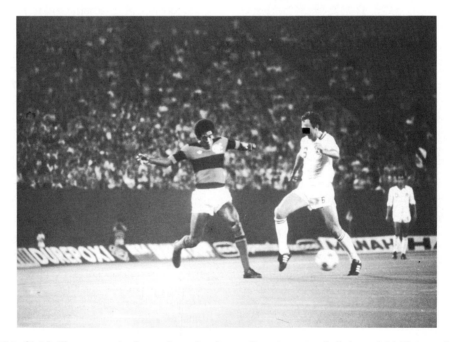

FIG. 65-54. Player severely plantar flexes his foot to direct incoming ball down field (dorsomedial aspect of foot—contact area with ball—faces new direction).

in any other sport. This syndrome occurs secondary to repetitive compression of the talus against the tibia at the extremes of motion. Lesions may be seen anteriorly or posteriorly. Anterior impingement is more common and results from repetitive hyperdorsiflexion of the ankle.[35,53] Marginal osteophytes are seen on the anteromedial aspect of the tibia and talus. Talotibial impingement syndrome is common among older soccer players. Posterior impingement occurs secondary to repetitive hyperplantar flexion (Fig. 65-54), and marginal exostoses develop on the posterolateral aspect of the talus and tibia.[24]

The soccer player with anterior impingement complains of chronic and severe anterior ankle pain, especially on "pushing off" of the affected foot. Examination reveals point tenderness over the anterior aspect of the ankle often with a palpable tender osteophyte and painful limitation of dorsiflexion. The soccer player with chronic ankle pain and limited dorsiflexion is often treated mistakenly for Achilles tendinitis; careful examination easily differentiates these entities. A standard lateral radiograph demonstrates hypertrophic, sclerotic osteophytes along the anterior margins of the talus and tibia (Figs. 65-55 and 65-56). Care should be taken to differentiate these findings from degenerative joint dis-

ease. Treatment consists of the use of a heel lift and NSAIDs. Open or arthroscopic debridement of the lesion should be considered for refractory cases.

Posterior impingement occurs in soccer players secondary to repetitive extreme plantar flexion that happens during the act of kicking (Fig. 65-57). There is often a history of recurrent plantar flexion sprains of the ankle, perhaps rendering the ankle more hypermobile. The athlete complains of posterior ankle pain, especially on kicking. Examination reveals painful limitation of plantar flexion and tenderness over the posterolateral aspect of the talotibial joint. Radiographs reveal marginal osteophytes along the posterior surface of the tibia and sclerosis or fragmentation of the lateral tubercle of the talus or os trigonum (if present) (Figs. 65-55, 65-56, and 65-58). This injury responds best to ankle taping to resist excessive plantar flexion. Recalcitrant cases may be considered for surgical exostectomy. There is probably some overlap between this condition and the os trigonum syndrome.[24]

Os Trigonum Syndrome

The os trigonum is an accessory ossicle that varies greatly in size and shape and is attached to the lateral

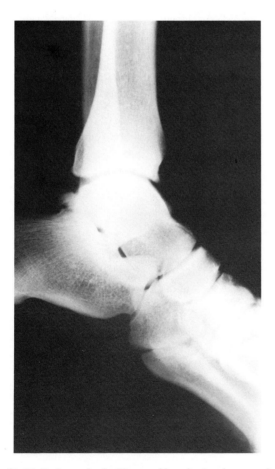

FIG. 65-55. Radiograph of a 30-year-old professional soccer player. Note fragmented osteophyte in anterior lip of tibia and osteophytes on neck and posterior tubercle of talus.

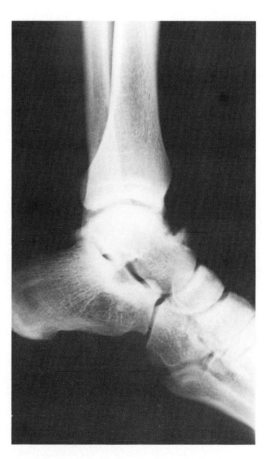

FIG. 65-56. Radiograph of 48-year-old professional soccer player and coach. Note advanced osteophytes in anterior edge of tibia and neck of talus. Note fragmentation of enlarged posterior tubercle of talus.

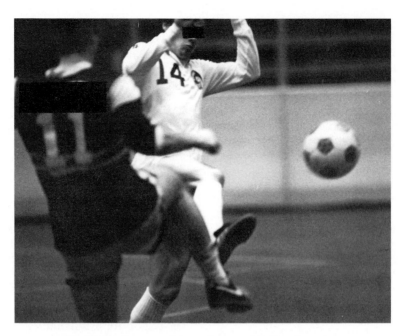

FIG. 65-57. Opponent injures dorsum of kicking foot.

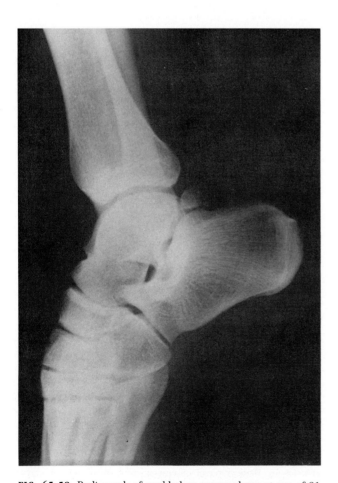

FIG. 65-58. Radiograph of world-class soccer player at age of 31. Note large os trigonum and changes on neck of talus.

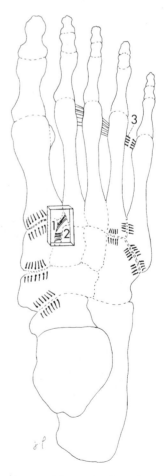

FIG. 65-59. Dorsal view of foot. *1*, Lisfranc ligament (cuneiform–second metatarsal ligaments); *2*, medial intercuneiform (interosseous) ligament; *3*, deep transverse metatarsal ligament.

tubercle of the posterior process of the talus.[2] It is present in only 7.7% of the general population. The os trigonum syndrome represents a stress fracture through the os trigonum, and this lesion can be seen in ballet dancers and athletes of jumping sports and soccer.[78] It can be considered a manifestation of posterior talotibial impingement syndrome and is caused by repetitive, forceful plantar flexion of the ankle. Patients have pain in the retrocalcaneal space during plantar flexion or walking on the toes. There is commonly a history of multiple ankle sprains, and radiographs reveal the presence of an os trigonum separated from the talus by a fracture line or complete displacement. The flexor hallucis longus runs just medial to the lateral tubercle as it crosses the posterior surface of the talus, and examination reveals pain on resisted plantar flexion of the great toe. Rest and a ½-inch heel lift eliminate the pain, but for the player wishing to return to his or her previous level of activity, the only effective treatment is excision of the os trigonum.

FOOT INJURIES

Foot injuries associated with soccer are common and may be severe. Several factors contribute to the frequency of these injuries. Like other running sports the feet of a soccer player are susceptible to the usual array of sprains, strains, and overuse syndromes endemic to these sports. Because soccer is a kicking sport, the foot is subjected to repetitive high torques that may result in unique patterns of injury. Last, soccer players tend to wear shoes that are up to one full size smaller than they usually wear, which predisposes them to a number of overuse injuries. Most players think that wearing a tight shoe allows for better ball control and a more effective kick. We believe that this benefit is mostly psychologic and that tight shoes do more harm than good. Unfortunately this belief is ingrained in players starting in the

youth leagues, and it is difficult to convince a player otherwise even after he or she has suffered an injury from, at least in part, constricting footwear.

Dorsal Foot Contusion

Contusion of the structures of the dorsum of the foot (Fig. 65-59) is caused by a direct blow either from kicking the ball or from an opponent stepping on the planted foot. The structures on the dorsum of the foot become swollen and tender. The injury prevents the player from running and kicking the ball. Radiographs of the foot should be taken to rule out fracture. Ice, elevation, and compression should be instituted. The injury responds promptly to conservative treatment, but the area remains tender on kicking. A felt pad should be applied over the tender area and incorporated into taping of the ankle joint until the area is completely healed and tenderness subsides.

Sprains

Acute sprains to the foot joints are common in soccer players because of the powerful forces generated by the act of kicking the ball or, unintentionally, the ground, which apply severe torque to the dorsal structures of the foot. Most of the sprains are located on the dorsum of the foot for two reasons. First, the plantar structures of the foot (the plantar capsule of the various joints, the plantar fascia, and the intrinsic muscles) are stronger in preventing hyperextension. Second, the nature of the kick is such that the dorsal structures are in tension, and any additional sudden force (ball contact) may produce sprain of the dorsal structures. Depending on the type of kick, different types of injury are observed.

Inside Kick

Inside kicks produce hyperflexion forces over the entire length of the foot and may result in dorsal capsular and ligamentous injuries of various joints (Fig. 65-59).

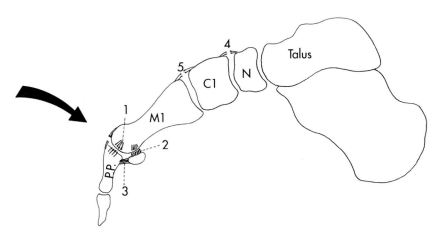

FIG. 65-60. Hyperflexion injuries to first metatarsophalangeal joint of foot, first cuneometatarsal joint (medial part of Lisfranc joint), and first cuneonavicular joint. *1,* Medial collateral ligament of first metatarsophalangeal joint; *2,* ruptured medial metatarsal sesamoid (suspensory) ligament; *3,* medial phalangeal sesamoid ligament; *4,* dorsal cuneonavicular ligament; *5,* dorsal cuneiform metatarsal ligament.

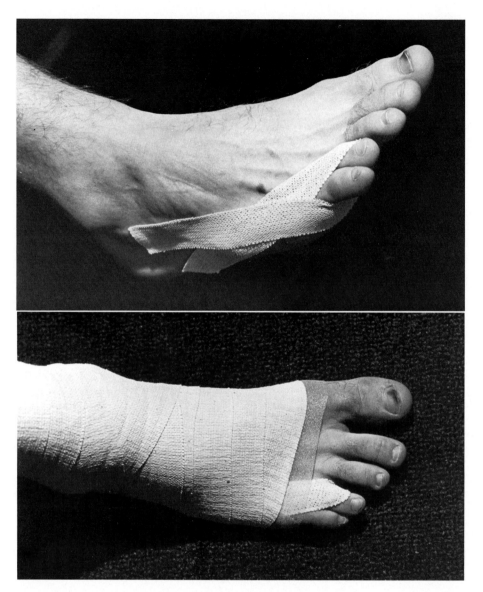

FIG. 65-61. Suggested taping of foot of soccer player for injury of deep transverse metatarsal ligaments between fourth and fifth toes, as depicted in Fig. 65-59.

Most commonly affected are the anterior capsule of the ankle, the anterior deltoid, the dorsal talonavicular ligament, Chopart's ligament, the cuneonavicular joint, the Lisfranc joint, and the metatarsophalangeal ligaments of the great toe (Fig. 65-60).

Outside Kick

Injuries produced by the outside kick are much less frequent, owing to the lower forces associated with this kick. The outside kick may result in dorsolateral injuries of multiple joints of the foot. Structures commonly injured include the anterior talofibular ligament, the calcaneocuboid joint, the cuneocuboid joint, and the metatarsophalangeal joints of the lesser toes (Fig. 65-61).

Hyperextension Injuries

Hyperextension injuries to the foot are mainly observed at the metatarsophalangeal joint of the great toe

and are known as turf toe. During a hyperextension injury of the first metatarsophalangeal joint, there is injury to the plantar capsule, the metatarsosesamoid ligament (because the sesamoids follow the proximal phalanx and are displaced with it and not with the metatarsal head),[65] and the LCL (Figs. 65-62 to 65-64). Predisposing factors to turf toe are hard-playing surfaces and wearing flexible shoes.[5]

Diagnosis

At the time of the injury the patient experiences pain in the foot. Early palpation of the foot helps determine which structures are injured. Swelling and discoloration ensue. Pain increases, and the player is unable to ambulate on the foot. Passive hyperflexion of the involved joint is painful and resisted. In turf toe, passive extension of the great toe produces discomfort. Radiographs should be taken to rule out any avulsion fractures.

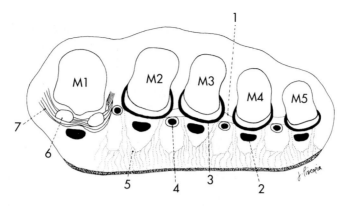

FIG. 65-62. Cross section through metatarsal head demonstrating deep transverse metatarsal ligament. *1,* Deep transverse metatarsal ligament; *2,* long flexor tendons; *3,* plantar plate; *4,* lumbrical tendon; *5,* arciform and perpendicular fibers; *6,* sesamoid; *7,* abductor hallucis.

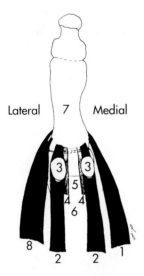

FIG. 65-63. Structures located on plantar aspect of plantar plate of first metatarsophalangeal joint. *1,* Abductor hallucis; *2,* medial and lateral heads of flexor hallucis brevis; *3,* medial and lateral sesamoids; *4,* longitudinal septa; *5,* plantar plate; *6,* first metatarsal; *7,* proximal phalanx; *8,* adductor hallucis.

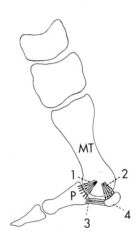

FIG. 65-64. Hyperextension injury to first metatarsophalangeal joint. *1,* Metatarsophalangeal ligament; *2,* medial metatarsal sesamoid (suspensory) ligament; *3,* medial phalangeosesamoid ligament; *4,* Sesamoid.

Treatment

Immediate elevation and application of ice to the foot are mandatory. A compression dressing should be applied between icing to reduce swelling. Weight bearing is restricted until discomfort is minimal or absent. Depending on the severity of the injury and the complaints, plaster immobilization may be used. As the injury heals, the player may start to walk in a pain-free gait, starting from flat-footed walking and progressing to a normal stride. Jogging is permitted when the athlete is pain free. When the patient is able to run at full speed, cutting maneuvers and kicking are allowed. Throughout rehabilitation the player is fitted with shoes modified to produce increased stability of the entire foot by supplying a firm insole (steel splint or Orthoplast), which should be used

for a minimum of 8 weeks.[10] The foot and toes are taped appropriately to prevent recurrence (Fig. 65-65).

Fractures and Dislocations

A plethora of avulsion-type fractures on the dorsum of the foot can be seen in soccer as a result of injuries to various joints. These injuries occur almost exclusively secondary to hyperflexion kicking forces. Although they may be seen in other sports, they are much more frequent in soccer.

Tibiotalar Joint

Avulsion fractures can occur on the tibial or corresponding superior surface of the neck of the talus. Avulsion fractures from the tibia occur along the anterome-

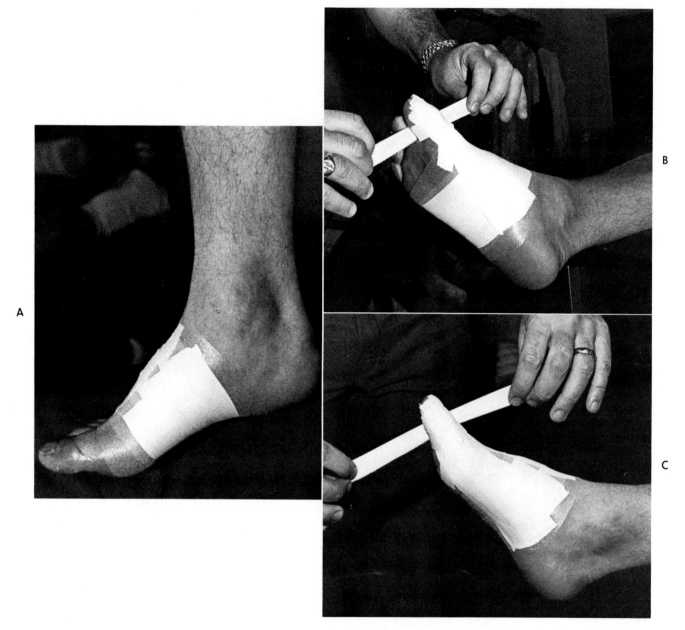

FIG. 65-65. Sequence of taping for turf toe in soccer players **A,** Anchors. **B,** Stirrups to limit motion of metatarsophalangeal joint. **C,** Final anchors.

dial portion of the plafond, usually at the site of the origin of the anterior tibiotalar portion of the deltoid ligament.

Avulsion fractures can also occur from the superior surface of the neck of the talus and are associated with severe plantar flexion. Treatment of these fractures, if they are symptomatic, is surgical excision and repair of the capsule through an anteromedial approach.[50]

Os Calcis

Avulsion fractures of the calcaneus can occur in the sustentaculum tali from the anterior border (from the origin of the superomedial calcaneonavicular ligament) or

from the posterior border (from the insertion of the medial talocalcaneal ligament). Avulsion fractures can also occur from the anterior process of the os calcis (Fig. 65-66) from Chopart's ligament and the dorsolateral calcaneocuboid ligament (Fig. 65-67).

The differential diagnosis of fracture of the sustentaculum tali includes posterior tibial tendinitis. The treatment of fractures of the sustentaculum, a weight-bearing area, includes elevation, ice, and a soft dressing. Weight bearing is delayed if the fragment is large and involves the middle calcaneal facet. Partial weight bearing is permitted at 6 to 8 weeks, progressing to full weight bearing at 10 to 12 weeks. Gradual athletic activities are sub-

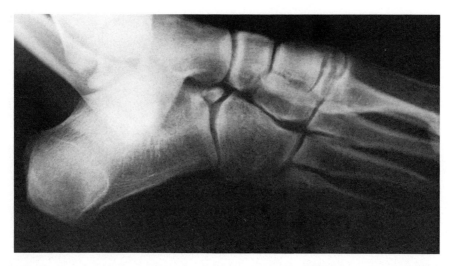

FIG. 65-66. Avulsion fracture of anterior calcaneal process of os calcis from avulsion of Chopart's ligament (lateral calcaneal navicular and medial calcaneal cuboid ligaments).

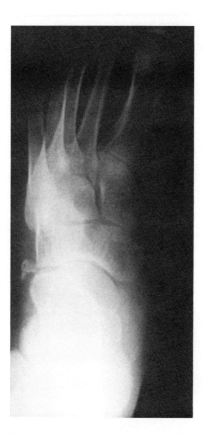

FIG. 65-67. Radiograph demonstrating avulsion fracture of os calcis attached to dorsolateral calcaneocuboid ligament.

sequently permitted. Painful nonunion necessitates surgical excision. Avulsion fractures of the anterior process are treated the same way except that early weight bearing is encouraged because this is not a weight-bearing surface. Excision of the anterior process is recommended in cases of symptomatic nonunion.

Talonavicular Joint

Fractures of the talonavicular joint usually involve the navicular and are the result of avulsion of the dorsal talonavicular ligament (Fig. 65-68). On physical examination after an acute injury, there is severe pain and tenderness over the dorsum of the foot. Ambulation is painful. Radiographic examination reveals the presence of an avulsed fragment from the navicular. Treatment is conservative. The patient ambulates without bearing weight for 10 days to 2 weeks and then gradually advances to full weight bearing. Gradual participation in athletics is permitted. The players who develop nonunion of these fractures are asymptomatic during ambulation or running, but they experience severe pain in the area of the fracture on attempting to kick the ball. The treatment of a symptomatic nonunion is surgical excision (Fig. 65-69). Ossification of the ligament is observed following removal of the fracture. Avulsion of the navicular tuberosity may occur from the forceful pull of the posterior tibialis tendon. Treatment is almost always symptomatic.

Lisfranc Joint

Injury to the Lisfranc joint (Fig. 65-70) may occur when a player inadvertently kicks the ground or kicks a ball blocked by another player. In soccer, injuries to the tarsometatarsal joint usually represent a sprain. Unlike those secondary to high-energy motor vehicle or industrial accidents, diastasis or dislocation is rare. The medial interosseous ligament between the first and second cuneiforms and the Lisfranc ligament between the first cuneiform and the base of the second metatarsal are usually stretched but intact. If these ligaments are disrupted, diastasis can occur. Right after the injury the player experiences pain in the foot. Physical examination reveals swelling and edema along the injured joint. Attempts at passive motion of the tarsometatarsal joint elicit severe pain. The player is unable to bear full weight on the foot. Suspected dislocation may be reduced on the field. Radiographs should be obtained, and if diastasis is sus-

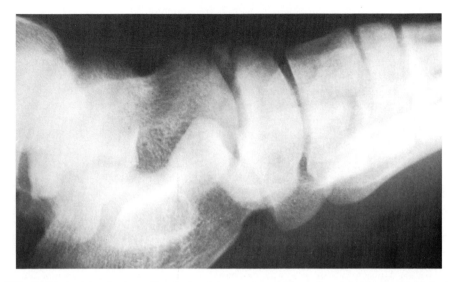

FIG. 65-68. Avulsion fracture of navicular. Injury occurred when player struck opponent's foot.

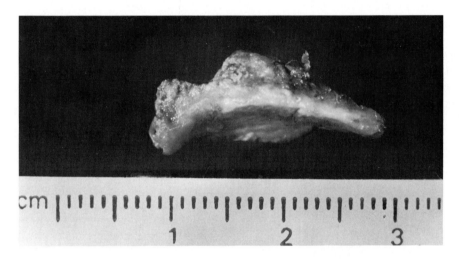

FIG. 65-69. Specimen of avulsed fracture of navicular in patient in Fig. 65-68.

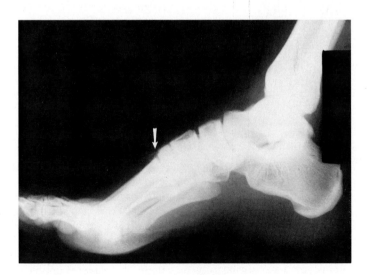

FIG. 65-70. Calcification in substance of cuneometatarsal ligament after dislocation of first cunei-form–metatarsal (Lisfranc) joint in soccer player who hit the ground instead of ball.

pected, comparison films should be obtained. The lateral view reveals an avulsion fracture, if present.

Sprains are treated with ice, a soft compression bandage, and a short period of limited weight bearing. Gradual return to activities is permitted when symptoms allow. Avulsion fractures are treated similarly; however, if they are associated with significant instability, a plaster cast worn for 2 to 3 weeks is warranted. Subsequently, the foot is treated with taping and is fitted with a steel shank shoe. Weight bearing is added gradually as tolerated. The player is able to run and kick the ball within 8 weeks after careful rehabilitation of the foot. In cases of rupture of the Lisfranc and medial interosseous ligaments, increased space can be seen between the first and second metatarsals and the first and second cuneiforms. Complete reduction of the diastasis with the patient under general anesthesia is necessary. Anatomic reduction is often impossible by closed means, and open reduction with internal fixation may be necessary. A short leg cast is applied for 6 weeks. Partial weight bearing can start in 8 to 10 weeks.

Metatarsophalangeal Joint

A metatarsophalangeal joint dislocation (Fig. 65-71) or fracture occurs secondary to the forefoot striking an immovable object, either the ground or a blocked ball. The direction of dislocation is usually dorsal, although plantar dislocation may occur. Dislocation of the lesser toes

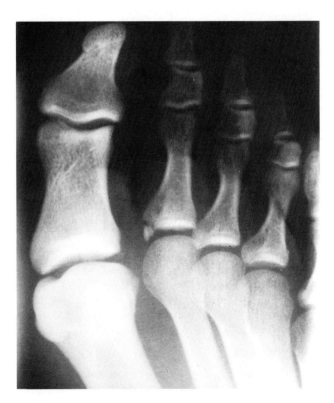

FIG. 65-71. Dislocation of first and second metatarsophalangeal joints following powerful inside kick while ball was blocked by opponent. Avulsion fragment from proximal phalanx of second metatarsophalangeal joint attached to medial collateral ligament is noted.

is rarely associated with fractures and is usually reduced on the field. Dislocation of the great toe is more commonly associated with intraarticular fractures and is somewhat more difficult to reduce. The vast majority of fractures are secondary to avulsion and reduce anatomically with concentric reduction of the joint. Once anatomic alignment has been restored, treatment involves rest, ice, immobilization, and the donning of a stiff-soled shoe. Running is allowed when pain and ligamentous instability resolve, usually in 4 weeks. The foot is protected with a stiff Orthoplast insert during athletic endeavor for the following 8 to 10 weeks.

Metatarsals

The most common fracture of the metatarsals is at the base of the fifth metatarsal. This injury represents an avulsion of either the insertion of the peroneus brevis or the origin of the abductor digiti minimi. Physical examination reveals swelling and tenderness over the base of the fifth metatarsal. Passive inversion or resisted eversion of the foot elicits pain at the base of the fifth metatarsal. Radiographs reveal a fracture of a portion of the metaphyseal base of the fifth ray. Treatment consists of ice and a soft-compression bandage. Unreliable players should be casted for 4 to 6 weeks. Running is resumed when there is clinical union upon examination. Nonunion is uncommon, and when it occurs, it is usually asymptomatic. For persistent, painful nonunion, surgical excision and reattachment of involved tendons is recommended.

This fracture should be differentiated from a diaphyseal fracture of the proximal fifth metatarsal. The incidence of delayed union of these injuries among young athletic individuals is unacceptably high with closed treatment. For the past several years we have treated these fractures acutely with compression screw fixation and have had excellent results.

Stress fractures of the metatarsals are also common among soccer players, particularly during preseason. The most common site for fatigue fracture is the proximal diaphysis of the fifth metatarsal. Symptoms consist of chronic forefoot pain, especially with running. On physical examination, there is tenderness over the affected ray. Swelling may be present, but ecchymosis is usually absent. Radiographs are helpful if positive, but sensitivity is poor. Bone scan is definitive. Treatment consists of avoidance of running and athletics for several weeks until pain and tenderness resolve, and then the athlete can gradually return to activity.

Sesamoid Bones

Sesamoid fracture (Fig. 65-72) can be observed in a soccer player who lands on a dorsiflexed metatarsophalangeal joint (Fig. 65-64). The sesamoid bones are located within the tendon of the flexor hallucis brevis, and they articulate with the inferior aspect of the metatarsal head. On physical examination, there is pain on weight bearing. There is tenderness on palpation of the sesamoid bones under the first metatarsal. Treatment should be non–weight bearing for a week to 10 days, and subsequently, the patient uses a metatarsal bar until the symptoms subside. This usually requires 4 to 5 weeks.

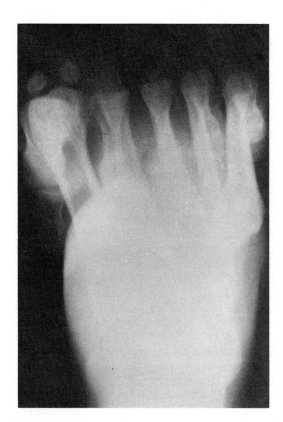

FIG. 65-72. Undisplaced fracture through lateral sesamoid.

If the symptoms persist for several months, surgical excision should be contemplated.

Soft-Tissue Afflictions
Heel Bruise

Contusion of the fat pad and subperiosteal bruise of the heel have been observed in soccer players. Injury occurs when the player lands on the heel after a jump, causing a crush injury to the fat pad. The heel is iced and is protected with a foam doughnut pad until complete recovery is achieved. A firm, well-fitting counter controls the fat pad and serves as a buffer to the force of impact.

Dorsal Foot Contusion Neuropathies

Traumatic neuropathy caused by contusion of the dorsum of the foot involves the dorsal cutaneous branches of the deep peroneal nerve. This nerve is especially susceptible at the tarsal metatarsal area where it lies superficially over a bony prominence. Numbness and paresthesias occur in the first web space. This injury may also involve the lateral dorsal cutaneous nerve, a continuation of the sural nerve distal to the lateral malleolus. This nerve is vulnerable to trauma behind the lateral malleolus and around the tubercle of the fifth metatarsal. Numbness and paresthesia over the lateral aspect of the forefoot and fifth toe are observed. It is believed that these neuropathies result, at least in part, from the tight-fitting shoes that soccer players insist on wearing. Treatment consists of restriction of activities until symptoms

abate and then appropriate padding over the areas of compression and shoewear modification.

Plantar Hyperkeratoses

Hyperkeratotic lesions (calluses) are a protective accumulation of the stratum corneum in response to local pressure over a long period produced by an imbalance of the weight distribution between toes and metatarsal heads. Calluses most frequently form on the ball of the foot under one or more metatarsal heads or the heel. The combination of callosities over the first metatarsal head and the tibial aspect of the great toe is common among soccer players. Callosities must be differentiated from a plantar wart. A symptomatic callus should be thinned, and orthotics (total-contact molded inserts) should be used to balance the distribution of weight-bearing forces.

Corns

A corn is an area of hyperkeratosis on the dorsum of the foot caused by excessive pressure. Pressure may occur interdigitally from a prominent condyle or exostosis or exteriorly from a tight shoe. Corns usually occur from a combination of these pressures. Hard corns are located on the dorsum of the forefoot, and soft corns are found in the web spaces. Corns are frequent among soccer players because of their tight footwear. Treatment consists of a doughnut-shaped pad to relieve the pressure over the area of the corn. Failing that, removal of the exostosis or partial condylectomy is advised.

Blisters

Blisters of the feet constitute the second most commonly seen condition affecting the skin, following abrasions. A blister is a shear injury with fluid accumulation separating the epidermal layer. Blisters can be the result of wearing new shoes or playing on artificial surfaces. Because of the increased stopping ability of a soccer player on artificial turf, the foot may slide forward and backward in the shoe.

If the blister is large and full of fluid, it should be drained under sterile conditions and covered overnight. The major objective in preparing the soccer player who has a blister on the foot for participation in a game is to remove or decrease the friction to which the area of the blister is exposed. First, the shoes must fit properly and give good support. A good protocol is to use Spenco's Second Skin affixed with cover roll. If the area is still tender, a doughnut-shaped pad may be placed over the periphery of the blister. To prevent formation of blisters, players should always wear the proper size shoes and absorbent socks. Topical benzoin is an excellent skin protectant for prophylaxis against blisters.

Hallux Rigidus

In hallux rigidus, dorsiflexion of the metatarsophalangeal joint of the great toe is severely limited and painful (Fig. 65-73). This is detrimental to the performance of the soccer player, who needs almost 90 degrees of hyperextension of the first metatarsophalangeal joint at push off. A stiff-soled or rocker-bottom shoe alleviates pain but may diminish performance. Rest, ice, and local

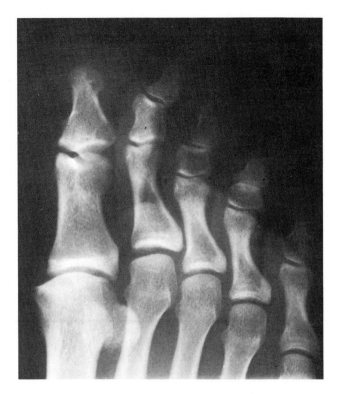

FIG. 65-73. Hallux rigidus in 34-year-old amateur soccer player.

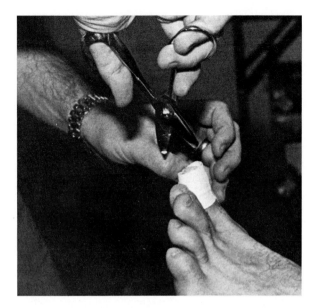

FIG. 65-74. Taping of avulsed nail.

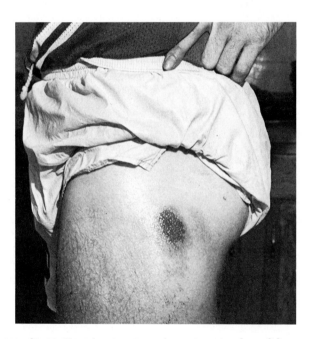

FIG. 65-75. Skin abrasions in trochanteric region from sliding on turf.

measures usually inhibit symptoms enough to allow play. Intraarticular steroid injections are not recommended. If conservative measures fail, surgery should be directed toward reestablishing motion by resecting the proliferative bone around the metatarsal head (cheilectomy).

Hallux Valgus

Athletes who suffer from hallux valgus usually complain of irritation of the bunion from the shoe and poor push-off; they rarely complain of pain. Treatment consists of an arch support to correct excessive pronation, supportive taping of the great toe in a more neutral position, and widening of the soccer shoe over the prominence of the bunion. If the player does not respond to conservative treatment, operative realignment with osteotomy of the first metatarsal may be considered.

Subungual Hematoma

Subungual hematoma is more common in soccer than in any other sport.[23] The average soccer player loses two to three toenails in a period of 1 year; some players lose up to six or seven toenails as a result of subungual hematoma. These injuries may be caused by jamming the longest toe against the toe box of the shoe or an opponent stepping on the toe. If the formation of the subungual hematoma is significant, it produces severe pain that often requires drilling through the center of the hematoma to relieve the pressure and alleviate the pain. The hole through the nail can be made with a specialized drill or by heating one end of a paper clip over a flame until it glows red and then pressing it against the nail to melt a hole through the center of the toenail. Oc-

casionally the toenail may be completely or partially avulsed. The avulsed toenail should be taped back into its original position until healing of the nail bed occurs and the new nail appears (Fig. 65-74). Replacing the avulsed nail is necessary to preserve the boundaries of the bed and protect it from injury.

ABRASIONS

The most common skin condition in soccer players is skin abrasion caused by sliding on synthetic turf or natural grass. The injury is usually the result of attempting a sliding tackle (a maneuver to kick the ball away from an opponent). The most commonly affected areas are the hip and buttock area (Fig. 65-75), the patella, the tibial tubercle, and the elbow. The presence of microorganisms on the turf subjects these injuries to possible infection. When an abrasion is suffered, the location and game situation dictate initial management. If the player can be attended to at halftime, the wound is cleaned with peroxide, covered with an antiseptic, and dressed with a nonstick pad. The area around the wound should be coated with a skin adherent. Cover Roll is then cut to the appropriate size and placed over the Telfa pad. At the conclusion of the game the wound is redressed and the bandage is left on overnight. The wound is examined for signs of infection with each daily dressing change. When the wound ceases to weep, the dressing may be discontinued and the abrasion is allowed to dry to the air. Protective covering for games and practice is continued until tenderness resolves.

REFERENCES

1. Adams RJ, Chandler FA: Osteitis pubis of traumatic etiology, *J Bone Joint Surg* 35A:685, 1953.
2. Bizarro AH: On sesamoid and supernumerary bones of the limbs, *J Anat* 55:256, 1921.
3. Blazina ME et al: Jumper's knee, *Orthop Clin North Am* 4:665, 1973.
4. Bostrom A: Fractures of the patella: a study of 422 patella fractures, *Acta Orthop Scand Suppl* 1:422, 1972.
5. Bowers DK Jr, Martin RB: Turf toe: a shoe-surface–related football injury, *Med Sci Sports Exerc* 8:81, 1976.
6. Brody DM: Running injuries, *Clin Symp* 32:24, 1980.
7. Burman M, Weinkel IN, Langston MJ: Adolescent osteochondritis of the symphysis pubis with a consideration of normal roentgenographic changes in the symphysis pubis, *J Bone Joint Surg* 16:649, 1934.
8. Butler JE, Eggert AW: Fracture of the iliac crest apophysis and unusual hip pointer, *Am J Sports Med* 3:192, 1975.
9. Clancy W, Foltz AS: Iliac apophysitis and stress fracture, *Am J Sports Med* 4:214, 1976.
10. Coker TP, Arnold JA, Weber DL: Traumatic lesions of the metatarsophalangeal joint of the great toe in athletes, *Am J Sports Med* 6:326, 1978.
11. Cooper DL: Hamstring strains, *Phys Sports Med* 6(8):104, 1978.
12. Dijan P et al: Surgical treatment of pubic pain in athletes, personal communication, 1993.
13. Ekstrand J: Incidence of soccer injuries and their relation to training and team success, *Am J Sports Med* 11(2):63, 1983.
14. Ekstrand J, Gillquist J, Sten-otto L: Prevention of soccer injuries: supervision by doctor and physiotherapist, *Am J Sports Med* 11:116, 1983.
15. Ekstrand J et al: The frequency of muscle tightness and injuries in soccer players, *Am J Sports Med* 10:75, 1982.
16. Ekstrand J et al: The avoidability of soccer injuries, *Int J Sports Med* 4:124, 1983.
17. Ellsasser JC et al: The nonoperative treatment of collateral ligament injuries of the knee in professional football players, *J Bone Joint Surg* 56A:1185, 1974.
18. Engstrom B, Johansson C, Tornkvist H: Soccer injuries among elite female players, *Am J Sports Med* 19:372, 1991.
19. Engstrom B et al: Does a major knee injury definitely sideline an elite soccer player? *Am J Sports Med* 18:101, 1990.
20. Fiore RD, Leard JS: A functional approach in the rehabilitation of the ankle and rear foot, *Athl Train* 231, 1980.
21. Freeman MAR: Treatment of ruptures of the lateral ligament of the ankle, *J Bone Joint Surg* 47B:661, 1965.
22. Gainor BJ et al: The kick: biomechanics and collision injury, *Am J Sports Med* 6:185, 1978.
23. Gibbs RC: Tennis toe, *JAMA* 228:24, 1974.
24. Hamilton WG: Stenosing tenosynovitis of the flexor hallucis longus tendon and posterior impingement upon the os trigonum in ballet dancers, *Foot Ankle* 3:74, 1982.
25. Hermans GPH: A new surgical approach to groin injuries in athletes, personal communication, October 1992.
26. Hoff G, Martin T: Outdoor and indoor soccer: injuries among youth players, *Am J Sports Med* 14:231, 1986.
27. Hollinshead WH: *Anatomy for surgeons: back and limb*, vol 3, ed 2, New York, 1969, Harper & Row.
28. Hoy K et al: European soccer injuries: a prospective epidemiologic and socioeconomic study, *Am J Sports Med* 20:318, 1992.
29. Huss CD, Paul JJ: Myositis ossificans of the upper arm, *Am J Sports Med* 8:419, 1980.
30. Imbert JC, Dupre-la-Tour L: Surgical treatment of groin pain in athletes: analysis of a series of 243 cases, personal communication, October, 1992.
31. Nicholas Institute for Sports Medicine and Athletic Trauma: Unpublished data.
32. Jackson DW: Managing myositis ossificans in the young athlete, *Phys Sports Med* 3(10):56, 1975.
33. Jackson DW, Feagin JA: Quadriceps contusions in young athletes, *J Bone Joint Surg* 55A:95, 1973.
34. Keller C, Noyes F, Buncher C: The medical aspects of soccer injury epidemiology, *Am J Sports Med* 15:230, 1987.
35. Kleiger B: Anterior talotibial impingement syndromes in dancers, *Foot Ankle* 3:69, 1982.
36. Leach RE, Dilorio E, Harney RA: Pathologic hindfoot conditions in the athlete, *Clin Orthop* 177:116, 1983.
37. Lewerentz H: Fotlederna och knana de svaga punkterna hos kvinnliga fotbollsspelare, *Lakaritidningen* 78:4448, 1981.
38. Lindenfeld TN et al: Incidence of injury in indoor soccer, *Am J Sports Med* 22(3):364, 1993.
39. Lockhart RD et al: *Anatomy of the human body*, Philadelphia, 1965, JB Lippincott.
40. Mariani PP, Puddu G, Ferrett A: *Jumper's knee*, Second Orthopedic Clinic, University of Rome
41. McMaster WC: Literary review on ice therapy in injuries, *Am J Sports Med* 5:124, 1977.
42. McMaster WC, Walter M: Injuries in soccer, *Am J Sports Med* 6:354, 1978.
43. McMurray TP: Footballer's ankle, *J Bone Joint Surg* 32B:68, 1950.
44. Mital M: Osgood-Schlatter's disease: the painful puzzler, *Phys Sports Med* 4:60, 1977.
45. Morris LH: "Athlete's ankle," *J Bone Joint Surg* 25A:220, 1943.
46. Nielson A, Yde J: Epidemiology and traumatology of injuries in soccer, *Am J Sports Med* 17:803, 1989.
47. Nilsson S, Roaas A: Soccer injuries in adolescents, *Am J Sports Med* 6:358, 1978.
48. Noble CA: Iliotibial band friction syndrome in runners, *Am J Sports Med* 8:232, 1980.
49. Norwood LA Jr, Cross MJ: Anterior cruciate ligament: functional anatomy of its bundles in rotary instabilities, *Am J Sports Med* 7:23, 1979.
50. O'Donahue DH: *Treatment of injuries to athletes*, ed 4, Philadelphia, 1984, WB Saunders.
51. Oka M, Hatanpaa S: Degenerative hip disease in adolescent athletes, *Br J Sports Med* 12:4, 1978.
52. Orava S, Puranen J: Exertion injuries in adolescent athletes, *Br J Sports Med* 12:4, 1978.
53. Parkes JC et al: The anterior impingement syndrome of the ankle, *J Trauma* 20:895, 1980.
54. Pierson EL: Osteochondritis of the symphysis pubis, *Surg Gynecol Obstet* 49:834, 1929.
55. Puranen J et al: Running and primary osteoarthritis of the hip, *BMJ* 5968:424, 1975.
56. Quigley TB, Scheller AD: Surgical repair of the ruptured Achilles tendon, *Am J Sports Med* 8:244, 1980.
57. Rachun A et al: *Standard nomenclature of athletic injuries*, Chicago, 1966, American Medical Association.
58. Renne JW: The iliotibial band friction syndrome, *J Bone Joint Surg* 57A:1110, 1975.

59. Ricklin P, Ruttiman A, Del Buono MS: *Meniscus lesions,* New York, 1971, Grune & Stratton.
60. Rispoli FP: Sindrome pubica dei calciatori socemiliana romagnola triveneta ortop, *Traumatol Atti* 8:331, 1963.
61. Risser JC: The iliac apophysis: an invaluable sign in the management of scoliosis, *Clin Orthop* 11:111, 1958.
62. Rockett J: Three-phase radionuclide bone imaging in stress injury of the anterior iliac crest, *J Nucl Med* 31:1554, 1990.
63. Roels J et al: Patellar tendinitits (jumper's knee), *Am J Sports Med* 6:362, 1978.
64. Sadat-Ali M, Sankaran-Kutty M: Soccer injuries in Saudi Arabia, *Am J Sports Med* 15:500, 1987.
65. Sarrafian SK: *Anatomy of the foot and ankle,* Philadelphia, 1983, JB Lippincott.
66. Schmidt-Olsen S et al: Injuries among young soccer players, *Am J Sports Med* 19:273, 1991.
67. Schneider R, Kaye JJ, Ghelman B: Adductor avulsion injuries near the symphysis pubis, *Radiology* 120:567, 1976.
68. Schwartzweller F: Kasuistischer beitrag zum krankheitsbild der sog "osteitis necroticans pubis," *Munich Med Wochenschr* 106:1, 1964.
69. Spinelli A: Nouva malattia sportive: la pubialgia degli schernitori, *Orthop Traumatol* 3:111, 1932.
70. Staples O: Ruptures of the fibular collateral ligament of the ankle, *J Bone Joint Surg* 57A:101, 1975.
71. Statistics on the 150 national associations of FIFA, *FIFA News* 235:528, 1982.
72. Steadman JR: Rehabilitation of first- and second-degree sprains of the medial collateral ligaments of the knee, *Am J Sports Med* 7:300, 1979.
73. Sullivan JA, Gross RH: Evaluation of injuries in youth soccer, *Am J Sports Med* 8:325, 1980.
74. Swift R, Hershman M, Wood C: Bilateral, spontaneous, concurrent patellar tendon rupture, *Br J Clin Pract* 44:730, 1990.
75. Tenvergert E, Ten Duis H, Klasen H: Trends in sports injuries, 1982-1988: an in-depth study on four types of sport, *J Sports Med Phys Fitness* 32:214, 1992.
76. Thompson TC, Doherty JH: Spontaneous rupture of tendon of Achilles: a new clinical diagnostic test, *J Trauma* 2:126, 1962.
77. Unverferth LJ, Olix ML: The effect of local steroid injections on tendon, *J Sports Med* 1:31, 1973.
78. Washington ZL: Musculoskeletal injuries in theatrical dancers: site, frequency, and severity, *Am J Sports Med* 6:75, 1978.
79. Wiley J: Traumatic osteitis pubis: the gracilis syndrome, *Am J Sports Med* 11:360, 1983.
80. Williams JCT: Limitations of hip joint movement as factor of traumatic osteitis pubis, *Br J Sports Med* 12:129, 1978.

CHAPTER 66 Cycling Injuries

James C. Holmes
Andrew L. Pruitt
Nina J. Whalen

The care and prevention of cycling injuries require a basic knowledge about the sport of cycling, an understanding of the equipment, and a working knowledge of cycling biomechanics. These three elements address what is unique to cyclists, that is, their level of participation and style of cycling, their equipment choices, and their individual biomechanics. Failing to address all of these elements when treating cyclists can result in prolonged injury and frustration.

Cyclists are susceptible to traumatic injuries and overuse injuries. **Traumatic injuries** result from falls and collisions.[3] Cyclists with traumatic injuries are typically treated either through the emergency medical system or by self-administering treatment to minor injuries. Repeated minor traumatic injuries such as abrasions or contusions can become problematic and may require medical or surgical intervention. **Overuse injuries** most commonly result from errors in training or bicycle fit. Technical errors and weather conditions (e.g., wind, cold, and dampness) can also contribute to the development of overuse problems; however, these causes are seen less frequently.[26] Cyclists often self-treat overuse injuries with bicycle adjustments, training modifications, soft-tissue manipulations, and over-the-counter antiinflammatory medications. Their efforts are usually unsuccessful and may aggravate injuries by delaying proper treatment.

RECENT DEVELOPMENTS

The sport of cycling has undergone many changes in the past 10 years. The number of people cycling on a regular basis has significantly increased since 1983 as a result of many factors, including a migration of runners to cycling, the baby boom, and an increased awareness of fitness. According to the Bicycle Institute of America, there has been nearly a 30% increase in cycling participation since 1983. This translates into approximately 93 million Americans who ride bicycles.* Included in this figure are an estimated 9.4 million cyclists over the age of 45,† 25 million cyclists who ride once a week,* 21 million mountain bicycle enthusiasts,‡ and 220,000 race participants.*

---

*Source: Bicycle Institute of America, 1990.
†Source: National Sporting Goods Association, 1991.
‡Source: National Off-Road Bicycling Association: estimated figures, 1992.

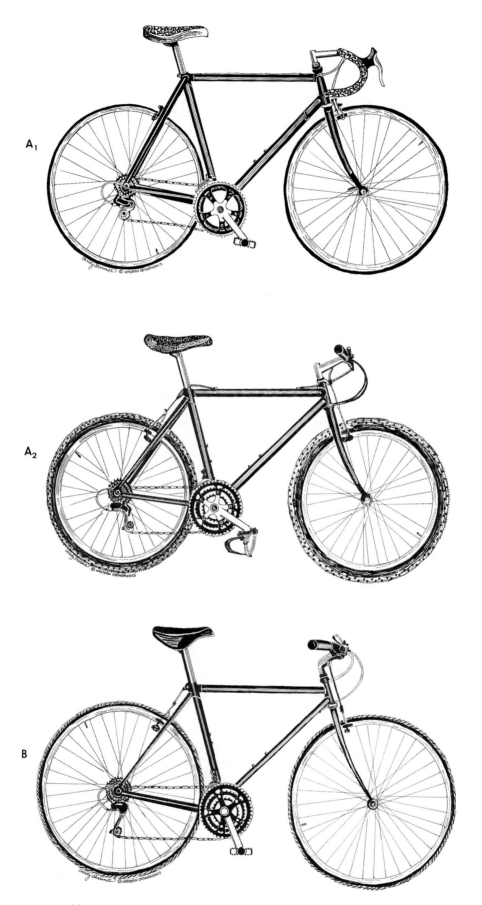

FIG. 66-1. A₁, Mountain bicycle compared with **A₂,** touring bicycle. **B,** Hybrid bicycle.

New Cycling Types

The addition of **mountain biking,** also called all-terrain cycling, has added a new dimension to the sport of cycling. In its purest form, mountain biking is performed on rugged, uneven terrain, necessitating a more durable and stable bicycle than the standard **touring bicycle** (Fig. 66-1, *A*). Agility and upper body strength are requirements of all-terrain cyclists and are not as critical to road or touring cyclists. Mountain bikes are popular among recreational and aerobic enthusiasts because they are more comfortable and stable. The **hybrid bike** is a road bike that is probably better recommended for the light recreational cyclist because it has smoother fat tires that make road cycling easier (Fig. 66-1, *B*). Understandably, traumatic type injuries are more common in the sport of all-terrain cycling; however, overuse injuries do occur. The incidence of overuse injuries of the lower extremities in all-terrain cyclists parallels the incidence in road cyclists with the knee being the most susceptible to overuse problems.

Pedal Systems

Another significant change in the sport of cycling has been in the area of pedal systems. These changes were directed at improving power transmission from the foot to the pedal. Early systems limited, but did not restrict, foot motion. These included **toe clips,** which used a slotted cleat on the bottom of the shoe and toe baskets (Fig. 66-2, *A* and *B*). Although these types of systems are nearly obsolete for serious road cyclists, most mountain bikes are still fitted with toe clips.

Clipless pedal systems first appeared around 1985. Their advantages included increased power transmission from the foot to the pedal, no straps, improved cornering clearance, lighter weight shoes that could be walked in, and easier entry and exit than toe clip systems.[2] The original clipless systems locked the cyclist's foot securely onto the pedal in one position through a shoe cleat–pedal interface mechanism similar to ski bindings (Fig. 66-2, *C*). This change in pedal systems necessitated a more rigid shoe material to ensure proper fixation of the foot to the pedal.

Most recently, manufacturers have introduced **floating clipless pedals.** These systems offer variable amounts of rotational foot movement on the pedal (Fig. 66-2, *D*), depending on the manufacturer, thereby allowing for individual kinematics. Floating clipless pedals are widely used today and are also available with controlled rotation, which provides a rotational end point according to the cyclist's needs. We have found floating pedal systems to be an important treatment option for those cyclists presenting with overuse injuries of the lower extremities related to anatomic variants or unusual kinematics.

BIOMECHANICS

The evaluation of cycling biomechanics in a clinical setting is used to determine the cyclist's optimum position based on anatomic variants, equipment choices, and level of participation to reduce his or her risk for overuse

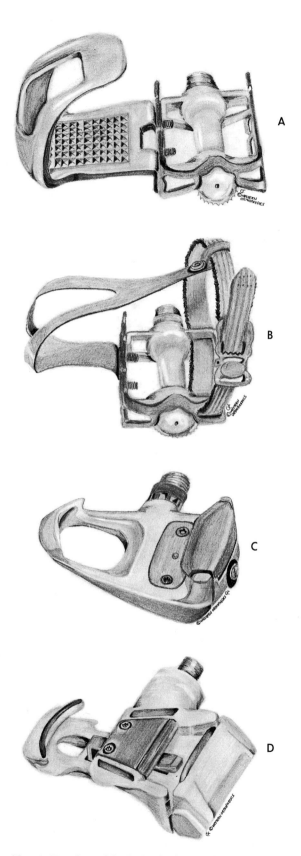

FIG. 66-2. A, Toe clip pedals. **B,** Toe basket pedals. **C,** Fixed clipless pedals. **D,** Floating clipless pedals.

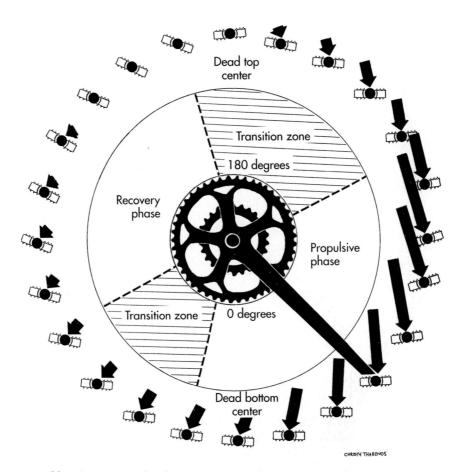

CHRISTY THARENOS

FIG. 66-3. Components of cycling gait. Arrows indicate direction and magnitude of force.

```
┌─────────────────────────────────────────┐
│                                           │
│         Phases of cycling gait            │
│                                           │
│     ■ Propulsive phase                    │
│     ■ Recovery phase                      │
│                                           │
└─────────────────────────────────────────┘
```

injuries. The concept of cycling gait is useful for evaluating individual kinematics. The first phase, the **propulsive phase,** begins just after dead top center (Fig. 66-3). This phase has a weight-bearing component that occurs when the power produced by the legs is transmitted through the foot to the pedal. As pressures in the foot increase, there is usually a compensatory pronation that is accompanied by internal rotation of the tibia and slight adduction of the hip (Fig. 66-4).[6] A significant decrease in pedaling force occurs just after the cyclist reaches the bottom of the pedaling stroke.[13] This signals the start of the **recovery phase.** During recovery, downward pedal forces are reduced or eliminated as the cyclist pulls up on the pedal to overcome gravity and inertia. Overuse injuries are more commonly associated with the propulsion phase of cycling gait because of the higher torque and loading of muscles, tendons, and joints. Additionally, any intrinsic (anatomic variants) or extrinsic (bicycle fit) factor that alters kinematics during propulsion can contrib-

ute to the development of overuse injuries.[14] Examples include excessive pronation of the foot, improper cleat position, incorrect saddle height, or a varus deformity of the lower leg.

BICYCLE FIT

Determining bicycle fit is a dynamic process based on each cyclist's unique biomechanics and equipment choices. Static bicycle fit formulas advocated by manufacturers and cycling celebrities often fail to address asymmetries and anatomic variants, but they can provide a starting point for fit.

Clinical Evaluation

The first step in the fitting process is determining the cyclist's normal off-bike alignment. Tibial rotation and foot orientation are easily evaluated by viewing the cyclist from the front while he or she is seated on an examination table. The knees should be approximately shoulder-width apart accompanied by a 90-degree angle of the hips, knees, and ankles (Fig. 66-5).

Cyclists should be evaluated for varus and valgus deformities while standing. Pronation and supination, which are active anatomic variants related to weight bearing, should also be assessed at this time.

Leg length inequalities, which may be tolerated with

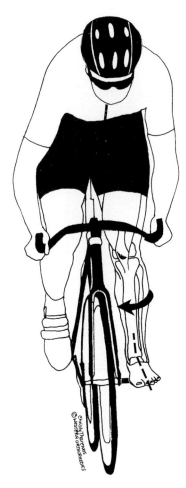

FIG. 66-4. Internal tibial rotation and pronation during weight-bearing phase of pedaling.

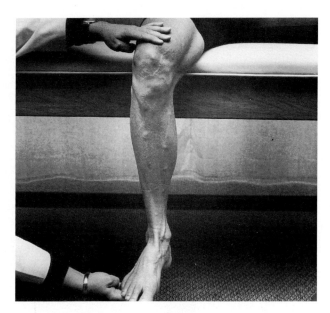

FIG. 66-5. Off-bicycle examination of cyclist's alignment.

walking or running, can become problematic with cycling because of the cyclist's fixation to the bike and a higher number of repetitions. It should be determined whether inequalities are functional or static, since corrections are specific for the type of length discrepancy. **Functional length differences** resulting from foot mechanics (i.e., they occur at the foot or ankle) are corrected primarily with orthotics and bicycle fit corrections.

Static length discrepancies may be present in the femur or the tibia. Scanograms, which can be done in the office, provide static segmental measurements and location of length differences (Fig. 66-6). Static inequalities can be treated with spacers, saddle, or foot position adjustments.

Functional length discrepancies can result from faulty foot mechanics. Radiographic evaluation with a standing anteroposterior view of the pelvis (performed on a level surface) can be used to detect functional length differences (Fig. 66-7).

Saddle Position

Saddle position is strongly related to a cyclist's ability to transmit power to the pedals. Unfortunately, for many

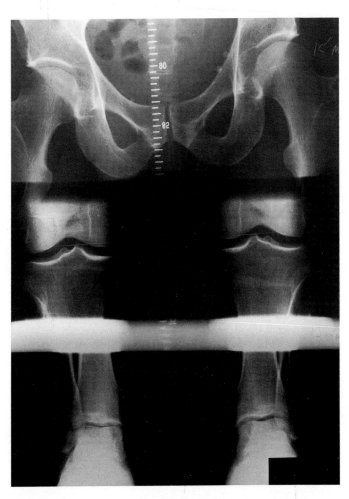

FIG. 66-6. Measurement of static leg length discrepancies using scanogram.

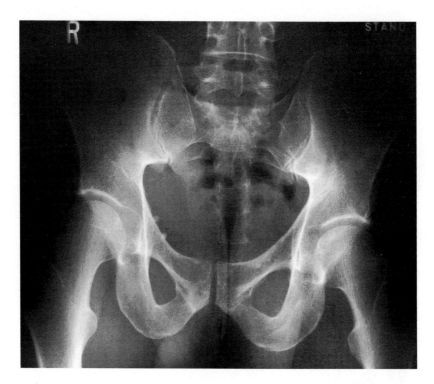

FIG. 66-7. Measurement of functional leg length discrepancies using standing anteroposterior x-ray study of pelvis.

cyclists the saddle positions that produce the most power are also stressful to the knee.[22]

Many formulas have been proposed to determine optimum saddle position.[20] The following recommendations based on clinical experience are designed primarily to reduce stress to the front of the knee while allowing for smooth power production.

Saddle Height

Saddle height is best determined by measuring degrees of knee flexion at dead bottom center of the pedaling stroke. Dead bottom center is the position of the crankarm at the bottom of the pedaling stroke (Fig. 66-8). The degree of knee flexion is easily measured using a goniometer placed on the greater trochanter, the lateral condyle of the knee, and the lateral malleolus of the ankle (Fig. 66-8). Clinically, we have found that **the optimum position that allows comfort while cycling and still produces a sensation of power is at 25 to 30 degrees of flexion at dead bottom center.** Furthermore, this position decreases anterior knee stress by reducing patellar compression. Saddles that are too high

can result in posterior knee pain, and saddles that are too low can produce anterior knee pain. Frequently, there is a delicate balance between these two. It is often the cyclist's tolerance to a particular saddle position that dictates the degree of change. The saddle height for cyclists with leg length discrepancies should always be adjusted to the long leg. Length corrections are then made on the shoe or pedal of the short leg or with fore-aft positioning of the feet if the length discrepancy occurs at the femur.

Tibial length discrepancies can easily be treated by using spacers to equalize lengths. These spacers can be placed between the shoe and the cleat or in the shoe for a touring cyclist using a noncleated shoe.

Femoral length discrepancies are more difficult to treat. We use a combination of spacers and an adjustment in the foot position on the pedal to provide correction for femoral length differences, although this method is anecdotal. For example, a 6-mm difference could be treated with a 3-mm shim placed between the shoe and cleat and by moving the foot of the short leg back 1 mm on the pedal and the foot of the long leg forward 1 mm on the pedal. Compensating for length differences through the use of a combination of asymmetric crankarms and elliptic chain rings is currently being investigated (Slocum T: Personal communication, October 22, 1992.) These systems are in the developmental phase and, to date, have not been evaluated for their effect on power production. Corrections for length should always slightly undercompensate the total difference because many cyclists slightly correct with "ankling" (exaggerated plantar or dorsiflexion). Length discrepancies of 4

Optimum saddle height

- 25 to 30 degrees of knee flexion at dead bottom center pedal position
- Too high → posterior knee pain
- Too low → anterior knee pain

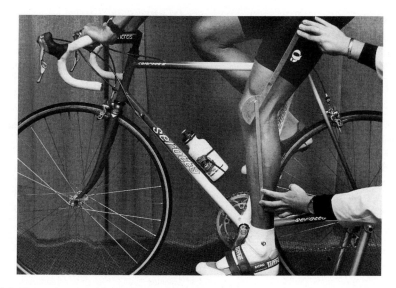

FIG. 66-8. Determining saddle height by measuring knee flexion at dead bottom center of pedaling stroke.

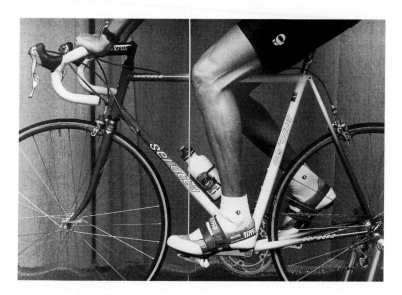

FIG. 66-9. Determining fore-aft saddle position using plumb line.

mm or less do not need correction unless the cyclist is symptomatic.

Fore-Aft Position

The fore-aft position of the saddle is determined by the length of the femur, crankarm, and foot, assuming that the ischial tuberosities are weight bearing and that the ball of the foot is over the pedal axle. Using the concept of a plumb line, the end of a string is placed on the front edge of the patella and dropped down toward the pedal. In the ideal fore-aft position the plumb line should fall at the end of the crankarm (Fig. 66-9).

Cleat Position

Cleat position should reflect any anatomic variants that were noted during the off-cycle examination. For example, a cyclist with external tibial rotation should be placed in a slightly externally rotated or toed out cleat position. This is especially critical for cyclists using fixed rather than floating cleat systems because there is no rotation to compensate for anatomic variants. The foot should be aligned over the pedal so that the metatarsal head of the great toe is over the axle of the pedal.

Cyclists who have marked pronation, excessive toeing out, or varus alignments may benefit from adding spacers between the pedal and the crankarm (Fig. 66-10). These can alleviate trauma to the medial malleolus for cyclists with excessive pronation and can improve hip-to-foot alignment for cyclists with varus alignment.

Torso Angle

The angle of the torso in relation to the cycle varies with the participation level of the cyclist (Fig. 66-11). Time trialists, for example, maintain an aggressive position of 45 degrees or less in relation to the top tube. A recreational mountain bike rider maintains a more upright position than a road racer. Reach length is determined by the length of the arms, arm strength, torso length, and low back strength. Cyclists typically adjust reach length by what is comfortable, their level of back conditioning, and what can be maintained for desired distances.

OVERUSE INJURIES

In our clinic the knee accounts for more overuse injuries in cyclists than any other area.[15] Injuries can best be classified as anterior, posterior, medial, or lateral problems (Table 66-1).

Anterior Knee

"Patellofemoral pain is a fairly common finding in young athletes, and the prudent physician recognizes

TABLE 66-1 Incidence of overuse knee injuries in 354 cyclists (may have more than one diagnosis)

	Level I (Elite)	Level II (Competitive)	Level III (Recreational)
Number of Cyclists	58	122	174
Anterior			
Chondromalacia	15	56	87
Patellar tendinitis	17	15	21
Quadriceps tendinitis	8	4	6
Patellofemoral disease	—	1	12
% Cyclists	68.9	62.3	72.4
Medial			
Medial capsule/plica	7	18	6
Medial retinaculum/ patellofemoral ligament	5	7	12
Plica and medial patellofemoral ligament	8	3	2
Pes anserinus	—	3	5
% Cyclists	34.5	25.4	14.4
Lateral			
Iliotibial band syndrome	13	26	46
% Cyclists	22.4	21.3	26.4
Posterior			
Hamstring	10	3	2
Posterior capsule	—	4	3
% Cyclists	17.2	5.7	2.9

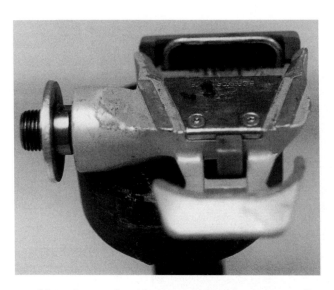

FIG. 66-10. Spacers placed between pedal and crankarm to widen cyclist's stance on bicycle.

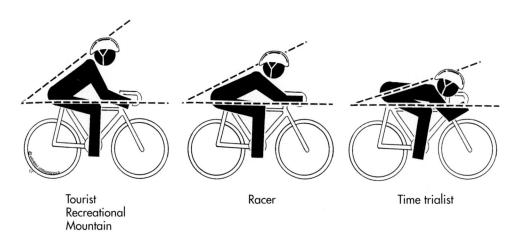

Tourist
Recreational
Mountain

Racer

Time trialist

FIG. 66-11. Torso angle variations in cyclists.

that there are a variety of clinical problems which can cause such pain."[10] Although chondromalacia is a frequent cause of patellofemoral pain, it is not the only cause. In cyclists, retinacular or synovial irritation and patellar or quadriceps tendinitis can also present as patellofemoral pain.

We have found that anterior knee injuries constitute the largest group of overuse knee problems in cyclists (Table 66-1). They are not inherent to the sport, as was once believed, but rather are a product of fit errors or training or preexisting anatomic abnormalities.

Chondromalacia

Etiology. In cycling, stress to the anterior knee results from overloading the extensor mechanism at angles of knee flexion that produce excess shear force between the patella and femur. Overtraining, excessive hill work, riding in too high of gears, inadequate training base, improper saddle position, and preexisting chondral changes can lead to symptomatic chondromalacia in cyclists.

Diagnosis. Cyclists with chondromalacia describe the onset of anterior discomfort with riding as that which eventually becomes bothersome with other patellofemoral loading activities (i.e., stair climbing, kneeling, or weight room activities). They may also describe subpatellar crepitus with flexion and extension of the knee. Physical examination may reveal static or dynamic patellofemoral malalignment, crepitus, and, in extreme cases, x-ray findings of patellofemoral joint space narrowing.

Treatment. In our experience the majority of cyclists with chondromalacia are able to continue cycling at some level, and most find it therapeutic if saddles are correctly adjusted. Treatment for chondromalacia in cyclists consists of the following:

1. Correct bicycle fit with special attention to saddle position (neutral fore-aft and 25 degrees of flexion at dead bottom center).
2. Restrict cycling activities to easy spinning (low resistance) and flat terrain rides until symptoms subside.
3. Encourage quadriceps muscle strengthening with terminal extension exercises (where shear force on the patellofemoral joint is minimal).
4. Maintain hip and calf strength without loading the patella.

Patellar Tendinitis

Etiology. Irritation to the patellar tendon from cycling is most likely caused by excess angular traction on the tendon while pedaling. According to Bassett, Soucacos, and Carr,[1] the site of tissue failure when the traction or tension threshold is exceeded depends on several factors:

1. Magnitude of the applied force.
2. Duration over which the load is applied.
3. The angle of knee flexion at the moment of loading.
4. The health and functional capacity of the involved tissues and their interfaces.
5. The degree of elastic deformation that the individual possesses (age).

6. The level of conditioning or fatigue of the extensor muscles of the extremity (ability to absorb kinetic energy).

Iatrogenic causes such as harvesting of the central one third of the patellar tendon for anterior cruciate ligament (ACL) reconstruction should also be considered when determining the cause of patellar tendinitis.

Cycling biomechanics that we believe contribute to the development of patellar tendinitis include internal tibial rotation and pronation because of the resultant medial and lateral patellar tendon stresses and saddles that are too low or too far forward, which produce excessive stress on the patellar tendon. Symptom onset is often related to a sudden increase in mileage, hill work, or a change in equipment and therefore is more commonly seen in the spring season. Off-season weight training can also contribute to patellar tendon irritation.

Factors that contribute to patellar tendinitis

- Internal tibial rotation
- Pronation
- Saddle too low
- Saddle too far forward
- Change in mileage
- Increased hill work
- Equipment change

Diagnosis. Cyclists with patellar tendinitis complain of significant patellar pain related to pedaling and other knee extension activities. Clinical examination may denote localized swelling at the inferior portion of the patella, crepitus, and fat pad irritation. Exquisite point tenderness is most commonly elicited on the lateral or medial inferior pole of the patella but may also occur at tibial insertion sites. Although midsubstance irritation of the patellar tendon is rare, it does occur.

Treatment. Patellar tendinitis is often recalcitrant to treatment. The need for *prolonged conservative measures, including rest,* should be strongly emphasized. Treatment for patellar tendinitis includes the following:

1. Evaluate and correct saddle position to 25 degrees of flexion at dead bottom center and a neutral fore-aft position.
2. Reflect any anatomic variants with cleat position, especially if there is evidence of internal tibial rotation or valgus alignment.
3. Treat excess pronation while pedaling with orthotics or lifts.
4. Permit only pain-free cycling.
5. Discourage extensor mechanism weight training activities.
6. Encourage frequent icing and use of nonsteroidal antiinflammatory drugs (NSAIDs).
7. Instruct the cyclist in friction massage (except at inferior pole).
8. Injection with local steroids has not been found effective in treating athletes for patellar tendinitis.[1]

Quadriceps Tendinitis

Quadriceps tendinitis may occur medially or laterally, but it is most often lateral in cyclists. It can be confused with chondromalacia or, in some cases, misdiagnosed as iliotibial band (ITB) syndrome.

Etiology. Symptom onset is insidious and usually related to an increase in training mileage, an increase in hill work, the lack of an adequate training base (e.g., in the early spring), riding into a head wind, or excessive weight training during the off season. Riding with too low of a saddle or with cleats that are too toed out or toed in can also contribute to quadriceps tendon irritation.

Diagnosis. Cyclists may indicate a diffuse area of tenderness at the lateral or medial suprapatellar area. Occa-

---

Factors that contribute to quadriceps tendinitis

- Increased training mileage
- Increased hill work
- Lack of training base
- Riding into a head wind
- Excessive off-season weight training
- Saddle position too low
- Cleats too toed out or in

---

sionally, a deficit can be palpated in the tendon. Other diagnoses such as ITB syndrome, chondromalacia, or medial retinacular pain must be ruled out before a diagnosis of quadriceps tendinitis can be made. Magnetic resonance imaging (MRI) can be used to confirm a tear in the quadriceps tendon (Fig. 66-12).

Treatment. Treatment for quadriceps tendinitis includes the following:

1. Correct saddle height to 25 to 30 degrees of flexion at dead bottom center and a neutral fore-aft position.
2. Reflect any off-bike anatomic variants with cleat position.
3. Reduce and modify training to easy spinning, or restrict cycling if symptoms are severe or if chondromalacia is also present.
4. Discourage weight training involving such exercises as squats and lunges.
5. Encourage frequent icing and use of NSAIDs.

Medial Knee

Over the past 10 years we have seen an increase in medial knee problems in cyclists. The medial peripatellar structures seem to be especially susceptible to overuse problems related to cleat position, saddle position, and mileage. The two most common medial knee problems seen in cyclists are irritation and fibrosis of the medial shelf (plica) and the medial patellofemoral ligament. The medial patellofemoral ligament is a distinct anatomic entity located within the medial retinaculum (Fig. 66-13). Anatomic studies have demonstrated variance in its size from mere wisps to well-developed structures.[25] Clinically, in a prospective study of 55 elite cyclists, we found a 72% incidence of palpable medial patellofemo-

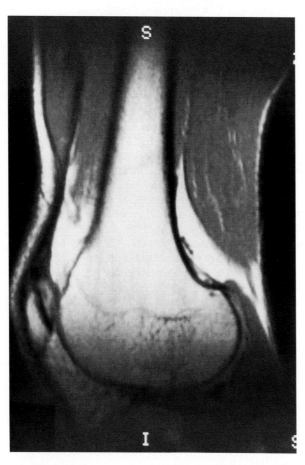

FIG. 66-12. Demonstration of quadriceps defect with magnetic resonance imaging.

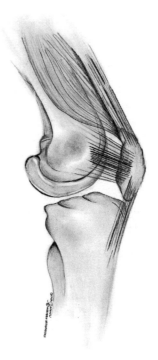

FIG. 66-13. Medial patellofemoral ligament.

ral ligaments with 49% exhibiting bilateral findings.* Interestingly, although clinical examination may only reveal one or the other of these structures, arthroscopy often reveals fibrosis and inflammation of both the medial patellofemoral ligament and the medial shelf. According to Fulkerson,[10] ". . . the aberrant mechanical factors that cause early retinacular strain and pain may ultimately lead to synovial inflammation." Despite difficulties in clinical differentiation, the treatment of these two entities is similar and therefore is discussed concurrently.

Medial Synovial Plica and Medial Patellofemoral Ligament

Etiology. High-mileage and high-intensity rides combined with improper cleat position, saddle position, or excessive pronation can precipitate the onset of medial knee pain in cyclists. Anatomic variants of valgus knees, internal tibial rotation, and excessive active pronation may contribute to medial knee stress while pedaling. Medial shelf irritation is most likely a result of friction of the medial plica across the medial femoral condyle with each pedaling stroke. Irritation of the medial patellofemoral ligament is related to excessive traction on this ligament as the patella is pulled laterally during pedaling.

Factors that contribute to medial knee pain

- High mileage ⎫
  ⎬ with ⎰ ■ Improper cleat position
- High intensity ⎭   ⎱ ■ Excessive pronation
                         ■ Improper saddle position

- Valgus knee
- Internal tibial torsion

Diagnosis. Cyclists often complain of disabling medial knee pain related to an intense ride or climb. Additionally, they may complain of a medial popping that occurs with each pedaling stroke. Exquisite point tenderness is often palpable at the medial margin of the patella. The presence of a medial patellofemoral ligament can sometimes be detected by displacing the patella medially (Fig. 66-14). Differentiating a medial patellofemoral ligament as the source of medial knee pain in the presence of a tender, medial plica may be difficult because of the close proximity of these two structures. Clinical diagnosis may be further obscured if chondromalacia is present.

Treatment. Local injection with steroids is unpredictable and therefore is usually not recommended because of the difficulty in identifying these distinct medial structures and because it has not proven effective for lasting symptom relief.[23] Nonoperative treatment includes the following:

1. Correct bicycle fit to reflect off-bike anatomy.
2. Correct or compensate for excessive active pronation with orthotics.

3. Modify cycling to pain-free participation, easy spinning, and no hills.
4. Encourage frequent icing (including ice massage) and use of NSAIDs.

Surgical intervention is indicated for failure of prolonged nonoperative measures or on occasion for the elite cyclist with professional or contractual obligations. We have found arthroscopic evaluation of the knee followed by complete medial wall synovectomy and excision or release of the medial patellofemoral ligament (Fig. 66-15), when indicated, to be effective for our population of high-level cyclists. Simple surgical division of the plica is

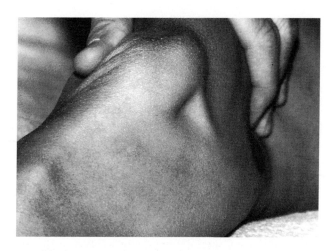

FIG. 66-14. Clinical examination for medial patellofemoral ligament.

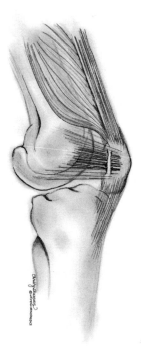

FIG. 66-15. Arthroscopic release of medial patellofemoral ligament.

---

*From unpublished data Holmes, Pruitt, Whalen, Evaluation of 55 elite cyclists for medial patellofemoral ligaments in the 1992 Tour Dupont

thought to be ineffective because symptomatic tissue may be left, resulting in recurrence of symptoms.[8]

Pes Anserine Irritation

The pes anserine is a confluence of the sartorius, gracilis, and semitendinosus tendons on the medial tibial flare. It is functionally described as a rotatory stabilizer and valgus restraint.

Etiology. External tibial rotation and pronation are probable causes of irritation to the pes anserine tendon; however, length discrepancies or too high of a saddle may also be contributing factors. Trauma to the medial knee from the bicycle frame can also result in pes anserine irritation.

Factors that contribute to pes anserine irritation

- External tibial rotation
- Pronation
- Leg length inequality
- Saddle too high
- Trauma from bicycle frame

Diagnosis. Cyclists with pes anserine irritation have localized pain and swelling at the pes anserine insertion. Pain can usually be reproduced by applying pressure to this area with active flexion and extension. Because improper biomechanics are usually the primary cause of this entity, it is especially important to observe the cyclist pedaling and to look specifically for external tibial rotation or pronation. Symptom relief with internal tibial rotation while pedaling may also be diagnostic.

Treatment. We have found injections of steroids to be beneficial on occasion. Other treatments include the following:

1. Correct or modify cycling biomechanics with orthotics to control excessive pronation.
2. Recommend controlled rotation of pedals, when appropriate, to prevent excess external tibial rotation.
3. Instruct in stretching exercises of the medial hamstrings and pes anserine muscles.
4. Encourage use of ice, NSAIDs, and friction massage.

Lateral Knee

ITB friction syndrome is the most common lateral overuse knee problem in cycling (Table 66-1). Lateral knee irritation commonly results from a combination of intrinsic (e.g., prominence of lateral femoral condyle or

---

Factors that contribute to iliotibial band friction syndrome

- Lateral femoral condyle prominence
- Tight iliotibial band (positive Ober test)
- Poor cleat position
- Inappropriate saddle height

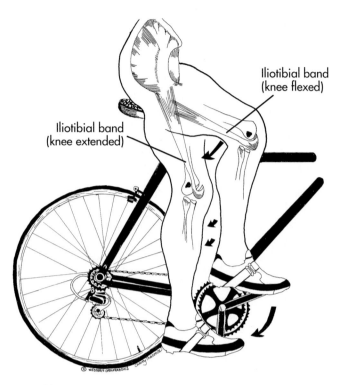

FIG. 66-16. Distal iliotibial band friction across lateral femoral condyle with pedaling.

tight ITB) and extrinsic (e.g., cleat position or saddle height) factors.

Iliotibial Band Friction Syndrome

Etiology. ITB irritation is the result of repetitive friction of the ITB across the lateral femoral condyle. Contact between the ITB and the lateral femoral condyle is most pronounced at approximately 30 degrees of knee flexion.[16] Cyclists are especially prone to this problem because, with each pedaling stroke, the ITB is pulled anteriorly on the downstroke and posteriorly on the upstroke (Fig. 66-16). The posterior fibers of the ITB are especially susceptible to this type of friction irritation because they contour more closely to the lateral femoral condyle than the anterior fibers. Abnormal friction may be caused by ITB tightness, active internal tibial rotation with external foot placement on the pedal, pronation, excessively internally rotated cleats, riding with the saddle too high, excessive hill work, or an inadequate training base.

Diagnosis. Cyclists typically complain of an acute onset of lateral knee pain that is often described as sharp or stabbing. Pain is usually rhythmic with each pedaling stroke and significantly reduces the cyclist's ability to transfer power to the pedal. Some cyclists also complain of pain radiating up the lateral thigh and down to Gerdy's tubercle.

Physical examination reveals point tenderness of the distal ITB over the lateral femoral condyle. Pain can be reproduced by applying pressure to the distal ITB at the lateral femoral condyle while extending the knee from 30 to 0 degrees of flexion. There may be associated dis-

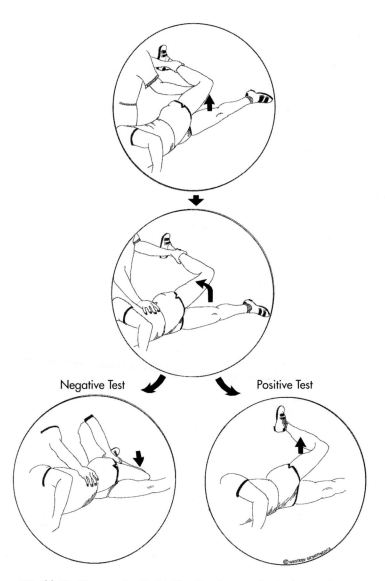

Negative Test   Positive Test

FIG. 66-17. Ober test for iliotibial band and tensor fasciae latae tightness.

comfort at the greater trochanter and Gerdy's tubercle. The Ober-type maneuver (Fig. 66-17) is diagnostic of tightness of the tensor fasciae latae and the ITB.[21]

Treatment. Because this is a friction problem, stretching exercises are of primary importance in the treatment plan. We recommend the Ober, modified Ober, crossover toe touch, and the lateral hip drop stretches (Fig. 66-18) to be done a minimum of twice daily. Other nonoperative interventions include the following:

1. Correct cleat position to reflect the cyclist's neutral anatomic alignment or a slight degree of external rotation. For cyclists using fixed pedal systems, a switch to floating pedals can be beneficial in the treatment of ITB friction syndrome.
2. Adjust stance width through the use of spacers placed between the pedal and the crankarm. These can reduce ITB stress by widening the cyclist's stance and thus improve hip-to-foot alignment.

3. Restrict cycling for cyclists with acute symptoms, and allow pain-free cycling only for subacute cases.
4. Instruct in focal icing and the use of NSAIDs.
5. Use deep-tissue massage proximal to the symptomatic area.
6. Physical therapy modalities of ultrasound and electric stimulation can be useful as adjunctive therapies.

For cyclists requesting immediate treatment because of racing or training obligations, the symptomatic area can be injected with cortisone. Stretching should be continued, and cycling can be resumed, if the athlete is pain free, after 3 to 7 days.

Surgical intervention should be considered when prolonged nonoperative measures fail. Percutaneous release has not proven to be an effective, long-term operative therapy in our hands. We have found an open release and excision of the distal ITB to be more effective in re-

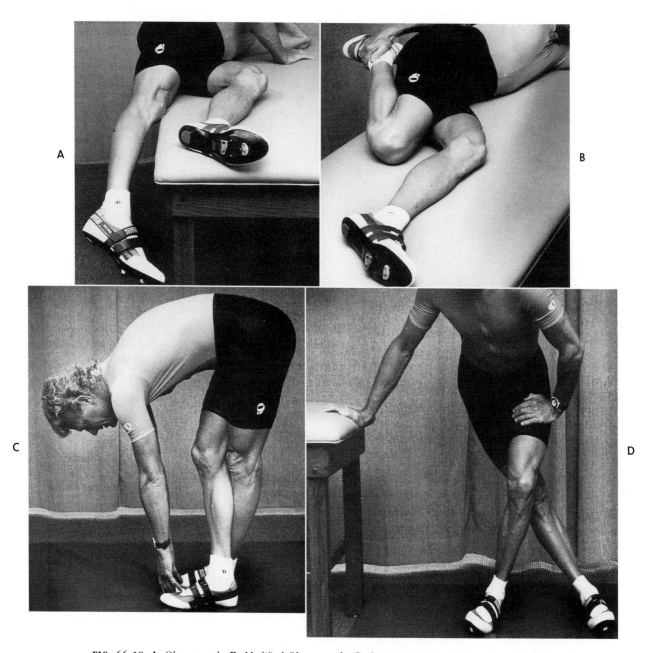

FIG. 66-18. A, Ober stretch. **B,** Modified Ober stretch. **C,** Crossover toe touch stretch. **D,** Lateral hip drop stretch.

lieving cyclists with ITB friction syndrome.[15,19] Our method involves excision of an elliptic piece of the distal ITB off the lateral femoral condyle (Fig. 66-19).

Postoperatively, on-bike biomechanics are evaluated and corrected. Cyclists are instructed in a gradual return to cycling and are encouraged to include ITB stretches as part of their daily routine.

Posterior Knee

Posterior knee complaints in cycling are rare. The most common posterior knee complaint is that of biceps tendinitis. Other posterior problems are most often a result of strain of the posterior capsule from excessive saddle height or a short leg.

Biceps Tendinitis

Etiology. Factors contributing to strain of the biceps femoris tendon include riding with the saddle too high, cleats that are excessively toed in, varus alignment of the knees, short leg length, and too aft of a saddle position. Cyclists should be questioned about recent changes in equipment, sudden increases in mileage or intensity, and previous diagnosis of length discrepancies.

Diagnosis. There is usually point tenderness of the biceps femoris tendinous attachment at the fibular head. Tenderness can often be elicited by strumming the biceps tendon as well. Differential diagnosis includes ITB friction syndrome, torn lateral meniscus, and popliteal tendinitis.

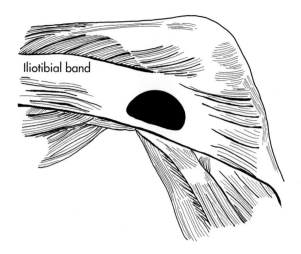

FIG. 66-19. Surgical release and excision of elliptic piece of distal iliotibial band off lateral femoral condyle.

Factors that contribute to biceps femoris tendinitis

- Saddle too high
- Cleats too toed in
- Varus knee alignment
- Short leg length
- Too aft saddle position
- Recent equipment change
- Sudden mileage increase

Treatment. Treatment should be focused on correcting bicycle fit errors to reflect off-bike anatomy. This includes the following:

1. Adjust saddle position to reflect a neutral fore-aft position and 30 to 35 degrees of flexion at dead bottom center to relieve the stretch on the biceps femoris at the bottom of the pedaling stroke.
2. Correct cleat position to reflect lower extremity alignment or a switch to a floating pedal system if lower extremity variants cannot be accommodated with fixed pedals.
3. Correct for leg length discrepancies with spacers, orthotics, or bicycle fit adjustments.
4. Encourage focal icing, passive stretching, and use of NSAIDs.

Surgery is rarely necessary except in cases that are resistant to nonoperative measures. The surgical debridement of the biceps tendon is done as an open procedure. The goal of surgery is to remove symptomatic scar tissue from the affected area and excise necrotic tissue from the biceps tendon.

Hips

Overuse injuries of the hip from cycling are typically strains resulting from prolonged positioning on the cycle.

Factors that contribute to trochanteric bursitis

- Tight iliotibial band
- Stance too narrow

Trochanteric Bursitis

Etiology. Overuse-related trochanteric bursitis is usually the result of a chronically tight tensor fasciae latae. Riding with too narrow of a stance width can cause excess tension across the trochanteric bursa.

Diagnosis. Cyclists should be evaluated for flexibility of the lateral hip using the Ober test (Fig. 66-17). The application of direct pressure to the trochanteric bursa elicits a positive pain response if the bursa is inflamed.

Treatment. Treatment of trochanteric bursitis includes the following:

1. Widen stance width on the bicycle, when indicated, with the use of crankarm spacers. The goal of adjusting the width is to produce a linear relationship between the hip, knee, and foot.
2. Instruct the cyclist in stretching exercises including the Ober, modified Ober, crossover toe touch, and lateral hip drop stretches.
3. Encourage use of ice and NSAIDs.

Ischial Tuberosity Irritation

Cyclists complaining of ischial tuberosity soreness are generally referring to discomfort at the insertion site of the hamstrings onto the ischial tuberosities.

Etiology. Saddle position, tilt, shape, texture, and prolonged sitting on the saddle can contribute to irritation of the ischial tuberosities.

Factors that contribute to ischial tuberosity irritation

- Saddle position
- Saddle tilt, shape, or texture
- Prolonged sitting on saddle

Diagnosis. Palpation of the hamstrings insertion site on the ischial tuberosities usually elicits a positive pain response.

Treatment. The primary treatment is to improve saddle position or type. (Saddle types include male, female, road, or mountain designs.) Saddle position should be carefully adjusted so that new problems do not appear from overcorrection.

Although hamstring stretching may be useful, rest from cycling is probably the most beneficial treatment.

Chronic Gluteal Muscle Strain

This can be an acutely debilitating and painful problem for any cyclist.

Etiology. Chronic irritation of the abductor gluteal muscle groups, often precipitated after a long ride or tour, may occur in the muscle belly, insertion, or origin. Symptom onset is usually after a long ride or a tour.

Diagnosis. Cyclists with chronic gluteal muscle strain complain of significant buttocks pain related to long rides or a recent tour. Differential diagnosis includes degenerative lumbar disk, degenerative joint disease of the low back, and sacroiliac discomfort. Physical examination is significant only for generalized soreness of the buttocks.

Treatment. Treatment for chronic gluteal muscle strain includes the following:

1. Provide the cyclist with a more upright position to reduce strain on the abductor muscles.
2. Encourage stretching of the abductor muscles.
3. Application of local heat may provide pain relief.
4. Advise the cyclist to restrict the length of rides until symptoms subside.

Back

Cyclists with healthy backs rarely develop overuse back problems related to cycling. Those cyclists with preexisting problems, however, can experience discomfort from the prolonged position of reaching or improper top tube stem combination. Mountain biking, which involves more impact than touring, can produce sacroiliac or low back discomfort.

Foot and Ankle
General Problems

Etiology. Overuse problems of the foot and ankle are generally caused by a combination of intrinsic (cavus or pes plantus deformities and overflexibility of the foot) and extrinsic (rigid or soft shoes and pedal systems) factors.

Diagnosis. Cyclists should be evaluated for active pronation and pes plantus. If the cyclist is also a runner, footwear should be evaluated for evidence of improper

---

Factors that contribute to foot and ankle overuse problems
■ Pes planus
■ Cavus foot
■ Rigid or soft shoes
■ Pedal systems

---

biomechanics. Foot and ankle mechanics can be assessed by viewing the cyclist both walking and pedaling.

Treatment. The treatment of foot and ankle problems often requires correction with cycling orthotics. Cycling orthotics differ from running orthotics in several ways (Fig. 66-20). Posting is aimed at forefoot correction because pedaling involves contact only of the forefoot with the pedal. The length of the cycling orthotic is substantially longer than the running orthotic because contact occurs under the metatarsal heads. Generally, cycling orthotics are made of polypropylene, which is a slightly more rigid material than the polyethylene used for running orthotics. Minor follow-up adjustments are often necessary to provide a comfortable proper fit of the orthotic in the cyclist's shoe.

Posterior Tibialis Tendinitis

Etiology. Posterior tibialis tendinitis can result from a pes planus foot, difficulty adapting to floating pedals, or excessively toed out cleats.

Diagnosis. Cyclists with posterior tibialis tendinitis usually complain of posterolateral ankle pain that worsens during cycling. The posterior tibialis tendon is usually tender to palpation.

Treatment. Treatment is directed at providing support with orthotics and correction of foot and ankle mechan-

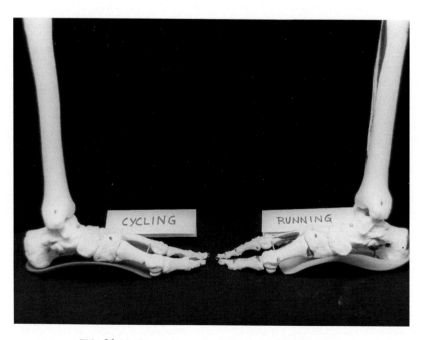

FIG. 66-20. Comparison of running vs. cycling orthotics.

Factors that contribute to posterior tibialis tendinitis

- Pes planus
- Floating pedals
- Toed out cleats

ics with either a temporary or permanent switch to fixed or controlled floating pedals. Treatment for posterior tibialis tendinitis includes the following:

1. Encourage use of ice and NSAIDs.
2. Use of physical therapy and stretching can be beneficial.

Achilles Tendinitis

Etiology. The foot is a flexible lever in running, but it acts as a rigid lever in cycling.[24] Achilles tendinitis in cyclists can result from excessive "ankling" while pedaling from an over flexible foot and a soft shoe or a foot that is placed too far behind the pedal spindle.

Factors that contribute to Achilles tendinitis

- Excessive "ankling"
  Flexible foot
  Soft shoe
- Foot too far back

Treatment. Treatment is directed at correction with orthotics or a more rigid supportive shoe and correction of foot placement on the pedal. In a neutral placement the metatarsal heads are just over the pedal axle. Placing the foot 1 to 3 mm forward of the axle can be a temporary or permanent treatment for Achilles tendinitis, depending on the cyclist's tolerance.

TRAUMATIC INJURIES

Traumatic injuries to the lower extremities from cycling consist mainly of abrasions, hematomas, and contusions from falls.[3] Occasionally, fractures may occur that require immobilization or surgery.

Abrasions

Abrasions from falls range from superficial to deep muscular. The most significant concern should be the depth of the abrasion, the amount of surface area involved, and how much gravel, dirt, or oil, is imbedded in the abraded area. Common sites for cycling-related abrasions are the hips, elbows, and lateral knees. Repeated abrasions and contusions to the greater trochanter can result in a bursitis.

Treatment of abrasions and contusions is directed at debridement of dirt and other matter, application of local antibiotics or anesthetics as necessary, and localized control of swelling with ice and compression.

Hematomas

Hematomas result from localized bleeding into a contused or injured area. They are perhaps one of the most undertreated traumatic injuries and can potentially result in a permanent disfigurement of soft-tissue areas such as Gerdy's tubercle or the lateral thigh. Treatment is directed at controlling bleeding and reducing swelling with local application of ice and pressure dressings. Long-term use of pressure dressings (up to 3 months) may be necessary to prevent fibrosis or myositis ossificans. Drainage or incision may be necessary on occasion.

Fractures

Hip and Pelvic Fractures

Etiology. Hip and pelvic fractures are the most common fractures of the lower extremities related to cycling. The mechanism of injury is usually a direct fall on the greater trochanter, resulting in a femoral neck, intertrochanteric, or acetabular fracture (Fig. 66-21).

Treatment. Hip fractures usually require surgical repair and fixation. Cyclists can often return to cycling less than 6 months after surgical repair, provided rehabilita-

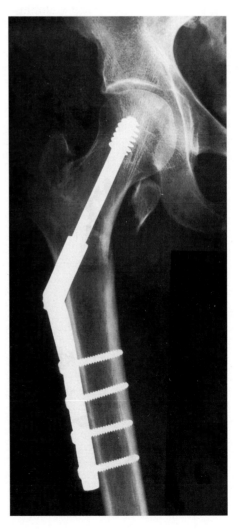

FIG. 66-21. Femoral neck fracture resulting from bicycle fall.

tion is aggressive and there were no surgical complications. Easy spinning can be resumed as soon as range of motion allows, provided that the fracture is stable. Increases in time and intensity are dependent on fracture healing. Hardware removal should be routinely contemplated for active cyclists because of friction irritation to the surrounding soft tissues.

Pelvic fractures should be treated according to the type of fracture either with operative or nonoperative treatment. Other lower extremity fractures are rare, although patellar fractures have been reported[3] and have been seen in our clinic.

INJURY PREVENTION

Bicycle fit, proper training routines, stretching, and education can assist the cyclist in preventing injuries.[18] Preseason evaluations of cyclists should include strength and flexibility testing. Cyclists often have zero degrees of hip extension as a result of their persistently flexed posture on the cycle. Ideally there should be 25 to 40 degrees of hip extension and more than 90 degrees of hip flexion from a supine position. Knee range of motion should be at least from 0 to 130 degrees. Back flexibility and strength should also be evaluated during the preseason evaluation. Complaints of chronic low back pain deserve orthopaedic evaluation with appropriate rehabilitation and bicycle adjustments. Cross training and preseason routines should be directed toward developing balanced strength and flexibility in all areas.

Helmets, gloves, and padded cycling shorts should be considered standard equipment for all cyclists. Additional protective clothing and padding are especially important to the mountain bicyclist to prevent minor traumatic injuries. All cyclists should be aware of the need for routine bicycle maintenance, especially concerning tires because unexpected flat tires during a ride can result in serious injury for any cyclist.

Injury prevention

- Bicycle fit
- Proper training routines
- Stretching
- Education
- Protective equipment
- Helmets
- Gloves
- Padded cycling shorts

REFERENCES

1. Bassett FH III, Soucacos PN, Carr WA: AAOS symposium on the athlete's knee, Hilton Head, SC, June 1978.
2. Berto F: A pedal revolution, *Bicycling* 30(3):172, 1989.
3. Bohlmann TJ: Injuries in competitive cycling, *Phys Sports Med* 9(5):117, 1981.
4. Burke ER: *Science of cycling*, Champaign, Ill, 1986, Human Kinetics.
5. Burke ER: Knees, *Bicycling* 31(8):72, 1990.
6. Burke ER, Newsom MM: *Medical and scientific aspects of cycling*, Champaign, Ill, 1988, Human Kinetics.
7. Dickson TB Jr: Preventing overuse cycling injuries, *Phys Sports Med* 13(10):116, 1985.
8. Dorchak JD et al: Arthroscopic treatment of symptomatic synovial plica of the knee, *Am J Sports Med* 19(5):503, 1991.
9. Fulkerson JP: Awareness of the retinaculum in evaluating patellofemoral pain, *Am J Sports Med* 10(3):147, 1982.
10. Fulkerson JP: The etiology of patellofemoral pain in young, active patients, *Clin Orthop* 179:129, 1983.
11. Fulkerson JP: Evaluation of the peripatellar soft tissues and retinaculum in patients with patellofemoral pain, *Clin Sports Med* 8(2):197, 1989.
12. Fulkerson JP, Hungerford DS: *Disorders of the patellofemoral joint*, ed 2, Baltimore, 1990, Williams & Wilkins.
13. Gregor RJ, Broker JP, Ryan MM: The biomechanics of cycling, *Exerc Sports Sci Rev* 19:127, 1991.
14. Hannaford DR, Moran GT, Hlavac HF: Video analysis and treatment of overuse knee injuries in cycling: a limited clinical study, *Clin Podiatr Med Surg* 3(4):671, 1988.
15. Holmes JC, Pruitt AL, Whalen NJ: Cycling overuse injuries, *Cycling Sci* 3(2):11, 1991.
16. Holmes JC, Pruitt AL, Whalen NJ: Iliotibial band syndrome in cyclists, *Am J Sports Med* 21(3):419, 1993.
17. Kelly C: At your own speed, *Denver Post* (suppl) September 6, 1992.
18. Koch C: The cycling docs, *Bicycle Guide* 7(7):46, 1990.
19. Martens M, Libbrecht P, Burssens A: Surgical treatment of the iliotibial band, *Am J Sports Med* 17(5):651, 1985.
20. Matheny F: Finding perfect saddle height, *Bicycling* 33(3):108, 1992.
21. Ober FR: The role of the iliotibial band and fascia lata as a factor in the causation of low back disabilities and sciatica, *J Bone Joint Surg* 18(1):105, 1936.
22. Pena N: The critical joint, *Bicycling* 32(5):74, 1991.
23. Rovere GD, Adair DM: Medial synovial shelf plica syndrome: treatment by intraplical steroid injection, *Am J Sports Med* 13(6):382, 1985.
24. Sanderson DJ: The biomechanics of cycling shoes, *Cycling Sci* 2(3):27, 1990.
25. Warren LF, Marshall JL: The supporting structures and layers on the medial side of the knee, *J Bone Joint Surg* 61A(1):56, 1979.
26. Weiss BD: Nontraumatic injuries in amateur long-distance bicyclists, *Am J Sports Med* 13(3):187, 1985.

Index

Hip—cont'd
strengthening exercises for, 978
Hip abduction exercise
in knee rehabilitation, 978
in patellofemoral joint treatment, 949, 952
in patellofemoral rehabilitation, 962
with Sport Cord, 979
Hip adduction exercise
in knee rehabilitation, 976, 978
in patellofemoral joint treatment, 949, 953
in patellofemoral rehabilitation, 962
with Sport Cord, 979
Hip drop stretch, 1571, 1572
Hip extension
in knee rehabilitation, 978
with Sport Cord, 979
strength testing of, 695
Hip flexion
contracture in, 200
exercises for
in knee rehabilitation, 978
in patellofemoral rehabilitation, 962
in patellofemoral joint treatment, 949, 952
with Sport Cord, 979
strength testing of, 695
Hip flexor
flexibility test for, 1221
in patellar tendinitis, 1417
strain of, 294
Hip pads
in pelvis and hip conditions, 1037
for protection, 309
Hip pointer
in football injuries, 1450
in iliac crest apophyseal avulsion, 1290
in pelvis and hip conditions, 1037
in soccer injuries, 1514-1515
Hip spica cast, 1298
Histamine
in inflammatory response, 82
infrared heating agents and, 214
HLNL; see Hydroxylysinonorleucine
Hockey, 311
Hodgkins lymphoma, 1337
Hoffa's disease, 1461
Home program in knee rehabilitation, 979, 981, 982
Hop test, 1050
Horizontal meniscal tear, 736, 738, 763-764
Hormone
in exercised ligaments, 33
in organ systems interaction, 95-96
in slipped capital femoral epiphysis, 1060, 1298
in stress fracture, 539
Horns of meniscus
lateral, 593
medial, 592
synovial vessels in, 588
Horseback riding
Duverney's fracture in, 1056
symphysis pubis in, 1055
Horseshoe pad
in ankle sprain, 239
in knee taping, 280
in sesamoid fracture, 1402, 1403
Hot air gun, 302, 303
Hot climate, 58
Hot spot in bone scintigraphy, 1160
HR; see Heart rate
Hughston technique
in knee radiography, 710
in patellofemoral reconstruction, 958
Hughston view, 946, 947
Hultkranz lines, 12
Human immunodeficiency virus, 873

Humphrey, ligament of; see Ligament of Humphrey
Hurdler
hamstring strains in, 1041
ischial apophyseal avulsion in, 1285
Hurdler's injury, 1047
Hyaline cartilage, 792-793
Hyaluronate, 17
Hyaluronic acid, 18
Hybrid bicycle, 1560, 1561
Hydration
of autograft, 869, 871
in heat cramps prevention, 295
Hydraulic amplifier mechanism, 1177
Hydrocollator heat pack machine, 302, 303
Hydrocollator packs, 213, 214
Hydrocortisone
in inflammatory process, 91
in patellofemoral joint cartilage, 948
in thoracolumbar spine treatment, 1166
Hydrogen
in cartilage, 10
in ligaments, 28
nuclei of, 112
proton of, 733
Hydrotherapy, 223
in strain treatment, 1043
Hydroxylysine, 15-16
Hydroxylysinonorleucine, 26-28
Hydroxyproline
in collagen, 12-13
excretion of, 53, 54
in muscle soreness, 43, 44
Hypaque, 412
Hyperdorsiflexion, 475-476
Hyperemia, 212, 214
Hyperextension
of anterior cruciate ligament, 1529, 1530
in cervical spine injuries, 1136
in knee taping, 280-284
in medial collateral and anterior cruciate ligament tears, 834, 835
one-leg test with
facet syndrome in, 1328
immature spine in, 1314-1315
thoracolumbar spine in, 1159
posterior cruciate ligament and, 890
in posterolateral complex, 856
radiculopathy in, 1117
in soccer injuries, 1548-1549, 1550
Hyperflexion
of ankle, 153
in first metatarsal, 1547
in hamstring injuries, 1454, 1455
posterior cruciate ligament and, 890
Hyperkalemia, 61
Hyperkeratosis, 1554
Hypermobility
patellar, 954
segmental, 1182
Hyperosmolar states, 57-58
Hyperphosphatemia, 61
Hyperplantar flexion, 483
Hyperplasia, 179
benign marrow, 752
Hyperpronation
in running, 1479, 1482-1483
in shin splints, 532-533
in soccer injuries, 1537, 1538
tenosynovitis in, 441
Hypertension, 791-792
Hyperthermia, 56
Hypertrophy, 154
muscle overload in, 178
in strength training, 100
Hyperuricemia, 56-57

I-32   Index (Vol. I, pp. 1-998; Vol. II, pp. 999-1576)

Hyperuricosuria, 56-57
Hypervolemia, 98
Hypocalcemia, 61
Hypokalemia, 57
Hyponatremia, 57
Hypothermia, 1502
Hypothyroidism, 1298
Hypovolemia, 98
Hypovolemic shock, 1089
Hysteresis
    of ligaments, 24-25
    in in vitro knee motion, 650

I

Ibuprofen, 89
Ice; *see also* Cryotherapy
    in ankle ligament injury, 427
    in ankle sprain, 239, 1424
    in hamstring injury, 284, 285, 290, 1012
    for hip pointer, 1515
    in inflammatory process, 88
    in knee rehabilitation, 972-973
    in lumbar spine injury, 1320
    massage with; *see* Ice massage
    in meniscal rehabilitation, 984
    in muscle rehabilitation, 984
    in muscle strain, 197
    in Osgood-Schlatter disease, 1263
    in patellar tendinitis, 923
    in quadriceps injury, 292
    in RICE treatment, 496
    for shin splints, 277, 533
    in stress injury, 75
    in thigh contusion, 199, 1452
    in thoracolumbar spine treatment, 1166
    wet, 211
Ice cream cone, 935, 936
    palpation of, 941
Ice hockey, 1040, 1282
Ice massage, 210
    deep, 285-286
        in quadriceps injury, 294
    for iliotibial band friction syndrome, 1490
    for osteitis pubis, 1524
    in patellofemoral pain syndrome, 1487, 1488
    in running routine, 1507
    in thigh rehabilitation, 1021
Idiopathic osteonecrosis, 785-789
IL; *see* Interleukin
Iliac apophysis
    iliotibial band tendinitis and, 149
    injury to, 1046
Iliac apophysitis
    in running injuries, 1498-1499
    in strain treatment, 1044
Iliac crest
    apophysitis of, 1514-1515
    fracture of, 1517
        apophyseal, 1289-1293
        stress, 1500
    in pelvis and hip injuries, 1046-1047
    in radiographic anatomy, 1279
    in soccer injuries, 1513-1515
Iliac fossa, 1026
Iliac spine
    fracture of, 1517
        apophyseal, 1287-1289
        avulsion, 1052
    in pelvis and hip injuries, 1047
Iliacus hematoma syndrome, 1037
Iliacus tendinitis, 1391-1392
Iliofemoral ligament, 1029, 1031
Iliolumbar ligament, 1027-1028
Iliopectineal bursitis, 1038-1039

Iliopsoas
    in dance injuries, 1391-1392
    in football injuries, 1450
    as hip flexor, 1034
    snapping of, 1039-1040
    in soccer players, 199-200
    strain of, 1282-1283
    stretches for, 1223
Iliopsoas tendon
    in iliopsoas muscle snapping, 1039
    strain of, 1042
Iliopubic eminence, 1026-1027
Iliotibial band, 1002
    in anterior cruciate ligament reconstruction, 851, 852
    flexibility test for, 1221
    of lateral knee, 607, 608
    snapping of, 1039, 1391
    stretches for, 974, 1224
    tendinitis of, 148-149
        in immature athlete, 1212-1213
        in knee physical examination, 685
Iliotibial band friction syndrome, 926-930
    in cycling injuries, 1570-1572, 1573
    as preventable adolescent injury, 1215
    quadriceps tendinitis versus, 1568
    in running injuries, 1489-1490
    in soccer injuries, 1534-1535
Ilium, 1026-1027
    fracture of, 1056
Illegal techniques in football, 1433
Imaging of muscle strains, 47-48
Imaging techniques, 109-125
    arthrography and, 109-110
    conventional radiography and, 109
    magnetic resonance, 111-123
        bone injuries in, 113-117, 118, 119
        soft-tissue injuries in, 118-123
        theory of, 112-113, 114, 115
    radionuclide, 110-111
    stress radiography and, 109
    tomography and, 110, 111
Immobilization
    in Achilles tendon rupture, 488, 573
    of ambulatory athlete, 1091
    cast
        in ankle ligament injury, 429
        for fibular stress fractures, 1397
        for knee ligament injury, 1395
    disuse atrophy in, 101
    of downed player, 1085
    halo-vest
        in atlantooccipital dislocation, 1121
        in atlas fractures, 1122
        in odontoid fractures, 1123-1124
        in traumatic spondylolisthesis of C2, 1125
    in medial collateral ligament treatment, 833-834, 838
    of musculotendinous unit, 529
    in osteochondritis dissecans, 778
    plaster
        of calcaneus fractures, 1237
        of immature talar dome fracture, 1242-1243
    in postoperative rehabilitation, 982
    principles of
        bone in, 184
        cartilage in, 29-32
        cartilage nutritional deficiency in, 19
        continuous passive motion in, 184-185
        duration of, 32
        healing in, 87-88
        ligament in, 29-32, 183-184
        muscle in, 182-183
        rehabilitation in, 181-185
        synovial joint in, 184
        transcutaneous electric nerve stimulation in, 184

Transforming growth factor
  in inflammatory response, 83-84
  in stress injury, 71-72
Transient ischemia, 48
Transient neuropraxia, 1333-1334
Transient neurologic deficits, 1446-1447
Transient quadriplegia
  in football injuries, 1446
  spinal cord neuropraxia and, 1119-1120
  syndrome of, 1103, 1104, 1106
Transient synovitis, 1062, 1302
Transitional movements, 1149
Translation
  anterior
    in knee-test devices, 664
    in patient evaluation, 669-670
    in in vivo knee motion, 658
  of joint, 826
  in meniscectomy, 654, 655
  of motion, 641-643
  posterior
    in knee-test devices, 664
    in in vitro knee motion, 656, 657, 658
    in in vivo knee motion, 658
  pure, 646, 647
Translational instability, 1120
Transmalleolar axis, 318
Transpatellar technique, 758-759
Transportation in cervical spine injuries, 1136
Transverse arch
  of foot, 321, 322
  metatarsal, 265
Transverse foramen of cervical spine, 1072
Transverse fractures of sacrum, 1056
Transverse friction, 230
Transverse ligament
  in burst fracture, 1121-1122
  of cervical spine, 1074
Transverse metatarsal ligament, 1548, 1549
Transverse plane
  in foot biomechanics, 337
  knee motion in, 616
Transverse process
  of lumbosacral spine, 1080
  of thoracic spine, 1076
  of vertebral arch, 1068
  visceral trauma and, 1331
Transverse relaxation time, 733
Transverse tarsal joint, 338
Transverse tear of menisci, 764
Transversus abdominis, 1176
Trauma
  of cervical spine, 1107
  in osteochondritis dissecans, 774
Traumatic arthritis, 907-908
Traumatic injury
  in cycling, 1559
  immature hip dislocation as, 1294-1298
  of knee, 675-677
Traumatic predeterminism, 1035
Traumatic spondylolisthesis, 1124-1126
Treadmill
  in knee rehabilitation, 981
  in runner evaluation, 1486
Trethowan's sign, 1298
Triangle in ankle radiography, 368
Triathlon runner, 1477
Triceps surae, 525
  in immature foot and ankle, 1231
  partial tears of, 1396
  stretches for, 1223
Trick knee, 844
Tricyclic antidepressants, 1144
Trigger toe, 1397, 1398, 1399

Trigone process fracture, 1240
Trigonitis, 1238
Tripartite patella, 715
Triple arthrodesis, 1233
Triple helix, 12-13
Triple-varus knee syndrome, 856
Tripping in dance injuries, 1406
Triradiate cartilage of pelvis, 1026
Trisomy 21, 1318
Tritium, 15
Trocar, 420
Trochanter, 1031
  apophysis of, 1280
  bursitis of
    in cycling injuries, 1573
    in pelvis and hip conditions, 1038
  fractures of, of immature femoral neck, 1301
  greater
    bursitis of, 1518
    contusion of, 1283
    iliotibial band tendinitis and, 148
    snapping over, 1391
  lesser
    apophysitis of, 1212, 1213
    avulsion fracture of, 1052
      in football injuries, 1450, 1451
    fracture of
      apophyseal, 1293-1294
      in soccer injuries, 1517
      stress, 1048-1049
    in pelvis and hip injuries, 1047-1048
Trochlea, femoral, 583
Trochlear groove, 948
Tropocollagen, 12
Tropomyosin, 40
Troponin, 40
Trunk, protective equipment for, 306-307
Trunk curl, 1081
Tube, nasogastric, 1089
Tubercle; *see also* Tibial tubercle
  Gerdy's, 582
    in anterior cruciate ligament reconstruction, 851
    iliotibial band tendinitis and, 149
Tuberosity
  ischial
    bursitis of, 1518-1519
    fracture of, 1517
    irritation of, 1573
  overgrown navicular, 1234-1235, 1236
  tibial, 1260, 1261-1262
Tumor
  imaging of, 405-407
  intramedullary, 1338-1339
  of pelvis and hip, 1036
    in immature athlete, 1302
    in running injuries, 1500
  radionuclide bone scan of, 136-137
  vertebral, 1337-1338
Tumor necrosis factor, 71-72
Tunnel
  for anterior cruciate ligament
    graft in, 878, 879
    in reconstruction, 883-884
  of flexor hallucis longus tendon, 442-443
  tarsal, 331, 398, 454-455
    in posterior tibial nerve entrapment, 1354-1355
Tunnel view, 699, 702
Turf, artificial
  in blisters, 1554
  in football injuries, 1433-1436
  footwear and, 518
  turf toe in, 455-456
Turf shoe in ankle sprain, 242